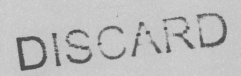

PRACTICAL
RHEUMATOLOGY

Commissioning Editor: Kim Murphy
Project Development Manager: Louise Cook
Project Manager: Cheryl Brant
Illustration Manager: Mick Ruddy
Design Manager: Jayne Jones
Illustrators: Robin Dean, Jenni Miller

THIRD EDITION
PRACTICAL RHEUMATOLOGY

Edited by

Marc C Hochberg MD MPH
Professor of Medicine, Head, Division of
Rheumatology and Clinical Immunology,
University of Maryland School of Medicine,
Baltimore, MD, USA

Alan J Silman MSc MD FRCP FMedSci
ARC Professor of Rheumatic Disease
Epidemiology; Director, Arthritis Research
Campaign Epidemiology Research Unit,
University of Manchester, UK

Josef S Smolen MD
Professor of Medicine, Chairman, Division of
Rheumatology, University of Vienna School of
Medicine and Chairman, Second Department of
Medicine, Centre for Rheumatic Disease, Lainz
Hospital Vienna, Austria

Michael E Weinblatt MD
Professor of Medicine, Harvard Medical School,
Division of Rheumatology, Immunology and
Allergy, Brigham and Women's Hospital, Boston,
MA, USA

Michael H Weisman MD
Director, Division of Rheumatology, Cedars-Sinai
Medical Center; Professor of Medicine, UCLA
School of Medicine, Los Angeles, CA, USA

NM Mosby

Philadelphia ■ Edinburgh ■ London ■ New York ■ Oxford ■ St Louis ■ Sydney ■ Toronto 2004

MOSBY
An affiliate of Elsevier Ltd

First edition 1995 © Times Mirror International Publishers
Second edition 1999
Third edition 2004

ISBN 0 323 02939 6

British Library Cataloguing in Publication Data
A catalogue record for this book is available from the British Library

Library of Congress Cataloging in Publication Data
A catalog record for this book is available from the Library of Congress

Notice
Medical knowledge is constantly changing. Standard safety precautions must be followed, but as new research and clinical experience broaden our knowledge, changes in treatment and drug therapy may become necessary or appropriate. Readers are advised to check the most current product information provided by the manufacturer of each drug to be administered to verify the recommended dose, the method and duration of administration, and contraindications. It is the responsibility of the practitioner, relying on experience and knowledge of the patient, to determine dosages and the best treatment for each individual patient. Neither the Publisher, editors nor contributors assume any liability for any injury and/or damage to persons or property arising from this publication.
The Publisher

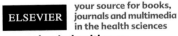
your source for books,
journals and multimedia
in the health sciences
www.elsevierhealth.com

Printed in China

The
publisher's
policy is to use
**paper manufactured
from sustainable forests**

CONTENTS

CONTRIBUTORS

Kristina Åkesson MD PhD
Associate Professor of Orthopaedics
Malmö University Hospital
Malmö, Sweden

Abdul-Wahab Al-Allaf MBChB MRCP(UK) MSC CCST Cert HE
Consultant Rheumatologist
Honorary Senior Lecturer
New Cross Hospital
Wolverhampton, UK

Roy D Altman MD
Professor of Medicine
Chief of Rheumatology and Immunology, University
   of Miami School of Medicine
Clinical Director, Geriatric Research, Education and
   Clinical Center
Miami Department of Veterans Affairs
Miami, FL, USA

Cynthia Aranow MD
Assistant Professor of Medicine
Albert Einstein College of Medicine
New York, NY, USA

Les Barnsley BMED(HONS) Grad Dip Epi PhD FRACP FAFRM(RACP)
Associate Professor of Medicine, Sydney University
Head, Department of Rheumatology, Concord Hospital
Sydney, NSW, Australia

Jill J F Belch MD (Hons) FRCP
Professor of Vascular Medicine
Ninewells Hospital and Medical School
Dundee, UK

Brian M Berman MD
Professor of Family Medicine
Director, The Complementary Medicine Program
University of Maryland School of Medicine
Baltimore, MD, USA

David G Borenstein MD
Clinical Professor of Medicine
The George Washington University Medical Center
Washington, DC, USA

Barry Bresnihan MD FRCP
Professor of Rheumatology and Consultant
   Rheumatologist
St Vincent's Hospital
Dublin, Ireland

Peter M Brooks MD FRACP FAFRM FAFPHM
Executive Dean, Faculty of Health Sciences
The University of Queensland Royal Brisbane Hospital
Herston, Brisbane, Queensland, Australia

Ian N Bruce MD FRCP
Consultant Rheumatologist and Honorary Clinical Lecturer
Rheumatism Research Centre
Central Manchester and Manchester Children's
   University Hospitals NHS Trust
Manchester, UK

Joseph A Buckwalter MD
Professor and Head, Department of Orthopedics,
   University of Iowa Hospitals,
   Iowa City, IA, USA

Juan J Canoso MD FACP
Adjunct Professor of Medicine, Tufts University, Boston
Rheumatologist, American British Cowdray Hospital
Mexico City, Mexico

Michael D Chard MB BS MD FRCP
Consultant Rheumatologist
Worthing Hospital
Worthing, West Sussex, UK

Milton L Cohen MB BS MD FRCP FFPMANZCA
Associate Professor of Rheumatology
Darlinghurst Arthritis and Pain Research Clinic
St Vincents Medical Centre
Sydney, NSW, Australia

Marta L Cuéllar MD
Associate Professor
Tulane Health Sciences Center
New Orleans, LA, USA

Seamus E Dalton MBBS FACRM FAFRM FACSP
Consultant in Rehabilitation and Sports Medicine
North Sydney Orthopaedic and Sports Medicine Centre
Sydney, NSW, Australia

Helen Emery MD
Professor of Pediatrics
Section Chief, Rheumatology
University of Washington Children's Hospital
Seattle, WA, USA

Paul Emery MA MD FRCP
ARC Professor of Rheumatology
Leeds General Infirmary
Leeds, UK

Bryan T Emmerson MD PhD FRACP
Emeritus Professor of Medicine
University of Queensland
Brisbane, Queensland, Australia

Luis R Espinoza MD
Professor and Chief, CSU Health Sciences Center
Louisiana State School of Medicine
New Orleans, LA, USA

John A Fairclough BM BS FRCS
Consultant Orthopedic Surgeon
Llandough Hospital
Penarth, Vale of Glamorgan, Wales

Adel G Fam MD FRCP(C) MRCP(UK) FACP
Professor of Medicine, University of Toronto
Sunnybrook and Women's College Health Sciences
   Center
Toronto, ON, Canada

David L George MD
Clinical Professor of Medicine, Pennsylvania State
   University
Associate Director of Medicine, Reading Hospital
Reading, PA, USA

Piet Geusens MD PhD
Professor of Rheumatology, Linburg University Center
University Hospital, Maastricht
Maastricht, The Netherlands

Terry Gibson MD FRCP
Consultant Physician, Guy's and St Thomas' Hospitals
   Trust
Department of Rheumatology, Guy's Hospital
London, UK

Ellen M Ginzler MD MPH
Professor of Medicine
Chief of Rheumatology, State University of New York –
   Downstate Medical Center
Brooklyn, NY, USA

Dafna D Gladman MD FRCPC
Professor of Medicine, University of Toronto
Deputy Director, Centre for Prognosis Studies in the
   Rheumatic Diseases and University of Toronto Lupus
   Clinic
Toronto Western Hospital
Toronto, ON, Canada

Don L Goldenberg MD
Professor of Medicine, Tufts University School of
   Medicine
Director, Arthritis – Fibromyalgia Center, Newton
   Wellesley Hospital
Chief of Rheumatology, Newton-Wellesley Hospital
Newton, MA, USA

Duncan A Gordon MD
Professor of Medicine, University of Toronto
Senior Rheumatologist
Toronto Western Hospital
Toronto, ON, Canada

Elena Gournelos BSC
The Complementary Medicine Program
University of Maryland School of Medicine
Baltimore, MD, USA

Geoffrey P Graham MB BS FRCS
Consultant Orthopaedic Surgeon
Llandough Hospital
Penarth, Vale of Glamorgan, Wales

Michael J Green MBChB MRCP
Consultant Rheumatologist
Academic Unit of Musculoskeletal Disease
Leeds General Infirmary
Leeds, UK

Ian Haslock MD MRCP
Consultant Rheumatologist, South Tees Hospitals
   Trust
Visiting Professor of Clinical Bioengineering, University
   of Durham
The James Cook University Hospital
Middlesborough, UK

David E Hastings MD
Professor of Surgery
University of Toronto
Toronto, ON, Canada

Brian L Hazleman MA MB FRCP
Consultant Rheumatologist
Clinical Director, Rheumatology Research Unit
Addenbrooke's Hospital
Cambridge, UK

Osvaldo Hübscher MD
Professor of Medicine
Section of Rheumatology and Immunology
CEMIC
Buenos Aires, Argentina

Laura K Hummers MD
Instructor of Medicine
Division of Rheumatology
The Johns Hopkins University
Baltimore, Maryland, USA

Richard A Kay MB ChB PhD ILTM
Senior Research Fellow and Honorary Senior Lecturer
Department of Cell and Molecular Biology
University of Dundee Dental School
Dundee, UK

Muhammad Asim Khan MD FRCP MACP
Professor of Medicine, Case Western Reserve University School of Medicine
Metro Health Medical Center
Cleveland, OH, USA

John R Kirwan BSc MD FRCP
Consultant and Reader in Rheumatology
University of Bristol Academic Rheumatology Unit
Bristol Royal Infirmary
Bristol, UK

George T Lewith MA DM FRCP MRCGP
Honorary Senior Research Fellow, University of Southampton
Complementary Medicine Research Unit, Royal South Hants Hospital
Southampton, UK

Lars Lidgren MD PhD
Professor of Orthopedics
Chairman and Professor, Department of Orthopedics
University Hospital of Lund
Lund, Sweden

Carlos J Lozada MD
Associate Professor of Medicine
Director, Rheumatology Training Program, Division of Rheumatology and Immunology
The University of Miami
Miami, FL, USA

Bernard Mazières MD
Professor of Rheumatology
University Hospital of Rangueil
Toulouse, France

Geraldine M McCarthy MD FRCPI
Consultant Rheumatologist, Mater Misericordiae Hospital
Honorary Senior Lecturer, Department of Clinical Pharmacology, Royal College of Surgeons in Ireland
Dublin, Ireland

Thomas A Medsger Jr MD
Gerald P. Rodnan Professor of Medicine
University of Pittsburgh School of Medicine
Pittsburgh, PA, USA

Chester V Oddis MD
Professor of Medicine
University of Pittsburgh School of Medicine
Pittsburgh, PA, USA

J David Perry MD FRCP
Consultant Rheumatologist
Royal London Hospital
London, UK

Mark A Quinn MBChB MRCP
Lecturer in Rheumatology
Academic Unit of Musculoskeletal Disease
Leeds General Infirmary
Leeds, UK

Dwight R Robinson MD
Professor of Medicine
Massachusetts General Hospital and Harvard Medical School
Boston, MA, USA

Philip N Sambrook MD FRACP
Professor of Rheumatology
Royal North Shore Hospital
St Leonards, Sydney
Australia

Peter H Schur MD
Professor of Medicine, Harvard Medical School
Director, Clinical Immunology Web
Brigham and Women's Hospital
Boston, MA, USA

Robert H Shmerling MD
Associate Professor of Medicine, Harvard Medical School
Beth Israel Deaconess Hospital
Boston, MA, USA

Allen C Steere MD
Professor of Medicine, Harvard Medical School
Director, Rheumatology
Massachusetts General Hospital
Boston, MA, USA

Auli Toivanen MD DrMeDsci
Professor of Medicine (Emerita)
Turku University
Turku, Finland

Murray B Urowitz MD FRCPC
Professor of Medicine, University of Toronto
Director, Centre for Prognosis Studies in The Rheumatic Diseases and University of Toronto Lupus Clinic
Toronto Western Hospital
Toronto, ON, USA

Fredrick M Wigley MD
Professor of Medicine
Associate Director, Division of Rheumatology
The Johns Hopkins University
Baltimore, Maryland, USA

Anthony D Woolf BSc MBBS FRCP
Professor of Rheumatology, Peninsula Medical School
Consultant Rheumatologist, Royal Cornwall Hospital
Truro, Cornwall, UK

PREFACE

Musculoskeletal disorders account for between 10 and 20% of all visits to primary care physicians. The primary care physician is faced with the task of determining whether the problem is a regional or generalized musculoskeletal disorder, inflammatory arthropathy, or diffuse connective tissue disease; this may involve laboratory tests and imaging procedures. The physician then has to develop a treatment plan that may include determining which patients are in need of referral to a specialist for further evaluation and management.

Practical Rheumatology has been specifically developed to help with this need. The first section of the book highlights recent information underpinning the scientific basis of rheumatology. The second and third sections provide a general introduction to the principles and practice of diagnosis and therapy of the musculoskeletal system. The remaining sections, which form the main part of the book, cover all the common disorders of the musculoskeletal system and include material on functional anatomy, pathophysiology, diagnosis and the latest information on treatment.

Practical Rheumatology is a derivative of the much larger text reference book Rheumatology 3e, that is designed for specialists and trainees with a special commitment to musculoskeletal disorders. Rheumatology 3e contains 209 chapters and 2199 pages and covers the scientific background to the rheumatic diseases and antirheumatic therapy, as well as many chapters on bone disorders and the less common forms of arthritis. The more clinically oriented chapters of Rheumatology 3e and those concerned with common musculoskeletal disorders have been included in Practical Rheumatology 3e, resulting in a book of only 46 chapters and 644 pages. The book is beautifully illustrated throughout, providing a valuable atlas of clinical signs and radiographic features of the rheumatic diseases, as well as numerous tables and figures that provide additional information to foster an understanding of these disorders and how to manage them.

The editors are proud of this book and confident that it will be an essential and practical guide on the diagnosis and management of musculoskeletal disorders for primary care physicians. We also owe a huge debt of gratitude to our publisher Kimberly Murphy and the excellent team of editors, illustrators, designers and producers who have been responsible for both books.

DEDICATION

We would like to dedicate this book to our parents (living or of blessed memory), wives and children:

Susan Hochberg, Francine and Jennifer Hochberg

Ruth Silman, Joanna, Timothy and Daniel Silman

Alice Smolen, Eva, Nina and Daniel Smolen, and Wanda and Stefan Smolen

Barbara Weinblatt, Hillary and Courtney Weinblatt

Betsy Weisman, Greg, Nicole and Mia Colette Weisman, Lisa, Andrew and David Temple Cope, and Annie Weisman

THE SCIENTIFIC BASIS OF RHEUMATIC DISEASE

1

The principles of adaptive immunity

Richard A Kay

- The adaptive immune system consists of T and B cells. They produce a large repertoire of T-cell receptors and immunoglobulins using somatic gene recombination. Clonal selection preserves those cells whose products prove useful

- The potential of this system to induce autoimmunity is usually controlled by a combination of deletional and regulatory mechanisms

- Immune receptor triggering involves the movement of membrane rafts containing the receptors and costimulatory molecules into special complexes followed by the assembly of enzyme cascades within the cells' interior

- Immune responses can become polarized into types 1 (cell-mediated) or 2 (humoral) and lymphocytes, in addition to helper T cells, reinforce this by specific cytokine secretion

- Immune polarization increases the severity of a reaction. Type 1 cytokines suppress type 2 effectors and *vice versa*. Polarization isolates effectors of one type from suppression by cells of the opposite polarity

- Lymphocyte subsets express different homing and chemokine receptors. These molecules direct lymphocyte migration, coordinate cellular interactions and reinforce the polarization of specific immune responses

- All of these processes may provide targets for the therapeutic manipulation of autoimmune diseases

INTRODUCTION

The immune system consists of a series of cells and soluble factors working in concert to maintain the host's individuality. It resists both external agents and internal mutations to preserve the biological integrity of the host and is only quiescent when these threats to the individual cease. However, when the immune system is chronically stimulated, those mechanisms that protect us in the short term often lead to significant morbidity and mortality in the long term – as is the case in autoimmune disease. Immune reactivity in most autoimmune diseases appears to be directed at a limited range of antigenic targets. So, while there may be a profoundly abnormal response to one antigen, immune responsiveness to other antigens is usually not compromised. The specific discrimination and control of pathogenic immune responses remains the central aim of workers in this field and as our understanding of basic immunology increases so does our appreciation of both the possibilities and complexities of achieving this aim. While later chapters will highlight the advances made in the therapeutic manipulation of the immune system, this chapter will focus on the basic mechanisms involved in T- and B-cell function.

THE ADAPTIVE IMMUNE SYSTEM

The adaptive immune system is capable of responding to and having specific memory of a wide variety of antigenic stimuli. In order to accom-

plish this, it more or less randomly generates a huge variety of receptors and effector proteins and relies on clonal selection to maintain only those cells that produce useful molecules. As a consequence, the system must be able to distinguish between self and non-self. Receptors or effector molecules that are potentially autoimmune have to be eliminated.

The two cells that make up the adaptive immune system are the T and B lymphocytes and the physiology of antigen recognition, cell development, effector function and migration of these cell types will be discussed further.

THE T CELL

The T cell is the principal regulator of the immune response. It distinguishes self from non-self by the use of a specific antigen receptor and targets the remainder of the immune system appropriately.

The T-cell receptor

The antigen receptor on T cells, also known as the T-cell receptor (TCR), is a clonally distributed cell-surface heterodimer. It is most frequently composed of an $\alpha\beta$ chain pairing but a significant minority of T cells (about 5% in peripheral blood) use a $\gamma\delta$ TCR. Each chain is a two-domain structure with a variable domain that determines antigen specificity and a constant domain that inserts into the cell surface. The TCR associates with four other invariant chains at the cell surface: the CD3 proteins γ, δ and ϵ and the ζ chain (Fig. 1.1). Collectively they are known as the TCR complex and are responsible for signaling receptor occupancy.

The TCR chain variable domain is so called because it contains areas where the peptide sequence varies greatly between TCRs on different cloned T cells and these form the complementarity determining regions (CDRs) that bind antigen/MHC complexes directly. The intervening domain sequence is much less variable between different receptors and serves as a framework to orientate the CDRs correctly. The diversity of the TCR variable domain arises through the way the genes that encode the receptor are organized in the genome.

A complex of subexonic gene segments located in discrete chromosomal areas encodes each TCR chain. The *TCRB* complex (encoding the β chain) is at 7q32–35, the *TCRG* complex (encoding the γ chain) is at 7p15 and the *TCRA* complex (encoding the α chain), which surrounds the much smaller *TCRD* (δ chain-encoding) is located at 14q11–12. Within these complexes there are multiple copies of two (α and γ) or three (β and δ) distinct types of subexonic gene segment, which are used to encode the variable domain. These subexonic gene segments are known as variable, diversity (δ and β chains only) and joining segments, respectively. One of each type of segment is recombined to form the functional gene that encodes each TCR variable domain. At the genomic level, this recombined V(D)J sequence remains separate and upstream from the gene segment that encodes the constant domain. It is at the RNA level that the intervening sequence is spliced out and the functional message encoding the final TCR is generated (Fig. 1.2).

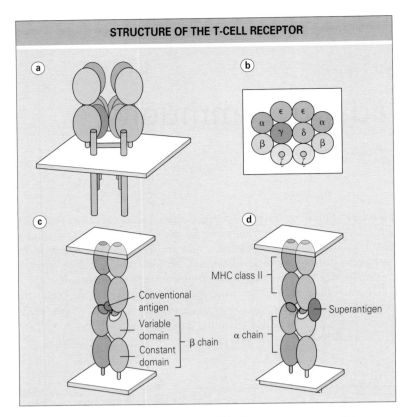

STRUCTURE OF THE T-CELL RECEPTOR

Fig. 1.1 Structure of the T-cell receptor. This diagram shows a possible arrangement of the TCR complex ($\alpha\beta$ TCR heterodimer, CD3 chains and ζ chain) inserted into the T-cell surface shown either from the side (a) or as a transmembrane view (b). Also shown is the interaction of the TCR with human leukocyte antigen (HLA) class II molecules and conventionally processed antigen (c) or superantigen (d).

The diversity of variable domains arises as a result of:

- the large numbers of each type of subexonic gene segment available for recombination; especially variable (between 70 and 90) and joining (61 functional) gene segments in the *TCRA* gene complex and variable gene segments (50 functional) in the *TCRB* complex
- the largely random recombination of these gene segments
- the templated and random insertions and deletions that occur during V–(D)–J gene segment recombination
- the limited amount of germline polymorphism that occurs in the variable gene segments particularly[1].

Somatic recombination occurs following the recognition of the heptamer/nonamer motifs that comprise the recombination signal sequences (RSS) that flank the coding regions of the gene segments. Recent studies have shown that the recombination activating gene (*RAG*) proteins 1 and 2, terminal deoxynucleotidyl transferase (TdT) and DNA-ligase IV, along with different non-homologous DNA end-joining components (XRCC4, Ku86, Ku70 and DNA-PK$_{CS}$) all play a role in either the cleavage, processing or rejoining of chromosomal DNA as part of the recombination process[2]. Gene segment selection depends on the accessibility of gene loci, which correlates with the differential expression of transcription factors and their interaction with enhancer and promoter elements during lymphopoiesis[3]. Inherited polymorphisms in the RSS[4] and promoter[5] sequences have been shown to influence the T-cell repertoire and some have been associated with the development of specific autoimmune disease[6].

Antigen recognition

T cells recognize complexes of peptide antigen presented in the context of major histocompatibility complex (MHC)-encoded HLA molecules.

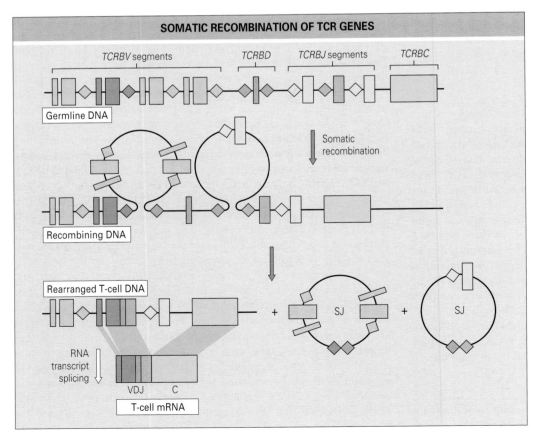

SOMATIC RECOMBINATION OF TCR GENES

Fig. 1.2 Somatic recombination of TCR genes. This is a diagrammatic representation of the *TCRB* gene complex, not drawn to scale, showing variable (*TCRBV*), diversity (*TCRBD*), joining (*TCRBJ*) and constant (*TCRBC*) gene segments, along with recombination site sequences (diamonds) where appropriate. TCR gene recombination randomly joins one of each gene segment together to form a variable domain-encoding gene subexon. Each recombination forms a coding joint (*BV* to *BD* and *BD* to *BJ*, with intervening random and templated nucleotide additions – not shown) and a signal joint (SJ). The final TCR β chain mRNA transcript is formed by RNA splicing.

MHC-encoded HLA antigens

Human leukocyte antigens (HLA) are cell-surface heterodimeric glycoproteins. There are two classes of MHC-encoded proteins: class I (e.g. HLA-A, -B and -C) and class II (e.g. HLA-DR, -DP and -DQ). The class I proteins consists of a three-domain α chain non-covalently complexed with β_2 microglobulin. They are expressed on the surface of all nucleated cells and bind the T-cell differentiation molecule CD8. The class II molecules consist of an α and a β chain. Each of these two class II chains has a two-domain structure. Class II molecules are constitutively expressed on professional antigen presenting cells (APCs) but can be induced on other cell types. They bind the T-cell co-receptor CD4. All the HLA molecules, therefore, have a four-domain structure with a peptide binding site formed between the two domains most distal from the cell surface (α_1 and α_2 for class I and α_1 and β_1 for class II molecules).

The peptide-binding groove, lying between two α helices and floored by a β-pleated sheet, shows degenerate binding specificity. Class I molecules bind peptides limited to about 8–10 amino acids in length, because of the pockets that anchor the peptide at the ends of the binding site. Class II molecules, free of this constraint, bind peptides of between 13 and 25 amino acids long.

The MHC spans some 4Mb on the short arm of chromosome 6. Each of the class I and II molecules is encoded by a separate gene locus within the complex. Each locus is highly polymorphic. Even although there is extensive linkage disequilibrium across the MHC and specific haplotypes may be reasonably common in particular ethnic backgrounds, it is uncommon for individuals to be identical across these loci. In short, it is the genetic diversity of the MHC loci that largely defines 'self' as recognized by the adaptive immune system. Polymorphic amino acid residues not only alter the shape of individual class I and II molecules themselves but may also affect the shape of the peptide-binding sites, altering both the epitopes and the range of peptides presented to TCRs.

Peptide processing for MHC molecules

The peptides lying in the class I and II molecular binding grooves come from different sources, are processed differently and are loaded into the MHC molecules in different intracellular compartments (Fig 1.3).

A significant proportion of the intracellular proteins newly synthesized in the ribosomes is released into the cytosol and degraded by the proteasome. The proteasome is a multiunit protein complex with a number of different proteolytic activities. Peptides generated by the proteasome are transported across the membrane of the endoplasmic reticulum by TAP (transporter associated with antigen-processing) proteins embedded within the membrane itself. Class I molecules also enter the endoplasmic reticulum and are chaperoned by calnexin until β_2 microglobulin binds. Once the molecule has been released by calnexin, other chaperones, including calreticulin and tapasin, stabilize and position it until a suitable peptide is loaded. The completed MHC/peptide complex is transported through the endoplasmic reticulum and the Golgi apparatus to the cell surface.

The peptides generated by this process vary with genetic background and the immune status of the individual. The proteasomal subunit composition and its resultant peptide repertoire is different in cells exposed to CD8[+] T cells and other bone marrow-derived cell cytokines. Similarly, inherited polymorphisms in the *TAP1* and *TAP2* genes that encode the TAP protein influence the repertoire of peptides presented by class I molecules[7,8].

Class II molecules present antigens internalized by the antigen presenting cells. Protein antigens taken up by phagocytosis, macropinocytosis, endocytosis and receptor-mediated endocytosis are taken into the endosomes. Peptides are generated from these proteins by a combination of protease digestion and decreasing pH in the endocytic compartment. MHC class II heterodimers, stabilized by their association with the invariant chain (Ii), are targeted to this endocytic compartment

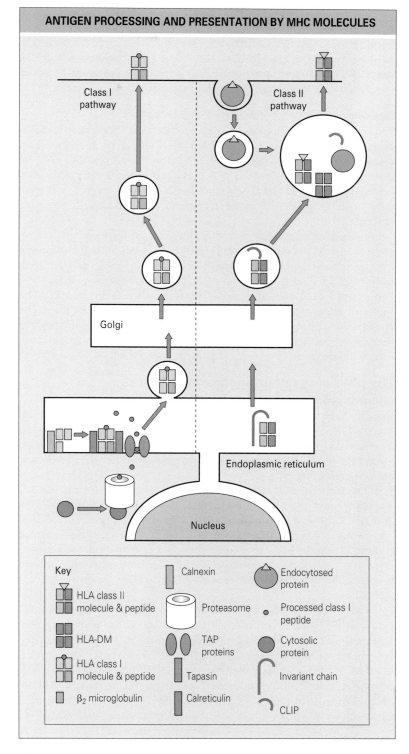

ANTIGEN PROCESSING AND PRESENTATION BY MHC MOLECULES

Class I pathway

Class II pathway

Golgi

Endoplasmic reticulum

Nucleus

Key

- HLA class II molecule & peptide
- HLA-DM
- HLA class I molecule & peptide
- β_2 microglobulin
- Calnexin
- Proteasome
- TAP proteins
- Tapasin
- Calreticulin
- Endocytosed protein
- Processed class I peptide
- Cytosolic protein
- Invariant chain
- CLIP

Fig. 1.3 Antigen processing and presentation by MHC molecules. Both class I and II antigen presentation pathways are shown. For detailed explanation, see text.

through a signal in the cytoplasmic tail of the invariant chain. Once there, the Ii is sequentially digested, leaving only a fragment (class-II-associated Ii peptide or CLIP) in the peptide-binding site. HLA-DM and HLA-DO (also encoded in the MHC class II region) then catalyze the exchange of CLIP for antigenic peptides, after which the antigen-loaded MHC class II molecules are transferred to the cell surface.

Once again, this process can be subtly modified according to the genetic background and immune status of the host. Cytokines can affect the protease and pH content of the endosomes and alter antigen processing[9]. Further, the peptides loaded into one HLA molecule can be altered if either antibodies or another HLA molecule have previously bound the antigen from which these peptides are derived[10]. This mechanism may help to explain both why some HLA backgrounds can be protective in autoimmune disease and a further mechanism by which autoantibodies may modify immune responsiveness.

Other molecules recognized by T-cell receptors

Two other groups of molecules may interact with TCRs. Firstly, superantigens (Fig. 1.1), the protein products of some bacteria and viruses, are capable of binding to class II molecules directly without the need for processing. They also bind the TCR β chain directly, usually at the loop between β strands D and E, and stimulate large numbers of T cells compared with the restricted range that respond to conventionally processed antigen[11].

CD1 consists of a group of molecules that associate with β_2 microglobulin on the cell surface, are divided on the basis of sequence homology into two groups and are capable of presenting lipids and glycolipids to $\alpha\beta$ and $\gamma\delta$ T cells. The group 1 CD1 family (comprising CD1a, -b, -c and -e) appears to present microbial antigens whereas the group 2 CD1d molecule appears to present self-antigens. The range of TCRs that CD1d appears to stimulate depends on its intracellular trafficking and, in particular, whether or not its has entered the late-endosome/lysosomal compartment[12].

The physiology of antigen recognition

Immune synapse formation

In order to be successfully activated, T cells require two signals. The first is cognate recognition of antigen through the TCR and the second may be delivered by co-receptor binding[13,14]. Both of these signals are generated at the so-called immunological synapse formed between T cells and antigen presenting cells.

In unstimulated T cells, TCRs and co-receptors are distributed homogeneously over the T-cell surface. At the synapse between T cells and APCs, however, supramolecular activation complexes (SMACs) are formed. In this complex, the TCR, MHC/peptide complexes and protein kinase C (PKC)-θ are enriched in a central circle, while integrins and the adhesion molecule ICAM-1 form an outer ring around this 'bullseye'. Formation of these SMACs correlate closely with T-cell activation[15,16].

Formation of these SMACs is an active process, involving the T cells' cytoskeleton, where receptors are brought into close proximity with sphingolipid/cholesterol-enriched membrane microdomains (rafts) that contain the protein tyrosine kinases (PTKs) necessary for signal transduction. A single contact between the TCR and the MHC/peptide complex is insufficient to stimulate T-cell triggering. In naive T cells, up to 20 hours continuous stimulation may be necessary to induce autonomous activation[16]. It is now thought that, within these SMACs, a few MHC/peptide complexes serially trigger many TCRs in order to maintain sustained levels of T-cell triggering. Each TCR sequentially binds antigen, phosphorylates its adapter signaling protein and disengages the MHC/peptide complex before the next TCR takes its place. Triggered TCRs are therefore phosphorylated and are consequently internalized and degraded within the cell's lysosomal compartments. A strong correlation has been shown between the capacity of an antigen to trigger and downregulate cell-surface TCRs and its ability to induce a strong T-cell response[16,17].

Signaling pathways in T cells

The biochemical pathways following TCR triggering are becoming increasingly understood. The earliest event following TCR crosslinking is the activation of the raft-associated Src-family PTK, Lck and Fyn, which phosphorylate the immunoreceptor tyrosine-based activation

motifs (ITAMs) in the CD3 and TCR ζ chains. Once phosphorylated, these motifs act as docking sites for another family (Syk) of PTK, ZAP-70. ZAP-70 itself is phosphorylated by the Src PTKs and recruits and activates the adapter signaling protein, LAT. LAT binds the adapter protein Gads, which in turn binds SLP-76. This trimer is now located to the membrane raft where ZAP-70 phosphorylates SLP-76, providing a binding site for the Tec kinase Itk. LAT also binds PLCγ1, which is activated by the dual actions of ZAP-70 and Itk. PLCγ1, which now lies in close proximity to its substrate, hydrolyzes PIP$_2$ to IP$_3$ and DAG. IP$_3$ leads to increases in cytosolic free calcium and the induction of the transcription factor NF-AT via calcineurin, and DAG activates PKC. Both calcineurin and PKC regulate the transcription factor NF-κB[18-20].

Activated LAT also binds Grb-2, which in turn recruits SOS to the plasma membrane, initiating the Ras–Raf–Mek–ERK signaling pathway that terminates in activation of the Fos transcription factor. The SLP-76/Gads complex that binds to LAT may also contribute to activation of PLCγ1 and the Ras–ERK pathway. SLP-76 also associates with Vav, promoting the formation of the SLP-76–Vav–Nck–Pak1 complex. Vav activates Rac-1. Rac-1, in combination with Pak1, can regulate actin polymerization but Rac-1, acting via JNK, also activates the transcription factor Jun[19-21] (Fig. 1.4).

Other receptors interact with these signaling pathways. CD4 and CD8 costimulation promotes TCR signaling, as they activate p56[Lck 22]. However, the effects that major costimulatory molecules, such as CD28, have on receptor signaling remains controversial. Likewise, the effect of inhibitory molecules, such as CTLA-4, are also unclear, although there

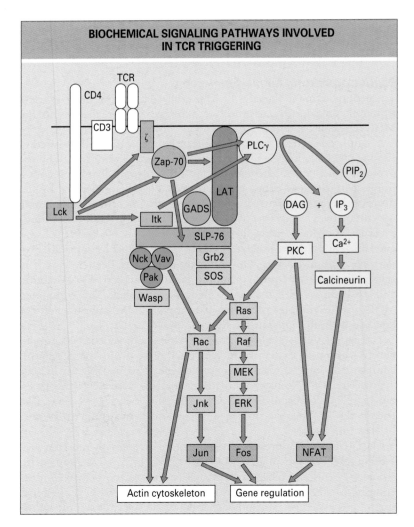

Fig. 1.4 Biochemical signaling pathways involved in TCR triggering.

are some data to suggest that inhibition involves the proximal molecules in the TCR triggering process[23].

Gene transcription in stimulated T cells

The result of all these signaling pathways is the translocation of transcription factors to the cell nucleus, where they interact with the regulatory regions of target genes. Transcriptional regulation of gene expression may operate locally or at a distance, by direct binding or by altering locus accessibility[24]. Regardless of how it is mediated, TCR triggering leads to the altered transcription of a large number of genes[25].

Identification of activation molecules or cytokines has been used as a means of identifying antigen-driven T cells *in vivo*. Unfortunately many of these markers are either too transiently expressed (e.g. CD69) or non-specifically induced (e.g. IL-2 or CD25) to be useful for this purpose. One exception may be the TCR genes themselves. All TCR variable genes have their own distinct promoter. This promoter becomes functional in rearranged genes because the rearrangement process brings it close enough to interact with the TCR enhancer, itself located near to the constant domain encoding gene segments. *TCRBV* (β chain variable gene segment) promoters have been most extensively studied. Recent data shows them to be capable of responding to a number of different transcription factors and being expressed in different amounts in a gene-specific manner[26–28]. Unlike other T-cell genes, *TCRBV* gene transcription appears to be an all-or-none event, independent of the form of antigen stimulating it and one that only occurs after direct stimulation with antigen. Identification of changes in the rate of *TCRBV* gene transcription in individual T cells appears to be a promising way of distinguishing antigen-driven T cells in unseparated lymphoid populations *in vivo*[28]. In common with many other antigen-stimulated T-cell genes, inhibition of *TCRBV* gene transcription may also prove a novel target in the search for selective immunosuppression.

Thymic development and T-cell selection

T-cell development occurs in the thymus[29] (Fig. 1.5). The most immature thymic T cell, the thymic lymphoid precursor (TLP), develops from the clonogenic common lymphoid precursor, itself differentiated from the hematopoietic stem cell. This TLP is the first triple-negative thymocyte (TN1), so-called because it lacks the cell surface proteins (CD3, CD4 and CD8). The TLP is positive for the adhesion molecule CD44 but is negative for the IL-2R β chain, CD25. The TLP passes through the TN2 (pro-T-cell) and TN3 (pre-T-cell) stages, acquiring CD25 and losing CD44 as it does so. Between these two stages, the gene loci encoding the TCR β, γ and δ chains undergo somatic rearrangement. If both TCR γ and δ chains undergo productive rearrangement then the T cell expresses this heterodimer and becomes committed to the γδ lineage. The majority of γδ T cells arise at this stage. If the β chain undergoes production rearrangement first, then the TCR β chain is expressed on the cell surface along with a surrogate α chain, the pre-Tα, the CD3 complex (at very low levels) and the ζ chain (TN3). Some of these T cells will carry productive rearrangements of either γ or δ TCR chains but not both. Expression of the pre-TCR suppresses further gene recombination, allowing these T cells to divide before further TCR gene rearrangements. Once completed, RAG expression increases and recombination recommences involving the γ, δ and α chains.

In cells carrying a productive γ or δ chain rearrangement, productive rearrangement of the complementary heterodimeric chain results in γδ T-cell development but successful α chain recombination results in the commitment to the αβ lineage. The majority of TN4 thymocytes (post-pre-TCR; CD25⁻CD44⁻) are αβ T cells. The thymocyte now acquires the CD4 and CD8 co-receptors and undergoes the selection process.

Positive selection allows the small percentage of the thymocyte population capable of recognizing MHC/peptide complexes to mature further, leaving the remainder to die by apoptosis. Until positive selection occurs, TCR α chain gene rearrangement continues, so some CD4⁺CD8⁺ thymocytes express two TCR α chains. Indeed, T cells with two TCR α chains can be found amongst mature T cells in the peripheral circulation[30]. Negative selection deletes T cells that bind self-peptide/MHC complexes so strongly as to be potentially autoimmune. The precise process by which signaling through the TCR mediates both positive and negative selection is poorly understood. However, the affinity and duration of TCR engagement, signaling pathways involving the TCR α chain, the C3δ chain, the guanine nucleotide exchange factor, Ras GDP and the signaling protein ERK, as well as the presence or

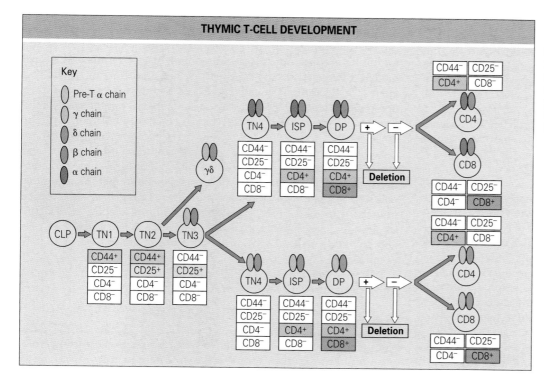

THYMIC T-CELL DEVELOPMENT

Fig. 1.5 Thymic T-cell development. Diagrammatic representation of T-cell development in the thymus showing the acquisition and loss of key surface markers, the ontogeny of the TCR and clonal deletion. Appropriately labeled arrows show positive and negative selection. CLP = common lymphoid precursor, TN = triple negative (lacking CD4, CD8 and CD3), ISP = immature single positive, DP = double positive.

absence of specific co-stimulation or thymic stromal cells, may all play a role in determining which outcome ensues[31–33].

During the final stage of development, CD4+CD8+ T cells suppress the expression of either their CD4 or CD8 co-receptors to give rise to single positive (SP), CD8+ or CD4+ mature thymocytes, respectively. T cells that express MHC class I restricted TCRs become CD8+ and lymphocytes that express MHC class II restricted TCRs become positive for the CD4 co-receptor alone. Co-receptor ligation, activation of the intracellular kinase p56^{Lck} and activation of the Ras–MAPK pathway promote CD4+ T-cell maturation, whereas signaling through the NOTCH transmembrane receptor favors CD8+ differentiation. It appears that these pathways may be integrated ultimately through their contrasting effects on the *Tcfe2a*-encoded transcription factor, E47[22]. It is at the end of this process that mature single positive thymocytes are finally released from the thymic medulla into the peripheral circulation.

Genetic manipulation using transgenic or knock-out mice has greatly increased our knowledge regarding the signaling pathways and transcription factors that contribute to the ontogeny of T cells throughout all stages of thymic development. The key role played by factors such as c-Myb, TCF-1 and LCF-1, E proteins and Id proteins, Ikaros and Notch, Nu77 and Nor1, MEF2 and NF-κB, to name but a few, lie outside the scope of this chapter but can be followed in a number of important review articles[34–36].

It can be seen that as well as acting as an environment for T-cell development, the thymus also acts as the principal source of autoreactive T-cell deletion and, as such, shapes the immune repertoire. However, may facets of thymic function still remain to be elucidated. For example, it is evident from animal models that, despite negative selection, pathogenic autoreactive T cells are still frequently present amongst mature thymic *émigrés*[37]. Also, the mechanism underlying how the mutation of the thymically-expressed transcription factor, AIRE, causes one of the human polyglandular autoimmune syndromes, APECED (autoimmune polyendocrinopathy candidiasis ectodermal dystrophy) remains unclear. These discoveries reinforce how much still remains to be understood of the full role of the thymus in autoimmunity.

Other mechanisms of tolerance

Given that self-reactive T cells are frequently present in peripheral circulation but that autoimmune disease is a relatively uncommon occurrence, there must be mechanisms of avoiding T cell activation and progression in the periphery. Mechanisms cited as responsible for peripheral tolerance include T-cell ignorance, peripheral deletion or exhaustion, T-cell anergy, immune deviation and regulatory T cells[38].

T-cell function

Once activated, T cells subserve different functions. They can provide help for cell-mediated or humoral immune systems, they can become cytotoxic or they can inhibit the activity of other effector T cells.

Helper T cells

CD4+ helper T cells are divided into Th1 and Th2 categories on the basis of their cytokine profile. Th1 cells secrete IL-2 and IFN-γ, circulate beyond the secondary lymphoid organs and promote macrophage activation. Th1 cells also secrete TNF-α and TNF-β, which contribute to the inflammatory cellular response and facilitate cell migration to the site of antigen encounter. Th2 cells produce IL-4, IL-5, IL-10 and IL-13, migrate less than Th1 cells, being commonly found in lymph nodes, and promote B-cell differentiation through antigen-mediated cognate interactions. Both types of Th cell secrete IL-3 and granulocyte–macrophage colony stimulating factor (GM-CSF).

Despite this, Th1 and Th2 cell responses represent the opposing poles of the Th immune response. This polarization occurs at the level of cell responses, Th differentiation and biochemical triggering. For example,

Th2 cytokines such as IL-10 promote humoral immunity but suppress Th1 and macrophage function. The cytokine IL-12, which promotes uncommitted helper T cells (Th0) to differentiate into Th1 effector cells, inhibits Th2 commitment. IL-4 acts in the reverse manner. Finally, the biochemical pathways involving Th1 or Th2 gene transcription are also distinct. GATA-3 is induced in Th2 cells and epigenetically alters chromatin structure to stabilize Th2 cytokine complex accessibility and permits Th2-specific transcription factors such as c-MAF to induce high levels of IL-4 secretion. A complementary pathway involving the transcription factor T-bet has now been described in Th1 cells that remodels IFN-γ chromatin and increases IFN-γ transcription. It appears that T-bet and GATA-3 may antagonize each other's expression, offering a further mechanism for Th polarization[39,40].

Cytotoxic T cells

While CD8+ cytotoxic T cells (Tc) can secrete cytokines, their main function appears to be inducing apoptotic cell death. For this they possess a number of mechanisms. They can release cytotoxins from lytic granules secreted at the site of target cell contact. These cytotoxins include a family of serine proteases, granzyme A, B and H, that are capable of inducing caspase-dependent and caspase-independent cell death. The role of another secreted cytotoxin, perforin, may be to form pores in the target cell membrane, facilitating granzyme entry into the cell. Perforin may also promote the endosomal release of endocytosed granzymes, allowing these enzymes increased access to the target cells' interiors[41].

Their second mechanism of inducing cell death is through Fas–FasL interactions. CD8+ T cells transiently upregulate FasL when stimulated through their TCRs. This induces apoptosis in any targets that are Fas-positive. Fas may be constitutively expressed in a number of tissues but its expression is also often induced as part of the inflammatory process[42].

Cytokine secretion patterns can be used to subdivide CD8+ T cells into Tc1 and Tc2 subsets. Like their helper cell counterparts, Tc1 cells secrete IFN-γ and IL-2, whereas Tc2s secrete IL-4 and IL-5. These cellular subsets can now also be distinguished by the expression of IL18R (type 1) or ST2L (type 2) surface markers[43].

Regulatory T cells

After several years of relative neglect, T cells capable of suppressing the activity of other effector T cells are once again receiving much attention. A subset of CD4+ T cells, called regulatory T cells or Treg, appears capable of suppressing the activity of effector T-cell responses and inhibiting autoimmune disease development in a number of animal models. Characteristically, these cells do not proliferate or secrete IL-2 after TCR ligation. Treg cells have been found to be both naturally occurring and inducible (Th3, Tr1 and anergic cells) but the precise relationship between these various types of regulatory cell remains to be established.

Naturally occurring CD4+CD25+ Treg can be found in human and murine thymuses and recent studies suggest that high-affinity interactions with thymic cortical epithelium might be important in the positive selection of the cells. A population of CD4+ CD25+ Treg cells can be induced from naive precursors after the administration of oral and intravenous antigen but, once again, the relationship between these cells and thymically derived cells of the same phenotype has yet to be fully examined.

Treg may secrete IL-10, TGF-β or both. However, some Treg require direct cell contact to achieve their inhibitory activity[44].

THE B CELL

Immunoglobulin (Ig) is the adaptive system's soluble effector molecule, produced as a result of terminal B-cell differentiation. As might be expected from a cell that originates from a common lymphoid precursor, many features of B lymphocyte physiology and biochemistry parallel those occurring in T cells.

Immunoglobulin

Immunoglobulin (Ig) or antibody can be either membrane-bound (acting as the B-cell antigen receptor) or a soluble effector molecule. The Y-shaped Ig molecule consists of four chains, two identical heavy chains and two identical light ones (Fig. 1.6). There are nine heavy-chain isotypes that determine both immunoglobulin class/subclass (α_1, α_2, δ, ϵ, γ_{1-4} and μ) and the effector mechanisms the antibody can elicit. There are two light-chain isotypes (κ and λ), which can associate with any heavy chain but do not influence effector function. When membrane-bound, each antibody molecule is coexpressed with an Igα and Igβ chain. Together these form a functional B-cell receptor (BCR) capable of signaling antigen recognition.

Each chain is folded into a number of domains. The light chain consists of a single variable and constant domain. The heavy chains also have a single variable domain but can have three (α, γ and δ) or four (ϵ and μ) constant region domains.

The gene complex encoding immunoglobulin heavy chain (IgH) is located on chromosome 14q32 and the κ and λ light-chain gene loci are located on chromosomes 2p12 and 22q11 respectively. Within these loci, subexonic Ig gene segments are distributed in a fashion analogous to that seen in the TCR gene complexes, the largest difference being the string of gene segments encoding the heavy-chain isotype constant regions lying downstream of the IgH J gene segments. As with the TCR, the Ig variable domains are encoded by a series of V(D)J somatic recombination events using essentially the same types of RSS and genetic machinery described for the T cell. Again, as for the T cell, promoter-enhancer interactions regulate the accessibility of the Ig gene locus chromatin to the recombination machinery.

However, there are several B-cell-specific differences in the way Ig genes are recombined and spliced compared with T cells. Firstly, mature naive B cells express both IgM and IgD with identical variable domains at their cell surface. This is accomplished by alternative RNA splicing. Either the transcribed RNA is truncated at the polyA site at the μ constant region to produce IgM or the μ region is deleted entirely from the primary transcript, leaving the δ constant region attached downstream of the rearranged VDJ transcript encoding IgD. RNA splicing is also used when the plasma cell produces secreted antibody. In this instance, the cytoplasmic tail sequence is spliced out of the constant region part of the RNA transcript (Fig 1.7).

Two other B-cell-specific genetic events are somatic hypermutation and class switching. Somatic hypermutation, where additional sequence variation is introduced into the recombined V(D)J sequence as part of affinity maturation and isotype switching where heavy-chain gene segments are looped out (Fig. 1.7) and deleted both appear to use some of the mechanisms seen in V(D)J recombination. Both events require B cell stimulation, active gene transcription, double-stranded DNA break repair mechanisms and appear to involve the activation-induced cytidine deaminase (AID) RNA editing enzyme[45,46].

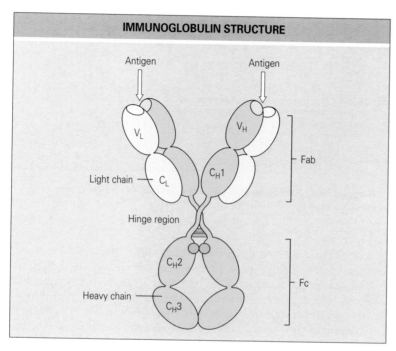

Fig. 1.6 Immunoglobulin structure. A model of IgG showing the globular domain structure. Carbohydrate units (blue circles) lie between the C_H2 domains.

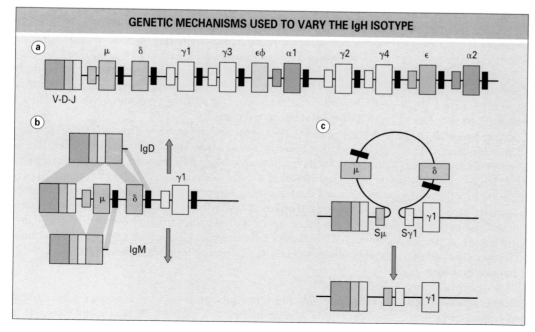

Fig. 1.7 Genetic mechanisms used to vary the IgH isotype. (a) The germline layout of the IgH constant region gene segments is as shown. The diagram includes an IgE pseudogene ($\epsilon\phi$). Shown also are the switch regions (small colored rectangles), the gene exons (large colored rectangles) and the polyA sites (black rectangles), where appropriate. (b) In mature naive B cells, IgD and IgM are co-expressed on the cell surface by differential splicing of the RNA transcript but class-switching is accomplished by an irreversible recombination between two switch regions (c) after which the intervening sequence (including any heavy chain gene exons) is lost. The gene segment that lies closest to the recombined VDJ sequence now encodes the IgH isotype.

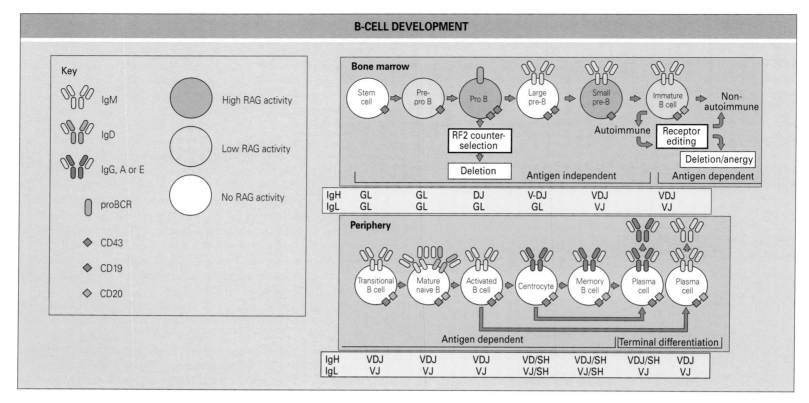

Fig. 1.8 B-cell development. Shown are the stages of B-cell development, the acquisition of the BCR, various developmentally regulated CD antigens and recombination status of the various heavy (IgH) and light (IgL) gene loci. GL = germline; SH = somatic hypermutation.

B-cell development

In adult life, B-cell maturation occurs in the bone marrow (Fig 1.8). B-cell development is dependent on both interacting with adhesion molecules on bone-marrow stromal cells and responding to the growth factors (e.g. IL-7 and stem cell factor) that these stromal cells produce. As with T cells, a number of transcription factors, including PU.1, Ikaros, EBF, E2A and Pax5, have been identified as key regulators of B-cell development[47].

The earliest committed B cell precursors are the pre-pro-B cells defined on the basis of surface molecule expression (Fig. 1.8). Pro-B cells begin rearrangement of the IgH genes and express the pro-BCR (calnexin complexed with Igα and Igβ). DJ rearrangements begin first and V to DJ rearrangements follow. Productively rearranged μ chains are expressed on the cell surface with a surrogate light chain (consisting of V-pre-B and λ5) and Igα and Igβ. This pre-BCR induces cell division and the generation of non-dividing small pre-B cells. It also suppresses further IgH gene recombination (allelic exclusion) by decreasing RAG expression and appears to make further V_H genes less accessible to the recombination machinery. Although the D_H segments are theoretically functional in any reading frame, reading frame 2 appears to encode a truncated form of mIgμ (Dm). When this forms part of pre-BCR, its function is defective and results in arrested pro-B development (RF2 counterselection) ultimately ending in either deletion or rescue by further gene recombination[48,49].

The small pre-B cells, resting in G1, re-express the RAG proteins and begin light-chain rearrangement. Productive rearrangement of the light chain leads to expression of the mature BCR, in which the surrogate light chain in the pre-BCR is replaced by a mature κ or λ chain. Expression of the BCR leads to suppression of further light-chain recombination; however, as with the TCR α chain, allelic exclusion at the light chain locus is 'leaky' and about 10% of B cells express two separate light chains. At this stage the lymphocyte becomes an immature B cell expressing IgM only and it is at this stage that tolerance induction

occurs. If the expressed Ig on these reacts with other cell surface self-antigen, such as glycoproteins, proteoglycans or glycolipids, then clonal deletion by apoptosis occurs. If the immature B cell binds to soluble self-antigens, such as proteins or glycoproteins, anergy (failure to proliferate upon stimulation with antigen or mitogen) ensues. Anergic B cells only survive briefly. However, a further tolerogenic mechanism, called receptor editing, in which Ig rearrangements continue even after assembly of a functional BCR, is now being recognized. This mechanism, in contrast to anergy or deletion, spares autoreactive B cells by replacing their receptors – a rare example of frugality by the adaptive immune system[48].

Immature B cells that emigrate from the bone marrow are known as transitional B cells. Only 10–30% of these cells enter the mature peripheral B cell compartment. The transitional cell pool appears to be variable and is homeostatically controlled to maintain mature B-cell numbers. Maturation from this stage depends on intact signaling pathways and accessory molecules[48]. Mature naive, IgM and IgD co-expressing B cells will survive between 3 and 8 weeks if they successfully enter primary follicles in secondary lymphoid tissues. This is where they will encounter specific antigen. If that happens, the B cell will interact with Th cells and become activated.

Some B cells will proliferate and differentiate directly into Ig-secreting plasma cells, others will enter into nearby primary follicles. These primary follicles become secondary follicles with germinal centers and the large proliferating B cells (centroblasts) undergo somatic hypermutation and class switching before becoming non-proliferating centrocytes. Activated B cells that have survived the affinity maturation process will home to other secondary lymphoid tissues or bone marrow and differentiate into plasma cells secreting IgG, IgA or IgE high-affinity antibodies; others will become quiescent, long-lived memory B cells.

B-1 B cells

B cells are divided into two groups, B-1 and B-2, based on cell surface and functional characteristics. B-1, cells which are mostly CD5+ (B-1a cells), but sometimes CD5⁻ (B-1b), express surface IgM and are characterized by the production of low-affinity antibodies against DNA, immunoglobulin, bacterial carbohydrate antigens and phosphatidyl choline. The origin of these cells is debated but the autoreactive nature of their receptors appears to be a factor in their development and also makes them of potential interest in autoimmune disease. Unlike the more usual B-2 cells, B-1 cells seem to rely on positive selection and BCR signaling to develop[48,49].

B-cell antigen recognition and B-cell receptor signaling pathways

Both the BCR and soluble Ig can bind both linear and conformational epitopes on a wide variety of molecules. Certain antigens (thymus-independent or TI antigens) can activate B cells without the need for helper T cells but many require T-cell help and are thymus-dependent (TD). TI-1 antigens bind other receptors besides the BCR and can induce proliferation of both mature and immature B cells. TI-2 antigens are typically composed repetitive epitopes and typically stimulate mature B-1 B cells.

B-cell receptor signaling pathways follow an essentially similar course to that seen in T cells (Fig. 1.9). BCR ligation activates the Src family of kinases that phosphorylate Syk, Btk and the ITAMs on the Igα and Igβ chains. Syk phosphorylates proteins, including SLP-65. This results in the formation of a complex containing SLP-65, Btk and PLCγ2. This appears to be targeted to membrane rafts by an unknown mechanism

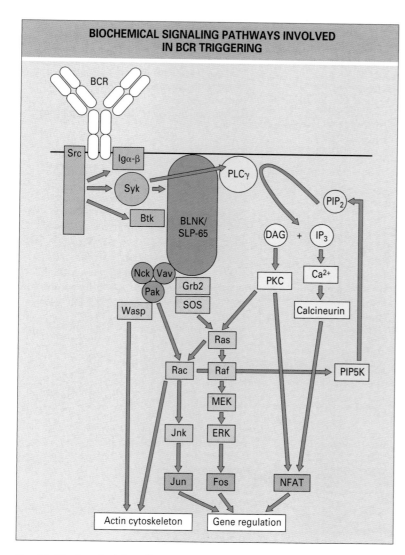

Fig. 1.9 Biochemical signaling pathways involved in BCR triggering.

where PIP2 hydrolysis to IP3 and DAG occurs with the same downstream consequences as in T cells. The complex also recruits Vav and can contribute to both cytoskeletal changes and Ca²⁺ mobilization via its action on Rac. The complex also recruits Grb2 and SOS which, in turn, activates the Ras–ERK pathway[50,51].

Modulation of signaling by B-cell co-receptors
The way in which costimulatory molecules can affect signaling pathways appears to be more fully characterized in B cells than in T cells[51,52]. CD19 acts to further enhance BCR signaling. It forms a non-covalent complex with CD21 (complement receptor type 2) and its coligation with the BCR is enhanced by antigens complexed with C3d. Upon phosphorylation, CD19 recruits PI-3K, Src PTKs and Vav and contributes to the activation of the MAPK pathways and Ca²⁺ mobilization. Negatively regulating co-receptors such as CD22, CD72 and FcRγIIB1 negatively regulate B-cell proliferation and Ca²⁺ mobilization. Their cytoplasmic immunoreceptor tyrosine-based inhibitory motifs (ITIMs) are phosphorylated upon BCR ligation via Lyn. CD22 and CD72 recruit SHP-1 and the Fc receptor recruits SHIP. Both inhibit BCR signaling. SHP-1 may phosphorylate signaling molecules such as Syk and SLP-65 and SHIP both inhibits PIP3 (indirectly preventing PLCγ and Ca²⁺ signaling) and binds RasGAP via the adaptor protein p62-Dok, making it unavailable for interaction in MAPK pathways.

B-cell function
The principal function of B cells is to differentiate into plasma cells and secrete antibody. Antibody has a number of functions. It can directly stimulate or neutralize its antigenic target or it can link antigen binding to innate effector mechanisms such as opsonization, complement activation or antibody-dependent cellular cytotoxicity (ADCC). The precise effector mechanisms activated depend on the Ig isotype and, in the case of cellular interaction, the commensurate distribution of specific Fc receptors.

B cells may also operate as specialist antigen presenting cells. However, another property of B cells, commonly overlooked, is their cytokine secretion. Recently data suggest that B cells, like Th and Tc cells, can be divided according to the range of cytokines they produce. Therefore B-cell cytokine secretion, like those of Th, Tc and other cell types, can be regarded as being polarized into, and positively reinforcing, a general type 1 or type 2 immune effector response[53].

LYMPHOCYTE MIGRATION

All the processes described in the foregoing paragraphs occur at specific anatomical locations. Lymphoid precursors arise in the bone marrow before migrating to the thymus. Mature naive T cells migrate to the T-cell areas of lymph nodes, adjacent to the primary follicles where the mature B lymphocytes have homed to following their emigration from the bone marrow. If dendritic cells are involved in an inflammatory process, they migrate in the afferent lymph from their location in the peripheral tissues, such as the skin, to the lymph node. Here they interact with naive T and B lymphocytes to induce both effector and memory cells. Once effector and memory cells have arisen by differentiation and proliferation from their naive precursors, depending on their function, they may migrate to either peripheral or secondary lymphoid tissues in order to either eliminate antigen or await further cognate encounters with it. In other words, the coordinated and regulated migration of lymphoid cells is essential for the development of the adaptive immune response and the ability of adaptive immune cells to respond anamnestically to subsequent antigenic encounters.

Cellular adhesion cascades
In the absence of inflammation, T cells are the predominant lymphocyte found in extracellular fluids. It is estimated that approximately

10^{10} T cells leave the blood, enter the tissues and return to the blood every 30 minutes[54]. In most tissues (except the lungs, liver and spleen), T-cell entry occurs via the postcapillary venules. Blood cells move extremely rapidly and cells that touch the endothelial walls are easily dislodged by the large shear stresses caused by the flowing blood. In order to overcome this, the T cells use adhesion molecules to bind ligands on the vessel wall (Table 1.1). Tissues (e.g. lymph nodes and Peyer's patches) whose vessels constitutively express these ligands and routinely have lymphocyte homing, do so on specialized endothelial cells (high endothelial vessels, HEVs). However, these adhesion molecule counter-receptors can also be induced on vascular endothelia in other tissues as part of the inflammatory process[55].

For extravasation of lymphocytes to occur, a cascade of adhesion molecule interactions must take place. Initial contact between the lymphocyte and endothelial cell, either directly or via bridging platelets, is made using the constitutively active selectins on each cell type (CD26L on lymphocytes, CD26E and CD26P on endothelium and CD26P on platelets) with the sialyl-Lewis^X components of the glycoprotein ligands on the opposing cell. For example, CD26L on lymphocytes can bind PNAd on endothelial cells and CD26E and P on endothelium may interact with PSGL-1 on lymphocytes. This selectin-mediated adhesion tethers the leukocyte to the cell wall but, because of the shearing forces applied by the flowing bloodstream, contact is lost on the upstream side and re-established with new selectins on the downstream side and the leukocyte begins to 'roll' down the vascular endothelium[55].

Rolling lymphocytes respond to signals from chemoattractants on the endothelial cell surface through specific seven-transmembrane, G-protein-coupled receptors. This activates them and induces rapid expression of the secondary adhesion molecules, the integrins. Some of these chemoattractants, such as the complement fragment C5a, leukotriene B4 and formyl peptides, are secreted or diffuse freely into the vessel lumen and some, such as chemokines, are expressed on the cell wall. The chemokines may be secreted as part of the inflammatory process but may also be constitutively expressed in some tissues[56]. Adhesion of the integrins with their targets arrests the rolling movement and allows diapedesis across the endothelium into the tissues along chemotactic gradients to begin.

The tissue distribution of these adhesion molecules varies. Where a particular molecule plays a dominant role in cell migration to a specific tissue it is referred to as an addressin. Its lymphocyte-borne

TABLE 1.1 ADHESION MOLECULES, THEIR LIGANDS AND THEIR ROLE IN MIGRATION

Adhesion molecule	Distribution	Ligand	Migratory function
Selectins		Sialyl-Lewis^x	
L-selectin (CD26L)	All leukocytes except effector and memory cells	PNAd, PSGL-1, MADCAM-1 E-selectin, etc.	Homing to lymph nodes and Peyer's patches
E-selectin (CD26E)	Activated endothelium	PSGL-1, ESL-1, CLA, glycoproteins, glycolipids	Homing of memory and effector cells to cutaneous and inflammatory sites
P-selectin (CD26P)	Activated endothelium and platelets	PSGL-1, CD24, PNAd	Homing of memory and Th1 effector cells to inflamed tissues
			Platelet interaction with PNAd-expressing venules
Selectin ligands			
P-selectin glycoprotein-1 (PSGL-1)	All leukocytes	All selectins	Binding to activated platelets
			Homing of Th1 memory and effector cells to inflamed tissues
Peripheral-node addressin (PNAd)	Lymph node HEVs Sites of chronic inflammation	L- and P-selectin	Homing of naive and central memory cells to lymph nodes
Cutaneous lymphocyte antigen (CLA)	Skin-homing T cells, dendritic cells, granulocytes	E-selectin	Homing of memory and effector cells to skin
Integrins			
α4β1 (VLA-4)	Leukocytes except neutrophils	VCAM-1, fibronectin	Homing to inflamed tissues, especially lung
α4β7	Lymphocytes, NK cells Mast cells, basophils, monocytes	MAdCAM-1, fibronectin VCAM-1 (weakly)	Homing to gut-associated lymphoid tissues (GALT)
αLβ2 (LFA-1)	All leukocytes	ICAM-1, 2, 3, 4 and 5	Homing to lymph nodes, Peyer's patches and inflamed tissues
			Adhesion to APCs
αMβ2 (Mac-1)	Myeloid cells, some activated T cells	ICAM-1, factor X, fibrinogen, C3b	Unknown
αXβ2 (p150,95)	Dendritic cells	Fibrinogen, C3b	Unknown
αDβ2	Monocytes, macrophages, eosinophils	ICAM-1 and -3, VCAM-1	Unknown
Immunoglobulin superfamily			
ICAM-1 (CD54)	Most cell types	LFA-1, Mac-1, fibrinogen	Endothelial ligand for β2 integrins
ICAM-2 (CD102)	Endothelial cells, platelets	LFA-1	Unknown
VCAM-1 (CD106)	Endothelial cells, bone marrow, dendritic cells, osteoblasts, mesothelium	VLA-4, α4β7, αDβ2	Homing to inflamed tissues
Mucosal addressin-cell adhesion molecule 1 (MAdCAM-1)	GALT HEVs, spleen Lamina propria, sites of chronic inflammation	α4β7, L-selectin	Homing of all lymphocytes to gut-associated lymphoid tissues

ligand is referred to as a homing molecule. One of the best examples of addressins determines whether naive T cells home to peripheral lymphoid tissue (PLT) or gut-associated lymphoid tissue (GALT). HEVs in PLT express peripheral node addressin (PNAd) whereas Peyer's patches and some mesenteric lymph nodes express the addressin mucosal-addressin-cell adhesion molecule (MAdCAM)-1. Both addressins are capable of binding CD26L but only in PLT is this interaction sufficient to initiate cell rolling. In the Peyer's patch, additional adhesion to MAdCAM-1 by the $\alpha 4\beta 7$ integrin is required for rolling to occur. Without this, T-cell activation, further integrin expression and extravasation do not occur. Homing to Peyer's patches is therefore a property of those naive lymphoid cells that express the $\alpha 4\beta 7$ integrin.

Chemokines

Just as the diversity and complexity of integrin and selectin expression may alter lymphocyte homing and consequent function, it is becoming apparent that the heterogeneity of the chemokine family plays a similar role in the development of adaptive immunity[55,57].

The chemokines are a group of small, structurally related, heparin binding cytokines named because of their ability to induce directed migration (chemotaxis) of various types of leukocyte. More than 50 chemokines and 18 specific receptors have now been identified (Table 1.2). The chemokines are classified into four groups on the basis of the arrangement of their amino-terminal cysteine residues, called CXC, CC, CX3C and C. The CXC group has been further divided according to whether or not there is a glutamic acid–leucine–arginine (ELR) motif immediately in front of the first cysteine residue. Functionally, the chemokines can be divided into inflammatory or immune (also known as homeostatic, constitutive or lymphoid) chemokine group, although this division is far from being absolute. LPS, IL-1 and TNF induce high levels of the classical inflammatory chemokines. Generally speaking, CXC chemokines are potent chemoattractants for neutrophils whereas CC chemokines recruit monocytes. However, these inflammatory chemokines display considerable redundancy with respect to function and receptor and ligand specificity.

The immune chemokines play a vital role in the development, maintenance and function of the immune system. However, their title is somewhat of a misnomer as they also play a role in non-lymphoid tissues and their expression is not only constitutive but also highly inducible under the appropriate conditions[57].

Chemokines and the development of primary lymphoid tissue

In bone marrow, interactions between SDF-1/CXCL12 expression and precursor cells bearing CXCR4 appear vital for normal B-cell development. However, chemokine receptor expression changes during B-cell development and the expression of the CCR7 receptor may allow SLC/CCL21 and ELC/CCL19 to control mature B-cell emigration into the peripheral circulation. In the thymus, SDF-1/CXCL12 attracts thymic precursors from the bone marrow, TECK/CCL25 interacting with CCR9 and TARC/CCL17 and MDC/CCL22, both binding CCR4, may be involved in later stages of thymocyte migration from the cortex to the medulla. As in B cells, late expression of CCR7 appears to be involved in emigration of mature naive T cells into the periphery[57].

Chemokines and immune response development

T and B cells are directed to the secondary lymphoid tissue by their expression of the chemokine receptor CCR7. There they home first to the T-cell areas and the B cells migrate further to the B-cell follicles because of their CXCR5-directed response to BLC/CXCL13 secretion by follicular dendritic cells (Fig. 1.10).

Monocytes and dendritic cells exit the blood into tissues. These cells express the inflammatory chemokine receptors CCR1, CCR2, CCR5, CXCR2 and CCR6. Upon exposure to inflammatory mediators LPS, IL-1 and TNF-α, dendritic cells express CD80 and CD86 (ligands for the costimulatory T-cell molecule CD28), downregulate their inflammatory chemokine receptors and express CCR7. This receptor guides dendritic cells to the T-cell areas of secondary lymphoid tissue, as it did for the naive T and B cells.

Cognate interactions between dendritic cells and naive T cells leads to production of effector and memory T cells. Th1 and Th2 effector cells not only secrete different cytokines but they also express different

TABLE 1.2 CHEMOKINES AND CHEMOKINE RECEPTORS			
Chemokine	Systematic name	Receptor	Major lymphocyte subset bearing receptor
CXC chemokines			
ELR motif chemokines			
Gro/MGSA-α	CXCL1	CXCR2	CD8 T cells, NK cells
Gro/MGSA-β	CXCL2	CXCR2	CD8 T cells, NK cells
Gro/MGSA-γ	CXCL3	CXCR2	CD8 T cells, NK cells
ENA-78	CXCL5	CXCR2	CD8 T cells, NK cells
GCP-2	CXCL6	CXCR1	CD8 T cells, NK cells
		CXCR2	CD8 T cells, NK cells
NAP-2	CXCL7	CXCR2	CD8 T cells, NK cells
IL-8	CXCL8	CXCR1	CD8 T cells, NK cells
		CXCR2	CD8 T cells, NK cells
Non-ELR motif chemokines			
PF-4	CXCL4	Unknown	
Mig	CXCL9	CXCR3	Th0/Th1 T cells
IP-10	CXCL10	CXCR3	Th0/Th1 T cells
I-TAC	CXCL11	CXCR3	Th0/Th1 T cells
SDF-1/PBSF	CXCL12	CXCR4	Naive > memory T cells
BLC/BCA-1	CXCL13	CXCR5	B cells, T$_{FH}$ cells
BRAK	CXCL14	Unknown	
CXCL16	CXCL16	CXCR6	CD8 T cells, NK cells

TABLE 1.2 (cont'd)

Chemokine	Systematic name	Receptor	Major lymphocyte subset bearing receptor
CC chemokines			
I-309	CCL1	CCR8	Th2 T cells
MCP-1	CCL2	CCR2	Activated T cells
MIP-1α	CCL3	CCR1	Memory > naive T cells
		CCR5	Th0/Th1 T cells
MIP-1β	CCL4	CCR5	Th0/Th1 T cells
RANTES	CCL5	CCR1	Memory > naive T cells
		CCR3	Th2 T cells
		CCR5	Th0/Th1 T cells
MCP-3	CCL7	CCR1	Memory > naive T cells
		CCR2	Activated T cells
		CCR3	Th2 T cells
MCP-2	CCL8	CCR3	Th2 T cells
		CCR5	Th0/Th1 T cells
Eotaxin	CCL11	CCR3	Th2 T cells
MCP-4	CCL13	CCR2	Activated T cells
		CCR3	Th2 T cells
HCC-1	CCL14	CCR1	Memory > naive T cells
HCC-2/leukotactin-1	CCL15	CCR1	Memory > naive T cells
		CCR3	Th2 T cells
HCC-4/LEC	CCL16	CCR1	Memory > naive T cells
		CCR2	Activated T cells
		CCR5	Th0/Th1 T cells
		CCR8	Th2 T cells
TARC	CCL17	CCR4	Th2 T cell, CLA+ cells
PARC/DC-CK1/AMAC-1	CCL18	Unknown	
ELC/MIP-3b/Exodus-3	CCL19	CCR7	B cells, naive T cells, T$_{CM}$
LARC/MIP-3a/Exodus-1	CCL20	CCR6	B cells, CLA+ cells, α4β7+ cells
SLC/6Ckine/Exodus-2	CCL21	CCR7	B cells, naive T cells, T$_{CM}$
MDC/STCP-1	CCL22	CCR4	Th2 T cells, CLA+ cells
MPIF-1	CCL23	CCR1	Memory > naive T cells
MPIF-2/Eotaxin-2	CCL24	CCR3	Th2 T cells
TECK	CCL25	CCR9	α4β7+ cells, IELs
Eotaxin-3	CCL26	CCR3	Th2 T cells
ILC/CTACK/Eskine	CCL27	CCR1O	CLA+ cells
MEC/CCL28	CCL28	CCR3	Th2 T cells
		CCR1O	CLA+ cells
CX3C chemokine			
Fractalkine	CX3CL1	CX3CR1	CD8 T cells, NK cells
C chemokine			
Lymphotactin/SCM-1/ATAC	XCL1,2	XCR1	CD8 T cells, NK cells

IELs, intra-epithelial lymphocytes; NK cells, natural killer cells; α4β7+, integrin-positive cells; CLA+, cutaneous-lymphocyte-antigen-positive cells; Th, helper T cells; T$_{CM}$, central memory T cells.

chemokine receptor profiles. The receptors that each helper cell type expresses respond to chemokines induced by the cytokines they secrete. Therefore, Th1 cells express CXCR3 and CCR5. The Th1 cytokine, IFN-γ, induces IP-10/CXCL10, Mig/CXCL9 and I-TAC/CXCL11, which bind CXCR3, and RANTES, which binds CCR5. CXCL10, CXCL9, CXCL11 and RANTES are secreted by a variety of cells, including keratinocytes, monocytes, fibroblasts, endothelium and T lymphocytes themselves. CCR5 receptors are also present on macrophages and natural killer (NK) cells. Together, this represents a positive feedback loop in which Th1 cells produce cytokines that induce chemokines in tissues that, in turn, recruit more cells that either produce or respond to

Th1 cytokines[57,58]. This tends to polarize immune reactions towards one specific effector phenotype (Fig. 1.10). Chemokines and chemokine receptors typical of this Th1 or delayed-type hypersensitivity (DTH)-like phenotype have been observed in the rheumatoid synovium and multiple sclerosis[59,60].

Similarly, Th2 cells express CCR3 and CCR8 chemokine receptors, among others. CCR3 is also present on eosinophils and basophils. The Th2 cytokines IL-4 and IL-13 induce secretion of the chemokines eotaxin-1/CCL11, eotaxin-2/CCL24, eotaxin-3/CCL26 and MCP-4/CCL13 by a variety of cells. These chemokines bind CCR3[57]. Once again, this positive feedback loop allows the accumulation and polarization of Th2

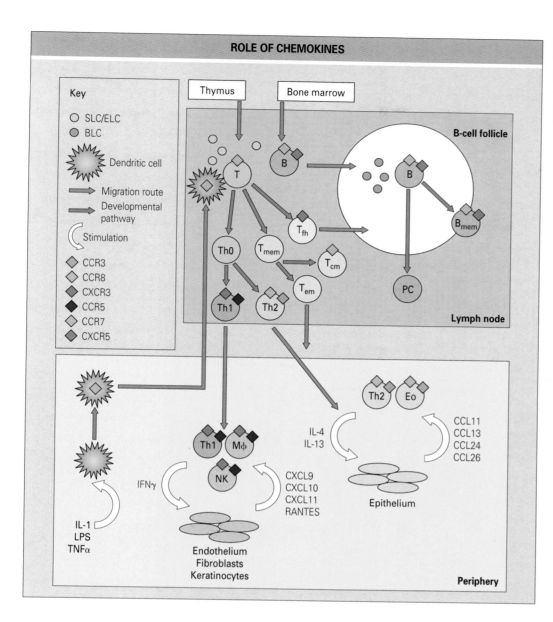

ROLE OF CHEMOKINES

Key

○ SLC/ELC
● BLC

Dendritic cell

→ Migration route
→ Developmental pathway

Stimulation

◇ CCR3
◇ CCR8
◆ CXCR3
◆ CCR5
◇ CCR7
◆ CXCR5

Thymus   Bone marrow

B-cell follicle

Lymph node

Th2 Eo

CCL11
CCL13
CCL24
CCL26

IL-4
IL-13

Epithelium

Th1 Mφ

NK

IFNγ

CXCL9
CXCL10
CXCL11
RANTES

IL-1
LPS
TNFα

Endothelium
Fibroblasts
Keratinocytes

Periphery

Fig 1.10 Role of chemokines in directing lymphocyte movement and immune response polarization. For detailed explanation see text. T_{CM} = central memory T cell, T_{EM} = effector memory T cell, T_{FH} = follicular homing helper T cell, Mφ = macrophage, NK = natural killer cell, Eo = eosinophil.

regulatory and effector T cells within lesions at particular anatomical sites (Fig. 1.10). In this way, chemokines not only control the migration of relevant cells to sites of ongoing immune response but they also segregate mutually antagonistic T cells that might impair the activity of one another.

A third Th-cell subset, the follicular homing cell T helper cell (T_{FH}) has recently been identified because of its expression of CXCR5. This receptor responds to CXCL13 and the T_{FH} cell homes to edge of the B-cell follicle in order to provide help for B-cell differentiation and antibody production[57,61].

Memory T cells can also be subdivided into effector memory and central memory cells, based on the expression of CCR7. CCR7+ central memory cells reside in the secondary lymphoid tissues whereas the effector memory T cells, which are CCR7-negative, are able to migrate through the peripheral tissues in search of cognate interactions with antigen[62].

SUMMARY

By its nature, the adaptive immune system potentially represents the most specific target for therapy in autoimmune diseases. From the foregoing brief sketch, I hope that it is clear that not only is our understanding increasing in specific details of immune physiology but the way the system is coordinated at the cellular, biochemical and, most recently, anatomical levels is also being radically dissected.

Many experiments are now revealing amplification loops by which specific adaptive immune responses are reinforced. One good example is the integration of immune response polarization by coordinated patterns of cytokine secretion by a variety of cell types. Another is the interplay between cytokines, chemokines and chemokine and homing receptor expression in the reinforcement of anatomic localization of specific immune responses. Clearly, therapeutic interruption of these feedback processes has and will continue to provide novel therapeutic agents.

Work on the negative regulation of these pathways is not yet so advanced but undoubtedly will follow. The resurgence of interest in regulatory T cells is the first step in this revival. It also raises the possibility that specific immunosuppression may be developed to retard the progress of autoimmune diseases without the complications of more generalized therapy.

Finally, despite huge advances, the regulation of repertoire formation, particularly in T cells, still represents a considerable mystery, especially in humans. Our understanding of that, ultimately, may allow us to selectively prevent the development of autoimmune disease in the first place.

REFERENCES

1. Kay RA. TCR gene polymorphisms and autoimmune disease. Eur J Immunogenet 1996; 23: 159–177.

2. Grawunder U, Harfst E. How to make ends meet in V(D)J recombination. Curr Opin Immunol 2001; 13: 186–194.

3. Schlissel MS, Stanhope-Baker P. Accessibility and the developmental regulation of V(D)J recombination. Semin Immunol 1997; 9: 161–170.

4. Posnett DN, Vissinga CS, Pambuccian C *et al*. Level of human *TCRBV3S1* (V beta 3) expression correlates with allelic polymorphism in the spacer region of the recombination signal sequence. J Exp Med 1994; 179: 1707–1711.

5. Kay RA, Snowden N, Hajeer AH *et al*. Genetic control of the human Vβ13.2 T cell repertoire: importance of allelic variation outside the coding regions of the *TCRBV13S2* gene. Eur J Immunol 1994; 24: 2863–2867.

6. Kay RA, Hutchings CJ, Ollier WER. A subset of Sjögren's syndrome associates with the *TCRBV13S2* locus but not the *TCRBV2S1* locus. Hum Immunol 1995; 42: 328–330.

7. Yewdell JW, Bennink JR. Cut and trim: generating MHC class I peptide ligands. Curr Opin Immunol 2001; 13: 13–18.

8. Quadri SA, Singal DP. Peptide transport in human lymphoblastoid and tumor cells: effect of transporter associated with antigen presentation (TAP) polymorphism. Immunol Lett 1998; 61: 25–31.

9. Watts C. Antigen processing in the endocytic compartment. Curr Opin Immunol 2001; 13: 26–31.

10. Watts, C. Capture and processing of exogenous antigens for presentation on MHC molecules. Annu Rev Immunol 1997; 15: 821–850.

11. Kay RA. The potential role of superantigens in inflammatory bowel disease. Clin Exp Immunol 1995; 100: 4–6.

12. Jayawardena-Wolf J, Bendelac A. CD1 and lipid antigens: intracellular pathways for antigen presentation. Curr Opin Immunol 2001; 13: 109–113.

13. Coyle AJ, Gutierrez-Ramos J-C. The expanding B7 superfamily: increasing complexity in costimulatory signals regulating T cell function. Nat Immunol 2001; 2: 203–209.

14. Watts TH, DeBenedette MA. T cell co-stimulatory molecules other than CD28. Curr Opin Immunol 2001; 11: 286–293.

15. Bromley SK, Burack WR, Johnson KG *et al*. The immunological synapse. Annu Rev Immunol 2001; 19: 375–396.

16. Lanzavecchia A, Sallusto F. From synapses to immunological memory: the role of sustained T cell stimulation. Curr Opin Immunol 2000; 12: 92–98.

17. Lanzavecchia A, Iezzi G, Viola A. From TCR engagement to T cell activation: a kinetic view of T cell behavior. Cell 1999; 96: 1–4.

18. Baldwin AS. The NF-κB and IκB proteins: new discoveries and insights. Annu Rev Immunol 1996 14: 649–681.

19. Pivniouk VI, Geha RS. The role of SLP-76 and LAT in lymphocyte development. Curr Opin Immunol 2000; 12: 173–178.

20. Myung PS, Boerthe NJ, Koretzky GA. Adapter proteins in lymphocyte antigen receptor signaling. Curr Opin Immunol 2000; 12: 256–266.

21. Rao A, Luo C, Hogan PC. Transcription factors of the NFAT family: regulation and function. Annu Rev Immunol 1997; 15: 707–747.

22. Basson MA, Zamoyska R. The CD4/CD8 lineage decision: integration of signalling pathways. Immunol Today 2000; 21: 509–514.

23. Chambers CA, Kuhns MS, Egen JG, Allison JP. CTLA-4 mediated inhibition in regulation of T cell responses: mechanisms and manipulation in tumor immunotherapy. Annu Rev Immunol 2001; 19: 565–594.

24. Agarwal S, Rao A. Long-range transcriptional regulation of cytokine gene expression. Curr Opin Immunol 1998; 10: 345–352.

25. Crabtree GR. Contingent genetic regulatory events in T lymphocyte activation. Science 1989; 243: 355–361.

26. Halle JP, Haus-Seuffert P, Woltering C *et al*. A conserved tissue-specific structure at a human T-cell receptor beta-chain core promoter. Mol Cell Biol 1997; 17: 4220–4229.

27. Deng X, Sun GR, Zheng Q, Li Y. Characterization of human TCR Vβ gene promoter: role of the duodecamer motif in promoter activity. J Biol Chem 1998; 273: 23709–23715.

28. Lennon GP, Sillibourne JE, Furrie E *et al*. Antigen triggering selectively increases *TCRBV* gene transcription. J Immunol 2000; 165: 2020–2027.

29. Kisielow P, von Boehmer H. Development and selection of T cells: facts and puzzles. Adv Immunol 1995; 58: 87–209.

30. Padovan E, Casorati G, Dellabona P *et al*. Dual receptor T-cells. Implications for alloreactivity and autoimmunity. Ann NY Acad Sci 1995; 756: 66–70.

31. Welen G, Hausmann B, Palmer E. A motif in the αβ T-cell receptor that controls positive selection by modulating ERK activity. Nature 2000; 406: 422–426.

32. Hogquist KA. Signal strength in thymic selection and lineage commitment. Curr Opin Immunol 2001; 13: 225–231.

33. Amsen D, Kruisbeek AM. Thymocyte selection: not by TCR alone. Immunol Rev 1998; 165: 209–229.

34. Kuo CT, Leiden JM. Transcriptional regulation of T lymphocyte development and function. Annu Rev Immunol 1999; 17: 149–187.

35. Osborne BA. Transcriptional control of T cell development. Curr Opin Immunol 2000; 12: 301–306.

36. Berg LJ, Kang J. Molecular determinants of TCR expression and selection. Curr Opin Immunol 2001; 13: 232–241.

37. Sagaguchi S. Animal models of autoimmunity and their relevance to human diseases. Curr Opin Immunol 2000; 12: 684–690.

38. Stockinger B. T lymphocyte tolerance: From thymic deletion to peripheral control mechanisms. Adv Immunol 1999; 71: 229–265.

39. Rengarajan J, Szabo SJ, Glimcher LH. Transcriptional regulation of Th1/Th2 polarization. Immunol Today 2000; 21: 479–483.

40. Reiner SL. Helper T cell differentiation, inside and out. Curr Opin Immunol 2001; 13: 351–355.

41. Trapani JA, Davis J, Sutton VR, Smyth MJ. Proapoptotic functions of cytotoxic lymphocyte constituents *in vitro* and *in vivo*. Curr Opin Immunol 2000; 12: 323–329.

42. Sabelko-Downes KA, Russell JH. The role of Fas ligand *in vivo* as a cause and regulator of pathogenesis. Curr Opin Immunol 2000; 12: 330–335.

43. Chan WL, Pejnovic N, Lee CA, Al-Ali NA. Human IL-18 receptor and ST2L are stable and selective markers for the respective type 1 and type 2 circulating lymphocytes. J Immunol 2001; 167: 1238–1244.

44. Read S, Powrie F. CD4+ regulatory T cells. Curr Opin Immunol 2001; 13: 644–649.

45. Kinoshita K, Honjo T. Unique and unprecedented recombination mechanisms in class switching. Curr Opin Immunol 2000; 12: 195–198.

46. Jacobs H, Bross L. Towards an understanding of somatic hypermutation. Curr Opin Immunol 2001; 13: 208–218.

47. O'Riordan M, Grosschedl R. Transcriptional regulation of early B-lymphocyte differentiation. Immunol Rev 2000; 175: 94–103.

48. Meffre E, Casellas R, Nussenzweig MC. Antibody regulation of B cell development. Nat Immunol 2000; 1: 379–385.

49. Hardy RR, Hayakawa K. B cell development pathways. Annu Rev Immunol 2001; 19: 595–621.

50. Schaeffer EM, Schwartzberg PL. Tec family kinases in lymphocyte signaling and function. Curr Opin Immunol 2000; 12: 282–288.

51. Leo A, Schraven B. Adapters in lymphocyte signalling. Curr Opin Immunol 2001; 13: 307–316.

52. Tsubata T. Co-receptors on B lymphocytes. Curr Opin Immunol 1999; 11: 249–255.

53. Mosmann T. Complexity or coherence? Cytokine secretion by B cells. Nat Immunol 2000; 1: 465–466.

54. Westermann J, Pabst R. Lymphocyte subsets in the blood: a diagnostic window on the lymphoid system? Immunol Today 1990 11: 406–410.

55. Von Andrian UH, Mackay CR. T-cell function and migration. N Engl J Med 2000; 343: 1020–1034.

56. Yoshie O, Imai T, Nomiyama H. Novel lymphocyte-specific CC chemokines and their receptors. J Leukocyte Biol 1997; 62: 634–644.

57. Yoshie O, Imai T, Nomiyama H. Chemokines in immunity. Adv Immunol 2001; 78: 57–110.

58. Mackay CR. Chemokines: immunology's high impact factors. Nat Immunol 2001; 2: 95–101.

59. Qin S, Rottman JB, Myers P *et al*. The chemokine receptors CXCR3 and CCR5 mark subsets of T cells associated with certain inflammatory reactions. J Clin Invest 1998; 101: 746–754.

60. Balashov KE, Rottman JB, Weiner HL, Hancock WW. CCR5 (+) and CXCR3 (+) T cells are increased in multiple sclerosis and their ligands MIP-1α and IP-10 are expressed in demyelinating brain lesions. Proc Natl Acad Sci USA 1999; 96: 6873–6878.

61. Mackay CR. Follicular homing T helper (Th) cells and the Th1/Th2 paradigm. J Exp Med 2000; 192: F31–F34.

62. Sallusto F, Lenig D, Foerster R *et al*. Two subsets of memory T lymphocytes with distinct homing potentials and effector functions. Nature 1999; 401: 708–712.

2 Inflammation

Dwight R Robinson

- Inflammation is an essential defense mechanism as well as an important pathologic process

- It is responsible for symptoms and tissue injury in a number of rheumatic and other diseases. The control of inflammatory processes is a major aim in therapy but achieving this goal is often difficult in practice

- Currently, a large number of biological agents are known or suspected to be involved in the pathogenesis of inflammation

- Inflammation is highly complex and probably involves many mediators and cell types in any disease state. Mediators appear to coordinate cellular infiltration and proliferation, the chemical modification of tissues and even tissue destruction

- Knowledge of the important biochemical mediators in any specific inflammatory process may lead to the rational development of new and more effective therapeutic agents

INTRODUCTION

Inflammation is a complex process that may be defined as the response of living tissues to injury[1]. The response only occurs in vascularized tissues, delivering essential molecules and cells to sites of inflammation in extravascular tissues. Inflammation is essential to protect the host from pathogenic microorganisms and to repair wounds from physical or chemical injury. The repair of injured tissues is an integral part of inflammation, after elimination of injurious organisms or matter.

In some forms of tissue injury, repair is the major beneficial result of inflammation, such as in the repair of 'clean' lacerations. In other cases, such as acute bacterial infections, the invaders may be removed and inflammation resolved with little tissue damage. However, in other infections, elimination of the invading microorganisms may be accompanied by significant tissue destruction. For example, in a bacterial abscess, extensive repair of tissues may be necessary, possibly with some degree of permanent functional impairment. This can occur with articular cartilage destruction in septic arthritis or with the formation of scar tissue in vital organs. In some cases, commonly in rheumatic disease, such tissue destruction and attempted repair may occur in the presence of chronic inflammation in which the cause is uncertain and no apparent microorganism or foreign material is present.

Here we review some of the mediators and cells that are currently thought to be important in the genesis of inflammatory reactions. It should be noted at the outset that in spite of extensive research in this area, inflammation is still not well understood. It seems likely that many different mediators and several cell types are required for any inflammatory reaction to occur. However, there is no inflammatory reaction for which a list of mediators and cells comprising all important components could be provided, much less determine the relative importance of each mediator and cell type. It should also be noted that establishing this kind of detailed information about inflammatory reactions is not just a theoretic academic exercise, since this information would serve as a basis for the rational design of therapeutic agents.

ACUTE AND CHRONIC INFLAMMATION

Inflammation may be either acute or chronic, although this division is arbitrary and elements of both are usually present at some time during the process[1]. The initial inflammatory response is usually acute, involving vascular responses, neutrophils and/or mast cells as the most prominent elements. Acute inflammation usually evolves into chronic forms, with or without a repair phase. Chronic inflammation is usually of longer duration and characterized by the presence of the mononuclear cell series, macrophages, lymphocytes and plasma cells, as well as the proliferation of connective tissue fibroblasts. Chronic inflammation may either follow the acute form or it may characterize the reaction from the beginning. Examples of chronic inflammatory reactions are those associated with persistent intracellular organisms, such as *Mycobacterium tuberculosis*, certain viruses, physical agents with low-grade toxicity, as in silicosis, and various autoimmune reactions. Acute inflammation is usually seen with highly virulent organisms, such as pyogenic bacteria, which may result in extensive neutrophil accumulation and tissue necrosis to form abscesses.

THE VASCULAR AND CELLULAR PHASES OF INFLAMMATION

The heat, redness and swelling of inflammatory reactions are a result of the vascular response to injury[1]. A transient period of vasoconstriction typically follows injury, after which vasodilatation of the arterioles occurs. Subsequently, there is increased permeability of the microvasculature, through gaps in the junctions between endothelial cells, resulting in exudation of plasma into the extravascular spaces. The plasma loss leads to increased blood viscosity and stasis of erythrocytes. Leukocytes then adhere to endothelium, a process called margination, migrate through the widened gap junctions and then through the basement membrane into the extravascular space (Fig. 2.1).

Infiltration of inflammatory cells is necessary for the development of all inflammatory reactions. Neutrophils are the primary cells in acute inflammation, eosinophils in inflammation secondary to immediate hypersensitivity reactions, and lymphocytes and monocytes for chronic inflammation. The migration of leukocytes from the vasculature into extravascular tissues is facilitated by a number of adhesion proteins, interacting molecules on the surfaces of leukocytes and endothelial cells[1]. These interactions are responsible initially for adhesion of leukocytes to endothelium, followed by their transmigration into tissues. The adhesion proteins are divided into four classes: selectins, immunoglobulins, integrins, and mucin-like glycoproteins (Table 2.1)

The selectins include E-selectin, located on endothelial cells, P-selectin, located on endothelial cells and platelets, and L-selectin, located on

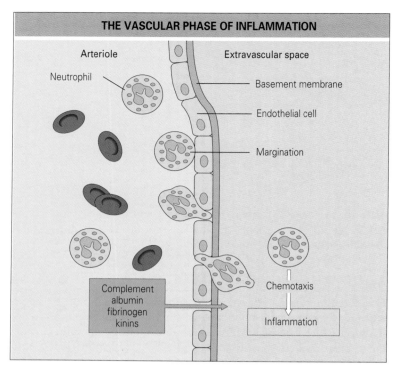

THE VASCULAR PHASE OF INFLAMMATION

Arteriole — Extravascular space

Neutrophil

Basement membrane

Endothelial cell

Margination

Complement
albumin
fibrinogen
kinins

Chemotaxis

Inflammation

Fig. 2.1 The vascular phase of inflammation.

leukocytes. The selectins bind to sialic acid in mucin-like glycoproteins on the surface of neutrophils, such as the sialyl–Lewis X molecule. Selectin binding is responsible for the initial step of adherence of leukocytes to endothelial cells, slowing the motion of leukocytes in the microcirculation, especially the venules, described as leukocyte rolling along the endothelial layer.

The immunoglobulin family here consists of two adhesion molecules on endothelial cells, intercellular adhesion molecule (ICAM)-1 and vascular cell adhesion molecule (VCAM)-1. Both these molecules bind to integrins on leukocytes.

Adhesion molecules are activated by inflammatory mediators in several ways. Some adhesion molecules, such as P-selectin, are stored in leukocyte granules and are transported to the surface on exposure of leukocytes to mediators such as histamine or platelet-activating factor (PAF). Other mediators, such as the cytokines interleukin (IL)-1 and tumor necrosis factor (TNF)-α, induce the synthesis and expression of adhesion proteins such as E-selectin, ICAM-1 and VCAM-1 on endothelium. Finally, certain adhesion proteins, especially the integrins, undergo conformation changes that increase their affinity for their ligands in the presence of chemotactic agents.

In summary, leukocyte migration into sites of inflammation appears to be initiated by endothelial activation leading to expression of E- and P-selectins, resulting in loose adherence of leukocytes to endothelial cells, or rolling. This is followed by firm adhesion of leukocytes to endothelium, which is mediated primarily by activation of integrins. Finally, transmigration of leukocytes into perivascular tissues occurs under the influence of integrins and other adhesion proteins. Certain human genetic diseases provide evidence for the importance of adhesion proteins in defense mechanisms. Patients with either leukocyte adhesion deficiency type 1, resulting in defective integrins, or leukocyte adhesion deficiency type 2, resulting in the absence of sialyl-Lewis X, suffer from recurrent bacterial infections.

PHAGOCYTOSIS

Neutrophils and monocytes identify noxious particles, such as bacteria, cell debris, crystals or foreign particles, and engulf these materials through phagocytosis[1,2]. Most microorganisms must be coated with serum components called opsonins in order to be recognized by phagocytes. Opsonins include immunoglobulin (Ig)G antibodies to antigens on the surface of microorganisms or the C3b fragment of the C3 complement component. These are recognized by specific receptors on the surfaces of phagocytes, which surround the invading particle with pseudopodia, eventually encasing it in a phagocytic vacuole. The vacuole fuses with lysosomes to form phagolysosomes, followed by discharge of the contents of the lysosome, usually resulting in degradation of the ingested particle. The phagocytosed particle is exposed to a variety of degradative enzymes, such as proteases, and chemical agents, such as oxygen free radicals. At the same time, however, some of these potent degrading agents escape from the phagocytic cell into the extracellular space, contributing to tissue injury.

CELLS AND MEDIATORS OF INFLAMMATION

The vascular and cellular events in inflammation briefly outlined above, as well as other events in inflammation, are induced and modulated by a large number of biochemical agents[1]. These agents include low-molecular-weight materials of a variety of chemical classes, and larger molecules including enzymes. These agents are produced by infiltrating inflammatory cells and by resident cells in the inflamed tissues. The synthesis and release of these agents is often a result of specific signaling mechanisms, usually as a consequence of interactions with specific cell receptors. Several dozens of mediators can be identified in any inflammatory exudate, and the complexity of the process is increased by synergistic or antagonistic effects, which exist between different mediators. The number of candidate compounds for important roles in inflammation increases with new research, and it is a major challenge to determine the functionally significant mediators in any given inflammatory reaction.

TABLE 2.1	ENDOTHELIAL CELL AND LEUKOCYTE ADHESION MOLECULES	
Endothelial molecule	**Leukocyte receptor**	**Function**
P-selectin	Sialyl-Lewis X	Partial adherence of leukocytes to endothelium
		Neutrophils, lymphocytes, monocytes
		Promotes rolling
E-selectin	Sialyl-Lewis X	Similar to P-selectin
ICAM-1	Integrins (CD11/CD18)	Firm adhesion and transmigration of all leukocytes
VCAM-1	Integrins (VLA4)	Adhesion of eosinophils, monocytes, lymphocytes
GlyCam-1 CD34	L-selectin	Rolling of lymphocytes, neutrophils and monocytes

ICAM, intracellular adhesion molecule; VCAM, vascular cell adhesion molecule.

We attempt to briefly review here the cells and mediators that have generally been considered to play important roles in inflammation, although important omissions are undoubtedly made. However, future research may almost certainly indicate new compounds that should be added to those discussed here.

Inflammatory cells

Inflammatory reactions require activation of several classes of leukocyte, including neutrophils, eosinophils, basophils, mast cells, monocytes and lymphocytes[1,2]. Most inflammatory cells arrive at sites of inflammation via the circulation, along with plasma components that contribute to inflammation. The neutrophil is the predominant cell in acute inflammation, especially with bacterial infections, but neutrophils are also prominent in vasculitis and in rheumatoid synovial fluid, in spite of their virtual absence in rheumatoid synovial tissue. Neutrophils and other leukocytes are guided to sites of inflammation by cell surface proteins called adhesion molecules, which interact with their ligands on endothelial cells and on extravascular sites.

Granulocytes

Neutrophils are attracted to sites of inflammation by chemotactic agents, where they may phagocytose bacteria, immune complexes or other particulate matter. Neutrophils contain surface receptors for the C3b fragment of the C3 complement component and the Fc portion of IgG immunoglobulin. Particulate matter that is coated with either complement, IgG, or both, is capable of being phagocytosed more rapidly than particles that do not contain these opsonins. Ingested material is then degraded by enzymes contained in lysosomes within the neutrophil.

Neutrophils contain two major types of lysosome, or granule – the azurophil granule and the specific granules (Fig. 2.2). The azurophil granules contain elastase, cathepsin G, glycosidases and lysozyme. The specific granules contain collagenase, lysozyme and lactoferrin. During phagocytosis, lysosomes fuse with the phagocytic vacuole and discharge their component enzymes into the vacuole. However, neutrophils may also discharge their lysosomal contents into tissues, which can lead to tissue injury or cell death. This may occur either during phagocytosis or when the cell encounters substances, such as immune complexes fixed to surfaces, that cannot be phagocytosed. In addition to degradative enzymes, phagocytosis or activating agents can elicit the production of

oxygen free radicals, hydrogen peroxide and hypochlorous acid from neutrophils, all of which may further contribute to tissue injury.

Other granulocytes that are important elements in inflammatory responses are eosinophils, mast cells and basophils. These cells release a variety of lipid and peptide mediators, as do neutrophils. The eosinophil appears to be particularly involved in host defense against parasitic infections, whereas mast cells and basophils are involved in the inflammatory response generated by allergic or immediate hypersensitivity reactions.

Macrophages

Macrophages are one of the most important cells in inflammatory reactions. They are especially important in chronic inflammation and play crucial roles in chronic inflammatory rheumatic diseases, such as rheumatoid arthritis (RA), chronic infections and atherosclerosis[1,3]. Macrophages are produced as monocytes in the bone marrow and travel to various tissue sites via the circulation taking up residence in peripheral tissues. Monocytes are long-lived and survive in tissues for periods of months or even years. Monocytes can then differentiate into active macrophages, which become capable of a variety of phagocytic and secretory functions in response to environmental stimuli.

Macrophages have several functions and produce a large number of biologically active substances. Among their most important functions are phagocytosis and the digestion of ingested material. In addition, soluble molecules, such as soluble immune complexes, are internalized by macrophages following attachment to surface receptors by a process termed pinocytosis. The ingested material is transported to the interior of the cell by either phagocytosis or pinocytosis in endocytotic vesicles, which then fuse with lysosomes, initiating degradation of the material. A large number of substances are produced and often secreted from macrophages, and these materials may contribute to inflammation and its consequences.

Enzymes capable of degrading proteins and other macromolecules include lysozyme, which degrades bacterial cell walls, and neutral proteinases, including plasminogen activator, elastase and collagenase. Other important proteins include IL-1, TNF-α and complement components. Activated macrophages produce active oxygen molecules, including free radicals, and a number of eicosanoids, including prostaglandin (PG)E$_2$, prostacyclin, thromboxane A$_2$ and leukotrienes (LT)B$_4$ and C$_4$. Some proteins that are produced may counteract the actions of other products, such as the protease inhibitor α_2-macroglobulin. The majority of the macrophage products serve to augment inflammation and destroy invading microorganisms but tissue injury may clearly result.

Finally, macrophages, along with dendritic cells, play a key role in the immune response by functioning as antigen-presenting cells. Antigenic material is ingested, degraded into low-molecular-weight fragments and presented on the cell surface bound to class II major histocompatibility complex (MHC) antigens. Here, the antigenic fragments are recognized by T cells in the context of the MHC antigens, leading to clonal expansion and activation of antigen-specific T cells.

Lymphocytes

Lymphocytes are important in identifying foreign (and auto-) antigens as well as in participating in the responses that lead to elimination of those antigens[1]. B cells recognize antigenic epitopes, proliferate and differentiate into antibody-forming plasma cells. T cells recognize antigens through their T cell receptors, which also leads to their proliferation.

The expanded T cell population contributes to inflammation in several ways. The CD4$^+$ T cell subset facilitates immune reactions by amplifying the B cell population through secretion of lymphokines, including IL-2, IL-4 and IL-5. CD4$^+$ cells also augment delayed hypersensitivity reactions based on the enhancement of antigen-specific cytotoxic T cells, which respond to viral antigens and other antigens. The

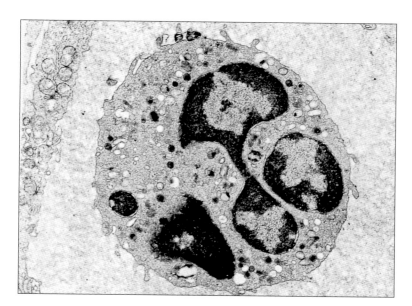

Fig. 2.2 The ultrastructure of a neutrophil. Note the presence of granules in the cytoplasm.

lymphokines secreted by CD4[+] cells also include interferon (IFN-γ), which activates macrophages and induces the expression of MHC antigens, IL-3 and granulocyte–macrophage colony stimulating factor (GM-CSF), which promote the growth and differentiation of bone marrow stem cells participating in inflammation and repair.

The CD8[+] cells, the other major T cell subset, carry out two important functions. These cells are cytolytic to cells bearing certain antigens in combination with class I MHC antigens, and are important in host defense against virus infected cells, as well as in rejection of alloantigens. The second important function of this T cell subset is the general suppression of immune responses.

Other T cells exist that belong to neither the CD4 nor the CD8 subset and they also carry out important functions. One of these classes of T cell comprises the natural killer (NK) cells, which recognize and eliminate neoplastic cells and are therefore important in immune surveillance of cancerous cells. Another T cell subset comprises cells expressing a different class of T cell receptor, containing γ–δ receptor chains instead of the α–β chains found on most T cells. The exact function of these cells is uncertain, but they are known to recognize antigens of *Mycoplasma* organisms, and thus may be important in host defense against this class of organism.

Mediators of inflammation

The coordination of vascular and cellular responses, and other events which are required for inflammation to take place, is dependent on a number of active mediators. These are derived either from the plasma, from migrating inflammatory cells or from cells comprising the local vasculature or other tissues at sites of inflammation. Several of the more important groups of inflammatory mediators are discussed below.

Complement

The ability of the immune system to function properly in host defense depends on a group of proteins called the complement system[1,2]. This system comprises over 20 proteins, which circulate in the plasma in inactive forms. Many complement components are converted into their active forms through selective proteolytic cleavage. The complement system is activated by a series of sequential proteolytic steps that are carried out by the complement components themselves, each of which

become active proteases following their own activation by proteolytic cleavage. The complement system has three important functions: the activation of inflammatory cells, the cytolysis of cells infected with invading microorganisms and the opsonization of foreign matter to facilitate phagocytosis.

Complement facilitates the elimination of harmful microorganisms as part of the system of innate immunity[2]. Immunity may be divided into two distinct systems, which cooperate to provide host defense and differ primarily in the mechanism by which they recognize foreign organisms. Phylogenetically, the oldest of these is the system of innate or natural immunity, which recognizes organisms by identifying them as harmful by their surface carbohydrate molecules, through the mannose receptors on macrophages, NK cells and complement. Thus the innate immune system distinguishes between foreign bacteria and the host through surface carbohydrates, resulting in recognition with a broad specificity. The system of acquired or specific immunity, on the other hand, is highly specific and recognizes foreign peptide antigens that are processed from proteins from microorganisms and bound to class I and class II antigens of the MHC on the surface of antigen-presenting cells. The recognition of protein fragments, as opposed to the carbohydrates that are recognized by the system of innate immunity, enables recognition of an almost infinite number of structures and of the genetically variable microorganisms. Cellular and soluble components (complement) of the innate immune system may also direct the specific immune system to assist in eliminating harmful organisms and distinguish them from autoantigens, to prevent autoimmune disease[2].

In order to carry out these functions, activation of the complement pathway takes place by two mechanisms, outlined in Figure 2.3. These two activation pathways each culminate in the activation of C3, which may either function as an opsonin or activate the remainder of the complement pathway by cleavage of C5, leading to formation of the membrane attack complex.

Classic complement cascade

The classic complement activation pathway is initiated when antigen–antibody complexes activate C1[1,2]. Active C1 cleaves both C4 and C2 to form the active C4bC2b complex, which is a C3 convertase, cleav-

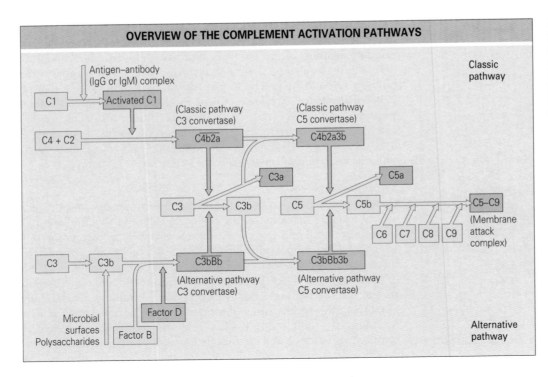

Fig. 2.3 Overview of the complement activation pathways. Activation of the classic pathway follows antigen–antibody complex binding to C1, and activation of the alternative pathway follows C3b binding to microbial agents or other surfaces. Both pathways act on C3a and C5 to generate the inflammatory components, C3, C5a and the C5–C9 attack complex. (Adapted from Abbas *et al.*[4])

OVERVIEW OF THE COMPLEMENT ACTIVATION PATHWAYS

ing C3 into C3a and C3b[1,2]. The C3b component binds to receptors on the surfaces of neutrophils, eosinophils and macrophages, facilitating adherence and phagocytosis of bacteria and other particles. The second function of C3b is to continue the activation of the complement sequence. The C3b component forms a complex with the C3 convertase, C4b2b, to form a specific protease which cleaves C5 into C5a and C5b. The larger fragment, C5b, becomes bound to cell membranes, where it is responsible for initiating assembly of the membrane attack complex, C5–C9, by the sequential addition of C6, C7, C8 and C9. This complex is inserted into cell membranes, perturbing them sufficiently to produce cell lysis.

Two of the products of the activation of the complement pathway, C3a and C5a, are termed anaphylatoxins, small peptides that cause histamine release from mast cells and smooth muscle contraction, thus mimicking an anaphylactic reaction. The C5a component is also a potent chemotactic factor for neutrophils; it triggers the neutrophil oxidative burst and stimulates LTB$_4$ synthesis.

Kinins and related proteins

The so-called contact system consists of a group of four proteins that circulate in the plasma in inactive forms and are activated to provide a host defense system[1]. The contact system consists of Hageman factor (also called coagulation factor XII), prekallikrein, high-molecular-weight kininogen (HMWK) and coagulation factor XI (plasma thromboplastin antecedent). Thus the contact system is closely related to the coagulation system.

The contact system is activated by contact with negatively charged surfaces, which may be found in a variety of substances, including monosodium urate and calcium pyrophosphate dihydrate crystals, collagen, vascular basement membranes, glycosaminoglycans and immune complexes. Activation is initiated by Hageman factor binding to negatively charged surfaces through positively charged amino acids near its amino-terminal end. Binding may be accompanied by a low level of activation by limited cleavage of Hageman factor to form active Hageman factor. The activation is accelerated by binding in the vicinity of bimolecular complexes of both prekallikrein and HMWK, and factor XI and HMWK. The active fragment of Hageman factor, HFa, then cleaves prekallikrein to release the active enzyme, kallikrein, and factor XI to produce active factor XIa. Factor XIa and kallikrein are capable of cleaving HMWK to release bradykinin (Fig. 2.4).

A kallikrein–kinin system also exists in the vascular wall, where it contributes to vasodilatation. Vascular tissues contribute substances that mediate vasodilatation, including endothelium-derived relaxing factor, now known to be nitric oxide (NO), endothelium-derived hyperpolarizing factor (EDHF), which causes vasodilatation by opening vascular smooth muscle K$^+$ channels, and prostacyclin.

Components of the contact system may function in several ways as mediators of inflammation. Active Hageman factor may increase vascular permeability and, when active Hageman factor is infused, it causes hypotension. Bradykinin is a peptide consisting of nine amino acids that causes vasodilatation, increases vascular permeability and also produces hypotension. In addition, it produces pain and causes leukocyte margination in blood vessels. It is inactivated by kininases, one of which (kininase II) is a dipeptidase, cleaving the two carboxy-terminal amino acids, and is identical to angiotensin-converting enzyme (ACE). Therefore ACE inhibitors not only promote vasodilatation, by inhibiting the conversion of angiotensin I to the more potent angiotensin II by ACE, but potentiate the vasodilatating effects of bradykinin by inhibiting bradykinin breakdown by kininase II.

Vasoactive amines and nitric oxide

There are two low-molecular-weight amines that are important inflammatory mediators: histamine and serotonin (5-hydroxytryptamine)[1].

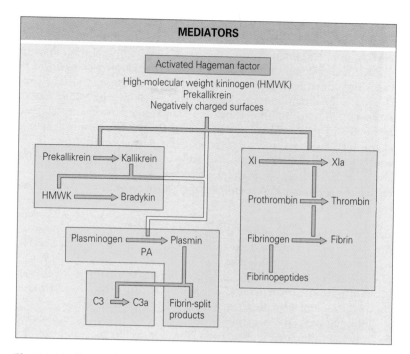

Fig. 2.4 Mediators. The figure shows interrelations between the four plasma mediator systems. Interrupted lines indicate that the pathway may not be physiologically important. PA, plasminogen activator. (Adapted from Cotran et al.[1])

Histamine

Histamine is the decarboxylation product of the amino acid histidine and is stored in mast cell granules. It is released on mast cell activation by substances such as IgE immunoglobulin, which promote immediate hypersensitivity reactions. The biological effects of histamine are mediated through its interactions with specific receptors. Histamine produces vasodilatation and enhanced permeability of postcapillary venules in addition to bronchoconstriction and the enhanced flow of bronchial mucus.

Serotonin

Serotonin is stored in the dense body granules of platelets. It is a vasoconstrictor, but also enhances microvascular permeability. Serotonin also promotes fibrosis by enhancing the synthesis of collagen by fibroblasts.

Nitric oxide

The discovery in 1987 that endothelial-derived relaxing factor was NO began an important new area of research with implications for inflammation and several other fields[1,5]. The synthesis of NO in endothelial cells is stimulated by bradykinin, thrombin and serotonin, and adenosine derived from platelets. The enzyme that catalyzes the release of NO from arginine is NO synthase, which exists in two forms. One form is a constitutive cytosolic enzyme, dependent on Ca^{2+} and calmodulin, that releases NO for short periods in response to various stimuli. The other form is induced by interactions of cytokines and other stimuli, including NO, with macrophages and endothelial cells. The inducible NO synthase is cytosolic, Ca^{2+}-independent and synthesizes NO for longer periods of time than the constitutive enzyme. It requires tetrahydrobiopterin and other cofactors. The induction of NO synthase is inhibited by glucocorticoids. The constitutive enzyme activates guanylate cyclase and causes vasodilatation and other physiologic responses. The inducible NO synthase acts as a cytotoxic molecule for invading microorganisms and tumor cells, and may have other consequences, including the vascular changes in inflammation.

The clotting system

As noted above, the contact and clotting systems are intimately related[1]. Activation of Hageman factor is the initial step in both of these systems and the end product of the clotting pathway, fibrin, is a component of many inflammatory reactions. The fibrinolytic system may also be considered to be a component of the clotting system, which also has an important role in inflammation. Fibrinopeptides, which are cleaved from fibrin by the fibrinolytic system, primarily plasmin, possess chemotactic activity and increase vascular permeability. Plasmin, in addition to lysing fibrin clots, is capable of activating Hageman factor and cleaving the C3 component of complement. Thus, components of the complement, kinin and clotting pathways interact to facilitate inflammation.

Activated forms of oxygen

Molecular oxygen is activated to form free radicals and other species, which are important in host defense against microorganisms[1,5–7]. However, active oxygen may react with several components of tissues, including lipids, proteins and other compounds, resulting in tissue injury during inflammatory reactions.

Molecular oxygen has a unique electron structure that is responsible for many of its biological properties. However, unlike most stable molecules, molecular oxygen has two unpaired electrons in its outer orbitals. In its fully reduced state with a valency of 2, as it exists in water and most stable organic molecules, each oxygen molecule may be considered to have gained four electrons. Reactive oxygen species are formed by partial reduction. Addition of a single electron to molecular oxygen yields the superoxide anion and reduction by two electrons yields the peroxide anion. Other reactive species are derived from superoxide and hydrogen peroxide; oxygen may also undergo electron rearrangement to form singlet oxygen, as described below.

Phagocytosis of bacteria, crystals or other particulate matter by neutrophils and macrophages is accompanied by a burst of oxygen consumption and by the production of several reactive oxygen species. The first reduction is due to a pyridine-nucleotide-linked oxidase, which reduces oxygen to the superoxide anion free radical. Superoxide is converted into hydrogen peroxide (H_2O_2) by the enzyme superoxide dismutase (equations 2.1 & 2.2):

$$2O_2 + NAD(P)H \text{ --- oxidase} \rightarrow 2O_2^- + NAD(P) + H^+. \qquad (2.1)$$

$$2O_2^- + 2H^+ \text{ --- superoxide dismutase} \rightarrow H_2O + O_2. \qquad (2.2)$$

Formation of H_2O_2 in neutrophils, however, probably cannot account for the bactericidal activity of these cells. The most important bactericidal agent in neutrophils appears to be hypochlorous acid, HOCl, formed from H_2O_2 by the enzyme myeloperoxidase. Macrophages lack this enzyme, probably using other reactive oxygen species to kill bacteria.

The superoxide anion (O_2^-) and hydrogen peroxide (H_2O_2) form the reactive hydroxyl radical (OH·) in the Haber–Weiss reaction (equation 2.3):

$$O_2^- + H_2O_2 \rightarrow O_2 + OH^· + OH^-. \qquad (2.3)$$

The reactive hydroxyl radical may actually result from two reactions catalyzed by ionic iron. First, the superoxide ion reduces ferric iron to ferrous iron, following which hydrogen peroxide is reduced to form a hydroxyl radical by ferrous iron (equations 2.4 & 2.5):

$$O_2^- + Fe^{3+} \rightarrow O_2 + Fe^{2+}. \qquad (2.4)$$

$$Fe^{2+} + H_2O_2 \rightarrow Fe^{3+} + OH^· + OH^-. \qquad (2.5)$$

The hydroxyl radical and singlet oxygen are highly reactive oxygen species and are able to induce lipid peroxidation and polypeptide chain cleavage, in addition to other reactions.

In its stable ground state with two unpaired electrons in the outer orbital, oxygen is referred to as a triplet state because of its electromagnetic behavior[6]. This triplet structure stabilizes oxygen, since, in order to be reduced by a two-electron donor, the donor electrons must also have parallel spins or, in molecular orbital terms, each electron must have the same spin quantum number. The electronic structure of singlet oxygen differs from that of the triplet state by having all electrons paired, leaving vacant the antibonding orbital, which has a single unpaired electron within the triplet molecule.

Singlet oxygen is formed in many reactions, such as enzymatic degradation of lipid peroxides, including the formation of PGH_2 from PGG_2 (Fig. 2.5), and by the one-electron oxidation of the superoxide anion by heavy metal anion-containing catalysts.

Arachidonic acid metabolites

A large number of biologically active metabolites are derived from the reactions of oxygen with arachidonic acid. These include the cyclo-oxygenase (COX) products (prostaglandins and thromboxanes) and lipoxygenase products, which include leukotrienes[1,9,10].

Arachidonic acid is a polyunsaturated fatty acid abundant in nearly all tissues. It is primarily found in ester linkage in the sn-2 or middle carbon position of the glycerol portion of phospholipids (Fig. 2.6). Before arachidonic acid can be metabolized, it must be released by phospholipases. There are two classes of phospholipases which account for most of the arachidonic acid that is hydrolyzed. Phospholipase A_2 hydrolyzes arachidonic acid from the ester group at the sn-2 position, producing arachidonic acid and lysophospholipids. The second route for arachidonic acid release is the hydrolysis of the glycerophosphate bond at the sn-3 carbon position by phospholipase C. This reaction produces the phosphoryl-base and diacylglycerols. Subsequently, lipases cleave arachidonic acid and other fatty acids from diacylglycerol.

Prostaglandins and thromboxane A_2

Cyclo-oxygenases, also called PGG/H synthases, are lipoxygenases which catalyze the addition of molecular oxygen to arachidonic acid to form, initially, the endoperoxide intermediate PGG_2. The same enzyme also possesses peroxidase activity and catalyzes reduction of the 15-hydroperoxy group of PGG_2 to form the 15-hydroxy compound, PGH_2. This endoperoxide (PGH_2) may then react with a number of enzymes, sometimes called isomerases, to become one of the prostaglandins or thromboxanes (Fig. 2.5).

The prostaglandins are characterized by a 5-membered ring, which determines the type of prostaglandin. In addition, PGH_2 can be converted into a 6-membered ring, thromboxane A_2. These compounds differ markedly in spite of the similarities in structure. For example, thromboxane A_2 is a powerful vasoconstrictor and causes platelet aggregation, whereas prostacyclin, or PGI_2, causes vasodilatation and opposes platelet aggregation.

Two prostaglandins, PGE_2 and PGI_2, are mediators of the vascular phases of inflammation and are both potent vasodilators. In addition, they act synergistically with certain other vasoactive mediators, such as histamine and kinins, to increase vascular permeability. Prostaglandins E_2 and I_2 also stimulate osteoclastic bone resorption, suggesting that bone erosion in chronic inflammatory diseases such as RA may be mediated, at least in part, by prostaglandins produced by inflamed tissues. In addition to their vascular effects, PGE_2 and PGI_2 elevate levels of cyclic 3',5'-adenosine monophosphate (cAMP) in cells; many of their biological effects may be related to this elevation of cAMP.

It is widely recognized that in addition to proinflammatory effects, PGE_2 (and probably PGI_2 as well) may have anti-inflammatory effects. One of the most prominent is their immunosuppressive effects in which both T cell activation and IL-2 formation, as well as the proliferation and maturation of B cells, may be inhibited by exposure to PGE_2. In

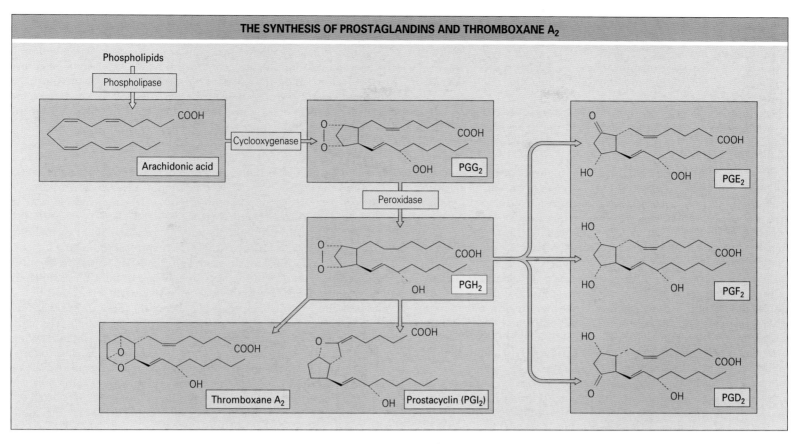

THE SYNTHESIS OF PROSTAGLANDINS AND THROMBOXANE A_2

Phospholipids

Phospholipase

COOH

Arachidonic acid

Cyclooxygenase

PGG$_2$

Peroxidase

PGH$_2$

PGE$_2$

PGF$_2$

PGD$_2$

Thromboxane A$_2$

Prostacyclin (PGI$_2$)

Fig. 2.5 The synthesis of prostaglandins and thromboxane A$_2$. (Adapted from Robinson[8].)

addition, several investigators have documented that PGE$_2$ may inhibit the secretion of inflammatory mediators by cells. This is especially prominent in the case of the synthesis of leukotrienes, which may be actively inhibited both *in vitro* and *in vivo*. Finally, it has been shown that administration of the E prostaglandins, or their derivatives, suppresses experimental inflammation in several model systems, although pharmacologic doses are often required. It is not well established whether endogenous production of PGE$_2$ acts as a suppressing agent in these pathologic models.

Two cyclo-oxygenase gene products

An important advance in prostaglandin biochemistry in recent years was the discovery that PGH synthase exists in two isoforms, PGHS-1 and PGHS-2, also called, respectively, COX-1 and COX-2[11]. These enzymes are the products of different genes but they have a large degree of amino acid homology and identity. Their kinetic parameters are similar and both enzymes are inhibited by non-steroidal anti-inflammatory drugs (NSAIDs). A major difference between the two enzymes is the regulation of their levels in cells. The levels of COX-1 are constitutive in most tissues; it is considered a 'housekeeping' enzyme, maintaining stable capacity for prostaglandin and thromboxane synthesis in tissues such as stomach, kidney, endothelial cells and blood platelets. In contrast, COX-2 is less widely distributed but it is an inducible enzyme and may be stimulated up to 80-fold by growth factors, cytokines or other agents. It may be considered a part of the inflammatory response and is produced in stimulated monocytes, synovial cells and fibroblasts.

Evidence for the roles of cyclo-oxygenases from gene deletion experiments

The genes for both COX-1 and COX-2 were deleted in separate experiments using stem cell technology, providing evidence for the roles of each of these enzymes in murine health and development and in inflammatory reactions[12–15]. Knockout mice for *COX2* had a shortened life span because of failure of normal kidney development. Myocardial fibrosis also occurred but the explanation for this finding is unknown. Female mice were infertile, indicating that COX-2 is required for ovulation. The results of experimental inflammatory reactions were somewhat unexpected, in that inflammations induced by either carrageenan or tetradecanoyl phorbol acetate (TPA) were similar in mice lacking the COX-2 gene and in the controls, and these agents were expected to be at least in part dependent on COX-2. Arachidonic acid-induced swelling was also similar in mice lacking COX-2 and in controls, but since this reaction occurs within 30 minutes of the application of arachidonic acid, any requirement for prostaglandins would be expected to be dependent on COX-1, since the induction of COX-2 requires longer time periods. In an additional model of inflammation, TNF-α-induced hepatotoxicity generated by the endotoxin lipopolysaccharide was reduced in mice lacking COX-2, suggesting that macrophage prostaglandin production contributes to this inflammatory reaction. In addition, the absence of COX-2 was associated with suppurative peritonitis, suggesting that COX-2 may confer protection against this bacterial infection[12,14].

Similar methods were used to delete the murine *COX1* gene[13]. Even though these mice have gastric PGE levels that are only about 1% of normals, they had no gastric pathology. The mice lacking COX-1 have reduced platelet aggregation as expected, since platelet thromboxane synthesis is essentially all from COX-1. Mice lacking COX-1 have a reduced inflammatory response to arachidonic acid applied to the skin, demonstrating that this response is dependent on COX-1. On the other hand, the inflammatory response to TPA in skin is normal, and thus these experiments and those described above demonstrate that this reaction is dependent on neither COX-1 nor COX-2. Although the fertility of mice lacking COX-1 is normal, few live births result from matings in which both males and females are homozygous for the COX-1 deletion. The lack of live births appeared to be based on impaired parturition in these animals, indicating that prostaglandin production by COX-1 is required for normal parturition. These models should be valuable in further determining the functions of COX-1 and COX-2 in health and in disease[12] (Table 2.2).

The presence of two isoforms of PGH synthase raises the important possibility that the enzymes may differ in their response to inhibitory drugs. That is, selective drugs might inhibit COX-2 in inflamed tissues while sparing COX-1 in the gastrointestinal tract, kidney and vasculature.

The older NSAIDs, such as aspirin and indomethacin (indometacin) and many others, are non-specific COX inhibitors, blocking prostaglandin synthesis by both COX isoenzymes. It was logical to assume that, if highly selective COX-2 inhibitors could be developed, these agents would be expected to be anti-inflammatory without side-effects on the gastric mucosa and other tissues. This expectation has been realized with the synthesis of the coxibs, and there are now four COX-2-selective inhibitors, celecoxib, valdecoxib, etoricoxib and rofecoxib, available for treatment of arthritis and other painful disorders (Table 2.3)[16].

Contrary to impressions left by advertising, the anti-inflammatory effectiveness of the non-selective COX-inhibitors and COX-2-selective inhibitors are comparable. The major advantage of the COX-2 inhibitors over non-selective inhibitors is the lack of adverse effects of the COX-2 inhibitors on the gastric mucosa (Table 2.4).

Since there is an approximately threefold increase in serious gastrointestinal toxicity in patients over the age of 65, it may be good practice for these patients to use non-specific NSAIDs only with cytoprotective agents, such as misoprostol, or proton pump inhibitors.

Non-specific NSAIDs should not be used in patients on anticoagulants. The COX-2-selective inhibitors are probably safe in this setting, but they may alter warfarin dosage.

Do selective COX-2 inhibitors increase the risk of cardiovascular events?

Prior to recent reports that have suggested the possibility that COX-2-selective inhibitors may increase the incidence of thrombotic cardiovascular events, theoretical considerations were consistent with this notion[16]. The selective COX-2 inhibitors are expected to inhibit prostaglandin production by vascular tissues, where the major product is prostacyclin, a compound that inhibits platelet aggregation and produces vasodilatation. At the same time, the COX-2-selective inhibitors have no effects on the formation of thromboxane from platelets, and the combination of these actions would be expected to favor vascular occlusion. On the other hand, non-selective COX inhibitors are also expected to inhibit prostacyclin formation from the vasculature, but this might be counterbalanced by inhibition of platelet thromboxane formation.

A recent meta-analysis of the results of several large trials concluded that the COX-2-selective inhibitors rofecoxib and celecoxib significantly increased the risk of myocardial infarction, transient ischemic attacks and stroke[17]. Two large, randomized post-marketing trials, as well as other cardiovascular prevention trials, were considered. In the VIGOR trial, in which aspirin was not allowed, the relative risk for thrombotic cardiovascular events for rofecoxib versus naproxen was 2.38, $p < 0.001$. Serious gastrointestinal events were approximately half as frequent in the refecoxib group as in the naproxen group. In the CLASS study, in which aspirin was allowed, there were no significant differences in the numbers of cardiovascular events in either of the three groups. The rate of complicated gastrointestinal events in patients taking celecoxib, however, was not significantly reduced compared to patients taking either diclofenac or ibuprofen.

However, in a meta-analysis of all randomized controlled trials of rofecoxib, there was no evidence of an increased risk of cardiovascular events in trials compared to placebo or other non-naproxen NSAIDs[18].

The meta-analysis of Mukheerjee et al. has limitations but may raise an important safety issue for the use of COX-2-selective inhibitors. A recent editorial thoroughly reviewed this topic and suggested that patients at risk for cardiovascular events should take low-dose aspirin in conjunction with COX-2-selective inhibitors[19].

Evidence for a role of cyclo-oxygenase products in neoplasia and Alzheimer's disease

Several lines of evidence indicates that cyclo-oxygenase products may play a role in neoplasia. Epidemiologic observations have shown that aspirin ingestion is associated with a reduction in the incidence of colon

---

TABLE 2.2 MAJOR DIFFERENCES BETWEEN THE TWO CYCLO-OXYGENASE ISOFORMS	
COX-1	**COX-2**
Maintains homeostasis; 'housekeeping' or protective functions	Promotes inflammation
Limited induction; baseline activity	Induced up to 100-fold in inflammation
Widespread distribution	Limited distribution; inflammatory cells
Protects the gastric mucosa	Minor role in stomach
Maintains renal blood flow	Contributes to renal function
Contributes to hemostasis	Contributes to vasodilatation

TABLE 2.3 COX-2-SELECTIVE INHIBITORS		
	Celecoxib (Celebrex)	**Rofecoxib (Vioxx)**
Dosing	100mg or 200mg bid	12.5mg or 25mg q.i.d.
Indications	RA, OA, familial adenomatous polyposis	RA, OA, pain, dysmenorrhea
Allergies	May cause allergies in sulfonamide-sensitive patients	Does not cause allergies in sulfonamide-sensitive patients

---

TABLE 2.4 MAJOR DIFFERENCES BETWEEN NON-SELECTIVE AND SELECTIVE COX-2 INHIBITORS	
Non-selective COX inhibitors	**Selective COX-2 inhibitors**
Cause erosive gastritis and gastroduodenal ulcers	No significant erosive gastritis; less likely to cause gastroduodenal ulcers
Cause fluid retention and may inhibit renal blood flow	Cause fluid retention
Inhibit platelet aggregation	Do not inhibit platelet aggregation
Anaphylaxis in aspirin-sensitive patients	Anaphylaxis in aspirin-sensitive patients
Less expensive	More expensive

cancer by 40–50%[20,21]. In experimental studies in rodents, NSAIDs inhibit carcinogen-induced colon tumors[21]. In humans, NSAIDs inhibit formation of adenomas in the colon, and these drugs induce apoptosis of intestinal epithelium in patients with familial adenomatous polyposis[8,22,23]. In addition, COX-2 mRNA and enzyme levels are increased in human adenocarcinomas of the colon[23,24]. Finally, rat intestinal epithelial cells that were transfected with the *COX2* gene expressed enhanced levels of COX-2 and were resistant to apoptosis. This enhanced proliferative response in the transfected cells was reduced by the NSAID sulindac sulfide. Thus, *in vitro* studies demonstrate that enhanced expression of the *COX2* gene is associated with a change in cell phenotype resembling neoplasia[25]. Evidence is thus accumulating that cyclo-oxygenase products may contribute to the development of cancer and that at least some of this effect may be modified by NSAIDs.

A possible benefit of cyclo-oxygenase inhibitors in Alzheimer's disease also has been reported[26].

Leukotrienes

Lipoxygenases other than PGG/H synthase also catalyze the addition of molecular oxygen to specific double bonds in polyunsaturated fatty acids, again primarily arachidonic acid[10]. The most important lipoxygenases are named for the position in the arachidonic acid molecule to which oxygen is added. The 5-lipoxygenase leads to the formation of leukotrienes, as illustrated in Figure 2.6. The addition of oxygen to the 5 position of arachidonic acid forms 5-hydroperoxyeicosatetraenoic acid (5-HPETE). The same molecule catalyzes the cyclization of the

hydroperoxy compound to form cyclic 5,6-epoxide (LTA_4). The LTA_4 intermediate undergoes two important reactions to form two different classes of leukotriene. In the first, the LTA_4 hydrolase reaction converts LTA_4 into the stereospecific dihydroxy derivative LTB_4. Alternatively, LTA_4 may react with glutathione to form LTC_4, which is further metabolized to LTD_4 and LTE_4 by elimination of a gammaglutamyl residue and, subsequently, a glycine residue. The three compounds LTC_4, LTD_4 and LTE_4 are collectively called the sulfidopeptide leukotrienes, compounds that account for the activity of the previously recognized slow-reacting substance of anaphylaxis, an important mediator of immediate hypersensitivity reactions.

Products of the 5-lipoxygenase pathway are important mediators of inflammation. For example, LTB_4 is a chemoattractant for leukocytes and promotes the adherence of leukocytes to endothelial cells. It also activates secretion of active oxygen species and degradative enzymes from neutrophils. In contrast, the sulfidopeptide leukotrienes LTC_4, LTD_4 and LTE_4 contract smooth muscle in vascular, respiratory and intestinal tissues. In addition, they cause vasoconstriction but increase microvascular permeability. They are important mediators of bronchial asthma because of their ability to cause bronchoconstriction and to increase the flow of bronchial mucus. Other organs may also be affected by these compounds. For example, the sulfidopeptide leukotrienes stimulate mesangial cell contraction and exert a negative inotropic and arrhythmogenic effect on the heart.

In addition to the leukotrienes, the lipoxygenases can also produce hydroperoxy derivatives of arachidonic acid, many of which have

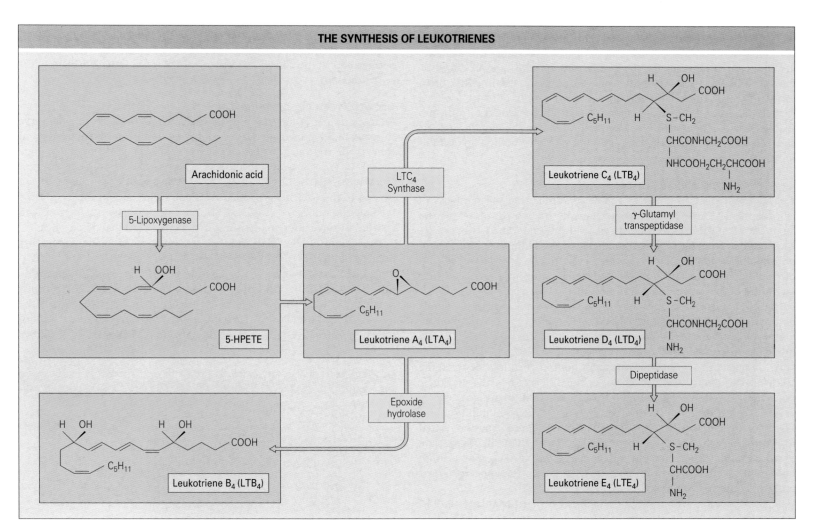

THE SYNTHESIS OF LEUKOTRIENES

Fig. 2.6 The synthesis of leukotrienes. (Adapted from Robinson[8].)

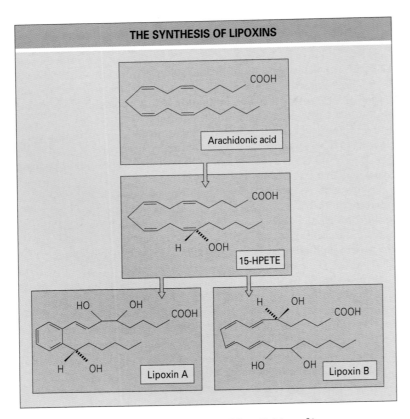

THE SYNTHESIS OF LIPOXINS

Fig. 2.7 The synthesis of lipoxins. (Adapted from Robinson[8].)

biological activity but have not been characterized in detail. Finally, the combined action of the 5- and 15-lipoxygenases produces triple lipoxygenation of the lipoxins (Fig. 2.7). These compounds are produced by neutrophils and by neutrophils interacting with certain other cells. Lipoxins have counter-regulatory properties; they tend to produce vasodilatation and are weakly chemotactic. Recent evidence indicates that lipoxin A_4 may also be involved in intracellular signaling through its capacity to activate protein kinase C. In addition, the lipoxins inhibit human NK cell cytotoxicity.

Regulation of eicosanoid synthesis

A large number of factors are capable of stimulating the synthesis of eicosanoids[9–11]. However, the mechanism by which these factors augment eicosanoid synthesis is not well understood. It is generally accepted that stimulation of eicosanoid synthesis requires stimulation of phospholipase activity. This is necessary to provide adequate quantities of free arachidonic acid for cyclo-oxygenase and lipoxygenase, since quantities of free arachidonic acid existing in resting cells are low.

The mechanism of inhibition of cyclo-oxygenase activity most familiar to physicians is inhibition by NSAIDs (see above). Vane and Botting proposed that the major therapeutic action of aspirin and other NSAIDs might be accounted for by the inhibition of the enzyme cyclo-oxygenase[9]. In part, this is based on reasonably good correlations between the relative anti-inflammatory potencies of the different NSAIDs and their potencies as cyclo-oxygenase inhibitors. In addition, many toxic effects of NSAIDs can also be accounted for by cyclo-oxygenase inhibition. For example, the tendency for NSAIDs to cause gastric ulcers may be related to elimination of the cytoprotective effects of PGE_2 in the gastric mucosa. While other pharmacologic effects of NSAIDs may also be important for their activity, cyclo-oxygenase inhibition appears to be a prominent mechanism of action of these agents.

Glucocorticoids also inhibit the synthesis of prostaglandins and leukotrienes but the mechanism of action differs from that of NSAIDs. Glucocorticoids appear to inhibit release of free arachidonic acid from phospholipids[9]. Several laboratories have provided evidence that glucocorticoids induce the synthesis of proteins called lipocortins, which in turn inhibit the hydrolysis of arachidonic acid from phospholipids. At least one of the lipocortins is similar to cytoskeletal proteins called capactins, which inhibit phospholipases by complexing phospholipids, effectively making phospholipids ineffective substrates for phospholipases. Other lipocortins apparently inhibit phospholipases directly. Glucocorticoids inhibit the formation of both cyclo-oxygenase and lipoxygenase products, whereas NSAIDs lack any important activity on lipoxygenases. In fact, under some conditions, NSAIDs may augment leukotriene synthesis.

The prostaglandins are ubiquitous and one or more of these compounds are produced by all cells with the exception of erythrocytes. Lipoxygenase products are more restricted and leukotrienes are only produced by inflammatory cells, neutrophils, monocytes and macrophages, mast cells, basophils and eosinophils. Eicosanoids act locally either on the cells from which they are produced (autocrine) or on neighboring cells (paracrine). The eicosanoids are labile in tissues, either because of chemical instability, as with the endoperoxide prostaglandins, prostacyclin and thromboxane A_2, or because of rapid enzymatic degradation such as occurs with PGE_2 and the leukotrienes.

Platelet activating factor

Platelet activating factor is the only phospholipid with potent biological activities[1]. It belongs to the class of ether phospholipids, having an O-alkyl ether residue in the *sn*-1 position of the glycerol moiety (Fig. 2.8). It is produced by neutrophils, macrophages and, to some extent, platelets. As the name implies, PAF causes platelet aggregation but, in addition, it has a wide range of biological activity. It induces chemotaxis, aggregation and granule secretion by neutrophils and macrophages, and it is also able to stimulate smooth muscle in the gut and lung. It induces microvascular permeability and is considered to be a mediator of immediate hypersensitivity reactions.

Growth factors or cytokines

A large number of polypeptides secreted by a number of cell types serve to regulate the growth, differentiation and activation of leukocytes and other cells involved in inflammation, as well as other pathologic states[27–29]. We will review the effects of some of these polypeptides that seem particularly important in the pathogenesis of inflammation. Several of these agents are called interleukins because of their ability to mediate the functions of leukocytes, but it is clear that this term is too restrictive, since interleukins affect many cells other than leukocytes.

The actions of IL-1, TNF and IL-6 are sometimes considered together because of their overlapping functions. These cytokines are produced in large quantities by monocytes. The numerous effects of IL-1 illustrate the pleiotropic activity of cytokines. It is an endogenous pyrogen, stimulating the synthesis of acute-phase proteins by the liver, augments the growth of T cells and facilitates B cell proliferation and immunoglobulin secretion. Also, IL-1 induces IL-6 secretion and potentiates the responses

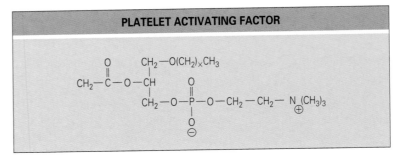

PLATELET ACTIVATING FACTOR

Fig. 2.8 The chemical structure of platelet activating factor.

of immature hematopoietic cells to macrophage-colony stimulating factor (M-CSF) and IL-3. It stimulates production of PGE$_2$ and collagenase, and augments the expression of adhesion molecules on endothelial cells, thus increasing the adherence of leukocytes.

Like IL-1, TNF-α is pyrogenic and promotes an acute phase reaction, stimulates PGE$_2$ and collagenase synthesis, and promotes osteoclast activation. It has also been called cachectin because it may mediate the wasting accompanying inflammatory and neoplastic states. The activation of synthesis of IL-1 and TNF-α in macrophages by bacterial endotoxin may account for tissue injury and shock produced by endotoxin. TNF-α acts synergistically with IFN-γ to enhance antiproliferative effects.

The actions of IL-6 include growth stimulation of a variety of cell types, including stem cells for neutrophils and monocytes, B cells and T cells. Also, IL-6 stimulates the synthesis of acute phase proteins by the liver.

Several interleukins augment the growth and activation of lymphoid cells, and therefore are of primary importance in immune reactions. IL-2 is produced by T-helper cells and stimulates the proliferation of T cells and the expression of IL-2 receptors on T cells. IL-4 also promotes the growth of T lymphocytes, and modifies the function of B cells, including the induction of immunoglobulin class switching and enhancement of IgE production. In addition to these effects, IL-4 increases the expression of class II MHC antigens on B cells and macrophages. It also stimulates the fusion of macrophages to form multinucleated giant cells and augments macrophage aggregation. IL-4 may thus participate in the development of the granulomatous response. Other interleukins are also pleiotropic growth factors including IL-3, IL-5 and IL-7. IL-3 promotes the growth and differentiation of hematopoietic stem cells, leading to the production of all blood cell types. IL-5 facilitates the growth and function of B cells and the growth of eosinophils. IL-7 is a growth factor for B cells and T cells. GM-CSF promotes the growth of neutrophils, macrophages, eosinophils, fibroblasts and endothelial cells. Another polypeptide, granulocyte-colony stimulating factor (G-CSF), is a more specific growth factor for neutrophils. IL-8 is a member of a family of low-molecular-weight, basic heparin-binding polypeptides. It causes chemotaxis and activation of neutrophils and produces inflammation on injection, as does IL-1 and TNF-α. A slightly larger form of IL-8 has been reported to have antichemotactic and anti-inflammatory effects.

The interferons were identified, on the basis of their antiviral activity, in three major forms, α, β and γ, based on their cells of origin[1]. IFN-γ, or immune interferon, is produced by activated T cells. It induces the expression of class II MHC antigens on several cell types, including connective tissue cells, monocytes and epithelial and endothelial cells. IFN-γ also activates macrophages for antigen presentation and for killing of intracellular parasites and tumor cells. It also acts synergistically with TNF-α in the lysis of tumor cells.

Proteinases and tissue injury

Proteinases are among the most important mediators of tissue injury and degradation[1,28,29]. Many proteinases are stored within the lysosomes of leukocytes, while others are synthesized and secreted in response to inflammatory stimuli. Proteinases may be divided into two classes, those active at acid pH and those active at neutral pH. The former enzymes probably function to degrade bacteria and cell debris at low pH within phagolysosomes, and it is doubtful that they have significant extracellular activity where the pH is near neutrality. Degradation of extracellular proteins in connective tissues is carried out by several neutral proteinases derived from neutrophils, monocyte–macrophages, fibroblasts and other cells.

Neutral proteinases include important enzymes. They may be divided into two groups, the metalloenzymes, which require metal ions such as Zn^{2+} as a cofactor, and the serine proteinases, which have a serine

hydroxyl group in their catalytically active sites. Collagenase initiates the degradation of extracellular or interstitial collagens. It is highly specific and cleaves five types of collagen, including type I, the most abundant type, and type II, which is the major form of collagen in articular cartilage. Collagenase cleaves a single specific peptide bond between the glycine–isoleucine residues 775–776, in each of the three polypeptide α-chains. Collagen must be in its native, triple-helical form to be cleaved by collagenase.

The products of collagen cleavage by collagenase are two fragments, the larger consisting of three-quarters of the original collagen molecule from the amino-terminal end, and the other quarter-length fragment containing the carboxyl-terminal end. The triple helices of each of these two products are more susceptible to thermal denaturation than the native collagen molecule and on denaturation become susceptible to proteolytic degradation by gelatinase and other proteinases. One form of collagenase is produced by fibroblasts, macrophages, synovial cells and endothelial cells, and a different form of collagenase is produced by neutrophils.

Gelatinases are enzymes that specifically degrade gelatin, which is denatured collagen. Their synthesis is regulated by many of the same factors that regulate collagenase synthesis. Gelatinases are produced by both macrophages and neutrophils. These enzymes cleave native collagens, types V and XI, as well as gelatin.

Proteoglycanase is an enzyme that is capable of degrading proteoglycans by cleaving the proteoglycan core protein. It has been found in articular cartilage and also may be produced by rheumatoid synovial tissue.

Several serine proteinases arise from the activation of inactive precursors in host defense systems that were discussed above. These include complement components, the coagulation cascade and the fibrinolytic system. Plasma kallikrein and plasmin both may activate collagenase, but the roles of other enzymes in these systems in degradation of connective tissue proteins remain unclear. Neutrophils produce elastase and cathepsin G, both of which are probably important in proteoglycan degradation. Elastase degrades elastin and may participate in collagen degradation by cleaving the telopeptide, non-helical portion containing collagen cross-links. Many serine proteinases are capable of degrading a variety of tissue proteins.

Regulation of proteolytic enzyme activity

It is clear that proteolytic enzymes are tightly regulated in order to avoid uncontrolled tissue degradation[27–29]. Some metalloproteinases are stored preformed in granules or lysosomes, such as both the specific granules and the azurophilic granules of neutrophils. Release of stored enzymes can be stimulated by many substances that activate neutrophils, such as C5a and LTB$_4$. Other proteolytic enzymes are synthesized in response to various stimuli. For example, IL-1 markedly augments synthesis of collagenase and gelatinase and secretion from synovial cells, chondrocytes and macrophages.

Metalloproteinases are often secreted as inactive precursors or proenzymes, which are activated by other proteolytic enzymes and certain chemical agents. For example, procollagenase is activated by plasmin, trypsin or a specific enzyme called procollagenase activator. Reactive oxygen species may activate human neutrophil collagenase.

Proteinase inhibitors

Inhibitors of proteolysis are normally abundant in plasma and tissues and are essential to prevent unwanted tissue degradation. Both metalloproteases and serine proteases are inhibited by a 720kDa α-macroglobulin, a large protein abundant in plasma. Another important inhibitor is called tissue inhibitor of metalloproteinases (TIMP), a 28kDa protein that inhibits proteases by complexing with them.

REFERENCES

1. Cotran RS, Kumar V, Collins T. Robbins pathologic basis of disease, 6th ed. Philadelphia, PA: WB Saunders; 1999.
2. Medhitov R, Janeway C. Advances in immunology. Innate immunity. N Engl J Med 2000; 343: 338–344.
3. Ross R. Atherosclerosis is an inflammatory disease. Am Heart J 1999; 138: S419–S420.
4. Abbas AK, Lichtmann AH, Jordan SP. Cellular and molecular immunology, 2nd ed. Philadelphia, PA: WB Saunders; 1994.
5. Squadrito GL, Pryor WA. Oxidative chemistry of nitric oxide: the roles of superoxide, peroxynitrite, and carbone dioxide. Free Radic Biol Med 1998; 25: 392–403.
6. Naqui A, Chance B. Reactive oxygen intermediates in biochemistry. Annu Rev Biochem 1986; 55: 137–166.
7. Kehrer JP. The Haber-Weiss reaction and mechanisms of toxicity. Toxicology 2000; 149: 43–50.
8. Robinson DR. Eicosanoids and related agents. In: Koopman WJ, ed. Arthritis and allied conditions, 13th ed. Baltimore, MD: Williams & Wilkins; 1997: 515–528.
9. Vane JR, Botting RM. New insights into the mode of action of anti-inflammatory drugs. Inflamm Res 1995; 44: 1–10.
10. Tilley SL, Coffman TM, Koller BH. Mixed messages: modulation of inflammation and immune responses by prostaglandins and thromboxanes. J Clin Invest 2001; 108: 15–23.
11. Leff AR. Regulation of leukotrienes in the management of asthma: biology and clinical therapy. Annu Rev Med 2001; 52: 1–14.
12. FitzGerald GA, Patrono C. Drug therapy: the coxibs, selective inhibitors of cyclooxygenase-2. N Engl J Med 2001; 345: 433–442.
13. Mukherjee D, Nissen SE, Topol EJ. Risk of cardiovascular events associated with selective Cox-2 inhibitors. JAMA 2001; 286: 954–959.
14. Dinchuk JE, Car BD, Focht RJ, et al. Renal abnormalities and an altered inflammatory response in mice lacking cyclooxygenase II. Nature 1995; 378: 406–409.
15. Langenbach R, Morham SG, Tiano HF et al. Prostaglandin synthase I gene disruption in mice reduces arachidonic acid-induced inflammation and indomethacin-induced gastric ulceration. Cell 1995; 83: 483–492.
16. Morham SG, Langenbach R, Loftin CD et al. Prostaglandin synthase 2 gene disruption causes severe renal pathology in the mouse. Cell 1995; 83: 473–482.
17. DeWitt D, Smith WL. Yes, but do they still get headaches? Cell 1995; 83: 345–348.
18. Konstam MA, Weir MR, Reicin A et al. Cardiovascular thrombotic events in controlled, clinical trials of rofecoxib. Circulation 2001; 104: 2280–2288.
19. Strand V, Hochberg MC. The risk of cardiovascular thrombotic events with selective cyclooxygenase-2 inhibitors. Arthritis Rheum 2002; 47: 349–355.
20. Giovannucci E, Rimm EB, Stampfer MJ et al. Aspirin use and the risk for colorectal cancer and adenoma in male health professionals. Ann Intern Med 1994; 121: 241–246.
21. Reddy BS, Rao CV, Rivenson A, Kelloff G. Inhibitory effects of aspirin on azoxymethane-induced colon carcinogenesis in F344 rats. Carcinogenesis 1993; 14: 1493–1497.
22. Pasricha PJ, Bedi A, O'Connor K et al. The effects of sulindac on colorectal proliferation and apoptosis in familial adenomatous polyposis. Gastroenterology 1995; 109: 994–998.
23. Steinbach G, Lynch PM, Phillips RK et al. The effect of celecoxib, a cyclooxygenase-2 inhibitor, in familial adenomatous polyposis. N Engl J Med 2000; 342: 1946–1952.
24. Eberhart CE, Coffey RJ, Radhika A et al. Up regulation of cyclooxygenase 2 gene expression in human colorectal adenomas and adenocarcinomas. Gastroenterology 1994; 107: 1183–1188.
25. Kargman S, O'Neill G, Vickers P et al. Expression of prostaglandin G/H synthase-1 and -2 protein in human colon cancer. Cancer Res 1995; 55: 2556–2559.
26. Maini RN, Taylor PC. Anti-cytokine therapy for rheumatoid arthritis. Annu Rev Med 2000; 51: 207–229.
27. Choy EHS, Panayi GS. Cytokine pathways and joint inflammation in rheumatoid arthritis. N Engl J Med 2001; 344: 907–916.
28. Yamanishi Y, Firestein GS. Pathogenesis of rheumatoid arthritis: the role of synoviocytes. Rheum Dis Clin North Am 2001; 27: 355–371.
29. Gravallese EM, Goldring SR. Cellular mechanisms and the role of cytokines in bone erosions in rheumatoid arthritis. Arthritis Rheum 2000; 43: 2143–2151.

EVALUATION, SIGNS AND SYMPTOMS

3 History and physical examination

Anthony D Woolf

- History taking is the most important skill needed in rheumatology.
- Examination is pivotal in confirming cause and effect of musculo-skeletal problems.
- Assessment of the musculoskeletal system should form part of any general medical examination as they are a frequent comorbidity.
- The consultation involves a patient-centered phase for their story, a physician-centered phase to clarify the story by interrogation and examination, and finally an interactive phase during which the patient and physician discuss their concerns, findings, conclusions and plans.
- The consultation must meet the expectations of the patient.
- Musculoskeletal conditions cause a broad range of problems, which need to be assessed by a multidisciplinary team to develop an appropriate plan of management.

INTRODUCTION

Musculoskeletal complaints are among the commonest and the cause and effect of them need to be established. The physician to whom the patient presents needs to identify any significant abnormality, establish the cause, develop a management plan, assess response to treatment and be able to recognize the lack of expected response. If the physician is not able to identify the problem, they must at least be able to describe the abnormality and recognize whether it is important and whether it requires a more skilled assessment. Musculoskeletal conditions are also frequent comorbidities that need to be identified and treated. Many common musculoskeletal problems are effectively managed within primary care but other less common or more serious problems will require specialist management, often within the context of a multidisciplinary team. This approach will require different competencies at the different levels of care. All physicians should be able to recognize abnormality of the musculoskeletal system and whether it is important by being able to perform a screening assessment in combination with basic knowledge of musculoskeletal conditions. More expert management will require a greater competency in clinical assessment and more detailed knowledge of the possible causes. Such an assessment will be made by a specialist physician.

This chapter considers first a basic screening assessment of the musculoskeletal system and second the more detailed evaluation that all specialists in musculoskeletal conditions should be competent in.

SCREENING ASSESSMENT

Musculoskeletal conditions should always be sought as part of any general history and examination by a routine screen. Once identified, a more detailed assessment is necessary to make a diagnosis, develop a plan of management and monitor the response to this. The minimum screening assessment of the musculoskeletal system should be sensitive to identifying the presence of any significant abnormality and feasible to perform as part of any general examination. The scheme proposed is a guide that can be adapted and the different components can be carried out at various stages of a general medical clerking. The scheme only takes a few minutes. It has been validated in a general medical setting and within undergraduate training[1].

Screening history

The common symptoms of any musculoskeletal condition are pain, stiffness and limitation of function. Joint disease is often associated with swelling. Function is frequently affected. Dressing without difficulty, including socks and shoes, is a complex activity that utilizes both upper and lower limbs and the ability to do so is a sensitive functional test. The ability to ascend and descend stairs without difficulty is sensitive to detecting abnormality in the lower limbs. If the only need is to establish quickly the presence or absence of major musculoskeletal problems, then these screening questions will suffice.

'Do you suffer from any pain or stiffness in your arms or legs, neck or back?'
'Do you have any swelling of your joints?'
'Do you have any difficulty with washing and dressing?'
'Do you have any difficulty with going up or down stairs or steps?'

Musculoskeletal conditions are often associated with systemic features and should not be considered in isolation. General enquiry should be made about the patient's health.

These questions should identify if there are any problems that might relate to the musculoskeletal system and need further evaluation.

Screening examination

Any significant abnormalities in the spine, arms or legs should be identified by inspection at rest and during certain movements with brief palpation and stress tests of selected joints. Good observation is essential. Normality is looked for in appearance, posture and resting position of the joints and in smooth movement through the expected normal range. When any joint is affected by a musculoskeletal condition, there is usually one movement that is nearly always affected and it is these movements that are assessed in this screen. For such a screen to be part of the routine examination of all patients, it has to be quick, simple and easy to annotate. This screen was developed to meet these criteria[1]. The gait, arms, legs and spine (G, A, L, S) should be assessed.

- **Gait.** The patient should be observed walking forwards for a few meters, turning and walking back again. Abnormalities of the different phases should be recognized: heel strike, stance phase, toe off and swing phases (Fig. 3.1). Look for abnormalities of movement of the arms, pelvis, hips, knees, ankles and feet during these phases.
- **Inspection of standing patient.** The patient should be viewed from the back, side and front, looking for any abnormalities, in particular of posture and symmetry. Examine for tenderness by applying pressure

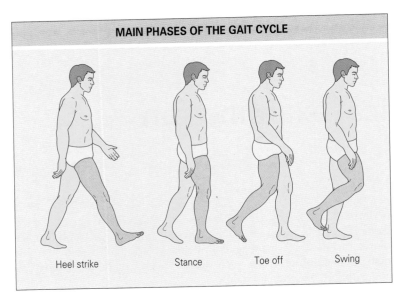

MAIN PHASES OF THE GAIT CYCLE

Heel strike   Stance   Toe off   Swing

Fig. 3.1 Main phases of the gait cycle. The phases related to the shaded leg.

in the midpoint of each supraspinatus and rolling an overlying skin fold.

- **Spine**. Ask the patient to flex the neck laterally to each side. Place several fingers on lumbar spinous processes and ask the patient to bend forward and attempt to touch their toes while standing with the legs fully extended, observing and feeling for normal movement.
- **Arms**. Ask the patient to place both hands behind their head with elbows right back. This is a sensitive test of many components of the shoulder apparatus. Straighten the arms down the side of the body and then inspect with elbows bent to 90° with palms down and fingers straight. Turn hands over and make a tight fist with each hand. Place in turn the tip of each finger on to the tip of the thumb. Squeeze the metacarpals from 2nd to 5th.
- **Legs**. With the patient reclining on a couch, flex each hip and knee in turn while holding and feeling the knee. Then passively rotate the hip internally. With the leg extended and resting on the couch, examine for tenderness or swelling of the knee by pressing down on the patella while cupping it proximally. Squeeze all the metatarsals and finally inspect the soles of the feet for callosities.

Such a screening examination should take a few minutes and identify abnormalities that then need fully assessing. These can be easily documented as:

G	✔	
	A (appearance)	M (movement)
A	✔	✗
L	✔	✔
S	✔	✗

Restricted movement left shoulder
Restricted movement cervical spine with crepitus

GENERAL PRINCIPLES

A complete medical history and examination are the most important steps in the evaluation of people with musculoskeletal problems. The whole person must be evaluated as many musculoskeletal conditions present with or develop symptoms and findings in other systems, and other conditions or therapy may be associated with manifestations in the musculoskeletal system. Gain the confidence of the person and establish a partnership between doctor and patient and a relationship of

trust. If their condition is chronic there is a dependency on the physician for their ongoing health and future quality of life. Their expectation of their condition and of the consultation must be identified early to achieve a satisfactory outcome. Are they expecting a cure or frightened of chronic disability? People, not surprisingly, find it difficult to accept chronic pain and fear long-term disability and they hope and look for cures. They may have already tried alternative or complementary therapies in an attempt to achieve this. The person should have a realistic, albeit optimistic, expectation of the likely outcome of their condition to avoid future dissatisfaction and difficulty in accepting their problem.

Any consultation should close with a full discussion of the findings and conclusions so that the person understands the cause, the treatment, what they can do to help themselves and what is the likely outcome. As many of these musculoskeletal conditions are chronic or recurrent, the patient will need more detailed explanation to enable them to actively participate in their own care. Other health professionals, written material, the Internet and patient support groups can give further support.

The cause of the problem should be considered in some framework. It is simplest to consider the structure affected and the mechanism of the problem. Is the cause related to the spine, joints, muscle, periarticular structures or bone? Is it a local or generalized musculoskeletal problem or a systemic condition? What is the underlying mechanism – is it vascular/ischemic, infectious, traumatic, autoimmune or immune-mediated, metabolic/toxic, inherited, neoplastic, congenital/developmental or degenerative? Musculoskeletal conditions are common and can coexist. It should not be assumed that each symptom relates to a single diagnosis. Each symptom should be evaluated individually and only interpreted once all the findings are collated.

The purpose of assessment is not only to establish the nature of the problem but is also to guide management. Musculoskeletal conditions affect the individual in a variety of ways and these must be identified. They are the commonest causes of chronic pain and physical disability and there is frequently depression and fatigue. The person may be unable to do their work. There is fear of the future. Their interpersonal relationships with family, carers and friends may be affected. A multi-disciplinary assessment is necessary to identify this broad range of problems to be able to develop an appropriate plan of management. There are many standardized assessments for musculoskeletal conditions to measure impact[2] and monitor response to treatment[3], which are considered within the relevant disease area elsewhere in this book.

Finally, clinical assessment requires good clinical skills combined with knowledge. Background knowledge is required of functional anatomy, of the features of common musculoskeletal conditions; of their differential diagnosis, risk factors and complications; and of their likely prognosis. Although specialist training ensures this, most musculoskeletal conditions are being managed in primary care or seen as a comorbid condition by other specialists and the general level of competency in the assessment and management of musculoskeletal conditions needs to be improved.

THE RHEUMATOLOGICAL CONSULTATION

The initial consultation should result in a clinical diagnosis (or at least offer a differential diagnosis) and provide an estimate of the severity and extent of the musculoskeletal condition and of the physical and psychosocial impact that it has on the life of the patient, their family and care givers. It should also give a clear idea of the patient's concerns. The consultation must fulfill the expectations of the patient as well as those of the physician (Table 3.1). The subsequent actions of investigation and management should follow logically from the findings of the consultation. Special investigations when dealing with a musculoskeletal problem are usually only necessary to confirm clinical suspicions regarding diagnosis and to help gauge disease activity, prognosis and choice of

TABLE 3.1 WHAT IS THE PURPOSE OF THE CONSULTATION?

Patient expectation	Clinician expectation
What is wrong?	Is there an abnormality?
What will happen?	What is the abnormality?
What can you do about it?	What effect is it having?
What can I do about it?	What is the cause?
Am I getting better?	Are there any predisposing or risk factors?
Am I receiving the best treatment, as I am not improving?	Are there any complications?
	What treatment is indicated?
	What has been the response to previous treatment?
	Is there a response to current treatment?
	What is the prognosis?

TABLE 3.2 PHASES OF THE CONSULTATION

Open phase	Listen: be interested and listen to their complaints, avoid interruption, understand their concerns Observe: appearance, manner, movement, abnormalities
History	Symptoms Chronology – temporal and anatomical pattern Impact Other aspects
Examination	Musculoskeletal system Systemic examination
Investigations	Diagnostic Monitoring
Conclusion	Analysis and interpretation Management plan Explanation and reassurance: communicate with the patient what is wrong, the cause, the prognosis, the treatment and its likely benefits and risks

treatment. The performance of unnecessary investigations may be avoided by this thoughtful sequence and by ensuring they are only performed if the results will influence decision-making. The use of investigations should be cost-effective just as cost-effectiveness is important for interventions. Further consultations will be more focused on monitoring response to treatment, with appropriate adjustment, and giving support to the patient with a chronic condition.

The process of the consultation can be divided into several phases (Table 3.2), which in practice overlap throughout the consultation process, with the physician continuously trying to piece together what the nature of the problem might be and directing their probing and examination accordingly.

History taking is by far the most important part of the evaluative process. It is an art that depends on experience but guidance can be given as to what information should be sought. Establish what has brought the person to you and characterize their problem. Explore for clues to make a diagnosis. Establish what their concerns and expectations are. The examination complements the history to confirm the cause and effect of the musculoskeletal problem.

It may be appropriate to concentrate relatively quickly and exclusively on the specific localized problem with which the person presents, but in the majority of cases it is necessary to make a full assessment, particularly as an apparently simple local problem may be the manifestation of a more generalized condition or the symptoms may be referred from a distant site. In addition the impact of the problem and expectations of the patient are central to developing a plan of management.

Open phase

The first part of a consultation is an open phase during which the patient should be listened to and observed.

Listening

The physician must first listen to what the patient has to say. The initial introductions should create a relaxed atmosphere and the history can begin with an open question, such as 'Tell me about it' – allowing the patient to tell their story uninterrupted. Some may need coaxing and encouragement, whereas others may need help and direction to get to the point. A few remarks will often help steer the conversation along the lines required, but nonverbal communication is often the key. The value judgment as to what is and is not relevant is in itself one of the crucial analytic skills employed by the physician. It is important to develop an understanding relationship with the patient during this phase. Avoid interruptions and specific questions, which can be answered with a 'yes' or 'no' or a simple factual statement which risk closing down the interview. This approach should help the patient bring out into the open the problems that really bother them and should also avoid the all too common complaint that 'the physician didn't listen to me'.

Observing

The first impressions are often the most revealing and careful observation is rewarding:

- **What is the overall appearance of the patient?** Estimate the approximate age. Note the gender. Note the body height and shape for evidence of body disproportion, such as obesity, cachexia, tallness (marfanoid habitus?), restricted growth or obvious skeletal deformity. Does the patient's appearance 'spell' illness or health, anemia, depression or emotional distress?
- **Are the patient's movements hesitant, labored, inhibited, painful or restricted?** Is the gait abnormal? Is a walking aid being used, or is the patient wheelchair-bound? How easily can they sit down and get up again? Watch them dressing, especially footwear.
- **How is the patient's manner?** Does the patient appear resentful, aggressive, unduly demanding, manipulative, argumentative or self-contradictory? How frustrated are they because of their problem? What about their affect? Is there a suggestion of anxiety or depression?

History

Taking the history should first clarify what has brought the patient to the consultation and what their expectations are. It should fully characterize the nature of the condition and its impact – the current symptoms, the chronology of the condition including the influence of any therapy and the impact of the disorder in both physical and psychological terms (Table 3.3). Then explore other factors that might influence this, such as clues to diagnosis from family or present and past general history, risk factors related to lifestyle or occupation and factors that may influence impact such as patients' expectations and their socioeconomic environment. Establish their concerns by simple questions such as 'What do you want to know?' and 'Do you have any worries?' and ensure that these are addressed by the end of the consultation. This should enable the physician to come to a diagnosis and plan of management. This requires background knowledge of the possible diagnosis, associated risk factors, expected effects of the condition and options for intervention to guide the interview.

This phase is more interrogative but use open questions, listening and steering the patient to give a clear account of the problem. The patient may need guiding to do this but very specific questions should be kept to the end of the interview, by which time the physician should have gained the patient's confidence.

What are the symptoms?

Musculoskeletal conditions affect the individual in a variety of ways. They are the commonest causes of chronic pain, there is often stiffness of the spine or limbs and there may be deformity. These symptoms are frequently accompanied by loss of function and mobility, which can limit activities and restrict participation. There is frequently depression related to chronic pain, poor-quality sleep and loss of function. Sleep deprivation, depression and inflammation result in fatigue. There is fear of the future. Interpersonal relationships may be affected. Assessment should be multidisciplinary to identify this broad range of problems associated with musculoskeletal conditions and to develop the management plan (Table 3.4).

Analysis of these symptoms helps the physician to differentiate a rheumatic complaint into six main types:

- inflammatory musculoskeletal disease
- mechanical joint or periarticular disorder
- bone disorder
- non-rheumatic disease causing musculoskeletal symptoms
- a functional disorder
- another of unknown cause.

TABLE 3.3 CHARACTERIZATION OF A MUSCULOSKELETAL PROBLEM

- What are the symptoms?
- Site and distribution of symptoms
- Chronology
- Associated symptoms
- Symptom response to health interventions
- Preceding factors
- What is its impact?

TABLE 3.4 SYMPTOMS OF A MUSCULOSKELETAL PROBLEM

- Pain
- Stiffness
- Swelling
- Deformity
- Weakness
- Instability
- Loss of function
- Fatigue and malaise
- Depression and fear
- Sleep disturbance
- Symptoms of systemic diseases

Pain

Characterizing the pain is important to identify its cause and effect (Table 3.5).

Where? – what is the site and distribution?

Knowing the site of pain helps to establish its origin. Description alone can be unreliable and the patient should be asked to demonstrate on themselves where the pain is felt and where it is most severe. Is the pain generalized or localized? How easily can it be localized? Articular and periarticular pain often radiates widely and presents far from its origin. Such referred pain is felt in the dermatome relating to the myotomal or sclerotomal origin of the affected structure (Table 3.6). Pain from bone and periosteum radiates little and is localized more reliably.

The distribution of pain should be characterized. Generalized pain all over can be due to fibromyalgia or polymyalgia rheumatica, whereas pain in the joints (arthralgia) indicates one of the many arthropathies. The typical patterns of the different arthropathies need to be recognized (see below, Table 3.15). Myeloma or metastatic malignancy must be considered with multiple sites of pain that are not just related to joints. The full differentiation of the anatomic site of origin of pain usually requires the examination of the patient.

What? – what are its characteristics and pattern?

The features of the pain, the time and mode of onset, diurnal pattern and evolution all provide diagnostic clues. Some typical descriptions of pain are the 'electric shock' and 'shooting pain' associated with a nerve entrapment, 'throbbing' vascular pain and the 'severe aching' sensation of joint pains. Severity is subjective but the extreme pain associated with acute gout is characteristic – just ask them if they would allow you to touch the joint when at its worst. However, neither the adjectives that people use to describe their pain nor their assessment of its severity is diagnostic alone although its perceived severity indicates the likely impact that it is having.

Certain musculoskeletal conditions are characterized by specific patterns of pain (Table 3.7). For example, gout usually begins in the middle of the night with a pricking sensation in the great toe, which

---

TABLE 3.5 QUESTIONS ABOUT PAIN

- Site and distribution
- Characteristics and pattern
- Preceding and precipitating factors
- Factors which worsen or improve symptoms
- Associated symptoms
- Symptom response to health interventions
- Impact

TABLE 3.6 COMMON PATTERNS OF REFERRED PAIN

Source of pain	Pattern of referral
Cervical spine	Occiput, shoulders
Shoulder	Lateral aspect of arm
Lateral epicondyle	Mid-forearm
Carpal tunnel	Radial fingers, occasionally forearm or arm
Lumbar spine	Sacroiliac joints, buttocks, posterior thigh, lower leg, foot
Hip joint	Groin, medial thigh, medial knee, greater trochanter, buttock above gluteal fold
Trochanteric bursa	Lateral thigh, buttock

TABLE 3.7 PATTERNS OF PAIN	
Bone pain – pain at rest and at night	Tumor Paget's Fracture
Mechanical joint pain – pain related to joint use only	Unstable joint
Osteoarthritic joint pain – pain on joint use, stiffness after inactivity, pain at end of day after use	
Inflammatory joint pain – pain and stiffness in the joints in the morning, at rest and with use	Inflammatory Infective
Neuralgic – diffuse pain and paresthesia in dermatome, worsened by specific activity	Root or peripheral nerve compression
Referred – pain unaffected by local movement	

quickly builds up into an intolerable persistent burning pain, whereas *osteoarthritis* is characterized by use-related pain and inactivity stiffness of the affected joints. *Mechanical pain* is generally related to use. *Inflammatory joint pain* is present at rest and with use and is usually worse at either end of the day. *Neuralgic pain* is diffuse, often worsened by a specific activity and associated with paresthesia in the dermatome. *Bone pain* is typically present at rest and at night. These give clues but are not diagnostic.

The pattern of evolution of the pain should be established in conjunction with the development of any other symptoms – how have they arrived at the present situation. For example the pain may have the characteristics of an inflammatory polyarthropathy but rheumatoid arthritis typically follows a gradual additive course whereas a viral arthropathy is of acute onset. These patterns should also be established when considering the development of the whole symptom complex.

When and why? – what precipitates, worsens or improves pain?
Establish any factors that precipitated the pain or affect it. Was there any preceding trauma, repetitive or unusual use? What kinds of activities induce pain – repetitive motion, climbing stairs, arising from a low chair, and so on. Periarticular problems are often induced by a specific type of activity. Mechanical pain and osteoarthritis are related to activity. Other disorders may also present with pain that has a specific relationship to activity; for example, when a twisting movement produces sharp pain and locking of the knee joint, it is likely that an internal derangement (such as a torn meniscus) is the problem; similarly it may be an easy task to diagnose spinal stenosis from the pain history when it is apparent that buttock and leg pain is activity-related and that walking downhill (which extends the spine) causes more pain than walking uphill or cycling. The buttock and leg pain related to spinal stenosis improves rapidly with rest only to recur after further activity.

The response to exercise in contrast to rest is a typical feature of sacroiliitis or spondylitis. Rest usually improves pain due to osteoarthritis but has little effect on inflammatory pain. The response to anti-inflammatory analgesics compared to simple analgesics can help distinguish an inflammatory cause of symptoms, such as ankylosing spondylitis, from mechanical back pain; the response of polymyalgia to glucocorticosteroids is also characteristic.

So what? – what is its impact
Pain is a subjective sensation that cannot be felt by others, cannot be remembered exactly and has psychological effects, including fear. It has quite different effects on different individuals. The response to pain and the degree to which it disrupts the person's life gives a more meaningful indication of severity. Does it affect their sleep? How has it affected their mood? What specific functions or activities does it limit? Understanding the problems it causes not only assists with its assessment but can also guide how to best manage their pain.

Stiffness
'Stiffness' means different things to different people and what it is being used to describe needs to be clarified with the individual patient. People often describe a generalized 'stiffness' after prolonged rest such as a long car journey, or the day after an unusual level of exercise, which is more common as people age. More specifically, patients often describe stiffness related to their symptomatic joints. An inflammatory joint disorder is generally associated with severe and prolonged morning and evening stiffness, whereas osteoarthritis is associated with short-lived but severe stiffness after inactivity. Inactivity 'gelling' of the osteoarthritic joint is mainly a difficulty in the initiation of movement, whereas morning stiffness in rheumatoid arthritis usually describes a more constant difficulty in moving the joints through any part of their range. 'Stiffness' can also be used to describe pain or aching in joints with movement, or to mean a reduced or limited range of movement. One of the disorders most characterized by morning stiffness is polymyalgia rheumatica, which can be so severe that it is virtually impossible to roll out of bed, although a few hours after getting up the patient may be virtually asymptomatic. The duration of morning stiffness can indicate the activity of rheumatoid arthritis or polymyalgia rheumatica. Simple questions such as 'What time do you wake?' followed by 'When are you as loose as you are going to get?' help pin down its duration (Table 3.8).

Stiffness of movement of the fingers can relate to tenosynovitis, sometimes with triggering, joint disease or tightening of the soft tissues such as in systemic sclerosis or with Dupuytren's contracture. 'Stiffness' can also be used by the patient to describe the difficulty in movement associated with muscle disease such as myositis and motor neurone disease. A careful examination is necessary to be certain as to the correct attribution of this symptom.

Locking of the joints, limbs or spine is a less common symptom. It describes the sudden inability to perform a particular movement and suggests a specific mechanical event in which some internal derangement actually causes the joint to lock in one position until a trick movement or help is used to free it up. This is a classic symptom of a loose body or torn meniscus of the knee joint, but it also occurs in the finger with triggering due to stenosing tenosynovitis.

TABLE 3.8 QUESTIONS ABOUT STIFFNESS
• What joints or muscles does it affect?
• When during the day?
• How long does it last?
• What makes it worse?
• What improves it?

TABLE 3.9 QUESTIONS ABOUT SWELLING AND DEFORMITY
• Did it follow an injury?
• Did it appear rapidly or slowly?
• Does it come and go?
• Is it gradually enlarging or progressing?
• Is it painful?

Swelling and deformity

Swelling is an important symptom and may be of the soft tissues, the joint or bone. Did it follow an injury? Did it appear rapidly or slowly? Is it painful? Does it come and go or is it gradually enlarging? (Table 3.9). Joint swelling is a sign of disease and examination is necessary to confirm whether it is related to the joint or a periarticular structure and to establish if it is due to an effusion, due to synovial proliferation or bony. Any other swelling will also need careful examination to establish its nature and cause. Imaging may be required.

Recognition of any deformity requires familiarity with the musculoskeletal system to separate normal variation from the abnormal and progressive. For instance a scoliosis needs to be recognized and treated at an early stage but short stature or wide hips just need reassurance.

Weakness and instability

Patients often describe weakness of limbs or of the whole body. This can be an important clue to a muscle disorder such as polymyositis or a neuropathy. The pattern of muscle weakness and its central or peripheral distribution should be established. Regional weakness is more likely to have a specific cause that needs identifying. However 'weakness' may be used by a patient to describe different things such as: general fatigue; difficulty with movement because of joint disease; the feeling of insecurity that is associated with a loss of proprioception, which accompanies many forms of joint disease; or the regional weakness of a joint or limb caused by the local muscle-wasting that can accompany joint damage. A joint may be unstable and suddenly give way because of muscle weakness or this may relate to the ligaments being ruptured, or lax in hypermobility. A sensation of 'giving way' and general instability of the lower limbs can result from weak quadriceps muscles.

Loss of function

The major impact of musculoskeletal conditions is the difficulty in performing various activities and this may be the presenting complaint. It is uncommon for these limitations to arise in the absence of a complaint of pain and/or stiffness but the painless loss of movement suggests a tendon rupture or a neurological cause. Enquiry should establish if any particular movements and functions are restricted and whether this relates to pain and stiffness or if it is a primary problem. The impact of musculoskeletal conditions, in other words how they affect activities and participation, should be fully explored.

Fatigue and malaise

Fatigue is a manifestation of most generalized rheumatic disorders, including rheumatoid arthritis, systemic lupus erythematosus (SLE) and most notably fibromyalgia. Fatigue may also be the consequence of poor sleep, often related to pain. It may be severely disabling, with a general sense of overwhelming tiredness making it impossible for the person to do anything. It is very distressing to the person but is often ignored by physicians or inappropriately passed off as being functional in origin. Although fatigue is sometimes functional and related to depression, the fatigue of rheumatoid arthritis or SLE is a good indicator of the systemic activity of the disease. The time at which fatigue becomes a problem is sometimes used, along with the duration of morning stiffness, as one of the monitors of disease activity.

People with inflammatory arthritis are often able to function well for several hours, only to suffer overwhelming fatigue in mid- or late afternoon. The fatigue of fibromyalgia is usually associated with lack of concentration and poor-quality sleep. Polymyalgia rheumatica is often associated with a feeling of sudden aging, with rapid rejuvenation with a moderate dose of corticosteroids.

Emotional lability

Fear and anxiety are common accompaniments of the first consultation. The degree of anxiety will be influenced by factors such as the severity of their symptoms, their knowledge of possible diagnosis, expectations of prognosis, personal experience of similar conditions affecting family or friends and their future aspirations. Fear of losing independence increases as people get older. Emotional lability, depression and other psychiatric disturbances can also be the direct result of a rheumatic disease, such as SLE. Sleep disturbance secondary to pain can also affect mood.

The consultation should establish the presence of anxiety and identify the concerns of the patient. At the same time the physician must allay their anxiety from an early stage of the consultation, responding to their fears and addressing them specifically and honestly in a reassuring and supportive manner.

Other presenting musculoskeletal symptoms

Patients with a rheumatic disorder occasionally present with a variety of other symptoms, including cracking or clicking of joints. Joint cracking is usually of no pathologic significance and patients should be reassured that it does not damage joints.

What is the pattern and chronology of symptoms?

The distribution and chronological pattern of each symptom needs to be established. Ask the simple questions, 'When were you last well?' and 'Exactly how did this begin?' to establish the onset, the first symptom and what was first affected. Was the onset sudden or gradual, spontaneous or after some specific event such as trauma or an infection (Table 3.10). The subsequent course should be established with respect to time and pattern of distribution of symptoms. If articular, is it peripheral small joints, large joints or axial? Has it followed an additive, intermittent or flitting course? Is it symmetric or asymmetric? The development and timing of any non-musculoskeletal symptoms or signs, the influence of drug therapy or any other interventions and the relationship of the symptoms to activities and life events should also be noted. Do the symptoms fit some recognized pattern? It is important, however, to avoid forcing the symptoms into a pattern – musculoskeletal conditions are common and different conditions can coexist.

A good history-taker will be able to draw a clear graphic representation of the chronology of the patient's illness and the anatomical pattern by the end of the consultation (Fig. 3.2). This has been discussed in part when considering pain (see Chapter 9).

The pattern of the problem is important in identifying the possible cause. For example, a traumatic condition obviously relates to a specific event, whereas a degenerative pathology usually presents in a slow, insidious fashion. Crystal-related inflammation is particularly rapid in onset and severe but self-limiting, whereas untreated sepsis causes a steadily worsening situation over a few days. Many of the idiopathic inflammatory or immunologic rheumatic diseases have a variable course with spontaneous remissions and exacerbations, whereas others, such as reactive arthritis, follow a more predictable course with the sequential development of mucocutaneous and joint inflammation over a period of a few weeks after the initiating event, which gradually subsides over a period of months. Other specific patterns include that of palindromic rheumatism, which, as the word implies, involves episodes of arthritis affecting one or two joints that come and go spontaneously over a few days.

TABLE 3.10 QUESTIONS ABOUT THE CHRONOLOGY OF THE DISORDER

- When did it start and the pattern that has developed with time?
- Where and how has it spread?
- What associated symptoms have developed and when?

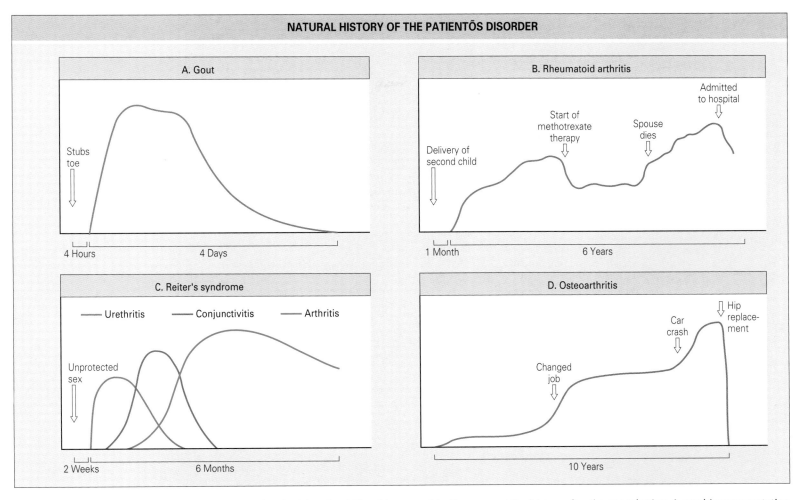

NATURAL HISTORY OF THE PATIENTŌS DISORDER

A. Gout

Stubs toe

4 Hours   4 Days

B. Rheumatoid arthritis

Admitted to hospital

Start of methotrexate therapy

Spouse dies

Delivery of second child

1 Month   6 Years

C. Reiter's syndrome

— Urethritis   — Conjunctivitis   — Arthritis

Unprotected sex

2 Weeks   6 Months

D. Osteoarthritis

Hip replace-ment

Car crash

Changed job

10 Years

Fig. 3.2 Natural history of the patient's disorder. The physician should be able to graphically represent the history after the consultation. A graphic representation is shown of (a) gout; (b) rheumatoid arthritis; (c) reactive arthritis and (d) osteoarthritis.

Associated symptoms and recent illnesses

Musculoskeletal conditions often have systemic features and systemic disorders often have musculoskeletal symptoms. The general review of other systems is very helpful in the differentiation of the many musculoskeletal conditions. There may have been a precipitating event. It is therefore important to ask about any recent trauma, illnesses, other medical problems and the presence of systemic symptoms, such as fever, night sweats or weight loss, which may indicate the presence of a serious systemic disorder such as a malignancy, infection or active inflammatory disease (Table 3.11).

The enquiry should be comprehensive but specific questions should be directed by knowledge of conditions under consideration. Specific patterns of association are common, for example a recent diarrheal illness, urethritis or psoriasis and mucocutaneous problems in the seronegative spondyloarthritides, dry eyes and mouth in sicca syndrome (although 'a dry mouth' is a common complaint) and a variety of systemic features in the connective tissue disorders, including rashes, mouth ulcers, Raynaud's phenomenon, neuropsychiatric disturbances and many others.

In practice it is often helpful to have a mental checklist of specific questions (such as, 'Have you ever had to see a physician or optician about your eyes for anything other than glasses?') for each of the common associations of a disorder that you consider likely when taking the history (Table 3.11). In addition, to gauge the relative importance of general or other-system-related problems, it may be useful to ask questions such as 'If you had no joint, muscle or back pain, would you feel well?'.

Previous health interventions and symptom response

Previous and present management should be reviewed. What has the patient been told, what knowledge and understanding do they have, which interventions have been tried and what was the response to them? Did they benefit or sustain any adverse effects? What is their attitude to and likely compliance with any treatment? Remember that patients often take 'alternative', 'complementary' or other over-the-counter medicines in addition to prescribed drugs and that they may be reticent about admitting this. Interventions include education and support as well as specific drug and non-drug treatments.

The influence of treatment on the course of a disease can also be of great relevance to the understanding of its nature and impact. Response to anti-inflammatory therapy is an important characteristic of many inflammatory disorders such as ankylosing spondylitis and a sudden and almost miraculous response to corticosteroids is typical of polymyalgia rheumatica. Drugs themselves may also be the cause of the problem, as in drug-induced lupus and thiazide diuretics in gout.

Preceding factors

The previous medical history may include past events that give clues to the present problem, such as a previous attack of unexplained epilepsy in someone with lupus, fetal loss or thrombosis in antiphospholipid syndrome, or a story of a swollen ankle in childhood in a young man with back pain who has now developed ankylosing spondylitis. In other cases, relevant previous medical events may relate to the associations between disorders, such as bronchiectasis preceding rheumatoid arthritis, or hypermobility in childhood and past joint trauma as risk factors for osteoarthritis.

TABLE 3.11 ASSOCIATED SYMPTOMS AND CONDITIONS

	Symptom	Possible diagnosis
Neurological	Headaches	SLE, temporal arteritis
	Numbness or paresthesia	Neuropathy – compression
	Weakness	Myositis, neuropathy
	Stroke	Antiphospholipid syndrome
	Epilepsy	SLE
Mouth	Dry mouth	Sjögren's syndrome
	Mouth ulcers	Reactive arthritis, Behçet's disease, inflammatory bowel disease
Eyes	Dry eyes	Sjögren's syndrome
	Red eyes	Spondyloarthropathy
	Visual loss	Temporal arteritis
Skin	Rashes	
	Psoriasis	Psoriatic arthritis
	Livedo reticularis	SLE
	Erythema nodosum	Acute sarcoid or erythema nodosum arthropathy
	Other	Viral
	Photosensitivity	Connective tissue disease
	Ulcers	Behçet's disease, vasculitis
	Raynaud's phenomenon	Connective tissue disease
	Nodules	Osteoarthritis, rheumatoid arthritis, gout, hyperlipidemia, SLE, rheumatic fever, polyarteritis nodosa, multicentric histiocytosis
	Alopecia	SLE
Respiratory	Pleuritis	Connective tissue disease
	Breathlessness	Pulmonary involvement with inflammatory disease eg systemic sclerosis, rheumatoid arthritis
Gastrointestinal	Indigestion, history of peptic ulcer	Non-steroidal gastritis or ulceration
	Diarrheal illness	Reactive arthritis, inflammatory bowel disease
Genitourinary	Renal stones	Gout
	Dysuria	Reactive arthritis, Behçet's disease, acute gonococcal arthritis
	Genital ulcers	Reactive arthritis, Behçet's disease, acute gonococcal arthritis
	Vaginal discharge	Reactive arthritis, Behçet's disease, acute gonococcal arthritis
Trauma	Fracture	
	Ligament rupture	
Non-specific symptoms	Malaise	Inflammatory disease, malignancy
	Fever	SLE, septic arthritis
	Weight loss	Inflammatory disease, malignancy
	Fatigue	Inflammatory disease
	Anorexia	Inflammatory disease, malignancy
	Aging	Polymyalgia rheumatica
Hematological	Thrombosis/thromboembolism	Antiphospholipid syndrome
	Anemia	
Obstetric history	Fetal loss – early and late	Antiphospholipid syndrome
	Intrauterine growth retardation	Antiphospholipid syndrome
	Pre-eclampsia	Antiphospholipid syndrome

Other relevant clues

The family history can help towards the differential diagnosis in some situations (Table 3.12), although almost everyone has a relative with arthritis and familial associations are seldom predictive. A family history also gives personal experience of the potential impact of a rheumatic condition and affects the person's anxieties about their own diagnosis and prognosis.

Useful clues include a recent flu-like illness in the family or other close contacts, raising the possibility of a viral arthritis; nodal arthritis affecting the mother when deciding if small-joint polyarthralgia of the hands is early rheumatoid arthritis or nodal osteoarthritis; a family history of ankylosing spondylitis, iritis or psoriasis in a young man presenting with back pain; or a family history of gout.

Lifestyle risk factors, such as smoking and alcohol intake, can be important in a few cases: smoking may be of great relevance in someone with rheumatoid arthritis who develops fibrosing alveolitis,

TABLE 3.12 IMPORTANCE OF FAMILY HISTORY

Family condition	Relevance to patient
Psoriasis	Psoriatic arthritis
Iritis	Spondyloarthropathy
Ankylosing spondylitis	Spondyloarthropathy
Fractures	Osteoporosis, osteogenesis imperfecta
Gout	Gout
Viral illness	Parvovirus or rubella arthropathy
Hypermobility	Hypermobility as cause of arthralgia
Nodal osteoarthritis	Nodal osteoarthritis as possible cause of early arthritis

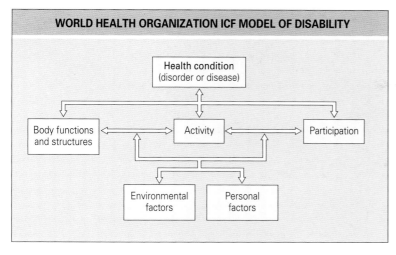

WORLD HEALTH ORGANIZATION ICF MODEL OF DISABILITY

Fig. 3.3 World Health Organization ICF model of disability. (Adapted from World Health Organization 2001[4].)

for example, and alcohol can be an important factor in the pathogenesis of gout. There are recognized risk factors for osteoporosis (see Chapter 44).

What is its impact?

The impact of the musculoskeletal condition must be assessed to understand the problems of the individual and to develop a plan of management that will try and address these. This impact will be affected by the patient's aspirations. This should be explored by listening and inquiring within the context of what to expect from knowledge and experience and against a framework such as the World Health Organization (WHO) International Classification of Functioning, Disability and Health (ICF)[4] (Fig. 3.3), which looks at the effect of any health condition on the functioning of an individual in terms of loss of function, limitation of activities and restriction of participation within the context of their life. There are two aspects to the context of an individual's life – environmental and personal. *Environmental factors* refer to all aspects of the extrinsic world that may have an impact on that person's functioning. These include the physical world and its features, the human-made physical world, other people in different relationships and roles, attitudes and values, social systems and services, and policies, rules and laws. *Personal factors* relate to the individual, such as age, gender, social status, life experiences and so on. The context of the person's life will interact with and affect the impact and progression of the disabling process at each stage. All these factors must be considered when assessing impact. Clearly identifying what contributes to the impact at all these different levels is essential to developing an effective plan for management.

Explore by watching, listening, talking through typical activities, think of restriction of expectations and aspirations as well as actual activities. It is often helpful to talk the person through a typical day – what time they wake, have they slept well, whether they can get to the toilet easily, any problems with washing and dressing, do they go to work, do they get out of the house much, do their own shopping and so forth. Potentially embarrassing or frustrating problems such as those associated with toilet difficulties or sexual dysfunction should be approached openly and frankly with simple direct questions.

Questions that can be used to explore current restrictions (Table 3.13) include 'Are there things that you cannot do now that you could do a year ago?'; to identify current aspirations, such as 'What do you most enjoy doing?'; and questions to identify the restriction of aspirations, such as 'What things do you find difficult that you would like to be able to do?' and 'What is it about your problem that you find most frustrating?' It is

important to look for the positive things as well as the negative ones. It is important to recognize and empathize with any emotionally charged issues. Psychosocial issues are just as important as the physical ones when considering the impact of a rheumatic disorder on a person.

Establish the amount of physical and emotional support the patient has from family, friends, other carers or from the social services. Does this meet their needs? How has their condition affected their economic situation? Are they working, have they had to change their employment, is their income reduced, or are they paying for help? Are they receiving any financial benefits to compensate for this? How are they getting around, since musculoskeletal conditions usually affect mobility, which can lead to practical difficulties of remaining independent, in addition to social isolation.

The effect on health-related quality of life can be formally assessed using various validated generic and disease specific questionnaires such as the HAQ[2].

Social history and occupation

Much of the most important information on the social history should be obtained when thinking about the impact of the condition. The personal and environmental context plays an important role in the impact

Occupation is important, as it is usually very informative. The person's occupation may have a causal role or an effect on the symptoms, or alternatively the symptoms may have an effect on occupation. Understanding the person's occupation can also give a clearer idea of the expectations they have and also of the impact of the condition. Unfortunately many people with musculoskeletal conditions have to change or modify their occupation.

Examination

The clinical examination complements the history and completes the clinical assessment. Examination of the musculoskeletal system should form part of the full general examination. A screening assessment to identify any significant abnormality of the musculoskeletal system has been described above. Once an abnormality has been identified it needs to be fully characterized. Much information will have been gained from a detailed history but a careful examination is also necessary to confirm clinical suspicions. Examination of the musculoskeletal system is principally an exercise in applied anatomy. Is the pain originating from the bone, muscle, joint or periarticular structures? Is the joint pain inflammatory or mechanical in origin? How painful is it to touch or move? How active is the synovitis? Examination may focus around the symptomatic structures but it is usually most informative to do this as part of a general examination of the musculoskeletal system and of the whole patient.

The recognition of abnormality is central to a good examination and this requires careful observation of structure, movement and function and also consistency with the history. This calls for much practice. The reproducible assessment of clinical abnormalities for the monitoring of the course of a condition, such as scoring joints for swelling and tenderness in rheumatoid arthritis or measuring spinal movement in ankylosing spondylitis, requires standardization of techniques and careful training.

TABLE 3.13 QUESTIONS ABOUT THE IMPACT OF THE CONDITION

- 'Are there things that you cannot do now that you could do a year ago?'
- 'What is it about your arthritis that you find most frustrating?'
- 'What do you most enjoy doing?'
- 'What things do you find difficult that you would like to be able to do?'
- 'How do you manage to get around the tasks which are difficult?'

TABLE 3.14 AIMS OF THE EXAMINATION
• Is it normal?
• What is the abnormality?
– What structures are involved?
– What is the nature of the abnormality?
• What is the pattern of distribution?
• What other features of clinical importance are there?

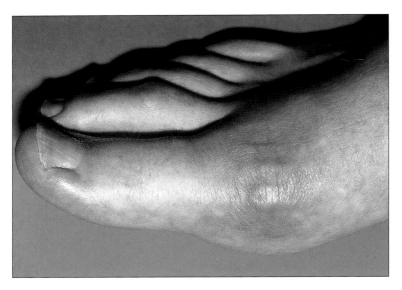

Fig. 3.5 Redness as seen in gout. This is a valuable indicator of the intensity of underlying joint inflammation.

Aims of examination

The aim of the examination of the musculoskeletal system is to answer four questions (Table 3.14) that, in combination with the history, should establish the differential diagnosis.

Is it normal?

The expected appearance and ranges of movement of the musculoskeletal system need to be recognized. Abnormalities can be observed as abnormal resting position, swelling or deformity with abnormal movement. There may be warmth, crepitus or tenderness on palpation with instability or weakness and muscle wasting.

What is the abnormality?

A careful examination and a thorough knowledge of surface and functional anatomy should enable the identification of the structure that is involved.

The nature of the abnormality needs to be established. Is there evidence of inflammation, damage, mechanical defects and/or biomechanical abnormalities? These are not mutually exclusive: a combination of them may be found.

Inflammation

An inflamed joint is characterized by pain and tenderness, warmth, redness and swelling. *Pain* is often apparent by observing movement and *tenderness* is elicited by gentle palpation. *Warmth* is mainly detectable in medium-sized and large joints, for example the knee, ankle and wrist joints (Fig. 3.4). *Redness* is uncommon but is encountered in gout, especially around the big toe (Fig. 3.5) and in sepsis.

Swelling of an inflamed joint is characterized by its articular origin, is fluctuant because of synovial proliferation or effusion and is tender, whereas there may be bony swelling along the joint line in osteoarthritis. There are a number of specific techniques for detection of synovitis and effusion at different joints (Fig. 3.6). Inflammation of periarticular structures such as bursae must be carefully distinguished from synovitis of the joint. Inflammation of muscle is characterized by tenderness.

Damage

Joint damage is recognized by the presence of deformity, crepitus, movement in an abnormal plane and loss of joint range of movement in the absence of features of current inflammation. *Crepitus* is an audible and palpable sensation resulting from the movement of one roughened surface on another. In osteoarthritis the crepitus has a fine quality. This should be distinguished from the coarser, clicking sensation encountered in normal joints, with which it may be confused.

Mechanical defects

There may be painful restriction of movement in a certain plane(s) in the absence of inflammation, due to mechanical defects such as a knee with an impacted meniscus tear or 'locking' of the spine in lumbar intervertebral disc prolapse. *Deformity* usually refers to malalignment or subluxation and is identified by abnormal posture, often more apparent on certain movements such as a developmental scoliosis of the spine. There may be movement in an abnormal plane of a severely damaged joint from rheumatoid arthritis or osteoarthritis. For example, the elbow is a simple hinge joint; hence its normal range is flexion/extension only and any other movement, such as elbow abduction, is abnormal and likely to indicate gross joint disruption. There may be bony deformity in Paget's disease.

Biomechanical abnormalities

For every joint there is a normal posture and a spectrum of normal range of joint motion, which varies with age, gender, genetic and ethnic origin. Outside this range there may be hypermobility or hypomobility. Biomechanical abnormalities can result in symptoms, such as scoliosis and back pain, joint hypermobility syndrome with joint pain, and foot pain is often caused by abnormal biomechanics. The joint range is reduced by joint inflammation (the bulk of inflamed synovium and the effusion) or by irreversible damage to the joint structures (articular cartilage). Movement is first lost from the extremes of

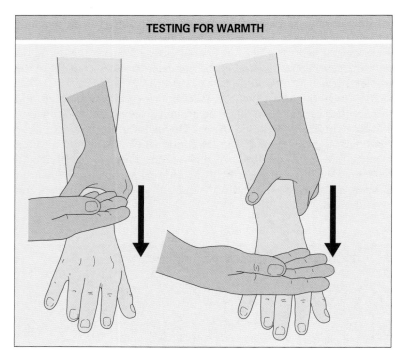

TESTING FOR WARMTH

Fig. 3.4 Testing for warmth, using the back of the hand.

THE BULGE SIGN IN THE KNEE

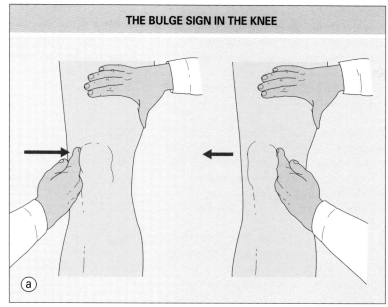

(a)

TESTING FOR SWELLING AND FLUCTUATION OF SMALL JOINT

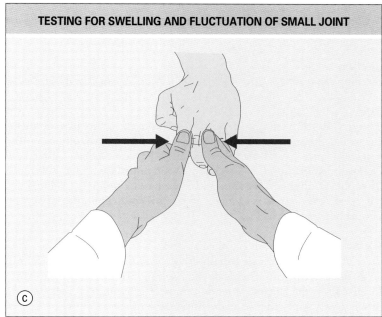

(c)

THE PATELLAR TAP

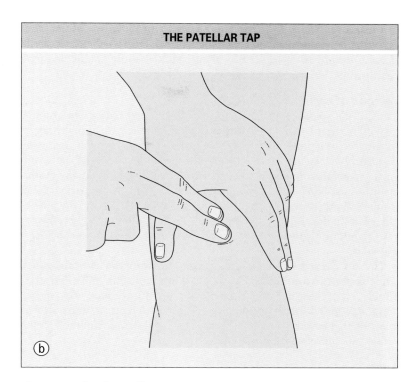

(b)

Fig. 3.6 Testing for swelling. (a) The bulge sign in the knee. The back of the hand gently pushes the fluid from one side of the knee to the other, filling out the 'dimples' on either side of the patella. This is most helpful in detecting small knee effusions. (b) The patellar tap. One hand is used to cup the patella and compress the suprapatellar pouch, and the fingers of the other hand press down on the patella to feel for cross-fluctuation. (c) Swelling/fluctuation of the small joints of the hand. Detect cross-fluctuation at the joint line with the index fingers and thumbs, with the examiner's fingers squeezing and feeling each side of the joint (as illustrated) or one index finger/thumb squeezing and feeling from side to side and the other from the palmar to the dorsal aspect ('interlocking C').

the range. Increasing joint damage results in a narrower range of motion about the neutral position. Complete loss of movement is described as ankylosis.

What is the pattern of distribution?
The distribution of involvement of the musculoskeletal structures is of crucial importance in the diagnosis of musculoskeletal conditions, as certain patterns are characteristic (Table 3.15 and Chapter 4). This

must be considered along with the course of the condition and the temporal pattern of the development of symptoms and signs. It is important to recognize that musculoskeletal conditions are common and there may be several different problems affecting an individual; the apparent pattern may be a false clue to the diagnosis. A careful examination is needed to confirm the pattern of distribution and to establish whether the various problems relate to a single diagnosis or to several coincident problems.

What other features of diagnostic importance are there?
Many musculoskeletal conditions are associated with systemic features (Table 3.11), which may be of diagnostic importance or of value in assessing severity. Many of them are easily visible as skin signs, such as skin laxity (joint hypermobility syndrome), rashes, nodules or vasculitic

TABLE 3.15 CHARACTERISTIC PATTERNS OF INVOLVEMENT OF THE MUSCULOSKELETAL SYSTEM

Diagnosis	Symmetry	Number of joints involved*	Large or small	Distribution	Upper or lower limbs
Rheumatoid arthritis	Symmetric	Polyarthritis	Large/small	Peripheral	Upper/lower
Ankylosing spondylitis	Asymmetric	Oligoarthritis	Large	Central and peripheral	Lower
Psoriatic arthritis	Asymmetric	Oligo/polyarthritis	Large/small	Peripheral	Upper/lower
Reactive arthritis	Asymmetric	Oligo/polyarthritis	Large/dactylitis	Peripheral	Lower
Gout	Asymmetric	Mono/oligoarthritis	Large/small	Peripheral	Lower/upper

*Oligoarthritis ≤ 5 joints affected; polyarthritis > 5 joints affected.

lesions, for example in rheumatoid arthritis (nodule, vasculitis), gout (tophi), dermatomyositis and psoriatic arthritis. Others will need a careful general examination to identify them, such as those characterizing a neuropathy.

Method of examination

Look at the whole person, their posture and movement. Then examine region by region, comparing one side with the other. It is usually necessary to examine the full musculoskeletal system to correctly assess the problem but placing most emphasis on the likely origins of the symptoms, remembering that pain is frequently referred and that any examination must consider all possible causes. Explain to the patient what you are about to do, ask them to inform you if they think any part of the examination is likely to be painful. To facilitate this, the examiner's eyes should study the patient's in order to anticipate discomfort before it happens.

The key elements of the examination to identify the clinical signs of musculoskeletal conditions (Table 3.16) are to look, feel, move and stress (Table 3.17). These are usually performed in an integrated way. Special tests may be necessary to identify specific problems. It must also be remembered that this should be part of a general examination to identify related and unrelated abnormalities.

Look

Attitude and spontaneous movement

Many of the abnormalities associated with musculoskeletal conditions can be noted by careful observation of the person undertaking various functional movements during the consultation. The way the person moves and performs activities and the attitude at which they hold the affected region may give clues to the underlying problem. An inflamed joint is most comfortable when the periarticular structures are at greatest laxity and the intracapsular pressure is least. Pain is most when intracapsular pressure is greatest. An indication of the severity of pain is given by the protection with which the person treats the affected region. There may be cracking of the joint as it is used, associated with hypermobility.

TABLE 3.16 CLINICAL SIGNS OF MUSCULOSKELETAL CONDITIONS

- Attitude
- Deformity
- Swelling
- Skin changes
- Muscle wasting
- Tenderness
- Movement restricted
- Crepitus
- Warmth
- Muscle weakness
- Instability
- Function limited

TABLE 3.17 SYSTEM FOR EXAMINATION OF THE MUSCULOSKELETAL SYSTEM

- Look – at rest, during movement
- Feel
- Move – active, passive, resisted, listen
- Stress
- Special tests

Deformities

Any deformity should be recorded. They are usually more apparent on weight-bearing or with use. A joint deformity is defined as malalignment of two articulating bones in relation to one another, whereas bone deformity is an abnormal shape of the bone(s) itself (themselves). There are a number of terms in common use to describe deformities.

- **Kyphosis:** a forward curvature of the thoracic spine
- **Scoliosis:** a lateral curvature of the spine
- **Dislocation:** articulating surfaces are displaced so that they are no longer in contact with one another
- **Subluxation:** partial dislocation
- **Fixed flexion:** loss of extension, so that the joint is permanently flexed
- **Valgus:** a lower limb deformity whereby the distal part is directed away from the midline (e.g. hallux valgus)
- **Varus:** a lower limb deformity whereby the distal part is directed towards the midline (e.g. genu varum).

Examination is necessary to determine if they are correctable.

Commonly encountered specific deformities of the spine and hand are shown in Figure 3.7.

Swelling

Swelling can be observed but palpation is necessary to characterize it.

Skin

The skin both overlying the affected region and generally should be inspected. Redness of the joint indicates marked inflammation and infection and crystal arthropathy must be considered. Other skin changes include psoriasis, ulceration, livedo reticularis and nodules such as tophi, erythema nodosum and rheumatoid nodules (Table 3.18). There are characteristic changes in the nailfold capillaries in certain connective tissue diseases.

Wasting

Loss of muscle bulk can usually be detected by careful inspection. Arthropathy can cause widespread wasting around the joint. More localized wasting suggests a tendon, muscle or peripheral nerve lesion. Swelling of a joint can give a false impression of loss of muscle.

Feel

Warmth

First feel gently for warmth. It is best elicited by using the back of the fingers and comparing to a normal structure (Fig. 3.4). It is a cardinal sign of inflammation but may only be detected over large joints.

Tenderness

The presence and localization of tenderness is important in identifying the cause of the problem (Table 3.19). Examine carefully to establish if it is the joint line or periarticular. Is it muscular, either generalized such as in myositis or localized such as the characteristic tender spots of fibromyalgia? Is it the temporal artery or temporomandibular joint? Is there no tenderness despite pain? Cautiously feel for tenderness, gradually increasing pressure while watching the person for any reaction and releasing as soon as the presence of tenderness is established. Only use pressure until blanching of the nail of the examining fingers. Percuss the vertebrae to detect localized tenderness.

Swelling

Characterize any swelling to determine its precise location and anatomical associations, if it is tender and whether it is fluid, soft tissue or bone.

SPINAL DEFORMATION

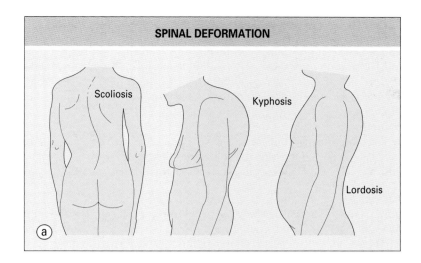

(a)

HAND DEFORMITY

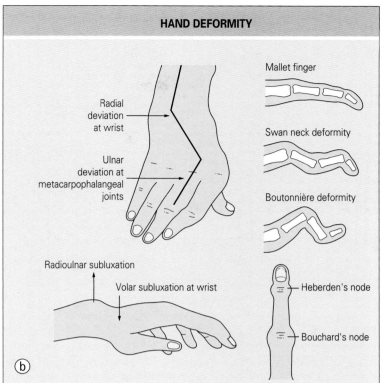

Radial deviation at wrist

Ulnar deviation at metacarpophalangeal joints

Radioulnar subluxation

Volar subluxation at wrist

Mallet finger

Swan neck deformity

Boutonnière deformity

Heberden's node

Bouchard's node

(b)

Fig. 3.7 Common deformities of (a) the spine and (b) the hand. These should be observed during examination. Spinal deformities are best observed from behind and from the side, with the patient in the erect posture.

TABLE 3.18 ASSOCIATED SKIN LESIONS		
Torso and limbs	Livedo reticularis	SLE, antiphospholipid syndrome, vasculitis
	Erythema ab igne	Sign of external heat applied to relieve pain
	Erythema migrans	Lyme arthritis
	Palpable purpura	Leukocytoclastic vasculitis
	Psoriasis	Psoriatic arthritis
	Erythema nodosum	Acute sarcoid
	Nodules	Heberden's
		Rheumatoid arthritis
		Gout
		Hyperlipidemia
		SLE
		Rheumatic fever
		Polyarteritis nodosa
		Multicentric histiocytosis
		Sarcoidosis
	Ulcers	Vasculitis, Behçet's disease, Crohn's disease?
	Calcinosis cutis	Scleroderma
Face and mouth	Butterfly rash	SLE
	Psoriasis	Psoriatic arthritis
	Heliotrope discoloration	Dermatomyositis
	Oral ulcers	SLE, reactive arthritis, Behçet's disease
	Telangiectasia	Limited cutaneous systemic sclerosis
Nails	Clubbing	Hypertrophic pulmonary osteoarthropathy
	Pitting	Psoriatic arthritis
	Onycholysis	Psoriatic arthritis
	Splinter hemorrhages	Small vessel vasculitis, endocarditis
Hands	Raynaud's phenomenon	SLE, scleroderma, mixed connective tissue disease
	Nail fold capillary abnormalities	Scleroderma, dermatomyositis
	Palmar erythema	Active rheumatoid arthritis, SLE
	Gottron's papules	Dermatomyositis
	Telangiectasia	Limited cutaneous systemic sclerosis
	Sclerodactyly	Limited cutaneous systemic sclerosis
	Vasculitic lesions	Rheumatoid arthritis, connective tissue diseases
Feet	Keratoderma blenorrhagica	Reactive arthritis

TABLE 3.19 POSSIBLE CAUSES OF TENDERNESS

Site	Possible cause
Joint line – generalized	Arthropathy or capsular disease
Joint line – localized	Abnormality of intracapsular structure, e.g. medial knee joint line tenderness with a meniscal tear
Periarticular	Bursitis Enthesiopathy Sarcoid
Muscular – generalized	Myositis
Muscular – localized	Myofascial lesion Fibromyalgia
Bone	Bone pathology – osteoporotic fracture or invasive lesion
Vertebral	Bone pathology – osteoporotic fracture or invasive lesion

Different types of swellings have typical characteristics at different sites. For example a knee effusion will initially fill the hollow on the medial aspect of the knee and then the suprapatellar pouch. Swelling of a joint is confined by the capsule and is most apparent at any weaknesses in this. Synovitis of the interphalangeal joints results in posterolateral swelling and an effusion of the knee may be associated with a popliteal cyst. Fluid and soft tissue is ballotable; this is the principle of the patellar tap and the interlocking-C examination of the interphalangeal joints (Fig. 3.6).

Movement

Feeling the joint and periarticular structures while moving it can give further information about pain and tenderness, as well as detecting crepitus from the joint or tendon sheaths.

Move

There are three methods of assessing joint movement – active, passive and against resistance.

- In examination of joints a combination of active and passive is recommended
- In detecting lesions in tendons or at tendino-osseous junctions, the against-resistance method is principally of use
- For measuring muscle power, the against-resistance method is, of course, the principal technique.

The recognition of abnormality requires familiarity with the normal ranges and planes of movement relevant to that particular joint. If the problem is unilateral, comparing the affected with the unaffected side can best assess the range of movement and establish if there is a loss. Formal measurement is of limited value.

Involvement of the joint, in particular synovitis, usually affects all movements, although some movements are more sensitive than others. Restriction of movement in one plane is characteristic of periarticular lesions, tenosynovitis and internal derangement of the joint.

The characteristics of joint pain on movement indicates the cause. Pain that increases towards the extremes of restricted movement with no or little pain in the midrange is described as stress pain. Its presence in all directions is a good sign for the presence of synovitis. Its presence in just one plane of movement indicates a localized articular or periarticular problem. Pain throughout the range of movement is more characteristic of mechanical problems such as osteoarthritis.

Movement against resistance measures power, although this is difficult to assess fully in the presence of pain. Resisted active movement is more valuable in identifying problems that relate to the muscle tendon or enthesis. This should be performed with the joint in a neutral position. The reproduction of pain indicates that it is originating from the muscle, tendon or tendon insertion relating to that movement. Passively stretching the tendon or ligament may also reproduce the pain.

Listening during joint movement may detect coarse crepitus due to cartilage damage, cracking associated with hypermobility or clonking due to a loose body or irregular surfaces such as severe damage.

Stress

Joint stability should be assessed, establishing if on stressing the joint there is any movement in abnormal planes for that joint. This can be abnormal due to generalized hypermobility, ligament rupture subsequent to trauma or inflammation, capsular inflammation, or loss of articular cartilage and bony changes due to osteoarthritis or rheumatoid arthritis.

Special tests

There are various special tests for specific diagnoses which are not within the scope of this overview but are considered elsewhere.

General examination

A full general examination forms an important part of the assessment of a person with a musculoskeletal problem. More frequent problems relate to the skin and nails (Fig. 3.7), neurological system and eyes.

Neurological examination is important because of the numerous neurological complications of rheumatic disorders, such as rheumatoid neuropathy, cervical myelopathy and radiculopathy, and lumbar nerve root compression resulting in foot drop. In addition muscle power is lost as a result of inhibition due to pain arising in adjacent inflamed joints. This effect forms the basis of the grip-strength test for assessing progress in rheumatoid arthritis.

It is important to recognize the symptoms and signs of nerve entrapment – carpal tunnel syndrome, ulnar neuritis, common peroneal nerve lesion, meralgia paraesthetica and tarsal tunnel syndrome. These peripheral nerve entrapment lesions are common and may be provoked by overuse injury. Careful attention to detection of neurological deficit in the territory of the trapped nerve will point to the correct diagnosis, which may be confirmed by a provocative sign such as tapping over the course of the median nerve (Tinel's sign) in the carpal tunnel syndrome or by neurophysiological tests.

The eyes are involved in a variety of musculoskeletal conditions and should be specifically examined. If there is any suspicion of dryness of the eyes, then this should be specifically assessed by a Schirmer test or rose Bengal staining by an ophthalmologist.

Regional examination of the musculoskeletal system

A systematic approach to examination should be taken but ensure to address any questions raised by the history (Tables 3.20 & 3.21). The sequence can vary but in general it is easiest to look at the patient as a whole walking and standing and then work from the head downwards and to compare one side with the other for each limb (Figs 3.8– 3.10).

Gait

The gait demonstrates the integrated function of the lower limbs and will reveal abnormalities of the neuromusculoskeletal system. Further assessment of the lower limbs will be necessary to identify the specific cause of any abnormality of gait. The full gait cycle should be observed as described in the screening examination (Fig. 3.1).

Certain abnormal patterns of gait are well recognized. Pain in one limb causes the avoidance of weight-bearing by that limb and shortening of that phase of the gait cycle. The cycle is asymmetric, with shorter steps

TABLE 3.20 THE EXAMINATION OF THE MUSCULOSKELETAL SYSTEM

- Watch the patient walk and undress
- Look at the posture with the patient standing undressed to their underwear
- Examine the
  - Neck
  - Spine and pelvis
  - Shoulders
  - Arms
  - Hands
  - Hips
  - Knees
  - Ankles and feet

TABLE 3.21 SYSTEM FOR EXAMINATION OF THE MUSCULOSKELETAL SYSTEM

Look	At rest for
	• Swelling
	• Deformity
	• Wasting
	• Attitude
	• Skin
	During movement
Feel for	Tenderness
	Swelling
	Movement – crepitus
	Temperature
Move	Active
	Passive
	Resistance
	Listen
Stress	Stability
Special tests	

on the painful limb and is described as an *antalgic gait*. Weakness of the hip adductors results in dipping of the pelvis to the other side when weight-bearing on the affected limb. During the gait cycle the person leans their upper body over the weak hip to compensate for this to keep their balance. This *Trendelenburg gait* is apparent as side-to-side movement of the shoulders when walking. Such movement of the shoulders is also seen if there is an inequality of leg length leading to tilting of the pelvis during the gait cycle. An alternative gait with leg length inequality is to flex the knee of the longer leg to clear the ground during the swing phase, with consequent dipping of the person up and down. A drop foot results in a *high-stepping gait* to avoid tripping on the toes during the swing phase.

Posture

The normal symmetry of the body helps identify abnormalities of posture. Look at the whole person standing undressed to their underwear and look for equality of height of landmarks – the shoulder tips, the scapulae, the pelvic brim, the crease of the buttock. Inspect the spine carefully for its normal curves and identify any scoliosis. Look at the feet for their normal posture.

Documentation

The history and examination need to be documented. The history should form a clear story that another clinician can read, assess and interpret. The examination is documented most easily on a

homunculus. A standardized approach is recommended to denote deformities, restricted movement, joint swelling and joint tenderness (Fig. 3.11).

There are various disease specific standardized assessments that can be used to evaluate conditions such as rheumatoid arthritis, ankylosing spondylitis or SLE. These are considered elsewhere (Chapter 28).

Investigation

The role of investigation in the assessment of the musculoskeletal system is usually to confirm suspicions from the history and examination. Investigations should only be performed if the results will influence decision-making. The acute-phase response can be used to confirm an inflammatory origin for the problem as well as to assess disease activity. Many investigations such as serum rheumatoid factor and antinuclear antibodies are not specific or sensitive enough to be diagnostic alone and they have to be interpreted in the context of the clinical picture. The specific investigations relevant for individual conditions are considered elsewhere.

Concluding the consultation

Interpretation

The aim of the consultation is to identify the cause of the person's problems, assess severity and response to any treatment, plan management and fully discuss this and the expected outcome with the patient.

Making a diagnosis requires the integration of the history and findings on examination with knowledge of the possible causes and results of appropriate investigations. Pattern recognition plays a key role. Knowing what is likely at different stages of life in different individuals and looking for clues throughout the consultation is important. As musculoskeletal conditions are common, it must be remembered that multiple pathologies are possible.

An important reason to make a specific diagnosis is to be able to give a prognosis from experience of similar cases and to plan management. Management also relates to the specific problems that the individual has relating to their condition and this will depend on them as well as the characteristics of the condition itself. That is why the full assessment of the individual, their expectations and the impact of the problem on them is so important.

The assessment of disease activity and severity is also essential for good management. How active is the inflammation related to the patient's rheumatoid arthritis? How much damage is there related to the person's SLE? Treatment needs to be adjusted accordingly and any assessment must separate out factors not specifically related to the inflammatory process to avoid treating the wrong target. Poor pain control due to depression will not respond well to disease-modifying therapy for rheumatoid arthritis. Careful assessment of the individual, understanding their problems and being able to relate to them all help to avoid these difficulties and ensure that management is aimed at their specific problems.

Communicating the findings

The most important part of the consultation, especially for the patient, is the communication of the findings and conclusions. That is why the patient is there. Establish what they want to know and what their worries are so that these can be addressed. Ensure that the person feels that all their problems have been listened to and their questions answered as far as is possible. It is sometimes difficult to explain all their symptoms with precise tissue-based causes and this can cause concern and loss of confidence in the physician. Concepts of mechanical back pain and fibromyalgia can be difficult for the person to grasp. This part of the consultation needs most time but is usually the most hurried part.

Cervical spine

Look	Look for hyperextension due to a thoracic kyphosis, or loss of normal lordosis.
Feel	Percuss the vertebrae for tenderness.
	Palpate the paraspinal muscles for spasm or tenderness.
Move	Actively turn head to right, left, flexion, extension, rotation to left and right and lateral flexion to left and right with examiner gently guiding the head to ensure maximum range is reached.
Special tests	Problems related to the cervical spine are often associated with neurological symptoms and signs which should be elicited.

Right rotation 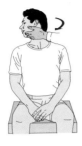 Left rotation 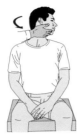 Right lateral flexion 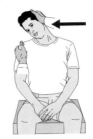 Left lateral flexion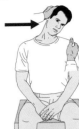

Flexion 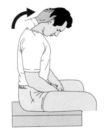 Extension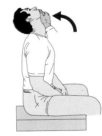

Temporomandibular joints

Feel	Palpate over the joint line for tenderness, crepitus or clicking. The joint can be palpated anterior to the tragus or from within the external auditory meatus. Feel for crepitus or clicking on movement.
Move	Open mouth wide.
	Deviate lower jaw side to side.

Mouth opening 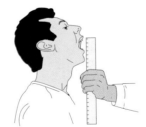 Side–to–side movement of jaw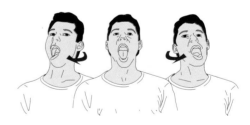

Dorsal spine

Look	Look for any kyphosis or scoliosis.
	Look for any asymmetry of scapulae
Feel	Percuss the vertebrae for tenderness.
	Palpate the paraspinal muscles for spasm or tenderness.
Move	Fix the pelvis by sitting and rotate the upper body to right and left with examiner gently guiding the shoulders to ensure maximum range is reached.

Left rotation 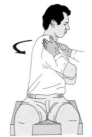 Right rotation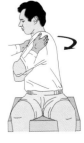

Fig. 3.8 The examination of the head, spine and pelvis.

Lumbar spine

Look	Look for a normal lordosis or any scoliosis. Look for any asymmetry of pelvic brim or the crease of the buttocks.
Feel	Percuss the vertebrae for tenderness.
	Palpate the paraspinal muscles for spasm or tenderness.
Move	While standing in an erect posture, bend forward as if trying to touch the toes, bend backwards to arch the back, and bend from side to side. Flexion can be more formally assessed by the Schober test with measurement of the extension of a line drawn when upright between 10cm above and 5cm below the level of the posterior iliac spines identified by the dimples of Venus.
Stress	Tests for tension of the lumbar roots should be performed.
	Femoral nerve stretch test
	With the person lying prone, hold their ankle and passively flex the knee as far as it will go. It is positive if pain is felt in the isolateral anterior thigh.
	Sciatic nerve stretch test
	With the person lying supine, gently raise the straight leg to the maximum angle achievable without significant pain and then dorsiflex the ankle. An increase in pain indicates sciatic nerve root tension.
Special tests	The lumbar spine houses the lumbar spinal nerve roots and neurological symptoms and signs should be elicited.

Lumbar flexion

Hypermobility

Lumbar extension

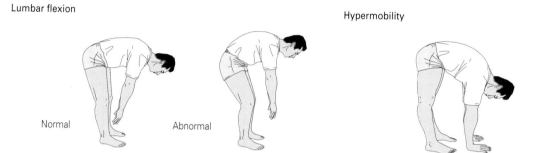

Normal   Abnormal

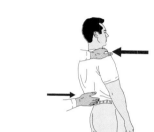

Right/left lateral flexion

Pelvis and sacroiliac joints

Look	Look for asymmetry of the pelvic brim and of the lower part of buttock.
Feel	Palpate for tenderness in the buttocks.
	Palpate the sacroiliac joints for tenderness.
Stress	Stress the sacroiliac joints for tenderness. There are various methods to compress or distract the joint to elicit tenderness such as pushing on both iliac wings when the person is lying on their back on the couch.

Test for cruralgia

Test for sciatica

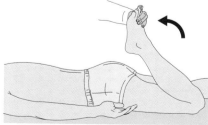

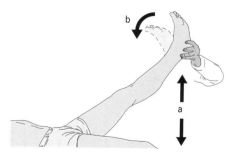

Fig. 3.8 (*continued*)

Shoulder

Look	Look for any asymmetry of scapulae, posture or muscle wasting.
Feel	Palpate over the midpoint of each trapezius and the supraspinatus to identify tender spots.
	Palpate over the acromioclavicular joint line, glenohumeral joint line and bicipital groove.
Move	Actively elevate arms into air.
	Actively place hands behind head.
	Actively place hands behind back.
	Steady scapula and with the elbow at 90° rotate internally and externally; then passively abduct, flex, internally and externally rotate the shoulder.
Special tests	There are several methods to establish if there is impingement – see Ch. 15

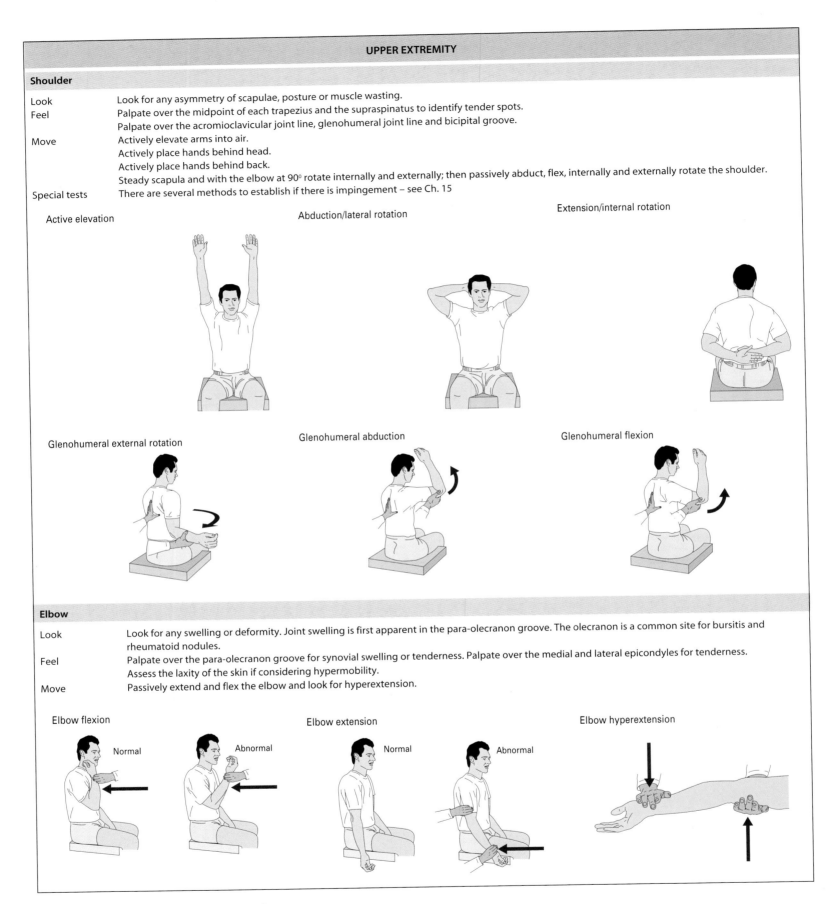

Active elevation

Abduction/lateral rotation

Extension/internal rotation

Glenohumeral external rotation

Glenohumeral abduction

Glenohumeral flexion

Elbow

Look	Look for any swelling or deformity. Joint swelling is first apparent in the para-olecranon groove. The olecranon is a common site for bursitis and rheumatoid nodules.
Feel	Palpate over the para-olecranon groove for synovial swelling or tenderness. Palpate over the medial and lateral epicondyles for tenderness. Assess the laxity of the skin if considering hypermobility.
Move	Passively extend and flex the elbow and look for hyperextension.

Elbow flexion

Normal

Abnormal

Elbow extension

Normal

Abnormal

Elbow hyperextension

Fig. 3.9 The examination of the upper extremity.

UPPER EXTREMITY

Wrist

Look	Look for any swelling or deformity.
	Swelling over the dorsum is of the joint or extensor tendon sheath. With active extension of the fingers, swelling of the extensor tendon sheath moves – the *tuck sign*.
	Look for squaring of the palm base because of swelling of the carpometacarpal joint seen in osteoarthritis. Typical deformities in established rheumatoid arthritis are volar subluxation and radial deviation at the wrist with dorsal subluxation of the ulnar styloid.
Feel	Palpate over the joint line for tenderness or synovial swelling.
Move	Passively flex and extend the wrist.
	Assess for hypermobility by passively moving the thumb towards the volar aspect of the forearm with the wrist in full flexion.
	Resisted flexion, extension or pronation if assessing epicondylitis at the elbow
Stress	Assess stability of the inferior radio-ulnar joint by demonstrating movement with pressing down on the radial head – the *piano key sign*

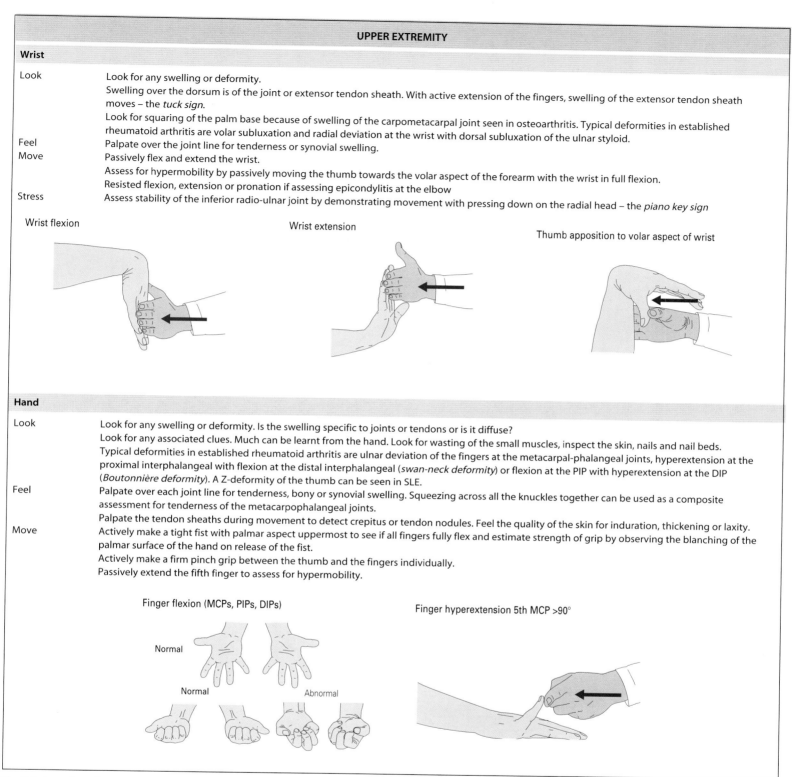

Wrist flexion

Wrist extension

Thumb apposition to volar aspect of wrist

Hand

Look	Look for any swelling or deformity. Is the swelling specific to joints or tendons or is it diffuse?
	Look for any associated clues. Much can be learnt from the hand. Look for wasting of the small muscles, inspect the skin, nails and nail beds.
	Typical deformities in established rheumatoid arthritis are ulnar deviation of the fingers at the metacarpal-phalangeal joints, hyperextension at the proximal interphalangeal with flexion at the distal interphalangeal (*swan-neck deformity*) or flexion at the PIP with hyperextension at the DIP (*Boutonnière deformity*). A Z-deformity of the thumb can be seen in SLE.
Feel	Palpate over each joint line for tenderness, bony or synovial swelling. Squeezing across all the knuckles together can be used as a composite assessment for tenderness of the metacarpophalangeal joints.
	Palpate the tendon sheaths during movement to detect crepitus or tendon nodules. Feel the quality of the skin for induration, thickening or laxity.
Move	Actively make a tight fist with palmar aspect uppermost to see if all fingers fully flex and estimate strength of grip by observing the blanching of the palmar surface of the hand on release of the fist.
	Actively make a firm pinch grip between the thumb and the fingers individually.
	Passively extend the fifth finger to assess for hypermobility.

Finger flexion (MCPs, PIPs, DIPs)

Finger hyperextension 5th MCP >90°

Normal

Normal

Abnormal

Fig. 3.9 (*continued*)

LOWER EXTREMITY

Observing the gait is an important part of assessing the lower limbs. Examination should be done with the person lying on a couch. Measure leg length if a pelvic tilt when standing suggests shortening. Pain in the hindquarter is often called 'hip pain' but can have many origins (Table 3.22) that need elucidating by examination.

Hip

Look	Observation of the person walking will have given some information about the hips. There may be wasting of the buttock or thigh muscles from disuse.
Feel	Palpation should be used to clarify the origin of any symptoms. The 'hip' is used to describe symptoms anywhere in the hind quarter. Tenderness is usually related to tendinitis or bursitis.
Move	With the person supine, passively flex the hip as far as possible with the knee in flexion.
	With the hip passively flexed to 90°, rotate it internally and externally by holding the foot, supporting the thigh and moving the lower leg inwards and outwards, careful to not inflict pain. Internal rotation is often affected first in disorders of the hip joint.
	With the person lying supine with the leg fully extended, hold the contralateral anterior superior iliac spine to prevent movement of the pelvis and passively abduct and adduct the leg.
	With the person lying prone or on their side, passively extend the straightened leg.

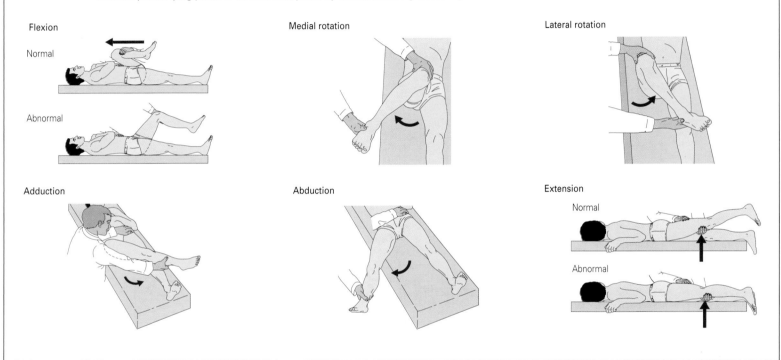

Knee

Look	Observation of the person walking will have given some information about the knees. There may be wasting of the thigh muscles from disuse. There may be instability. Look for any swelling and its exact site as it may relate to the joint or peri-articular structures. Look for any deformity. Typical deformities are fixed flexion, valgus or varus.
Feel	Palpate for tenderness or swelling and establish the affected structures. Palpate the joint line for tenderness. Assess for articular swelling and effusion by the *bulge sign* or *patella tap* (Fig. 3.6). Palpate for a popliteal cyst.
Move	With the person supine, passively flex the knee as far as possible with the hip in flexion. If the hip is also abnormal, hang the leg over the side of the couch to examine flexion of the knee without hip flexion.
	With the person lying supine, fully extended the leg in an attempt to touch the back of the knee onto the couch. Assess passively if the knee will hyperextend.
Stress	Anterior and posterior stability should be tested to assess the cruciate ligaments
	Medial and lateral stability should be tested to assess the collateral ligaments and for loss of joint space.

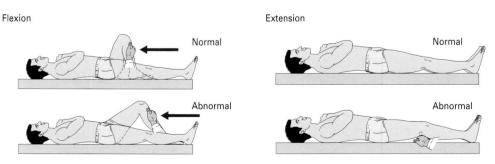

Fig. 3.10 The examination of the lower extremity.

LOWER EXTREMITY

Foot and Ankle

Look
Observe the feet when standing and during walking. Look for a normal longitudinal arch and during the gait cycle look for normal heel strike and take off from the forefoot. Look for any callosities beneath the metatarsal heads and for any swelling and redness of the toes. Swelling of the metatarsophalangeal joints can separate the toes and daylight becomes visible between them. Look for any deformities. Deformities include pes planus (flattening of the longitudinal arch), pronation of the foot, valgus deformity of the hindfoot (eversion of the sub-talar joint, pes cavus (high longitudinal arch), talipes equinovarus, hallux valgus, subluxation of the metatarsophalangeal joints, and claw, hammer and mallet deformities of the toes.

Feel
Symptoms may relate to the joint; the periarticular bone; the tendons, their sheaths and insertions; or bursae. Palpate for tenderness or swelling and establish the affected structures. Squeeze across the metatarsus and if there is tenderness, examine the metatarsophalangeal joints individually.

Move
Passively flex and extend the ankle.

Passively deviate the heel medially (inversion) and laterally (eversion) by grasping the heel between the examiner's thumb and index finger of one hand and moving it while anchoring the lower leg with the other hand.

Passively rotate the forefoot on the hindfoot by grasping the forefoot between the examiner's thumb and fingers while anchoring the heel with the other hand to assess the midtarsal joint.

See if they are able to stand on their toes which requires an intact posterior tibialis tendon.

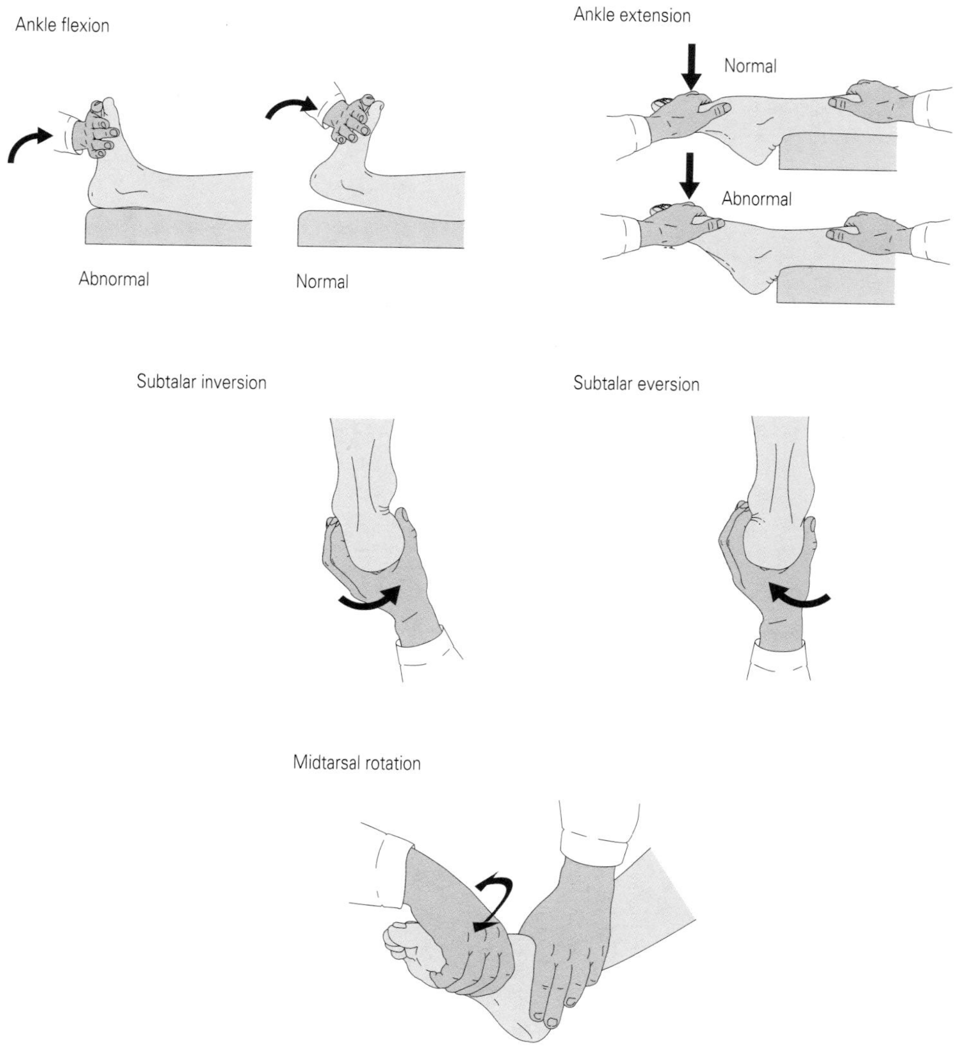

Ankle flexion

Ankle extension

Normal

Abnormal

Abnormal   Normal

Subtalar inversion

Subtalar eversion

Midtarsal rotation

Fig. 3.10 (*continued*)

TABLE 3.22 'HIP' PAIN

- Lumbosacral spine
- Sacroiliac joint
- Hip joint
- Adductor tendon
- Gluteal tendon
- Trochanteric bursa
- Iliopectineal bursa
- Ischiogluteal bursa
- L3 root
- Lateral cutaneous nerve of the thigh (meralgia paraesthetica)
- Inguinal or femoral hernia

ANNOTATING THE EXAMINATION FINDINGS

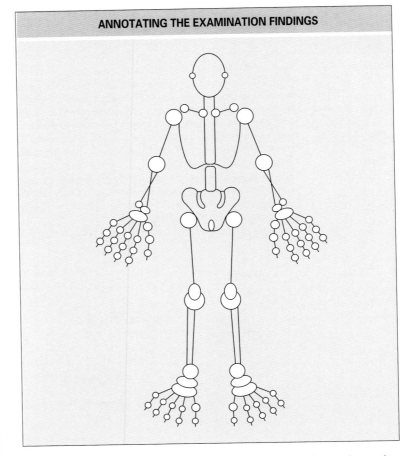

Fig. 3.11 Annotating the examination findings. A homunculus can be used to annotate the abnormal findings made during examination.

A specialist nurse can supplement the information that the person wants, and there is a lot of material available about musculoskeletal conditions from support organizations, such as the Arthritis Foundation or Arthritis Care, and from the Internet.

REFERENCES

1. Doherty M, Dacre J, Dieppe P, Snaith M. The 'GALS' locomotor screen. Ann Rheum Dis 1992; 51: 1165–1169.
2. Fries JF, Spitz PW, Kraines RG, Holman HR. Measurement of patient outcome in arthritis. Arthritis Rheum 1980; 23: 137–145.
3. Van der Heijde DMFM, van't Hof MA, van Riel PLCM, van de Putte LBA. Development of a disease activity score based on judgement in clinical practice by rheumatologists. J Rheumatol 1993; 20: 579–581.
4. World Health Organization. International Classification of Functioning and Health. Geneva: WHO; 2001.

FURTHER READING

Doherty M, Hazleman BL, Hutton CW *et al.* Rheumatology examination and injection techniques, 2nd ed. London: WB Saunders; 1999.

McRae R. Clinical orthopaedic examination, 4th ed. Edinburgh: Churchill Livingstone; 1997.

4 Pattern recognition in arthritis

Osvaldo Hübscher

- Pattern recognition is the key to diagnosis of the rheumatic disorders: the central questions that need to be asked are:
  - Is there a locomotor problem or a disease of another system?
  - Is the condition articular or periarticular?
  - Is the condition mechanical (arthrosis) or inflammatory?
  - Does it affect appendicular or axial structures or both?
- These questions can be answered from a synthesis of data from the history and examination, in particular:
  - From the *history* – the mode of onset, the sequence of development of different features and the duration and pattern of the symptoms
  - From the *examination* – the number, distribution and pattern of the affected joints or periarticular structures and the nature of any systemic involvement.

INTRODUCTION

The history and physical examination are the two most important components of the diagnostic process for patients complaining of musculoskeletal pain, stiffness or other rheumatic symptoms[1]. Clinical judgment in interpreting findings elicited from the history and physical examination should allow the physician to answer several key questions:

- Do the symptoms originate in the locomotor system or do they reflect diseases primarily affecting other systems (e.g. neurologic disorders, vascular disease, Pancoast's syndrome)?
- Is it an articular or non-articular process? A substantial number of patients will have localized mechanical problems or non-specific soft tissue conditions. Muscular syndromes or pain originating in periarticular foci can often mimic an articular origin (sometimes affecting more than one site). Examples are uni- or bilateral anserine bursitis resembling an intra-articular knee joint disorder, and extensor tendinitis of the thumb (de Quervain's tenosynovitis) mimicking wrist involvement. Primary bone conditions (e.g. Paget's disease, osteoid osteoma) as well as infiltrative (e.g. lymphomas) and lytic (e.g. metastatic disease) lesions may also provoke pain referred to a joint. Bone infarction or infection and stress fractures may also generate confusion.
- Does the patient have arthralgias or arthritis? *Arthralgia* is used to refer to pain localized in a joint whereas *arthritis* refers to the objective evidence of an inflammatory or degenerative change of the joint. Arthritis is a much more specific sign of an articular disorder.
- Is there evidence of other organ involvement (e.g. systemic connective tissue disorders) or does it appear to be a disorder restricted to the musculoskeletal system (e.g. osteoarthritis)?
- Is the articular problem inflammatory, degenerative or something else?
- Does the disease affect axial or appendicular structures, or both?

Once the physician establishes that the disorder originates in the joints, several other aspects of the history and physical examination should be considered in order to delineate a diagnostic pattern of arthropathy (Table 4.1). The attributes of joint involvement that will be considered in this section focus on those dominating the clinical picture during the early phases of rheumatic disorders, when treatment could be of greater benefit. Moreover, the diagnostic value of pattern recognition will be considered without taking into account other characteristics of the patient (e.g. gender, age, family history) or the presence or absence of extra-articular features of disease normally contributing to diagnostic certainty.

MODE OF ONSET AND DURATION OF SYMPTOMS

Some arthropathies typically present with an acute onset of pain with the peak intensity reached within hours or a few days[2], whereas in others maximum severity is reached gradually (over several weeks or months). Variations may occur and the same disorder may have a sudden onset in some patients and be gradual in others. Rheumatoid arthritis (RA), for instance, may present as an acute polyarthritis (especially in the elderly) and psoriatic arthropathy as an acute monoarthritis resembling gout, whereas in most cases both disorders begin insidiously. Examples of an acute onset also include bacterial arthritis, rheumatic fever, reactive arthritis, palindromic rheumatism and crystal-induced arthritis (the best example being nocturnal attacks of gout). Arthritogenic virus (in particular parvovirus B19, rubella virus and hepatitis B virus) may also cause acute synovitis. An insidious pattern is common in early-onset pauciarticular juvenile chronic arthritis (EOPA-JCA), as well as in the polyarticular-onset type and in osteoarthritis (OA), hypertrophic

TABLE 4.1 MAJOR DIAGNOSTIC FEATURES OF JOINT DISORDERS	
Mode of onset	Acute
	Insidious
Duration of symptoms	Self-limiting
	Chronic
Number of affected joints	Monoarthritis
	Oligoarthritis (2–4 joints)
	Polyarthritis
Distribution of joint involvement	Symmetric
	Asymmetric
Localization of affected joints	Axial
	Appendicular
	Both
Sequence of involvement	Additive
	Migratory
	Intermittent
Local pattern of involvement (in individual joints)	

osteoarthropathy, mycobacterial and fungal arthritis and most cases of neuropathic arthropathy (Charcot's joints).

Arthritic disorders lasting less than 4–6 weeks are considered to be self-limiting in practical terms, while those lasting longer are considered to be chronic. In self-limiting arthritic disorders the duration of symptoms and signs may be a valuable discriminating feature. Early episodes of monoarticular gout tend to subside spontaneously after 3–10 days and resolution is complete; acute or subacute pseudogout attacks of calcium pyrophosphate dihydrate crystal deposition disease (CPPD) may last from 2–3 days to 3–4 weeks; most articular or periarticular episodes of palindromic rheumatism disappear within hours to several days with no articular sequelae. A steady inflammation in an individual joint for more than a few days or a week in children is highly unlikely to be due to rheumatic fever.

THE NUMBER OF AFFECTED JOINTS

The clinical pattern may be monoarticular or polyarticular. Although almost any individual arthropathy may begin as monoarthritis, the initial pattern of some disorders is characteristically monoarticular regardless of the subsequent course. In particular, patients with an acute painful synovitis of a single joint and varying degrees of overlying redness represent a challenging subset in clinical rheumatology[3,4].

Although redness may occur in any acute arthritis regardless of the etiology, its presence usually evokes a restricted list of possible diagnoses (Table 4.2). The most common diagnoses are crystal-induced synovitis (including acute calcific periarthritis[5]), bacterial infectious arthritis (Fig. 4.1), traumatic conditions, psoriatic arthritis and palindromic rheumatism (in which the joint may reach a dark, bluish redness). Very occasionally, rheumatologists are confronted with rare causes of acute monoarthritis such as synovitis associated with pancreatic disease or with unusual findings in the synovial fluid examination (e.g. lipid microspherulites).

Owing to the frequency of the underlying disease, it should be remembered that the uncommon occurrence of a red-hot joint in the context of RA may be due to superimposed infectious synovitis and not to the disease process itself[6]. None the less, a syndrome of acute sterile arthritis mimicking articular infection may occur in RA patients and respond to anti-inflammatory therapy[7]. Although systemic lupus erythematosus (SLE) causes a number of articular problems, the occurrence of monoarthritis suggests infection or osteonecrosis.

Chronic monoarthritis is often the presenting manifestation of a variety of joint disorders (Table 4.3); histologic elucidation may be necessary to make the correct diagnosis[8]. In a substantial number of patients the cause remains undetermined[9].

Involvement of two to four separate joints is referred to as oligoarthritis. In general, rheumatic disorders manifesting as monoarthritis may also be oligoarticular. Despite this overlap, there are examples in which involvement of two or three joints (rather than one) may significantly narrow the diagnostic spectrum. As an example, lower limb oligoarthritis (especially of the knees and ankles) in an asymmetric fashion is reminiscent of the HLA-B27-associated seronegative spondylarthopathies[10]. An asymmetric oligoarthritis affecting scattered distal interphalangeal (DIP) and proximal interphalangeal (PIP) finger joints and metacarpophalangeal (MCP) joints characterizes a common subgroup of patients with psoriatic arthropathy.

TABLE 4.2 THE RED-HOT JOINT	
Infectious	Bacterial
	Neisserial (may be preceded by transient polyarticular disease)
	Mycobacterial
	Virus
	Lyme disease
Crystal-induced	Gout
	CPPD (pseudogout type)
	Hydroxyapatite (acute calcific periarthritis)
Traumatic	
Palindromic rheumatism	
Psoriatic arthropathy	
Reactive arthritis	
Bacterial endocarditis	

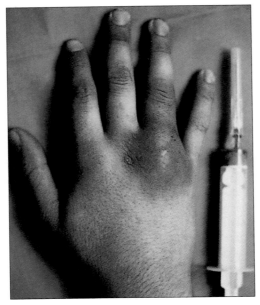

Fig. 4.1 The red hot joint. Septic arthritis of the ring finger metacarpophalangeal joint showing swelling and intense redness of the skin.

TABLE 4.3 SELECTED CAUSES OF CHRONIC MONOARTHRITIS	
Infectious arthritis	Mycobacterial, fungal, bacterial, viral, Lyme disease
Inflammatory arthritis	Crystal-induced
	Monoarticular RA
	EOPA-JCA
	Seronegative spondyloarthopathies (ankylosing spondylitis, reactive arthritis, inflammatory bowel disease arthritis, undifferentiated)
	Psoriatic arthropathy
	Foreign body synovitis (e.g. plant thorn synovitis)
	Sarcoidosis
Non-inflammatory arthritis	Osteoarthritis
	Internal derangement
	Osteonecrosis
	Synovial osteochondromatosis
	Reflex sympathetic dystrophy
	Hemarthrosis (e.g. coagulopathy, anticoagulants)
	Neuropathic (Charcot joint)
	Stress fracture
	Transient regional osteoporosis
	Juvenile osteochondroses
Tumors	Pigmented villonodular synovitis
	Lipoma arborescens
	Synovial metastasis from solid tumors
	Synovial sarcoma
Undiagnosed	

TABLE 4.4 DISTRIBUTION OF SELECTED OLIGO- AND POLYARTHRITIS	
Symmetric	**Asymmetric**
Inflammatory	
RA; JCA (systemic and polyarticular types)	Ankylosing spondylitis
Adult-onset Still's disease	Reactive arthritis
Systemic lupus erythematosus	Psoriatic arthropathy
Mixed connective tissue disease	(oligoarticular type)
Polymyalgia rheumatica	Enteropathic arthritis
Rheumatic fever (adult onset)	Undifferentiated
Jaccoud's arthritis	spondyloarthropathy
	JCA (pauciarticular types)
	Palindromic rheumatism
Degenerative/crystal-induced	
Osteoarthritis (primary generalized,	Gout (especially oligoarthritis)
erosive and nodal types)	CPPD (pseudogout-type)
CPPD (pseudo-RA type)	
'Milwaukee shoulder'	
Hemochromatosis arthropathy	
Infectious	
Viral arthritis	Bacterial arthritis
	Bacterial endocarditis
	Lyme disease (late phase)
Miscellaneous	
Hypertrophic osteoarthropathy	'Cancer polyarthritis'
Amyloid arthropathy	Pancreatic disease-associated
Myxedematous arthropathy	arthritis
Sarcoid arthritis (acute type)	
Most asymmetric arthritides may be, or are characteristically, initially monoarticular	

TABLE 4.5 CHRONIC ARTHROPATHIES WITH PERIPHERAL AND AXIAL INVOLVEMENT	
Inflammatory	
Spondyloarthropathies	Ankylosing spondylitis
	Reactive arthritis
	Psoriatic arthropathy (a subset of
	patients)
	Enteropathic arthritis
	Undifferentiated
Juvenile chronic arthritis	
Adult-onset Still's disease	Systemic and polyarticular onset
Syndrome of SAPHO (synovitis, acne, pustulosis, hyperostosis and osteitis)	
Non-inflammatory	
Osteoarthritis	
Diffuse idiopathic skeletal hyperostosis	
Acromegaly	
Ochronosis	
Spondyloepiphyseal dysplasia	

The third articular pattern is the one in which polyarticular involvement dominates the clinical picture. A wide variety of inflammatory and non-inflammatory disorders, both common and uncommon, may present as polyarthritis[11] (Table 4.4).

IS IT A SYMMETRIC OR AN ASYMMETRIC DISORDER?

This distinction is very helpful in the differential diagnosis of oligo- and polyarticular conditions, with RA being the classic example of symmetric arthritis. Symmetry is not necessarily strict in the hands; the same MCP or PIP joint may not be equally affected in both extremities of RA patients. Erosive inflammatory OA, parvovirus arthritis and many cases of SLE may resemble RA, whereas reactive arthritis, psoriatic arthropathy and polyarticular gout usually present with asymmetric involvement of appendicular joints. An acute asymmetric seronegative polyarthritis with predilection for lower limbs has been rarely described in association with neoplasias[12].

This feature of the articular pattern has obvious limitations; every patient with a symmetric disorder may have an initial asymmetric phase. Table 4.4 lists a number of conditions classified according to the most characteristic pattern.

LOCALIZATION OF AFFECTED JOINTS

Axial involvement

Axial structures include, apart from the spine, centrally located joints such as the sacroiliac, sternoclavicular and manubriosternal joints and the rest of the chest wall and sometimes shoulders and hips.

In the presence of peripheral arthritis one of the most helpful clues in the differential diagnosis is to determine the presence of concomitant axial involvement. While some rheumatic conditions rarely affect the axial segments (e.g. gout, SLE, systemic vasculitis), a combined pattern is often seen in others (Table 4.5). Osteoarthritis of the spine often coexists with appendicular involvement. Patients with ankylosing spondylitis, psoriatic arthropathy, reactive arthritis (following both enteric and sexually transmitted infection) and arthritis accompanying inflammatory bowel disease may also exhibit varying degrees of combined axial and peripheral involvement. Polyarticular and systemic-onset juvenile chronic arthritis (JCA), as well as adult-onset Still's disease, commonly affect the apophyseal joints of the cervical spine in addition to peripheral joints. The SAPHO syndrome (synovitis, acne, pustulosis, hyperostosis and osteitis) is a further example among the much less frequent arthritides[13].

Involvement of the cervical spine structures is frequent in RA patients whereas the dorsal and lumbar segments are spared. Persistent pain in these areas should lead to other diagnoses (e.g. insufficiency fractures of the spine, sacrum or iliac bones)[14].

Peripheral involvement

Although a large number of related and unrelated rheumatic diseases may eventually affect any individual joint, tendon sheath or bursae, the general pattern of joint involvement may be of predominance in the lower or upper limbs. Moreover, some specific joints are closely associated with an individual disease or group of diseases. Understandably, these topographic characteristics refer to the early phases when diagnostic clues are much needed. Most arthritides may later expand to other articular segments, rendering the clinical scenario less clear.

Common examples in clinical rheumatology include the following.

Upper limbs
- Bilateral and symmetric involvement of small and large joints is typical of RA. The MCP and PIP joints of the fingers and wrists are commonly affected with a striking absence of DIP joint disease. Patients with SLE or other systemic rheumatic diseases may occasionally present with a 'rheumatoid' pattern of disease. The small joints of the upper extremities are by far the most commonly affected in parvovirus-associated arthritis.
- Exclusive inflammatory DIP joint involvement of the fingers is a relatively infrequent, although important, clue to the diagnosis of a subset

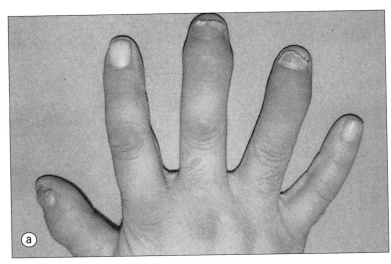 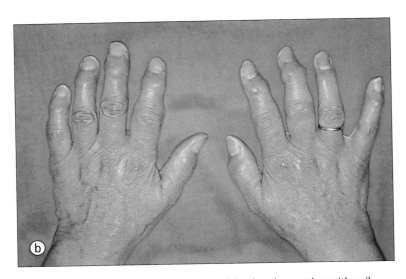

Fig. 4.2 Rheumatic disorders affecting the DIP joints. (a) Psoriatic arthropathy of two DIP joints and the interphalangeal joint of the thumb, together with nail dystrophy. (b) Osteoarthritis is the commonest disorder affecting this segment (Heberden's nodes).

of patients with psoriatic arthropathy (Fig. 4.2). Nodal OA (Heberden's nodes) is the most frequently encountered disorder affecting this segment.

- Bilateral bony enlargement of the second and third MCP joints with restricted motion is characteristic of hemochromatosis arthropathy[15].
- Severe proximal pain (neck and shoulders) with minimal objective findings in an appropriate setting is highly indicative of polymyalgia rheumatica, although the onset of RA in the elderly may be difficult to differentiate from this entity[16].
- Acute involvement of a sternoclavicular joint (one of the less frequently involved joints) suggests septic arthritis in intravenous drug abusers[17].
- Bilateral shoulder disease with striking joint enlargement (shoulder pad sign) is very typical of amyloid arthropathy.

Lower limbs

- Podagra and pseudopodagra: the MTP joint of the big toe is typically affected in acute gouty attacks (Fig. 4.3). Less frequently, CPPD and other crystalline disorders[18], as well as OA, psoriatic arthropathy and a wide variety of conditions, may mimic the podagra of gout[19]. The

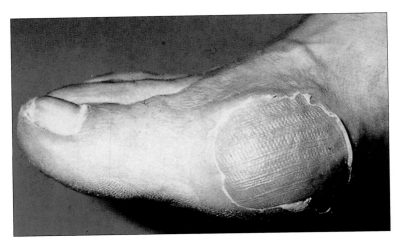

Fig. 4.3 Acute gout. The first MTP joint is involved at some time in approximately 75% of patients. Desquamation of the skin often occurs.

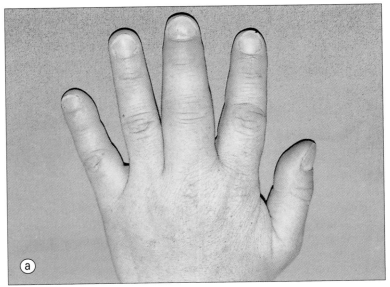 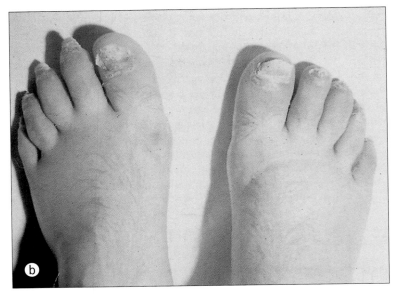

Fig. 4.4 Sausage fingers and toes. (a) Psoriatic arthropathy – dactylitis at the third finger. (b) Reactive arthritis – dactylitis more evident at the second and third left toes and nail dystrophy.

occurrence of 'pseudopodagra' is one of the best examples of how the specific site of the index joint, although helpful, can only suggest the diagnosis.

- Pain and swelling of knees and ankles (often asymmetric) may be seen in the seronegative spondyloarthropathies, including *Chlamydia*-associated arthritis and postenteric arthritis[10,20]. In both of the latter conditions, reactive arthritis involvement of the toes is also frequent and the clinical appearance of dactylitis (sausage toe) is most typical.
- Juxta-articular pain and tenderness (symptoms of inflammatory enthesopathies) may dominate the clinical picture in some patients with seronegative spondyloarthropathies. An enthesopathy is a pathologic process at the sites of tendinous, ligamentous or articular capsule attachment to bone and can be inflammatory, degenerative, crystalline or metabolic[21]. Achilles tendon and plantar fascia insertions into the calcaneum (heel pain) are principally involved. The costosternal areas, iliac crests, ischial tuberosities, greater trochanters and manubriosternal joint may be also affected. The finding of an enthesopathic digit or dactylitis strongly suggests psoriatic arthropathy or reactive arthritis (Fig. 4.4).
- Intermittent synovitis of the knee is a relevant feature of late Lyme disease and seldom becomes chronic. Chronic arthritis of the knee and/or ankle is also the commonest joint involvement in early EOPA-JCA.

SEQUENCE OF JOINT INVOLVEMENT

Clinical involvement of joints may follow three major patterns: additive, migratory and intermittent. An additive pattern refers to the involvement of more joints while the previous joints remain symptomatic. Polyarticular OA, reactive arthritis and RA are typical examples of this progressive sequence.

A migratory pattern means that the process ceases or abates in one joint while simultaneously or immediately after starting in a previously normal joint. Neisserial arthritis may present as a migratory arthritis and tenosynovitis, while the fleeting arthritis of rheumatic fever in children is a classic example.

In the intermittent rheumatic disorders there is complete remission of symptoms and signs until the next recurrence in the same or other joints. No evidence of active disease or residual signs can be detected during intervals. Crystal-induced arthritis, familial Mediterranean fever, the arthritis seen in Whipple's disease and palindromic rheumatism usually follow this pattern for years with asymptomatic periods that vary in length. Patients with SLE often show complete resolution of synovitis (commonly polyarthritis) and follow a discontinuous pattern of arthropathy. Adult-onset Still's disease may also run a polycyclic clinical course[22].

LOCAL PATTERN OF JOINT DISEASE

Some local signs may be of great diagnostic help. In the same manner as the presence of redness often suggests a particular group of diagnoses (see above), the occurrence of skin desquamation when inflammation declines is suggestive of acute gouty monoarthritis. Additional findings which may be of diagnostic value include the following.

- Enlargement of a given individual joint may be symmetric or asymmetric. This physical sign is more obvious in the finger joints. Fusiform swelling of PIP joints in RA is the best example of symmetric involvement, as opposed to Heberden's nodes, erosive OA, chronic sarcoidosis and tophaceous gout, which often produce asymmetric enlargement of the affected joint.
- The local signs of inflammation may extend beyond the anatomic limits of the joint. This feature may be a major diagnostic contribution, as illustrated by the presence of dactylitis, a characteristic sign of

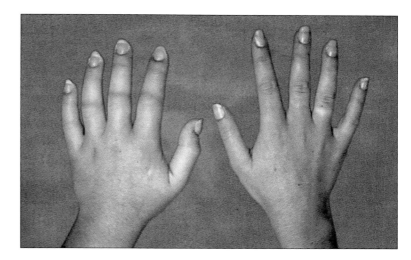

Fig. 4.5 Reflex sympathetic dystrophy syndrome. There is diffuse edematous swelling of the entire left hand.

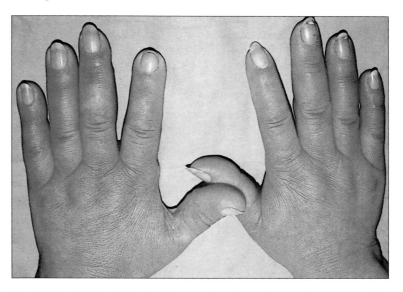

Fig. 4.6 Swollen hands in mixed connective tissue disease. The presence of symmetric puffy hands is a common early finding. Similar changes are often seen in the early stages of scleroderma.

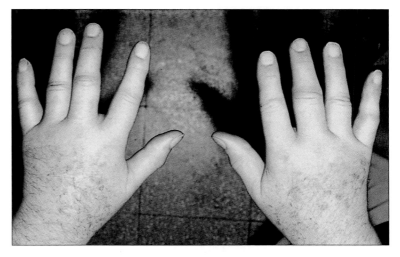

Fig. 4.7 Remitting seronegative symmetric synovitis with pitting edema. Massive acute painful edema of both hands in an 80-year-old man.

an enthesopathic process (see above). A diffusely painful swollen hand or foot may indicate reflex sympathetic dystrophy syndrome in that extremity (Fig. 4.5). Bilateral symmetric puffy swelling of hands and fingers (and sometimes the feet) may be seen in the early phases of systemic sclerosis and mixed connective tissue disease (Fig. 4.6). In a totally different clinical context, diffuse swelling of both hands with pitting is a conspicuous feature of the so called 'syndrome of remitting seronegative symmetric synovitis with pitting edema' (RS3-PE syndrome)[23] (Fig. 4.7). These findings have occasionally been noted in the hands and feet of patients with polymyalgia rheumatica, RA and other arthropathies[23]. Unilateral painless swelling of the dorsum of one hand (extending to a variable degree to the elbow) with pitting edema due to lymphatic obstruction is an infrequent finding in RA patients[24].

- Symmetric enlargement of hands and feet associated with variable degrees of pain is seen from time to time by rheumatologists[25]. Digital clubbing and local signs of inflammation may or may not be prominent. Hypertrophic osteoarthropathy, pachydermoperiostosis, acromegaly and the rare thyroid acropachy should be considered when encountering these cases.

- A striking painful thickening of the palmar area of the hands with flexion contractures of the fingers and marked decreased active and passive mobility (Fig. 4.8) may occasionally be seen. This palmar fasciitis may occur in association with neoplastic conditions (especially ovarian carcinoma)[26]. Diabetic patients may also develop painless contractures of the finger joints[27]. Transient reddening and indurative edema of hands and feet is also a characteristic early feature of Kawasaki disease.

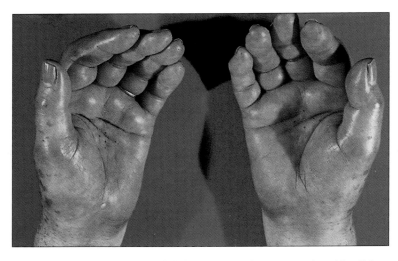

Fig. 4.8 Flexion contractures of all fingers in carcinoma-associated fasciitis. A 50-year-old woman developed painful swelling and contractures of both hands secondary to marked hardening and thickening of the palmar fascia. Palmar erythema is also present. Investigations revealed an ovarian carcinoma, the most commonly associated neoplasm in these patients.

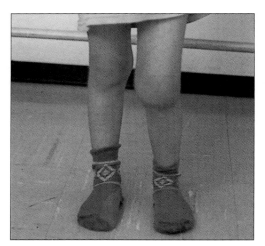

Fig. 4.9 EOPA-JCA in a young girl with monoarthritis. This patient had associated asymptomatic iridocyclitis. In some cases a synovial biopsy is mandatory to exclude other disorders.

THE CLINICAL VALUE OF PATTERNS OF ARTHROPATHY

Evidence of some distinct articular patterns focuses the spectrum of diagnostic options and reduces unnecessary diagnostic testing[28]. These patterns are not diagnostic *per se* and they must always be viewed as a rough guide only for various reasons.

First, unrelated arthropathies may share one or more clinical patterns. As an example, EOPA-JCA, tuberculous arthritis and foreign body arthritis (e.g. plant thorn synovitis)[29] may all present as a gradual-onset chronic monoarthritis of the knee (Fig. 4.9). Both gout and pseudogout can mimic septic arthritis in the setting of febrile acute mono- or polyarthritis[30].

Second, some major arthritides have more than one mode of onset. It should be remembered, for example, that chronic or intermittent mono- and oligoarthritis (with no involvement of the small joints of the hands) may occasionally dominate the early course of RA before a symmetric polyarthritis evolves. The same presentation may also precede the appearance of typical inflammatory low back pain in patients with ankylosing spondylitis. Moreover, CPPD has many clinical patterns, pseudogout and pseudo-osteoarthritis being the most frequent[31]. Among the unusual conditions, arthritis in association with pancreatic disease may have multiple modes of onset and also a variable course[32].

Third, the articular pattern may change with time in the course of a single disorder. In these cases the correct diagnosis is facilitated when the patient is seen during the 'typical' phase of the disease and may be hampered during the 'atypical' phases. Early gout, for instance, is an acute, intermittent, monoarticular arthropathy; as the disease progresses, however, the patient may present with a chronic additive, relatively symmetric, polyarticular disease leading to confusion with RA on physical examination[33]. Finally, a single clinical pattern of joint disease may correspond to more than one diagnosis. Chronic gout superimposed on Heberden's nodes[34] and the coexistence of crystals and infection in cases of subacute monoarthritis[35] are examples of this clinical situation (Fig. 4.10).

The combination of features analyzed above can often contribute to the accurate diagnosis of an arthropathy. A deeper knowledge of each of the individual disorders is necessary to enhance the specificity of the diagnostic process. However, this may require the addition of laboratory studies, joint fluid examination, imaging techniques and other tests to refine the analysis. The more varied the articular patterns possible in a given arthropathy, the more necessary complementary studies become. Systemic vasculitis, SLE, bacterial endocarditis, HIV infection, solid tumors and leukemia, Behçet's syndrome, sickle cell disease and relapsing polychondritis are examples of disorders in which several patterns of arthropathy have been described and which may require a panoply of investigations in addition to the physical findings. However, a careful history and physical examination remains the cornerstone of a diagnostic evaluation for all patients who present with rheumatic complaints.

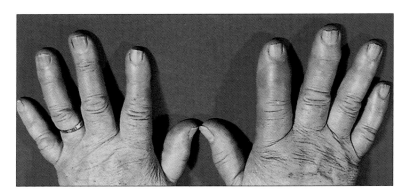

Fig. 4.10 Gouty attack superimposed on a Heberden's node. The clinical combination may be found in elderly patients treated with diuretics as seen in the distal interphalangeal joint of the right index finger in this 78-year-old woman. Note mild desquamation of the overlying skin.

REFERENCES

1. American College of Rheumatology Ad Hoc Committee on Clinical Guidelines. Guidelines for the initial evaluation of the adult patient with acute musculoskeletal symptoms. Arthritis Rheum 1996; 39: 1–8.
2. Carias K, Panush R. Acute arthritis. Bull Rheum Dis 1994; 43: 1–4.
3. Rogachefsky RA, Carneiro R, Altman RD et al. Gout presenting as infectious arthritis. J Bone J Surg 1994; 76A: 269–273.
4. Baker DG, Schumacher HR. Acute monoarthritis. N Engl J Med 1993; 329: 1013–1020.
5. McCarthy GM, Carrera G, Ryan L. Acute calcific periarthritis of the finger joints. A syndrome of women. J Rheumatol 1993; 20: 1077–1080.
6. Goldenberg DL. Infectious arthritis complicating RA and other chronic rheumatic disorders. Arthritis Rheum 1989; 32: 496–502.
7. Singleton JD, West S, Nordstrom D. 'Pseudoseptic' arthritis complicating RA. J Rheumatol 1991; 18: 1319–1322.
8. Fletcher M, Scott JT. Chronic monarticular synovitis. Ann Rheum Dis 1975; 34: 171–176.
9. Blocka K, Sibley JT. Undiagnosed chronic monarthritis. Clinical and evolutionary profile. Arthritis Rheum 1987; 30: 1357–1361.
10. Dougados M, Van Der Linden S, Juhlin R et al. The European Spondyloarthropathy study group preliminary criteria for the classification of spondyloarthropathy. Arthritis Rheum 1991; 34: 1218–1227.
11. Pinals RS. Polyarthritis and fever. N Engl J Med 1994; 330: 769–774.
12. Naschitz J. Rheumatic syndromes: clues to occult neoplasia. Curr Opin Rheumatol 2001; 13: 62–66.
13. Kahn MF. Why the 'SAPHO' syndrome? J Rheumatol 1995; 22: 2017–2019.
14. Speed C. Stress fractures. Clin Rheumatol 1998; 17: 47–51.
15. Von Kempis J. Arthropathy in hereditary hemochromatosis. Curr Opin Rheumatol 2001; 13: 80–83.
16. Bahlas S, Ramus-Remus C, Davis P. Clinical outcome of 149 patients with PMR and GCA. J Rheumatol 1998; 25: 99–104.
17. Rosenthal J, Bole GG, Robinson WD. Acute nongonococcal infectious arthritis. Arthritis Rheum 1980; 23: 889–897.
18. Fam A, Stein J. Hydroxyapatite pseudopodagra in young women. J Rheumatol 1992; 19: 662–664.
19. Bomalaski JS, Schumacher HR. Podagra is more than gout. Bull Rheum Dis 1984; 34: 77–84.
20. Inman R, Whittum-Hudson J, Schumacher HR. Chlamydia and associated arthritis. Curr Opin Rheumatol 2000; 12: 254–262.
21. McGonagle D, Gibbon W, Emery P. Classification of inflammatory arthritis by enthesitis. Lancet 1998; 352: 1137–1140.
22. Cush J, Medsger T, Christy W et al. Adult-onset Still's disease. Arthritis Rheum 1987; 30: 186–194.
23. Dudley J, Gerster D, So A. Polyarthritis and pitting edema. Ann Rheum Dis 1999; 58: 142–147.
24. Sant S, Tormey V, Freyne P et al. Lymphatic obstruction in rheumatoid arthritis. Clin Rheumatol 1995; 14: 445–450.
25. Kirsner R, Goodless D, Kerdel F et al. Enlargement of the hands and feet in a chronic smoker. Arthritis Rheum 1993; 36: 569–571.
26. Elkhoff E, Van der Lubbe P, Breedveld F. Flexion contractures associated with a malignant neoplasm. Clin Rheumatol 1998; 17: 157–159.
27. Kapoor A, Sibbitt WL. Contractures in diabetes mellitus: the syndrome of limited joint mobility. Semin Arthritis Rheum 1989; 18: 168–180.
28. Solomon D, Shmerling R, Schun P et al. A computer based intervention to reduce unnecessary serologic testing. J Rheumatol 1999: 26: 2578–2584.
29. Reginato A, Ferreiro JL, Riester O'Connor C et al. Clinical and pathologic studies of 26 patients with penetrating foreign body injury to the joints, bursae and tendon sheaths. Arthritis Rheum 1990; 33: 1753–1762.
30. Ho G, DeNuccio M. Gout and pseudogout in hospitalized patients. Arch Intern Med 1993; 153: 2787–2790.
31. Chuzhin Y, Panush RS. CPPDDD: what is it and why is it underrecognized? Bull Rheum Dis 1995; 44: 3–5.
32. Shbeeb M, Duffy J, Bjornsson J et al. Subcutaneous fat necrosis and polyarthritis associated with pancreatic disease. Arthritis Rheum 1996; 39: 1922–1925.
33. Talbott J, Altman RD, Yu T. Gout arthritis masquerading as rheumatoid arthritis or vice versa. Semin Arthritis Rheum 1978; 8: 77–114.
34. Lally E, Zimmermann B, Ho G et al. Urate-mediated inflammation in nodal osteoarthritis: clinical and roentgenographic correlations. Arthritis Rheum 1989; 32: 86–90.
35. Zyskowski L, Silverfield J, O'Duffy JD. Pseudogout masking other arthritides. J Rheumatol 1983; 10: 449–453.

5 Laboratory tests in rheumatic disorders

Peter H Schur and Robert H Shmerling

- Acute phase reactants include the erythrocyte sedimentation rate, C-reactive protein, and other proteins that typically reflect inflammation. Monitoring levels may be helpful in some diseases

- Antinuclear antibodies (ANAs) are associated with many connective diseases, especially systemic lupus erythematosus (SLE), scleroderma, mixed connective tissue disease, Sjögren's disease and others – as well as being found in normals. Identifying specific ANAs such as anti-DNA, Sm, RNP, Ro, La, Scl-70 and others can facilitate diagnosis of SLE, Sjögren's, scleroderma and mixed connective tissue disease

- Antineutrophil cytoplasmic antibodies (ANCAs) represent antibodies relatively specific to Wegner's granulomatosis and various forms of vasculitis. Monitoring titers to cANCA may be useful in assessing activity of Wegner's

- Rheumatoid factors are antibodies found in many chronic inflammatory diseases and in elderly people. However, the presence of high titers of rheumatoid factors in a patient with arthritis is suspicious of rheumatoid arthritis

- Antiphospholipid antibodies are antibodies to protein–lipid complexes that predispose individuals to thromboembolic disease, as well as thrombocytopenia and midtrimester miscarriage

- Antistreptolysin-O (ASLO) is an antistreptococcal antibody typically elevated after a streptococcal infection

- Lyme disease can often be recognized by a blood test. It is important, however, to not diagnose Lyme disease after just a screening enzyme-linked immunosorbent assay (ELISA) test, but to perform a confirmatory Western blot test demonstrating the requisite number of Centers for Disease Control (CDC)-defined bands

- Complement levels can be elevated during acute and chronic inflammation. However, levels can be depressed through complement fixation by immune complexes – thus clearance is greater than synthesis

- Human leukocyte antigen (HLA) genetic markers are associated with various rheumatic diseases, e.g. DR4 with rheumatoid arthritis and B-27 with the spondyloarthropathies

- Uric acid levels are often elevated in patients with renal disease and especially with gout. Demonstration of urate crystals in a joint facilitates the diagnosis of gout

- Synovial fluid analysis is useful to discriminate infectious arthritis from inflammatory arthritis from non-inflammatory arthritis

INTRODUCTION

The interpretation of laboratory tests in rheumatic disorders follows the traditional interpretation of any laboratory test. They help in the diagnosis of a particular disease, and are sometimes helpful in monitoring the activity of disease. Critical in the interpretation of any test is determining its sensitivity (e.g. that proportion of patients with the target disorder who have a positive test), specificity (e.g. that proportion of patients who are free of the target disorder and have negative or normal test results) and positive and negative predictive values (which calculate the likelihood that disease is present or absent based on test results using the test's sensitivity, specificity and the probability of disease before the test is performed – pretest probability). Similar information can be derived from a nomogram using pretest probability and likelihood ratios[1,2].

Contingent on making these calculations is data based on the study of an adequate number of patients and controls (with both related and unrelated diseases, as well as normals), using standardized, reproducible tests. Unfortunately, adequate information about many tests is not always available.

This chapter reviews the available information regarding a number of tests that are frequently used in the diagnosis and evaluation of patients with rheumatic disorders.

Use of *p* values

The methods used to assess statistical significance are also critical. Most straightforward population studies of disease association use odds ratio analysis to compare the frequency of a particular variable in the patient population to its frequency in a control population. If the *p* value is less than 0.05, the association is said to be statistically significant; this means that the chance of this association occurring by chance alone is less than 1 in 20.

However, if one is analyzing dozens of different variables for possible association, it becomes likely that one or more variables will result in a spurious association in which *p* is less than 0.05 simply because of the many comparisons being made. As a result, the *p* value must be corrected for the number of tests performed. For instance, if one studies 10 different DR alleles for association with a particular disease, the *p* value for each one must be multiplied by 10. Thus, if the uncorrected *p* value is 0.05, the corrected value (p_c) becomes 0.5, or statistically non-significant. If, on the other hand, the original *p* value is 0.0005, the corrected value of $p_c = 0.005$ is still significant.

ACUTE PHASE PROTEINS

The acute phase response is a major pathophysiologic phenomenon that accompanies inflammation[3]. Despite its name, the acute phase response accompanies both acute and chronic inflammatory states. It can occur in association with a wide variety of disorders, including infection, trauma, infarction, inflammatory arthritides and various neoplasms.

Acute phase proteins are defined as those proteins whose plasma concentrations change by at least 25% during inflammatory states. These changes largely reflect their production by hepatocytes.

Acute phase proteins that increase with inflammation are called positive reactants; they may vary from approximately 50% (e.g. ceruloplasmin and several complement components) to 1000-fold (e.g. C-reactive protein – CRP – and serum amyloid A). Other positive acute phase proteins include fibrinogen, α_1-antitrypsin, haptoglobin and ferritin, while negative reactants (ones that decrease with inflammation) include albumin, transferrin and transthyretin.

Clinical relevance of acute phase reactants

Despite the lack of diagnostic specificity, the measurement of serum levels of acute phase proteins is useful because it may reflect the presence and intensity of an inflammatory process. Currently, the most widely used indicators of the acute phase protein response are the erythrocyte sedimentation rate (ESR) and CRP. The ESR depends largely upon the plasma concentration of fibrinogen.

These tests may be useful both diagnostically, in helping to differentiate inflammatory from non-inflammatory conditions, and prognostically. In addition, they may aid in monitoring activity of disease, since they may reflect the response to therapeutic intervention and a need for closer monitoring. As an example, serial measurements of CRP concentrations may provide prognostic information in rheumatoid arthritis. It is important for physicians to be aware that some laboratories report CRP concentrations as milligrams per liter while others employ milligrams per deciliter.

Comparison of erythrocyte sedimentation rate and C-reactive protein

Compared to measurement of CRP, the ESR has the advantages of familiarity, simplicity and an abundant literature compiled over the last seven decades. However, the ESR has a number of disadvantages compared to the CRP determination:

- The ESR is only an indirect measurement of plasma acute phase protein concentrations; it can be greatly influenced by the size, shape, and number of red cells, as well as by other plasma constituents. Thus, results may be imprecise and sometimes misleading.
- As a patient's condition worsens or improves, the ESR changes relatively slowly; by comparison, the CRP concentrations change rapidly.
- The range of abnormal values for CRP is greater than for the ESR, with accompanying clinical implications: as an example, among patients with CRP concentrations greater than 1omg/dl (100mg/l), 80–85% have bacterial infections.
- ESR values steadily increase with age (to approximately age in years divided by 2)[4] but plasma CRP concentrations do not.
- Normal values for the ESR are slightly higher among women than men.

For most clinical purposes, CRP values less than 0.1 or 0.2mg/dl can be regarded as normal and values over 1.0 as indicating clinically significant inflammation. However, although CRP is a sensitive reflection of inflammation, it is not specific. Values between 0.2 and 1.omg/dl may reflect minor degrees of inflammation but may also reflect obesity, cigarette smoking, diabetes mellitus or other non-inflammatory causes.

Rationale for employing multiple tests

Although elevations in multiple components of the acute phase response commonly occur together, not all happen uniformly in all patients. Discordance between concentrations of different acute phase proteins is common, perhaps because of differences in the production of specific cytokines or their modulators in different diseases.

Discrepancies between ESR and CRP are found with some frequency, the clinical significance of which is unclear. Measurement of any acute phase reactant should take into account how the results will affect management, since history and physical examination are generally more reliable reflections of disease activity. In addition, knowing which acute phase reactant has best correlated with an individual's disease in the past is helpful in choosing the test to follow over time.

Specific applications

The assessment of acute phase reactants may be most helpful in patients with rheumatoid arthritis (RA), polymyalgia rheumatica and giant cell arteritis. Reports also raise the possibility of other applications, such as non-invasive assessment of the prognosis of patients with malignancy, or whether an infectious process (such as abscess, osteomyelitis or endocarditis) has been eradicated.

Rheumatoid arthritis

Although acute phase reactants are usually of little use in distinguishing between early RA, osteoarthritis and systemic lupus erythematosus (SLE), they may be helpful in monitoring disease activity in RA. The ESR is more widely used; however, CRP levels correlate somewhat better with activity than does ESR[5].

While CRP levels average 2–3mg/dl (20–30mg/l) in RA patients with moderate disease activity[6], there is considerable variation: approximately 10% of patients have values in the normal range while a few patients with severe disease activity have very high concentrations.

Measurements of the levels of acute-phase reactants are also of value in assessing the progression and prognosis of patients with RA:

- elevations in both CRP and ESR are associated with radiographic progression at 6 and 12 months after study entry
- time-integrated values of ESR and CRP correlate significantly with disease progression over periods of up to 20 years
- Acute-phase reactant levels are significantly associated with early synovitis and erosions as detected by MRI, with synovial cellular infiltrates, with osteoclastic activation and reduced bone mineral density, and with work disability on long-term follow-up.

These findings have suggested to some clinicians that normalization of acute-phase reactants should be a major goal in the treatment of RA. However, these data can alternatively be interpreted to indicate that patients with worse, more resistant disease have higher, more resistant acute phase reactants. In addition, progressive joint damage can occur despite improvement in acute phase reactants. As a result, it is doubtful that physicians should change therapy, in patients who are otherwise doing well on a given regimen, solely because acute-phase reactants continue to be elevated.

Polymyalgia rheumatica and giant cell arteritis

Although polymyalgia rheumatica and giant cell arteritis are frequently accompanied by markedly elevated levels of the ESR (often higher than 100mm/h), such elevated levels should not be regarded as a *sine qua non* for these disorders. As many as 7–20% of patients with polymyalgia rheumatica have normal ESRs. It has been suggested that patients with polymyalgia rheumatica who have relatively low ESRs at onset require lower doses of steroids, for shorter periods of time, than those with high values.

In patients with these diseases, CRP and ESR have been regarded as having nearly equal value in assessing disease activity. More recently, however, reports suggest that CRP levels may be more sensitive for detection of active disease. In addition, the uncertainty as to what ESR values are 'normal' in the elderly implies that CRP levels may be more valuable in this population.

Systemic lupus erythematosus

Systemic lupus erythematosus represents an exception to the generalization that CRP concentrations correlate with the extent and severity of inflammation in patients with rheumatic disorders. Many patients with active SLE do not have elevated CRP concentrations, although they may have marked increases in concentrations during bacterial infection. This finding can be applied to the differential diagnosis of fever in patients with SLE but one must remember that CRP concentrations may be high in some patients with active lupus serositis or chronic synovitis.

ANTINUCLEAR ANTIBODIES

Antinuclear antibodies[7] (ANAs) were initially discovered in the 1940s using the LE cell test. This test is no longer performed because of lack of sensitivity, specificity and predictive value – as well as difficulty of performance. It has been replaced by immunofluorescent techniques for the detection of ANAs in general and solid-phase immunoassays (e.g. enzyme-linked immunosorbent assay, ELISA) for the detection of specific antinuclear antibodies, although immunodiffusion, immuno-blotting and radio-immunoassays are occasionally performed. There is currently no standardized assay for ANA measurement; therefore, each laboratory must perform careful quality control measures to ensure appropriate cut-off values for considering the ANA to be positive so that false-positive and false-negative test results are minimized.

The immunofluorescent ANA test is especially useful as an initial screen for patients clinically suspected of having SLE, but is also useful for the evaluation of patients with other rheumatic conditions, including Sjögren's syndrome, mixed connective tissue disease, drug-induced lupus erythematosus and scleroderma, juvenile arthritis and auto-immune hepatitis. However, the presence of an ANA does not mandate the presence of illness, since these antibodies may also be found in otherwise normal individuals.

The sensitivity of the ANA for a particular systemic autoimmune disease can widely vary (Table 5.1).

Other well-recognized disorders associated with a positive ANA titer include chronic infectious diseases, such as mononucleosis, subacute bacterial endocarditis, tuberculosis and some lymphoproliferative diseases. ANAs have also been identified in up to 90% of patients taking certain drugs, especially procainamide and hydralazine; however, most of these patients do not develop drug-induced lupus. Likewise, TNF-blocking agents can lead to development of ANAs but the occurrence of drug-induced lupus is rare.

False-positive ANAs (i.e. ANAs in the absence of autoimmune disease) are more commonly found in normal women and in elderly patients (usually in low titer) but may also be detected in persons with infections or other non-rheumatic inflammatory disease.

Most laboratories currently use HEp-2 cells (human epithelial cell tumor line), or murine (rat or mouse) liver or kidney. HEp-2 cells offer a standardized substrate with larger nucleoli. They also provide better sensitivity for antibodies to centromere antigens. In addition, ANA titers are almost always higher when measured on HEp-2 cells. However, the increased sensitivity achieved by using HEp-2 cells is offset by the decreased specificity (and predictive value) for SLE.

Interpretation

An ANA with titer, in combination with a full history and physical examination, can be extremely useful in the diagnosis and exclusion of connective tissue disease.

Usefulness of ANA titer

- The presence of high concentrations of antibody (titer >1:640) should increase the suspicion that an autoimmune disorder is present. However, its presence alone is not diagnostic of disease. If no initial diagnosis can be made, it is our practice to watch the patient carefully over time for the development of an ANA-associated disease.
- The combination of low titers of antibody (<1:80) and no or few signs or symptoms of disease portend a much smaller likelihood of an autoimmune disease. As a result, these patients need to be reevaluated less frequently.

False positives

Positive ANAs are commonly found in the normal population, including first-degree relatives of persons with ANA-associated rheumatic disease. When HEp-2 cells are used as a substrate, one study of 125 normal individuals found an ANA titer above 1:40 in 32%, above 1:80 in 13% and above 1:320 in 3%. No patient had anti-double-stranded DNA antibodies.

False negatives

A patient with a negative ANA and strong clinical evidence of a systemic autoimmune disorder may require specific antibody assays to accurately diagnosis a rheumatic disease.

Types and usefulness of staining pattern

Antinuclear antibodies produce a wide range of different staining patterns. The nuclear staining pattern has been recognized to have a relatively low sensitivity and specificity for different autoimmune disorders. At present, tests that detect the presence of antibodies directed at specific nuclear and cytoplasmic antigens have largely supplanted the use of ANA patterns (Fig. 5.1)

- The homogeneous or diffuse pattern represents antibodies to the DNA–histone complex, also called ribonucleoprotein or nucleosome
- The peripheral or rim pattern is produced by antibodies to DNA
- The speckled pattern is produced by antibodies to Sm, RNP, Ro/SSA, La/SSB, Scl-70, RNA polymerase II and III and other antigens
- The nucleolar pattern is produced by antibodies to nucleolar RNA
- The centromeric pattern is produced by antibodies to centromeres.

Types of antinuclear antibody

The different types of ANA are defined by their target antigen, including single- and double-stranded DNA, individual nuclear histones, non-histone nuclear proteins and RNA–protein complexes.

- Anti-Sm, RNP, Ro (SSA), La (SSB), Scl-70, and Jo-1 antibodies are detected by immunoblotting, ELISA, and occasionally immunodiffusion
- Antibodies to dsDNA may be measured by ELISA, radioimmunoassay or immunofluorescence
- Antibodies to histones are generally detected by ELISA
- Antibodies to centromere are detected directly on Hep-2 cells.

TABLE 5.1 SENSITIVITY OF THE ANA IN AUTOIMMUNE AND NON-RHEUMATIC DISEASE

Disease	Sensitivity (%)
Autoimmune disease	
Systemic lupus erythematosus	95–100
Scleroderma	60–80
Mixed connective tissue disease	100
Polymyositis/dermatomyositis	61
Rheumatoid arthritis	52
Rheumatoid vasculitis	30–50
Sjögren's syndrome	40–70
Drug-induced lupus	100
Discoid lupus	15
Pauciarticular juvenile chronic arthritis	71
Non-rheumatic disease	
Hashimoto's thyroiditis	46
Graves' disease	50
Autoimmune hepatitis	100
Primary autoimmune cholangitis	100
Primary pulmonary hypertension	40

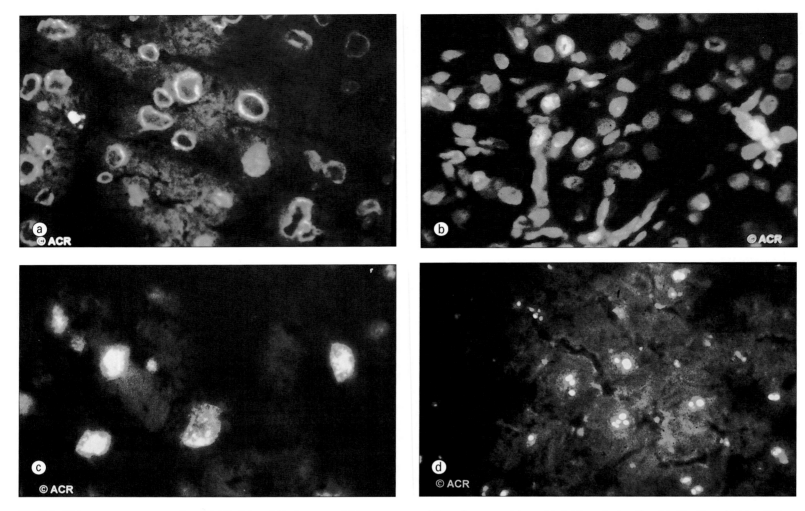

Fig. 5.1 ANA patterns on mouse liver. (a) Peripheral (rim) pattern; (b) homogeneous (diffuse) pattern; (c) speckled; (d) nucleolar. (Provided by Peter H Schur MD for this publication as well as to UpToDate.)

The ANA is reliable and reproducible, if laboratories use commercially available tissue culture cell substrates and participate in proficiency testing.

Antibodies to DNA

Antibodies to DNA[8,9] can be primarily divided into two groups: those reactive with single-stranded DNA (ssDNA); and those recognizing double-stranded DNA (dsDNA).

Anti-single-stranded DNA

Antibodies that identify ssDNA are probably reacting with the purine and pyrimidine bases that are accessible on ssDNA but are buried within the beta helix of dsDNA. Thus, anti- ssDNA antibodies do not cross react with dsDNA. Antibodies to ssDNA have the following general properties.

- They have been eluted from the kidneys of lupus patients with proliferative nephritis and may therefore be of pathogenic significance
- They are much less specific for SLE than antibodies to dsDNA. Anti-ssDNA antibodies have been reported in rheumatoid arthritis, drug-related lupus, healthy relatives of patients with SLE, and, less commonly, in other rheumatic diseases (see Table 5.2); thus, anti-ssDNA has limited usefulness for the diagnosis of SLE or other rheumatic diseases
- They do not correlate well with disease activity and are therefore not useful for disease management.

Anti-double-stranded DNA

- Anti-dsDNA antibodies are specific (95%) though not highly sensitive (30–70%) for SLE, making them very useful for diagnosis when positive[9] (Table 5.1). They are occasionally found in other conditions, including rheumatoid arthritis, juvenile arthritis, drug-induced lupus, autoimmune hepatitis and even normal persons
- Titers of anti-dsDNA antibodies often fluctuate with disease activity and are therefore useful in many patients for following the course of SLE
- There is a well recognized association of high anti-dsDNA titers with active glomerulonephritis; there also appear to be highly enriched amounts of anti-dsDNA antibodies in the glomerular deposits of immune complexes found in patients with lupus nephritis. These observations have led many investigators to believe that anti-dsDNA antibodies are of primary importance in the pathogenesis of lupus nephritis.

Measurement of anti-dsDNA antibodies

These tests measure both high- and low-avidity antibodies:

- the Farr assay (a radioimmunoassay)
- the *Crithidia luciliae* assay (using indirect immunofluorescence)
- the ELISA technique.

Antibody titer and correlation with activity

Titers of anti-dsDNA antibodies are important in the management of some patients with SLE. Titers rise when disease is active, and usually fall (generally into the normal range) when the flare subsides. Early studies reported a tight correlation between high-titer anti-dsDNA antibodies and nephritic activity, particularly in the setting of hypocomplementemia. More recent studies, however, have reported exceptions to this correlation; for example, some patients have elevated titers of anti-dsDNA antibodies in the setting of inactive or minimally active lupus.

The association between anti-DNA antibodies and other disease manifestations of SLE is far less clear. For example, there is no relationship between antibody titer and disease activity in neuropsychiatric SLE.

Distinguishing active lupus manifestations from infectious complications or toxic effects of drugs, and from unrelated disease, is always a challenge. Anti-DNA antibodies may be helpful in some patients in making this distinction.

Anti-Smith and anti-ribonucleoprotein antibodies

The anti-Smith (anti-Sm) and anti-ribonucleoprotein (anti-RNP) systems[8] are considered together since they coexist in many patients with SLE and bind to related but distinct antigens.

The Smith antigen is a nuclear non-histone protein that consists of a series of proteins: B, B′, D, E, F and G, complexed with small nuclear RNAs; U1, U2, U4-6 and U5, which can be characterized by Western and Northern blots. These complexes of nuclear proteins and RNAs are called small nuclear ribonucleoprotein particles (snRNPs); they are important in the splicing of precursor messenger RNA.

Anti-Smith antibodies are found in only 10–40% of patients with SLE but infrequently in patients with other conditions, i.e. they are not sensitive but are highly specific (Table 5.2). Measurement of anti-Sm titers may be useful diagnostically, particularly at a time when anti-DNA antibodies are undetectable. Given their relatively low sensitivity, however, a negative value in no way excludes the diagnosis.

Anti-ribonucleoprotein antibodies bind to antigens that are different from but related to Sm antigens. These antibodies bind to proteins containing only U1-RNA. The U1-RNP particle is involved in splicing heterogeneous nuclear RNA into messenger RNA.

Methods of measurement

While anti-Sm antibodies and anti-RNP antibodies can be detected by immunodiffusion or counterimmunoelectrophoresis in agarose gels, these methods are relatively insensitive and difficult to quantitate. Most clinical laboratories now employ ELISA to detect these antibodies.

Usefulness

The prevalence of anti-Sm antibodies in SLE using the ELISA assay varies depending upon whether Sm is measured alone or in combination with RNP. Generally accepted rates of anti-Sm antibody positivity in SLE are in the range of 10–30% in Caucasians and 30–40% in Asians and Afro-Americans. Anti-Sm antibodies correlate with disease activity and specific disease manifestations in some but not all studies, perhaps because of the use of different immunoassays.

Anti-ribonucleoprotein antibodies are found in about 40–60% of patients with SLE but are not specific for SLE, being a defining feature of mixed connective tissue disease and occurring in low titers and low frequencies in other rheumatic diseases, including RA and scleroderma (Table 5.2).

Anti-Ro/SSA and anti-La/SSB antibodies

Anti-Ro/SSA and anti-La/SSB[10] have been detected in high frequency in patients with Sjögren's syndrome and in SLE.

Antibodies to Ro are detected clinically by immunodiffusion, ELISA or Western blot. ELISA and Western blots are the most sensitive assays for detecting these antibodies. There are also non-blotting anti-Ros. Some experts believe that the best methods to characterize anti-Ro/La are the immunoprecipitation methods, such as Ouchterlony and CIE.

Anti-Ro/anti-SSA antibodies

These antinuclear antibodies recognize cellular proteins with molecular weights of approximately 52kDa and 60kDa.

Anti-Ro/SSA antibodies are primarily found in patients with SLE and Sjögren's syndrome but also in patients with photosensitive dermatitis. They are rarely found in other connective tissue diseases such as scleroderma, polymyositis, mixed connective tissue disease, juvenile rheumatoid arthritis, chronic active hepatitis and rheumatoid arthritis. There is a strong link between anti-Ro antibodies, a genetic deficiency of the C2 or C4 complement component and the HLA-DR3 genotype. Anti-Ro antibodies may be detectable in 0.1–0.5% of healthy adults, some of whom may demonstrate enhanced sensitivity to ultraviolet light.

Clinical significance in systemic lupus erythematosus

Anti-Ro/SSA antibodies are found in approximately 50% of patients with SLE (Table 5.2). They have been associated with photosensitivity, subacute cutaneous lupus, cutaneous vasculitis (palpable purpura), interstitial lung disease, neonatal lupus and congenital heart block.

Clinical significance in Sjögren's syndrome

Anti-Ro/SSA antibodies are found in approximately 75% of patients with primary Sjögren's syndrome (Table 5.2), and high titers of these antibodies are associated with a greater incidence of extraglandular features, especially purpura and vasculitis. By contrast, Ro/SSA antibodies are present in only 10–15% of patients with secondary Sjögren's syndrome associated with rheumatoid arthritis. Therefore, the presence of Ro/SSA or anti-La/SSB antibodies in patients with suspected primary Sjögren's syndrome strongly supports the diagnosis.

TABLE 5.2 ANA DISEASE ASSOCIATIONS

	SLE		Drug-induced lupus		RA		Scleroderma		PM/DM		Sjögren's syndrome	
	Sen (%)	Spec (%)	Sen (%)	Spec (%)	Sen (%)	Spec (%)	Sen (%)	Spec (%)	Sen (%)	Spec (%)	Sen (%)	Spec (%)
dsDNA	70	95		1–5		1		<1		<1		1–5
ssDNA	80		80	50	Mod	Mod		Low		Low	Mod	Mod
Histone	30–80	50	95	High	Low			<1		<1	Low	Low
Nucleoprotein	58	Mod	50	Mod	25	Low	<1		<1		Mod	Mod
Sm	25–30	Mod	1		1		<1		<1		1–5	
RNP	45	99			47		20				5–60	
Ro	40	87–94	Low		Low				Low		8–70	87
La	15		Low		Low						14–60	94

PM/DM, polymyositis/dermatomyositis; Sen, sensitivity; Spec, specificity.
Other associations – RNP: mixed connective tissue disease; Ro: subacute cutaneous lupus erythematosus, biliary cirrhosis, vasculitis, coronary heart block.
Sensitivity and specificity of different antinuclear antibodies. (Adapted from Barland and Wachs[7].)

Relationship to 'ANA-negative systemic lupus erythematosus'

In the 1970s there were several reports of patients who met the American College of Rheumatology (ACR) criteria for SLE but were persistently negative for ANA, using rodent cells, and had anti-Ro antibodies. However, the substitution of HEp-2 cells (a human cell line) resulted in only a small number of patients with SLE who consistently had a negative ANA. The explanation for this difference is that rodent tissue is poor in Ro and HEp-2 cells are rich in Ro. Detection of anti-Ro in the absence of a positive ANA may make one suspect the presence of a connective tissue disease.

Anti-La/SSB antibodies

Approximately 50% of patients with SLE who have anti-Ro antibody also have anti-La antibody, a closely related RNA-protein antigen. Similarly, most patients with Sjögren's syndrome also have anti-La (SSB) antibodies. It is exceedingly rare to find patients with anti-La antibodies without anti-Ro antibodies.

Clinical associations of anti-La

Anti-La/SSB antibodies are found in the following circumstances:

- isolated anti-La/SSB antibody activity has been seen in some patients with primary biliary cirrhosis and autoimmune hepatitis
- antibodies to the La/SSB antigen are present in 40–50% of patients with primary Sjögren's syndrome, and in 15% of patients with SLE, but are rarely seen in other connective tissue diseases.

In our opinion, the indications for ordering an anti-Ro/SSA and anti-La/SSB antibody tests are:

- women with SLE who are pregnant or may become pregnant in the future
- women who have a history of giving birth to a child with heart block or myocarditis
- patients with a history of unexplained photosensitive skin eruptions
- patients strongly suspected of having SLE but who have a negative ANA test
- patients with symptoms of xerostomia, keratoconjunctivitis sicca and/or salivary and lacrimal gland enlargement

Anti-centromere antibodies

Anti-centromere antibodies[11] (ACA) are found almost exclusively in patients with limited cutaneous systemic sclerosis, especially in those with the CREST syndrome (calcinosis, Raynaud's, esophageal dysmotility, sclerodactyly and telangiectasias). ACA has been observed in 57% of patients with CREST but has also been seen in patients with other conditions, including in some patients with Raynaud's phenomenon alone. ACA are typically detected by the characteristic immunofluorescent pattern on HEp-2 cells.

Anti-Scl-70 (topoisomerase-1) antibodies[12]

Approximately 15–20% of patients with scleroderma have antibodies to a 70kDa protein (topoisomerase-1), subsequently named Scl-70. The usual method for detection was immunodiffusion but most laboratories now detect it by ELISA. The presence of these antibodies appears to increase the risk for pulmonary fibrosis among patients with scleroderma and is quite specific for the disease.

Antiribosomal P protein antibodies[13]

Serum from patients with SLE may have antibodies to ribosomes. These antibodies react with three phosphoproteins (P proteins) located on the 60S subunit of ribosomes.

Clinical associations

All published studies agree on the specificity of antiribosomal P protein antibodies for SLE, which is not found using conventional assays in normal controls or in patients with other rheumatic diseases (e.g. rheumatoid arthritis, scleroderma and myositis).

Antiribosomal P protein antibodies have been detected in 10–20% of patients with SLE; however, they have been reported in 40–50% of Asian patients.

Antiribosomal P protein antibodies may be highly specific for lupus-associated psychosis, although not all studies have confirmed this. Depression, renal and liver involvement in lupus patients have also been associated with antiribosomal P protein antibodies in some small studies.

Antihistone antibodies[14]

Antihistone antibodies are present in more than 95% of cases of drug-induced lupus (Table 5.3), particularly those taking procainamide,

TABLE 5.3 CLINICAL ASSOCIATIONS OF AUTOANTIBODIES IN SLE		
Antigen specificity	**Clinical associations**	**Sensitivity (%)**
dsDNA	Marker for active disease, titers fluctuates with disease activity, correlates best with renal disease	40–70
ssDNA	Non-specific, no clinical utility	80
Ro/SSA	Subacute cutaneous lupus (75%), photosensitivity, neonatal lupus, complement deficiencies	40
La/SSB	With Ro; low prevalence of renal disease; neonatal lupus (75%)	15
RNP (U1-RNP)	SLE generally in conjunction with Sm; in mixed connective tissue disease, required for diagnosis	45
Sm	Highly specific; not generally useful in management; may be associated with central nervous system disease	25–30
Phospholipids	Hypercoagulable state in some patients, no clinical significance in others. Thrombocytopenia, late trimester abortions	30
Histones	>95% in drug-related lupus. Also present in RA, SLE, reported in systemic sclerosis with pulmonary fibrosis	30–80
Ribosomal P	Initially associated with psychosis in SLE, more recently with depression	10–40
KU	SLE, mixed connective tissue disease (European, American population); scleroderma/myositis overlap (Japanese population)	≤19, ≤39
PCNA		3

(With permission from Reichlin M. Measurement and clinical significance of antinuclear antibodies. In: Rose B, Schur PH, eds. UpToDate. Wellesley, MA: UpToDate; 2003. Copyright © 2003 UpToDate, Inc. For more information, visit www.uptodate.com.)

hydralazine, chlorpromazine and quinidine; other autoantibodies are uncommon in this disorder. Antihistone antibodies are also seen in up to 80% of patients with idiopathic lupus; however, patients with SLE also form a variety of other autoantibodies, including those directed against DNA and small ribonucleoproteins.

The autoantibodies in drug-induced lupus are primarily formed against a complex of the histone dimer H2A–H2B and DNA[15] and, with hydralazine, to the H1 and H3–H4 complex. DNA is required either to stabilize the complex or perhaps to contribute part of the antigenic epitope[15]. Although the drugs that can cause drug-induced lupus are markedly heterogeneous, there may be a common pathway for disease induction since the autoantibodies produced are in most, but not all, cases nearly identical[15]. In contrast, the antihistone antibodies in idiopathic lupus are primarily directed against the H1 and H2B histone subunits.

The development of IgG antibodies to the complex of H2A–H2B and DNA soon after starting procainamide is associated with a high risk of developing drug-induced lupus; by comparison, autoantibodies to single-stranded DNA or histones alone do not distinguish between symptomatic or asymptomatic individuals. It is not known if these observations apply to other causes of drug-induced lupus.

It is important to note that while up to 80% of patients taking procainamide for 1–2 years will develop a positive ANA, most do not develop drug-induced lupus. Thus, screening for these antibodies in the absence of symptoms and stopping the drug if antibodies develop are not recommended.

Miscellaneous antinuclear antibodies[12]

Other autoantibodies reactive with nuclear and perinuclear antigens have been described in association with connective tissue diseases:

- anti-RNA polymerase I, II, and III: scleroderma
- anti-fibrillarin (U3 nucleolar RNP): scleroderma
- anti-nucleolus organizer region (NOR 90): not scleroderma
- antinucleolar RNA helicase (Gu): scleroderma, SLE, watermelon stomach
- anti-DNA-associated acidic protein (Ku): scleroderma–polymyositis overlap
- anti-signal recognition protein: dermatomyositis
- anti-Mi-2: dermatomyositis
- anti-Jo-1 (an antisynthetase antibody): dermatomyositis
- antinucleosomal high mobility group proteins (HMG): juvenile RA
- anti-major nucleolar phosphoprotein (B23):antiphospholipid antibody syndrome
- anti-annexin XI (56K): 4–10% of connective tissue diseases

anti-heterogeneous nuclear ribonucleoprotein antibodies (hnRNP): RA, SLE, scleroderma.

These antibodies are not routinely assayed in clinical laboratories and may have more limited specificity or sensitivity than other antinuclear antibodies.

ANTINEUTROPHIL CYTOPLASMIC ANTIBODIES (ANCA)

Two different immunofluorescence patterns can be seen when the patient's serum is incubated with ethanol-fixed, normal human neutrophils.

- Cytoplasmic ANCAs (cANCAs) stain the cytoplasm diffusely; these antibodies are almost always directed against a serine protease called proteinase (PR)3. cANCA with anti-PR3 specificity is found primarily in patients with Wegener's granulomatosis and microscopic polyarteritis, and occasionally in other diseases (Table 5.4; Fig. 5.2)[16,17].

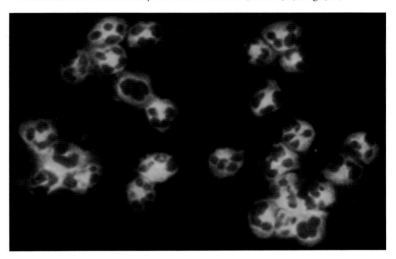

Fig. 5.2 cANCA pattern. Demonstration of cytoplasmic antineutrophil cytoplasmic antibodies (cANCAs) by indirect immunofluorescence with normal neutrophils. There is heavy staining in the cytoplasm while the multilobular nuclei (clear zones) are non-reactive. These antibodies are usually directed against proteinase 3 and most patients have Wegener's granulomatosis. (Courtesy of Dr Helmut Rennke.)

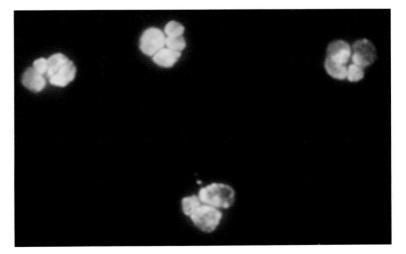

Fig. 5.3 pANCA pattern. Demonstration of perinuclear antineutrophil cytoplasmic antibodies (pANCAs) by indirect immunofluorescence with normal neutrophils. Staining is limited to the perinuclear region and the cytoplasm is non-reactive. Among patients with vasculitis, the antibodies are usually directed against myeloperoxidase. However, a pANCA pattern can also be seen with autoantibodies against a number of other antigens, including lactoferrin and elastase. Non-MPO pANCA can be seen in a variety of non-vasculitic disorders. (Courtesy of Dr Helmut Rennke.)

TABLE 5.4 SIGNIFICANCE OF cANCA DIRECTED AGAINST PROTEINASE 3

Disease	Frequency (%)
Wegener's granulomatosis	90
Microscopic polyarteritis	50
Polyarteritis nodosa	5–10
Churg–Strauss angiitis	10
Hypersensitivity vasculitis	Rare
Henoch–Schönlein purpura	Rare
Immunoglobulin A nephropathy	Rare
Postinfectious glomerulonephritis	Rare
Systemic lupus erythematosus	Rare
Kawasaki disease	+
Controls	±

+, reported to be present; ±, occasionally present.

- Perinuclear ANCAs (pANCAs) are usually directed against myelo-peroxidase (MPO). The pANCA fluorescence pattern represents an artifact of ethanol fixation; with ethanol, positively charged granule constituents rearrange around and upon the negatively charged nuclear membrane. Antigens other than MPO can induce pANCA production (see below; Fig. 5.3).

Perinuclear ANCAs identified by indirect immunofluorescence techniques using ethanol-fixed neutrophils must be distinguished from ANAs. Serum containing pANCAs in ethanol-fixed neutrophils produce diffuse granular cytoplasmic staining with formalin-fixed polymorphonuclear cells, thus allowing distinction from ANAs. In addition, the concurrent use of formalin- and ethanol-fixed polymorphonuclear cells permits pANCA and ANA to be distinguished from each other in serum containing both antibodies.

Immunoblotting techniques or ELISA are more accurate than immunofluorescence studies and enable the identification of the target antigens associated with these autoantibodies. The identification of anti-MPO antibodies is particularly important, since pANCAs directed against non-MPO molecules such as elastase, cathepsin G, lactoferrin, lysozyme and azurocidin have lower clinical specificity as they may occur in a variety of non-vasculitic disorders (see below).

Perinuclear ANCAs directed primarily against MPO have been described in patients with a variety of rheumatic autoimmune diseases (Table 5.5), while non-MPO pANCAs have been associated with several rheumatic and non-rheumatic diseases (Table 5.6)[16]. In addition, ANCA testing that includes ELISA testing for anti-PR3 and anti-MPO has a reported specificity for vasculitis of 99.5% among patients with connective tissue disease[16]. Although patients with rheumatic diseases have an increased frequency of vasculitis, data suggesting that ANCA positivity enhances the risk of vasculitis are contradictory. Non-vasculitic aspects of rheumatic disease activity, severity and chronicity also fail to consistently correlate with ANCA status. As a result, there is little clinical utility for ANCA testing in patients in whom the presence of an ANCA-associated systemic vasculitis is not suspected on clinical grounds.

How accurate is the ANCA for diagnosis?

In Wegener's granulomatosis, the reported sensitivity of cANCA, pANCA, anti-PR3 and anti-MPO in one large trial[18] was 64%, 21%, 66% and 24% respectively. In microscopic polyarteritis, the sensitivities were 23%, 58%, 26% and 58% respectively. These results confirm a relative association of anti-PR3 with Wegener's granulomatosis and anti-MPO with microscopic polyarteritis. In idiopathic rapidly progressive

TABLE 5.6 SIGNIFICANCE OF pANCA DIRECTED AGAINST LACTOFERRIN, CATHEPSIN G, ELASTASE, AND LYSOZYME

Disease	Frequency (%)
Giant cell arteritis	+
Rheumatoid arthritis	+
Systemic lupus erythematosus	25
Sjögren's	+
Inflammatory bowel disease	+
Ulcerative colitis	+
Crohn's disease	10–27
Primary sclerosing cholangitis	+
Unaffected relatives of patients with ulcerative colitis or primary sclerosing cholangitis	25–30
Chronic active hepatitis	+
Primary biliary cirrhosis	+

+, reported to be present.

glomerulonephritis, the sensitivities were 36%, 45%, 50% and 64% respectively.

The combination of indirect immunofluorescence and ELISA testing resulted in increased sensitivity and specificity. The sensitivity of either cANCA plus anti-PR3 or pANCA plus anti-MPO was 73%, 67% and 82% for Wegener's granulomatosis, microscopic polyangiitis and rapidly progressive glomerulonephritis respectively. Specificity was 99% for both combinations[18].

Combination testing consisting of cANCA immunofluorescence plus anti-PR3 ELISA and pANCA immunofluorescence plus anti-MPO ELISA was therefore much more accurate than immunofluorescence or ELISA alone.

As with any test, the predictive value of ANCA testing depends upon the clinical presentation of the patient in whom the test is performed. As an example, the finding of an elevated ANCA titer in a patient presenting with acute or rapidly progressive glomerulonephritis predicts the presence of Wegener's granulomatosis, microscopic polyarteritis or idiopathic necrotizing glomerulonephritis with an accuracy that can reach 98%[19,20]. However, the accuracy of ANCA, even cANCA, is substantially less in patients referred for evaluation for the possible diagnosis of vasculitis and in those presenting with sinusitis alone[19]. cANCA is much more specific than pANCA, probably because cANCA is almost always due to anti-PR3 while pANCA may be related to less specific antigens. It is therefore recommended that a positive pANCA always be followed by an antigen-specific assay to document the presence of anti-MPO antibodies. Whether a positive cANCA should routinely be checked for anti-PR3 is less clear.

Although controversial, some investigators feel that, in the appropriate clinical setting, treatment may be instituted among patients with a presumptive diagnosis of systemic vasculitis and a positive ANCA (particularly cANCA or one with anti-PR3 or anti-MPO specificity) without the traditional reliance upon invasive biopsy procedures to confirm the diagnosis. In this setting, the diagnosis must be reconsidered if there is a poor response to appropriate treatment. However, others feel that confirmation of the diagnosis by biopsy of an affected tissue is still indicated despite the presence of strong circumstantial evidence of an underlying ANCA-associated vasculitis, since currently available therapies are toxic.

Utility of sequential ANCA studies

Persistent high titers or rising titers of ANCA (anti-MPO or anti-PR3) are often associated with relapse from remission in patients with microscopic polyarteritis or Wegener's granulomatosis. However, this associa-

TABLE 5.5 SIGNIFICANCE OF pANCA DIRECTED AGAINST MYELOPEROXIDASE

Disease	Frequency (%)
Microscopic polyarteritis	50–70
Idiopathic necrotizing glomerulonephritis	50–85
Churg–Strauss syndrome	70–85
Goodpasture's syndrome (anti-GBM)	10–30
Wegener's granulomatosis	5–10
Polyarteritis nodosa	+
Polyangiitis overlap	+
Systemic lupus erythematosus	+
Hydralazine-induced crescenteric glomerulonephritis	+
Kawasaki disease	+
Ill children	+

+, reported to be present.

tion may not occur in one-third or more of those with such ANCA profiles during 1 or more years of follow-up. The use of an elevation in ANCA titer as the sole parameter to justify immunosuppressive therapy cannot be endorsed, since that strategy would place approximately one-third of patients at risk of unnecessary toxicity. Therapy should only be instituted based upon unequivocal clinical (or even pathologic) evidence of relapse. What role sequential ANCA studies should play in patient care, after the diagnosis is established, is still unclear. If titers are sequentially followed and an increase is noted in an asymptomatic patient, surveillance should be increased to help detect a possible relapse. It is presently unknown whether it is cost-effective or prudent to sequentially follow ANCA titers.

Drug-associated ANCA

The administration of certain drugs has been reported to induce ANCA reactivity in association with varying symptoms. These include:

- hydralazine-induced lupus with anti-MPO and anti-elastase antibodies
- hydralazine-associated vasculitis and anti-MPO and antilactoferrin antibodies
- minocycline-induced arthritis, fever and livedo reticularis with anti-MPO antibodies
- propylthiouracil-induced vasculitis and positive ANCA specificities to several different target antigens, including PR3, MPO and elastase.

Anti-glomerular basement membrane antibody disease

Anti-glomerular basement membrane (GBM) antibody disease, which has similar renal and pulmonary manifestations to Wegener's granulomatosis, may be associated with ANCA in 10–38% of cases.

The clinical significance of combined ANCA and anti-GBM antibodies is uncertain. Some patients have findings that are uncommon in anti-GBM antibody disease alone, suggesting that there is a concurrent systemic vasculitis. These include purpuric rash, arthralgias, granulomas in the kidney and a more favorable renal prognosis.

RHEUMATOID FACTORS

Rheumatoid factors[21] are antibodies directed against the Fc portion of IgG. The rheumatoid factor (RF) as currently measured in clinical practice is an IgM RF, although other immunoglobulin types, including IgG and IgA, have been described.

The presence of RF can be detected by agglutination of IgG-sensitized sheep red cells or bentonite or latex particles coated with human IgG, radioimmunoassay, ELISA or nephelometry. Measurement of RF is not standardized in many laboratories and no one technique has clear advantages over others. Testing for RF is primarily used for the diagnosis of rheumatoid arthritis; however, RF may also be present in other rheumatic diseases and chronic infections[21].

Clinical disorders associated with rheumatoid factor positivity

Rheumatic disorders

Patients may have detectable serum RF in a variety of rheumatic disorders, many of which share similar features, such as symmetric polyarthritis and constitutional symptoms. These include[21,22]:

- rheumatoid arthritis: 26–90% (see below)
- Sjögren's syndrome: 75–95%
- mixed connective tissue disease: 50–60%
- mixed cryoglobulinemia (types II and III): 40–100%
- systemic lupus erythematosus: 15–35%
- polymyositis/dermatomyositis: 5–10%.

TABLE 5.7 RHEUMATOID FACTOR IN NON-RHEUMATIC DISEASES

Condition		Frequency of RF (%)
Aging (>age 60)		5–25
Infection	Bacterial endocarditis*	25–50
	Hepatitis B or hepatitis C*	20–75
	Tuberculosis	8
	Syphilis*	Up to 13
	Parasitic diseases	20–90
	Leprosy*	5–58
	Viral infection*	15–65
Pulmonary disease	Sarcoidosis*	3–33
	Interstitial pulmonary fibrosis	10–50
	Silicosis	30–50
	Asbestosis	30
Miscellaneous diseases	Primary biliary cirrhosis*	45–70
	Malignancy*	5–25
After multiple immunizations		10–15

* Disorders that may cause symptoms suggestive of rheumatoid arthritis.
(Reprinted From American Journal of Medicine, Vol. 91, Shmerling, RH, Delbanco, TL. The rheumatoid factor: an analysis of clinical utility, pp. 528–534, © 1991, with permission from Excerpta Medica Inc.)

The reported sensitivity of the RF test in RA has been as high as 90%. However, population-based studies, which include patients with mild disease, have found much lower rates of RF-positive RA (26–60%). This difference may reflect classification criteria that lead published series of patients with RA to be biased toward more severe (and more seropositive) disease, thereby overestimating the sensitivity of RF in RA.

Non-rheumatic disorders

Non-rheumatic disorders characterized by chronic antigenic stimulation (especially with circulating immune complexes or polyclonal B lymphocyte activation) commonly induce RF production (Table 5.7). Included in this group are[22]:

- indolent or chronic infection, as with subacute bacterial endocarditis or hepatitis B or C virus infection. As an example, hepatitis C infection, especially when accompanied by cryoglobulinemia, is associated with a positive RF in 70–76% of cases. RF production typically ceases with resolution of the infection in these disorders
- inflammatory or fibrosing pulmonary disorders, such as sarcoidosis
- malignancy
- primary biliary cirrhosis.

Healthy individuals

Rheumatoid factors have been found in up to 5% of young, healthy individuals. The reported incidence may be higher in elderly subjects without rheumatic disease, ranging from 3% to 25%. Part of this wide range may be explained by a higher incidence of RF among the chronically ill elderly as compared to healthy older patients. RF is typically present in low to moderate titer (1:40–1:160) in individuals with no demonstrable rheumatic or inflammatory disease.

When is it useful to measure rheumatoid factor?

Population-based studies have shown that some healthy people with a positive RF develop RA over time. However, most of these subjects do not progress to RA; as a result, measurement of RF is a poor screening test for future rheumatic disease.

Predictive value

The predictive value of RF testing has not been widely studied. As noted above, the sensitivity of RF in RA has ranged from 26% to 90%. The specificity is reported as high as 95%, but the positive predictive value for RA has been noted to be only 24%, and 34% for any rheumatic disease. On the other hand, a negative test had a negative predictive value for RA and for any rheumatic disease of 89% and 85% respectively.

Rheumatoid factor titer

The titer of RF should be considered when analyzing its utility. The higher the titer, the greater the likelihood that the patient has rheumatic disease. There are, however, frequent exceptions to this rule, particularly among patients with one of the chronic inflammatory disorders noted above. Furthermore, the use of a higher titer for diagnosis decreases the sensitivity of the test at the same time as it increases the specificity.

Prognostic value

Rheumatoid-factor-positive patients with RA may experience more aggressive and erosive joint disease and extra-articular manifestations than those who are RF-negative. Similar findings have been observed in juvenile rheumatoid arthritis. These general observations, however, are of limited utility in an individual patient because of wide interpatient variability. In this setting, accurate prediction of the disease course is not possible from the RF alone.

ANTI-CCP ANTIBODIES

A new class of autoantibodies associated with rheumatoid arthritis has been described over the last two decades[23–29]. Originally called antikeratin antibodies and antiperinuclear factor[23–27], both of these antibodies target filaggrin antigen, a modified form of the amino acid citrulline. Now called anticyclic citrullinated protein (anti-CCP), these antibodies have a reported sensitivity of 30 to 60% and a specificity of 95 to 98% among patients meeting criteria for rheumatoid arthritis[23–28]. This test may identify some RF-negative patients with RA and could be most helpful in the evaluation of patients with suspected RA for whom uncertainty persists after full evaluation. The absence of anti-CCP antibodies may also identify some RF-positive patients who do not have RA, e.g. patients with hepatitis C and cryoglobulins[24]. Finally, one study[29] found that anti-CCP antibodies may be present years before the development of RA, a finding reminiscent of the RF in RA. The precise role for anti-CCP testing among patients with arthralgia and the role of this antibody in the pathogenesis of RA remain uncertain.

ANTIPHOSPHOLIPID ANTIBODIES

Antiphospholipid antibodies[30] (APL) are antibodies directed against either phospholipids or plasma proteins bound to anionic phospholipids. Patients with these antibodies may have a variety of clinical manifestations, including venous and arterial thrombosis, recurrent fetal losses and thrombocytopenia. Patients with these antibodies have either the 'primary antiphospholipid antibody syndrome (APS)' when it occurs alone, or the secondary APS when it is seen in association with SLE or other rheumatic or autoimmune disorders.

Major types of antiphospholipid antibody

Four major types of antiphospholipid antibodies have been characterized:

- false positive serologic test for syphilis
- lupus anticoagulants
- anticardiolipin antibodies
- anti-β_2-glycoprotein-I antibodies.

False positive serologic test for syphilis

Some patients, especially those with SLE, have a false positive serologic test for syphilis. Such patients have been noted to have fewer successful pregnancies and an increased number of thrombotic events, livedo reticularis and migraine headaches, although this may be related to the presence of other antiphospholipid antibodies.

The false-positive serologic test for syphilis should not be used to screen for APL since it has a low sensitivity and specificity and because this antibody has little independent association with clinically relevant events (clotting or obstetric problems).

Lupus anticoagulants

Lupus anticoagulants are antibodies directed against plasma proteins bound to anionic phospholipids. The lupus anticoagulant blocks the *in vitro* assembly of the prothrombinase complex, resulting in a prolongation of *in vitro* clotting assays such as the activated partial thromboplastin time (aPTT), the dilute Russell viper venom time (RVTT), the kaolin clotting time and, rarely, the prothrombin time. These abnormalities are not reversed when the patient's plasma is diluted 1:1 with normal platelet-free plasma, a procedure that will correct clotting disorders due to deficient clotting factors[31]. The abnormal clotting test results can be largely reversed by incubation with a hexagonal-phase phospholipid, which neutralizes the inhibitor[31]. Although these changes suggest impaired coagulation, patients with a lupus anticoagulant have a paradoxical increase in frequency of arterial and venous thrombotic events.

Anticardiolipin antibodies

Anticardiolipin antibodies (aCL) react with phospholipids such as cardiolipin and phosphatidylserine. There is approximately 85% concordance between the presence of a lupus anticoagulant and aCL. In many cases, however, the lupus anticoagulant is a separate population of antibodies from aCL[31]. Thus, testing should be performed for both lupus anticoagulant and aCL if APS is clinically suspected. Lupus anticoagulant positivity is probably associated with a somewhat greater risk for thrombosis than aCL.

Different immunoglobulin isotypes are associated with aCL, including IgG, IgA and IgM. Elevated levels of IgG aCL incur a greater risk of thrombosis than do other immunoglobulin isotypes.

Anti-β_2-glycoprotein-I antibodies

Antibodies to β_2-glycoprotein I, a phospholipid-binding inhibitor of coagulation, are found in a large percentage of patients with primary or secondary APS. Although antibodies to β_2-glycoprotein I are commonly found in those with other antiphospholipid antibodies, they are the sole antiphospholipid antibody found in approximately 11% of patients with APS.

The importance of β_2-glycoprotein I as a pathogenic cofactor in at least some patients with aCL and lupus anticoagulant has been demonstrated by the following observations:

- In one group of patients with SLE, antibodies directed against free β_2-glycoprotein I were found in 35 of 39 patients with symptoms of the APS versus only two of 55 without such symptoms. Patients with syphilis and other infections (e.g. malaria, human immunodeficiency virus, Q fever) do not form anti-β_2-glycoprotein-I antibodies, which may explain why they are not hypercoagulable even although they may have anticardiolipin antibodies.
- Antibodies to β_2-glycoprotein I correlate better with symptoms of APS than do antibodies to cardiolipin alone.

Prevalence of antiphospholipid antibodies

Although antiphospholipid antibodies are associated with a propensity for thrombosis and with various autoimmune disorders, they are found in up to 2–5% of normal individuals.

Associated disorders

Antiphospholipid antibodies have been noted in increased frequency in patients with SLE: approximately 31% of patients have a lupus anticoagulant and 40–47% have an aCL. On the other hand, roughly 50% of patients with a lupus anticoagulant have SLE. Antiphospholipid antibodies also occur with increased frequency (5–10%) in women with more than three spontaneous recurrent abortions.

Both lupus anticoagulant and aCL have also been found in patients with a variety of autoimmune and rheumatic diseases including:

- hemolytic anemia
- idiopathic thrombocytopenic purpura (up to 30%)
- juvenile arthritis
- rheumatoid arthritis (7–50%)
- psoriatic arthritis (28%)
- scleroderma (25%), especially with severe disease
- Behçet's syndrome (20%)
- Sjögren's syndrome (25–42%)
- mixed connective tissue disease (22%)
- polymyositis and dermatomyositis
- polymyalgia rheumatica (20%)
- chronic discoid lupus erythematosus
- Raynaud's phenomenon.

Antiphospholipid antibodies have also been noted in patients with infections and after the administration of certain drugs. These are usually IgM aCL antibodies, which are less commonly associated with thrombotic events. Furthermore, the antibodies do not appear to have anti-β_2-glycoprotein-I antibody activity. The infections that have been associated with these antibodies include hepatitis A, mumps, bacterial septicemia, human immunodeficiency virus, syphilis, HTLV-I, malaria, *Pneumocystis carinii*, infectious mononucleosis and rubella. Among the drugs that have been implicated are phenothiazines (chlorpromazine), phenytoin, hydralazine, procainamide, quinidine, quinine, valproate, amoxicillin, propranolol, cocaine, sulfadoxine, pyrimethamine and streptomycin.

ANTISTREPTOLYSIN-O

In the evaluation of a patient suspected of having acute rheumatic fever, the antistreptolysin-O (ASLO)[32] is useful to demonstrate evidence of a preceding streptococcal infection. Adequate evidence of infection includes:

- increased antistreptolysin O or other streptococcal antibodies
- positive throat culture for group A β-hemolytic streptococci
- recent scarlet fever.

Throat cultures are usually negative by the time rheumatic fever appears but an attempt should be made to isolate the organism. Streptococcal antibodies are more useful for the following reasons:

- they reach a peak titer at about the time of onset of rheumatic fever
- they indicate true infection rather than transient carriage
- by testing for several different antibodies, any significant recent streptococcal infection can be detected.

Titers of antistreptolysin vary with age, season and geography. Healthy children of elementary (primary) school age commonly have titers of 200–300 Todd units per milliliter. After streptococcal pharyngitis, the antibody response peaks at about 4–5 weeks, which is usually during the second or third week of rheumatic fever (depending upon how early it is detected). Thus, it is useful to take one serum specimen when the diagnosis of acute rheumatic fever is first suspected and another 1 or 2 weeks later for comparison. Antibody titers fall off rapidly in the next few months and then decline more slowly after 6 months. Titers cannot be used as a measure of rheumatic activity.

Only 80% of patients with documented acute rheumatic fever show a rise in the titer of antistreptolysin. Thus, a negative titer should incite testing for other antistreptococcal antibodies such as anti-DNase B, anti-DNase and anti-streptococcal hyaluronidase (ASH).

Acute rheumatic fever is an inflammatory condition; thus, acute-phase reactants are typically increased. Both the CRP concentration and the ESR are usually abnormal during the active rheumatic process, if not suppressed by antirheumatic drugs. When treatment has been discontinued or is being tapered, the CRP may increase again.

TESTING FOR LYME DISEASE

Serologic testing with an ELISA and Western blot may be used to confirm exposure to *Borrelia burgdorferi*, the spirochete that causes Lyme disease[33]. The American College of Physicians recently published three position papers, two on laboratory evaluation in the diagnosis of Lyme disease and a third on test-treatment strategies for patients suspected of having Lyme disease[34]. The conclusions of all three reports can be briefly summarized as follows.

- The clinician should not test or treat the patient in whom the clinical assessment does not suggest that there is at least a moderate probability of Lyme disease.
- The clinician should not diagnose Lyme disease on the basis of testing; instead, the diagnosis is based upon the presence of specific historical information and objective clinical findings.

The US Food and Drug Administration supports this position and again emphasizes that serologic testing is not a primary diagnostic modality for Lyme disease. In addition, standardization of assays will be particularly important when the OspA vaccine begins to be used more commonly.

Techniques
Enzyme-linked immunosorbent assay
The ELISA is currently the most common initial test to serologically confirm exposure to *B. burgdorferi*.

There are, however, false-positive results with this assay (see below); results that are positive or equivocal by ELISA should be confirmed by Western (immuno) blot analysis. 'False seropositivity' is defined as a positive ELISA with a negative Western blot, analogous to the false-positive test for syphilis.

Western blot
Western blot allows detection of antibodies to individual components of the organism and can therefore be much more specific than the ELISA. Antibodies have been detected against: a 41kDa flagellin; multiple outer surface proteins, of which ospA (31kDa), ospB (34kDa) and ospC (23kDa) are the best-studied; heat shock proteins (60kDa and 66kDa); and other prominent proteins, including those at 39kDa, 75kDa and 83kDa. Studies correlating clinically diagnosed Lyme disease with patterns of reactivity in immunoblot have allowed criteria to be proposed by the Centers for Disease Control and Prevention (see Chapter 27).

Cautions to be used in interpretation
There are a number of issues that must be taken into account when evaluating the significance of a positive or negative serologic test for the presence of antibodies to *B. burgdorferi*.

False positives with ELISA
Cross-reacting antibodies can occur in patients with other borrelial diseases (relapsing fever), spirochetal diseases (syphilis, leptospirosis, pinta, yaws), viral illnesses, autoimmune diseases (lupus, rheumatoid arthritis) and infectious diseases (including Epstein–Barr virus, malaria

and endocarditis). Finally, it is estimated that 5% or more of the normal population may test positive for Lyme disease by the ELISA because of cross-reacting antibodies elicited by other infections or by the immune response to normal flora. In determining a 'normal' range that by definition includes 95–97% of normal individuals, it can be anticipated that 3–5% of normal subjects will test positive in this or similar assays. The optimal approach to a possible subclinical infection (i.e. asymptomatic true seropositivity defined by positive immunoblot) remains uncertain and is not a reason to screen asymptomatic patients.

Lack of sensitivity in early disease
IgM antibodies directed against Borrelial antigens typically appear 2–4 weeks after erythema migrans, peak at 6–8 weeks, and decline to low levels after 4–6 months. IgG appears after 6–8 weeks, peaks at 4–6 months and often remains elevated indefinitely despite therapy and resolution of symptoms.

Because most patients with early Lyme disease will not yet have produced detectable antibodies, those with clinically definite erythema migrans need not be serologically tested. If the true nature of the skin lesion is in doubt, serologic testing may be helpful, but a negative result does not rule out disease and should not necessarily discourage treatment in settings of high clinical suspicion. Serologic testing is clearly not cost-effective if treatment is to be administered independent of testing results.

In comparison to the findings in early disease, almost all untreated patients are antibody-positive in the later stages.

Effects of antibiotic therapy
The administration of antibiotics in early disease may abort seroconversion, even if inadequate therapy is given. This concern does not apply in patients with long-standing Lyme disease who have recently received antibiotics; these patients should have been seropositive on the basis of their chronic infection. The test will remain positive for some time after treatment is begun even although antibody production has ceased. However, some patients continue to make antibodies and therefore remain seropositive for long periods of time (see below).

Follow-up testing
- **Interlaboratory variation.** Results of ELISA tests from different laboratories may vary because of technique; therefore, it is best to compare results from the same laboratory.
- **Persistence of positivity.** As mentioned above, high levels of IgG are commonly sustained despite adequate therapy and resolution of symptoms. For this reason, follow-up serologic testing is of no value in assessing the patient who is cured or slowly improving.

The one setting in which follow-up testing may be helpful is the patient in whom there is either worsening of Lyme disease or the appearance of new features of possible Lyme disease (as with a patient with erythema migrans who is treated, and months later develops monoarthritis). In this clinical setting, if sequential immunoblots, performed in the same laboratory, demonstrate the appearance of new 'bands' (i.e. reactivity with proteins not previously recognized), the clinician should consider the possibility of ongoing infection. However, the immune response does not immediately cease simply because antibiotic therapy is begun, and new reactivity on immunoblot may appear despite effective antibiotic therapy. Thus, an expanding repertoire cannot be interpreted as reflecting ongoing infection unless worsening and/or evolution of the clinical signs is present.

Usefulness of serologic tests
- If the test is used in a clinical setting in which Lyme disease is likely, such as isolated monoarthritis or bilateral facial nerve palsy in an endemic area, a positive test is likely to confirm the clinical suspicion of Lyme disease.

- In disease of long duration, such as tertiary neuroborreliosis or Lyme arthritis, seroreactivity by ELISA and immunoblot is virtually universal. Absence of seroreactivity in such a patient, unless there is a plausible explanation, should raise significant doubts about the diagnosis of Lyme disease. In other words, the negative predictive power of a test in such a patient is high.
- In patients with inflammatory joint disease or central nervous system disease, testing the synovial or cerebrospinal fluids for the presence of antibodies to *B. burgdorferi* and then comparing the results with serum is invaluable in assuring that the closed-space inflammation is due to *B. burgdorferi*, not merely a coincidence.

COMPLEMENT

Complement levels can be evaluated either by functional or antigenic assays[35]. The most frequently used are immunoassays (antigenic assays) for C3 and C4 and the total hemolytic complement (CH50), which measures activation of the entire classical pathway.

Clinical significance
Although complement activation accompanies many infectious or inflammatory processes, static levels are either increased or normal and are rarely helpful clinically. It should be remembered that static levels results from both production and consumption effects. Depressions in serum complement levels, however, are often informative. Hypocomplementemia may be present in disorders associated with excessive levels of immune complexes, such as SLE and mixed cryoglobulinemia. In addition, inherited complement deficiencies predispose to the development of autoimmune syndromes.

Any disease associated with circulating immune complexes may cause acquired hypocomplementemia. Measurement of complement can assist in the diagnosis of a limited number of illnesses but more often provides an index of disease activity.

Measurement of total hemolytic complement and individual components
Individual complement components may be assessed either to follow the progression of a disease state or to verify the presence of a deficiency. For example, assays of static levels of C1q, C4, C3 and factor B may be valuable in following the course of certain diseases.

- Classical pathway activation is indicated by low levels of C4 and C3 and normal levels of factor B.
- Alternative pathway activation is indicated by decreased factor B and C3, and normal levels of C4.
- Activation of the classical and alternative pathways is indicated by decreased levels of early components of each pathway such as C4 and factor B.

Decreased levels of individual components may result either from *in vivo* consumption (in which there is a varying reduction in multiple complement components) or from an inherited complement deficiency (in which there is fixed absence of a single complement component). Elevated levels of C3, C4 and factor B are common in many diseases associated with inflammation and represent an increase in hepatic synthesis as part of the acute phase response.

CH50
The CH50 assesses the ability of the test serum to lyse sheep erythrocytes optimally sensitized with rabbit antibody. All nine components of the classical pathway (C1 through C9) are required to give a normal CH50.

CH50 is a useful screening tool for detecting a deficiency of the classical pathway, either of a single component or of several components (as may be seen in SLE). The CH50 can also detect a homozygous deficiency of classical pathway components as indicated by a value of close to 0 units/ml. In contrast, with activation-induced reduction, several components, such as C4 and C3, will be decreased. In this setting, the CH50 is rarely less than 10 units/ml.

The CH50 assay requires appropriate collection, processing and storage of specimens, since several of the complement proteins are unstable. As a result, a common cause of a depressed CH50 is improper specimen handling. Serum samples should be assayed the day of collection or stored frozen at −70°C.

Plasma C3 and C4 levels

Plasma C3 and C4 levels are usually measured in nephelometric immunoassays. These assays are helpful in following patients, such as those with SLE, who present with low levels and then undergo treatment.

Inherited complement deficiency

A genetic deficiency of a single component is indicated by the fixed absence of a single component combined with normal levels of other complement components. This can usually be confirmed by noting 50% of normal levels in the patient's parents.

Inherited C4 deficiency is more complicated, because there are four genes which code for the protein and deficiencies of one, two, or three genes occur in 20–40% of the population. In addition, persons with C4 deficiency are predisposed to SLE, which may in turn lower C4 levels. The question of a partial inherited C4 deficiency usually arises when the C4 level is persistently lower than is commensurate with the clinical activity of the underlying disease. In this setting, genetic analysis and serial evaluations may be necessary to diagnose C4 deficiency. Measurement of split products also can be helpful.

C1 inhibitor deficiency

A functional deficiency of C1 inhibitor (C1-Inh) produces the clinical syndrome of hereditary angioedema. In contrast to 'allergic' angioedema, the edematous lesion lasts several days, is non-pruritic and non-erythematous and is not associated with hives.

C1 inhibitor deficiency can be acquired or inherited in an autosomal dominant fashion. The acquired form is caused by either an autoantibody to C1-Inh or by excessive usage (usually in the setting of malignancy).

A deficiency of functional C1 inhibitor prevents the proper regulation of activated C1. As a result, plasma levels of C4 and C2, the substrates of C1, are chronically reduced in most patients even between attacks and uniformly reduced during an attack.

HUMAN LEUKOCYTE ANTIGEN

There is a substantial literature describing the association of various rheumatic diseases with certain human leukocyte antigen (HLA) class I or class II alleles. However, the clinical relevance of this literature is limited. In addition, associations of certain HLA types with disease states in populations may confer some increased risk of disease to an individual, but the absolute risk is generally quite small[36].

For example, RA is associated with HLA-DR4, but that designation encompasses many different alleles, some of which are RA-associated and some of which are not; as a result, the associations are generally weaker than initially reported. Ethnic differences must be taken into account. Thus, DRB1*0401 and DRB1*0404 are associated with RA in most Caucasians, while DR1 is associated with RA in Israelis.

In addition, HLA B27 is strongly associated with ankylosing spondylitis, especially with the subtype B*2705, but also, to a lesser extent, with the subtypes B*2702, 2703, 2704, 2707 and 2710. Some 30% of the susceptibility to ankylosing spondylitis appears to be encoded by HLA-B27 genes. Despite the strong association with spondylitis, the clinical utility of testing for HLA-B27 in patients with low back pain is low.

Definition of the patient group is also responsible for some differences among studies. It now seems clear, for example, that in studies of patient groups acquired from tertiary medical center practices, associations with these alleles are much stronger than studies in which the patients come from primary care practices, presumably because of clinical differences in patient populations.

URIC ACID

Uric acid determination[37] may be helpful in certain clinical settings, particularly in suspected gout, or with monitoring urate-lowering therapy. Since most patients with asymptomatic hyperuricemia will never develop gout or related problems, screening patients for hyperuricemia is not recommended. While the findings of an elevated or high–normal uric acid has little predictive value with respect to gout, patients with 'low–normal' uric acid levels (e.g. 5.5mg/dl or less) rarely develop gout.

If hyperuricemia is persistent, a thorough history, physical examination and laboratory work should be performed, directed at discovering potential causes of hyperuricemia that may mandate treatment. As an example, lympho- and myeloproliferative disorders, polycythemia vera, vitamin B_{12} deficiency, pre-eclampsia and lead nephropathy (or lead-exposure) may all lead to hyperuricemia and warrant treatment of the underlying disease.

Urinary collections of uric acid over a 24 hour period may be useful in the evaluation of nephrolithiasis, to classify a patient with gout as an overproducer or underexcreter, or if uricosuric therapy is under consideration.

SYNOVIAL FLUID

Synovial fluid analysis is inexpensive and may be diagnostic in patients with bacterial infections or crystal-induced synovitis. According to the ACR clinical guidelines committee, this analysis should be performed in the febrile patient with an acute flare of established arthritis to rule out superimposed septic arthritis as well as any patient with an undiagnosed acute, inflammatory monoarthritis[38]. In other situations, its main value is to permit classification into an inflammatory, non-inflammatory or hemorrhagic category and to monitor a condition (e.g. to determine whether an infection is clearing).

The white cell count, differential count, cultures, Gram stain and polarized light microscopy are the most valuable studies[39,40]. Non-inflammatory fluids generally have fewer than 2000 white blood cells/mm³, with fewer than 75% polymorphonuclear leukocytes (Table 5.8)[40]. An unexplained inflammatory fluid, particularly in a febrile patient, should be assumed to be infected until proven otherwise.

Examination of synovial fluid

Normal joints contain a small amount of synovial fluid with the following characteristics:

- highly viscous
- clear
- essentially acellular
- protein concentration approximately one-third that of plasma
- glucose concentration similar to that in plasma.

If a synovial effusion is present and arthrocentesis is indicated, joint fluid should be routinely analyzed for volume, clarity, color, viscosity, cell count with differential, Gram stain, culture and crystals. In certain clinical settings, such as partially treated septic arthritis, synovial fluid glucose and protein may have utility as well.

Synovial fluid is subsequently categorized as normal, non-inflammatory, inflammatory, septic or hemorrhagic based upon the clinical and laboratory analysis (Table 5.8). The differential diagnosis of each of these specific categories is broad, and not necessarily exclusive:

- The most common causes of a **non-inflammatory** joint effusion include degenerative joint disease (osteoarthritis), trauma, mechanical derangement (ligament or cartilage injury), neuropathic arthropathy, subsiding or early inflammation, hypertrophic osteoarthropathy and aseptic necrosis
- The most common causes of **inflammatory** effusions include rheumatoid arthritis, acute crystal-induced synovitis, and spondyloarthropathy; SLE may be associated with an inflammatory or non-inflammatory effusion.
- **Septic** effusions may be due to bacteria, mycobacteria or fungus
- **Hemorrhagic** effusions may be caused by hemophilia or other hemorrhagic diathesis, calcium pyrophosphate deposition disease (pseudogout), trauma with or without fracture, mechanical derangement, neuropathic arthropathy, excessive anticoagulation, pigmented villonodular synovitis or other neoplasm.

Infections

Septic effusion

Synovial fluid is normally sterile, acellular and of minimal volume. With joint infection, synovial fluid accumulates, turns cloudy and becomes less viscous to varying degrees depending upon the immunocompetence of the host and the nature of the infection. The cornerstone of the diagnosis of septic arthritis is synovial fluid Gram stain and culture. Any bacteria seen on smear and any growth on culture should be considered pathologic, providing that the observations are reliable, the specimen has been collected and prepared properly, and contamination can be ruled out.

Other findings are helpful but not diagnostic[40]. Infected fluid is usually purulent with a leukocyte count (most of which are neutrophils) of over 50 000 cells/mm³. However, lower cell counts may be observed among immunocompromised patients and in infections due to mycobacterial, some neisserial and several Gram-positive organisms. Chemistry studies such as the concentrations of glucose, lactate dehydrogenase or protein have only limited value: a reduction in glucose concentration and elevation in lactate dehydrogenase concentration are consistent with bacterial infection but are not sufficiently sensitive or specific[40].

Synovial fluid Gram stain

The Gram stain of synovial fluid is easily performed and can provide immediate, useful information concerning the diagnosis and therapy (Gram-positive versus Gram-negative coverage) of septic arthritis. In addition to identifying common organisms, Gram stain may be the only evidence of infection with fastidious organisms that do not grow in culture. Of note, most patients with gonococcal septic arthritis will have negative Gram stain (and culture) when synovial fluid is tested; positive microbiologic test results are much more likely to be found with genital, pharyngeal, rectal or blood specimens (see below).

Despite its utility, the sensitivity of synovial fluid Gram stain is not known. In some cases, the Gram stain results are classic and easy to identify, as with multiple Gram-positive cocci aspirated from an acutely swollen knee. However, common problems include:

- clumps of stain or cellular material and other debris simulating bacteria, which may give false-positive Gram stains
- incorrect blanching, so that Gram-positive organisms appear Gram-negative or, rarely, *vice versa*
- the presence of crystals in the synovial fluid; although this finding is often indicative of crystal-induced arthritis (as in gout), some patients have coexisting crystal and septic arthritis.

Routine culture

The synovial fluid samples are routinely sent for culture of the common non-gonococcal causes of bacterial arthritis: staphylococci followed by streptococci and Gram-negative bacteria. These organisms are easily grown on routine culture media in the absence of concomitant antibiotic therapy. The diagnostic yield may be improved by inoculation of blood culture bottles, although the efficacy of this approach is controversial.

A positive synovial culture should be indicative of septic arthritis in 100% of cases if laboratory error and contamination can be excluded. However, the sensitivity of synovial culture is not precisely known because of the lack of an alternative gold standard (and rarity of synovial biopsy prior to antibiotic treatment). It is difficult to prove that infection is present if synovial fluid cultures are negative.

False-negative cultures can be seen with fastidious organisms, poor laboratory techniques or prior antibiotic therapy. False-positive results are less common, most often resulting from contamination of the synovial fluid with organisms from the skin.

Gonococcal arthritis

Gonococcal arthritis is a common cause of septic arthritis in which the organism cannot be cultured on routine culture media.

The joint aspirate should be cultured for *Neisseria gonorrhoeae* when the history is suggestive. The yield can be increased if plates of chocolate

Measure	Normal	Non-inflammatory	Inflammatory	Septic	Hemorrhagic
Volume, knee (ml)	<3.5	Often >3.5	Often >3.5	Often >3.5	Usually >3.5
Clarity	Transparent	Transparent	Translucent–opaque	Opaque	Bloody
Color	Clear	Yellow	Yellow to opalescent	Yellow	Red
Viscosity	High	High	Low	Variable	Variable
WBC (/mm³)	<200	200–2000	2000–50 000	>50 000*	200–2000
PMNs (%)	<25	<25	>50	>75	50–75
Culture	Negative	Negative	Negative	Often positive	Negative
Total protein (g/dl)	1–2	1–3	3–5	3–5	4–6
LDH (compared to levels in blood)	Very low	Very low	High	Variable	Similar
Glucose (mg/dl)	Nearly equal to blood	Nearly equal to blood	>25, lower than blood	<25, much lower than blood	Nearly equal to blood

TABLE 5.8 CATEGORIES OF SYNOVIAL FLUID (BASED UPON CLINICAL AND LABORATORY FINDINGS)

* Lower with infections caused by partially treated or low-virulence organisms.

LED, lactate dehydrogenase; PMNs, polymorphonuclear leukocytes; WBC, white blood count.

(With permission from Sholter DE, Russell AS. Synovial fluid analysis and the diagnosis of septic arthritis. In: Rose B, Schur PH, eds. UpToDate. Wellesley, MA: UpToDate; 2003. Copyright © 2003 UpToDate, Inc. For more information, visit www.uptodate.com.)

agar or Thayer–Martin medium are inoculated with synovial fluid at the bedside along with cultures from the pharynx, urethra, cervix, rectum and skin lesions (if present). Blood cultures are often positive in patients presenting with tenosynovitis and skin lesions alone but are frequently negative if a joint effusion is present.

Cultures of synovial fluid tend to be positive in less than 50% of cases of gonococcal arthritis. Use of polymerase chain reaction (PCR) techniques to detect gonococcal DNA in synovial fluid can increase the yield in culture-negative cases and permits monitoring of the response to therapy. However, this technique is not yet widely available and its cost-effectiveness remains unproven.

When should cultures be sent for unusual organisms?

The history may reveal clues suggesting the possibility of an unusual cause of septic arthritis:

- a history of tuberculosis exposure
- a history of trauma or an animal bite
- travel to or living in an area endemic with fungal infections or Lyme disease
- the presence of immune suppression
- a monoarthritis that is refractory to conventional therapy.

Synovial fluid crystal analysis

Aspiration of synovial fluid from the affected joint and analysis of the fluid by polarized light microscopy permits identification of sodium urate crystals in the great majority of instances of acute gouty arthritis. Joint aspiration is also helpful in distinguishing acute gout from pseudo-gout (calcium pyrophosphate crystal deposition – CPPD – disease), although occasionally both crystals may be identifiable in the synovial fluid of patients in whom these disorders coexist. In contrast, arthritis or periarthritis due to the deposition of basic calcium phosphate crystals cannot usually be diagnosed with certainty by polarized microscopy

because the crystalline aggregates are below the resolution of standard light microscopy. In these circumstances, transmission electron microscopy, and more recently atomic force microscopy and X-ray powder diffraction, have been successfully used in the identification of these crystals.

Gout crystals are needle-shaped and display strongly negative birefringence (i.e. they are yellow when parallel to the axis of the polarizer). CPPD crystals are pleomorphic, often in the shape of rhomboids, with blunt ends, and are weakly positively birefringent (they appear blue when parallel to the axis of the polarizer). The clinical significance of intracellular crystals is often said to be greater than when they are extracellular, although no convincing evidence supports this suggestion.

The sensitivity of polarized microscopy in demonstrating negatively birefringent crystals in patients with acute gouty arthritis is at least 85%, and the specificity for gout is 100% if the results are unequivocal. However, gouty arthritis may occasionally coexist with another type of joint disease, such as septic arthritis or pseudogout. In some cases, needle-shaped crystals may be evident on a slide without polarized microscopy, especially when the crystals are abundant.

- Even during the asymptomatic intercritical period, extracellular urate crystals are identifiable in synovial fluid from previously affected joints in virtually all untreated gouty patients and approximately 70% of those administered uric acid lowering therapy. This allows late establishment of the diagnosis in the majority of patients in whom the diagnosis was not made in the acute setting.
- Demonstration of urate crystals in aspirates of tophaceous deposits provides a convenient and specific means to corroborate the diagnosis in the small proportion of gouty individuals with tophi. Since these patients are typically treated with lifelong urate-lowering therapy, identification of tophaceous gout has significant therapeutic impact.

REFERENCES

1. Griner PF, Mayewski RJ, Mushlin AI, Greenland P. Selection and interpretation of diagnostic tests and procedures. Principles and applications. Ann Intern Med 1981; 94: 557–592.
2. Sackett DL, Strauss S. On some clinically useful measures of the accuracy of diagnostic tests. ACP J Club 1998; 129: A17.
3. Kushner, I. Acute phase proteins. In: Rose B, Schur PH, eds. UpToDate. Wellesley, MA: UpToDate; 2001.
4. Sox HC Jr, Liang MH. The erythrocyte sedimentation rate. Guidelines for rational use. Ann Intern Med 1986; 104: 515–523.
5. Cohick CB, Furst DE, Quagliata S et al. Analysis of elevated serum interleukin-6 levels in rheumatoid arthritis: correlation with erythrocyte sedimentation rate or C- reactive protein. J Lab Clin Med 1994; 123: 721–727.
6. Cush JJ, Lipsky PE, Postlethwaite AE et al. Correlation of serologic indicators of inflammation with effectiveness of nonsteroidal antiinflammatory drug therapy in rheumatoid arthritis. Arthritis Rheum 1990; 33: 19–28.
7. Barland P, Wachs J. Measurement and clinical significance of antinuclear antibodies. In: Rose B, Schur PH, eds. UpToDate. Wellesley, MA: UpToDate; 2001.
8. Wachs J, Barland P. Antibodies to DNA; SM; and RNP in systemic lupus erythematosus. In: Rose B, Schur PH, eds. UpToDate. Wellesley, MA: UpToDate; 2001.
9. Hahn BH. Antibodies to DNA. N Engl J Med 1998; 338: 1359–1368.
10. Barland P, Wachs J. Clinical significance of anti-Ro/SSA and anti-La/SSB antibodies. In: Rose B, Schur PH, eds. UpToDate. Wellesley, MA: UpToDate; 2001.
11. Denton CP, Black CM. Classification of scleroderma. In: Rose B, Schur PH, eds. UpToDate. Wellesley, MA: UpToDate; 2001.
12. Wachs, Barland P. Miscellaneous antinuclear antibodies. In: Rose B, Schur PH, eds. UpToDate. Wellesley, MA: UpToDate; 2001.
13. Wachs J, Barland P. Antiribosomal P protein antibodies. In: Rose B, Schur PH, eds. UpToDate. Wellesley, MA: UpToDate; 2001.
14. Schur PH, Rose BD. Drug-induced lupus. In: Rose B, Schur PH, eds. UpToDate. Wellesley, MA: UpToDate; 2001.
15. Rubin RL, Bell SA, Burlingame RW. Autoantibodies associated with lupus induced by diverse drugs target a similar epitope in the (H2A-H2B)-DNA complex. J Clin Invest 1992; 90: 165–173.
16. Rose BD, Hoffman GS. Clinical sprectrum of antineutrophil cytoplasmic antibodies. In: Rose B, Schur PH, eds. UpToDate. Wellesley, MA: UpToDate; 2001.
17. Merkel PA, Polisson RP, Chang Y et al. Prevalence of antineutrophil cytoplasmic antibodies in a large inception cohort of patients with connective tissue disease. Ann Intern Med 1997; 126: 866–873.
18. Hagen EC, Daha MR, Hermans J et al. for the EC/BCR Project for ANCA Assay Standardization. Diagnostic value of standardized assays for anti-neutrophil cytoplasmic antibodies in idiopathic systemic vasculitis. Kidney Int 1998; 53: 743–753.
19. Rao JK, Weinberger M, Oddone EZ et al. The role of antineutrophil cytoplasmic antibody (cANCA) testing in the diagnosis of Wegener granulomatosis. A literature review and meta-analysis. Ann Intern Med 1995; 123: 925–932.
20. Jennette JC, Wilkman AS, Falk RJ. Diagnostic predictive value of ANCA serology. Kidney Int 1998; 53: 796–798.
21. Shmerling RH. Origin and utility of measurement of rheumatoid factors. In: Rose B, Schur PH, eds. UpToDate. Wellesley, MA: UpToDate; 2001.
22. Shmerling, RH, Delbanco, TL. The rheumatoid factor: an analysis of clinical utility. Am J Med 1991; 91: 528–534.
23. Hoet RMA, Boerbooms AM, Arends M et al. Antiperinuclear factor, a marker antibody for rheumatoid arthritis: colocalisation of the perinuclear factor and profilaggrin. Ann Rheum Dis 1991; 50:611–618.
24. Kessel A, Rosner I, Zukerman E et al. Use of antikeratin antibodies to distinguish between rheumatoid arthritis and polyarthritis associated with hepatitis C infection. J Rheumatol 2000; 27:610–612.
25. Palosuo T, Lukka M, Alenius H et al. Purification of filaggrin from human epidermis and measurement of antifilaggrin autoantibodies in sera from patients with rheumatoid arthritis by an enzyme-linked immunosorbent assay. Int Arch Allergy Immunol 1998; 115:294–302.
26. Schellekens GA, de Jong BA, van den Hoogen FH et al. Citrulline is an essential constituent of antigenic determinants recognized by rheumatoid arthritis-specific autoantibodies. J Clin Invest 1998; 101:273–281.
27. Paimela L, Palosuo T, Aho K et al. Association of autoantibodies to filaggrin with an active disease in early rheumatoid arthritis. Ann Rheum Dis 2001; 60:32–35.
28. Lee DM, Schur PH. Clinical utility of the anti-CCP assay in patients with rheumatic diseases. Ann Rheum Dis. 2003; 62:870–874.
29. Rantapää-Dahlqvist S, de Jong BAW, Berglin E et al. Antibodies against cyclic citrullinated peptide and IgA rheumatoid factor predict the development of rheumatoid arthritis. Arthritis Rheum 2003; 48: 2741–2749.

30. Bermas BL, Schur PH, Rose BD. Clinical manifestations and diagnosis of the antiphospholipid antibody syndrome. In: Rose B, Schur PH, eds. UpToDate. Wellesley, MA: UpToDate; 2001.

31. Roubey, RA. Immunology of the antiphospholipid antibody syndrome. Arthritis Rheum 1996; 39: 1444–1454.

32. Gibofsky A, Zabriskie JB. Clinical manifestations and diagnosis of acute rheumatic fever. In: Rose B, Schur PH, eds. UpToDate. Wellesley, MA: UpToDate; 2001.

33. Sigal LH. Laboratory confirmation of the diagnosis of Lyme disease. In: Rose B, Schur PH, eds. UpToDate. Wellesley, MA: UpToDate; 2001.

34. American College of Physicians. Guidelines for laboratory evaluation in the diagnosis of Lyme disease. Ann Intern Med 1997; 127: 1106–1108.

35. Liszewski MK, Atkinson JP. Inherited and acquired disorders of the complement system. In: Rose B, Schur PH, eds. UpToDate. Wellesley, MA: UpToDate; 2001.

36. Nepom B. HLA: A roadmap. In: Rose B, Schur PH, eds. UpToDate. Wellesley, MA: UpToDate; 2001.

37. Becker MA. Clinical manifestations and diagnosis of gout. In: Rose B, Schur PH, eds. UpToDate. Wellesley, MA: UpToDate; 2001.

38. Sholter DE, Russell AS. Synovial fluid analysis and the diagnosis of septic arthritis. In: Rose B, Schur PH, eds. UpToDate. Wellesley, MA: UpToDate; 2001.

39. American College of Rheumatology Ad Hoc Committee on Clinical Guidelines. Guidelines for the initial evaluation of the adult patient with acute musculoskeletal symptoms. Arthritis Rheum 1996; 39: 1–8.

40. Shmerling RH, Delbanco TL, Tosteson AN, Trentham DE. Synovial fluid tests. What should be ordered? JAMA 1990; 264: 1009–1014.

6 Aspiration and injection of joints and periarticular tissues

Juan J Canoso

- Synovial aspiration is a basic diagnostic tool in rheumatology
- Synovial fluid analysis allows distinction between inflammatory and non-inflammatory conditions and provides direct proof of crystal arthropathy, infection and hemarthrosis
- Major diagnostic errors can be made by simply assuming the nature of an effusion
- Corticosteroid injections and infiltrations are basic treatment tools in rheumatology, orthopedics, physiatry and general medicine
- Synovial aspiration and corticosteroid injections and infiltrations carry minimal risk to the patient when properly indicated and performed
- Technical difficulties vary; some of these procedures require specialized knowledge for optimal results

TABLE 6.1 INDICATIONS FOR ASPIRATING OR INJECTING JOINTS	
Diagnosis	Mandatory if septic arthritis suspected
	Strongly advised if crystal arthritis or hemarthrosis suspected
	Differentiation of inflammatory from non-inflammatory arthritis
	Imaging studies – arthroscopy and arthrography
	Synovial biopsy
Therapy	To remove tense effusions to relieve pain and improve function
	To remove blood or pus from a joint
	For injection of corticosteroids and other intra-articular therapies
	For tidal lavage of joints

Joints and periarticular structures such as bursae and tendon sheaths may need aspiration for diagnostic or therapeutic purposes. In addition, corticosteroids and other drugs are often injected in and around soft tissue periarticular lesions to treat regional pain syndromes (Table 6.1). The principles and practice of inserting a needle into either a joint cavity or periarticular lesion are very similar.

INDICATIONS FOR ASPIRATING OR INJECTING MUSCULOSKELETAL TISSUES

Aspirating fluid for diagnostic or therapeutic purposes

In patients in whom sepsis, crystal synovitis or bleeding is the suspected cause of a joint, bursal or tendon sheath lesion, aspiration and analysis of the fluid is essential for diagnosis[1–3]. In addition, in patients who have poorly defined forms of arthritis, knowledge of the nature of the synovial fluid, particularly the inflammatory cell content, will complement findings from the history and physical examination and help provide the basic framework for diagnosis and treatment. In patients with tense joint effusions, aspiration of synovial fluid provides prompt relief of pain and permits the patient to move or bear weight on the affected joint. Finally, in hemarthrosis or septic arthritis, the blood and pus within a synovial cavity may be damaging to the joint cartilage and synovial membrane, so evacuation of the fluid is necessary to avoid permanent joint damage. Large articular effusions should be drained as fully as possible to decrease pressure, improve synovial circulation and prevent muscle atrophy.

Synovial fluid should be aspirated into sterile syringes, which are either capped or immediately aliquoted into sterile containers. Anticoagulants can help avoid the formation of fibrin clots, making the fluid easier to handle and allowing analyses of the cellular content. If unusual or chronic infections are suspected it may be prudent to inoculate some of the fluid into appropriate growth media (such as chocolate agar for gonococcal infections) immediately after aspiration. The fluid should be inspected for the presence of blood and to see how opaque it is, which is a rough guide to cell content. Three laboratory investigations should then be carried out on all fluids aspirated for diagnostic purposes:

- the total and differential cell count
- examination for organisms (gram stain, culture, etc.)
- compensated polarized light microscopy for the presence of urate or pyrophosphate crystals.

TABLE 6.2 SYNOVIAL FLUID FINDINGS				
	Normal	Osteoarthritis	Rheumatoid and other inflammatory arthritis	Septic arthritis
Gross appearance	Clear	Clear	Opaque	Opaque
Volume (ml)	0–1	1–10	5–50	5–50
Viscosity	High	High	Low	Low
Total white cell count/mm³	<200	200–10 000	500–75 000	>50 000
% polymorphonuclear cells	<25	<50	>50	>75

Knee joint synovial fluid findings in common forms of arthritis.

As crystal synovitis and infections can coexist it is never wise to rely on one of these investigations alone. The cellular content is indicative of the type of arthritis (Table 6.2). Other special investigations that can be of value include cytology and the assay of a variety of biochemical markers of connective tissue turnover, such as products of the synthesis and degradation of cartilage aggrecan.

Practical procedure and aftercare

Technical considerations

Some joints are easier to enter than others. There is a rank order of technical difficulty in which knee aspiration stands as the easiest procedure and sacroiliac joint injection[4] as the most difficult. Because sacroiliac joint injection, facet joint injection[5] and epidural block[4,6] fall in the field of interventional radiology they are not discussed further in this chapter.

The procedure

Aspiration or injection of joints or soft tissues is an outpatient procedure that does not require specialized equipment (Table 6.3). Universal precautions must be followed during the procedure; gloves are recommended, and are required by medical practice regulations in many countries.

The patient should be placed in a comfortable supine or recumbent position (in case of possible fainting, as well as to aid relaxation), and the procedure must be fully explained. Prior to cleaning the skin, bony and other landmarks need to be identified by palpation and the needle site marked in some way, such as with a thumbnail imprint in the skin. The skin must then be carefully cleaned with antiseptic agents. For local anesthesia, the skin and subcutaneous tissues can be infiltrated down to the level of the periarticular lesion or joint capsule using 1% or 2% lidocaine without epinephrine (adrenaline) and a small-bore needle. However, physicians experienced with the procedure often prefer to use topical ethyl chloride or no anesthetic at all. This is often appropriate for joint aspiration, as it is difficult to anesthetize the capsule, so a single, simple, quick needle thrust may be much less painful than the local anesthesia. With the proper technique, the needle passes freely through the extra-articular tissues and a 'pop' is felt as the needle enters the joint. The ease with which fluid can be withdrawn depends on the needle size used, viscosity of the fluid, degree of effusion and presence of any fibrin clots or 'rice bodies' in the joint fluid. Free flow of fluid is often suddenly interrupted because of clogging of the needle end by the synovial membrane or debris. Rotating the needle, withdrawing it slightly or even re-injecting a little of the fluid will often help unclog the needle and allow additional fluid to be withdrawn. If corticosteroids or other substances are to be injected, this can be done through the same needle, but removing the aspirating syringe from the needle hub may be difficult and require forceps.

At the end of any procedure, the needle should be swiftly withdrawn, and light pressure should be put on the needle site in the skin. The application of a simple adhesive plaster for a few hours is all that is usually required thereafter.

Aftercare

There is a great deal of variation in the advice given to patients after aspiration or therapeutic injection of joints or soft tissues. Some doctors give no specific instructions, others recommend a prolonged period of rest[7] to help facilitate the best possible therapeutic response. In most cases, it is sensible for patients to rest the affected joint for 24–48 hours after a therapeutic injection, to minimize leakage of the therapeutic agent and improve the anti-inflammatory response. However, this advice must depend on the patient's circumstances.

CONTRAINDICATIONS AND COMPLICATIONS

Contraindications

There are few absolute contraindications to joint or soft tissue aspirations and injections; if infection is suspected then fluid should always be aspirated from a joint. In other indications, the procedures should probably be avoided if there is infection of the overlying skin or subcutaneous tissues or if bacteremia is suspected. The presence of a significant bleeding disorder or diathesis or with severe thrombocytopenia may also preclude joint aspiration. However, if it is deemed necessary for diagnosis or therapy, the procedure may be carried out after an injection of factor VIII in a hemophiliac for example, or with other appropriate cover for the bleeding disorder. Warfarin anticoagulation with international normalization ratio values in the therapeutic range is not a contraindication to joint or soft tissue aspiration or injection[8]. Aspiration of a joint with a prosthesis in it carries a particularly high risk of infection and is often best left to surgeons using full aseptic techniques.

Lack of response to previous injections may be a relative contraindication to therapeutic injections and, if there is any suspicion of infection being the underlying cause of the musculoskeletal problem, corticosteroids must not be injected for fear of exacerbating the infection.

Complications

There are surprisingly few complications of these procedures. The most significant issue is the risk of infection, and care must always be taken to use sterile 'no-touch' techniques, as well as avoiding corticosteroids in those who could have existing sepsis. It is estimated that the risk of a septic arthritis following aspiration or corticosteroid injection is in the order of 1 per 15 000 procedures[9]. Patients who have severe immunodeficiency problems, as well as those with implants, may be at greater risk.

Other complications can arise from misplaced injections. The best described problem is tendon rupture following corticosteroid injections for tendinitis. The risk can be minimized by avoiding injection into the tendon itself, and no therapeutic agent should be injected against any unexpected resistance. Occasionally, nerve damage can also result from a misplaced injection, for example median nerve atrophy following attempted injections for a carpal tunnel syndrome.

TABLE 6.3 EQUIPMENT REQUIRED FOR JOINT AND SOFT TISSUE INJECTIONS	
Skin preparation	Antiseptic solution (povidone–iodine), alcohol swabs, 4×4 gauze pads
Local anesthetic	1% lidocaine
Needles	23–27 gauge needles for local anesthetic, 18 gauge for large to moderate-sized joints (knees, shoulders, ankles, etc.), 23–25 gauge for smalll joints (wrists, metacarpophalangeal joints, etc.)
Syringes	3ml or 5ml syringe for anesthetic–steroid injection and 10–50ml syringe for joint aspiration
Miscellaneous	Gloves; forceps for removing needles from syringe; specimen tubes/plates for cultures and fluid studies

All the required supplies should be assembled in advance. Very importantly, the needle must be long enough to reach the intended place and have a caliber adequate to the nature of the fluid. While standard needle lengths work well in thin patients, longer needles and even a spinal needle may be required in obese patients. On the other hand, a 1ml syringe with a half-inch no. 27 needle is particularly useful to infiltrate superficial structures such as the interphalangeal, metacarpophalangeal and metatarsophalangeal joints, digital flexor tendon sheaths, the carpal tunnel, de Quervain's tenosynovitis and the elbow joint through the lateral approach. Purulent effusions require no. 18 or no. 16 needles. A failure to fully drain a septic joint indicates large debris or loculation and calls for tidal lavage (see below), arthroscopy or arthrotomy

CORTICOSTEROID INJECTIONS

Corticosteroid injections are frequently used to achieve local anti-inflammatory activity. The indications for their use include the presence of persistent inflammation at a single site in the absence of a contra-indication, such as suspicion of infection (see below). Synovial joints and other cavities should generally be injected with a long-acting crystalline form of corticosteroid such as triamcinolone hexacetonide or methylprednisolone acetate. These agents are taken up by the synovial lining cells, allowing continued local release into the targeted area. Only a relatively small proportion escapes into the general circulation but, during the first 24 hours after injection, patients may experience flushing or other evidence of a corticosteroid 'pulse'. For periarticular injections, particularly subcutaneous bursae and de Quervain's tenosynovitis, methylprednisolone acetate should be used, as the less soluble (and therefore more potent) triamcinolone hexacetonide is likely to induce skin atrophy.

Local anesthetic is sometimes mixed with corticosteroids for such injections. In the case of some periarticular lesions, for example rotator cuff lesions around the shoulder, this can have the advantage of confirming the correct placement of the injection, as the local anesthetic should result in almost immediate relief of the problem if the injection is correctly placed. An additional indication for intra-articular corticosteroids is the reduction of pain following arthroscopic surgery[10].

Corticosteroid doses vary with the structure injected. For each of the described procedures below a dose range is shown based on the use of methylprednisolone acetate 40mg/ml. If the more potent triamcinolone hexacetonide 20mg/ml is used, the lower figure of the range should be chosen.

Corticosteroid injections are used in joints, bursae, tendon sheaths and entheses[11]. Some of these procedures are easy to perform while others are technically demanding or have dubious results. The simple procedures include infiltrations for trigger finger[12,13], carpal tunnel syndrome[14,15], ganglia, olecranon bursitis[16], rotator cuff tendinitis, trochanteric bursitis, anserine bursitis[17] and 'trigger points'. The technically demanding group includes injections for de Quervain's tenosynovitis[18], lateral epicondylitis (tennis elbow)[19], medial epicondylitis (golfer's elbow), frozen shoulder[20], suprascapular nerve block[21,22], iliopsoas bursitis[23], ischial 'bursitis', Achilles tendinitis, retrocalcaneal bursitis[24], plantar fasciitis, posterior tibialis tenosynovitis and Morton's neuroma[25]. Intracavitary position of the needle can be ascertained by withdrawing some articular fluid or checking to see if the cavity distends as fluid is injected. In the soft tissues, correct positioning may be ascertained by elimination of pain by a preceding lidocaine infiltration. Rest of the injected site for 48 hours following the procedure is generally recommended. Additional rest may lead to better results and should be considered under special circumstances[7].

Complications of corticosteroid injections and infiltrations

- **Facial flushing.** Very common, occurring in perhaps 40% of cases. Transient and inconsequential, it may nevertheless worry patients who have not been warned.
- **Postinjection flare.** Corticosteroid-crystal-induced synovitis occurs in about 5% of intra-articular injections. Pain appears several hours following the procedure and may last from a few hours to 1 day. Persisting pain and mounting swelling may indicate missed or iatrogenic infection; these joints should be re-aspirated for Gram stain and aerobic and anaerobic cultures. Tennis elbow infiltrations are often followed by protracted pain, which may last several weeks. Repeated tennis elbow infiltrations are believed to contribute to the development of chronic pain.
- **Skin atrophy.** This is a frequent complication of superficial infiltrations and olecranon bursa injections. The condition is characterized by cigarette-paper-like skin, recurrent ecchymosis and chronic pressure pain. Postinjection atrophy is more likely to develop in elderly individuals.
- **Skin hypopigmentation.** Superficial corticosteroid infiltrations such as those used in de Quervain's tenosynovitis often cause a hypopigmented patch which may be quite disfiguring in people with dark skin. The condition resolves in a few months to 2 years.
- **Infection.** This is an extremely rare complication of corticosteroid injections, except for injections in the olecranon bursa. Postinjection septic bursitis may occur from exacerbation of a missed infection (infections of superficial bursae may be quite subdued) or may be caused by contamination of a sterile bursa through the needle track. The skin at the elbow tip has little recoil. Taps made at the bursal apex, where the skin is maximally stretched, often create a leaking point that may act as a portal of entry.
- **Tendon rupture.** A ruptured tendon following a corticosteroid injection may indicate abuse of the procedure, intratendinous injection or coincidental rupture caused by the very condition that led to the injection. Conditions that lead to spontaneous tendon rupture include dorsal wrist tenosynovitis and posterior tibialis tenosynovitis in rheumatoid arthritis (RA), chronic subacromial impingement damaging the rotator cuff and the long biceps tendon, senile changes in the supraspinatus or long biceps tendon, chronic corticosteroid use, overuse Achilles tendinopathy, fluoroquinolone-induced Achilles tendinopathy, uremia, hyperparathyroidism and systemic lupus erythematosus.
- **Corticosteroid arthropathy.** Abuse of intra-articular injections may result in a Charcot's-like arthropathy similar to the one described in calcium pyrophosphate crystal deposition disease.
- **Osteonecrosis.** This is a reported complication of abused articular or soft tissue corticosteroid infiltrations.
- **Corticosteroid-induced osteoporosis.** Patients who have been serially injected, for recurrent tendinitis, for example, are at an enhanced risk of osteoporosis during the injection period, particularly if additional factors are present such as prolonged bed rest or a low calcium intake. Intra-articular corticosteroids are said to have less effect on bone than oral corticosteroids[26]. However, the relative safety of the intra-articular route has not been shown in clinical trials.
- **Other systemic complications.** Corticosteroid injections cause transient pituitary inhibition, lasting up to several days[27,28]. Serial infiltrations may cause adrenal suppression and result in acute adrenal crisis[29]. Anaphylactic shock, albeit exceedingly rare, may also occur[30].

Associated procedures

A number of other agents apart from corticosteroids have been used for intra-articular or periarticular therapy via injection. Examples include the radioactive colloids such as yttrium-90, which can irradiate the synovium to achieve a form of chemical synovectomy, other sclerosing agents, long-acting local anesthetics, sometimes used alone to help sort out the origin of musculoskeletal pain, and hyaluronan for pain relief in osteoarthritis.

- **Imaging joints with contrast agents.** Injection of contrast agents with or without air can help image soft tissue and cartilage lesions in joints using radiography (arthrography)
- **Joint lavage.** Tidal lavage of joints with saline, through a simple percutaneous cannula, or during arthroscopy can result in lasting relief of pain and inflammation in osteoarthritis
- **Synovial biopsy.** Synovial biopsy can be of diagnostic value, and is essential for the diagnosis of pigmented villonodular synovitis and

other neoplastic lesions, as well as sometimes being necessary to diagnose chronic infections such as tuberculosis and foreign body synovitis. This can be done percutaneously, using a 'Parker Pearson' needle, or through arthroscopy which has the advantage of providing larger and targeted samples.

● **Needle arthroscopy and 'chondroscopy'.** Full arthroscopic examination and surgery is largely the province of the orthopedic surgeon. However, arthroscopic examination of some joints, especially the knee, can be carried out under local anesthesia, particularly if modern small-bore arthroscopes (needlescopes) are used. This can be of value in examining the synovium and cartilage (chondroscopy) and in joint lavage, as well as allowing biopsy under direct vision.

THE WRIST AND HAND

Finger and metacarpophalangeal joints

Indications. Injection in RA, psoriatic arthritis, active Bouchard's nodes.

Corticosteroid dose. 10–15mg methylprednisone acetate (no. 25 or no. 27 needle).

Approach. Dorsolateral with the digit in semiflexion (Figs 6.1 & 6.2). Corticosteroid injection produces circumferential distention of the joint. Multiple joints may be injected in one session.

Precautions. Do not overdistend joint(s). Fluid has a tendency to back up; keep firm pressure with a sterile gauze for at least 5 minutes following the procedure.

Complications. Joint hyperlaxity, capsular calcification (frequent but inconsequential).

Flexor tendon sheaths

Indications. Injection in trigger finger; flexor tenosynovitis in RA, psoriatic arthritis.

Corticosteroid dose. 15–20mg methylprednisone acetate mixed with 1–2ml lidocaine (no. 25 or no. 27 needle or no. 23 butterfly).

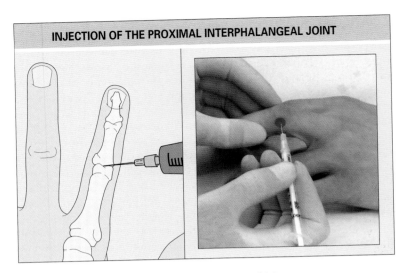

Fig. 6.2 Injection of the proximal interphalangeal joint.

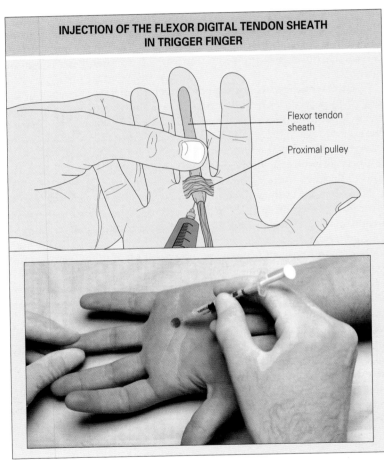

Fig. 6.3 Injection of the flexor digital tendon sheath in trigger finger.

Approach. Just distal to palmar crease of thumb, proximal palmar crease (index), distal palmar crease (long, ring and little fingers) with needle held at a 45° distal inclination (Fig. 6.3).

Precautions. Avoid intratendinous injection. Reciprocal needle movements upon gentle finger motion indicate tendon engagement; back up by the millimeter, free the needle and inject. Up to three injections given 3 weeks apart are allowed.

Complications. Superficial extravasation may produce asymptomatic focal palmar fat atrophy. Large published series comment on a lack of tendon rupture and iatrogenic infection.

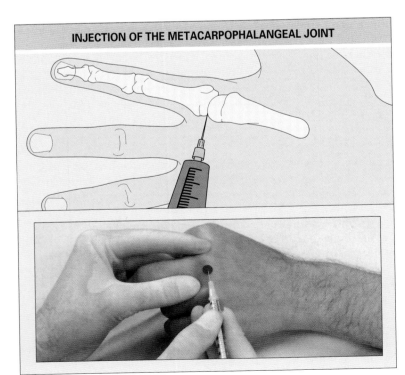

Fig. 6.1 Injection of the metacarpophalangeal joint.

De Quervain's tenosynovitis

Indications. Most instances of inflammation of the common sheath of the abductor pollicis longus and extensor pollicis brevis result from hand overuse. Corticosteroid injections are highly successful in these cases.

Corticosteroid dose. 20–30mg methylprednisolone acetate (no. 25 or no. 27 needle).

Approach. The needle is aimed towards the radial styloid, which underlies the sheath. The needle is then pulled back by the millimeter and injection is attempted. Successful injections distend the sheaths of both abductor pollicis longus and extensor pollicis brevis.

Precautions. Make sure that the corticosteroid remains within the sheath. Do not infiltrate grossly thickened sheaths, as mycobacterial infection may be present.

Complications. As mentioned previously, skin hypopigmentation frequently complicates this procedure. Skin atrophy, leading to recurring ecchymosis, is particularly prevalent in elderly patients.

Carpal tunnel syndrome

Indications. Injection treatment is indicated in all etiologies of carpal tunnel syndrome except acute cases due to fracture, hemorrhage, infection and carpal tunnel syndrome of late pregnancy.

Corticosteroid dose. 30–40mg methylprednisolone acetate mixed with 2–3ml lidocaine (no. 22, no. 25 or no. 27 needle or no. 23 butterfly).

Approach. Just distal to the distal wrist crease and just medial to palmaris longus tendon (Fig. 6.4). If the palmaris longus tendon is absent (25% of people lack it), use the midline. The needle is inserted to a depth of 1cm with a 45° distal inclination and a 45° lateral inclination.

Precautions. Paresthesias indicate median nerve engagement; if they occur, reposition the needle. Reciprocal needle motion upon gentle finger motion (which should be rehearsed beforehand) indicates tendon engagement; again, reposition the needle.

Complications. Transient increase of paresthesias.

Note: A properly made resting splint to hold the wrist in the neutral position provides the lowest pressures within the carpal tunnel.

FIRST CARPOMETACARPAL JOINT

Indications. Painful osteoarthritis (OA). The patient presents with a 'square hand' with grating and tenderness at the prominence.

Corticosteroid dose. 15–30mg methylprednisone acetate (no. 23, no. 25 or no. 27 needle).

Approach. Within the anatomic snuffbox. After localizing the joint line at the base of the first metacarpal, the joint is entered at the anatomic snuffbox between the common sheath of the abductor pollicis longus and extensor pollicis brevis anteriorly and the extensor pollicis longus posteriorly. To optimally expose the joint the thumb is flexed across the palm towards the little finger.

Precautions. Avoid the radial artery. The course of this vessel varies and may encircle the joint line.

Complications. None, as long as the radial artery is avoided.

Wrist

Indications. For diagnosis in acute arthritis. Most cases of acute wrist arthritis are due to calcium pyrophosphate dihydrate pseudogout, gout and septic arthritis. For injection in RA, other sterile synovitides and OA such as is associated with chondrocalcinosis and hemochromatosis.

Corticosteroid dose. 30–40mg methylprednisone acetate (no. 25 or no. 27 needle). Aspiration should be attempted before injection. For aspiration alone use a no. 20 or no. 18 needle.

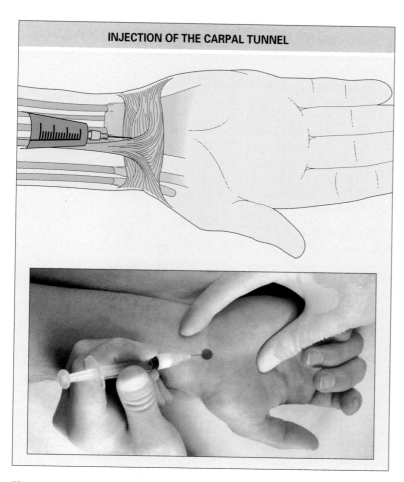

Fig. 6.4 Injection of the carpal tunnel.

INJECTION OF THE CARPAL TUNNEL

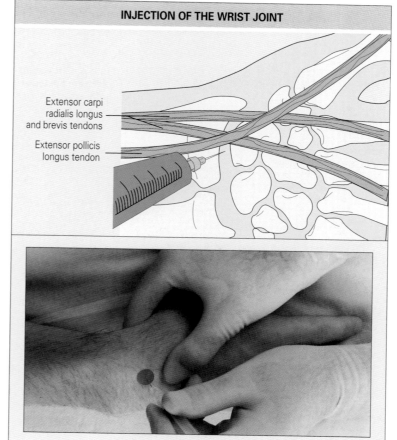

INJECTION OF THE WRIST JOINT

Extensor carpi radialis longus and brevis tendons

Extensor pollicis longus tendon

Fig. 6.5 Injection of the wrist joint.

Approach. Dorsal, just distal to Lister's tubercle (a bony prominence in the dorsal distal radius where the extensor pollicis longus bends radially to reach the thumb), just ulnar to the extensor pollicis longus tendon (Fig. 6.5). The wrist should be slightly palmar flexed to facilitate the procedure.

Precautions. There are no important neurovascular structures of concern at this site.

Complications. None.

Ganglia

Indications. Local corticosteroids are highly effective in the treatment of routine dorsal ganglia. Ganglia within the carpal tunnel that impinge on neurovascular structures, or those larger than 3cm in diameter, should be treated surgically.

Corticosteroid dose. Depends on the lesion; usually 15–20mg methylprednisone acetate (no. 20 or no. 18 needle; thinner needles may be clogged).

Approach. The needle is aimed to the center of the lesion, which is aspirated prior to injection. Ganglia contain a very viscous, translucent fluid. Fluids with other characteristics indicate that the lesion is not a ganglion; they should therefore be cultured and inspected for crystals.

Precautions. In wrist ganglia, rule out radial artery aneurysm, which mimics a ganglion. These lesions are expansile with the pulse, as opposed to the focal pulsation caused by a normal adjacent radial artery.

Complications. None.

THE ELBOW REGION

Elbow

Indications. Aspiration in acute arthritis, injection in RA and psoriatic arthritis.

Corticosteroid dose. 30–40mg methylprednisone acetate (no. 22, no. 25 or no. 27 needle). Aspiration should be attempted before injection. For aspiration alone use a no. 20 or no. 18 needle, depending on the suspected diagnosis.

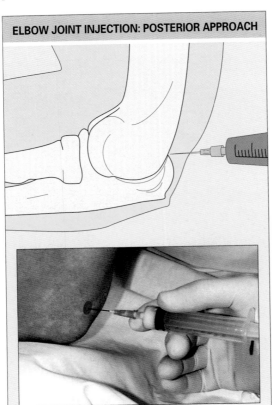

Fig. 6.6 Elbow joint injection: posterior approach.

ELBOW JOINT INJECTION: POSTERIOR APPROACH

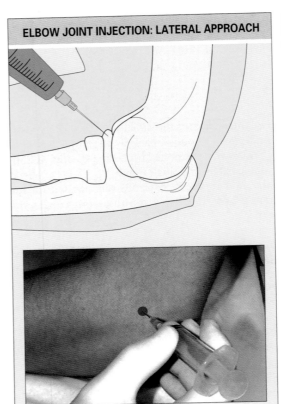

ELBOW JOINT INJECTION: LATERAL APPROACH

Fig. 6.7 Elbow joint injection: lateral approach.

Approach. There are three commonly used entries. For all entries the elbow is held flexed at 90°.

- *Posterior approach.* The depression in the midline between the two halves of the triceps tendon is palpated at the back of the elbow. The needle is then passed perpendicular to the skin into the olecranon fossa (Fig. 6.6).
- *Inferolateral approach.* The midpoint cleft between the olecranon tip and the lateral epicondyle is palpated. The needle is then inserted perpendicularly, aiming at the center of the joint.
- *Lateral approach.* The radiocapitellar joint may be entered from the side, just proximal to the radial head. The needle is passed tangentially between the two bones rather than directly (Fig. 6.7).

Precautions. There are no neurovascular structures in the vicinity.

Complications. None.

Olecranon bursa

Indications. For diagnosis of effusion and for treatment of aseptic bursitis (traumatic or idiopathic) in cases that are refractory to conservative treatment. A negative bursal fluid culture is required for the procedure to be performed.

Corticosteroid dose. 20mg methylprednisolone acetate (no. 22 needle). Aspiration should be attempted before injection. For aspiration alone use a no. 20 needle.

Approach. Lateral through normal skin, aiming at the center of the bursa.

Precautions. Taps at the tip of the bursa may create a chronic leak. Medial entries may damage the ulnar nerve.

Complications. Skin atrophy, pain on leaning and septic bursitis are recognized complications of the intrabursal administration of 20mg of triamcinolone hexacetonide[13]. The injection of 20mg of methylprednisolone acetate has not caused complications[14].

Note: In traumatic or idiopathic olecranon bursitis conservative treatment is recommended, namely avoiding leaning on the elbow for 3

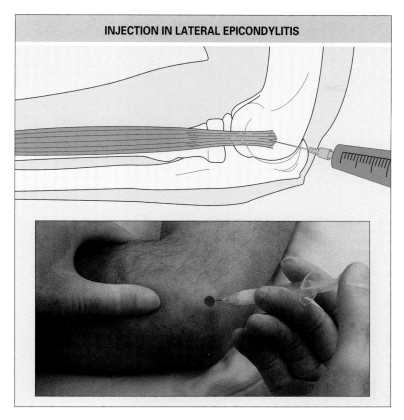

INJECTION IN LATERAL EPICONDYLITIS

Fig. 6.8 Injection in lateral epicondylitis. Injection of corticosteroid and local anesthetic into the common extensor tendon origin at the lateral humeral epicondyle.

months. Intrabursal corticosteroids may be tried in cases that fail to resolve.

Tennis elbow

Indications. Failure of conservative treatment. To shorten symptomatic period (long-term outcome is similar in injected and uninjected patients). To speed up recovery in high-performance athletes, although this is a controversial procedure.

Corticosteroid dose. 10–20mg methylprednisone acetate (no. 25 or no. 27 needle).

Approach. At the most tender point (Fig. 6.8). Pass the needle to periosteal contact and infiltrate with 2–3ml lidocaine. Failure to eradicate pain on resisted wrist dorsiflexion indicates the wrong injection site; reposition needle and reinfiltrate with lidocaine. The corticosteroid should be infiltrated deeply, at the tenoperiosteal junction.

Precautions. Avoid injecting too superficially.

Complications. Transient increase in pain in 20–40% of patients. Repeated corticosteroid infiltrations may result in chronic pain.

Note: Lack of improvement with lidocaine infiltration suggests an alternative diagnosis such as compressive neuropathy of the deep branch of the radial nerve or cervical radiculopathy.

THE SHOULDER REGION

Shoulder (glenohumeral joint)

Indications. Aspiration in acute arthritis; injection in RA, spondyloarthropathy, the initial stages of frozen shoulder; OA.

Corticosteroid dose. 40–60mg methylprednisone acetate (no. 22 needle). Aspiration should be attempted before injection. In the frozen shoulder, injection into the joint may be difficult on account of the capsular restriction. For aspiration alone use a no. 20 or larger needle.

Approach. Two entries are described, the posterior approach, which is preferred because it causes less apprehension and pain and the needle is farther away from neurovascular structures, and the anterior approach.

- *Posterior approach*. The patient should be sitting. The posterior margin of the acromion is palpated. The needle is then inserted posteroanteriorly 1cm below and 1cm medial to posterior corner of the acromion, aiming towards the coracoid process until bone is touched at the articular space (Fig. 6.9).
- *Anterior approach*. Again, the patient should be sitting (landmarks are lost in the recumbent position) with the arm hanging at the side of the body, elbow flexed 90°, and forearm in the sagittal plane. The needle is entered anteroposteriorly 1cm distal and 1cm lateral to the coracoid process (Fig. 6.10). Prior to each advancement of the needle some lidocaine is injected, so the needle is moving through an anesthetized front. Once the bone is touched (which happens soon after the capsular toughness is felt) the forearm is very gently and passively brought into internal rotation as the needle is pushed into the articular space.

Precautions. Use a chair with armrests; have an assistant present; watch for fainting.

Complications. Vasovagal syndrome. Prior to the procedure patients should be asked about previous fainting upon venipuncture or other minor procedures. Any such experience dictates a posterior approach. Misplaced anterior injections may encounter neurovascular structures.

Note: Glenohumeral joint aspiration may be difficult. In cases of acute arthritis in which a 'dry tap' results, the procedure should be repeated under fluoroscopic or echo control.

Subacromial bursa

Indications. Injection may be indicated in subacromial impingement and some cases of calcific tendinitis.

Corticosteroid dose. 30–40mg methylprednisone acetate (no. 22 or no. 25 needle).

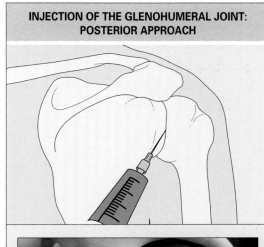

INJECTION OF THE GLENOHUMERAL JOINT: POSTERIOR APPROACH

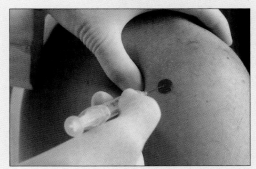

Fig. 6.9 Injection of the glenohumeral joint: posterior approach.

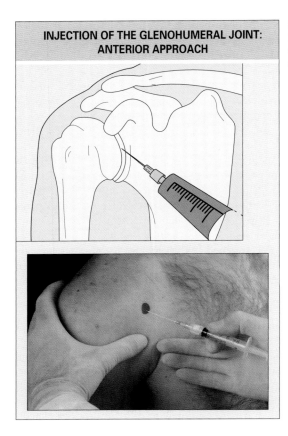

Fig. 6.10 Injection of the glenohumeral joint: anterior approach.

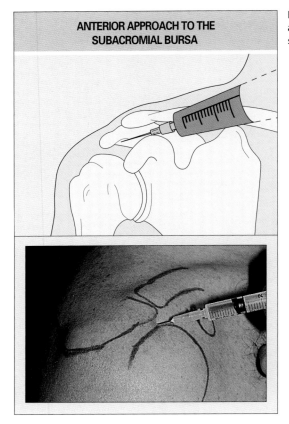

Fig. 6.12 Anterior approach to the subacromial bursa.

Approach. There are several possible entries. Two are described here, the posterolateral approach and the anterior approach. Adequate muscle relaxation is important, as it allows a better palpation of the gap between the acromion and humeral head.

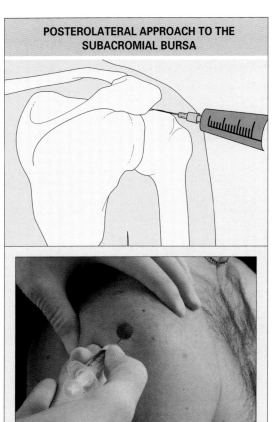

Fig. 6.11 Posterolateral approach to the subacromial bursa.

- *Posterolateral approach*. The needle is aimed anteromedially ensuring that it passes under the acromion (Fig. 6.11). Easy flow indicates bursal injection.
- Anterior approach. A front of lidocaine is required in this approach. The needle is aimed anteroposteriorly flush with the inferior surface of the acromion, 1cm lateral to the acromioclavicular joint (Fig. 6.12). Once the tough coracoacromial ligament is passed, tissue resistance to the lidocaine ceases. Easy flow indicates a bursal location of the needle.

Precautions. Use a chair with armrests; have an assistant present; watch for fainting.

Complications. None.

Note: Subacromial bursa injections are technically difficult. Only about 50% of injections fall on target. However, even if the bursal sac is not entered, the results may be excellent.

Acromioclavicular joint

Indications. Aspiration in acute arthritis, injection in OA, RA and spondyloarthropathy.

Corticosteroid dose. 10–20mg methylprednisone acetate (no. 23 butterfly or no. 22, no. 25 or no. 27 needle). Aspiration should be attempted before injection. For aspiration alone use a no. 20 needle.

Approach. Aim the needle perpendicular to the articular cleft; advance it by 0.5cm; aspirate or inject to distend joint.

Precautions. The procedure is difficult because the acromioclavicular joint is very narrow and has a partial meniscus. Septic acromioclavicular arthritis should be suspected in drug addicts and in patients who have, or have recently had, an indwelling subclavian catheter. If sepsis is suspected, corticosteroids should not be injected.

Complications. None.

Bicipital tendinitis

Indications. Bicipital tenosynovitis. This is a tenuous indication, as most cases of bicipital tendinitis are caused by subacromial impingement.

INJECTION INTO THE BICIPTAL GROOVE

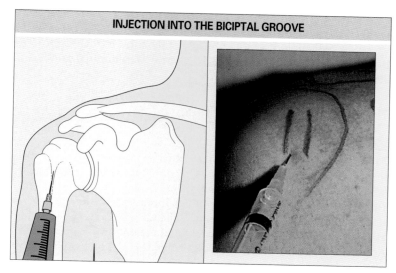

Fig. 6.13 Injection into the bicipital groove.

INJECTION OF THE HIP JOINT

Fig. 6.14
Injection of the hip joint.

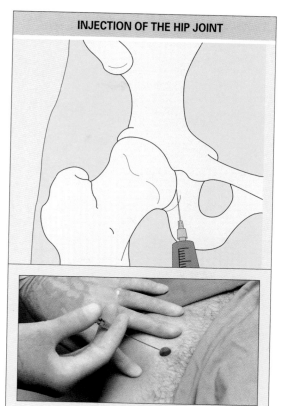

Corticosteroid dose. 15–20mg methylprednisone acetate (no. 22 or no. 25 needle).

Approach. The bicipital tendon should be palpated and a mark made on the skin. The needle is then directed somewhat superiorly, tangentially to the tendon (Fig. 6.13). A deeper injection is also possible if easy flow of fluid is obtained.

Precautions. Inject under low pressure.

Complications. The integrity of the biceps tendon may be already compromised by the usual underlying condition, subacromial impingement. Thus, the relatively common postinjection ruptures may reflect this underlying damage as much as a direct effect of the corticosteroid on the tendon. For this reason, I do not favor direct injection of the bicipital tendon sheath.

THE SPINE

Interspinous ligaments

Indications. Reactive arthritis, ankylosing spondylitis with interspinous ligament enthesopathy.

Corticosteroid dose. 15–20mg methylprednisone acetate (no. 25 needle).

Approach. Posteroanterior at the midline between the vertebral spinous processes; infiltrate ligament and its attachments. Several levels may have to be treated.

Precautions. This is an intraligamentous infiltration and a fair amount of pressure is required. There is no need to infiltrate deeper than 1.5cm; this precaution should keep the needle away from the dural sac.

Complications. None.

THE HIP REGION

Hip

Indications. Diagnosis of septic arthritis of the hip, including the differential diagnosis of septic arthritis versus aseptic loosening in a prosthetic hip.

Corticosteroid dose. Although the procedure is generally performed for diagnosis, there are proponents of hip injection in advanced hip osteoarthritis as a temporizing procedure.

Approach. Hip aspiration is performed with the patient lying supine and the affected leg in external rotation. The femoral neck projection follows a line bisecting the angle between the inguinal ligament and the femoral artery. The needle is inserted cephalad medially, one finger breadth lateral to the femoral artery and two finger breadths distal to the inguinal ligament (Fig. 6.14).

Precautions. The danger of injuring the femoral neurovascular bundle is averted by using an imaging procedure as control.

Complications. None.

Note: Hip aspiration belongs in the realm of orthopedics and radiology. The yield of the procedure can be maximized by using fluoroscopic, ultrasound or computed tomography guidance.

Iliopsoas bursa

Indications. Painful iliopsoas bursitis.

Corticosteroid dose. 30–40mg methylprednisone acetate mixed with 3ml of 1% lidocaine (no. 22 needle). Aspiration should be attempted before injection.

Approach. As for hip aspiration. Once the femoral head is contacted, the needle is withdrawn by the millimeter and small amounts of a contrast medium are injected until the iliopsoas bursa is outlined. At this time the corticosteroid is injected.

Precautions. The use of a contrast medium is essential for injecting intrabursally, rather than within the joint or in more superficial planes.

Complications. None.

Trochanteric 'bursa'

Indications. Trochanteric 'bursitis' syndrome.

Corticosteroid dose. 30–40mg methylprednisolone acetate mixed with 3ml of 1% lidocaine (no. 22 1.5 inch needle; a spinal needle may be required in obese patients).

Approach. With the patient lying on his/her opposite side, the greater trochanter is identified by distal to proximal palpation along the femur. The point of maximal tenderness is usually located at the posterior corner of the greater trochanter. The needle is inserted vertically to make periosteal contact (Fig. 6.15).

- *Step 1.* Lidocaine should then be infiltrated radially to cover the base of a cone 3cm in diameter, half on bone and half in the proximal soft tissues.

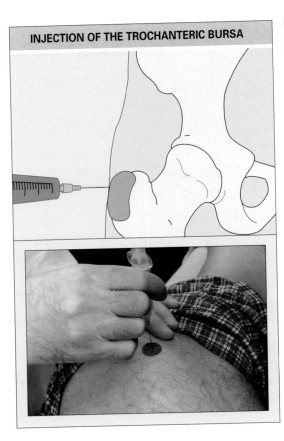

INJECTION OF THE TROCHANTERIC BURSA

Fig. 6.15 Injection of the trochanteric bursa.

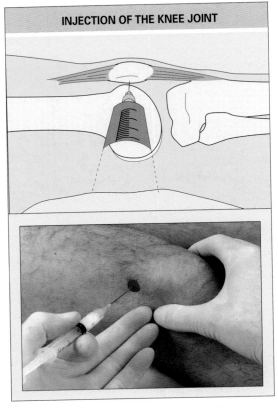

INJECTION OF THE KNEE JOINT

Fig. 6.16 Injection of the knee joint. Lateral approach.

- Step 2. If pain is relieved, the mixture of corticosteroid and lidocaine (to increase the volume of injection) is infiltrated in the same area. Experienced physicians may skip Step 1.

Precautions. The needle should be of sufficient length to reach the bone.
Complications. None.

Note: Rather than bursitis, this process represents a stress tendinopathy at the gluteus medium and minimus insertion. The cause of the excessive pull should be sought (foot, knee, hip or back disorder, a discrepant leg length, increased tension of the iliotibial band) and addressed to achieve sustained relief.

THE KNEE REGION

Knee

Indications. For diagnosis in any joint effusion. For corticosteroid injection in RA, spondyloarthropathies, OA, occasionally in crystal-induced synovitis.
Corticosteroid dose. 40–60mg methylprednisone acetate (no. 22 needle). Aspiration should be attempted before injection. For aspiration alone use a no. 20 or no. 18 needle, depending on the clinical suspicion.
Approach. Lateral, aiming needle to the patellar undersurface mid-distance between the upper and lower poles of the patella (Fig. 6.16). A lateral approach is preferred because a thick medial intra-articular fat pad may result in a 'dry tap' in some patients. There are, however, many possible entries to the knee and the choice is very personal.
Precautions. Beware of superimposed septic arthritis in RA patients. Postpone the injection of an acutely inflamed joint until a negative synovial fluid culture result becomes available.
Complications. None.

Note: If synovial fluid analysis has not been performed, any fluid removed during the procedure should be studied for cell count, differential, crystals and culture. Because corticosteroid crystals remain in joints for weeks and even months, an erroneous diagnosis of gout or pseudogout can be made in a previously injected patient.

Baker's cyst

Aspiration or injection of the cyst is unnecessary. In adults, Baker's cysts develop in connecting gastrocnemius–semimembranosus bursae and depend for their persistence and growth on excessive synovial fluid produced in the knee. Baker's cysts are best treated by correcting the causative knee disorder with systemic treatment, corticosteroid injection or surgery such as arthroscopic meniscectomy or synovectomy.

Anserine 'bursitis'

Indications. The syndrome of anserine bursitis.
Corticosteroid dose. 20–30mg methylprednisone acetate mixed with 2–3ml of lidocaine (no. 22 needle).
Approach. The injection site is best determined by following the medial tendinous border of the thigh (semitendinosus tendon), with the knee in semiflexion, to the tibia, where a mark is placed. The knee is then brought to extension and the needle is entered perpendicularly to tibial contact. An area 3cm in diameter is infiltrated adjacent to the periosteum.
Precautions. Paresthesias extending along the medial leg indicate engagement of the saphenous nerve; reposition needle.
Complications. None.

Note: Because anserine bursitis is almost always secondary (genu valgum, patellofemoral OA, etc.) the condition is expected to recur unless the primary process has been addressed. A vigorous program of isometric quadriceps exercises should be initiated at once.

THE ANKLE AND FOOT

Ankle

Indications. As for the knee.
Corticosteroid dose. 40–60mg methylprednisone acetate (no. 22 or no. 25 needle). Aspiration should be attempted before injection. For aspiration alone use a no. 20 needle.

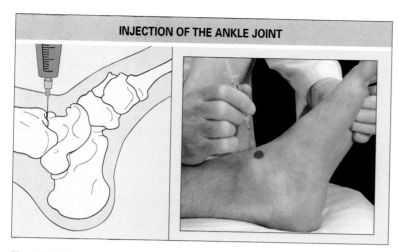

INJECTION OF THE ANKLE JOINT

Fig. 6.17 Injection of the ankle joint.

Approach. With the patient supine on the examination table, seek the cleft between tibia and talus by gently flexing and extending the foot. Insert the needle vertically medial to the anterior tibialis tendon (Fig. 6.17).

Precautions. Avoid the dorsalis pedis artery.

Complications. None.

Subtalar joint

Indications. As for the knee.

Corticosteroid dose: 20–30mg methylprednisone acetate (no. 22 needle). Aspiration should be attempted before injection. For aspiration alone use a no. 20 needle.

Approach. By gently inverting and everting the foot find the soft cleft (sinus tarsi) anterior to the lateral malleolus. Insert the needle perpendicularly towards the tip of the medial malleolus (Fig. 6.18). Aspiration of fluid proves an articular insertion. Inject under low pressure.

Precautions. None.

Complications. None.

Posterior tibialis tendon sheath

Indications. Posterior tibialis tenosynovitis in RA and spondyloarthropathies; tarsal tunnel syndrome.

Corticosteroid dose. 20–30mg methylprednisolone acetate (no. 22 or no. 25 needle).

Approach. Patient lies supine with the injected leg resting on the contralateral knee. Have patient invert the foot to identify the posterior tib-

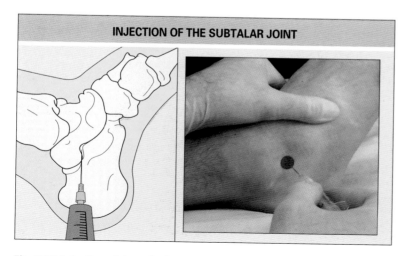

INJECTION OF THE SUBTALAR JOINT

Fig. 6.18 Injection of the subtalar joint.

ialis tendon. The needle is inserted at a 45° angle, three finger breadths proximal to the tip of the medial malleolus and flush with the posterior border of tibia, to a depth of about 1.5cm. Inject under low pressure. Fluid may be felt distending the sheath.

Precautions. Aspirate first to make sure that the posterior tibial artery has not been punctured. Plantar paresthesias indicate engagement of the posterior tibial nerve. Avoid intratendinous injection by assuring free flow of the corticosteroid. *This procedure should only be performed by rheumatologists, orthopedists or other health professionals with a thorough knowledge of anatomy.*

Complications. The posterior tibialis tendon is prone to spontaneous rupture in RA. A misplaced (intratendinous) injection enhances this tendency.

Retrocalcaneal bursa

Indications. Refractory Achilles tendon enthesitis in the spondyloarthropathies; RA.

Corticosteroid dose. 15–20mg methylprednisone acetate (no. 22, no. 25 or no. 27 needle or butterfly). Aspiration should be attempted before injection. Presence of fluid (usually a trace) proves intrabursal location. *Do not inject if the intrabursal position of the needle cannot be shown.*

Approach. Patient lies prone on examination table with foot outside mattress. Allow calf relaxation.

- *Posterior approach.* The needle is advanced vertically, transtendinous, aiming at the posterior superior calcaneal angle. Touch the bone and back up 1mm.
- *Lateral approach.* An alternative is a lateral approach. Bursal pressures may be decreased by keeping the foot in a slight plantar flexion.

Precautions. Do not inject large volumes; high pressures produce back flow as the needle is removed. The distal leg and foot should be placed in a cast for 10 days to achieve maximal anti-inflammatory effect. *This procedure should only be performed by rheumatologists, orthopedists, or other health professionals with a thorough knowledge of anatomy.*

Complications. Tendon rupture is possible and more than one reinjection is discouraged. A period of 2–3 weeks should elapse between the initial injection and the first (and last) reinjection.

Plantar fascia calcaneal enthesis

Indications. Refractory plantar fasciitis in the spondyloarthropathies.

Corticosteroid dose. 20–30mg methylprednisone acetate diluted with 2ml of lidocaine (no. 22 needle).

Approach. Medial, needle parallel to the plantar skin 2cm deep to plantar surface. Aim the needle into the medial plantar tubercle of the calcaneus. Resilience indicates a fascial location. Relocate the needle and inject deeply and superficially to the fibrous fascia.

Precautions. *This procedure should only be performed by rheumatologists, orthopedists or other health professionals with a thorough knowledge of anatomy.*

Complications. Repeated infiltrations result in fat atrophy and pressure plantar heel pain. Discourage more than one reinjection (2–3 weeks after the initial injection).

Morton's neuroma

Indications. Morton's neuroma.

Corticosteroid dose. 20–30mg methylprednisolone acetate mixed with 1ml lidocaine (no. 22 or no. 25 needle).

Approach. Dorsal between metatarsal heads. The needle must be advanced plantarly about 2cm and pass through the intermetatarsal ligament, which is indicated by tough fibrous resistance.

Precautions. Inject under low pressure. *This procedure should only be performed by rheumatologists, orthopedists or other health professionals with a thorough knowledge of anatomy.*

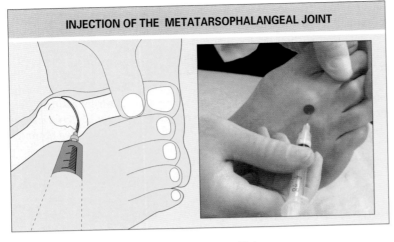

INJECTION OF THE METATARSOPHALANGEAL JOINT

Fig. 6.19 Injection of the metatarsophalangeal joint.

Metatarsophalangeal joints

Indications. Aspiration for the diagnosis of gout (usually the first metatarsophalangeal). Injection in hallux rigidus, RA and the spondyloarthropathies.

Corticosteroid dose. 10–20mg methylprednisolone acetate (no. 22, no. 25 or no. 27 needle). Attempt aspiration before injection. For aspiration alone use a no. 22 needle.

Approach. Dorsal, lateral or medial to extensor tendon. Slight passive plantar flexion facilitates the procedure (Fig. 6.19).

Precautions. None.

Complications. None.

Trigger points in the myofascial syndromes

Indications. Acute cases if pressure on a point or nodule consistently reproduces pain.

Corticosteroid dose. 3–5ml of lidocaine or bupivacaine (no. 22 needle). Do not use corticosteroids.

Approach. Aim at a tender point or the center of a nodule, which should be infiltrated radially throughout the indurated area.

Precautions. None.

Complications. None.

Complications. None are expected; up to two reinjections 2–3 weeks apart are allowed.

REFERENCES

1. Cohen AS, Goldenberg D. Synovial fluid. In Cohen AS, ed. Laboratory diagnostic procedures in the rheumatic diseases, 3rd ed. Orlando, FL: Grune & Stratton; 1985: 1–54.
2. Schumacher HR Jr, Reginato AJ. Atlas of synovial fluid analysis and crystal identification. Philadelphia, PA: Lea & Febiger; 1991: 1–257.
3. Canoso JJ, Yood RA. Reaction of superficial bursae in response to specific disease stimuli. Arthritis Rheum 1979; 22: 1361–1364.
4. Aesbach A, Mekhail NA. Common nerve blocks in chronic pain management. Anesthesiol Clin North Am 2000; 18: 1–18.
5. Carette S, Marcoux S, Truchon R et al. Facet joint injection of corticosteroids in chronic low back pain: a randomized double-blind placebo controlled trial. N Engl J Med. 1991; 325: 1002–1007.
6. Carette S, Leclaire R, Marcoux S et al. Epidural corticosteroid injections for sciatica due to herniated nucleus pulposus. N Engl J Med 1997; 336: 1634–1640.
7. McCarty DJ, Harman JG, Grassanovich JL, Qian C. Treatment of rheumatoid joint inflammation with intrasynovial triamcinolone hexacetonide. J Rheumatol 1995; 22: 1631–1635.
8. Thumboo J, O'Duffy JD. A prospective study of the safety of joint and soft tissue aspirations and injections in patients taking warfarin sodium. Arthritis Rheum 1998; 41: 736–739.
9. Hollander JL. Intrasynovial steroid injections. In: Hollander JL, McCarty DL Jr, eds. Arthritis and allied conditions. Philadelphia, PA: Lea & Febiger; 1972: 517–534.
10. Wang J-J, Ho S-T, Lee S-C et al. Intraarticular triamcinolone acetonide for pain control after arthroscopic knee surgery. Anesth Analg 1998; 87: 1113–1116.
11. Neustadt DH. Local corticosteroid injection therapy in soft tisssue rheumatic conditions of the hand and wrist. Arthritis Rheum 1991; 34: 923–926.
12. Murphy D, Failla JM, Koniuch MP. Steroid versus placebo injection for trigger finger. J Hand Surg 1995; 20A: 628–631.
13. Lambert MA, Morton RJ, Sloan JP. Controlled study of the use of local steroid injection in the treatment of trigger finger and thumb. J Hand Surg 1992; 17B: 69–70.
14. Kay NRM. A safe, reliable method of carpal tunnel injection. J Hand Surg 1992; 17A: 1160–1161.
15. Dammers JWHH, Veering MM, Vermeulen M. Injection with methylprednisolone proximal to the carpal tunnel: randomised double blind trial. Br Med J 1999; 319: 884–886.
16. Smith DL, McAfee JH, Lucas LM et al. Treatment of nonspecific olecranon bursitis. A controlled, blinded prospective trial. Arch Intern Med 1989; 149: 2527–2530.
17. Larsson L-G, Baum J. The syndrome of anserina bursitis: An overlooked diagnosis. Arthritis Rheum 1985; 28: 1062–1065.
18. Moore JS. De Quervain's tenosynovitis. J Occup Environ Med 1997; 39: 990–1002.
19. Hay EM, Paterson SM, Lewis M et al. Pragmatic randomised trial of local corticosteroid injection and naproxen for treatment of lateral epicondylitis of elbow in primary care. Br Med J 1999; 319: 964–968.
20. Van der Windt DAWM, Koes BW, Deville W et al. Effectiveness of corticosteroid injections versus physiotherapy for treatment of painful stiff shoulder in primary care: randomised trial. Br Med J 1998; 317: 1292–1296.
21. Jones DS. Suprascapular nerve block for the treatment of frozen shoulder in primary care: a randomized trial. Br J Clin Pract 1999; 49: 39–41.
22. Dahan TH. Double blind randomized clinical trial examining the efficacy of bupivacaine suprascapular nerve blocks in frozen shoulder. J Rheumatol 2000; 27: 1464–1469.
23. Fortin L, Bélanger R. Bursitis of the iliopsoas: four cases with pain as the only clinical indicator. J Rheumatol 1995; 22: 1971–1973.
24. Canoso JJ, Wohlgethan JR, Newberg AH, Goldsmith MR. Aspiration of the retrocalcaneal bursa. Ann Rheum Dis 1984; 43: 308–312.
25. Greenfield J, Rea J Jr, Ilfeld FW. Morton's interdigital neuroma. Indications for treatment by local injections versus surgery. Clin Orthop 1984; 185: 142–144.
26. Emkey RD, Lindsay R, Lyssy J et al. The systemic effect of intraarticular administration of corticosteroids on markers of bone formation and bone resorption in patients with rheumatoid arthritis. Arthritis Rheum 1996; 39: 277–282.
27. Lazarevic MB, Skosey JL, Djordjevic-Denic G et al. Reduction of cortisol levels after single intra-articular and intramuscular steroid injection. Am J Med 1995; 99: 370–373.
28. Huppertz HI, Pfuller H. Transient supression of endogenous cortisol production after intraarticular steroid therapy for chronic arthritis in children. J Rheumatol 1997; 24: 1833–1837.
29. Wicki J, Droz M, Cirafici L, Valloton MB. Acute adrenal crisis in a patient treated with intraarticular steroid therapy. J Rheumatol 2000; 27: 510–511.
30. Mace S, Vadas P, Pruzanski W. Anaphylactic shock induced by intraarticular injection of methylprednisolone acetate. J Rheumatol 1997; 24: 1191–1194.

7 Skin and rheumatic disease

David L George

- Skin lesions often provide valuable diagnostic clues for a number of rheumatic diseases
- The spectrum of dermatoarthropathies ranges from primary immunologic syndromes to infectious, metabolic and neoplastic disorders
- The principal types of skin lesion seen in patients with arthritis are exanthems, papulosquamous rashes, nodules, vesicles and bullae, ulcers and purpura

INTRODUCTION

The diagnosis of rheumatic diseases is commonly based on pattern recognition. The skin is the most accessible organ and often provides valuable diagnostic clues that may lead to a specific diagnosis or limit the list of possibilities[1,2]. For example, a diagnosis of psoriatic arthritis might be based upon the presence of distal interphalangeal joint synovitis, erythematous scaling plaques over extensor surfaces and nail pitting. Conversely, unrelated skin lesions may occasionally mislead the clinician. For example, incorrect diagnosis of systemic lupus erythematosus (SLE) might be made in a patient with a symmetric polyarthritis who manifests the facial rash of acne rosacea.

Pattern recognition of skin lesions is based upon the type (Table 7.1), configuration, distribution and evolution of the lesions. Selective laboratory techniques may further assist diagnosis. This chapter focuses on the cutaneous diseases most relevant in patients with rheumatic complaints (Table 7.2) and emphasizes characteristic features that will allow the physician to distinguish those cutaneous lesions commonly associated with musculoskeletal syndromes from entities with which they are often confused.

EXANTHEMS

An exanthem is a diffuse rash with fever and systemic symptoms, which is usually due to a viral, allergic or primary immunologic illness but certain bacterial infections must be considered.

Dermatomyositis, SLE, Lyme disease and rheumatic fever may have characteristic cutaneous lesions in association with acute systemic disease and are discussed later in this chapter. Characteristic exanthems are also seen in Still's disease and Kawasaki's disease (Fig. 7.1).

The patient with Still's disease develops discrete pink to salmon-colored macules or slightly elevated papules several millimeters in size on the trunk and extremities, although lesions may occur on the face and rarely on the palms and soles[3,4]. The lesions are maximal during episodes of fever and are prominent in areas of minor skin trauma (Köebner's phenomenon). Still's lesions are irregular in shape and have no associated purpura or vesicles. They are asymptomatic or only mildly pruritic. The lesions do not spread and last only minutes to hours. When the rash recurs, lesions are in new locations. No oral lesions accompany the rash. Such a rash in the presence of quotidian

TABLE 7.1 IMPORTANT DERMATOLOGIC TERMS	
Macule	Flat lesion differentiated from surrounding skin by its color
Papule/nodule	Raised solid lesion less than/greater than 1cm in diameter respectively
Vesicle/bulla	Raised fluid-filled lesion less than/greater than 0.5cm respectively
Pustule	Vesicle filled with purulent exudate
Wheal (urticaria)	Pale, erythematous papule or plaque resulting from upper dermal edema
Ulcer	Lesion resulting from destruction of the epidermis and at least the upper dermis
Petechia/purpura	Intradermal hemorrhage less than/greater than 3mm in diameter respectively
Desquamation (scaling)	Abnormal shedding or accumulation of the stratum corneum
Sclerosis	Hardening or induration of the skin
Pathergy (Köebnerization)	Induction of skin lesion in location of minor trauma

fever, diffuse palpable lymphadenopathy and polyarthritis is diagnostic of Still's disease.

Kawasaki's disease presents with a polymorphous rash (morbilliform, scarlatiniform, pustular or erythema-multiforme-like rash), which is notable for early erythema of the palms and soles with desquamation days later, along with scarlet-fever-like oral mucosal changes, including strawberry tongue, dry, red, fissured lips and conjunctival congestion[5]. The rash is often prominent in the diaper area. Such a rash in the setting of prolonged fever, pronounced lymphadenopathy and polyarthralgias or arthritis in a child would strongly favor the diagnosis of Kawasaki's disease.

Bacterial infections with exanthems include acute and chronic meningococcemia. A non-specific, measles-like eruption may antedate the petechial and purpuric lesions of acute meningococcemia. This diagnosis should be considered in a child or young adult who presents with prostration, fever and morbilliform rash. Early polyarthralgia or polyarthritis during the bacteremic phase has been observed and reactive pauciarthritis may occur days later[6]. Periodic fever, maculopapular skin rash and arthritis may occur with chronic meningococcemia[7]. Lesions are often distributed near involved joints or over areas of pressure. They are variable in appearance but are most often macules or papules that later develop central hemorrhage. Petechiae, pustules and erythema-nodosum-like lesions may also be seen.

Rocky Mountain spotted fever, a rickettsial disease, may have a maculopapular eruption before becoming purpuric. Diagnosis is

	Lesion type					
Disorder	Macular/papular	Papulonodular	Vesicular/bullous	Pustular	Ulcerating	Petechial/purpura
Primary immune disease						
Systemic lupus erythematosus	•	•	•		•	•
Scleroderma		•			•	
Dermatomyositis	•	•				•
Rheumatoid arthritis		•			•	•
Still's disease	•					
Sjögren's syndrome					•	
Erythema nodosum		•				
Pyoderma gangrenosum				•	•	
Sarcoid	•	•				
Inflammatory bowel disease	•		•	•	•	•
Psoriatic arthritis	•			•		
Reiter's syndrome	•			•		
Behçet's syndrome	•	•	•	•	•	•
Multicentric reticulohistiocytosis		•				
Serum sickness	•					•
Neutrophilic dermatoses	•	•	•	•	•	
Kawasaki's disease	•		•	•		
Necrotizing venulitis	•	•	•			•
Polyarteritis nodosa		•			•	•
Wegener's granulomatosis	•	•	•		•	•
Lymphomatoid granulomatosis	•	•			•	
Infections						
Neisserial infections	•		•	•		•
Rheumatic fever	•					•
Subacute bacterial endocarditis						•
Hydradenitis suppurative/acne conglobata				•		
Syphilis	•	•				
Lyme disease	•				•	
Rickettsial infections	•		•			
Viral infections	•		•	•		•
Fungal infections			•		•	
Mycobacterial infections	•	•			•	
Other conditions						
Diabetes mellitus		•	•		•	
Thyroid disease	•	•				
Hyperlipidemia (type II)		•				
Crystal disease		•				
Neoplasms	•	•			•	•

TABLE 7.2 TYPES OF CUTANEOUS LESION OBSERVED IN DISEASES WITH RHEUMATIC EXPRESSION

aided by a characteristic evolution that begins in the distal parts of extremities and spreads centrally. This infection is often associated with arthralgias and myalgias, and rarely with severe muscle weakness, but not generally with arthritis[8,9]. Secondary syphilis should be considered in the sexually active patient with fever and diffuse maculopapular eruption, especially that involving palms and soles[10]. Toxic shock syndrome may express a scarlatiniform eruption similar to that of Kawasaki's disease, and also a reactive arthropathy accompanied by fever and hypotension secondary to toxin-producing staphylococcal infection[11]. *Streptobacillus moniliformis* infection manifests as a non-specific, diffuse maculopapular eruption with arthritis of large joints that occurs within a few days to 1 week after a bite from an infected rat or ingestion of contaminated rat excretions[12]. Where endemic, lepto-spirosis should be considered in the patient with unexplained fever, arthralgia and myalgia. Erythematous macules over the tibia are an important diagnostic clue[13].

Viral infections[14] and drug reactions are the illnesses most commonly confused with exanthem-associated primary rheumatic disorders. Some viral rashes have a characteristic pattern and course. Rubella rash classically begins on the face and spreads rapidly to the neck, arms, trunk and legs, and resolves in the same order. The rash is of short duration, only 2–3 days, and arthritis usually develops as the rash fades. Human parvovirus B19 infection (erythema infectiosum) may be associated with a similar rash; the slapped cheek appearance and a lace-like body rash are more common in children than in adults[15]. Hepatitis B virus may commonly be associated with polyarthritis and rash but, in addition to erythematous papules, urticarial lesions are commonly observed. The presence of an enanthema, petechiae or vesicles and localized lymphadenopathy may also suggest a viral illness, although mononucleosis, cytomegalovirus infection and acute human immunodeficiency virus infection[16] may be associated with diffuse lymphadenopathy and diffuse maculopapular rash. Arthralgias rather than frank arthritis are usually seen with these illnesses.

Drug eruptions usually develop almost simultaneously over the entire body, although the intensity may increase with time. The initial appearance may be in the flexure creases before becoming generalized. Fever generally resolves within 3 days of stopping the drug. Erythema multiforme[17] may result from drug allergy or infection. The skin findings

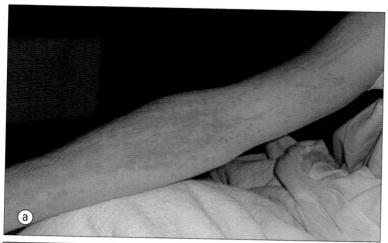

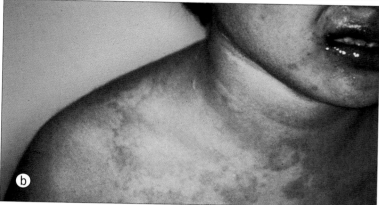

Fig. 7.1 Exanthems. (a) Still's rash. (b) Kawasaki's disease. (© 1972–1999 American College of Rheumatology Clinical Slide Collection. Used with permission.)

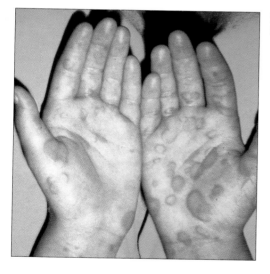

Fig. 7.2 Erythema multiforme.

Rare disorders with rash, fever and arthritis include familial Mediterranean fever[19], in which a characteristic erysipelas-like rash may exist on the lower extremity in conjunction with an acute monoarthritis and fever. Angioimmunoblastic lymphadenopathy[20] should be considered in the adult with fever, generalized morbilliform rash, polyarthritis and diffuse lymphadenopathy. Schnitzler's syndrome includes chronic urticaria, intermittent fever, bone pain, arthralgia or arthritis, and monoclonal IgM gammopathy[21].

PAPULOSQUAMOUS LESIONS

Rheumatic diseases notable for papulosquamous lesions include psoriatic arthritis, reactive arthritis and lupus erythematosus (subacute and discoid). Scale formation in patients with inflammatory cutaneous papules or plaques results from accumulation of the stratum corneum.

The characteristic lesions of psoriasis are sharply demarcated inflammatory plaques with a silvery scale, most commonly present on extensor surfaces of the elbows and knees as well as the scalp, ears and presacral area (Fig. 7.3). Nail abnormalities are common. Pustular psoriasis results from a greater collection of neutrophils. The lesions of keratoderma blennorrhagicum and pustular psoriasis are histologically identical but patients with reactive arthritis usually have lesions restricted to the palms and soles (Fig. 7.4) and are identified by other clinical characteristics, such as conjunctivitis and urethritis.

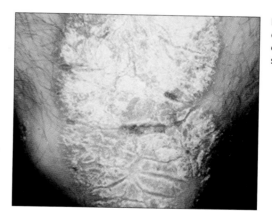

Fig. 7.3 Psoriatic plaque on elbow with characteristic silver scale.

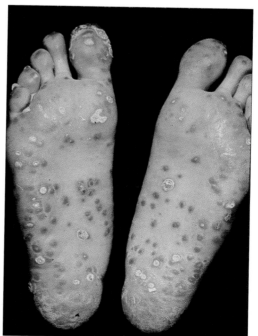

Fig. 7.4 Keratodermia blennorrhagicum on the soles of a patient with reactive arthritis.

are characterized by round erythematous lesions which are symmetrically distributed, involving the palms, soles and oral mucosa. The presence of target lesions is helpful diagnostically (Fig. 7.2). The milder form of the disease, erythema multiforme minor, may be associated with fever and polyarthralgias. High fever and polyarthritis are common in erythema multiforme major (Stevens–Johnson syndrome), and this illness must be distinguished from Kawasaki's disease. Inspection of the oral mucosa may help in this clinical differential diagnosis (see Oral Lesions, below).

Other potentially serious drug reactions associated with joint symptoms include hypersensitivity and serum-sickness-like reactions[18].

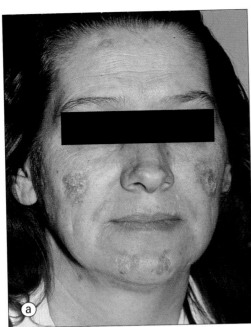

Fig. 7.5 Discoid lupus involving (a) the face and (b) the ear.

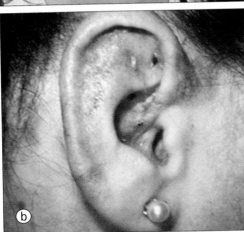

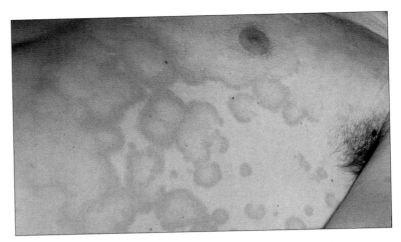

Fig. 7.6 Erythema marginatum. (© 1972-1999 American College of Rheumatology Clinical Slide Collection. Used with permission.)

secondary to gold or D-penicillamine therapy, and pityriasis rosea may be seen secondary to gold or antimalarial drug therapy[24]. Diffuse papulosquamous lesions and arthralgias may occur in T-cell lymphoma[25] or secondary syphyllis[10].

ANNULAR LESIONS

Three rheumatic illnesses, rheumatic fever, SCLE and Lyme disease, are suggested by characteristic annular or arciform skin lesions in which the central portion has a distinctive appearance compared with the border.

In rheumatic fever, migratory polyarthritis may be accompanied by erythema marginatum, an annular eruption with a round or serpiginous border that may be flat or slightly raised and is usually present on the trunk or proximal extremities (Fig. 7.6). Lesions migrate rapidly over a period of hours. The rash typically develops in crops lasting hours to several days[26].

The annular variety of SCLE (Fig. 7.7) is non-migratory and has the same distribution as the papulosquamous variety[23]. Raised, erythematous, plaque-like lesions with central clearing have been described in Japanese patients with anti-Ro-antibody-positive Sjögren's syndrome[28].

The primary lesion of erythema migrans, which is nearly pathognomonic of acute Lyme disease[29], is at the site of the tick bite, most often the axilla, groin, thigh or buttocks (Fig. 7.8). The primary lesion migrates outward, much more slowly than that of erythema marginatum, and reaches an average size of 15cm. The central area may

Scale formation is also a prominent feature of discoid lupus (Fig. 7.5) and the papulosquamous variety of subacute cutaneous lupus erythematosus (SCLE). In addition to an adherent scale, characteristic features of discoid lesions include follicular plugging, hyper- or hypopigmentation, atrophy (loss of skin markings), sclerosis and telangiectasia. Lesions are most common on the face (but sparing the nasolabial folds), scalp, neck and ears. Lesions may occur elsewhere on the body only if also present above the neck[22,23]. Lesions of SCLE do not reveal signs of follicular plugging, pigmentary change or scarring and are distributed primarily on the shoulders, the extensor surface of the forearm and the upper back and upper chest. The face and scalp are generally spared and lesions below the waist are rare. In the papulosquamous form of SCLE, papules may commonly enlarge and coalesce, leading to a reticulate pattern. Histopathologic studies are diagnostic, although immunofluorescence is not routinely positive in SCLE[23].

Lichen planus and pityriasis rosea may be confused with papulosquamous rashes due to rheumatic disease but have features that allow their differentiation. Lichen planus is a pruritic eruption with violet-colored, polygonal, flat-topped lesions with thin white scales often present on flexor aspects of the wrists and ankles, the presacral area, glans penis and mucous membranes. Pityriasis rosea is manifested by erythematous papules with thin scaly borders following truncal lines of cleavage (Christmas tree pattern). The initial lesion, or herald spot, is larger than subsequent lesions. Lichen planus may occur

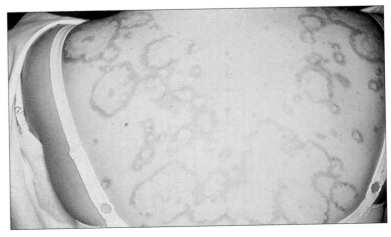

Fig. 7.7 Annular variety of subacute cutaneous lupus. (With permission from Sontheimer et al.[27])

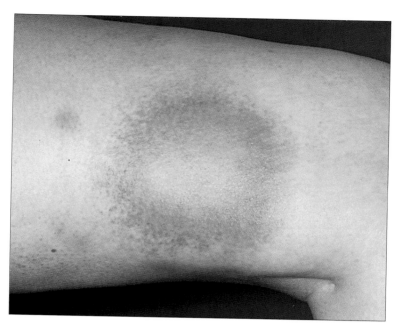

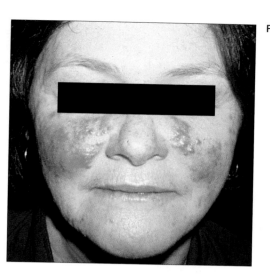

Fig. 7.9 Acne rosacea.

Fig. 7.8 Erythema migrans. This annular, erythematous lesion developed over a period of 3 weeks around the site of a tick bite. (With permission from McKee.[30])

reveal blue discoloration, vesicles, purpura, necrosis or ulceration. A target lesion may form. Secondary lesions are smaller, migrate less and have less indurated centers. Erythema migrans spares the palms, soles and oral mucosa and commonly accompanies constitutional symptoms, headache and arthralgias. Recurrent erythema migrans may be coincident with pauciarthritis.

Other distinctive annular lesions include elastosis perforans serpiginosa, which is seen as a side effect of D-penicillamine therapy. Annular rashes may be observed in cutaneous granuloma annulare, cutaneous T-cell lymphoma, secondary syphilis, sarcoid, erythema multiforme and psoriasis[31], and the clinical picture and histopathology are distinctive.

FACIAL LESIONS AND PHOTOSENSITIVE SKIN RASH

In a patient with polyarthritis, photosensitive dermatitis involving the face prompts consideration of a diagnosis of SLE and, less commonly, dermatomyositis.

As described above, discoid lupus has a virtually diagnostic appearance and distribution. Facial lesions that mimic discoid lesions[32–34] are described in Table 7.3. In addition to the clinical features, which may help discriminate these lesions, histopathology and immunofluorescence studies may be required[23]. It should be noted that some immunofluorescent deposits may be found at the dermal–epidermal junction in polymorphous light eruption, Jessner's lymphocytic eruption, seborrheic dermatitis and acne rosacea (Fig. 7.9), and that early discoid lesions may lack this finding.

The malar rash of acute lupus is a photosensitive dermatitis that may be flat (malar blush) or raised (butterfly eruption)[22]. There is no atrophy or sclerosis and little scale. Nasolabial folds are not involved. This rash may resolve over hours or it may persist for days. The facial rash of acute lupus may be more widespread than the malar area. The chin is often involved but the area below the chin is spared. Features of dermatomyositis rash (Fig. 7.10) that might allow discrimination from lupus include occasional nasolabial fold involvement, prominent heliotrope and extrafacial involvement including erythema over the interphalangeal joints rather than the extensor surface of skin between phalangeal joints (Fig. 7.11), erythema following the course of extensor tendons and scaling and fissuring of lateral aspects of the fingers (mechanic's hands). The presence of papules with erythema over the interphalangeal joints, Gottron's papules, is pathognomonic for dermatomyositis[35].

TABLE 7.3 FACIAL LESIONS – MIMICS OF DISCOID LUPUS	
Diagnosis	**Discriminating features**
Polymorphous light eruption (occasional)	Large papule/edematous plaque without follicular plugging, scar or telangiectases following early-season sun exposure
Benign lymphocytic infiltration of Jessner (rare)	Red, slightly raised discoid appearance without follicular plugging or scar
Seborrheic dermatitis (common)	Erythema with yellow greasy scale involving nasolabial folds, eyebrows and hairline
Acne rosacea (common)	Erythematous papules and plaques involving nasolabial folds; presence of pustules
Tinea faciei (occasional)	Localized dermatophyte infection; scale present but no follicular plugging; positive fungal scraping; may coexist with discoid lupus lesion
Lupus vulgaris tuberculosus (rare)	Solitary papule/nodule slowly extends leaving atrophy and scar but not follicular plugging; smooth, yellow-brown (apple jelly) nodules at periphery by diascopy
Lupus pernio sarcoida (rare)	Small nodules on the nose or nodules/plaques on cheeks and ears associated with upper respiratory involvement and pulmonary fibrosis

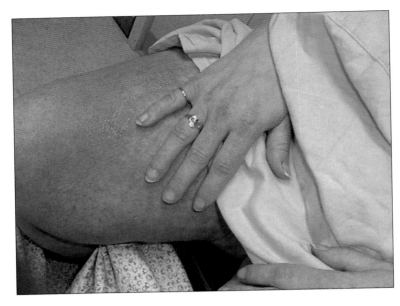

Fig. 7.10 Dermatomyositis.

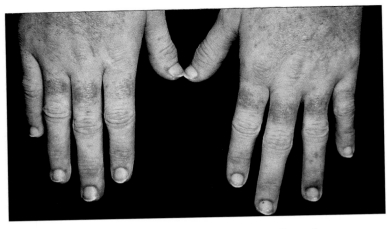

Fig. 7.11 Acute lupus (hand). (© 1972-1999 American College of Rheumatology Clinical Slide Collection. Used with permission.)

Misdiagnosis of acute lupus may occur in patients expressing other photosensitive eruptions[36,37] and in those with conditions that produce vascular dilation (Table 7.4). Facial lesions of erysipelas (Fig. 7.12), porphyria cutanea tarda, and human parvovirus infection[39] have rarely been confused with the malar rash of lupus. Clinical history and examination are usually sufficient to discriminate these processes, but rarely histopathology and immunofluorescence are indicated.

URTICARIA

Diseases that might be considered in the setting of urticaria and arthritis include hepatitis B infection[40], serum sickness[41], primary urticarial vasculitis, mononucleosis and C1q complement deficiency[42].

Leukocytoclastic vasculitis is the pathologic process in a small number of patients with urticaria (urticarial vasculitis)[43]. Such urticaria is more likely to be associated with symptoms of burning or pain rather than pruritus, tends to resolve more slowly (generally in not less than 4 hours and up to about 72 hours) and may have a purpuric component. Secondary skin changes of pigmentation, scaling or purpura may be found after resolution of the urticaria.

Arthralgias may be observed in chronic urticaria resulting from processes other than leukocytoclastic vasculitis but arthritis generally suggests underlying vasculitis. The erythrocyte sedimentation rate is nearly always elevated in patients with urticarial vasculitis, and early components of complement are depressed in about 50% of cases of primary urticarial vasculitis.

NODULAR LESIONS

The character and distribution of cutaneous and subcutaneous nodules are critical in the evaluation of patients with diseases such as rheumatoid arthritis (RA), rheumatic fever, crystal deposition diseases, atypical infections, panniculitis, vasculitis and malignancy.

TABLE 7.4 FACIAL LESIONS – MIMICS OF ACUTE LUPUS	
Diagnosis	**Discriminating features**
Dermatomyositis* (occasional)	Heliotrope version more common; rash often involves nasolabial folds; rash has a distinctive pattern at other body locations
Photoallergic/phototoxic drug reactions* (common)	Clinical history of exposure to drugs including sulfa, thiazides, phenothiazines, tetracycline, piroxicam (phototoxic within days of first exposure), naproxen (porphyria-like)
Polymorphous light eruption* (common)	Small papule/papulovesicle variety; occasionally on face and commonly on forearms, chest or thighs, very pruritic, fewer recurrences with further sun exposure over the season
Porphyria* (rare)	Vesicular/bullous lesions and skin fragility in photosensitive distribution; may coexist with SLE
Pellagra* (rare)	Mucosal erythematous patches and ulcers antedate rash; associated gastrointestinal and psychological disturbances
Early acne rosacea	Malar erythema involving nasolabial folds
Carcinoid (rare)	Episodic flushing associated with other systemic symptoms, including diarrhea
Erysipelas (rare)	Bridge of nose and one or both cheeks involved with raised, rapidly spreading, warm erythematous rash, which may later vesiculate and crust in the febrile patient
Parvovirus infection (occasion)	Episodic flushing associated with other systemic symptoms, including diarrhea
*Photosensitive processes.	

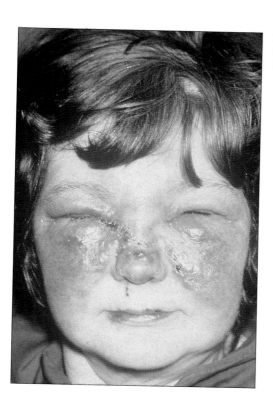

Fig. 7.12 Erysipelas. (With permission from Farrar et al.[38])

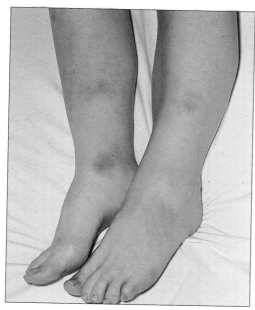

Fig. 7.13 Erythema nodosum – tender subcutaneous nodules on the lower legs. (Courtesy of St Mary's Hospital Medical School, London.)

Rheumatoid nodules[44] are firm, non-tender, flesh-colored subcutaneous lesions about 0.5–4cm in diameter that may be movable or fixed to periosteum or deep fascia. They are observed most commonly over areas of pressure and are found in about 20% of patients with RA and a small fraction of lupus patients[45]. Nearly all of these patients are observed to be serologically positive for rheumatoid factor.

Rheumatoid nodules may be pathologically indistinguishable from necrobiosis lipoidica diabeticorum or granuloma annulare but these disorders do not present a problem of clinical differential diagnosis since necrobiosis lipoidica diabeticorum is most commonly observed as a pretibial subcutaneous nodule in the diabetic patient and granuloma annulare is usually intracutaneous rather than subcutaneous. However, generalized granuloma annulare is more commonly seen in patients with RA and lupus[46].

Rheumatic-fever-associated nodules are also firm, non-tender lesions in areas of pressure but tend to be smaller, usually less than 1cm, and

shorter-lived (the average duration is 4–6 days and the lesions rarely last longer than 1 month). Rheumatic nodules at the elbow tend to occur at the point of the olecranon rather than several centimeters distal as with rheumatoid nodules. Rheumatic nodules are rare. When they occur the nodules tend to form in crops late in the course of the illness in patients who also manifest signs of carditis.

Tophi secondary to uric acid deposits may produce subcutaneous nodules with a distribution similar to those of rheumatoid nodules. Helpful discriminating features include asymmetry, distal interphalangeal joint involvement, involvement of the helix of the ear, origin at the joint margin rather than adjacent tissue, yellow appearance, overlying erythema, history of recurrent monoarthritis, asymmetric joint involvement and absence of a positive rheumatoid factor. Such signs should prompt joint aspiration and possible nodule biopsy to define the histopathology. A portion of the pathologic specimen should be placed in ethanol rather than formaldehyde to prevent dissolution of monosodium urate crystals.

Periarticular deposits of calcium crystals (pyrophosphate dihydrate, hydroxyapatite and oxalate) may rarely produce subcutaneous nodules and inflammatory or mechanical joint symptoms[47–49]. In oxalosis, miliary intradermal papules of calcium are more characteristic than nodule formation.

Achilles tendinitis in association with subcutaneous nodules of cholesterol at the tendon may be observed in the homozygous and heterozygous forms of type II hyperlipoproteinemia. In the homozygous state patients may also develop subcutaneous nodules over extensor surfaces of the knees and elbows and a migratory polyarthritis of large joints[45].

Multicentric reticulohistiocytosis[50] is a rare disorder associated with a destructive polyarthritis and multiple nodules. These nodules are usually cutaneous rather than subcutaneous, light copper to red-brown and often involve the hands, forearm and face. Periungual lesions, 'coral beads', are also characteristic. Unlike RA, multicentric reticulohistiocytosis commonly involves the distal interphalangeal joint. This entity is frequently associated with occult malignancy. Fibroblastic rheumatism[51] describes a rare entity associated with seronegative polyarthritis and flesh-colored dermal nodules, which are commonly located adjacent to involved hand joints. Sclerodactyly may be another clue to this diagnosis.

Red and tender subcutaneous nodules may occur in panniculitis, arteritis, atypical infections and metastatic tumor. The location of nodules, their propensity to scar and their histopathology assist differential diagnosis[52,53].

Erythema nodosum lesions are red or violet subcutaneous nodules, 1–5cm in diameter, without associated epidermal abnormalities (Fig. 7.13). The pathology shows a septal panniculitis without vasculitis. Usually, erythema nodosum nodules develop in pretibial locations and resolve spontaneously over several weeks without ulceration or scarring. The lesions may develop less frequently on the thighs, arms, face, neck and trunk. Whether idiopathic or associated with a known precipitant, erythema nodosum lesions are often accompanied by acute polyarthralgias or arthritis predominantly in large joints of the lower extremities. A diagnosis of erythema nodosum should prompt consideration of primary immune processes (e.g. sarcoidosis – Lofgren's syndrome, inflammatory bowel disease, Behçet's syndrome), the effects of drugs (sulfa, birth control pills), pregnancy, and infections (post-β-hemolytic streptococcus, Mycobacterium tuberculosis or M. leprae, fungus, Yersinia, Chlamydia, etc.)

Erythematous subcutaneous nodules that are unusually painful, develop in locations other than the pretibial region, ulcerate or scar, persist for more than several weeks, or are not in association with the above diseases, may be expressions of a different pathologic entity. Weber–Christian disease is an idiopathic lobular panniculitis with fever, polyarthralgias and painful subcutaneous nodules that are more widespread than in erythema nodosum and often ulcerate or scar (secondary to fat necrosis). Panniculitis with pancreatitis or pancreatic carcinoma may manifest similar skin lesions and polyarthritis. Serum lipase levels are often elevated. Excisional biopsy will reveal a lobular panniculitis, often with characteristic 'ghost-like' fat cells, presumed to be due to the enzyme effects upon the adipose cell.

Lupus profundus[23] is a lobular panniculitis found on the face, upper arms or buttocks. Overlying cutaneous involvement with discoid lesions is common. The lupus band test in the overlying skin is positive in about 70% of cases. This entity usually follows a chronic course associated with local scarring.

Diffuse granulomas in the subcutaneous tissue may also produce lobular panniculitis in sarcoidosis, although the septal panniculitis of erythema nodosum is a much more common expression[54].

Erythema induratum (nodular panniculitis) is a lobular panniculitis with local vasculitis which may be idiopathic or associated with tuberculosis. Unlike erythema nodosum nodules, the nodules of erythema induratum are commonly on the calf and tend to ulcerate. Erythema nodosum leprosum lesions tend to be more widespread, and upper extremity joint involvement is seen more often than in primary erythema nodosum[55].

Necrotizing arteritis such as polyarteritis nodosa and Wegener's granulomatosis may be associated with painful cutaneous and subcutaneous nodules. These lesions tend to be smaller than those of erythema nodosum. They develop in crops and are found most commonly on the lower legs and feet, especially along the course of arteries, although they may have a widespread distribution. Other skin lesions, such as purpura and livedo reticularis, may also be present[56].

Polyarthralgias may accompany erythema elevatum diutinum[57], nodular skin lesions secondary to leukocytoclastic vasculitis. These vasculitic lesions have a predilection for extensor surfaces of joints as well as skin overlying the buttocks and Achilles tendons.

Nodules adjacent to an inflammatory joint or tendon sheath should prompt consideration of local infections, such as sporotrichosis (Fig. 7.14), atypical mycobacterial infection and treponemal infections[45]. Ulceration develops frequently.

Cutaneous and subcutaneous nodules may also result from infiltration of metastatic tumor cells. When there are multiple nodules, hematologic malignancies are most common.

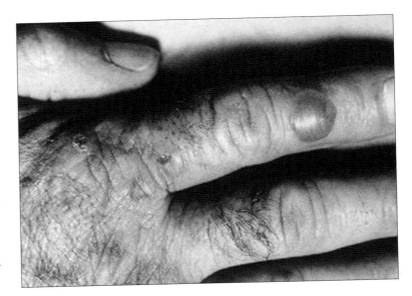

Fig. 7.15 Porphyria cutanea tarda.

VESICLES AND BULLAE

Vesicles and bullae result from a disturbance of intraepidermal coherence or dermal–epidermal adherence. A host of pathologic mechanisms may lead to blistering of the skin. Two blistering eruptions are seen in SLE[58]. First, a generalized bullous eruption may develop in normal appearing or erythematous skin (bullous eruption of SLE). This eruption is bullous-pemphigoid-like and has histologic similarities to dermatitis herpetiformis: it may be dapsone-responsive. Unlike dermatitis herpetiformis, it is not pruritic and is more widespread. Immunofluorescence and electron microscopic studies may be helpful diagnostically. Second, blistering may be seen in areas of photosensitive dermatitis. Such lesions must be distinguished from the rash of porphyria cutanea tarda, which is seen occasionally in the lupus patient (Fig. 7.15)[59].

Some primary immune skin disorders have been described with increased frequency in a number of rheumatic diseases[60]. Bullous pemphigoid is significantly more common in the rheumatoid patient and has been described in SLE, polymyositis and primary biliary cirrhosis. Dermatitis herpetiformis is commonly associated with autoimmune thyroid disease and has been reported in RA, Sjögren's syndrome, dermatomyositis and ulcerative colitis. Pemphigus has been described in patients with SLE, RA, Sjögren's syndrome and lymphomatoid granulomatosis. Pemphigus foliaceous may result from a D-penicillamine reaction.

Vesicles and bullae may accompany more characteristic lesions in patients with necrotizing vasculitis, ecthyma gangrenosum and disseminated intravascular coagulation. Blistering may also be a prominent feature in erythema multiforme major, and short-lived bullae may be seen in staphylococcal scalded skin syndrome. Musculoskeletal symptoms may accompany each of these entities.

Localized or generalized vesicles may also be seen in varicella or herpes viral infections. Tzanck test or culture may be helpful. Lesions of erythema migrans may vesiculate centrally.

Pseudoporphyria has been described with several non-steroidals, especially naproxen.[61]

PUSTULAR LESIONS

Pustular skin lesions in patients with rheumatic disease include pustular vasculitis associated with several bowel-associated processes, Sweet's syndrome, Behçet's syndrome, disorders with palmar and plantar pustular skin lesions and disorders associated with severe forms of acne. In addition,

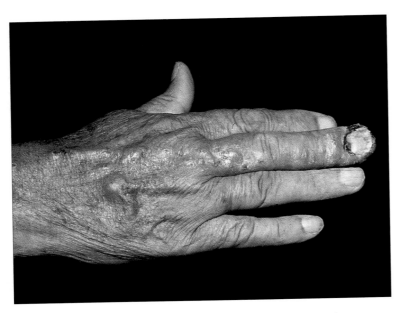

Fig. 7.14 Sporotrichosis. Several secondary nodules are apparent along lymphatic channels. (Courtesy of Dr TF Sellers Jr.)

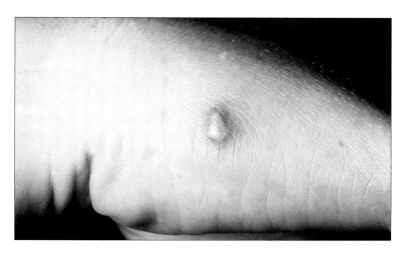

Fig. 7.16 Gonococcemia. Pustules are commonly found on the hands and feet. (With permission from McKee[30] and courtesy of Dr RN Thin, St Thomas' Hospital, London, UK.)

disseminated gonococcemia (Fig. 7.16), chronic meningococcemia, disseminated viral infections, such as varicella and disseminated herpes simplex, and reactions to drugs (especially sulfa drugs, hydantoins and halogen compounds) may produce disseminated pustular lesions.

A syndrome of cutaneous pustules, fever and polyarthritis is seen in patients with inflammatory bowel disease and those having undergone Billroth II surgery, thus prompting the descriptive term bowel-associated dermatosis–arthritis syndrome[62]. Episodic painful cutaneous pustules on a purpuric base are seen primarily on the upper extremities and upper trunk.

Patients with Sweet's syndrome (acute febrile neutrophilic dermatosis) may also present with painful papulonodules or pustules[63] (Fig. 7.17). Although painful oral and genital ulcers are most characteristic of Behçet's syndrome, pustular skin lesions, especially at sites of minor trauma (e.g. needlestick pathergy), should also lead to its consideration. The arthritis is frequently pauciarticular in these disorders. Histology of pustular skin lesions may be similar in Behçet's syndrome, Sweet's syndrome and bowel-associated dermatitis–arthritis[62].

Isolated palmar and plantar pustulosis, pustular psoriasis and keratoderma blennorrhagicum are identical pathologically. Patients with psoriasis and keratoderma blennorrhagicum may have symptoms of spondyloarthropathy. An association of palmar pustulosis with sternal

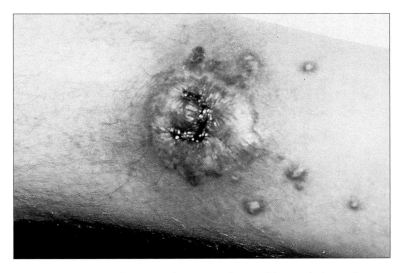

Fig. 7.17 Sweet's syndrome. Erythematous plaque with pustulation and ulceration. (Courtesy of Dr Kenneth DeBenedictus.)

clavicular hyperostosis and chronic recurrent multifocal osteomyelitis has been described[64].

Severe forms of acne have also been associated with rheumatic illnesses[65]. Acne fulminans has also been associated with sternal clavicular hyperostosis and chronic recurrent multifocal osteomyelitis. The patients described have usually been young, white males who become acutely ill with fever, weight loss, arthralgias, myalgias and multiple inflammatory skin lesions with ulceration on the back and chest. Acne conglobata and related illnesses exhibit extensive cystic and nodular acne on the buttocks, thighs and upper arms as well as the conventional locations of acne vulgaris. Some of these patients, most notably young black males, have a higher frequency of spondyloarthropathy and sternal clavicular hyperostosis. Isotretinoin, a vitamin A derivative used for severe acne, has been associated with mild myalgias and arthralgias, which often resolve spontaneously without cessation of therapy, and with axial skeletal hyperostoses.

PURPURA

Purpura, non-blanching erythematous lesions, should be evaluated by size and palpability[31,66]. Petechiae are characteristic of platelet disorders. They result from leakage of erythrocytes from dermal capillaries where platelet plugs serve as the major source of coagulation. Larger collections of blood form ecchymoses that are due to leakage from arterioles or venules at sites of minor trauma; ecchymoses are also common in platelet and other bleeding disorders. These lesions are not usually palpable unless bleeding occurs into an unrelated inflammatory lesion.

Non-palpable purpura result from extravasation of erythrocytes in the absence of inflammation. Causes of non-palpable purpura in the patient with rheumatic complaints include: platelet deficiency states such as immune thrombocytopenia; vascular fragility as observed in primary amyloid, scurvy and genetic disorders of collagen formation; reduced integrity of supportive connective tissue as observed in corticosteroid therapy; and vessel thrombosis or non-septic emboli such as thrombotic thrombocytopenic purpura, antiphospholipid syndrome, cholesterol emboli and marantic endocarditis[31].

In primary amyloid, vascular fragility results from infiltration of the vessel with amyloid light chain protein. Purpura is most common in the periorbital region, at skin folds and in areas of minor trauma (pinch purpura). Patients may manifest polyarthritis secondary to amyloid infiltration of synovium. In scurvy, altered collagen formation probably contributes to vascular fragility[67] and the lesions are rarely palpable. Perifollicular hemorrhage with central corkscrew hairs on the lower extremities is characteristic. Hemorrhage into muscle or joints may occur. Cholesterol emboli, a consequence of severe atherosclerotic vessel disease, may mimic vasculitis and characteristically involves the lower extremity with purpura, livedo reticularis, nodules and ischemic ulcers[31,68]. Rickettsial and certain viral illnesses (echovirus and Coxsackie virus infections) may show petechial lesions in the course of the illness.

Palpable purpura

Petechiae and flat purpuric lesions are rarely observed in necrotizing angiitis[69] because vascular inflammation leads to increased permeability. Palpable hemorrhagic lesions of the dermis should suggest vasculitis or embolus associated with an infectious agent.

Palpable purpura in dependent locations (areas with increased orthostatic pressure, such as the buttocks or lower extremities) is the most common presentation of necrotizing venulitis (Fig. 7.18). Lesions are round or oval secondary to radial diffusion of erythrocytes from the postcapillary venules of the upper vascular plexus of the dermis[69]. The differential diagnosis includes chronic bacterial infection[70], acute hepatitis B infection, drug reaction, associated lymphoproliferative disorder, associated rheu-

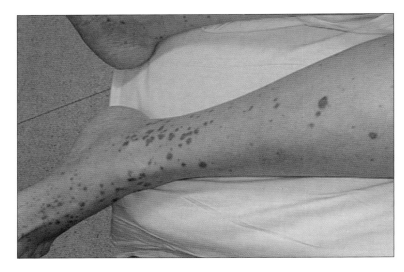

Fig. 7.18 **Palpable purpura of necrotizing venulitis.**

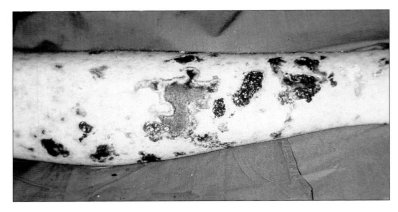

Fig. 7.20 **Purpura fulminans with secondary skin necrosis.** (With permission from Farrar *et al.*[38])

matic disease and Henoch–Schönlein purpura. Biopsy within 24–48 hours helps define the inflammatory nature of the lesion. The presence of IgA immunofluorescent deposits at the dermal–epidermal junction supports the presence of Henoch–Schönlein purpura. In isolated leukocytoclastic vasculitis the prognosis is generally good; nevertheless, necrotizing venulitis may be associated with larger-vessel vasculitis and should prompt a careful search for systemic necrotizing arteritis[72]. Signs of necrotizing arteritis include irregularly outlined purpura, since inflammation and thrombosis of deep dermal and subcutaneous vessels result in areas of hemorrhage and infarction[69]. Cutaneous nodules, livedo reticularis, digital infarcts and deep cutaneous ulcers (Fig. 7.19) are also seen.

Acute onset of purpuric lesions in the febrile patient is sepsis until proved otherwise[73]. Acute meningococcemia begins as small, irregular, often palpable purpura, which are more widely distributed and less symmetric than leukocytoclastic vasculitis. The lesions may progress rapidly over hours to extensive bullous and irregular hemorrhagic lesions with central necrotic gunmetal gray patches (Fig. 7.20). The vascular lesions result from direct invasion of the organism as well as being secondary to disseminated intravascular coagulation.

Gram-negative infection may embolize to the skin (ecthyma gangrenosum) and also seed the joint. The skin lesions are erythematous wheals or papules with irregular areas of purpura followed by necrosis and ulceration. The morphology of wheal or papule containing an irregular purpuric area is a specific sign of septicemia with Gram-negative organisms including gonococcus, meningococcus, *Klebsiella* spp., *Pseudomonas* spp. and *Escherichia coli*[74].

ULCERS

Vascular, infectious and tumor-associated causes must be considered in the patient with cutaneous ulceration and musculoskeletal symptoms. Ulcerations secondary to ischemia may result from vasospasm in Raynaud's phenomenon, vascular thrombosis in antiphospholipid syndrome or paraproteinemia and vascular necrosis in necrotizing venulitis or arteritis. Other skin findings and associated systemic signs and symptoms differentiate among these causes.

Lower extremity ulcers in the debilitated rheumatoid patient[75–78] present a common diagnostic dilemma. The differential diagnosis includes vasculitis, pyoderma gangrenosum, pressure sores, infection and vascular insufficiency. Pyoderma gangrenosum (Fig. 7.21) is observed more commonly in patients with RA, inflammatory bowel disease, Behçet's syndrome, Wegener's granulomatosis, paraproteinemias or chronic active hepatitis[79].

Pyoderma gangrenosum is a rare ulcerating lesion of unknown cause, which begins as a nodule or hemorrhagic pustule that breaks down to form a painful ulcer with an irregular, undermined, raised violaceous border. The lesion is usually single and is most commonly observed in the lower extremities, buttock or abdomen. Such lesions often develop at sites of previous minor trauma. Pathologic specimens may be suggestive of this entity but are not diagnostic. Differential diagnosis of the lesion includes necrotizing arteritis and infectious causes, including atypical mycobacterial

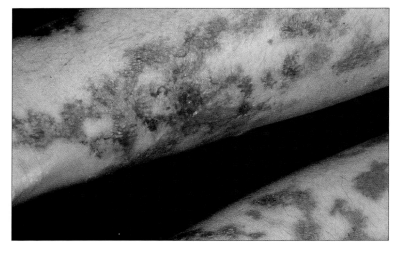

Fig. 7.19 **Polyarteritis nodosa with irregular purpura, livedo reticularis and necrosis.** (With permission of the American Academy of Dermatology. All rights reserved.)

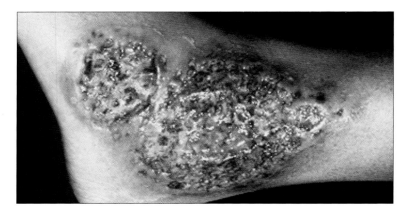

Fig. 7.21 **Pyoderma gangrenosum.**

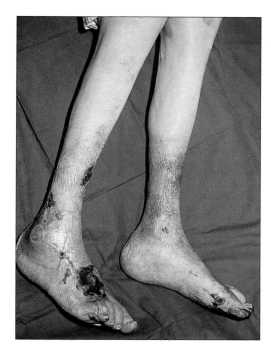

Fig. 7.22 Rheumatoid vasculitic ulceration in various stages of evolution. (With permission from Dieppe PA *et al.* Slide atlas of clinical rheumatology. London: Gower Medical Publishing 1983.)

or fungal infection, amoebiasis, tropical ulcer and anaerobic bacterial synergistic gangrene (Meleney's ulcer)[31].

Rheumatoid vasculitic ulcers classically develop suddenly on the calves or dorsum of the foot[80]. They are multiple, painful, have a 'punched out' appearance and an indurated base, and may enlarge rapidly (Fig. 7.22). They are most often seen in patients with long-standing erosive nodular RA, especially those with Felty's syndrome or other signs of vasculitis. Chronic superficial leg or sacral ulcers are also observed in rheumatoid patients with other signs of vasculitis, but these lesions are less specific.

Venous stasis ulcers are most common in the ankle area, especially near the medial malleolus, and are painless unless there is secondary infection. These ulcers are shallow and wide and have an irregular outline. They are often surrounded by thick and hyperpigmented skin secondary to the chronic venous insufficiency. Venous insufficiency ulcers are common in the rheumatoid patient because of reduced skin integrity, increased venous stasis due to inactivity and possibly reduced venous muscle pump activity secondary to reduced ankle mobility[81].

Painful ulceration with pale edges on the toes and dorsum of the foot, or the heel, and poor granulation tissue in a leg with trophic changes and reduced peripheral arterial pulse pressures suggest arterial insufficiency ulcers on an atherosclerotic basis. Vasculitis may reduce the threshold of pressure or atherosclerotic disease that will produce ischemia and ulceration.

Other ulcerating lesions may be of assistance in differentiating various immune diseases. For example, perianal ulcers secondary to cutaneous granulomatous disease may be seen in Crohn's disease[82]. Genital ulcers are often a sign of Behçet's syndrome.

DERMAL SCLEROSIS

Fibrosis of the skin producing visible and palpable thickening is a characteristic feature of scleroderma (see Chapter 35). Attention to the appearance, distribution and histopathology of the involved skin can be helpful in distinguishing between patients with scleroderma and those with scleroderma-like abnormalities[83,84] (Table 7.5). The distribution of involvement helps to distinguish the limited form of scleroderma (formerly the CREST – calcinosis cutis, Raynaud's phenomenon, esophageal dysfunction, sclerodactyly and telangiectasia – syndrome) variant from progressive systemic sclerosis. The CREST variant does not generally produce scleroderma of the proximal extremities or of the trunk and has a more benign prognosis.

TELANGIECTASES

Telangiectases result from dilated venules, capillaries and arterioles. Periungual telangiectases and broad lesions called mat telangiectases are important types to identify because of their specificity for scleroderma (Fig. 7.23). Mat telangiectases are broad, oval or polygonal macules

TABLE 7.5 MIMICS OF SCLERODERMA	
Diagnosis	**Discriminating features**
Eosinophilic fasciitis	Cutaneous sclerosis of extremities sparing hands and feet, which often lack Raynaud's phenomenon, nailfold abnormalities and body telangiectases; fascial inflammation on biopsy
Diabetes mellitus	Bound-down skin over hands with joint contractures in the chronic diabetic
Scleredema	Benign skin tightening developing rapidly over the neck and upper back in the non-insulin-dependent diabetic
Monoclonal gammopathy (POEMS syndrome)	Polyneuropathy, organomegaly, endocrinopathy, M protein and skin changes (POEMS) – skin is thickened and may be hyperpigmented but is not bound down
Primary amyloid	Scleroderma-like skin changes are rare: waxy cutaneous papules are more characteristic
Scleromyxedema	Induration of hands, face, arms (trunk and lower extremities to a lesser degree) with multiple fine waxy papules (may be associated with monoclonal gammopathy)
Carcinoid	Scleroderma-like lesions of lower extremities in association with other carcinoid symptoms
Palmar fasciitis/polyarthritis paraneoplastic syndrome	Bound-down palmar or plantar fascia associated with internal malignancy
Reflex sympathetic dystrophy (late phase)	Tight dystrophic skin of extremity following period of vasomotor instability, altered sympathetic nerve function

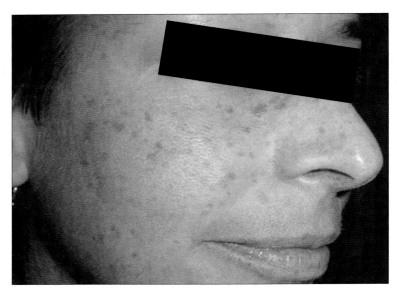

Fig. 7.23 Mat telangiectases in a patient with a limited form of scleroderma.

2–7mm in diameter and are found on the face, mucous membranes and hands. These lesions are clinically distinguishable from the broad, often palpable telangiectases of hereditary hemorrhagic telangiectasia. In this latter disease, telangiectases are actually arteriovenous malformations and are associated with epistaxis and gastrointestinal bleeding (Osler–Rendu–Weber disease)[85].

Linear telangiectases are non-specific and may be seen in sun damage, acne rosacea, venous hypertension (lower extremities), carcinoid and hypercorticism. When linear telangiectases are present on the face, malar erythema may result which can be confused with a non-raised malar rash of lupus.

Nailfold telangiectases observed by the naked eye or, preferably, by capillary microscopy are quite specific for the presence of systemic rheumatic disease, especially scleroderma (Fig. 7.24), dermatomyositis and occasionally lupus (Fig. 7.25), and may occur in as many as two-thirds of patients with such conditions. They may be helpful as early markers of these diseases[86]. The characteristic pattern of scleroderma and dermatomyositis is dilated capillaries frequently bordered by avascular areas. In SLE a tortuous pattern of capillaries without avascular areas is characteristic. In dermatomyositis and lupus, periungual erythema is commonly present as well.

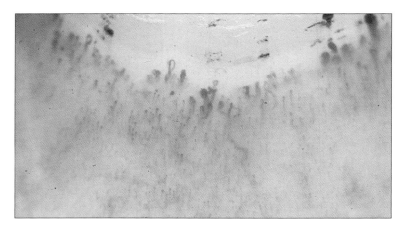

Fig. 7.24 Nailfold capillary pattern in a patient with scleroderma. Notice the avascular areas. (Courtesy of Dr Hildegard Maricq.)

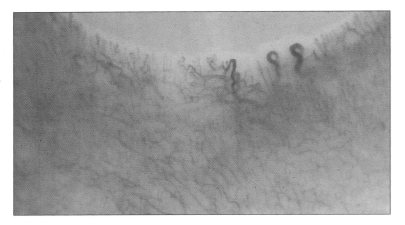

Fig. 7.25 Nailfold capillary pattern in a patient with discoid lupus erythematosus. (Courtesy of Dr Hildegard Maricq.)

HYPERPIGMENTATION

Pigmentary changes of the skin may be a clue to diagnosis in patients with rheumatic complaints[31]. Joint pain and diffuse hyperpigmentation may be seen in primary biliary cirrhosis, hemochromatosis and Whipple's disease. Rarely, diffuse hyperpigmentation may antedate the more characteristic skin changes of scleroderma. Generalized hyperpigmentation has also been reported rarely in SLE. Hyperpigmentation may also be present without dermal sclerosis in patients with POEMS syndrome, but arthritis occurs infrequently.

Brown to blue-gray discoloration of the skin secondary to drug deposition may occur in rheumatoid patients treated with gold (chrysiasis). Diffuse yellow discoloration is observed frequently with quinacrine therapy, and bluish-black pigmentation of the pretibial area, face and nailbeds is associated with the use of antimalarial drugs[87]. A diagnosis of ochronosis should be considered in the osteoarthritic patient with pigmentary changes overlying cartilage and tendons.

ORAL LESIONS

A careful evaluation of the mouth and pharynx is helpful in the evaluation of rheumatic disease. Findings of ulceration, xerostomia and gingivitis, and an assessment of tongue size and color, may all be of diagnostic importance.

Oral ulcers are common findings in Behçet's syndrome, Crohn's disease, reactive arthritis and SLE. Oral ulcerations of Behçet's syndrome and Crohn's disease may be indistinguishable from those of recurrent aphthous stomatitis. Patients with Behçet's syndrome or Crohn's disease may experience painful, shallow, round to oval ulcers with discrete borders, which often occur in crops. These lesions tend to occur on mucosa not bound to periosteum as opposed to the lesions of recurrent intraoral herpes which tend to be present upon the hard palate and gingiva. Histopathology of the lesions of Behçet's syndrome or Crohn's disease is not helpful for differential diagnosis, and other clinical signs and symptoms are required to distinguish between these illnesses. In contrast, the lesions of reactive arthritis are painless, have an irregular border and are commonly located upon the palate or dorsum of the tongue.

Oral ulcers are common in patients with active lupus and may herald a disease flare. Lesions are usually painless, but may occasionally be painful, and are most common on the hard palate[23]. Discoid lesions may produce irregularly shaped white scars upon the mucosa that may be confused with lichen planus or leukoplakia. Histopathology and immunofluorescence studies are diagnostic of these discoid lesions. Non-specific oral ulcers frequently develop in patients receiving non-steroidal anti-inflammatory drugs or disease-modifying drugs such as gold, D-penicillamine, methotrexate and azathioprine.

Gingivitis secondary to immune disease has been described rarely in lupus and may also be seen as an early manifestation of Wegener's granulomatosis[88].

Kawasaki's disease and erythema multiforme major may both reveal signs of fever, conjunctivitis and oral mucosa lesions as well as a polymorphic skin eruption. In Kawasaki's disease diffuse erythema of the oral cavity is seen, as well as erythema of the lips followed by dryness, fissuring and surface erosions, which contrast to the bloody, crusting lips of a patient with erythema multiforme major. Erythema of the tongue with prominent ungual papillae leads to the strawberry tongue of Kawasaki's disease, which can be seen in scarlet fever but not in erythema multiforme major.

REFERENCES

1. Lawley TJ, Yancey KB. Approach to the patient with a skin disorder. In: Braunwald E, Fauci AS, Kasper DL et al., eds. Harrison's principles of internal medicine, 15th ed. New York: McGraw-Hill; 2001: 305–309.
2. Mallia C, Uitto J, eds. Rheumaderm. Current Issues in Rheumatology and Dermatology. New York: Kluwer Academic/Plenum; 1999.
3. Schneider R, Laxer RM. Systemic onset juvenile rheumatoid arthritis. Baillière's Clin Rheumatol 1998; 12: 245–271.
4. Schachua L, Littlejohn GO. Adult-onset Still's disease: a concise review of clues to an important rare syndrome. Aus N Z J Med 1999; 29: 98–99.
5. Bradley DL, Glode MP. Kawasaki disease. The mystery continues. West J Med 1998; 168: 23–29.
6. Kidd BG, Hart HH, Gregor RR. Clinical features of meningococcal arthritis: a report of four cases. Ann Rheum Dis 1985; 44: 790–792.
7. Apicella MA. Neisseria meningitidis. In: Mandell GL, Bennett JE, Dolin R, eds. Principles and practice of infectious diseases, 5th ed. London: Churchill Livingstone; 2000: 2234.
8. Krober MS. Skeletal muscle involvement in Rocky Mountain spotted fever. South Med J 1978; 71: 1575–1576.
9. Case records of the Massachusetts General Hospital. N Engl J Med 1971; 288: 1400–1404.
10. Gerster JC, Weintraub A, Vischer TL, Fallet GH. Secondary syphilis revealed by rheumatic complaints. J Rheumatol 1977; 4: 197–200.
11. Gertner E, Inman RD. Aseptic arthritis in a man with toxic shock syndrome. Arthritis Rheum 1986; 29: 910–916.
12. Washburn RG. Streptobacillus moniliformis (Rat-bite fever). In: Mandell GL, Bennett JE, Dolin R, eds. Principles and practice of infectious diseases, 5th ed. London: Churchill Livingstone; 2000: 2423.
13. Kreisberg RA. Clinical problem solving. An abundance of options. N Engl J Med 1993; 281–283.
14. Mangi RJ. Viral arthritis – the great masquerader. Bull Rheum Dis 1994; 43: 5–6.
15. Scroggie DA, Carpenter MT, Cooper RI, Higgs JB. Parvovirus arthropathy outbreak in the southwestern United States. J Rheumatol 2000; 27: 2444–2448.
16. Lapins J, Gaines H, Lindback S et al. Skin and mucosal characteristics of symptomatic primary HIV-1 infection. AIDS Patient Care and STDs 1997; 11: 67–70.
17. Huff JC, Weston WL, Tonneson MG. Erythema multiforme: a critical review of characteristics, diagnostic criteria and causes. J Am Acad Dermatol 1983; 8: 763–775.
18. Roujeau JC, Stern RS. Severe adverse cutaneous reactions to drugs. N Engl J Med 1994; 331: 1272–1285.
19. Samuels J, Aksentijevich I, Torosyan Y et al. Familial Mediterranean fever at the millennium. Medicine 1998; 77: 268–297.
20. Layton MA, Musgrove C, Dawes PT. Polyarthritis, rash and lymphadenopathy: case reports of two patients with angioimmunoblastic lymphadenopathy presenting to a rheumatology clinic. Clin Rheumatol 1998; 17: 148–151.
21. Lipsker D, Veran Y, Grunenberger F et al. The Schnitzler syndrome. Medicine 2001; 80: 37–44.
22. Yell JA, Mbuagbaw J, Burge SM. Cutaneous manifestations of systemic lupus erythematosus. Br J Dermatol 1996; 135: 355–362.
23. Sontheimer RD, Provost TT. Lupus erythematosus. In: Sontheimer RD, Provost TT, eds. Cutaneous manifestations of rheumatic disease. Baltimore: Williams & Wilkins; 1996: 1–71.
24. Wintroub BU, Stern R. Cutaneous drug reactions: pathogenesis and clinical classification. J Am Acad Dermatol 1985; 13: 167–179.
25. Piette WW. An approach to cutaneous changes caused by hematologic malignancies. Dermatol Clin 1987; 7(3): 467–479.
26. Ansell BM. Rheumatic disorders in childhood. London: Butterworths; 1980: 155–156.
27. Sontheimer RD, Maddison PJ, Reichlin M et al. Serologic and HLA associations in subacute cutaneous lupus erythematosus, a clinical subset of lupus erythematosus. Ann Intern Med 1982; 97: 664–671.
28. Provost TT, Watson R. Mucocutaneous manifestations of Sjögren's syndrome. In: Sontheimer RD, Provost TT, eds. Cutaneous manifestations of rheumatic disease. Baltimore: Williams & Wilkins; 1996: 157–169.
29. Shapiro ED, Gerber MA. Lyme disease. Clin Infect Dis 2000; 31: 533–542.
30. McKee PH. Pathology of the skin, 2nd ed. London: Mosby Wolfe; 1996.
31. Bolognia J, Braverman I. Skin manifestations of internal disease. In: Braunwald E, Fauci AS, Kasper DL et al., eds. Harrison's principles of internal medicine, 15th ed. New York: McGraw-Hill; 2001: 315–330.
32. Almeida L, Grossman M. Widespread dermatophyte infections that mimic collagen vascular disease. J Am Acad Dermatol 1990; 23: 855–857.
33. Braverman IM. Skin signs of systemic disease, 2nd ed. Philadelphia: WB Saunders; 1981: 255–377.
34. Zax RH, Callen JP. Sarcoidosis. Dermatol Clin 1989; 7: 505–514.
35. Callen JP. Dermatomyositis. Lancet 2000; 355: 53–57.
36. Taylor CR, Hawk JLM. Recognizing photosensitivity. Ann Rheum Dis 1994; 53: 705–707.
37. Bickers DR. Photosensitivity and other reactions to light. In: Braunwald E, Fauci AS, Kasper DL et al. eds. Harrison's principles of internal medicine, 15th ed. New York: McGraw-Hill; 2001: 342–348.
38. Farrar WE et al. Infectious diseases: text and color atlas, 2nd ed. London: Gower; 1992.
39. Nesher G, Osborn TG, Moore TL. Parvovirus infection mimicking systemic lupus erythematosus. Semin Arthritis Rheum 1995; 24: 297–303.
40. McElgunn PS. Dermatologic manifestations of hepatitis B virus infection. J Am Acad Dermatol 1983; 8: 539–548.
41. Bielory L, Gascon P, Lawley TJ et al. Human serum sickness: a prospective analysis of 35 patients treated with equine anti-thymocyte globulin for bone marrow failure. Medicine 1988; 67: 40–57.
42. Burrall BA, Halpern GM, Huntley AC. Chronic urticaria. West J Med 1990; 152: 268–276.
43. Black AK. Urticarial vasculitis. Clin Dermatol 1999; 17: 565–569
44. Kaye B, Kaye D, Bobrove A. Rheumatoid nodules. Am J Med 1984; 76: 279–292.
45. Moore CP, Willkens RF. The subcutaneous nodule: Its significance in the diagnosis of rheumatic disease. Semin Arthritis Rheum 1977; 7: 63–79.
46. Dabski K, Winkelman RK. Generalized granuloma annulare: clinical and laboratory findings in 100 patients. J Am Acad Dermatol 1989; 20: 39–47.
47. Reginato AJ, Kurnik B. Calcium oxalate and other crystals associated with kidney diseases and arthritis. Semin Arthritis Rheum 1989; 18: 198–224.
48. Resnick C. Tumoral calcinosis. Arthritis Rheum 1989; 32: 1484–1486.
49. Leisen JC, Austard ED, Bluhm GB, Sigler JW. The tophus in calcium pyrophosphate deposition disease. JAMA 1980; 244: 1711–1712.
50. Rapini RP. Multicentric reticulohistiocytosis. Clin Dermatol 1993; 11: 107–111.
51. Fam A, Hanna W, Mak V, Assaad D. Fibroblastic rheumatism: clinical and histologic evolution of cutaneous manifestations. J Rheumatol 1998; 25: 2262–2266.
52. Diaz Cascajo C, Borghi S, Weyes W. Panniculitis: definition of terms and diagnostic strategy. Am J Dermatopathol 2000; 22: 530–549.
53. Garcia-Porrua, Gonzalez-Gay MA, Vazquez-Caruncho M et al. Erythema nodosum. Arthritis Rheum 2000; 43: 584–592.
54. Kalb RE. Sarcoidosis with subcutaneous nodules. Am J Med 1988; 85: 731–736.
55. Albert DA, Weisman MH, Kaplan R. The rheumatic manifestations of leprosy. Medicine 1980; 59: 442–448.
56. Francis C, Huong LT, Piehe J et al. Wegener's granulomatosis. Dermatological manifestations in 75 cases with clinicopathologic correlation. Arch Derm 1994; 130: 861–867.
57. Gibson LE, el-Azhary RA. Erythema elevatum diutinum. Clin Dermatol 2000; 18: 295–299.
58. Mascaro JM, Herrero C, Hausmann G. Uncommon cutaneous manifestations of lupus erythematosus. Lupus 1997; 6: 122–131.
59. Kutz DC, Bridges AJ. Bullous rash and brown urine in a systemic lupus erythematosus patient treated with hydroxychloroquine. Arthritis Rheum 1995; 38: 440–443.
60. Callen J. Internal disorders associated with bullous disease of the skin. J Am Acad Dermatol 1980; 3: 107–119.
61. Checketts SR, Morrison KA, Baughman RD. Nonsteroidal anti-inflammatory-induced pseudoporphyria: is there an alternative drug? Cutis 1999; 63: 223–225.
62. McNeely MC, Jorizzo JL, Solomon AR et al. Primary idiopathic cutaneous pustular vasculitis. J Am Acad Dermatol 1986; 14: 939–944.
63. Daniel SU, Fett DL, Gibson LE, Pittelkow MR. Sweet syndrome: acute febrile neutrophilic dermatosis. Sem Dermatol 1995; 14: 173–178.
64. Laxer RM, Shore AD, King S et al. Chronic recurrent multifocal osteomyelitis and psoriasis: a report of a new association and review of related disorders. Semin Arthritis Rheum 1988; 17: 260–270.
65. Knitzer RH, Needleman BW. Musculoskeletal syndromes associated with acne. Semin Arthritis Rheum 1991; 20: 247–255.
66. Schreiner DT. Purpura. Dermatol Clin 1989; 7: 481–489.
67. Reuler JB, Broudy VC, Cooney TG. Adult scurvy. JAMA 1985; 253: 803–807.
68. Cappiello RA, Espinoza LR, Adelman H et al. Cholesterol embolism: a pseudo-vasculitis syndrome. Semin Arthritis Rheum 1989; 18: 240–246.
69. Braverman IM. Skin signs of systemic disease, 2nd ed. Philadelphia: WB Saunders; 1981: 378–452.
70. Millikan LE, Flynn TC. Infectious etiologies of cutaneous vasculitis. Clin Dermatol 1999; 17: 509–514.
71. Kraft DM, McKee D, Scott C. Henoch–Schönlein purpura: a review. Am Fam Phys 1998; 58: 405–408.
72. Callen JP. Cutaneous vasculitis. What have we learned in the past 20 years? Arch Dermatol 1998; 134: 355–357.

73. Spencer LV, Callen JP. Cutaneous manifestations of bacterial infections. Dermatol Clin 1989; 7: 579–589.
74. Braverman IM. Skin signs of systemic disease, 2nd ed. Philadelphia: WB Saunders; 1981: 809–922.
75. Cawley MI. Vasculitis and ulceration in rheumatic disease of the foot. Baillière's Clin Rheumatol 1987; 1: 315–333.
76. Vollersten RS, Conn DL. Vasculitis with rheumatoid arthritis. Rheumatol Dis Clin North Am 1990; 16: 445–461.
77. Jorizzo JL, Daniels JC. Dermatologic conditions reported in patients with rheumatoid arthritis. J Am Acad Dermatol 1983; 8: 439–457.
78. Levine JM. Leg ulcers: differential diagnosis in the elderly. Geriatrics 1990; 45: 32–42.
79. Callen JP. Miscellaneous disorders that commonly affect both skin and joints. In: Sontheimer RD, Provost TT, eds. Cutaneous manifestations of rheumatic disease. Baltimore: Williams & Wilkins; 2001: 257–283.
80. Bacon DG, Tribe CR. Systemic rheumatoid vasculitis: a clinical and laboratory study of 50 cases. Medicine 1981; 60: 288–297.
81. Gaylarde PM, Dodd HJ, Sarlcony I. Venous leg ulcers and arthropathy. Br J Rheumatol 1990; 29: 142–144.
82. Burgdorf W. Cutaneous manifestations of Crohn's disease. J Am Acad Dermatol 1981; 5: 689–695.
83. Tuffanelli DL. Systemic sclerosis. In: Sontheimer RD, Provost TT, eds. Cutaneous manifestations of rheumatic disease. Baltimore: Williams & Wilkins; 2001: 115–139.
84. Greenberg AS, Falanga V. Localized cutaneous sclerosis. In: Sontheimer RD, Provost TT, eds. Cutaneous manifestations of rheumatic disease. Baltimore: Williams & Wilkins; 2001: 141–155.
85. Braverman IM. Skin signs of systemic disease, 2nd ed. Philadelphia: WB Saunders; 1981: 532–565.
86. Minkin W, Rabhan NB. Office nail fold microscopy using ophthalmoscope. J Am Acad Dermatol 1982; 7: 191–193.
87. Bailin PL, Matkaluk RM. Cutaneous reactions to rheumatological drugs. Clin Rheum Dis 1982; 8: 493–516.
88. Hen SF, Tomak KJ. Wegener's granulomatosis: cutaneous and oral mucosal diseases. J Am Acad Dermatol 1993; 28: 710–718.

PRINCIPLES OF MANAGEMENT

8 Principles of management of patients with rheumatic disease

Peter M Brooks and Joseph A Buckwalter

Management of chronic rheumatic disease

- Diagnosis should include the assessment of activity, prognosis and goal setting
- Treatment is adjusted in the light of evaluation of the response
- Coordination of a multidisciplinary approach and re-evaluation of disease are essential

Therapeutic issues

- Which drugs should be used and when?
- What surgical procedures and when?
- Which physical therapies are appropriate?
- Continuing re-evaluations of the patient's disease status, disability and expectations and requirements are essential

INTRODUCTION

Management of patients with rheumatic disease remains a significant challenge and one that requires careful consideration, judgment and an adherence to the principles of evidence-based medicine[1]. Some rheumatic diseases are acute and settle completely with early and appropriate treatment. These include infectious arthritis and gout – diseases for which we are well aware of the pathogenesis and treatment. Even in these conditions, however, damage may occur to the joint during the acute phase that can lead on to progressive degenerative arthritis later in life. The process is complex because of:

- the chronicity of these diseases and the need for ongoing monitoring of disease activity
- functional status and patient response to the disease and treatment
- the need to coordinate a multidisciplinary therapeutic approach, including a variety of medical specialties as well as allied health-care providers.

The doctor providing rheumatologic management must coordinate specialist input in a variety of areas and must be knowledgeable about management options, their applications and their risks and benefits. Patients treated continuously by subspecialist rheumatologists demonstrate a slower progression of disability than those treated intermittently or by those not seeing a rheumatologist[2]. Orchestrating these various approaches and monitoring their efficacy requires knowledge of what each offers but, as importantly, requires the doctor to think in terms of the influence of life stages on disease and treatment and how they may relate to disease expression and modulation (e.g. the effect of aging on drug metabolism and toxicity). Of great importance here is the establishment of realistic goals for the various treatments. Although doctors can give patients information on the likely outcomes of treatment, the final decision on a particular therapy should be made in consultation with the patient. It is generally recognized that the goals of the patient and the physician are often different, and this must be acknowledged by the treating 'team'. The ability to communicate with patients is extremely important when caring for any patient with a chronic disease, particularly a rheumatic condition, and emphasizes the importance of attainment of these communication skills in undergraduate and postgraduate education[3].

The problem of involving the patient in therapeutic decisions is the very different experiences of the doctor and the patient. The doctor can appreciate the long-term disability that is likely to result if the disease is not treated immediately, whereas the patient has little understanding of what is likely to occur in 10 or 20 years. The patient is much more likely to be influenced by the potential for immediate adverse consequences of a therapy (an adverse drug reaction, risks of surgery or anesthetic) than by a 'potential' reduction of disability (decreased pain or joint erosion) in 10 years time. Optimal management of patients will increasingly involve them in making decisions regarding musculoskeletal risk factors such as weight, exercise and a range of lifestyle modifications.

TABLE 8.1 THERAPEUTIC STRATEGIES IN RHEUMATIC DISEASES	
Pharmacotherapy	**Non-pharmacologic**
● Analgesics	Rehabilitation
● Non-steroidal anti-inflammatory drugs	Education
● Antirheumatic drugs	● Knowledge
● Corticosteroids	– General
● Immunosuppressive agents	– Specific
● Biological modifiers	● Behavioral modification
● Specific antigout preparations	– Relaxation techniques
● Radiotherapy	– Stress management
– Direct	Physical therapy
– Radiopharmaceutical	● Exercise
	– General preventive
	– Specific therapeutic
Surgery	● Rest
● Reconstruction	● Light
– Tendon	– Ultraviolet
– Ligament	– Laser
● Arthroplasty	● Heat/cold
● Arthrodesis	● Hydrotherapy
● Synovectomy	● Electricity
● Osteotomy	– Transcutaneous nerve stimulation
● Joint debridement	● Ultrasound
● Decompression	● Mobilization/manipulation
– Spinal cord	● Devices
– Peripheral nerve	– Splints
	– Orthoses
	– Household modifications
	– Home/work/walking devices

Pharmacologic interventions, rehabilitation, orthoses and other devices, non-pharmacologic modalities and surgery should be considered to influence both disease and the patient, and these are mutually interdependent. They cannot be seen as isolated intervention points in a disease process because they may significantly alter the course of the disease – and the patient – sometimes permanently. Other life issues that are very important and have to be considered in treatment include the changes associated with age and development, be they those of childhood or adolescence, and the influence of occupations such as school, work and home tasks. Rheumatic diseases are invariably chronic and are characterized by unpredictable remissions and relapses. The course of these diseases can be influenced by many factors, including biological processes, family and societal interactions, education and treatment. Good management requires acknowledgment of all and attention to most. A critical concept to remember is that expectations as to what a therapy will or will not do may differ substantially between the treating health-care professional and the patient[4,5]. Great care must be taken to inform patients of the benefits and risks of various therapies and to respect their ultimate treatment choices.

The major therapeutic strategies in rheumatic diseases are shown in Table 8.1. It is very rare in chronic rheumatic diseases that these interventions are used singly, and a critical issue in good management comes with the timing of each of the interventions. This is particularly so with drug therapy and with surgery, where a decision to use one modality may preclude others. Surgical management may also be complicated by multiple joint involvement and the need to consider surgery on some joints before others.

ASSESSMENT OF DISEASE AND MANAGEMENT

A range of outcome measures[6,7] has been proposed for the assessment of rheumatic diseases and is summarized in Table 8.2. The outcome measures will vary with the disease under review. Although primarily designed for use in clinical trials, they do have applications in everyday

clinical practice. These outcomes should be measured in a reliable and valid way, but just how many should be included in any particular study will depend on a variety of factors, including the study objectives, the interests of the investigator, registration requirements and budget. With the increasing number of scales to measure outcome, it is important that those selected are reliable, valid and able to detect a clinically important change.

Professional groups such as the American College of Rheumatology (ACR) and the International League of Associations for Rheumatology, the OMERACT group and the Osteoarthritis Research Society have recently addressed some of the problems of lack of consistency in trials and have developed core sets of end points for rheumatic diseases such as rheumatoid arthritis (RA), osteoarthritis (OA), osteoporosis and ankylosing spondylitis. For rheumatoid arthritis[6], OMERACT and the American College of Rheumatology have recommended a core set of outcomes, which include clinician and patient global assessment, a disability measure, an acute phase reactant, joint counts both tender and swollen, a visual analog pain scale and radiographs for long-term studies. The American Academy of Orthopedic Surgeons and the Council of Musculoskeletal Specialty Societies have developed instruments to assess outcomes of treatment based on region-specific musculoskeletal function, including instruments for the upper extremities, the spine and the lower extremities[8–10]. These groups have also developed a specific outcome instrument for children with musculoskeletal injuries and disorders. Currently these instruments are being used to collect data in the USA on outcomes of a variety of musculoskeletal diseases and injuries.

Some of these outcomes will also be useful in clinical practice for routinely monitoring patients. Because clinical disagreement and observer variability are common throughout medicine, clinicians need to recognize the necessity for explicit, objective criteria for clinical outcomes of interest. Training can help reduce the level of clinical disagreement but in clinical trials the criteria should be applied by observers who are unaware of whether the patient is being treated with an active compound or not.

PRINCIPLES OF MANAGEMENT STRATEGIES

The timing and type of intervention used in rheumatic diseases will depend on the disease and the therapy.

Non-pharmacologic treatment

Non-pharmacologic treatments can be relatively harmless but are costly in terms of time and resources. Their efficacy needs to be assessed like any other treatment. If outcome measures and quality of life are not improved, the therapy should be discontinued or not used. Non-pharmacologic treatments vary in their sophistication from massage of a painful area in soft tissue rheumatism to careful mobilization of a lumbar apophyseal joint by a well-trained manipulative physical therapist for acute and chronic back pain. Educational activities can be generic or specific and may involve the imparting of new knowledge or a specific behavioral modification program[11]. Exercises, again, may be specific for particular muscles or muscle groups or they may be generalized. The importance of low-impact general exercise programs is seen throughout life; even the elderly can benefit, in terms of musculoskeletal symptoms, from a general aerobic exercise program[12]. A variety of devices for patients afflicted by musculoskeletal disease assist in performing activities of daily living, ranging from turning on faucets, getting on and off a toilet and opening jars to remaining mobile.

Pharmacotherapy

Pharmacotherapy is disease-specific. In metabolic diseases such as hyperuricemia, drugs to lower the serum uric acid (allopurinol or a uricosuric agent) can be combined with a specific anti-inflammatory

TABLE 8.2 OUTCOME MEASURES IN RHEUMATIC DISEASES

Attribute	Example
Death	Mortality rate
Disease	Imaging • Computed tomogram • Radiograph Biochemical Serologic • C-reactive protein • Rheumatoid factor • DNA binding
Distress	Pain assessment Joint count Range of motion
Disability	Health Assessment Questionnaire Western Ontario McMaster Arthritis Impact Measurement Scale
Dysfunction	Psychosocial questionnaires
Disposition	Risk factor assessment
Debt	Cost of disease/therapy Resource consumption
Drug effect/toxicitiy	Side effects/toxicity index
Disharmony	Family function scales

drug (e.g. colchicine or a non-steroidal anti-inflammatory drug (NSAID)) to suppress pain and inflammation. In OA, pure analgesic agents such as acetaminophen (paracetamol) are often more appropriately used. Despite this, patients with OA prefer anti-inflammatory drugs over pure analgesic drugs in terms of pain relief and greater mobility[13]. The advent of specific cyclo-oxygenase (COX)-2 inhibitors with anti-inflammatory analgesic activity but reduced gastrointestinal adverse events provides a useful alternative in patients with OA who have risk factors for gastrointestinal complications. In OA, advice on changes in lifestyle, such as weight reduction and exercise, may be extremely beneficial when combined with simple analgesics.

'Aggressive' pharmacotherapies

Rheumatoid arthritis and the other major inflammatory connective tissue diseases require aggressive therapies. There is increasing evidence that, in conditions such as RA, damage to cartilage occurs at an early stage, which is when the disease should be aggressively treated[14]. Indeed, there is a good argument now for treating RA from the outset (at least at diagnosis) with specific antirheumatic drugs and/or corticosteroids. A recent study has shown that early treatment of RA (within 6 months of disease onset) reduces the odds of disability 5 years later to a level comparable with that of patients judged clinically as not requiring treatment[15]. In RA it is important continually to re-assess the patient and determine whether disease activity is really being suppressed in order to prevent development of significant deformity.

Combinations of pharmacologic agents tend to be the norm now in the management of many inflammatory rheumatic diseases, but a frequent review of therapy is required to ensure that the drugs being used actually suppress disease activity. Of interest is a recent study from tenWolde et al., which assesses whether patients with RA who have a good response to long-term treatment with antirheumatic drugs would benefit from continuation of therapy[16]. In this 12-month study the cumulative incidence of a flare was 38% for patients continuing on placebo and 22% for those continuing on their specific antirheumatic drug. A number of other studies in the literature have also suggested that patients with RA on long-term treatment are not able to continue on a single agent for long periods of time, either because they develop side effects or because the disease becomes active again[17] (Fig. 8.1). In practice, very few patients achieve either complete or a clinically significant remission on antirheumatic drugs and the disease (RA) continues its inexorable progression to long-term disability.

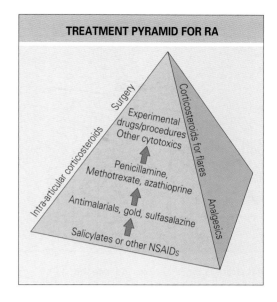

Fig. 8.2 Treatment pyramid for RA.

The 'pyramid' and 'step-down' or 'sawtooth' approaches

As important as the individual or combined action of drugs used is the way in which they are used in the clinical setting. In RA, for example, the conventional 'pyramid' approach (Fig. 8.2) has been largely superseded by the 'step-down' (Fig. 8.3) or 'sawtooth' models (Fig. 8.4). Although both have considerable merit[18,19], these novel approaches need to be assessed in formal clinical trials. In a recent study of the 'sawtooth' strategy in patients with early RA, Möttönen et al.[20] demonstrated that, over a 6-year period, 32% of 142 patients attained ACR remission criteria[21]. Boers et al.[22] have shown that, in a randomized study, a combined 'step-down' regimen of prednisone (prednisolone), methotrexate and sulfasalazine is more effective than sulfasalazine alone in slowing radiologic progression in a group of patients with early RA.

Surgery

In the chronic rheumatic diseases, physicians should work closely with surgeons in attempting optimally to time surgical intervention. Modified interventions such as arthroscopic debridement, tendon synovectomy and synovectomy need to be reviewed carefully to see if they could reduce the need for arthroplasty in the future. Timing of surgery

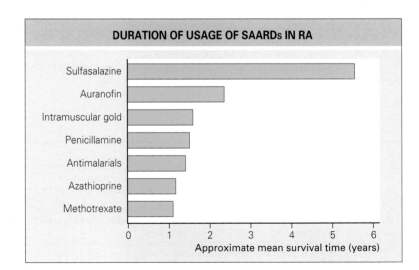

Fig. 8.1 Duration of usage of disease-modifying antirheumatic drugs (SAARDs) in RA. Approximate median survival time for seven drugs. (With permission from Wolfe[17].)

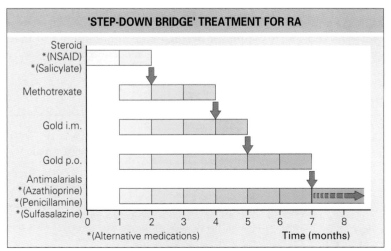

Fig. 8.3 'Step-down bridge' treatment for RA. (With permission from Wilske and Healey[18].)

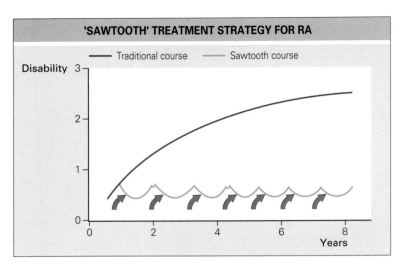

Fig. 8.4 'Sawtooth' treatment strategy for RA. Arrows indicate the administration of slow-acting antirheumatic drugs singly or in combination. (Modified with permission from Fries[19].)

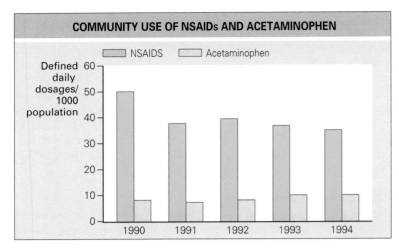

Fig. 8.5 Community use of NSAIDs and acetaminophen (paracetamol) in Australia 1990–94. (McManus P *et al.* Pattern of non-steroidal anti-inflammatory drug use in Australia 1990–1994. Med J Aus 1996; 164:589–592. © 1996. The Medical Journal of Australia, reproduced with permission.)

needs to be assessed carefully and, in particular, the sequence of surgery performed on various joints, particularly in the chronic rheumatoid patient, needs to be carefully evaluated. Joint replacement, however, remains one of the most cost-effective surgical interventions available.

Alternative medicine

Alternative and traditional medications are used by an extraordinarily large number of patients with musculoskeletal conditions (see Chapter 12). A recent study from Australia has estimated the cost to the Australian population of alternative medicine in 1993 to be in excess of Aus$621 million and that of alternative therapists to be in excess of Aus$300 million[23]. This combined amount is nearly three times the total amount of patient contributions for all classes of pharmaceutical drugs purchased in Australia for 1992/93. These data should be viewed in the light of the few properly evaluated safety or efficacy data for the vast majority of these therapies, although a recent study of glucosamine in osteoarthritis demonstrated not only decrease in pain but a suggestion of a decrease in radiologic progression.

CHANGING THERAPEUTIC PRACTICES

Management of rheumatic diseases has changed dramatically over the past 10 years. There has been much less emphasis on the use of NSAIDs, particularly in OA and soft tissue disorders, although this may change with the advent of COX-2 inhibitors. This is reflected by data[24] from Australia showing a significant decrease in community use of these drugs over the years 1990–1994 (Fig. 8.5). The reduction in NSAID use is

due to a number of factors, including recognition of the toxicities of NSAIDs[25], earlier and more aggressive use of slow-acting antirheumatic drugs in the treatment of RA and data suggesting that, for OA, acetaminophen (paracetamol) should be used initially before commencing a NSAID. It has also been appreciated over the past few years that different NSAIDs vary in their potential for gastrointestinal toxicity: ibuprofen is least likely to be associated with this adverse event[26].

The advent of specific COX-2 inhibitors[27] has reduced the use of traditional NSAIDs, although the total market has increased. More aggressive approaches to the early treatment of inflammatory arthritis and the use of specific biological agents such as tumor necrosis factor antagonists is also impacting significantly on management strategies. Evolving surgical approaches – with arthroscopic surgery, early intervention and new prostheses with different fixations and use of biomaterials – will also change practices. Changes in health-care systems, including a much greater emphasis on the evaluation of interventions and on cost-effectiveness, are also beginning to influence the way we treat patients and have led to the development of a series of guidelines for the management of OA[28] and RA[29] and the monitoring of antirheumatic therapy[30]. These guidelines will need to be reviewed continually and updated as therapeutic advances are made.

CONCLUSIONS

We are at an exciting stage in the therapy of rheumatic diseases, with a vast array of interventions to help patients cope better with their disease. We still need to think carefully how we use these interventions and continually reassess their efficacy.

REFERENCES

1. Cochrane's legacy (editorial). Lancet 1992; 340: 1131–1132.
2. Ward MM, Leigh JP, Fries JF. Progression of functional disability in patients with rheumatoid arthritis – associations with rheumatology subspecialty care. Arch Intern Med 1993; 153: 2229–2237.
3. Brooks PM. Undergraduate education in rheumatology. Br J Rheumatol 1996; 35: 203–204.
4. Lorig K, Cox T, Cuevas Y *et al.* Converging and diverging beliefs about arthritis: Caucasian patients, Spanish speaking patients and physicians. J Rheumatol 1984; 11: 76–79.
5. Donovan J. Patient education and the consultation: the importance of lay beliefs. Ann Rheum Dis 1991; 50: 418–421.
6. Boers M, Tugwell P, Felson D *et al.* WHO–ILAR core endpoints for symptom modifying antirheumatic drugs in RA clinical trials. J Rheumatol 1994; 41(suppl): 86–89.
7. LeQuesne M, Brandt K, Bellamy N *et al.* Guidelines for testing slow acting drugs in OA. J Rheumatol 1994; 41(suppl): 65–74.

8. American Academy of Orthopaedic Surgeons/Council of Musculoskeletal Speciality Societies. Disabilities of the arm, shoulder and hand outcomes data collection package (Version 1.3). Rosemont, IL: American Academy of Orthopaedic Surgeons, 1996: 1–7.
9. American Academy of Orthopaedic Surgeons/Council of Musculoskeletal Speciality Societies. Lower Limb Outcomes Data Collection Package (Version 1.3). Rosemont, IL: American Academy of Orthopaedic Surgeons, 1996: 1–40.
10. American Academy of Orthopaedic Surgeons/Council of Musculoskeletal Speciality Societies/Council of Spine Societies. Spine Outcomes Data Collection Package (Version 1.3). Rosemont, IL: American Academy of Orthopaedic Surgeons, 1996: 1–25.
11. Hawley DJ. Psycho-educational interventions in the treatment of arthritis. Baillière's Clin Rheumatol 1995; 9: 803–823.
12. Fiatrone M, Marks BC, Ryan ND *et al.* High intensity strength training on nonagenarians. JAMA 1990; 263: 3029–3034.

13. Pincus T, Swearingen C, Cummins P, Callaghan LF. Preference for non steroidal anti-inflammatory drugs versus acetaminophen and concomitant use of both types of drugs in patients with osteoarthritis. J Rheumatol 2000; 27: 1020–1027.

14. Wiles NJ, Lunt M, Barrett EM *et al.* Reduced disability at five years with early treatment of inflammatory polyarthritis: result from a large observational cohort, using propensity models to adjust for disease severity. Arthritis Rheum 2001; 44: 1033–1042.

15. Emery P. The optimal management of early rheumatoid arthritis: the key to preventing disability. Br J Rheumatol 1994; 33: 765–768.

16. TenWolde S, Breedveld FC, Hermans J *et al.* Randomised placebo-controlled study of stopping second-line drugs in rheumatoid arthritis. Lancet 1996; 347: 347–352.

17. Wolfe F. The epidemiology of drug treatment failure in rheumatoid arthritis. Baillière's Clin Rheumatol 1995; 9: 619–632.

18. Wilske KR, Healey LA. Remodelling the pyramid – a concept whose time has come. J Rheumatol 1989; 16: 565–567.

19. Fries JF. Re-evaluating the therapeutic approach to rheumatoid arthritis: the 'saw tooth' strategy. J Rheumatol 1990; 17(Suppl 22): 12–15.

20. Möttönen T, Paimela L, Ahonen J *et al.* Outcome in patients with early rheumatoid arthritis according to the 'saw tooth' strategy. Arthritis Rheum 1996; 39: 996–1005.

21. Pinals RS, Masi AT, Larsen RA. The Subcommittee for Criteria of Remission in Rheumatoid Arthritis of the American Rheumatism Association Diagnostic and Therapeutic Criteria Committee. Preliminary criteria for clinical remission in rheumatoid arthritis. Arthritis Rheum 1981; 24: 1308–1315.

22. Boers M, Verhoeven AC, Markusse HM *et al.* Randomised comparison of combined step-down prednisolone, methotrexate and sulphasalazine with sulphasalazine alone in early rheumatoid arthritis. Lancet 1997; 350: 309–318.

23. MacLennan AH, Wilson PH, Taylor AW. Prevalence and cost of alternative medicine in Australia. Lancet 1996; 347: 569–573.

24. McManus P, Primrose JG, Henry DA *et al.* Pattern of non-steroidal anti-inflammatory drug use in Australia 1990–1994. Med J Aust 1996; 164: 589–592.

25. Somervaile K, Faulkner G, Langman M. Non-steroidal anti-inflammatory drugs and bleeding peptic ulcer. Lancet 1986; 1: 462–464.

26. Henry D, Kim L-Y, Garcia-Rodriquez LA *et al.* Variability in risk of gastrointestinal complications with individual non-steroidal anti-inflammatory drugs: results of a collaborative meta-analysis. Br Med J 1996; 312: 1563–1566.

27. Richardson CE, Emery P. New cyclo-oxygenase and cytokine inhibitors. Baillière's Clin Rheumatol 1995; 9: 731–758.

28. American College of Rheumatology Subcommittee on Osteoarthritis Guidelines. Recommendations for the medical management of osteoarthritis of the hip and knee. Arthritis Rheum 2000; 43: 1905–1915.

29. American College of Rheumatology Ad Hoc Committee on Clinical Guidelines. Guidelines for management of rheumatoid arthritis. Arthritis Rheum 1996; 39: 713–722.

30. American College of Rheumatology Subcommittee on Rheumatoid Arthritis Guidelines. Guidelines for the management of rheumatoid arthritis 2002 update. Arthritis Rheum 2002; 46: 328–346.

9

Principles of pain and pain management

Milton L Cohen

- Pain is best appreciated in a biopsychosocial framework, which identifies nociceptive, neuropathic, cognitive–perceptual and socioenvironmental determinants

- Pain is the major contributor to the morbidity, disability and socioeconomic costs of musculoskeletal disorders

- The fundamental clinical feature in the assessment of pain is the phenomenon of tenderness (correctly, allodynia and hyperalgesia), which allows inference of the anatomic origin and mechanism of production of pain

- Management of pain includes influencing nociception where possible, treating the pain itself as a distressing symptom and addressing the consequences of pain on mood, beliefs and behavior

- Treatment modalities include non-opioid, opioid and adjuvant analgesic drugs, physical programs and a variety of cognitive and behavioral approaches, tailored to the individual

TABLE 9.1 BIOPSYCHOSOCIAL MODEL FOR PAIN

Biopsychosocial hierarchy	Clinical determinants	Example
Society	Socioenvironmental	Unemployment
Interperson	Cognitive–perceptual	Depression
Person	Cognitive–perceptual	Inability to write or type
Nervous system	Neuropathic	Pain
Tissue	Nociceptive	Arthritis of hands

INTRODUCTION – MUSCULOSKELETAL PAIN IN A BIOPSYCHOSOCIAL FRAMEWORK

The cardinal clinical feature of musculoskeletal problems is pain. The International Association for the Study of Pain[1] defines pain as an unpleasant sensory and emotional experience associated with actual or potential tissue damage or described in such terms. This links pain not only to nociception (the detection of tissue damage) but also to the threat or apprehension of nociception, thus involving factors governed by perception or belief. Despite the tradition of clinical method as a quest for an underlying disease process of which the pain is merely a symptom, some clinical problems characterized by arthralgia and myalgia, such as various forms of 'soft-tissue rheumatism' or 'non-specific spinal pain', do not resolve into clear pathologic entities. This is also reflected in the well-documented but poorly applied discordance between radiologic signs of altered musculoskeletal anatomy and the clinical picture. This is a challenge to the biomedical model of illness that, if not addressed, can lead to inappropriate assessment, labeling and therapy. Furthermore, the morbidity, disability and socioeconomic costs of rheumatologic disorders are attributable largely to the pain that characterizes them.

Pain may be driven by nociception initially but may persist in situations where nociception is no longer readily detectable. Pain then becomes not only a problem in its own right as a form of distress but also a source of disability or loss of function. These concerns underline the importance of a biopsychosocial framework for analyzing rheumatologic disorders. This embraces both the somatic reductionist direction (considering the person as a collection of organs, tissues, cells and molecules) and the broader psychosocial direction (reflecting the emotional and cognitive functions of a person and the interaction of the person with family, friends, workplace, local community, national community and the biosphere itself)[2].

A simplified approach (Table 9.1) identifies, in ascending biopsychosocial hierarchical order:

- tissue damage (nociceptive level)
- processing of nociceptive information by the nervous system (neuropathic level)
- the whole person in terms of affect, cognition and behavior (cognitive–behavioral level)
- society at large (social and environmental levels).

This chapter presents a framework for appreciating rheumatologic disorders as problems of pain, from the somatic basis for nociception through understanding the clinical phenomenon of tenderness (allodynia) to appreciating the role of disrupted psychological and social functioning arising out of the attendant distress.

NOCICEPTION IN MUSCULOSKELETAL TISSUES

Basic outline of nociception

Nociception is signaled by primary afferent neurons, which respond to noxious (tissue-damaging) stimuli and as such are characterized by high thresholds for activation.[3] Cutaneous nociceptors have been the best described and in humans include those subserved by lightly myelinated (Aδ) and non-myelinated (C) fibers. Mechanoheat receptors, served by Aδ afferent fibers, are considered to transduce pain of sharp, pricking quality as experienced initially following insult, while polymodal nociceptors, served by the more slowly conducting C afferents, are responsible for the dull, deep quality of prolonged pain following injury. As nociceptive afferents enter the spinal cord, those of smaller diameter segregate laterally and terminate in the more superficial layers of the dorsal horn (laminae I and II); the larger non-nociceptive afferents segregate medially and terminate in deeper laminae (Fig. 9.1). Of the many neuropeptides that are candidates for transmitter function in primary nociceptive afferents, substance P and excitatory amino acids such as glutamate and aspartate have received most attention.

In the dorsal horn, primary afferent neurons interact with interneurons and descending supraspinal pathways to modulate incoming nociceptive information. The interneurons comprise both nociceptive-specific and

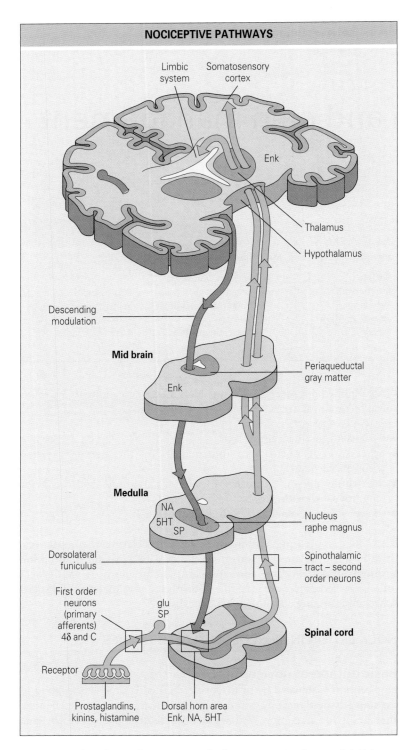

NOCICEPTIVE PATHWAYS

Fig. 9.1 Nociceptive pathways. 5HT, 5-hydroxytryptamine (serotonin); Enk, enkephalins and other opioids; glu, glutamate and other excitatory amino acids; NA, norepinephrine (noradrenaline); SP, substance P and other tachykinins.

wide-dynamic-range cells, the latter in particular receiving convergent input from cutaneous and deep structures, providing a substrate for the phenomenon of referred pain. The pharmacology of this interaction is complex, serotonin, norepinephrine (noradrenaline) and enkephalin in particular being described in descending inhibitory pathways.

The myelinated axons from the majority of second-order nociceptive neurons terminate in the contralateral thalamus via the anterolateral quadrant of the spinal cord. A minor spinothalamic projection ascends ipsilaterally. Spinothalamic axons terminate in several distinct thalamic nuclei: the lateral (ventrobasal) nuclei project to the somatosensory

cortex while the medial nuclei, which also receive input from the reticular formation, project to wide areas of the ipsilateral cortex. This division is held to underlie respectively the sensory–discriminative and motivational–affective aspects of pain.

Receptors and primary afferents in joint, bone and muscle

Animal studies have been the predominant source of information concerning nociception in musculoskeletal tissues[4,5]. Mammalian joints have a rich array of receptors potentially able to signal nociception. Nociceptors homologous with polymodal cutaneous nociceptors subserved by unmyelinated C afferent fibers are found in a diffuse lattice throughout the joint capsule, while free nerve endings found in internal and external joint ligaments correspond to high-threshold Aδ cutaneous nociceptors. These receptors may also respond to non-noxious mechanical and chemical stimuli. Joint cartilage does not contain such receptors. The human synovium itself is now known to contain postganglionic sympathetic efferent fibers and unmyelinated C nociceptive afferents[6]. These fibers may be relevant in the process of neurogenic inflammation, if not also in signaling nociception.

Little is known about bone nociception. Structurally, the periosteum and bone marrow have been shown to be richly innervated in normal rats by fibers containing neuropeptides, suggesting that they may be nociceptive.

Pain in muscle may be difficult to localize and is often referred to other deep somatic structures. Specific nociceptors are probably present in skeletal muscle, of which the majority may be free nerve endings, again subserved by Aδ and C afferents. As with cutaneous nociceptors, there appears to be considerable heterogeneity of muscle nociceptors. A relatively high proportion of slowly conducting muscle afferents are non-nociceptive, responding to low-threshold mechanical stimuli including muscle contractions. Similar endings are present in tendons. These receptors may signal pressure, force or movement.

Mechanically insensitive afferents (MIAs), which do not normally respond even to noxious mechanical stimulation, have been described in feline joints. In the presence of an experimental arthritis, these MIAs acquire new response properties, characterized by spontaneous activity and discharge during non-noxious movement. No such receptors have been found in skeletal muscle.

Spinal and supraspinal connections

At the spinal cord level, nociceptive-specific and wide-dynamic-range neurons in the dorsal horn receive nociceptive inputs from articular tissues and may also respond to non-noxious mechanical stimulation of limb joints. These dorsal horn neurons receive convergent inputs from cutaneous, muscle and visceral afferents. Dorsal horn neurons responding exclusively to activation of muscle nociceptors are very rare.

Noxious joint and muscle inputs can reach thalamic and cortical levels. In models of experimental arthritis, the populations of neurons and ascending pathways activated by inflamed joints appear to be different from those signaling noxious cutaneous inputs. Tonic descending inhibitory influences have been described on dorsal horn neurons that receive convergent input from deep tissues. Such inhibition affects both the excitability of dorsal horn neurons in response to external stimuli and the degree of convergence from different sources.

Biochemistry of musculoskeletal nociception

The major role of activation and sensitization of joint afferents appears to be played by prostaglandins, in a manner similar to that of inflammation itself. Prostaglandin (PGE) reverses the depressing effect of cyclooxygenase inhibitors on the spontaneous and movement-evoked activity of nociceptive afferents from inflamed joints. Leukotrienes sensitize nociceptors in animals and humans. Bradykinin, serotonin and histamine also activate these afferents, although the effects are of short duration. These inflammatory mediators may act synergistically: bradykinin, PGE$_2$ and serotonin enhance responsiveness of joint afferents to mechanical stimuli. Substance P may stimulate the release of prostaglandins from synovial cells[3,5].

Muscle nociceptors are activated particularly by mechanical stimulation and by bradykinin. They can be sensitized by increase in temperature, increase in acidity and exposure to substances such as bradykinin, serotonin and PGE$_2$. Once irritated by a noxious mechanical stimulus, muscle nociceptors develop sensitivity to epinephrine (adrenaline).

Clinical correlates

In microneurographic studies in humans, Aδ and C afferents subserving muscle nociceptors have been found, which respond to local pressure and to algesic substances similarly to receptors in animals. Repetitive electrical stimulation of these muscle afferent units has been associated with cramp-like sensations; however, it remains difficult to assess whether different types of muscle nociceptor mediate different qualities of muscle pain. Intrafascicular microstimulation of single joint afferents has been associated with innocuous deep sensations in humans.

The degree of convergence of deep afferents at the spinal level provides an anatomic basis for the poor localization and discrimination that may attend joint and muscle pain, and the referral of pain and hyperalgesia that may accompany pathology.

PATHOPHYSIOLOGY OF MUSCULOSKELETAL PAIN AND HYPERALGESIA

Hyperalgesia, allodynia and sensitization

The cardinal clinical phenomenon attending musculoskeletal pain is tenderness, which encompasses two clinicopathologic phenomena: hyperalgesia and allodynia. Consistent with the definition of pain above, hyperalgesia is defined as increased pain in response to a noxious stimulus[1], allodynia as pain in response to an innocuous stimulus[1]. In clinical examination, both hyperalgesia and allodynia can be elicited, depending on the nature and intensity of the stimulus used: for example, palpation (pressure) is potentially noxious; light touch or brushing is not.

The clinical characteristics of hyperalgesia and allodynia are:

- decreased threshold to noxious stimuli (which may include responding to innocuous stimuli)
- increased pain from suprathreshold stimuli
- spontaneous pain.

The neurophysiologic correlates of these phenomena at the receptor or afferent fiber level, called sensitization, are:

- decreased response threshold
- increased response to suprathreshold stimuli
- spontaneous activity.

In the context of cutaneous injury, the most extensively studied model, two types of allodynia/hyperalgesia have been described. Primary allodynia/hyperalgesia occurs in an area of injury while secondary allodynia/hyperalgesia may be found in the undamaged tissue surrounding the injury. The psychophysical characteristics and mechanisms of these two types are distinct[7] (Table 9.2).

Primary hyperalgesia – peripheral sensitization

The main mechanism of primary cutaneous hyperalgesia to thermal stimuli is sensitization of Aδ and C fiber afferents. Primary mechanical hyperalgesia may be attributable to sensitization of some nociceptors to mechanical stimuli or to enlargement of the mechanical receptive field of the primary afferent nociceptor, although sensitization of central nociceptive pathways may also be relevant (see below).

Sensitization of joint nociceptors has been shown in both cat and rat models of joint inflammation: MIAs and afferents previously responding only to intense joint movement develop increased resting activity and begin to respond to non-noxious movements[5]. Experimental myositis in these animals is associated with an increase in resting discharge in both presumed nociceptors and receptors responding to weak mechanical stimuli, with an increased proportion of the latter[4].

Neurogenic inflammation

The involvement of the nervous system in inflammation[8,9] has been recognized since the demonstration of the 'axon reflex', localized vasodilatation and exudation that can be induced by antidromic stimulation of primary C nociceptive afferent fibers, which release neuropeptides at their peripheral terminals. These peptides are synthesized proximally in cell bodies in the dorsal root ganglia and are transported distally as well as centrally. They include substance P, calcitonin-gene-related peptide, somatostatin, vasoactive intestinal peptide, neurokinin A and neurokinin B. As a group, they exert a variety of influences on inflammation, including changes in vascular tone and permeability, activation of neutrophils, proliferation and function of T and B lymphocytes, release of cytokines, production of oxygen-free radicals and release of prostaglandins.

Neurogenic inflammation contributes to acute and chronic arthritis. Intra-articular injection of substance P in rats induces local inflammation, while capsaicin, which selectively depletes substance P from primary afferent fibers, attenuates the development of experimental arthritis in the rat. In animal models of chronic arthritis, injection of substance P increases the local severity of inflammation, and the severity of arthritis

TABLE 9.2 DISTINCTION BETWEEN PRIMARY AND SECONDARY HYPERALGESIA/ALLODYNIA IN SKIN

	Primary	Secondary
Clinical	Tissue inflamed or damaged Allodynia in region of inflammation or damage	Absence of obvious tissue inflammation or damage Provocable hyperesthesias (including allodynia) in region of pain
Psychophysical	Reduced threshold to stimulation Reduced tolerance to thermal and mechanical stimulation	Normal threshold to stimulation Reduced tolerance to mechanical stimulation only
Mechanism	Sensitization of nociceptors (thermal; possibly mechanical) Enlarged receptive fields (mechanical)	'Axon reflex' Sensitization of central nociceptive pathways

and the density of substance-P-containing nociceptive afferents are directly related.

In humans, immunohistochemical techniques reveal at least substance P and calcitonin-gene-related peptide in synovium, found in patterns suggesting local release in inflammatory arthritis compared with osteoarthrosis. Clinically, afferent or sympathetic interruption influences inflammatory joint disease. These observations together establish the relevance of the efferent influence of primary nociceptive afferents on joint inflammation.

Secondary hyperalgesia – central sensitization

Allodynia occurring outside an area of tissue damage or inflammation ('secondary hyperalgesia') is usually defined by the response to mechanical stimuli. There are three potential mechanisms:

- peripheral sensitization (nociceptor level)
- central sensitization (spinal level)
- reduced descending inhibition (supraspinal level).

Microneurographic studies in humans have provided some evidence for the first of these.

The major mechanism invoked to explain secondary allodynia/hyperalgesia is the phenomenon of neural plasticity at the spinal cord level. This refers to the changes in connectivity resulting from persistent nociceptive input (injury, noxious stimulation or C-fiber afferent electrical stimulation), characterized by increased activity, enhanced responsiveness to peripheral stimuli and enlarged receptive field size of dorsal horn cells[10]. The clinical correlates of this are spontaneous pain, allodynia, hyperalgesia and an increase in the size of the region from which pain can be elicited.

In rats, changes in dorsal horns following peripheral nerve injury, including trans-synaptic degeneration and reorganization with the formation of new synaptic connections, provide an anatomic basis for the phenomenon of sensitization. Its proposed biochemical basis is the release of neuropeptides and excitatory amino acids (EAAs) into the dorsal horn, leading to slow depolarization, then persistent changes in excitability and ultimately excessive depolarization with EAA-induced cytotoxicity. This cell dysfunction, with possible loss of inhibitory mechanisms, could lead to persistence of changes in the absence of further noxious input[11].

Central changes in experimental arthritis and myositis

Acute or chronic arthritis or myositis can induce changes in central nociceptive pathways (dorsal horn, thalamus and primary somatosensory cortex), manifest as increased background discharge and enhanced responsiveness to afferent activity both from the site of inflammation and from other convergent inputs[4,5]. Reduction in tonic descending inhibition of spinal cord neurons that receive articular afferent input has been shown in association with acute feline arthritis.

Initiation and maintenance of central sensitization

An extensive literature, both in animals and clinically and experimentally in humans, supports the concept that sustained C-afferent nociceptive input from peripheral inflammation or nerve damage is associated with central hyperexcitability[12]. In humans, duration and extent of secondary allodynia/hyperalgesia in skin are dependent on the intensity of the initiating nociceptive stimulus. It has been suggested that central excitability may be a physiologic accompaniment of ongoing nociception. Whether central sensitization needs ongoing afferent 'drive' or may become autonomous has yet to be determined.

ASSESSMENT OF PAIN AT THE SOMATIC LEVEL

At the clinical level the presenting feature is pain. A rational approach is to determine:

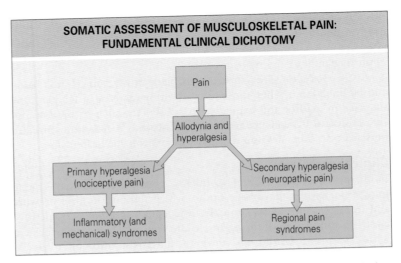

Fig. 9.2 Somatic assessment of musculoskeletal pain: fundamental clinical dichotomy.

- what is the anatomic origin of pain
- what are the mechanisms of pain production
- is there an associated disease process?

The first two can be addressed through dissection of the accompanying allodynia and hyperalgesia: whether primary (implying peripheral sensitization) or secondary (implying central changes) (Fig. 9.2).

Primary hyperalgesia: nociceptive pain – inflammatory and mechanical models

Conceptually, inflammation may be seen as the combination of:

- pain, attributable to activation of nociceptors
- primary allodynia/hyperalgesia, due to sensitization of nociceptors
- swelling, which reflects the vascular effects of neuropeptide release.

This conceptualization accounts for inflammation occurring in response to both immunologic and neurogenic processes[8]. This inflammatory model accounts for most (but not all) of the pain and allodynia/hyperalgesia of active (but not inactive) inflammatory disease. As inflammation is known to sensitize nociceptors and MIAs, a scenario for subsequent persistent sensitivity to movement of damaged joints and muscles may well be created.

Nociceptors and mechanoreceptors in musculoskeletal tissues may also be activated by increased intra-articular pressure or abnormal posture of joints. Although not usually considered to transduce nociception, mechanoreceptors may become involved in the generation and maintenance of spinal cord plasticity such that mechanoreceptive information is processed as noxious.

The relevant clinical observation is that joints that do not move properly (hypomobile, less commonly hypermobile) may be painful whether or not they are anatomically abnormal. This model implies that changes in joint biomechanics *per se* may be responsible for pain and primary hyperalgesia without invoking inflammatory processes. It follows that mechanical nociception may be particularly relevant in joints that have been damaged by a pathologic process (e.g. osteoarthritis), especially if nociceptors have been sensitized by prior influences.

Secondary hyperalgesia: neuropathic model

The well-recognized phenomenon of referred pain is considered to depend on neuroanatomic convergence at a spinal level and on perceptual divergence at thalamic and cortical levels. The finding of (mechanical) allodynia in regions of referred pain argues in favor of altered central function as well: the psychophysical characteristics of referred pain are those of secondary hyperalgesia[7,10].

Referred pain is recognized in chronic arthropathy. For example, pain from an osteoarthritic hip is commonly referred to the knee. Considering the chronicity of many rheumatologic diseases and the attendant potential for sustained nociception over time, the role of altered function of central nociceptive pathways in the pathogenesis of musculoskeletal pain should be considered. Clinically this would be expressed as regions of secondary allodynia/hyperalgesia.

The constructs of fibromyalgia and related syndromes (Chapter 20) are built on the assumption that peripheral musculoskeletal pathology accounts for the pain. In the absence of convincing evidence for such pathology, the concepts of secondary allodynia/hyperalgesia and central sensitization must be invoked for physiologic plausibility of this construct and to avoid circular arguments.

In humans, however, the question remains of how the perception of these presumed central changes may in turn influence them. The occurrence of clinical allodynia in the absence of 'hard' signs has led to considerable controversy. On one side of the debate are the proponents of specific clinical entities such as 'fibromyalgia syndrome' and 'myofascial pain syndrome' (Chapter 20); the critics on the other side describe these as examples of 'pseudoneuropathies' of implied psychogenic origin[13]. This debate is difficult to resolve, as primary psychogenic hypotheses are untestable and the human central nociceptive system is at present only indirectly accessible. In these situations of joint and muscle pain where the pathology is not readily attributable to (peripheral) nociception, the role of perception by conscious, sentient humans confronted with a nociceptive event that fails to settle must be taken into account. Clinical assessment may then depend even more on understanding the biopsychosocial hierarchical levels of 'nervous system' and above (Table 9.1).

ASSESSMENT OF PAIN AT THE COGNITIVE–BEHAVIORAL AND SOCIOENVIRONMENTAL LEVELS

Pain disrupts the life of the individual in terms of self-esteem and self-image, relationships with others, ability to complete tasks of daily living and to work and function as a member of the community. Identification of the somatic processes leading to musculoskeletal pain forms only part of the clinical picture. The consequences of pain for function and for mood are of at least equal importance, especially with respect to the person's ability to cope with the usual demands of life. In chronic musculoskeletal illnesses where the pathology is known and

TABLE 9.3 FACTORS IN THE COGNITIVE–PERCEPTUAL AND SOCIOLOGIC ASSESSMENT OF PAIN	
Affective	Anxiety Anger Depression
Behavioral	Posture and usage patterns Reinforcement of inactivity Role changes Interference with sleep Interpersonal relationships Treatment-seeking: doctor-shopping; drug usage
Cognitive	Beliefs and expectations regarding causation, pathology and prognosis Influence of industrial, financial and legal issues Intercurrent stressors

rational therapy available, such as the inflammatory joint diseases, the three major determinants of overall health are psychologic status, physical functioning and pain itself[14]. Anxiety and depression are common in cohorts of patients with rheumatoid arthritis, persistent low back pain and persistent neck pain, their development being related more to socioeconomic than to clinical indices. Disability is strongly correlated with attitude to illness: these considerations underlie the importance of assessing patients' beliefs regarding the nature and prognosis of their pain[15–17].

Assessment of the person with pain at this cognitive–behavioral level includes effects on mood, activity and rest patterns and the consequences of pain for ability to work and to function socially, for self-esteem and for beliefs (Table 9.3). Of the many instruments that have been developed for the assessment of these aspects of pain[18], the Westhaven Yale Multidimensional Pain Inventory (WHYMPI) has been most used. Cognitive factors, such as pain coping strategies, modulate health status in both inflammatory and non-inflammatory musculoskeletal disease. A number of these instruments correlate with changes in pain intensity and physical functioning and respond to cognitive–behavioral therapy[19].

These outcome measures can be used in assessing the efficacy of a variety of interventions, including pharmacologic ones, and may also be used in determining prognosis, especially in musculoskeletal diseases where impairment may not always be reflected in disability for which, in turn, there is no simple single measure.

TABLE 9.4 PRINCIPLES OF PAIN MANAGEMENT		
Aims	Minimize distress Maximize function	
Modalities	Pharmacologic (see Table 9.5)	Analgesics Anti-inflammatories Adjuvant analgesics
	Physical	Ergonomic analysis of posture and function Exercise regimens Avoidance of passive treatments
	'Psychological' (cognitive–behavioral)	Validation Goal-setting Pacing of activity Self-regulatory skills (relaxation, distraction) Stress-management skills Problem-solving skills

MANAGEMENT OF PAIN

A management plan based on an understanding of physical and psychosocial contributions is optimal for the patient with musculoskeletal pain. In both inflammatory and non-inflammatory conditions, it has been shown that prognosis may be affected as much by cognitive, behavioral and socioeconomic factors as by specific treatments. With respect to persistent musculoskeletal pain, however, both nociception (peripheral or central) and the pain itself (as a problem in its own right) need to be addressed. A rational approach to pain management includes treatments directed at the mechanisms of nociception, at the affective and cognitive components of the pain, aspects of the underlying disease and at the consequences in terms of personal and social function (Table 9.4).

Treatment of mechanisms of nociception

The traditional approach to the management of inflammatory disease has included the use of a range of drugs, often prescribed in a rather hierarchical fashion. Non-steroidal anti-inflammatory drugs (NSAIDs) tend to be used initially, followed after some period of time by the use of second-line agents (see Chapters 10 and 11). Specific antagonists to non-prostaglandin mediators have yet to be developed for the clinical setting.

The role of altered central nociception in the production of pain and (secondary) allodynia/hyperalgesia in chronic musculoskeletal disorders awaits further elucidation. This phenomenon does suggest the usefulness of agents that may interfere with excitatory EAAs and monoamines in these conditions, where sensitization of dorsal horn neurons is highly likely to have occurred. Currently available agents include anticonvulsant and tricyclic antidepressant drugs.

Two interacting groups of neurochemical mediators, colocalized to the terminals of fine primary afferent fibers in the dorsal horn, are held to be responsible for the mechanism of plasticity induced by noxious stimulation. These include C-fiber neuropeptides and EAAs – L-glutamate, L-aspartate, N-methyl-D-aspartate (NMDA)[10]. Antagonists to these mediators have been shown in experimental animals to suppress or prevent sensitization of dorsal horn neurons in response to nociceptive input. In humans, experience is limited to postoperative and experimental pain.

Treatment of pain itself

The use of non-opioid and opioid analgesics is rational in these disorders, to reduce the distress of pain itself, over and above the physical consequences of disease (Table 9.5). Acetaminophen (paracetamol) is an undervalued effective analgesic agent. Its mechanism of action remains poorly understood, although there is evidence for direct effects on the central nervous system[20]. A major advantage is its lack of upper gastrointestinal toxicity, especially ulceration and bleeding. The well-known hazard of hepatotoxicity, seen virtually only with drug overdose, is increased with liver disease and alcoholism, and the daily dose should be carefully monitored in these situations. The risk for nephrotoxicity with chronic dosing remains uncertain but is probably very small.

The role of opioids in the management of chronic, moderate to severe musculoskeletal pain remains controversial. A diverse literature supports the clinical experience that patients with nociceptive and neuropathic chronic pain syndromes may benefit from long-term opioid therapy while those with idiopathic pain syndromes fare less well.[21] Although they are considered to work mainly through opiate receptors in the central nervous system, by inhibition of transmission of nociceptive messages to higher centers or through activation of descending antinociceptive pathways[22], increasing evidence points to peripheral analgesic actions of opioids, especially in conditions characterized by inflammatory (primary) hyperalgesia[23]. As toxicity and addiction remain concerns in both clinical and administrative spheres, guidelines for the prescription of opioids in chronic non-malignant pain have been published[24]. The essential features of such guidelines, which advocate the use of written treatment contracts, include:

- multidisciplinary biopsychosocial assessment, especially to establish a diagnosis, to identify psychosocial amplifiers of pain and to consider psychological stability and prior history of substance abuse
- consideration of the role of physical and cognitive modalities of treatment and the use of non-opioid analgesic drugs and to tricyclic antidepressant and/or membrane-stabilizing drugs
- the sole prescribing doctor to have an established therapeutic relationship with the patient
- opioids prescribed initially on a trial basis, with agreed outcome goals.

It is emphasized that opioid therapy in this context is not an end in itself but a passport to increased activity and quality of life.

Antidepressant drugs may enhance the analgesia induced by other drugs. The presumed site of action is at the spinal cord level (as for their putative effect on central sensitization), although their beneficial effect on sleep and on mood, where appropriate, suggests action elsewhere in the neuraxis. Debate continues over possible modes of action and whether or not these drugs induce analgesia in the absence of depression in chronic pain generally[25].

TABLE 9.5 RATIONAL PHARMACOTHERAPY FOR PAIN		
Target	**Drug**	**Proposed action**
Inflammation; peripheral sensitization	NSAID	Antiprostaglandin
	Corticosteroids (systemic or local)	Vascular and cellular effects
Neuropathic pain; central sensitization	Tricyclic antidepressants	Effects on monoamine (serotonin and norepinephrine (noradrenaline))-mediated central pathways
	Anticonvulsants	Suppression of paroxysmal discharges
	Local anesthetics (oral)	Non-depolarizing neural blockade
	Neuropeptide antagonists*	Opposition to substance P, calcitonin-gene-related peptide (CGRP), etc.
	NMDA receptor antagonists*	Opposition to EAAs
Pain itself	Acetaminophen (paracetamol)	Central
	Opioid agonists	Activation of μ receptors (brain), δ and κ receptors (spinal cord); possible peripheral action

* Under development.

Physical therapy

The goals of physical therapy include increasing and maintaining muscle strength and endurance, increasing joint motion, reducing joint instability and improving capacity to perform activities of daily living. As with pharmacologic agents, physical prescriptions should be individualized, ideally based on a biopsychosocial evaluation, to take into account comorbidity, issues of pain control and compliance. Although a recent review found little evidence that any specific therapy had long-term efficacy greater than placebo, there is evidence of the effectiveness of most forms of physical therapy during the treatment phase[26]. Physical therapy has an important cognitive as well as behavioral dimension in chronic pain.

Cognitive–behavioral therapy and pain clinics

Chronic pain management programs emphasize therapies that seek to change behavior and belief systems. The recognition that the clinical problem of chronic pain should be processed in a biopsychosocial framework (Table 9.1) has led to the development of multidisciplinary management programs that incorporate both physically and psychologically based components. The latter include operant deconditioning, cognitive restructuring, problem-solving, coping skills training, relaxation and biofeedback.

Cognitive–behavior therapy in arthritis has been associated with significant reductions in pain behavior and anxiety and, in the case of rheumatoid arthritis, with reduction in disease activity[27]. A meta-analysis of 25 controlled studies of cognitive behavior therapy in mixed examples of chronic pain found that active psychological treatments were effective, especially in the domains of pain experience, enhancing positive coping measures and reducing behavioral expression of pain.

However this review also noted that such studies, being based on volunteers and having strict criteria for participation, may not be generalizable to patients in community practice, while it was not possible to distinguish between the effects of different protocols[28].

Many publications proclaim the effectiveness of interdisciplinary pain programs, a meta-analysis of 65 such studies concluding that the benefits can extend to variables such as return to work and use of the health-care system[29.] However there remains diversity among pain centers with respect to diagnostic and etiologic frames of reference, professional background of staff, selection criteria used and treatment modalities offered. The factors responsible for improvement in the context of multidisciplinary programs require further clarification: efficacy may be related to changes in belief and cognitive coping strategies rather than to the use of specific techniques such as exercise, suggesting that improvements may be more closely associated with what patients think about their pain than with what they do about it[30].

SUMMARY

An understanding of the neurobiology and the sociobiology of pain is integral to the practice of rheumatological medicine. Recognition of the interaction of the somatic components (nociception and its central transmission) with the cognitive components (belief, mood and behavior) provides a framework for comprehensive assessment and management. At the somatic level, this includes insight into the mechanisms of the fundamental clinical phenomena of allodynia and hyperalgesia, while at the cognitive–behavioral level, it may be appreciated that not all the observed distress need be nociceptive. A combination of pharmacologic and cognitive–behavioral (including physical) therapies, appropriate to the individual patient, is recommended.

REFERENCES

1. Merskey H, Bogduk N, eds. Classification of chronic pain, 2nd ed. Seattle: IASP; 1994.
2. Steig RL, Williams RC. Chronic pain as a biosociocultural phenomenon: implications for treatment. Semin Neurol 1983; 3: 370–376.
3. Portenoy RK. Basic mechanisms. In: Portenoy RK, Kanner RM, eds. Pain management: theory and practice. Philadelphia: FA Davis; 1996: 19–39.
4. Graven-Nielsen T, Mense S. The peripheral apparatus of muscle pain: evidence from animal and human studies. Clin J Pain 2001; 17: 2–10.
5. Schaible H-G, Grubb BD. Afferent and spinal mechanisms of joint pain. Pain 1993; 55: 5–54.
6. Mapp P. Innervation of the synovium. Ann Rheum Dis 1995; 54: 398–403.
7. Koltzenburg M. Neural mechanisms of cutaneous nociceptive pain. Clin J Pain 2000; 16(suppl): S131–S138.
8. Matucci-Cerini M, Partsch G. The contribution of the peripheral nervous system and the neuropeptide network to the development of synovial inflammation. Clin Exp Rheumatol 1992; 10: 211–215.
9. Levine JD, Goetzl EJ, Basbaum AI. Contribution of the nervous system to the pathophysiology of rheumatoid arthritis and other polyarthritides. Rheum Dis Clin North Am 1987; 13: 369–383.
10. Coderre TJ, Katz J, Vaccarino AL, Melzack R. Contribution of central neuroplasticity to pathologic pain: review of clinical and experimental evidence. Pain 1993; 52: 259–285.
11. Mannion RJ, Woolf CJ. Pain mechanisms and management: a central perspective. Clin J Pain 2000; 16(suppl): S144–S156.
12. Dubner R Neural basis of persistent pain: sensory specialization, sensory modulation and neuronal plasticity. In: Jensen TS, Turner JA, Wiesenfeld-Hallin Z, eds. Proceedings of the 8th World Congress on Pain. Seattle: IASP Press; 1997: 243–258.
13. Ochoa JL. Essence, investigation and management of 'neuropathic' pains: hopes from acknowledgement of chaos. Muscle Nerve 1993; 16: 997–1008.
14. Kazis LE, Meenan RF, Anderson JJ. Pain in the rheumatic diseases: investigations of a key health status component. Arthritis Rheum 1983; 26: 1017–1022.
15. McFarlane AC, Brooks PM. An analysis of the relationship between psychological morbidity and disease activity in rheumatoid arthritis. J Rheumatol 1988; 15: 926–931.
16. Weiser S, Cedrashi C. Psychosocial issues in the prevention of chronic low back pain – a literature review. Baillière's Clin Rheumatol 1992; 6: 657–684.
17. Radanov BP, Sturzenegger M, Di Stefano G. Long-term outcome after whiplash injury. A 2-year follow-up considering features of injury mechanism and somatic, radiologic and psychosocial findings. Medicine (Baltimore) 1995; 74: 281–297.
18. Turk DC, Melzack R, eds. Handbook of pain assessment. New York: Guilford Press; 1992.
19. Parker JC, Bradley LA, DeVellis RM et al. Biopsychosocial contributions to the management of arthritis disability. Arthritis Rheum 1993; 36: 885–889.
20. Prescott LF. Paracetamol: past, present and future. Am J Therapeutics 2000; 7: 143–147.
21. Graven S, de Vet HCW, van Kleef M, Weber WEJ. Opioids in chronic non-malignant pain: a criteria-based review of the literature. In: Devor M, Rowbotham MC, Wiesenfeld-Hallin Z eds. Proceedings of the 9th World Congress on Pain. Seattle: IASP Press; 2000: 965–972.
22. Twycross RG. Opioids. In: Wall PD, Melzack R, eds. Textbook of pain, 4th edn. Edinburgh: Churchill Livingstone; 1999: 1187–1214.
23. Stein C. The control of pain in peripheral tissues by opioids. N Engl J Med 1995; 332; 1685–1690.
24. Graziotti PJ, Goucke CR. The use of oral opioids in patients with chronic non-cancer pain. Med J Aust 1997; 167: 30–34.
25. McQuay HJ, Tramer M, Nye BA et al. A systematic review of antidepressants in neuropathic pain. Pain 1996; 68: 217–227.
26. Feine JS, Lund JP. An assessment of the efficacy of physical therapy and physical modalities for the control of chronic musculoskeletal pain. Pain 1997; 71: 5–23.
27. Bradley LA, Alberts KR. Psychological and behavioral approaches to pain management for patients with rheumatic disease. Med Clin North Am 1999; 25: 215–232.
28. Morley S, Eccleston C, Williams A. Systematic review and meta-analysis of randomized controlled trials of cognitive behavior therapy and behavior therapy for chronic pain in adults, excluding headache. Pain 1999; 80: 1–13.
29. Flor H, Fydrich T, Turk DC. Efficacy of multidisciplinary pain treatment centers: a meta-analytic review. Pain 1992; 49: 221–230.
30. Jensen MP, Turner JA, Romano JM. Correlates of improvement in multidisciplinary treatment of chronic pain. J Consult Clin Psychol 1994; 62: 172–179.

10 Non-steroidal anti-inflammatory drugs

Peter M Brooks

- Non-steroidal anti-inflammatory drugs (NSAIDs) continue to provide 'background' anti-inflammatory therapy for rheumatic diseases
- Newer NSAIDs with specific inhibition of cyclo-oxygenase (COX)-2 (inducible) enzyme are associated with a lower incidence of gastrointestinal adverse events
- Variability in response to NSAIDs is seen both in terms of anti-inflammatory activity and adverse events

INTRODUCTION

Non-steroidal anti-inflammatory drugs (NSAIDs) remain the principal pharmacologic agents for symptom relief in patients with the rheumatic diseases. They constitute the largest single group of drugs used worldwide and annually have total sales in excess of $US14 billion. The NSAIDs are prescribed in the full range of rheumatic diseases and in many countries can now be purchased over the counter for symptomatic relief of headaches, dysmenorrhea and sports injuries. Over the past few years there has been a broadening in the traditional use of NSAIDs with their prescription for such things as renal and biliary colic, headache and other painful disorders. NSAIDs – both non-selective and selective – have also been shown to be beneficial in the management of Alzheimer's disease, colon cancer and hereditary polyposis coli.

The number of NSAIDs available continues to proliferate and, although subtle differences exist in pharmacokinetics, adverse reaction profiles and mechanisms of action, none of these parameters alone explains the marked variability in response noted with these agents in clinical practice. The question as to how many NSAIDs are required is a vexed one but is continually asked by rheumatologists, pharmaceutical manufacturers and drug regulators. Quite marked differences exist internationally in the availability of NSAIDs, with only six or seven NSAIDs being available in many Scandinavian countries and up to 40 in Italy. Despite the fact that the disease-modifying antirheumatic drugs (DMARDs) are being used earlier in the management of inflammatory rheumatic diseases, NSAIDs will continue to provide symptomatic relief in the foreseeable future.

In this chapter we explore new insights into the mechanism of action of NSAIDs, including specific cyclo-oxygenase (COX)-2 inhibitors, cover the range of drugs available, discuss their major pharmacokinetic and pharmacodynamic differences and raise some of the issues relevant to variability in response to these drugs. Adverse drug reactions produced by NSAIDs still pose a major problem, and strategies for reducing these to a minimum, together with practical prescribing points, are discussed.

MECHANISM OF ACTION

Inflammation in the rheumatic disease is extremely complex, involving a multiplicity of interactions between cells, mediators and other factors.

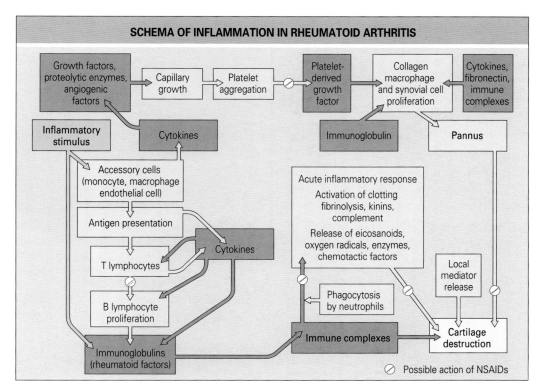

Fig. 10.1 Schema of inflammation in rheumatoid arthritis. The possible sites of action of NSAIDs are indicated.

SCHEMA OF INFLAMMATION IN RHEUMATOID ARTHRITIS

⊘ Possible action of NSAIDs

Over the past few years it has been realized that the traditional principal mechanism of action of NSAIDs, i.e. inhibition of COX, only partly explains their success in suppressing inflammatory responses. A simple schema of the inflammatory process in rheumatoid arthritis (RA) is shown in Figure 10.1, along with the sites of possible action of NSAIDs[1]. It is now clear that prostaglandins have significant influences on many of the cells and other mediators involved in the immune response. Interfering with prostaglandin synthesis will, therefore, have far-reaching effects on these activities, and NSAIDs can be said to have some mild immunomodulatory activity. In this respect the differentiation between NSAIDs, DMARDs and immunosuppressive drugs is becoming less clear.

The major actions of NSAIDs are summarized in Table 10.1. The effect of NSAIDs on prostaglandin production is well known, but it is interesting to note that non-acetylated salicylate, which has little effect on this parameter, is as effective in patients with RA as aspirin (a potent prostaglandin synthesis inhibitor)[2]. NSAIDs differ in their affects on neutrophils, lymphocytes and chondrocytes[3].

Recently it has been shown that COX has two distinct isoenzymes – a constitutive form (COX-1) and an inducible form (COX-2) found at sites of inflammation[4] (Fig. 10.2). COX-1 is responsible for maintaining normal gastric mucosal function. Specific COX-2 inhibition has the advantage of reducing gastric adverse events[5].

The available NSAIDs come from a variety of chemical classes and differences in their physicochemical parameters may influence the pharmacokinetics and give rise to differences in their beneficial and adverse effects. For example, the more lipid-soluble NSAIDs, such as ketoprofen, naproxen and ibuprofen, penetrate the central nervous system (CNS) more easily and are associated with mild changes in mood and cognitive function. The majority of NSAIDs are weakly acidic and will preferentially concentrate in inflamed tissues.

PHARMACOKINETICS

The pharmacokinetic parameters of a drug are dependent on its absorption and bioavailability, its distribution throughout the body and its half-life. An understanding of the pharmacokinetics of a drug is only relevant to patient care if the therapeutic response and adverse reactions are related to the plasma concentrations achieved with that drug[7]. Dose- and/or plasma concentration-response relationships have been demonstrated in RA for a number of NSAIDs, including naproxen, carprofen and ibuprofen[3,7]. As can be seen from Figure 10.3, the percentage of patients responding to naproxen increases with the plasma concentra-

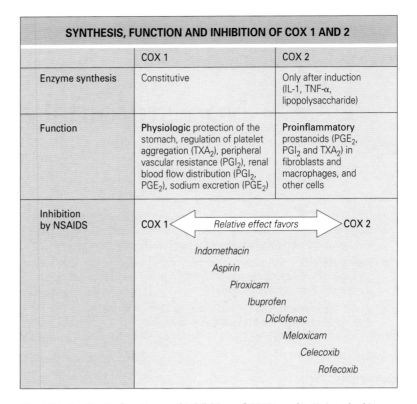

Fig. 10.2 Synthesis, function and inhibition of COX 1 and 2. IL, interleukin; PG, prostaglandin; TNF, tumor necrosis factor; TX, thromboxane. (Adapted from Frölich[6].)

	COX 1	COX 2
Enzyme synthesis	Constitutive	Only after induction (IL-1, TNF-α, lipopolysaccharide)
Function	**Physiologic** protection of the stomach, regulation of platelet aggregation (TXA$_2$), peripheral vascular resistance (PGI$_2$), renal blood flow distribution (PGI$_2$, PGE$_2$), sodium excretion (PGE$_2$)	**Proinflammatory** prostanoids (PGE$_2$, PGI$_2$ and TXA$_2$) in fibroblasts and macrophages, and other cells
Inhibition by NSAIDS	COX 1 ← *Relative effect favors* → COX 2	

Indomethacin
Aspirin
Piroxicam
Ibuprofen
Diclofenac
Meloxicam
Celecoxib
Rofecoxib

TABLE 10.1 PROCESSES INFLUENCED BY NSAIDs

- Prostaglandin synthesis
- Leukotriene synthesis
- Superoxide radical production
- Superoxide scavenging
- Lysosomal enzyme release
- Cell membrane activities
  - Enzymes: Nicotinamide adenine dinucleotide phosphate (NADPH) oxidase Phospholipase
  - Transmembrane anion transport
  - Uptake of prostaglandin precursor
- Neutrophil aggregation and adhesion
- Lymphocyte function
- Rheumatoid factor production
- Cytokine production
- Cartilage metabolism
- Synthesis of nitric oxide

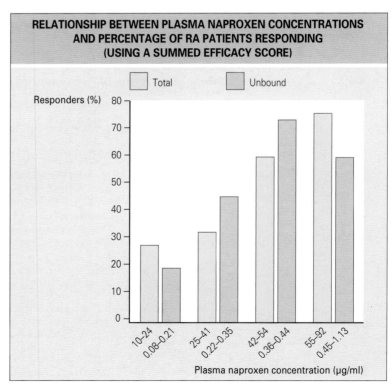

Fig. 10.3 Relationship between plasma naproxen concentrations and percentage of RA patients responding (using a summed efficacy score). (Adapted from Tonkin and Wing[24].)

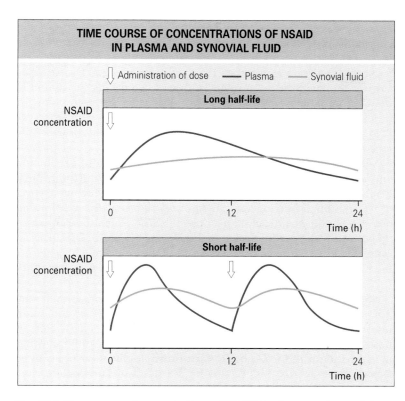

Fig. 10.4 Time course of concentrations of NSAID in plasma and synovial fluid.

tion. Linear relationships between plasma concentration of NSAIDs and toxicity have also been demonstrated.

Most NSAIDs are completely absorbed from the gastrointestinal tract but this can be slowed by food. NSAIDs are now generally presented as enteric-coated tablets or as a sustained-release preparation. These have been developed together with the longer half-life NSAIDs in an attempt to provide more stable plasma concentrations throughout a 24-hour period. It should be appreciated, however, that NSAIDs diffuse more slowly into synovial fluid and that the synovial fluid concentrations are much more stable and show fewer fluctuations than plasma concentrations, even for short half-life drugs (Fig. 10.4). This fluctuation in synovial fluid concentrations may in part be responsible for the dosing interval of short half-life drugs being longer than their plasma half-lives[8].

Non-steroidal anti-inflammatory drugs are highly bound to plasma proteins, and the amount of free drug (the active component) is relatively small. The binding of NSAIDs to plasma proteins can be reduced in various diseases, or in subjects with hypoalbuminemia. For most NSAIDs the unbound fraction does not change in relation to the plasma concentration but naproxen, phenylbutazone and salicylate do have dose-dependent protein binding, unbound concentrations increasing proportionally with dose. Binding of some NSAIDs, for example naproxen, decreases in elderly patients and in patients with RA, emphasizing the importance of correlating unbound concentrations with effect rather than total plasma concentrations. The NSAIDs can be divided into two groups on the basis of their plasma elimination half-life (Table 10.2). Those drugs with a long half-life, such as piroxicam and tenoxicam, take a long time to reach steady state in the body and, therefore, a longer period of treatment is required before a maximum clinical response can be expected.

The clearance of NSAIDs is predominantly by hepatic metabolism, with production of inactive metabolites. These inactive metabolites are then excreted in the urine. The clearance of some NSAIDs, including diflunisal, ketoprofen, fenoprofen, naproxen and indomethacin, is decreased in renal failure.

Some NSAIDs, such as aspirin, nabumetone, fenbufen and sulindac, are converted into active metabolites, which produce the major anti-inflammatory pharmacologic effect. Sulindac is particularly interesting since the active metabolite (the sulfide) is produced in the large intestine and the process seems to be reversible. Conversion of the active sulfide metabolite into the inactive sulindac occurs in the kidney and has been proposed as the explanation for the reported renal sparing effects of this drug. Enterohepatic recycling of certain NSAIDs, particularly indomethacin and sulindac, can occur.

Some of the NSAIDs of the propionic acid class, including ibuprofen, ketoprofen, fenoprofen, naproxen, tiaprofenic acid and flurbiprofen, exist as two optical isomers, or enantiomers. Interestingly, it is only the S enantiomer that inhibits cyclooxygenase, while the R enantiomer is inactive. Unidirectional conversion of the R into the S form of the NSAID can occur to a variable degree in vivo, depending on the drug and the individual subject. Naproxen is marketed as the S enantiomer only but the other arylpropionic acids, such as ibuprofen, ketoprofen and flurbiprofen, exist as equal mixtures of the inactive R and active S.

The pharmacokinetics of most NSAIDs can be affected to some extent by liver disease, renal disease or old age[9]. NSAIDs should be used with care in these situations.

CLINICAL EVIDENCE FOR VARIABILITY IN RESPONSE

Comparative trials of NSAIDs rarely show any clinically significant difference between agents, although this might be due in part to inadequate trial design, insensitive measurements and suboptimal data analysis. The first demonstration of variability in response to NSAIDs was made by Huskisson et al.[10], who compared fixed doses of ibuprofen, fenoprofen, ketoprofen and naproxen in patients with RA. Although only minor differences in mean values of disease activity variables were demonstrated between the drugs, marked variations in individual response, with preferences for particular NSAIDs, were noted. A number of other workers have also demonstrated individual differences in response to NSAIDs, although the basis for this variability in response is still not clear[3]. It may be due to a number of factors:

- physicochemical parameters
- dosage selection and timing of dose
- pharmacokinetic variation
- pharmacodynamics (i.e. variability in anti-inflammatory activity)

TABLE 10.2 HALF-LIVES OF NSAIDs			
Short (<6h)		**Long (>12h)**	
NSAID	Half-life (h)	NSAID	Half-life (h)
Aspirin	0.25	Azapropazone	15.0
Diclofenac	1.1	Carprofen	12.0
Etodolac	6.0	Celecoxib	12.0
Fenoprofen	2.5	Diflunisal	13.0
Flufenamic acid	1.4	Fenbufen	11.0
Flurbiprofen	3.8	Meloxicam	20.0
Ibuprofen	2.1	Nabumetone	26.0
Indomethacin	4.6	Naproxen	14.0
Ketoprofen	1.8	Oxaprozin	58.0
Mefenamic acid	2.0	Phenylbutazone	86.0
Pirprofen	3.8	Piroxicam	57.0
Suprofen	2.5	Rofecoxib	17
Tolmetin	1.0	Salicylate	2.0–15.0
Tiaprofenic acid	3.0	Sulindac	14.0
		Tenoxicam	60.0

● intersubject variability in pathophysiology of various rheumatic diseases
● different adverse reactions.

Although differences in pharmacokinetics between so-called responders and non-responders would seem to be reasonable explanation, this does not appear to be the case[3].

ADVERSE DRUG REACTIONS

Adverse drug reactions to NSAIDs are frequently reported to drug evaluation authorities[11] and cover a broad spectrum of reactions, from the common gastrointestinal problems to rare side effects such as aseptic meningitis[12] (Table 10.3). Gastrointestinal adverse events are usually mild but are seen most often (in approximately 10% of patients on NSAIDs), followed by renal events, skin rashes and CNS reactions. Serious adverse reactions to NSAIDs are relatively rare but they do assume importance since up to 30% of the elderly population are taking these drugs on a regular basis. Fries et al. have suggested that NSAIDs may have a toxicity equal to DMARDs and this should be another argument for early use of disease modifying drugs[13].

Gastrointestinal

Gastrointestinal reactions to NSAIDs include gastric erosions, peptic ulcer formation and perforation, upper and lower gastrointestinal hemorrhage, and inflammation and changes in permeability of the small and large bowel. With the increased prescribing of NSAIDs, there has been a rapid rise in the incidence of reported deaths from gastrointestinal hemorrhage and perforation. The true relationship between NSAID use and serious gastrointestinal complications is hard to estimate. The

absolute risk of serious gastrointestinal adverse effects varies from approximately 2 cases per 10 000 person months of prescription to an increased risk of hospitalization of over seven times in patients with RA[14]. These data suggest that the syndrome of NSAID-associated gastropathy might be responsible for over 16 500 deaths per annum in the USA in patients with RA and OA[15]. Particular risk factors for the development of NSAID-associated peptic ulceration in RA are age (>65 years), a past history of peptic ulceration, concomitant corticosteroid ingestion and multiple organ dysfunction[15].

All NSAIDs have the ability to suppress prostaglandin production and are likely to share the potential for inducing gastrointestinal hemorrhage. There is now emerging data to support a differential effect of NSAIDs on gastric mucosa. Studies have shown a clear relationship between bleeding peptic ulcer and dose of NSAID, but also a suggestion that NSAIDs such as ibuprofen and diclofenac might be less likely to cause peptic ulceration than others[16]. One of the problems with assessing the incidence of side effects is the fact that, in patients with RA, up to 50% of peptic ulcers are asymptomatic.

NSAID-induced ulcers should be treated like any other gastric lesion. The ulcers may be treated with H_2-receptor antagonists, proton pump inhibitors such as omeprazole or prostaglandin analogs such as misoprostol[17,18]. Data is not yet available as to the use of antiulcer drugs in association with COX-2 but on first principles the ulcer needs to be treated on its merits. Risk factors for NSAID-associated peptic ulcer complications include age over 65, prior ulcer disease, high dose and multiple NSAIDs, concurrent steroid therapy and duration of therapy. Smoking, alcohol and infection with Helicobacter pylori may also play a role. Prophylaxis with histamine receptor antagonists, prostaglandin analogs and proton pump inhibitors reduces ulcer formation and other gastrointestinal complications as well[18]. If a patient with peptic ulceration is known to be infected with H. pylori, this should be treated although there is no data to support widespread elimination of H. pylori at this time. In summary, peptic ulceration should be treated with NSAIDs withdrawal if possible. Prophylaxis with a proton pump inhibitor or misoprostol should be offered to those at-risk patients who genuinely require long-term NSAIDs. In patients who develop abdominal symptoms or are at risk for ulcer disease the non-selective NSAID should be ceased and a COX-2-specific agent substituted.

Renal and cardiac

Since prostaglandins modulate many of the physiologic activities of the kidney, including renal blood flow and glomerular filtration, renin release, tubular ion transport and water exchange, it is not surprising that NSAIDs commonly produce renal toxicity[19]. These prostaglandin-driven renal functions are of particular importance in patients with underlying renal disease, and great care must be taken in prescribing NSAIDs to people with even mild renal dysfunction. NSAIDs can cause reversible impairment of glomerular function, edema, interstitial nephritis and papillary necrosis, acute renal failure and hyperkalemia.

Although there is a strong link between analgesic intake and renal disease, this involves compound analgesic agents rather than NSAIDs. It is quite common to see a transient rise in the serum creatinine level within 2 weeks of commencing an NSAID, but this returns to normal despite continuation of the drug. The particular risk factors for NSAID-induced renal disease are a past history of renal disease, volume depletion in association with diuretic therapy or hypoalbuminemia, and hepatic disease.

It has been suggested that sulindac might have a lesser effect on renal function but it is clear that no NSAID can be prescribed with absolute safety with respect to renal adverse effects. Sodium retention, edema and hypertension are often precipitated by NSAIDs, and NSAIDs might also interfere with the action of a number of antihypertensive and diuretic

TABLE 10.3 ADVERSE REACTIONS TO NSAIDs	
Gastrointestinal	Indigestion
	Gastroesophageal reflux
	Erosions
	Peptic ulcer
	Gastrointestinal hemorrhage and perforation
	Small and large bowel ulceration
Hepatic	Transaminitis
	Hepatocellular cholestasis
Renal	Transient rise in serum creatinine
	Hyponatremia
	Acute renal failure
	Interstitial necrosis
	Hyperkalemia
	Analgesic nephropathy
Hematologic	Thrombocytopenia
	Neutropenia
	Red cell aplasia
	Hemolytic anemia
Cutaneous	Photosensitivity
	Erythema multiforme
	Urticaria
	Toxic epidermal necrolysis
Respiratory	Bronchospasm
	Pneumonitis
Central nervous system	Headache
	Dizziness
	Personality change
	Aseptic meningitis

medications, NSAIDs interfere with blood pressure control on an individual basis, and patients commenced on these drugs should have their blood pressure monitored at regular intervals[20]. There is no clear evidence that COX-specific agents are significantly different from non-selective NSAIDs in their effects on the renal and cardiovascular systems. There is now emerging evidence that non-selective NSAIDs are associated with a significant incidence of renal and cardiac failure in the community, particularly in elderly patients[21,22]. This may well be so for the specific COX-2 agents as well.

Hepatic

A transient rise in liver enzyme levels is commonly seen with NSAIDs but this usually settles despite continuing therapy. Occasionally, significant hepatitis may occur, and this is seen particularly with aspirin in association with acute viral illnesses (Reye's syndrome). Cholestasis is associated with sulindac and diclofenac therapy but is usually mild[23].

Hematologic

A broad spectrum of hematologic adverse reactions to NSAIDs has been described, including anemia, thrombocytopenia, neutropenia and aplastic anemia. Aplastic anemia has a high mortality but is rarely associated with NSAIDs, except with phenylbutazone or oxyphenbutazone. Thrombocytopenia has been associated with most NSAIDs, while all NSAIDs will interfere with platelet aggregation. With aspirin this effect on platelet function is irreversible and is seen throughout the life of the platelet but with other NSAIDs the effect is most often seen while the drug is present in the bloodstream in significant quantities. From a practical point of view, this means that platelet function will return to normal approximately three half-lives after an NSAID is ceased, and approximately 4 days after aspirin is ceased. COX-specific agents do not affect platelet function.

Dermatologic

Most dermatologic side effects, including macular eruptions, urticaria and rarely pseudoporphyria, are relatively mild and settle quickly once

TABLE 10.4 INTERACTIONS BETWEEN NSAIDs AND OTHER DRUGS			
Drug affected	**NSAID implicated**	**Effect**	**Approach to management**
Oral anticoagulants	Phenylbutazone Oxyphenbutazone Azapropazone	Inhibition of metabolism of S-warfarin, increasing anticoagulant effect	Avoid NSAIDs if possible. Careful monitoring where unavoidable
Lithium	Probably all NSAIDs	Inhibition of renal excretion of lithium, increasing lithium serum concentrations and risk of toxicity	Use sulindac or aspirin if NSAID unavoidable. Careful monitoring of lithium concentration and appropriate dose reduction
Oral hypoglycemic agents	Phenylbutazone Oxyphenbutazone Azapropazone	Inhibition of metabolism of sulfonylurea drugs, prolonging half-life and increasing risk of hypoglycemia	Avoid this group of NSAIDs if possible; if not, monitor blood sugar closely
Phenytoin	Phenylbutazone Oxyphenbutazone	Inhibition of metabolism of phenytoin, increasing plasma concentration and risk of toxicity	Avoid this group of NSAIDs if possible; if not, intensify therapeutic drug monitoring
	Other NSAIDs	Displacement of phenytoin from plasma protein, reducing total concentrations for the same unbound (active) concentration	Avoid aspirin; close monitoring of plasma concentration if other NSAID used
Methotrexate	Probably all NSAIDs	Reduced clearance of methotrexate (mechanism unclear) increasing plasma concentration and risk of severe toxicity	This is only relevant to high-dose methotrexate used in cancer chemotherapy
Sodium valproate	Aspirin	Inhibition of valproate metabolism increasing plasma concentration	Avoid aspirin; close monitoring of plasma concentration if other NSAID used
Digoxin	All NSAIDs	Potential reduction in renal function (particularly in very young and very old) reducing digoxin clearance and increasing plasma concentration	Avoid NSAIDs if possible; if not, frequent checks of digoxin plasma concentration and plasma creatinine
Aminoglycosides	All NSAIDs	Reduction in renal function in susceptible individuals, reducing aminoglycoside clearance and increasing plasma concentration	Close plasma concentration monitoring and dose adjustment
Antihypertensive agents: beta-blockers, diuretics, ACE inhibitors, vasodilators	Indomethacin Other NSAIDs	Reduction in hypotensive effect, probably related to inhibition of renal prostaglandin synthesis (producing salt and water retention) and vascular prostaglandin synthesis (producing increased vasoconstriction)	Avoid all NSAIDs in patients with cardiac failure; monitor clinical signs of fluid retention
Diuretics	Indomethacin Other NSAIDs	Reduction in natriuretic and diuretic effects; may exacerbate congestive cardiac failure	Avoid NSAIDs in patients with cardiac failure; monitor clinical signs of fluid retention
Anticoagulants	All NSAIDs	Gastrointestinal tract mucosal damage, together with inhibition of platelet aggregation, increasing risk of gastrointestinal bleeding in patients on anticoagulants	Avoid all NSAIDs if possible
Hypoglycemic agents	Salicylate (high dose)	Potentiation of hypoglycemic effects (mechanism unknown)	Monitor blood sugar level
ACE, angiotensin converting enzyme.			

the drug is ceased but fatal reactions, including erythema multiforme, have been described with most NSAIDs. Dermatologic side effects seem to be most commonly associated with those NSAIDs that have long half-lives.

Respiratory

Asthma is most common with salicylate but may be precipitated or exacerbated by NSAIDs. Symptoms may be mild or severe, and fatal attacks of bronchospasm have been precipitated by a single dose of NSAID. If aspirin-sensitive asthmatic patients require an NSAID, then a low dose should be administered in a controlled environment equipped with facilities to reverse bronchospasm. Pulmonary alveolitis has also recently been reported with NSAID therapy and, although rare, should be considered when an illness suggestive of pulmonary infection but failing to respond to antibiotic therapy develops in a patient on an NSAID. Early data suggests that COX-2-specific agents can be used safely in asthmatics. Non-acetylated salicylates are often used in this situation.

Adverse reactions in the central nervous system

Side effects in the CNS are probably more common with NSAID therapy than is normally appreciated. Headaches might occur with indomethacin, and an aseptic, meningitis-like picture has been described with ibuprofen in systemic lupus erythematosus. Many patients report drowsiness and alteration in mood. Aspirin has effects on the electro-encephalogram and it might be that some of the non-ulcer dyspepsia (nausea) commonly seen in association with NSAIDs has its basis in the CNS rather than the gastrointestinal tract. Tinnitus is commonly seen in patients on salicylate therapy and can be used as a method of monitor-ing treatment. This particular side effect has recently been shown to be dose-related.

DRUG INTERACTIONS

Since NSAIDs are commonly taken by the elderly, who generally have many diseases, the potential for drug interaction is enormous. The common interactions of NSAIDs are shown in Tables 10.4 and 10.5. Interactions can be pharmacokinetic or pharmacodynamic, as described by Tonkin and Wing[24]. The most important potential interactions occur between NSAIDs and diuretic and hypotensive agents, anticonvulsants, lithium and anticoagulants. The potential interaction with methotrexate and NSAIDs is not seen with the low doses of methotrexate prescribed for RA or seronegative arthropathies. With care, most significant interactions can be avoided.

CYCLO-OXYGENASE-2-SPECIFIC AGENTS

The COX-2-specific agents have been developed to maintain anti-inflammatory and analgesic activity without the side effects associated with other NSAIDs. Their mechanism of action and regulation is described in Figure 10.5. There are three currently available specific COX-2 inhibitors – celecoxib, rofecoxib and valdecoxib. Other drugs of this class that are in development include etoricoxib, paracoxib, and a number of others.

Efficacy

A number of clinical trials have been published showing that celecoxib and rofecoxib are as efficacious as the comparator non-selective NSAIDs

TABLE 10.5 INTERACTIONS BETWEEN NSAIDs AND OTHER DRUGS: DRUGS AFFECTING NSAIDs

Drug implicated	NSAID affected	Effect	Approach to management
Antacids	Indomethacin Other NSAIDs	Variable effects of different preparations: Aluminum-containing antacids reduce rate and extent of absorption of indomethacin Sodium bicarbonate increases rate and extent of absorption of indomethacin that have enteric coating or slow-release profile	No action required unless marked reduction in absorption results in poor response to NSAID; dose may need to be increased in this case. Not as important with those NSAIDs
Probenecid	Probably all NSAIDs	Reduction in metabolism and renal clearance of NSAIDs and acyl glucuronide metabolites, which are hydrolyzed back to parent drug	May be used therapeutically to increase the response to a given dose of NSAID
Cholestyramine	Naproxen and probably other NSAIDs	Anion exchange resin binds NSAIDs in gut, reducing rate (and extent) of absorption	Separate dosing times by 4h; may need larger than expected dose of NSAID
Metoclopramide	Aspirin	Increased rate and extent of absorption of aspirin in patients with migraine	May be used therapeutically

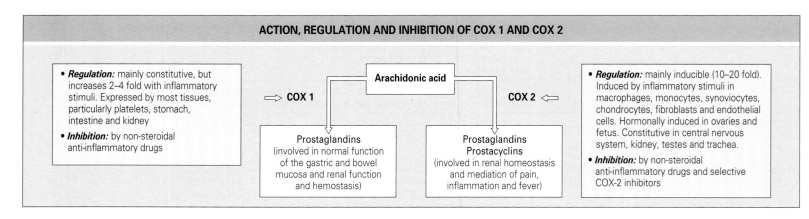

ACTION, REGULATION AND INHIBITION OF COX 1 AND COX 2

- **Regulation:** mainly constitutive, but increases 2–4 fold with inflammatory stimuli. Expressed by most tissues, particularly platelets, stomach, intestine and kidney
- **Inhibition:** by non-steroidal anti-inflammatory drugs

Arachidonic acid

COX 1

Prostaglandins (involved in normal function of the gastric and bowel mucosa and renal function and hemostasis)

COX 2

Prostaglandins Prostacyclins (involved in renal homeostasis and mediation of pain, inflammation and fever)

- **Regulation:** mainly inducible (10–20 fold). Induced by inflammatory stimuli in macrophages, monocytes, synoviocytes, chondrocytes, fibroblasts and endothelial cells. Hormonally induced in ovaries and fetus. Constitutive in central nervous system, kidney, testes and trachea.
- **Inhibition:** by non-steroidal anti-inflammatory drugs and selective COX-2 inhibitors

Fig. 10.5 Action, regulation and inhibition of Cox 1 and Cox 2. (Modified from Brooks and Day[5].)

in acute pain (third molar tooth extraction, dysmenorrhea and post-orthopedic surgical pain). In osteoarthritis of the hip and knee, rheumatoid arthritis and ankylosing spondylitis, celecoxib, rofecoxib and valdecoxib have demonstrated similar efficacy in terms of pain relief, increased function and anti-inflammatory activity as non-selective NSAIDs[5]. The major differences between the two widely available coxibs are shown in Table 10.6.

Adverse effects

The significant differences between rofecoxib and celecoxib and the other NSAIDs are seen in the incidence of gastrointestinal adverse events. A number of short- and medium-term trials have demonstrated that the coxibs are associated with a significantly lower incidence of endoscopically proven ulcers than with comparator NSAIDs such as naproxen, diclofenac, ibuprofen or nabumetone. Two major gastrointestinal outcome studies (CLASS and VIGOR) have been published[25,26]. Each of these studies had around 8000 patients on rofecoxib or celecoxib and similar numbers on comparator NSAIDs. In the CLASS study, between 3 days and 6 months, celecoxib 400mg b.d. was associated with a significantly lower incidence of upper gastrointestinal ulcer complications than ibuprofen 2.4g daily or diclofenac 150mg daily in patients with rheumatoid arthritis or osteoarthritis. In the VIGOR study[26] there was a significant reduction in all upper GI events with rofecoxib compared to naproxen in patients with rheumatoid arthritis over a 12-month period.

Full data sets for these two studies have recently been posted on the Food and Drug Agency website[27]. Review of these data shows that the gastrointestinal benefits of celecoxib disappear at 12 months and also raises questions about the cardiovascular effects of COX inhibitors. Differences between the CLASS and VIGOR trials are well summarized by Fitzgerald and Patrono[28]. Significant questions remain to be answered about the use of the specific COX-2 inhibitors – particularly in relation to cardiovascular and renal disease. On the evidence thus far presented, COX-2-specific inhibitors do increase blood pressure and can be associated with fluid retention[29]. Particular care needs to be taken in treating patients who have underlying cardiovascular disease or the potential to develop thromboses, such as those with antiphospholipid antibody syndrome. There are already a number of patients with this condition in whom thromboses have been associated with treatment with specific COX-2 inhibitors[30]. Low-dose aspirin (81mg) has been recommended to be taken concurrently with COX-2 inhibitors in patients at risk for cardiac or vascular disease because of the lack of effect of the coxibs on platelet aggregation.

PRACTICAL PRESCRIBING

Patients with rheumatic disease continue to show variability in their response to NSAIDs. The therapeutic challenge in each case is to find the right NSAID in terms of providing pain relief without significant adverse reactions. The vast majority of patients will respond to an NSAID within 7–10 days of commencing therapy, and if this does not occur the NSAID should be ceased and another one commenced. To date there is no evidence that combinations of NSAIDs are more efficacious than adequate doses of single agents. Because NSAIDs are primarily anti-inflammatory, they should be reserved for those patients who do have evidence of inflammation and not used long-term in those with non-inflammatory degenerative disease. The dose of NSAID should be kept to a minimum, possibly with supplementation of analgesics such as acetaminophen (paracetamol). Patients on NSAIDs should be continually assessed for the development of adverse drug reactions and to establish whether or not they are continuing to respond to the NSAIDs. When NSAIDs are ceased, this should be done over a period of a few days to prevent any rebound in pain and inflammation. COX-2 inhibitors can be prescribed for patients with rheumatoid arthritis, osteoarthritis and a range of acute and chronic pain conditions who are not responding to conventional NSAIDs or are at risk of gastrointestinal toxicity because they:

● have had previous NSAID-associated gastrointestinal toxicity
● are elderly
● have severe arthritic or multisystem disease
● are taking high doses of NSAIDs.

Patients taking these drugs are still at risk of renal and cardiovascular adverse events and great care should be taken in prescribing COX-2 inhibitors to those patients with underlying cardiovascular disease or an increased risk of thrombosis.

TABLE 10.6 PHARMACOLOGICAL PROFILE OF CELECOXIB AND ROFECOXIB

Action	Metabolism
At therapeutic plasma concentrations, coxibs block COX 2 but do not significantly interfere with COX 1	Celecoxib: by cytochrome P450; half-life 12h; protein binding 97% Rofecoxib: by metabolic reduction; half-life 17h; protein binding 85%

Onset of action	Adverse effects
Analgesia: 1h Anti-inflammatory effect: less than 2 weeks after starting therapy	Reduction in gastrointestinal events (ulcers, bleeds, erosions) compared with non-selective NSAIDs
Dosing Celecoxib, 200–400mg orally once or twice daily Rofecoxib, 12.5–50mg orally once daily	Effects on renal function (potential for mild fluid retention, renal insufficiency in renally compromised patients and those taking ACE inhibitors) similar to those of non-selective NSAIDs

Drug interactions	Celecoxib	Rofecoxib	Effect	Clinically significant
Warfarin	Yes	Yes	Increased prothrombin time	Yes
Lithium	Yes	Yes	Increased lithium levels	Yes
ACE inhibitors	Yes	Yes	Reduced antihypertensive effects (potential for renal impairment)	Yes
Inhibitors of CYP2C9*	Yes	No	Increased plasma concentrations of celecoxib	Yes
Substrates of CYP2D6†	Yes	No	Increased plasma concentrations of substrate	Probably
Furosemide and thiazides	Yes	Yes	Reduced diuretic effect	Yes

*Amiodarone, cimetidine, fluoxetine, fluconazole, metronidazole, fluvastatin
† Beta-blockers, antidepressants (amitriptyline, desipramine, clomipramine, fluoxetine), antipsychotics (haloperidol, thioridazine), perhexiline
ACE, angiotensin converting enzyme.

REFERENCES

1. Forrest M, Brooks PM. Mechanism of action of nonsteroidal anti-inflammatory drugs. Baillière's Clin Rheumatol 1985; 2: 275–294.
2. Preston SJ, Arnold MH, Beller EM et al. Comparative analgesic and anti-inflammatory properties of sodium salicylate and acetyl salicylic acid (aspirin) in rheumatoid arthritis. Br J Clin Pharmacol 1989; 27: 607–611.
3. Brooks PM, Day RO. Non-steroidal anti-inflammatory drugs differences and similarities. N Engl J Med 1991; 324: 1716–1725.
4. De Witt DL, Meade EA, Smith WL. PGH synthase isoenzyme selectivity: the potential for safe non steroidal anti inflammatory drugs. Am J Med 1993; 95: 40S–44S.
5. Brooks PM, Day RO. COX-2 inhibitors. Med J Aust 2000; 173: 433–436.
6. Frölich JC. Prostaglandin endoperoxide synthetase isoenzymes: the clinical relevance of selective inhibition. Ann Rheum Dis 1995; 54: 942–943.
7. Day RO, Graham GG, Williams KM. Pharmacokinetics of non-steroidal anti-inflammatory drugs. Baillière's Clin Rheumatol 1988; 2: 363–393.
8. Graham GG. Pharmacokinetics and metabolism of non-steroidal anti-inflammatory drugs. Med J Aust 1980; 147: 597–602.
9. Verbeek RK. Pathophysiologic factors affecting the pharmacokinetics of non-steroidal anti-inflammatory drugs. J Rheumatol 1988; 15: 44–57.
10. Huskisson EC, Woolf PC, Baume HW et al. Four new anti-inflammatory drugs – responses and variations. Br Med J 1974; 1: 1084–1089.
11. Committee on Safety of Medicines Update. Non-steroidal and anti-inflammatory drugs on serious gastrointestinal adverse reactions. Br Med J 1986; 292: 614.
12. Brooks PM. Side effects of non-steroidal anti-inflammatory drugs. Med J Aust 1988; 148: 248–281.
13. Fries JF, Williams CA, Ramey DR, Bloch DA. The relative toxicity of alternative therapies for rheumatoid arthritis: implications for the therapeutic progression. Semin Arthritis Rheum 1993; 23(suppl 1): 68–73.
14. Langman MJS. Epidemiological evidence on the association between peptic ulceration and anti-inflammatory drugs use. Gastroenterology 1989; 96: 640–646.
15. Wolfe MM, Lichtenstein DR, Singh G. Gastrointestinal toxicity of non steroidal anti-inflammatory drugs. N Engl J Med 1999; 340: 1888–1899.
16. Rodriguez LAG, Jick H. Risk of upper gastrointestinal bleeding and perforation associated with individual non-steroidal anti-inflammatory drugs. Lancet 1994; 343: 769–772.
17. Lichtenstein DR, Syngal S, Wolfe MM. Non-steroidal anti-inflammatory drugs and the gastrointestinal tract. Arthritis Rheum 1995; 1: 5–18.
18. Silverstein FE, Geis GS, Struthers BJ and the Mucosa Study Group. NSAIDs and gastrointestinal injury: clinical outcome. The Mucosa Trial. Gastroenterol 1994; 106: A180.
19. Schlondorff D. Renal complications of non-steroidal anti-inflammatory drugs. Kidney Int 1993; 44: 643–653.
20. Pope JE, Anderson JJ, Felson DT. A meta analysis of the effects of non-steroidal anti-inflammatory drugs on blood pressure. Arch Intern Med 1993; 153: 477–484.
21. Henry D, Page J, Whyte, I, Nanra R, Hall C. Consumption of non-steroidal anti-inflammatory drugs and the development of functional renal impairment in elderly subjects. Results of a case control study. Br J Clin Pharmacol 1997; 44: 85–90.
22. Heerdink ER, Leufkens HG, Herings RMC et al. NSAIDs associated with increased risk of congestive cardiac failure in elderly subjects taking diuretics. Arch Intern Med 1998; 158: 1108–1112.
23. Carson JL, Strom BL, Duff A et al. Safety of non-steroidal anti-inflammatory drugs with respect to acute liver disease. Arch Intern Med 1993; 153: 1331–1336.
24. Tonkin AL, Wing LMH. Interactions of non-steroidal anti-inflammatory drugs. Baillière's Clin Rheumatol 1988; 22: 455–483.
25. Silverstein FE, Faich G, Goldstein JL et al. Gastrointestinal toxicity with celecoxib vs non steroidal antiinflammatory drugs for osteoarthritis and rheumatoid arthritis: the class study: a randomised controlled trial. Celecoxib long-term arthritis safety study. JAMA 2000; 284: 1247–1255.
26. Bombardier C, Laine L, Reicin A et al. A comparison of upper gastro-intestinal toxicity of rofecoxib and naproxen in patients with rheumatoid arthritis. N Engl J Med 2000; 343: 1520–1528.
27. www.fda.gov/cder/audiences/acspage/arthritismeetings1.htm#Past%20Meetings.
28. Fitzgerald GA, Patrono C. The coxibs, selective inhibitors of cyclooxygenase-2. N Engl J Med 2001: 345; 433–442.
29. Brater DC, Harris C, Redfern JS, Gertz BJ. Renal effects of COX-2 selective inhibitors. Am J Nephrol 2001: 21; 1–15.
30. Crofford LJ, Oates JC, McCune WJ et al. Thrombosis in patients with connective tissue diseases treated with specific cyclooxygenase-2 inhibitors: a report of 4 cases. Arthritis Rheum 2000; 43: 1891–1896.

PRINCIPLES OF MANAGEMENT

11 Systemic glucocorticoids in rheumatology

John R Kirwan

- Glucocorticoids act generally through specific cytoplasmic receptors and control of gene transcription but may also have non-genomic effects at higher doses
- Glucocorticoid treatment increases lipocortin production and induces changes in lymphocyte function, Fc receptor suppression and downregulation of many proinflammatory enzymes produced by macrophages
- Low-dose oral glucocorticoids only transiently reduce symptoms of inflammation in rheumatoid arthritis but inhibit bony erosion in the longer term
- In polymyalgia rheumatica the main pitfalls are the use of too high an initial dose of glucocorticoid and too rapid a reduction in treatment thereafter
- The potential adverse effects of glucocorticoids require careful consideration before initiating high-dose or long-term therapy

MECHANISM OF ACTION

Structure

The principal glucocorticoid hormone of the human adrenal cortex is cortisol (hydrocortisone), derived from hydroxylation of cortisone (Fig. 11.1). The 11β and 17α hydroxyl groups are important for glucocorticoid activity and prednisone, a synthetic analog of cortisone, is also hydroxylated before becoming biologically active. The additional double bond in ring A of the resultant prednisolone enhances glucocorticoid activity without increasing mineralocorticoid activity, an effect that is increased by 6α methylation (to produce methylprednisolone) or 9α fluorination (triamcinolone) or both (dexamethasone)[1].

Plasma levels

Plasma cortisol is normally maintained at a concentration of $5-25\mu g/ml$ by the hypothalamic–pituitary–adrenal feedback control mechanism. Most (80%) is bound to the α-globulin transcortin and some (10%) to albumin[2]. The remaining 10% provides biological activity. Synthetic analogs do not compete for transcortin binding sites, are less extensively bound to albumin and are able to diffuse into tissues more completely.

Glucocorticoid receptors

Free cortisol diffuses into individual cells where specific receptor proteins are found in the cytoplasm of glucocorticoid-responsive tissues (Fig. 11.2). The human glucocorticoid receptor is a 95kDa phosphorylated protein with glucocorticoid-binding, DNA-binding and strongly antigenic regions, each of roughly equal size. It belongs to a superfamily of regulatory proteins that includes receptors for thyroid hormones and retinoic acid[3].

The glucocorticoid and receptor form a complex that undergoes a conformational change, moves to the nucleus and binds reversibly to specific DNA promotor or suppressor sites. This results in the production of mRNA, which codes for enzymes or other proteins that produce the hormonal effects. Most cellular responses to glucocorticoids can be detected within 2 hours of glucocorticoid exposure and some within 10 minutes[2]. In general, glucocorticoid response is not observed if RNA synthesis is inhibited. In addition, the concentration of a specific glucocorticoid required for optimal response is lower when it has a higher affinity for the glucocorticoid receptor. However, when glucocorticoid concentrations are higher, sufficient glucocorticoid and receptor complexes accumulate in the cytoplasm to initiate non-genomic effects by direct interaction with other cellular processes. Further, when glucocorticoid receptors become saturated, such as occurs after treatment with very high doses of glucocorticoid (see below), the free glucocorticoid molecules dissolve in the cell membrane, initiating other 'non-genomic' changes in cell metabolism and responsiveness[4].

Action through protein synthesis

Although reduced protein synthesis has been recognized in some tissues (e.g. lymphoid cells, muscle, bone and skin), the main glucocorticoid effect seemed to be through increased rates of synthesis of certain proteins, especially lipocortin. The anti-inflammatory effect of lipocortin is mediated through its inhibition of the enzyme phospholipase A_2, which converts membrane-bound phospholipids into arachidonic acid, with the subsequent intracellular production of prostaglandins, leukotrienes and oxygen radicals (Fig. 11.3)[5]. These products leave the cell and are themselves able to stimulate the release of phospholipase A_2 from adjacent cells. By stimulating lipocortin production, glucocorticoids inhibit proinflammatory cytokine production, including that of interleukin (IL)-1, IL-2, the IL-2 receptor, interferon (IFN)-α[6], tumor necrosis factor (TNF)[7] and, perhaps, various colony stimulating factors (CSFs) such as IL-3[6].

In addition, glucocorticoids even in very low concentrations inhibit the synthesis of a variety of proinflammatory enzymes, including the macrophage products collagenase, elastase and plasminogen activator[8]. Glucocorticoids also stimulate the production of a protein that controls the cyclo-oxygenase (COX)-2 gene and downregulate COX-2 activation in inflammatory cells[9].

Lymphocyte function

Although glucocorticoids inhibit the expression of murine major histocompatibility complex (MHC) class II antigens and may inhibit antigen presentation by human monocytes, there seems to be no relation in man between the reduction in class II expression and suppression of antigen presentation[10]. Lymphocyte proliferation *in vitro* and delayed-type hypersensitivity *in vivo* are inhibited by glucocorticoids, although information about the differential effects of glucocorticoids on particular T-cell subsets is scarce.

Information about glucocorticoid effects on B lymphocytes and antibody production in man is contradictory. A 5-day course of methylprednisolone (96mg/day) lowered serum immunoglobulin levels by 20%[11]

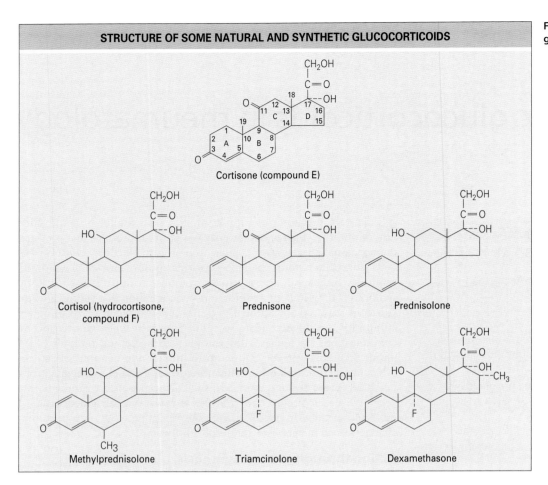

Fig. 11.1 Structure of some natural and synthetic glucocorticoids.

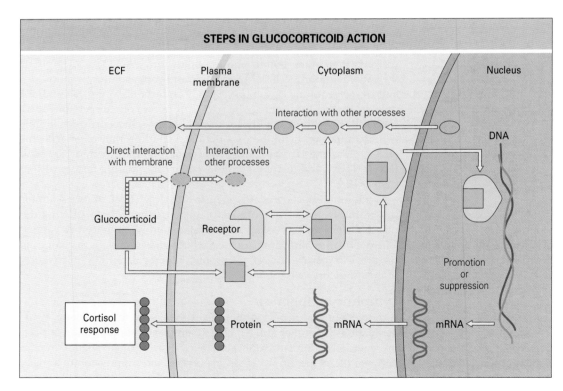

Fig. 11.2 Steps in glucocorticoid action. Unbound glucocorticoid diffuses across the cell membrane and binds to the glucocorticoid receptor. The glucocorticoid–receptor complex moves to the nucleus, promoting or suppressing gene expression. When there are many glucocorticoid-receptor complexes, they may directly interact with other (non-genomic) cellular processes. When all receptors are occupied, free glucocorticoid dissolves in the cell membrane, interacting with other cell processes.

but in more chronic experiments specific antibody production was not reduced in glucocorticoid-treated patients[12]. Also, *in vitro* immunoglobulin production by cells taken from patients on high-dose glucocorticoids is decreased, although B cells from normal subjects given a bolus of glucocorticoids actually produce more immunoglobulins[13].

Fc receptor suppression

Many cells, including red blood cells, carry a surface receptor for the Fc portion of immunoglobulin – the Fc receptor. Glucocorticoids inhibit expression of this receptor[14], which may explain the prompt improvement seen when patients with autoimmune hemolytic anemia

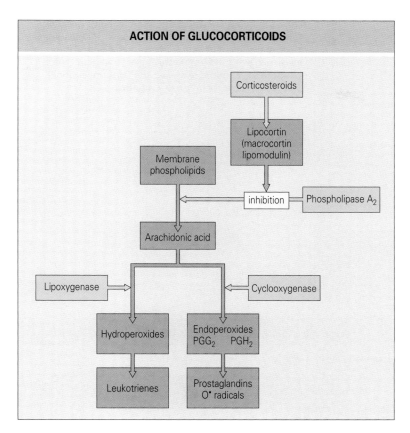

ACTION OF GLUCOCORTICOIDS

Corticosteroids

Lipocortin (macrocortin lipomodulin)

Membrane phospholipids

inhibition — Phospholipase A_2

Arachidonic acid

Lipoxygenase   Cyclooxygenase

Hydroperoxides   Endoperoxides PGG_2 PGH_2

Leukotrienes   Prostaglandins $O^{\bullet}$ radicals

Fig. 11.3 Action of glucocorticoids. Glucocorticoids induce the synthesis of lipocortin, which inhibits the enzyme phospholipase A_2. Arachidonic acid release from membrane phospholipids is blocked and the production of proinflammatory substances via cyclooxygenase and lipoxygenase is reduced. Glucocorticoids also suppress cyclooxygenase production in inflammatory cells.

or autoimmune thrombocytopenia are given glucocorticoids. By inhibiting the Fc receptor (and C3 receptors) in the mononuclear–phagocyte (reticuloendothelial) system, the clearance of antibody-coated red blood cells and platelets is reduced.

Changes in white cell traffic

Large intravenous doses of glucocorticoids given to normal human volunteers increase the numbers of circulating neutrophils but decrease peripheral lymphocytes, eosinophils and monocytes[15]. These changes reach their maximum in 4–6 hours and generally return to normal by 24 hours. Most of these effects reflect changes in patterns of cell traffic rather than changes in bone marrow function. Neutrophilia, for example, results from a combination of increased release of immature cells from the bone marrow, an increase in circulating half-life, reduced neutrophil egress from blood and reduced vascular margination of cells.

Pharmacokinetics and pharmacodynamics

All glucocorticoids bind to the same glucocorticoid receptor and their relative potencies relate to their structure and plasma half-life (Table 11.1). Prednisolone is rapidly absorbed from the gastrointestinal tract and is reversibly bound to plasma proteins. At low or normal plasma concentrations, binding is largely to globulins, but at higher concentrations there is an increase in albumin-bound and free glucocorticoid. Prednisolone is rapidly metabolized in the liver, conjugated and excreted in the urine. It disappears from the blood within 1.5–3 hours, having a half-life of about 1 hour[16]. However, its action at the tissue level lasts considerably longer.

Drug interactions with glucocorticoids may occur. Enhancement of the rate of metabolism of some glucocorticoids has been noted with concurrent administration of phenobarbital, phenytoin and rifampin (rifampicin), probably by inducing hepatic microsomal drug-metabolizing enzymes[17]. Giving aspirin and glucocorticoids concurrently decreases salicylate levels by causing an increased rate of salicylate metabolism. A reduction in glucocorticoid dosage in such patients may result in increased plasma salicylate levels with symptoms of salicylate overdosage[18]. This interaction is relevant in children receiving salicylates and glucocorticoids for the therapy of juvenile inflammatory arthritis. Glucocorticoids may make control of diabetes mellitus with insulin or oral hypoglycemic drugs more difficult and potassium loss may be increased by giving glucocorticoids and thiazides or related diuretics concurrently.

NOMENCLATURE

The current terminological confusion in the description of glucocorticoid doses is exemplified by the different interpretations of the various terms used (very low, low, mild, mild to moderate, moderate, high, very high, ultra-high and mega doses) and by the great variation in interpretation of the terms 'low-dose therapy', 'high-dose therapy' and 'pulse therapy'. A recent proposal[19] made through the European League Against Rheumatism argues that 'glucocorticoid' is the collective name of choice for these agents, and that an appropriate description of a given glucocorticoid therapy regime should follow this example: 'Initially Xmg prednisone orally once a day (at 8am) for 2 weeks, then reduced to Ymg prednisone per day, followed by … (describe each step of reduction in terms of milligrams and time) … reaching zero after (for example) 1 year (overall duration). The cumulative dose was Zmg prednisone.' Conventional terms for glucocorticoid therapy are proposed, based on mechanisms of action and apparent clinical effects, as follows:

- low dose $\leq$ 7.5mg prednisone equivalent per day
- medium dose >7.5mg but $\leq$ 30mg
- high dose >30mg, but $\leq$ 100mg
- very high dose >100mg
- pulse therapy > 250mg for one or a few days.

TABLE 11.1 SOME COMMONLY USED GLUCOCORTICOIDS

Glucocorticoid	Equivalent oral dose (mg)	Plasma half-life (min)	Relative anti-inflammatory effect	Relative mineralocorticoid effect
Cortisol	20	90	1	1
Prednisolone	5	200	4	0.8
Methylprednisolone	4	200	5	0.5
Triamcinolone	4	200	5	0
Dexamethasone	0.75	300	25	0

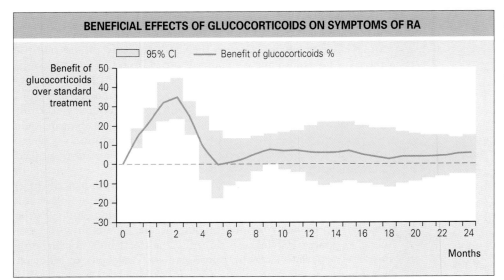

Fig. 11.4 Beneficial effect of glucocorticoids on symptoms of RA. Taking five studies together[21–25], this summary chart of the mean benefit (as percentage clinical improvement) achieved shows that the improvement in clinical symptoms is about 35% greater than on conventional therapy but lasts for only a few months.

EFFICACY

Glucocorticoids in rheumatoid arthritis

Glucocorticoids are the only drugs that reliably, effectively and rapidly suppress synovitis in rheumatoid arthritis (RA). This effect was demonstrated long before their mechanism of action was investigated and cannot yet be fully explained by the factors described earlier. In a recent review[31] of the main clinical trials in RA it was concluded that glucocorticoids are effective anti-inflammatory agents, significantly better than placebo in the relief of pain and stiffness and superior to non-steroidal anti-inflammatory drugs (NSAIDs). However, benefits are not sustained[21–25] unless increasingly high doses are employed (Fig. 11.4) so that side effects and adrenal suppression preclude their long-term use in RA except in specific circumstances.

In early studies there was a suggestion that glucocorticoids might be able to reduce the rate of radiologic progression[26]. Uncontrolled long term follow-up of some of these patients appeared to show the inhibition of continued erosion development over a 4 year treatment period[27]. A randomized, placebo-controlled trial of the addition of a fixed daily dose of 7.5mg prednisolone to existing standard treatment was conducted in 128 patients with active disease of less than 2 years duration[24]. Most patients received NSAIDs and specific antirheumatoid drugs in addition to their study medication, and clinical symptoms improved in both groups. Symptoms improved more rapidly in the prednisolone group, but this added benefit of glucocorticoid treatment lasted only 6–9 months. There was no difference between the groups in changes in the acute phase response (although measurements were not made during the first 3 months of treatment). No significant short-term glucocorticoid-related adverse effects were reported.

The development of erosions and radiological progression were assessed by changes in the Larsen score. After 2 years the Larsen score had shown very little change in the prednisolone-treated patients while the placebo group had substantial joint destruction ($p = 0.004$). This effect was lost during the 1-year blinded post-treatment follow-up (Fig. 11.5). In addition, there was an effect on preventing the onset of erosions, as well as their progression. In placebo patients 46% of hands that did not have erosions at the start of the study developed them, while the figure was 22% for prednisolone-treated patients.

In a study from The Netherlands (the COBRA study[25]), 76 test and 79 control patients received continuous sulfasalazine. The test subjects were also treated with methotrexate for 40 weeks and prednisolone for 28 weeks. The daily prednisolone dose was 60mg, 40mg, 25mg, 20mg, 15mg and 10mg each for 1 week then 7.5mg thereafter. Both methotrexate

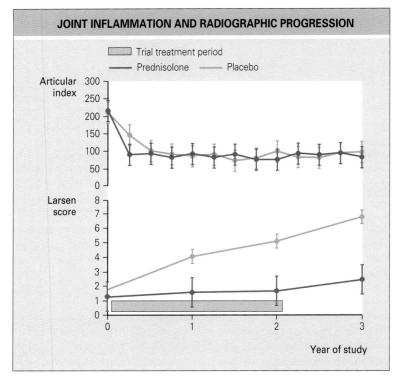

Fig. 11.5 Joint inflammation and radiographic progression. Mean values for joint inflammation (articular index) and radiographic damage (Larsen score) in the ARC Low Dose Glucocorticoid Study[24,28].

and prednisolone were discontinued gradually. Erosive progression was prevented during the period of treatment with prednisolone and methotrexate in addition to sulfasalazine. In this study the benefits of the prednisolone seemed to persist for several weeks after treatment was discontinued, but erosive progression resumed between 56 and 80 weeks.

The report of a double-blind randomized controlled clinical trial by Rau and colleagues[29] compared 5mg of prednisolone with placebo in 196 patients with RA of only 2 years duration. All patients also received co-medication with auranofin or methotrexate. Scored by a modified Sharp method, erosions progressed three times faster in the control group compared to prednisolone.

Treating patients with very early disease, van Everdingen and colleagues[30] tested prednisolone 10mg daily without additional specific

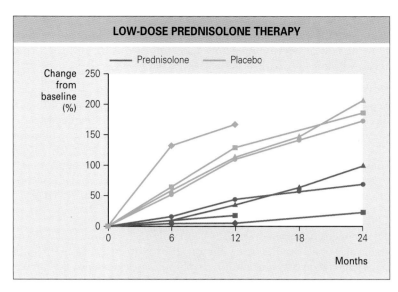

Fig. 11.6 Low-dose prednisolone therapy. Efficacy of low-dose prednisolone therapy for the prevention or reduction of progressive joint destruction in rheumatoid arthritis. Proportion change in erosion scores in four trials of prednisolone in early rheumatoid arthritis. Red, placebo; yellow, prednisolone; diamond, Boers[25]; square, Kirwan[24]; circle, Rau[29]; triangle, van Everdingen[30].

antirheumatoid treatment. This reduced the rate of radiological progression by half.

As most of the studies summarized here included patients of similar severity and disease duration, it is reasonable to directly compare their results. Figure 11.6 shows such a comparison, based on the proportionate change from baseline. The cumulative magnitude and consistency of these findings supports a significant protective effect of glucocorticoids on joint destruction. In view of these findings, treatment can be advocated for 2 years in patients early in the disease and probably for patients who have had arthritis for up to 4 years. Non-erosive patients who have had the diagnosis for more than 2 years are unlikely to ever develop erosions and therefore do not require prednisolone therapy. Patients will experience a 'bonus' of short-term symptomatic control but should be warned that this will eventually subside even though the glucocorticoids will continue to protect against joint destruction at least for the 4-year period. Longer periods of treatment would raise the specter of adverse events such as osteoporosis and atherosclerosis (see below).

Pulsed glucocorticoids

Pulse therapy involves the intravenous infusion of a large dose of glucocorticoid (usually 1g of methylprednisolone) over a short time – perhaps 60–90 minutes. Many current regimens entail a course of three pulses on alternate days, followed by a resting phase of around 6 weeks. This form of treatment was first used in renal transplants but gradually spread to the treatment of other renal disorders, most notably lupus nephritis, where glomerular inflammation responded rapidly and for prolonged periods. Controlled studies were performed in RA that suggested beneficial effects lasting 6–12 weeks with relatively few adverse effects. These trials are small, however, and therefore limited in statistical power.

Methylprednisolone has been used in a number of studies to produce an early initial response in RA patients commencing second-line agents, thus attempting to bridge the gap between initiation and response with these agents. A review[31] of the use of pulsed methylprednisolone stresses the impressive favorable risk:benefit ratio of this therapy with few or minor adverse effects. Most of the serious adverse effects – cardiovascular collapse, myocardial infarction, severe infection – have occurred in patients with compromised cardiovascular or immune systems as a result of their disease, or due to concomitant drug treatment. The

minimal effective dose of methylprednisolone is uncertain at present. It has been reported that doses as low as 320mg may be as effective as 1g[32] although others[33] have concluded that using only 500mg results in substantial loss of efficacy. If equivalent oral doses are as effective as intravenous treatment[34], this will allow pulsed treatment to become an outpatient procedure with reduced costs and less patient discomfort, although Choy[35] found that intramuscular methylprednisolone was superior to equivalent oral doses in their study of glucocorticoids and gold therapy.

Glucocorticoids in vasculitis

In experimental models of vasculitis, such as serum sickness, circulating immune complexes activate platelets, deposit in blood vessel walls fixing complement and induce chemotaxis and phagocytosis by polymorphonuclear leukocytes with the release of enzymes that cause tissue damage. Aggregates of activated platelets form a nidus for blood coagulation and release thromboxane, which itself propagates further platelet activation, vasoconstriction and thrombus formation. In some vasculitides, such as Kawasaki syndrome and Takayasu's disease, there is evidence of such a coagulopathy with hyperfibrinogenemia and hypofibrinolytic activity, which may result in luminal occlusion[36] Glucocorticoids are widely used to treat systemic vasculitis in RA, systemic lupus erythematosus (SLE) and other autoimmune diseases and are clearly powerful inhibitors of the inflammatory processes. However, glucocorticoids may not inhibit subsequent organization of the platelet and fibrin thrombus and induction of endothelial cell and smooth muscle cell proliferation. Thus, in spite of clinical and laboratory improvement after glucocorticoid treatment, patients may go on to develop evidence of progressive ischemia, such as blue digits. Conn et al.[36] suggest that where there is no clinical evidence of active inflammation indicated by fever, myalgia, arthralgias or active skin lesions, and no laboratory evidence of inflammation such as elevation of the erythrocyte sedimentation rate (ESR), a more plausible management strategy would be the use of vasodilators and inhibitors of platelet activation. They postulate that glucocorticoids fail to control the generation of platelet-derived thromboxane (possibly because platelets do not possess a nucleus and cannot form lipocortin), but it may be that this deficiency is often offset by the concomitant, widespread use of (platelet suppressing) NSAIDs.

Glucocorticoids in polymyalgia rheumatica and temporal arteritis

The signs and symptoms of polymyalgia rheumatica and temporal arteritis overlap and can often be confused, but both are treated with glucocorticoids. No trials have been conducted that allow an adequate definition of the best treatment regimen, but four substantial cohorts of patients have been reported in the literature[37–40]. Although there are some differences, the overall pattern suggests the need to treat polymyalgia rheumatica initially with about 15mg prednisolone daily, reducing slowly over 18–24 months. About two or three times that dose will be required to treat coexisting or separate temporal arteritis and for perhaps 6 months longer. All series reported a few complications, including some patients with polymyalgia rheumatica who become more definite cases of temporal arteritis while on treatment. The main pitfalls seem to be the use of too high a dose of glucocorticoids initially, with a too rapid reduction in treatment thereafter[41]. This criticism could also be directed towards some recent controlled trials of treatment that have shown disappointing results[42,43].

VARIABILITY OF RESPONSE

Bioavailability

Enteric-coated prednisolone is often prescribed on the assumption that it reduces gastrointestinal adverse reactions, although there is no clear documentation of this in the literature. Bioavailability may be variable and dissolution of the plant extract coating may be affected by factors such as food intake and gastrointestinal motility, hence absorption of enteric-coated preparations may be unreliable[44].

Antilipocortin antibodies

Hirata[45] observed that a high proportion of patients with chronic rheumatic diseases had autoantibodies to lipocortin, whereas disease-free people did not. Levels were particularly high in patients with SLE and RA. This has led to the concept that the presence of these autoantibodies may contribute to the etiology of these diseases by removing 'protective' proteins that regulate eicosanoid generation.

Using recombinant human lipocortin-1 as a target, Podgorski *et al.*[46] devised an assay for measuring antilipocortin autoantibodies. They confirmed the presence of both IgG and IgM antilipocortin autoantibodies in patients with SLE and RA. They observed that in patients with SLE the antibodies were present whether or not the patient had already received any glucocorticoid therapy but, in the group with RA, significantly raised titers were only seen in patients who had received oral glucocorticoid therapy. In both groups, high titers of autoantibodies correlated strongly with the clinical phenomenon of glucocorticoid 'resistance'. This was not seen with other inflammatory diseases for both those who were receiving glucocorticoids or those who were 'glucocorticoid-resistant'.

The idea that administration of glucocorticoids may stimulate the formation of autoantibodies to lipocortin in certain susceptible groups, and possibly glucocorticoid resistance, may have important implications for glucocorticoid therapy.

ADVERSE DRUG REACTIONS

General

The clinical complications that may occur during the use of glucocorticoid therapy are protean and have been further elaborated in recent observational studies[47]. Glucocorticoids induce alterations of fat distribution that account for the classic cushingoid appearance. These include truncal obesity, 'buffalo hump' and moon face, which occur in 13% of patients who receive glucocorticoids for 2 months and almost half of patients treated for 5 years or more. Other localized fat deposits may be found in the mediastinum and temporal fat pads. Obesity and cushingoid features often resolve rapidly when patients are switched to alternate-day therapy.

Exogenous glucocorticoids also influence glucose, protein and electrolyte metabolism, and hepatic enzyme function, resulting in a tendency towards hyperglycemia and insulin resistance, protein catabolism in muscle and bone, sodium retention and potassium loss.

Infections

Glucocorticoid therapy seems to predispose to a wide range of infections. Staphylococcal, Gram-negative, tuberculous and *Listeria* infections appear most frequently associated, and certain viral and fungal infections also occur. Data to support a large increase in the risk of infection are harder to obtain. In many published clinical trials, patients also have diseases that predispose to infection and are exposed to atypical organisms in a hospital environment[48]. The putative association between glucocorticoid therapy and reactivation of tuberculosis provides a good example. In large studies of patients receiving glucocorticoids in low doses over long periods of time for chest conditions, no increased risk of developing active tuberculosis has been observed. Likewise, cohorts of patients with positive tuberculin skin tests have been followed up for prolonged periods without development of active disease. Those studies reporting an increased risk of tuberculosis in patients treated with glucocorticoids have often included patients treated with several immunosuppressive agents or with diseases predisposing to infection. These findings have led many authors to conclude that the risk of developing active tuberculosis during glucocorticoid therapy is much lower than initially suspected[49].

Peptic ulceration

Peptic ulceration is not a common occurrence in endogenous Cushing's disease yet it is widely held that glucocorticoid therapy is frequently complicated by the appearance or reactivation of peptic ulcers. The basis for this view resides in a number of anecdotal reports but the evidence from controlled studies suggests that an increased risk of peptic ulceration – if it exists at all – is considerably lower than is widely believed. However, glucocorticoids may exacerbate the ulcerogenic properties of NSAIDs[50].

Osteoporosis

The bone loss associated with glucocorticoid therapy principally affects trabecular bone. Studies using photon absorptiometric measurement of bone mineral density have shown that bone loss is greater in the lumbar spine, less in the proximal femur and least in the forearm. Vertebral wedge and crush fractures are a frequent complication of glucocorticoid-treated RA, with prevalence rates from 11% to 20% reported[51].

The increased risk of fractures at other skeletal sites in such patients, however, remains unclear. In a case-control study of hip fracture in the UK[52], current use of glucocorticoids was associated with a doubled hip fracture risk. Studies of bone loss in patients treated with glucocorticoids do not clearly suggest a threshold dose below which osteoporosis can be avoided. Bone loss has been reported with prednisolone doses of 10mg daily, reducing to zero over 20 weeks[53], other studies suggest maintenance of bone stock on doses up to 7.5mg daily[54]. The relationship between doses above 7.5mg daily and increased rate of bone loss appears to be consistent.

Rheumatoid arthritis patients on glucocorticoids tend to have more severe disease and so are at greater risk of osteoporosis due to the disease itself and the associated functional disability. The improved function resulting from glucocorticoid treatment would reduce the rate of bone loss because of increased functional activity, which has a positive effect on bone density. Finally, even if low-dose glucocorticoid treatment does cause increased bone loss in RA it is not entirely clear how this translates into clinically important fractures, even although there is evidence that fracture risk is partially related to the total cumulative steroid dose. Treatment with bisphosphonates and/or hormone replacement therapy may retard bone loss with the potential to reduce the frequency of fractures[55]. In general, for patients who are expected to receive more than 7.5 mg prednisolone for longer than 6 months, one should identify and treat modifiable risk factors, and if one or more major non-modifiable risk factor is present, consider treatment with bisphosphonates (Fig. 11.7).

Atherosclerosis

Several studies of mortality in RA and other connective tissue diseases have detected an increased cardiovascular mortality among sufferers, suggesting an approximate doubling in the death rate from ischemic heart disease. Although data on glucocorticoid use in these studies are often incomplete, one study reported an excess of coronary artery deaths in a glucocorticoid-treated group when compared with a non-glucocorticoid-treated control group[56]. The evidence linking glucocorticoid therapy with atherosclerosis falls far short of proof[21] but, if true, even a small effect would have considerable clinical significance.

Pulsed intravenous therapy

Reports of complications following pulsed glucocorticoid therapy[21] have usually arisen in renal transplant patients. Most important among these is sudden death, most probably arising as a result of ventricular dysrhythmia and consequent myocardial infarction. In three

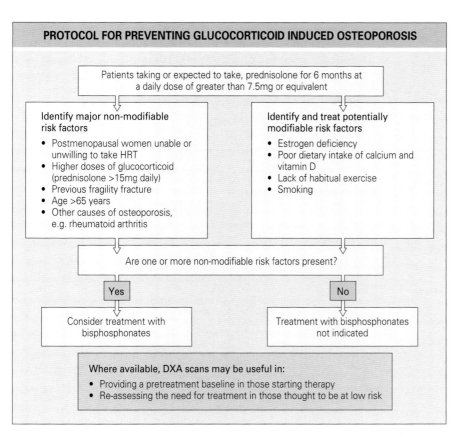

PROTOCOL FOR PREVENTING GLUCOCORTICOID INDUCED OSTEOPOROSIS

Patients taking or expected to take, prednisolone for 6 months at a daily dose of greater than 7.5mg or equivalent

Identify major non-modifiable risk factors
- Postmenopausal women unable or unwilling to take HRT
- Higher doses of glucocorticoid (prednisolone >15mg daily)
- Previous fragility fracture
- Age >65 years
- Other causes of osteoporosis, e.g. rheumatoid arthritis

Identify and treat potentially modifiable risk factors
- Estrogen deficiency
- Poor dietary intake of calcium and vitamin D
- Lack of habitual exercise
- Smoking

Are one or more non-modifiable risk factors present?

Yes → Consider treatment with bisphosphonates

No → Treatment with bisphosphonates not indicated

Where available, DXA scans may be useful in:
- Providing a pretreatment baseline in those starting therapy
- Re-assessing the need for treatment in those thought to be at low risk

Fig. 11.7 One protocol for preventing glucocorticoid-induced osteoporosis. DXA, dual X-ray absorptiometry; HRT, hormone replacement therapy.

such cases, the intravenous bolus was administered rapidly (in one case over only 20 seconds) and all were taking furosemide, which may have induced hypokalemia. It has been suggested that increasing the infusion time to at least 30 minutes might prevent such events. Nevertheless, the incidence of such sudden death appears to be extremely low, given that well over 10 000 renal transplant patients are likely to have been treated with pulse glucocorticoids. Other reported complications include transient arthralgias and synovitis, hyperglycemia, pancreatitis, gastrointestinal bleeding, visual disturbance and acute psychosis.

Severe fatal infections have also been reported. However, these are rare, and have occurred in transplant patients on daily doses of azathioprine, often following continued, long-term use of 1g pulses. *In vitro* studies indicate, however, that methylprednisolone pulses fail to reduce bacterial phagocytosis or killing by human neutrophils.

PRACTICAL PRESCRIBING TIPS

General approach

It may be helpful to consider the prescription of glucocorticoids in three broad dose ranges. Low to medium daily doses, in the region of 15mg prednisolone or less, are used to treat polymyalgia, symptomatic arthritis and relatively quiescent SLE. Medium to high doses (20–60mg daily) are helpful in vasculitis (particularly involving larger arteries as in temporal arteritis or polyarteritis nodosa) or active, systemic SLE. Very high doses and pulse therapy are used to treat severe acute crises such as widespread vasculitis or nephritis.

Glucocorticoids in children

Growth retardation may occur in children receiving glucocorticoids as these agents inhibit linear bone growth and delay epiphyseal closure. Regular daily administration of more than 7.5mg prednisolone is associated with inhibition of linear growth. The mechanism of action is unknown, although suppression of growth hormone secretion and other

metabolic effects may contribute. Alternate-day administration of the same total dose may reduce this effect[57] and is now preferred.

Reducing the dose

High doses of glucocorticoids are often used for only short periods and can be reduced rapidly with little adverse effect provided the underlying disease remains controlled. The precise pattern of reduction will depend upon the particular clinical circumstances under consideration, but control of short, severe exacerbations of, for example, vasculitis can be achieved with high doses over several days to a week or two followed by rapid reduction to more moderate levels (15–20mg daily). Patients treated in the longer term with moderate or low doses of glucocorticoid may develop a 'glucocorticoid withdrawal syndrome' if their treatment is then reduced. This constellation of symptoms includes myalgia, fatigue, malaise, anorexia, nausea and weight loss[58] and has been reported in as many as 70% of patients treated with 30mg prednisone daily for longer than 3 months. There appears to be no correlation between symptoms and adrenal function. In certain clinical settings, however, such as polymyalgia rheumatica and polymyositis, it may be difficult to differentiate from poor control of the primary disease.

One approach to avoiding this is to reduce the glucocorticoid treatment only slowly – perhaps by as little as 2.5mg daily every 6–10 weeks down to 7.5 mg daily, then by about 1mg daily over the same time interval, and in some patients by 1mg on alternate days to gradually stop the final few milligrams.

Glucocorticoid-sparing agents

This term is used to describe drugs that are prescribed in order to make it easier to reduce the glucocorticoid dose while at the same time controlling the underlying disease. Azathioprine, cyclophosphamide and methotrexate are each used for this purpose, commonly in doses lower than when used as single agents (e.g. azathioprine maybe prescribed at 50mg daily rather than the 2.5mg/kg/day target dose used to treat RA). This use of 'combination' therapy to reduce adverse reactions is well recognized in other fields of medicine.

FUTURE DIRECTIONS

Glucocorticoids, acting through their receptor molecule, clearly play a central role in the control of the inflammatory process. The primary and tertiary structures of human phospholipase A_2 have been determined[59], raising the prospect of designing specific inhibitors for the active site that may be more powerful than lipocortin. Evidence is now emerging that some rheumatic diseases may in themselves blunt the normal anti-inflammatory response of the hypothalamic–pituitary–adrenal axis, resulting in inappropriately low glucocorticoid levels[60]. Attempts are also being made to develop tissue-specific effects which may reduce potential adverse reactions[61]. Many developments can be expected in this field.

REFERENCES

1. Jenkins D. Pharmacology of prednisone, prednisolone, 6-CH$_3$ prednisone and prednisolone and triamcinolone. In: Mills LC, Mayer JE, eds. Inflammation and disease of connective tissue. A Hakremann Symposium. Philadelphia, PA: WB Saunders; 1961: 328–335.
2. Baxter HD, Forssham PH. Tissue effects of glucocorticoids. Am J Med 1972; 53: 573–589.
3. Gehring U. Genetics of glucocorticoid receptors. Mol Cell Endocrinol 1986; 48: 89–96.
4. Buttgereit F, Wehling M, Burmester GR. A new hypothesis of modular glucocorticoid actions. Glucocorticoid treatment of rheumatic diseases revisited. Arthritis Rheum 1998; 41: 761–767.
5. Rothbut B, Russo-Marie F. Novel concepts in the mode of action of anti-inflammatory steroids. Agents Actions 1984; 14(suppl): 171–180.
6. Grabstein K, Dower S, Gillis S et al. Expression of interleukin-2, interferon-gamma and the IL-2 receptor by human peripheral blood lymphocytes. J Immunol 1986; 136: 4503–4508.
7. Beutler B, Krochen N, Milsark IW et al. Control of cachetin (TNF) synthesis mechanism of endotoxin resistance. Science 1986; 232: 977–980.
8. Werb Z. Biochemical actions of glucocorticoids on macrophages in culture-specific inhibition of elastase, collagenase and plasminogen activator secretion and effects on other metabolic functions. J Exp Med 1978; 147: 1695–1712.
9. Santine G, Patrignani P, Sciulli MG et al. The human pharmacology of monocyte cyclooxygenase 2 inhibition by cortisol and synthetic glucocorticoids. Clin Pharmacol Ther 2001; 70: 475.
10. Gerrard TL, Volkman DJ, Jurgensen CH et al. Activated human T cells can present antigens but cannot present soluble antigens. Cell Immunol 1985; 95: 65–74.
11. Butler WT, Rossen RD. Effects of glucocorticoids on immunity in man. 1. Decreased serum IgG concentrations caused by 3 or 5 days of high doses of methylprednisolone. J Clin Invest 1973; 52: 2629–2640.
12. Tuchinda M, Newcomb RW, Devald BL. Effect of prednisone treatment on the human immune response to keyhole limpet haemocyanin. Int Arch Allergy Appl Immunol 1972; 42: 533–544.
13. Cupps TR, Edgar LL, Thomas CA et al. Multiple mechanisms of B cell immunoregulation in man after administration of in-vivo glucocorticoids. J Immunol 1984; 132: 170–175.
14. Crabtree GR, Munck A, Smith KA. Glucocorticoids inhibit expression of Fc receptors on the human granulocytic cell line, HL-60. Nature 1979; 279: 338–339.
15. Parillo JE, Fauci AS. Mechanisms of glucocorticoid action on immune processes. Annu Rev Pharmacol Toxicol 1979; 19: 179–201.
16. Oluhy RG, Newmark SR, Lauler DR et al. Pharmacology and chemistry of adrenal glucocosteroids in steroid therapy. In: Azarnoff DL, ed. Philadelphia, PA: WB Saunders; 1975: 8.
17. Brooks SM, Werk EE, Ackerman SJ et al. Adverse effects of phenobarbital on glucocorticoid metabolism in asthmatics. N Engl J Med 1972; 286: 1125.
18. Klinenberg JR, Mullen R. Effect of glucocorticoids on blood salicylate concentrations. JAMA 1965; 194: 601.
19. Buttgereit F, da Silva JA, Boers M et al. Standardised nomenclature for glucocorticoid dosages and glucocorticoid treatment regimens; current questions and tentative answers in rheumatology. Ann Rheum Dis 2002; 61: 718–722.
20. Saag KG, Criswell LA, Sems KM et al. Low-dose corticosteroids in rheumatoid arthritis. A meta-analysis of their moderate-term effectiveness. Arthritis Rheum 1996; 39: 1818–1825.
21. Empire Rheumatism Council. Multi-centre controlled trial comparing cortisone acetate and acetyl salicylic acid in the long-term treatment of rheumatoid arthritis. Ann Rheum Dis 1955; 14: 353–367.
22. Joint Committee of the Medical Research Council and Nuffield Foundation. A comparison of prednisolone with aspirin or other analgesics in the treatment of rheumatoid arthritis. Ann Rheum Dis 1959; 18: 173–187.
23. Van Gestel AM, Laan RFJM, Haagsma CJ et al. Low-dose oral steroids as bridge therapy in rheumatoid arthritis patients starting with parenteral gold. A randomized double-blind placebo-controlled trial. Br J Rheumatol 1995; 34: 347–351.
24. Kirwan JR and the Arthritis and Rheumatism Council Low-Dose Glucocorticoid Study Group. The effect of glucocorticoids on joint destruction in rheumatoid arthritis. N Engl J Med 1995; 333: 142–146.
25. Boers M, Verhoeven AC, Markusse HM et al. Randomised comparison of combined step down prednisolone, methotrexate and sulphasalazine with sulphasalazine alone in early rheumatoid arthritis. Lancet 1997; 350: 309–318.
26. Bryon MA, Kirwan JR. Glucocorticoids in rheumatoid arthritis: is a trial of their disease modifying potential feasible? Ann Rheum Dis 1986; 46: 171–173.
27. West HF. Rheumatoid arthritis. The relevance of clinical knowledge to research activities. Abstr World Med 1967; 41: 401–417.
28. Hickling P, Jacoby RK, Kiwan JR and the Arthritis and Rheumatism Council Low-Dose Glucocorticoid Study Group. Joint destruction after glucocorticoids are withdrawn in early rheumatoid arthritis. Br J Rheumatol 1998; 37: 930–936.
29. Rau R, Wassenberg S, Zeidler H; LDPT-Study Group. Low dose prednisolone therapy (LDPT) retards radiographically detectable destruction in early rheumatoid arthritis–preliminary results of a multicenter, randomized, parallel, double blind study. Z Rheumatol 2000; 59(suppl 2): II/90–96.
30. Van Everdingen AA, Jacobs JWG, van Reesema DRS, Bijlsma WJ. Low-dose prednisone therapy for patients with early active rheumatoid arthritis: clinical efficacy, disease-modifying properties, and side effects. Ann Intern Med 2002; 136: 1–12.
31. Weusten BLAM, Jacobs JWG, Bijlsma JWJ. Glucocorticoid pulse therapy in active rheumatoid arthritis. Semin Arthritis Rheum 1993; 23: 183–192.
32. Radia M, Furst DE. Comparison of three pulse methylprednisolone regimens in the treatment of rheumatoid arthritis. J Rheumatol 1988; 15: 242–256.
33. Shipley ME, Bacon PA, Berry H et al. Pulsed methylprednisolone in active early rheumatoid disease: a dose ranging study. Br J Rheumatol 1988; 15: 242–246.
34. Needs CJ, Smith M, Boutagy J et al. Comparison of methylprednisolone (1 gram IV) with prednisolone (1 gram orally) in rheumatoid arthritis: a pharmokinetic and clinical study. J Rheumatol 1988; 15: 224–228.
35. Choy EHS, Kingsley G, Corkhill MM, Panayi GS. Intramuscular methylprednisolone is superior to pulse oral methylprednisolone during the induction phase of chrysotherapy. Br J Rheumatol 1993; 32: 734–739.
36. Conn D, Tomkins RB, Nichols WL. Glucocorticoids in the management of vasculitis – a double edged sword? J Rheumatol 1988; 15: 1181–1183.
37. Salvarini C, Macchioni PL, Tartoni PL et al. Polymyalgia rheumatica and giant cell arteritis: a 5-year epidemiologic and clinical study in Reggio Emilia, Italy. Clin Exp Rheumatol 1987; 5: 205–215.
38. Delecoeuillerie G, Joly P, de Lara AC, Paolaggi JB. Polymyalgia rheumatica and temporal arteritis: a retrospective analysis of prognostic features and different glucocorticoid regimens (11 year survey of 210 patients). Ann Rheum Dis 1988; 47: 733–739.
39. Lundberg I, Hedfors E. Restricted dose and duration of glucocorticoid treatment in patients with polymyalgia rheumatica and temporal arteritis. J Rheumatol 1990; 17: 1340–1345.
40. Kyle V, Hazleman BL. Treatment of polymyalgia rheumatica and giant cell arteritis. II. Relation between steroid dose and steroid associated side effects. Ann Rheum Dis 1989; 48: 662–666.
41. Kirwan JR. Treatment of polymyalgia rheumatica. Br J Rheumatol 1990; 29: 316.
42. Dasgupta B, Gray J, Fernandes L, Olliff C. Treatment of polymyalgia rheumatica with intramuscular injections of methylprednisolone. Ann Rheum Dis 1991; 50: 942–945.
43. Jover JA, Hernandez-Garcia C, Morado IC et al. Combined treatment of giant-cell arteritis with methotrexate and prednisone. a randomized, double-blind, placebo-controlled trial. Ann Intern Med 2001; 134: 106–114.
44. Henderson RG, Wheatlev T, English J et al. Variation in plasma prednisolone concentrations in renal transplant recipients given enteric-coated prednisolone. Br Med J 1971; 1: 1534–1536.
45. Hirata F. The regulation of lipomodulin, a phospholipase inhibitory protein in rabbit neutrophils by phosphorylation. J Biol Chem 1981; 256: 7730–7733.
46. Podgorski MR, Goulding NJ. Hall ND et al. Autoantibodies to recombinant lipocortin in RA and SLE. Br J Rheumatol 1987; 26(suppl 2): 54–55.
47. Weisman MH. Glucocorticoids in the treatment of rheumatologic diseases. Curr Opin Rheumatol 1995; 7: 183–190.
48. Grieco MH. The role of glucocorticoid therapy in infection. Hosp Pract 1984; 18: 131–143.
49. Haanaes QC, Bergman A. Tuberculosis in patients treated with glucocorticoids. Eur J Respir Dis 1983; 64: 294–297.
50. Piper JM, Ray WA, Daughery JR, Griffen MR. Glucocorticoid use and peptic ulcer – role of non-steroidal anti-inflammatory drug. Ann Intern Med 1991; 114: 735–740.
51. Cooper C, Kirwan JR. The risk of local and systemic glucocorticoid administration. Baillière's Clin Rheumatol 1990; 4: 305–332.
52. Cooper C, Barker DJP, Wickham C. Physical activity, muscle strength and calcium intake in fracture of the proximal femur in Britain. Br Med J 1988; 297: 1443–1446.
53. Laan RFJM, Van Reil PLCM, van de Putte LBA et al. Low dose prednisolone induces rapid reversible axial bone loss in patients with rheumatoid arthritis: a randomized controlled study. Ann Intern Med 1993; 119: 963–968.
54. Sambrook PN, Eisman JA, Yeates MG et al. Osteoporosis in rheumatoid arthritis: Safety of low dose glucocorticoids. Ann Rheum Dis 1986; 45: 950–953.
55. Adachi JD, Papaioannou A. Corticosteroid-induced osteoporosis: detection and management. Drug Saf 2001; 24: 607–624.
56. Million R, Poole P, Kellgren JH et al. Long-term study of management of rheumatoid arthritis. Lancet 1984; 1: 812–816.
57. Reimer LG, Morris HG, Ellis EF. Growth of asthmatic children during treatment with alternate-day steroids. J Allergy Clin Immunol 1975; 55: 224–231.
58. Dixon R, Christy N. On the various forms of glucocorticoid withdrawal syndrome. Am J Med 1980; 68: 224–230.
59. Wery JP, Schevitz RW, Clawson DK et al. Structure of recombinant human rheumatoid arthritis phospholipase A_2 at 2.2Å resolution. Nature 1991; 352: 79–82.
60. Chikanza IC, Petrou P, Kingsley G et al. Defective regulation of the hypothalamic–pituitary–adrenal axis in rheumatoid arthritis is not a consequence of chronic inflammation per se. Br J Rheumatol 1992; 31(suppl 2): 28.
61. Messina OD, Barreira JC, Zanchetta JR et al. Effect of low dose deflazacort rheumatoid vs prednisolone on bone mineral content in premenopausal rheumatoid arthritis. J Rheumatol 1992; 19: 1520–1526.

12 Complementary and alternative medicine

Brian M Berman, Elena Gournelos and George T Lewith

- The majority of rheumatology patients use some form of complementary and alternative medicine (CAM).
- Acupuncture, herbal medicine, nutriceuticals and homeopathy are among the most commonly used CAM treatments
- The evidence for the efficacy of these therapies is limited
- The majority of research on traditional Chinese medicine in the West has focused on acupuncture
- Studies have shown acupuncture to be effective for specific types of pain reduction
- Some herbal therapies may be as effective as analgesics and anti-inflammatories for rheumatic and musculoskeletal conditions
- Nutriceuticals, in particular glucosamine and chondroitin, appear effective in the treatment of osteoarthritis and in preventing long-term joint damage
- Homeopathy has not been definitively proven to work for rheumatologic conditions
- Moderate evidence exists for the effectiveness of mind-body therapies as adjuncts in the treatment of rheumatoid and osteoarthritis
- Physicians should consider that CAM can be integrated into the conventional management of rheumatological conditions in a thoughtful, professional and co-operative manner

OVERVIEW

Complementary, alternative and integrative medicine are blanket terms that comprise a large variety of health treatments clustered together because they exist outside the parameters of conventional treatment (i.e. neither taught widely in medical schools nor generally available in hospitals[1]). They include whole systems of medicine as well as individual treatment options. The terms complementary, alternative and integrative refer not to the particular modalities used but to the manner in which health care is obtained; in other words, people can obtain health care from a non-conventional practitioner in conjunction with conventional care (*complementary*), instead of conventional care (*alternative*) or from a provider or group of providers that have blended conventional and non-conventional care in their practice (*integrative*). Moreover, the status of any therapeutic practice is in constant flux; many therapies once considered complementary or alternative may gain acceptance and be slowly incorporated in to mainstream practice while others may prove ineffective or dangerous.

While it is commonly known that the traditional medical systems of Asia have been practiced for thousands of years, the history of complementary and alternative medicine (CAM) in the West, although well documented[2], is not always discussed. CAM use in the West is not a recent phenomenon; rather, many of the alternative systems of medicine being used today (e.g. herbalism, chiropractic, naturopathy and homeopathy) have evolved alongside allopathic medicine. While the medicinal use of Western herbs predates history, herbalism as it is practiced today was first developed in the late 18th century. Homeopathy was developed during the same time period, while chiropractic, osteopathy and naturopathy followed in the late 19th century. In addition, Asian systems of medicine were formally introduced to the West as early as 1683, when the first European text on acupuncture and arthritis was written[3], the first journal articles on acupuncture appeared in the 1820s[4,5]. Over time, as these medical systems developed and the needs of the population continuously changed, the popularity of CAM ebbed and flowed accordingly[6].

In recent years, CAM use has been on the rise. In the USA, a 1997 survey[7] estimated that over 40% of the general population made over 629 million visits to CAM practitioners, a 45% increase since a similar survey in 1990[1]. Although there is no compelling evidence to suggest that the use of CAM among rheumatology patients has increased dramatically over the last 15 years[8], usage rates among this subpopulation are still higher than average. Studies have reported usage rates as high as 94%[9] but recent surveys report that, on average, 44–66% of rheumatology patients use CAM[10–12]. However, the usage rate of fibromyalgia patients is particularly high, at 91%[13].

Because of the chronic nature of rheumatic disease, as well as the palliative nature and adverse effects associated with conventional care for this condition, it is not surprising that so many rheumatology patients are using CAM. Eisenberg *et al.*[7] found that four out of 10 CAM users do so to treat chronic disease. A 1996 British survey found that patients turned to CAM because:

- they valued the emphasis of treating the whole person
- they believed that CAM would be more effective than conventional treatment
- they wanted to take an active role in their health
- conventional treatment was not effective for their problem[14].

Another survey in the USA, however, found that dissatisfaction with conventional medicine was no more prevalent among CAM users than among non-users; rather, the study found that people were more likely to choose CAM if it was congruent with their own values, beliefs and philosophical orientations toward health and life[15]. Still, this study reported that chronic problems such as low back pain, chronic pain, anxiety and generally poor health status were predictors of CAM use.

WIDELY USED COMPLEMENTARY AND ALTERNATIVE MEDICINE SYSTEMS AND THERAPIES

Surveys indicate that chiropractic, copper bracelets, magnets, herbs, topical treatments, electrical stimulators, neutraceuticals, homeopathy, massage, acupuncture, diet therapies, relaxation and spiritual healing are all therapies used by rheumatology patients[8,12]. This section aims to give a brief introduction to the philosophy and practice of a few main, commonly used modalities; in particular, therapies that are supported by evidence are discussed. Moreover, these examples have been chosen to illustrate the complexity of CAM systems as well as to introduce the reader to some of the main clinical, philosophical and research issues that must be confronted if integration of these therapies into mainstream medical practice is to occur. Table 12.1 provides a glossary of CAM therapies.

Traditional Chinese medicine and acupuncture
Philosophy and history

Traditional Chinese medicine (TCM) is the product of thousands of years of philosophical, political, spiritual and scientific evolution. Although its exact origin remains controversial, it is generally accepted that the first true Chinese medical texts emerged around 200BC[17]. Today,

TABLE 12.1 GLOSSARY OF COMMON COMPLEMENTARY AND ALTERNATIVE MEDICINE THERAPIES

Category and select modalities	Description
I. Alternative medical systems	Complete systems of diagnosis and practice that are based on a unique theoretical framework and are developed independently of biomedicine
Traditional Chinese medicine	Originating in China over 2000 years ago, this system uses acupuncture, herbs, massage and meditative exercise (*qi gong*) to restore balance within the body and with nature. It is based on the eight principles of *yin*, *yang*, hot, cold, external, internal, deficiency and excess
Ayurveda	The traditional medical system of India, which uses herbs, massage, yoga and therapeutic elimination to restore balance within the body and with nature. It is based on balancing the three *doshas*: *vata*, *pitta* and *kapha*
Homeopathy	A system of medicine developed in Germany in the late 1700s. Homeopathy is based on the law of similars, in which compounds that *cause* a set of symptoms in large doses can purportedly cure the same symptoms when given in minute doses
Naturopathy	A system of medicine founded on the healing power of nature. Naturopathy uses a combination of therapies from the sciences of clinical nutrition, herbal medicine, homeopathy, physical medicine, exercise therapy, counseling, stress management, acupuncture, natural childbirth and hydrotherapy
II. Mind–body interventions	Therapies that employ techniques designed to facilitate the mind's capacity to affect bodily function and symptoms[16]
Meditation	Intentional self-regulation of attention, or a systematic mental focus on particular aspects of inner or outer experience. Most meditation practices were developed within a religious/spiritual context and held as their ultimate goal some type of spiritual growth, personal transformation and/or transcendental experience. However, it has been argued that, as a health-care intervention, meditation can be effective regardless of an individual's cultural or religious background
Relaxation techniques	Practices that are specifically designed to elicit a psychophysiological state of hypoarousal. They may be aimed at reducing sympathetic nervous system activity and blood pressure, easing muscle tension, slowing metabolic processes or altering brain wave activity
Guided imagery	The use of mental images to promote relaxation and wellness or to facilitate healing of a particular ailment (e.g. cancer, psychological trauma). The images can involve any of the senses and may be self-directed or guided by a practitioner
Hypnosis	A state of attentive and focused concentration in which people can be relatively unaware of, but not entirely unconscious of, their surroundings. Hypnotized individuals becomes absorbed in the images presented by the hypnotherapist and tend not to register experiences as a part of their conscious awareness
Biofeedback	The use of mechanical devices that amplify physiological signals (e.g. blood pressure, muscle activity) in order to teach methods of regulating these physiological processes through intention
III. Biologically-based therapies	Natural and biologically based practices, interventions and products
Herbalism	The use of plants to treat disease and promote health
Orthomolecular therapies	The use of molecules normally found in the body (e.g. hormones, vitamins, and nutrients), to treat disease and promote health
Diet therapies	Specialized dietary regimens (e.g. Gerson therapy, Kelley regimen, macrobiotic diet, Ornish diet, Pritikin diet) for the treatment or prevention of a specific disease (e.g. cancer, cardiovascular disease) or for the promotion of general health
Biological therapies	The use of substances (e.g. shark cartilage) or molecules (e.g. SAM-e, glucosamine) naturally occurring in animal physiology to treat specific diseases
IV. Body-based therapies	Manipulation or movement of the body for healing purposes
Chiropractic	Manipulation of bones and joints based on the relationship between structure (e.g. the spine) and function (i.e. central nervous system) in order to restore balance to the body
Massage	Manipulation of body tissues to promote wellness and reduce pain and stress
Rolfing	Manipulation and stretching of the fascias in order to re-establish a healthy alignment of bone and muscle
Reflexology	Application of manual pressure to specific areas of the foot that theoretically correspond to different organs or systems of the body
Postural re-education	The use of movement and touch to help patients relearn healthy posture. The therapies seek to release habitual, harmful ways of holding the body by focusing on awareness through movement
V. Energy therapies	Therapeutic practices that focus on energy fields originating either within the body (biofields) or from external sources (electromagnetic fields)
Magnets	The placement of magnets on the body to ease pain
Pulsed electrical field	Injured body parts are placed in an induced electrical field to facilitate healing
Reiki	A technique of Japanese origin where a practitioner channels energy through his/her body and into a patient's body to promote healing
Therapeutic touch	Often referred to as 'laying on of hands' even though actual touch is not required, this therapy uses the healing energy of the therapist to identify and repair imbalances in a patient's biofield
External *qi gong*	A subset of Chinese medical *qi gong* practice in which a master healer uses the energy of his/her own biofield to bring another person's energy into balance

CAM therapies have been organized into five major groups by the National Center for Complementary and Alternative Medicine: (I) alternative medical systems, (II) mind–body interventions, (III) biologically based interventions, (IV) manual therapies and (V) energy therapies.

TCM is an intricate medical system based on ancient philosophies, symptom-based clinical practice, a complicated individualized diagnostic system and a variety of treatment modalities including various types of acupuncture, massage (*tui na*) and herbal medicines. Like many CAM systems, TCM is based on a belief in the existence of a life force or vital energy that runs through the body and affects its functioning. This energy takes the form of the vital substances: *qi, blood, essence* and *body fluids*. People are healthy when their energy is unobstructed, balanced and harmonious; it is the practitioner's aim to restore this energetic state through the manipulation of the vital essences. Imbalances are diagnosed into syndrome patterns according to a number of complex yet subtle theories that provide the basis for treatment. Central to this is the theory of *yin* and *yang* (Fig. 12.1). The terms and concepts within TCM have no Western equivalents; at best, they are roughly translated and therefore easily misinterpreted. For example, concepts such as *blood* or *kidney* may seem familiar but their meaning in the context of TCM encompasses more and differs significantly from the Western biomedical model. Learning TCM without stepping out of a Western framework is like trying to edit a Chinese text with English grammar rules.

Treatment

The TCM system encompasses many different treatment modalities, each used to shift the vital energy of the body. Many of these techniques stimulate specific points on the body in order to alter the flow of *qi*; usually, these points are located on meridians (specific channels that carry *qi* though the body; Fig. 12.2). Acupuncture, the most well known, involves the insertion of thin, stainless steel needles into these points (Fig. 12.3). Similarly, moxibustion (the burning of a specific variety of the herb *Artemisia vulgaris*), cupping (the use of suction) and acupressure (manual stimulation) all stimulate acupuncture points. Internal

remedies are a vital component of TCM; a materia medica of over 10 000 herb and animal compounds has been developed. These herbal remedies are always given in combination and are chosen to complement and balance each other. Additionally, TCM incorporates a unique system of massage called *tui na* and uses meditative exercises such as *qi gong*.

The TCM approach to rheumatic disease is very different than that of conventional modern medicine. First, the concept of rheumatic disease as it is understood in the West does not exist in TCM. Rather, the majority of rheumatic disorders fall into the general classifications of painful obstructions (*bi* syndrome). Within this general diagnosis, the particular energetic characteristics that a patient expresses (e.g. *hot, cold,* yin *deficiency, blood stagnation, wind, damp*) will determine diagnosis and treatment. Thus, TCM treatment of rheumatic disorders, as with many CAM disciplines, is individualized; patients with the same conventional diagnosis may receive different TCM diagnoses and treatments.

Evidence

Although herbal combinations and other treatments are used in conjunction with acupuncture in clinical practice, the vast majority of research on TCM in the West focuses on acupuncture. A large body of evidence exists for the underlying physiological mechanisms of acupuncture in the treatment of pain[18]. Most basic research in acupuncture focuses on mechanisms for acupuncture analgesia; these include neural, humoral and bioelectric components[19]. Numerous studies show that various levels of the nervous system are involved in acupuncture analgesia from the afferent pathways to the thalamus[20–22]. Moreover, the endorphin system is implicated in acupuncture physiology[23]; endorphin levels in cerebrospinal fluid rise after acupuncture[24]; caudate, arcuate, pre-optic and limbic regions appear to mediate acupuncture analgesia; and central nervous system naloxone administration blocks acupuncture analgesia in some cases[19]. The serotonergic and cholinergic systems have also been implicated in acupuncture analgesia; this may account for the partial naloxone inhibition[25]. In addition, functional magnetic resonance imaging research indicates that activity in numerous brainstem, midbrain and cortical structures is affected by acupuncture; the magnitude of the effect is dependent on the level of needle stimulation[26]. Also, acupuncture points have been shown to correspond with areas of low electrical resistance on the body[27]; the conductance of these points varies with pathogenesis[28,29].

However, evidence for the efficacy of acupuncture in the treatment of rheumatic and musculoskeletal disorders is mixed. Different systematic reviews of the clinical effects of acupuncture analyzed many of the same, rather poor-quality, randomized controlled trials and, while agreeing about the paucity of research in this field, have come to different conclusions with respect to its clinical effectiveness[30–33]. Ezzo *et al.*[34] reviewed seven trials of acupuncture for OA and found limited evidence that acupuncture is more effective than waiting lists or usual treatment, strong evidence that acupuncture is more effective than sham for pain and inconclusive evidence for function. However, another study by Ernst *et al.*[30] reviewed 11 OA randomized controlled trials; seven trials reported positive results but were of poor quality. A review of the randomized controlled trials of acupuncture for fibromyalgia[32] ($n = 7$) found positive but limited evidence that acupuncture affects pain, stiffness and global improvement ratings[35]. Van Tulder *et al.*[33] reviewed 11 randomized controlled trials of acupuncture in the treatment of low back pain; they found 'no evidence that acupuncture was more effective than no treatment, moderate evidence that acupuncture is not more effective than trigger point injection and transcutaneous electrical nerve stimulation, and limited evidence that acupuncture is not more effective than placebo or sham acupuncture'. However, a meta-analysis ($n = 9$) by Ernst *et al.*[36] found evidence that acupuncture is more effective than active controls for low back pain (odds ratio = 2.3). A review of

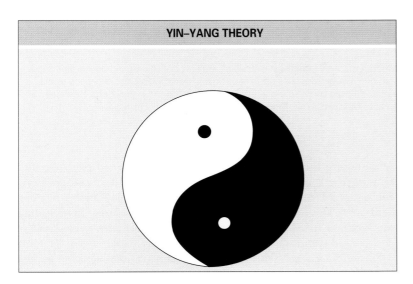

YIN–YANG THEORY

Fig. 12.1 *Yin–yang* theory. The concept of *yin* and *yang* is of utmost importance in traditional Chinese medicine, as well as in other styles of oriental medicine and acupuncture. *Yin* and *yang* are two dynamic parts of a whole; they are opposing, interchangeable forces that contain and define each other. They are always in flux and both are always present: one cannot exist without the other. *Yin* is characteristically cool, heavy, dark, moist, condensing, descending and still; *yang* is bright, expansive, creative, hot, light, ascending and active. *Yin* is associated with the earth while *yang* is associated with the sun and the heavens. All people contain a balance of *yin* and *yang*; when this balance is disrupted, health may be affected. For example, *yin* deficiency/*yang* excess may manifest as hot, dry inflammation with restlessness while *yin* excess/*yang* deficiency could manifest as heavy, dull pain that is exacerbated by cold and accompanied by general listlessness. *Yin–yang* theory is the basis for more detailed diagnostic theories such as the 'eight principles' and *zhang-fu* organ differentiation. According to ancient Chinese philosophy, *yin–yang* theory is an elegant model for all of nature and the universe.

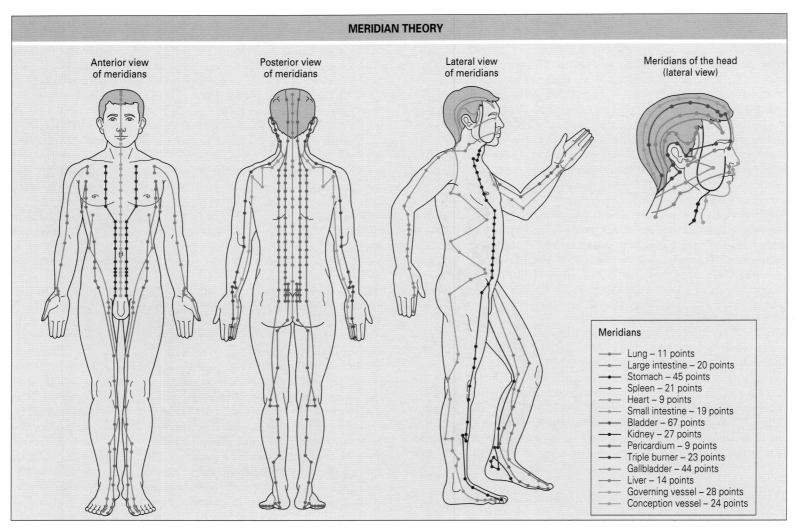

Anterior view of meridians

Posterior view of meridians

Lateral view of meridians

Meridians of the head (lateral view)

Meridians

- Lung – 11 points
- Large intestine – 20 points
- Stomach – 45 points
- Spleen – 21 points
- Heart – 9 points
- Small intestine – 19 points
- Bladder – 67 points
- Kidney – 27 points
- Pericardium – 9 points
- Triple burner – 23 points
- Gallbladder – 44 points
- Liver – 14 points
- Governing vessel – 28 points
- Conception vessel – 24 points

Fig. 12.2 Meridian theory. Qi is believed to run through the body in channels called meridians; although most meridians are associated with a major organ of the body (e.g. kidney, spleen), they each govern a much broader range of emotional/physiological functions. Although they flow inside the tissue and organs of the body, the meridians are accessible from the surface in some areas; thus, the *qi* can be manipulated by needling acupuncture points on the meridians. However, *qi* flow is not restricted to specific channels; there are numerous acupuncture points that are not located on meridians.

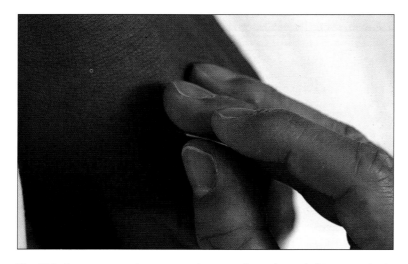

Fig. 12.3 Acupuncture. Acupuncture is one tool a traditional Chinese medical doctor uses to shift a person's vital energy. It involves the insertion of thin, solid, stainless-steel needles into specific points on the body. There are numerous styles of acupuncture, including Japanese, Korean, five-element and six energetic levels. Acupuncture points can also be stimulated manually without the use of needles; this approach may be better suited for children or the elderly.

acupuncture for chronic pain ($n = 51$) found limited evidence that acupuncture is more effective than no treatment and inconclusive evidence that it is more effective than placebo, sham acupuncture or standard care[31]. There are very few randomized controlled trials investigating acupuncture for rheumatoid arthritis (RA); preliminary evidence is positive and suggests that more research is warranted[37].

The differing conclusions from these systematic reviews may in part be caused by the standard rating scales used (e.g. Jadad scale), which strongly favor placebo-controlled trials. Acupuncture has no true placebo, so many valid randomized controlled trials may be given low methodological scores[38]. Important methodological improvements must guide further research. First, most acupuncture trials use formulaic acupuncture treatments that are applied to all patients; however, because acupuncture treatments are highly individualized in clinical practice, this study design tests acupuncture outside of its therapeutic context[39]. Regardless of whether investigators choose a standardized, individualized or hybrid design, an appropriate number of treatments must be administered; positive results are significantly correlated with trials that include six or more treatments[31]. Also, appropriate acupuncture points must be chosen: because there is no standard protocol for any given condition[40], the knowledge and skill of the investigators is of the utmost importance. Furthermore, appropriate controls must be used. Because placebo-controlled trials are difficult, numerous sham procedures have been developed; however, there is no single design that will control for all non-specific effects[39].

With these questions in mind, the Universities of Maryland and Southampton are conducting large multicenter trials. The University of Maryland is involved in a study ($n = 570$) of acupuncture for osteoarthritis (OA) of the knee (to be published in 2003) and the University of Southampton is involved in a study ($n = 150$) of chronic mechanical neck pain (to be published in 2002).

Despite the lack of clear efficacy data, the safety of acupuncture is well documented in both ancient and modern literature[41]. From 1965–99, only 202 cases of acupuncture complications were reported; 46.5% of these were hepatitis infections resulting from inadequate needle sterilization[41]. Clean needling techniques mandated in the mid-1980s have significantly reduced such adverse effects, dropping the incidence by over two-thirds between 1975–1985 and 1986–1999. Other complications include contact dermatitis ($n = 7$), pneumothorax ($n = 26$) and spinal cord injury ($n = 13$); often, these cases were due to practitioner negligence[41]. However, when it is considered that there were an estimated 9–12 million visits to acupuncturists in 1993 in the USA alone[42], the number of adverse events due to acupuncture is quite small.

Herbalism

Philosophy and history

Although herbs are the most popular and ancient CAM modality[7], herbalism is one of the least understood systems of medicine. For example, herbs are commonly used in isolation with expectations that they will treat a particular disease or symptom; however, herbs are very rarely used in isolation by professional herbalists. Also, when a herb is shown to be effective for a specific condition, the herb tends to be narrowly categorized and its other therapeutic properties are ignored; traditionally, herbs are used in multiple organ systems and are applicable to many different conditions. Furthermore, herbal treatment protocols are highly individualized and indications for herbs may be very specific. Sometimes, herbs are used in an overtly dangerous manner. The majority of herb users self-medicate without informing their doctors[7], and inappropriate selection or combinations of herbs can cause adverse events that may mimic, magnify or oppose the effects of pharmaceuticals[43,44] (Table 12.2). Moreover, serious adverse effects are often the result of intentional and inappropriate marketing of potent herbs, as in the case of ephedra (*ma huang*) for weight loss and energy. Traditionally used to treat asthma in China, ephedra is a powerful sympathetic nervous system stimulant that has caused cardiovascular and CNS events such as hypertension and stroke[45].

The practice of traditional herbalism (TCM or *ayurveda*) is plant-centered and requires the use of whole plant material as it is found naturally. On an energetic level, the whole plant is believed to contain a unique life force that is essential for treatment; on the biochemical level, the whole plant is needed to ensure that all the possible complex and unidentified, synergistic compounds within the plant are included with the known active constituents.

Treatment

Herbs are usually prescribed in combination and treatment is individualized. A herbalist approaches the body as a whole system and formulates treatments that address underlying physiological problems as well as acute symptoms. Treatments are usually given orally but may be prescribed as external salves. The bulk of a herbal formula is composed of alteratives, antirheumatics and anti-inflammatories such as sarsaparilla, black cohosh, celery, meadowsweet, nettle, turmeric, boswellia, wild yam, devil's claw and ginger (Fig. 12.4 & Table 12.3). Often, blends will contain diuretics, immune stimulants, circulatory stimulants and digestive tonics as well; only a small portion of the blend addresses symptoms through analgesic action. Nutritional approaches are frequently combined with herbs; ideally, herbs are woven into the daily diet as spices and foods.

Evidence

To date, systematic and meta-analytic reviews of the literature in rheumatology indicate that a number of herbs may be effective treatments for rheumatic and musculoskeletal conditions[47–50]. Four randomized controlled trials have shown that devil's claw (*Harpagophytum procumbens*) may significantly reduce pain associated with OA[51,52] and low back pain[53,54]; two randomized controlled trials indicate that willow bark extract improves WOMAC pain scores in OA patients[49,55]. Six randomized controlled trials of the herbal mixture Phytodolor (golden rod, aspen leaf/bark and ash bark) showed significantly decreased pain[49,56,57], increased function[56] and decreased rescue medication[58,59] for mixed rheumatic disorders, including OA; there was no significant difference between Phytodolor and piroxicam[49]. Four randomized controlled trials investigated topical capsaicin (cayenne) for the treatment of OA[60–63], collectively, meta-analysis of these data indicate that capsaicin is an effective therapy for pain, tenderness and range of motion[50,64].

There are also a handful of single studies but, although they were of adequate quality, one study is insufficient to draw conclusions about the efficacy of any intervention. For instance, one small study ($n = 27$) showed that topical application of nettle leaf reduced pain and disability[65] and another herbal combination, Reumalex, significantly reduced pain in arthritic patients but was not significantly efficacious in OA patients alone[66]. Numerous herbs rich in gammalinolenic acid have also been shown to have positive effects on RA symptoms: treatment with evening primrose oil resulted in less rescue medication and greater well-being[67]; blackcurrant seed oil improved tenderness[68]; and borage seed oil improved tenderness, swelling, stiffness and functioning[69,70]. However, to date, single studies of ginger[71] and the herbal combinations Eazmov[72] and Gitadyl[73] have not produced evidence of efficacy.

Because of the paucity of quality trials, many herbs traditionally used by professional herbalists have not been adequately investigated (if at all). Further research is clearly needed.

Neutraceuticals

The term neutraceuticals is a general classification that refers to the wide array of biologically based products available to health practitioners and consumers; they include vitamins, minerals, neurotransmitters, hormones, animal products such as shark cartilage and glandulars, and other naturally occurring substances such as glucosamine and *S*-adenosyl-methionine (SAM-e). The sheer number of these products can be overwhelming to practitioners and consumers alike; to date, the efficacy and safety of most of these therapies have not been thoroughly investigated. However, there are a few neutraceuticals for which a substantial evidence base is beginning to emerge in the treatment of rheumatic and musculoskeletal diseases, most notably glucosamine and chondroitin, SAM-e and essential fatty acids.

Glucosamine and chondroitin

Numerous narrative and meta-analytic reviews indicate that glucosamine, either combined with chondroitin or alone, is an effective treatment for OA[74–76]. Towheed *et al.*[76] reviewed 16 randomized double-blind studies and found glucosamine to be significantly more effective than placebo (ES = 1.4) and more effective than or equal to non-steroidal anti-inflammatory drugs (NSAIDs) with minimal adverse effects (approximately 6%). McAlindon *et al.*[75] reviewed randomized trials of both glucosamine and chondroitin and found moderate to large effect sizes (0.44 and 0.78 respectively); modest yet positive effective sizes (0.3 and 0.4 respectively) were found when methodologically weak studies were excluded and results were recalculated for outcomes at 4 weeks. A narrative review of six trials by Delafuente[74] also supports the

TABLE 12.2 REPORTED POTENTIAL HERB–DRUG INTERACTIONS RELEVANT TO RHEUMATOLOGY PRACTICE[43,44]

Herb	Pharmaceutical	Effect	Mechanism/comment
Asian herbal mixtures:	Prednisone		
Sho-saiko-to		Decreased AUC	Contains *Glycyrrhiza glabra*, *Bupleurum falcatum*, *Pinellia ternate*, *Scutellaria abaicalensis*, *Zizyphus vulgaris*, *Panax ginseng*, *Zingiber officialis*
Saiboku-to		Increased AUC	Same as above, with addition of *Poria cocos*, *Magnolia officinalis* and *Perillae frutescens*
Betel nut (*Areca catechu*)	Prednisone, albuterol (salbutamol)	Inadequate control of asthma	Arecoline challenge caused dose-related bronchoconstriction
Cayenne (*Capsicum* spp.)	ACE inhibitors	Cough	Capsaicin depletes substance P
	Theophylline	Increased absorption and bioavailability	
Devil's claw (*Harpagophytum procumbens*)	Warfarin	Purpura	
Dan shen (*Salvia miltlorrhiza*)	Warfarin	Increased INR, prolonged PT/PTT	Decreased elimination of warfarin in rats
	Aspirin	Spontaneous hyphema	Inhibition of platelet adhesion factor
	Warfarin	Intracerebral hemorrhage	
	Paracetamol and ergotamine/caffeine	Bilateral subdural hematoma	May be due to gingko alone
	Thiazide diuretic	Hypertension	Gingko alone is not associated with hypertension
GLA-rich herbs (evening primrose, blackcurrant, borage)	Drugs that lower seizure threshold	Increased side effects	Decreased seizure threshold
Licorice (*Glycyrrhiza glabra*)	Prednisone	Glycyrrhizin decreases plasma clearance, increases AUC, increases plasma concentrations of prednisolone	Glycyrrhizin and its metabolite, glycyrrhetinic acid, are inhibitors of $5\alpha,5\beta$-reductase and 11β-dehydrogenase (converts endgenous cortisol to cortisone
	Hydrocortisone	Glycyrrhetinic acid potentiates cutaneous vasoconstrictor response	
	MAOIs	Increased side effects	Glycyrrhizin is an MAOI
	Oral contraceptives	Hypertension, edema, hypokalemia	Oral contraceptives may increase sensitivity to glycyrrhizin
Nettles (*Urtica dioica*)	NSAIDs	Increased therapeutic effect	Potentiation of anti-inflammatory activity
Panax ginseng	Warfarin	Decreased INR	
	Phenelzine	Headache and tremor, mania	
	Corticosteroids	Increased side effects	Similar side effects
	Estrogen replacement	Postmenopausal bleeding or mastalgia	
Papaya (*Carica papaya*)	Warfarin	Increased INR	
St John's wort (*Hypericum perforatum*)	Paroxetine	Lethargy/incontinence	
	Trazodone	Mild serotonin syndrome	Can occur with St John's wort alone
	Sertraline	Mild serotonin syndrome	
	Nefazodone	Mild serotonin syndrome	
	Theophylline	Decreased theophylline concentrations	
	Digoxin	Decreased AUC, decreased peak and trough concentrations	Most studies indicate that St John's wort inhibits cytochrome P450 isoenzymes
	Phenprocoumon	Decreased AUC	
	Cyclosporin	Decreased concentrations in serum	
	Oral contraceptives	Breakthrough bleeding	
Tamarind (*Tamarindus indica*)	Aspirin	Increased bioavailability of aspirin	
Yohimbe (*Pausinystalla yohimbe*)	Tricyclic antidepressants	Hypertension	Yohimbe alone is associated with hypertension; combination with tricyclics lowers active yohimbe dose

ACE, angiotensin converting enzyme; AUC, area under the curve; INR, international normalized ratio; GLA, gammalinolenic acid; MAOI, monoamine oxidase inhibitor; NSAID, non-steroidal anti-inflammatory drug; PT, dilute prothrombin time; PTT, partial thromboplastin time.

It is impossible to summarize all drug–herb interactions. Clinical data is sparse, uncontrolled and often unreliable; most data is in the form of case reports, and issues of dosage, temporal relations, contamination and concomitant drug/herb use are often unreported. Moreover, the majority of herb–drug interactions described in the literature are theoretical in nature and have not been shown to occur in clinical practice; thus, only clinically reported interactions are summarized here. In addition, the effects may depend on mode of ingestion; for example, effects may be stronger if an extract is used (e.g. standardized allicin) as compared with incorporation of herbs in to the diet (e.g. garlic cloves in food).

use of glucosamine for OA of the knee; although optimal dosage has not yet been determined, a dose of 500mg three times daily is generally used. A randomized controlled trial (*n* = 212) published since the above reviews[77] has shown that patients taking 1500mg of oral glucosamine sulfate daily over 3 years experienced no significant joint-space loss and minimum joint-space narrowing compared to patients on placebo. There has been some concern raised, however, about overinterpretation of the radiographic results because of the radiographic views used in this

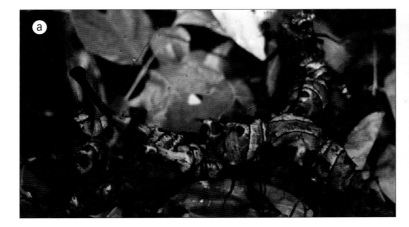

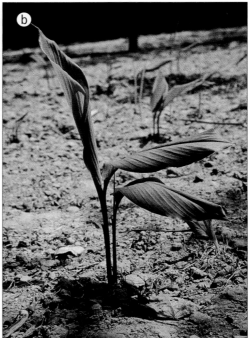

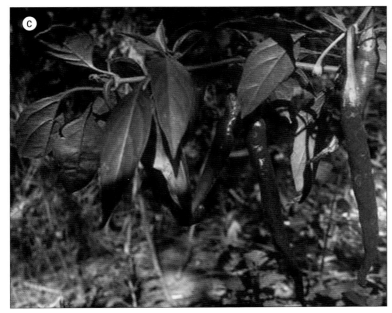

Fig. 12.4 Examples of herbs used in rheumatologic conditions. (a) Sarsaparilla (*Smilax rotundifolia*); the root is used medicinally. (b) Turmeric (*Curcuma longa*); the root is used medicinally. (c) Cayenne (*Capsicum annuum*); the fruit is used medicinally. (Courtesy of M. Moore, Southwest School of Botanical Medicine.)

TABLE 12.3 MECHANISMS OF PHYTO-ANTI-INFLAMMATORY DRUGS

Herb	Cyclo-oxygenase	Lipoxygenase	Cytokine release	Antioxidant
Devil's claw	Inhibition	Inhibition	Inhibition	?
Stinging nettle	Inhibition	Inhibition	Inhibition	?
Willow bark	Inhibition	Inhibition	?	Yes
Black currant seed	Inhibition	Inhibition	?	?
Black currant leaf	Inhibition	Inhibition	?	Yes
Evening primrose seed	Inhibition	Inhibition	?	?
Borage seed	Inhibition	Inhibition	?	?
Goldenrod leaf, aspen leaf/bark, and ash bark	Inhibition	Inhibition	?	Yes

Known anti-inflammatory mechanisms of medical plants have been summarized by Chrubasik and Roufogalis[46].

study. No differences in safety were noticed between the placebo and treatment groups.

Current research suggests that glucosamine and chondroitin may be chondroprotective agents[78]. Both are constituents of connective tissue and are capable of increasing proteoglycan synthesis in articular cartilage[78,79]. Moreover, despite controversy in this area, both substances appear to be absorbed intact in the digestive tract[80–82].

S-adenosyl-methionine

Originally used to treat depression[83,84], the effects of SAM-e on joint pain were discovered serendipitously when they were observed as side effects in clinical trials. Produced from L-methionine and adenosine triphosphate, SAM-e is a methyl donor involved in a wide variety of metabolic processes throughout the body[85]. Although the mechanism of action is not completely understood, SAM-e has been shown to have anti-inflammatory and analgesic effects without gastrointestinal damage in animal models[86]; *in vitro*, SAM-e has exhibited chondroprotective effects via the stimulation of chondrocytes and the subsequent increase in new cartilage production[87].

A recent meta-analysis of 13 trials investigating SAM-e in the treatment of OA[88] indicated that SAM-e is comparable to ibuprofen (ES = 0.16) and superior to placebo (ES = 0.36); however, demonstrated efficacy was not related to dosage or length of intervention. SAM-e has no known side-effects[84] but the long-term effects are unknown.

Essential fatty acids

Essential fatty acids, including omega-6 fatty acids – linolenic acid (LA) and gamma linolenic acid (GLA) – and omega-3 fatty acids – alpha-linolenic acid (ALA), eicosapentaenoic acid (EPA) and docosahexaenoic acid (DHA) – are the first components of a physiological cascade that results in prostaglandin, leukotriene and thromboxane production[89]. Specifically, the presence of omega-3 fatty acids can antagonize the cellular biosynthesis of prostaglandins E_2 and LTB4, interleukin-1β, leukotriene B4 and tumor necrosis factor[90,91]; these lipids play an important role in the pathophysiology of RA[92]. Moreover, omega-3 fatty acids may inhibit the platelet-activating factor synthesis pathway, the cyclo-oxygenase pathway and the 5-lipoxygenase pathway[93].

Omega-3 fatty acids have been shown in numerous reviews to improve RA symptoms[91,94,95]. Studies have consistently shown that omega-3 supplementation reduces the number of tender joints and morning stiffness; effects are modest but clear[91,94,96]. In addition, multiple studies indicate that omega-3 supplementation can reduce dependence on NSAIDs and antirheumatic drugs[97–100]; however, additional studies are needed before definitive conclusions can be made[91]. No significant toxicities have been associated with their use[101].

Omega-3 fatty acids are found in fish oils (EPA, DHA), leafy green vegetables (ALA) and plant oils such as flaxseed, rapeseed and walnuts (ALA); while all forms are important, EPA and DHA are more easily utilized by the body[102]. To date, most studies have investigated the effects of fish oils; these show that a minimum daily dosage of 3g of EPA and DHA is required for clinical efficacy; benefits become apparent after a minimum of 12 weeks[91].

In addition, there is evidence for the efficacy of certain omega-6 fatty acids[89]; these, however, are generally administered in the form of herbal extracts of evening primrose, borage or blackcurrant[67,68,103] (see above).

Homeopathy

Homeopathy is probably one of the most widespread, and certainly one of the most controversial, treatments within CAM. It involves the prescription of often very dilute, indeed in some cases ultramolecular, doses of usually herbal products that have been shaken and serially diluted. Homeopathy was developed by Samuel Hahnemann, a German physician, some 200 years ago. The first principle of homeopathy is that of similars: this states that patients who present with particular signs and symptoms can be cured if they are given a homeopathic medication that produces the same signs and symptoms in a healthy individual. In other words, homeopathy is designed around the concept of picture-matching the patient's symptoms with a drug picture produced by a homeopathic remedy and the idea of 'like cures like' is derived from this concept. The second, and probably the most confusing principle to orthodox physicians, is that serial dilutions of a medication, often until the medication has no molecules of the original product, will result in the medication still retaining its homeopathic effects even though it is diluted beyond the Avogadro number. Homeopathy therefore confronts conventional science at its core, and many believe that homeopathy can have no more than a placebo effect. Our reason for including homeopathy in this chapter is not to provide conclusive evidence that it 'works' in arthritic conditions but to illustrate some of the problems that face us within CAM research[104].

Evidence

Linde et al.[105] provide an excellent systematic review of homeopathy. This contains six studies on musculoskeletal complaints which include sprains, strains and cramps, and seven further studies specifically looking at rheumatology. The studies in rheumatology indicate an odds ratio that, overall, significantly favors homeopathy but would suggest, as indeed does the whole of Linde et al.'s systematic review, that there is currently inadequate evidence to make specific claims about homeopathy in any particular condition but overall evidence that homeopathy is probably more than a simple placebo effect.

Of particular interest in the context of these seven studies is that of Gibson et al. in 1980[106]. This was the first study of individualized homeopathy published in the recent medical literature. It involved 48 patients with RA who were randomized to receive either placebo or a specific homeopathic remedy appropriate to their complaints, and who were then followed up over a period of 6 months. Gibson's study suggested that homeopathy was effective for RA and as such became the focus of great interest, both among homeopaths and conventional physicians interested in investigating homeopathy scientifically. The second study, which was both innovative and thoughtful, was that by Fisher et al. published in the British Medical Journal in 1989[107]. In this study, patients with a defined diagnosis (fibromyalgia) were entered with a dual allocation process. Patients were entered if they fulfilled the diagnostic criteria for fibromyalgia, but a second inclusion criteria involved them in only being entered into the double-blind, randomized, controlled trial if they also fulfilled the specific requirements for the prescription of a particular homeopathic remedy, Rhus tox. Fisher's study indicates that individualized treatment need not be a bar to entry and therefore evaluates a particular homeopathic remedy against placebo in a well-defined, conventional complaint.

Homeopathy therefore provides us with excellent examples of both individualized treatment and innovative study methodology as far as CAM is concerned. If homeopathy is effective, and can be proved to be so, this must represent an interesting and complex challenge to modern pharmacology.

Mind–body interventions

Mind–body therapies (MBTs) do not constitute a system of medicine in and of themselves. Rather, it is a general classification that encompasses a wide spectrum of interventions from many different medical paradigms; in both traditional and modern practice, MBTs are often used as adjunctive or preventative therapies. They include more conventional Western therapies such as psychotherapy, cognitive–behavioral therapy and hypnosis as well as techniques native to Asian medical systems and cultures such as yoga, qi gong and meditation. In addition, MBTs include techniques such as relaxation response, guided imagery and biofeedback as well as more controversial therapies such as art, music and dance therapies, prayer and distant healing.

While these techniques are all based on their own underlying philosophies and vary widely in their complexity, they are linked together by a fundamental concept. They not only assume that the mind and body are inextricably linked, they are based on the idea that the mind can be trained to improve the functioning of the body. Common characteristics of MBT include self-regulation of attention, focused concentration and development of self-awareness and mental equanimity[108]. Sometimes, as in the cases of yoga and qi gong, this process is facilitated by physical movements specifically developed for this purpose. In other therapies, the mind–body connection is developed through external cues. For example, biofeedback uses a mechanical device that amplifies physiological indicators (e.g. blood pressure) in order to help patients become 'tuned in' to the functioning of their body; when the mind has been 'trained' to consciously regulate these physiological indicators, the device is no longer needed as patients are able to independently alter their physiological state. Other more traditional MBTs (e.g. meditation and prayer) were developed as a part of religious or spiritual practice. Some controversial therapies, such as distant healing, may even be able to establish a mind–body connection between people who are not in immediate contact[109].

Evidence

Moderate evidence suggests that MBTs are effective adjuncts in the treatment of RA and OA. A meta-analytic comparison ($n = 47$) of psychoeducational interventions (i.e. biofeedback, relaxation, coping skills, information, behavioral instruction, social support) and NSAID treatment found that psychoeducational components provided additional benefits over NSAID treatment alone[110]. While the effect sizes for MBT were not large, they provided an additional: 20–30% relief of pain in OA and RA, 40% increase in functional ability in RA and 60–80% decrease in joint tenderness in RA over NSAID treatment alone. The Arthritis Self-Management Program (ASMP) may be particularly effective for arthritis[111](especially OA)[112,16].

In addition, a meta-analysis of similar MBTs for RA found small but significant effect sizes for pain (ES = 0.22), disability (ES = 0.36) and depression (ES = 0.17)[113]. Moreover, a meta-analysis of behavioral therapies for chronic low back pain[114] found that there was strong evidence that MBTs have a moderately positive effect on pain (ES = 0.62) and a small positive effect on both functional status (ES = 0.35) and behavioral outcomes (ES = 0.40) as compared to inactive controls; there was moderate evidence, however, that MBTs do not improve outcomes as adjunct treatments for low back pain.

The current evidence for efficacy of MBT for fibromyalgia is equivocal: a review of 13 randomized controlled trials found limited evidence that MBTs are more effective than waiting list, usual care and placebo for some outcomes, inconclusive evidence for MBTs when compared to education/attention controls and limited evidence that moderate/high-intensity exercise is more effective than MBTs[115].

The current evidence indicates that MBTs are particularly suited to improving quality of life by decreasing pain, disability and depression[113] and improving mood, coping and social function[116]. However, MBT research is still in its early stages, and issues such as the relative efficacy of different MBTs for specific medical conditions, as well as synergistic effects of multiple MBTs, have not been adequately examined. Moreover, while some studies have suggested that MBTs may be cost-effective[117–120], no definitive data currently exist and conclusions are premature[16].

REFERRAL AND PROFESSIONAL PRACTICE

Above all, physicians need to initiate an open dialogue with their patients about CAM therapies; more than 70% of patients who use CAM do not inform their physician that they are doing so[1]. When discussing CAM use with patients, it is important to remain neutral, as negative attitudes or labels such as 'unorthodox' may discourage the patient from discussing CAM use[121]. Moreover, issues of safety and efficacy (of both conventional and CAM options) should always be reviewed, and patient preferences and expectations should be discussed and documented. From here, patients and physicians can make responsible decisions about treatment options and monitor progress together with the CAM provider. Table 12.4 provides information about the licensing and professional training of CAM practitioners in the USA.

TABLE 12.4 LICENSING AND TRAINING OF MAJOR COMPLEMENTARY AND ALTERNATIVE MEDICINE THERAPIES IN THE USA

Therapy	Licensure as of 2000	Appropriate training	Professional organizations
Acupuncture	All states except Alabama, Delaware, Kansas, Kentucky, Michigan, Mississippi, Nevada, Oklahoma, South Dakota and Wyoming	Minimum 3-year master's or doctorate degree, variable postgraduate training for medical providers Board exams	American Association of Oriental Medicine American Academy of Medical Acupuncture National Acupuncture Foundation Accreditation Commission for Acupuncture and Oriental Medicine National Certification Commission for Acupuncture and Oriental Medicine
Chiropractic	50 states	3–4-year doctorate program at an accredited university Board exams	American Chiropractic Organization Foundation for Chiropractic Education and Research
Massage therapy	Alabama, Arkansas, Connecticut, Delaware, District of Columbia, Florida, Hawaii, Iowa, Louisiana, Maine, Maryland, Mississippi, Missouri, Nebraska, Nevada, New Hampshire, New Jersey, New Mexico, New York, North Carolina, Ohio, Oregon, Rhode Island, South Carolina, Tennessee, Texas, Utah, Virginia, Washington, West Virginia and Wisconsin	Minimum of 500 hours, usually from an accredited program Board exams	American Massage Therapy Association Commission on Massage Training Accreditation National Certification Board for Therapeutic Massage and Bodywork
Herbalism	None; often practiced under another health-care license	Apprenticeship program or 3-year degree	American Herbalist's Guild American Botanical Council Herb Research Foundation
Naturopathy	Arkansas, Arizona, Connecticut, Hawaii, Maine, Montana, New Hampshire, Oregon, Utah, Vermont and Washington	4-year accredited doctorate program Board exams	American Association of Naturopathic Physicians North American Board of Naturopathic Examiners
Homeopathy	Arizona, Connecticut and Nevada; often practiced under another health-care license	Naturopathic program, post-graduate training for medical providers, homeopathic universities abroad	National Center for Homeopathy American Board of Homeotherapeutics Homeopathic Academy of Naturopathic Physicians Council for Homeopathic Certification

Licensing laws vary widely from state to state in terms of eligibility, examination, scope of practice and autonomy; moreover, many states have introduced statutes that have yet to take effect. Training is highly variable; the minimum training required for professional competency is listed here. Contact the appropriate professional organization for information on qualified practitioners in your area.

It is impossible to provide specific guidelines for the training and practice of CAM on a worldwide basis. As a consequence, we have provided some general questions that should be asked by physicians thinking of referring patients to CAM or patients thinking of seeking CAM treatment.

How do I know the therapist is competent?

● Do you think that the practitioner is technically competent? This usually means, are they a member of an appropriate organization and have they adequate training in the field in which they practice?
● Might they advise the patient to change their conventional medical treatment without seeking the advice of their doctor?
● Can the proposed treatment be provided safely? If you are discussing referral to a herbalist, are you sure the herbalist is aware of the potential cross-reactions between herbal medicine and your conventional medications?
● Will the complementary practitioner set guidelines at the first appointment for how the practitioner thinks the treatment should progress? Should the patient expect a response to treatment after three or four acupuncture sessions or would it be more reasonable to assess the treatment after eight or 10 sessions?

Is the therapist a professional?

● Is the environment in which treatment is provided safe and appropriate?
● Does the therapist have professional indemnity?
● Do therapists have a code of ethics, is the data they hold legally protected and will they treat the information given to them in a confidential manner?

● Do therapists have an organization that employs a process of self-regulation and will it remove members from their lists if they are not behaving ethically?
● Are therapists aware of, and do they have a process of reporting, adverse reactions to the treatments they provide?

Is complementary and alternative medical treatment appropriate?

● Has a clear diagnosis of the problem been made? If such a diagnosis cannot be made, have other common problems been excluded? Is the patient missing out on an appropriate conventional medical treatment?
● If the patient has a chronic condition which is relatively stable, then it may be reasonable to try a CAM approach, either to help symptoms or minimize the use of potentially damaging long-term conventional medications.
● You may know a competent complementary therapist to whom you regularly refer; are you sure that the therapist is a safe, professional and competent person?
● You may wish to refer a patient to another doctor practicing some form of CAM; this kind or referral should be treated in exactly the same manner as referral to any other properly medically qualified specialist.

In general, we have so little information about whether complementary medicine works that it is usually impossible to make an evidence-based decision. In our view, it is reasonable to embark on CAM treatment as long as it is safe and provided in the context of proper professional practice associated with clear clinical guidelines.

REFERENCES

1. Eisenberg DM, Kessler RC, Foster C et al. Unconventional medicine in the United States. Prevalence, costs, and patterns of use. N Engl J Med 1993; 328: 246–252.
2. Jonas W, Levin J, eds. Essentials of complementary and alternative medicine. Philadelphia, PA: Lippincott Williams & Wilkins; 1999.
3. Gwei-Djen L, Needham J. Celestial lancets: history and rationale of acupuncture and moxa. London: Cambridge University Press; 1980.
4. Saks M. The flight from science? The reporting of acupuncture in mainstream British medical journals from 1800 to 1990. Complement Med Res 1991; 5: 178–182.
5. Bache F. Cases illustrative of the remedial effects of acupuncture. North Am Med Surg J 1826; 1: 31–321.
6. Wood M. Vitalism : the history of herbalism, homeopathy and flower essences. Berkeley, CA: North Atlantic Books; 2000.
7. Eisenberg DM, Davis RB, Ettner SL et al. Trends in alternative medicine use in the United States, 1990–1997: results of a follow-up national survey. JAMA 1998; 280: 1569–1575.
8. Ernst E. Usage of complementary therapies in rheumatology: a systematic review. Clin Rheumatol 1998; 17: 301–305.
9. Kronenfeld J, Wasner C. The use of unorthodox therapies and marginal practitioners. Soc Sci Med 1982; 16: 1119–1125.
10. Anderson DL, Shane-McWhorter L, Crouch BI, Andersen SJ. Prevalence and patterns of alternative medication use in a university hospital outpatient clinic serving rheumatology and geriatric patients. Pharmacotherapy 2000; 20: 958–966.
11. Boisset M, Fitzcharles MA. Alternative medicine use by rheumatology patients in a universal health care setting. J Rheumatol 1994; 21: 148–152.
12. Rao JK, Mihaliak K, Kroenke K et al. Use of complementary therapies for arthritis among patients of rheumatologists. Ann Intern Med 1999; 131: 409–416.
13. Pioro-Boisset M, Esdaile JM, Fitzcharles MA. Alternative medicine use in fibromyalgia syndrome. Arthritis Care Res 1996; 9: 13–17.
14. Vincent C, Furnham A. Why do patients turn to complementary medicine? An empirical study. Br J Clin Psychol 1996; 35: 37–48.
15. Astin JA. Why patients use alternative medicine: results of a national study. JAMA 1998; 279: 1548–53.
16. Astin JA, Shapiro SL, Eisenberg DE. Mind–body medicine: state of the science, implications for practice. submitted.
17. Ergil K. China's traditional medicine. In: Micozzi M, ed. Fundamentals of complementary and alternative medicine. New York: Churchill Livingstone; 1996: 185–223.
18. Stux G, Hammerschlag R, eds. Clinical acupuncture: scientific basis. Berlin: Springer-Verlag; 2001.
19. Sims J. The mechanism of acupuncture analgesia: a review. Complement Ther Med 1997; 5: 102–111.
20. Melzack R, Jeans ME. Acupuncture analgesia. A psychophysiological explanation. Minn Med 1974; 57: 161–166.
21. Chang H. Neurophysiological basis of acupuncture analgesia. Sci Sinica 1978; 21: 829–846.
22. Levy B, Matsumoto T. Pathophysiology of acupuncture: nervous system transmission. Am Surg 1975; 41: 378–384.
23. Acupuncture: National Institutes of Health Consensus Development Conference statement. Dermatol Nurs 2000; 12: 126–133.
24. Sjolund B, Terenius L, Eriksson M. Increased cerebrospinal fluid levels of endorphins after electro-acupuncture. Acta Physiol Scand 1977; 100: 382–384.
25. Han J, Tang J, Fan S. Central 5-hydroxytryptamine, opiate-like substances and acupuncture analgesia. Research on acupuncture, moxibustion, and acupuncture anaesthesia. Beijing: Science Press; 1986: 309–316.
26. Cho Z, Na C, Wang E et al. Functional magnetic resonance imaging of the brain in the investigation of acupuncture. In: Stux G, Hammerschlag R, eds. Clinical acupuncture: scientific basis. Berlin: Springer-Verlag; 2001: 83–95.
27. Zhu Z. Research advances in the electrical specificity of meridians and acupuncture points. Am J Acupuncture 1981; 9: 203–216.
28. Oleson TD, Kroening RJ, Bresler DE. An experimental evaluation of auricular diagnosis: the somatotopic mapping or musculoskeletal pain at ear acupuncture points. Pain 1980; 8: 217–229.
29. Saku K, Mukaino Y, Ying H, Arakawa K. Characteristics of reactive electropermeable points on the auricles of coronary heart disease patients. Clin Cardiol 1993; 16: 415–419.
30. Ernst E. Acupuncture as a symptomatic treatment of osteoarthritis. A systematic review. Scand J Rheumatol 1997; 26: 444–447.
31. Ezzo J, Berman B, Hadhazy VA et al. Is acupuncture effective for the treatment of chronic pain? A systematic review. Pain 2000; 86: 217–225.
32. Berman BM, Ezzo J, Hadhazy V, Swyers JP. Is acupuncture effective in the treatment of fibromyalgia? J Fam Pract 1999; 48: 213–218.
33. Van Tulder MW, Cherkin DC, Berman BM et al. The effectiveness of acupuncture in the management of acute and chronic low back pain. Spine 1999; 24: 1113–1123.
34. Ezzo J, Hadhazy V, Birch S et al. Acupuncture for osteoarthritis of the knee: a systematic review. Arthritis Rheum 2001; 44: 819–825.
35. Deluze C, Bosia L, Zirbs A et al. Electroacupuncture in fibromyalgia: results of a controlled trial. Br Med J 1992; 305: 1249–1252.
36. Ernst E, White AR. Acupuncture for back pain: a meta-analysis of randomized controlled trials. Arch Intern Med 1998; 158: 2235–2241.

37. Berman BM, Swyers JP, Ezzo J. The evidence for acupuncture as a treatment for rheumatologic conditions. Rheum Dis Clin North Am 2000; 26: 103–115.

38. Birch S. Systematic review of acupuncture – are there problems with these? Clin Acupunct Orient Med 2001; 2: 17–22.

39. Lao L, Ezzo J, Berman B, Hammerschlag R. Assessing clinical efficacy of acupuncture: considerations for designing future acupuncture trials. In: Stux G, Hammerschlag R, eds. Clinical acupuncture: scientific basis. Berlin: Springer-Verlag, 2000: 187–209.

40. Birch S. An exploration with proposed solutions of the problems and issues in conducting clinical research in acupuncture. Exeter: University of Exeter; 1997.

41. Lao L. Safety issues in acupuncture. J Altern Complement Med 1996; 2: 27–31.

42. Lytle C. An overview of acupuncture. Washington, DC: Center for Devices and Radiological Health, FDA, PHS, DHHS; 1993.

43. Hardy M. Herb–drug interactions: an evidence based table. Alter Med Alert 2000; June: 64–69.

44. Fugh-Berman A. Herb–drug interactions. Lancet 2000; 355: 134–138.

45. Haller CA, Benowitz NL. Adverse cardiovascular and central nervous system events associated with dietary supplements containing ephedra alkaloids. N Engl J Med 2000; 343: 1833–1838.

46. Chrubasik S, Roufogalis B. Herbal medicinal products for the treatment of pain. Special Interest Group on Rheumatic Pain Newsletter 1999; Nov.

47. Little C, Parsons T. Herbal therapy for treating rheumatoid arthritis. In: The Cochrane Library, Issue 1. Oxford: Update Software; 2001.

48. Little C, Parsons T. Herbal therapy for treating osteoarthritis. In: The Cochrane Library, Issue 1. Oxford: Update Software; 2001.

49. Ernst E, Chrubasik S. Phyto-anti-inflammatories. A systematic review of randomized, placebo-controlled, double-blind trials. Rheum Dis Clin North Am 2000; 26: 13–27.

50. Long L, Soeken K, Ernst E. Herbal medicines for the treatment of osteoarthritis: a systematic review. Rheumatology. 2001; 40: 79–793.

51. Guyader M. Les plantes historique et pharmacologique, et étude clinique du nebulisat d'Harpagophytum procumbens DC chez 50 patients arthrosiques suivis en service hospitalier. Paris: Université Pierre et Marie Curie; 1984.

52. Lecomte A, Costa J. Harpagophytum dans l'arthrose: études en double insu contre placebo. Le Magazine 1992; 15: 27–30.

53. Chrubasik S, Junck H, Breitschwerdt H et al. Effectiveness of Harpagophytum extract WS 1531 in the treatment of exacerbation of low back pain: a randomized, placebo-controlled, double-blind study. Eur J Anaesthesiol 1999; 16: 118–129.

54. Chrubasik S, Zimpfer C, Schutt U. Effectiveness of Harpagophytum procumbens in treatment of acute low back pain. Phytomedicine 1996; 3: 1–10.

55. Schaffner W. Antiarrheumatikum der modernen Phytotherapie? In: Chrubasik S, Wink M, eds. Rheumatherapie mit Phytopharmaka. Stuttgart: Hippokrates-Verlag; 1997: 125–127.

56. Hahn S, Hubner-Steiner U. Behandlung schmerzhafter rheumatischer Erkrankungen mit Phytodolor im Vergerch zur Placebo und Ammuno-behandlung. Rheum Schmerz Entzundung 1988; 8: 55–58.

57. Schreckenberger F. Die Behandlung von Epicondylitiden mit Phytodolor. Österreich Zeitschr Allgemeinmed 1988; 42: 1638–1644.

58. Schadler W. Phytodolor zur Behandlung aktivierter Arthrosen. Rheuma 1988; 8: 280–290.

59. Von Huber B. Therapie degenerativer rheumatischer Erkrankungen. Fortschr Med 1991; 109: 248–250.

60. Schinitzer T, Morton C, Coker C, Flynn P. effectiveness of reduced applications of topical capsaicin (0.025%) in osteoarthritis. Arthritis Rheum 1992; 35: S132.

61. Altman R, Aven A, Holmburg C et al. Capsaicin cream 0.025% as monotherapy for osteoarthritis: a double blind study. Semin Arthritis Rheum 1994; 23(suppl): 25–33.

62. Deal CL, Schnitzer TJ, Lipstein E et al. Treatment of arthritis with topical capsaicin: a double-blind trial. Clin Ther 1991; 13: 383–395.

63. McCarthy GM, McCarty DJ. Effect of topical capsaicin in the therapy of painful osteoarthritis of the hands. J Rheumatol 1992; 19: 604–607.

64. Zhang WY, Li Wan Po A. The effectiveness of topically applied capsaicin. A meta-analysis. Eur J Clin Pharmacol 1994; 46: 517–522.

65. Randall C, Randall H, Dobbs F et al. Randomized controlled trial of nettle sting for treatment of base-of-thumb pain. J R Soc Med 2000; 93: 305–309.

66. Mills SY, Jacoby RK, Chacksfield M, Willoughby M. Effect of a proprietary herbal medicine on the relief of chronic arthritic pain: a double-blind study. Br J Rheumatol 1996; 35: 874–878.

67. Belch JJ, Ansell D, Madhok R et al. Effects of altering dietary essential fatty acids on requirements for non-steroidal anti-inflammatory drugs in patients with rheumatoid arthritis: a double blind placebo controlled study. Ann Rheum Dis 1988; 47: 96–104.

68. Leventhal LJ, Boyce EG, Zurier RB. Treatment of rheumatoid arthritis with blackcurrant seed oil. Br J Rheumatol 1994; 33: 847–852.

69. Zurier RB, Rossetti RG, Jacobson EW et al. Gamma-linolenic acid treatment of rheumatoid arthritis. A randomized, placebo-controlled trial. Arthritis Rheum 1996; 39: 1808–1817.

70. Leventhal LJ, Boyce EG, Zurier RB. Treatment of rheumatoid arthritis with gammalinolenic acid. Ann Intern Med 1993; 119: 867–873.

71. Bliddal H, Rosetzky A, Schlichting P et al. A randomized, placebo controlled, cross-over study of ginger extracts and ibuprofen in osteoarthritis. Osteoarthritis Cartilage 2000; 8: 9–12.

72. Biswas N, Biswas K, Pandey M, Pandey R. Treatment of osteoarthritis, rheumatoid arthritis, and non-specific arthritis with an herbal drug: a double-blind, active drug controlled parallel study. JK Pract 998; 5: 129–132.

73. Ryttig K, Schlamowitz P, Warnoe O, Wilstrup F. Gitadyl versus ibuprofen in patients with osteoarthritis. The results of a double-blind, randomized crossover study. Ugeskr Laeger 1991; 153: 2298–2299.

74. Delafuente JC. Glucosamine in the treatment of osteoarthritis. Rheum Dis Clin North Am 2000; 26: 1–11.

75. McAlindon TE, LaValley MP, Gulin JP, Felson DT. Glucosamine and chondroitin for treatment of osteoarthritis: a systematic quality assessment and meta-analysis. JAMA 2000; 283: 1469–1475.

76. Towheed T, Anastassiades T, Shea B et al. Glucosamine therapy for treating arthritis. In: The Cochrane Library, Issue 1. Oxford: Update Software; 2001.

77. Reginster JY, Deroisy R, Rovati LC et al. Long-term effects of glucosamine sulphate on osteoarthritis progression: a randomised, placebo-controlled clinical trial. Lancet 2001; 357: 251–256.

78. Bassleer C, Henrotin Y, Franchimont P. In-vitro evaluation of drugs proposed as chondroprotective agents. Int J Tissue React 1992; 14: 231–241.

79. Uebelhart D, Thonar E, Zhang J, Williams J. Protective effect of exogenous chondroitin 4,6-sulfate in the acute degradation of articular cartilage in the rabbit. Osteoarthritis Cartilage 1998; 6(suppl A): 6–13.

80. Ronca F, Palmieri L, Panicucci P, Ronca G. Anti-inflammatory activity of chondroitin sulfate. Osteoarthritis Cartilage 1998; 6(suppl A): 14–21.

81. Setnikar I, Giacchetti C, Zanolo G. Pharmokinetics of glucosamine in the dog and in man. Arzneimittelforschung 1986; 36: 729–735.

82. Conte A, Volpi N, Palmieri L et al. Biochemical and pharmacokinetic aspects of oral treatment with chondroitin sulfate. Arzneimittelforschung 1995; 45: 918–925.

83. Gaster B. S-adenosylmethionine (SAMe) for treatment of depression. Alter Med Alert 1999; 2: 133–135.

84. Bressa GM. S-adenosyl-L-methionine (SAMe) as antidepressant: meta-analysis of clinical studies. Acta Neurol Scand Suppl 1994; 154: 7–14.

85. Baldessarini RJ. Neuropharmacology of S-adenosyl-L-methionine. Am J Med 1987; 83: 95–103.

86. Stramentinoli G. Pharmacologic aspects of S-adenosylmethionine. Pharmacokinetics and pharmacodynamics. Am J Med 1987; 83: 35–42.

87. Harmand MF, Vilamitjana J, Maloche E et al. Effects of S-adenosylmethionine on human articular chondrocyte differentiation. An in vitro study. Am J Med 1987; 83: 48–54.

88. Soeken KL, Lee WL, Bausell RB et al. Safety and efficacy of s-Adenosylmethionine (SAMe) for osteoarthritis: a meta-analysis. J Fam Prac 2002; 51: 425–430.

89. Belch J, Hill A. Evening primrose oil and borage oil in rheumatologic conditions. Am J Clin Nutr 2000; 71(suppl 1): 352s–356s.

90. Cleland L, Hill C, James M. Diet and arthritis. Boiler's Clin Rheumatol 1995; 9: 771–785.

91. Kremer J. ω-3 fatty acid supplements in rheumatoid arthritis. Am J Clin Nutr 2000; 71(suppl 1): 349s–351s.

92. Salinas A, Berchuk M, Welch V et al. Omega-3 fatty acids supplementation for treating rheumatoid arthritis. In: The Cochrane Library, Issue 1. Oxford: Update Software; 2001.

93. Sperling R. Omega-3 fatty acids: effects on lipid mediators of inflammation and rheumatoid arthritis. Rheum Dis Clin North Am 1991; 17: 373–389.

94. James MJ, Cleland LG. Dietary ω-3 fatty acids and therapy for rheumatoid arthritis. Semin Arthritis Rheum 1997; 27: 85–97.

95. Fortin P, Liang M, Beckett L et al. A meta-analysis of the efficacy of fish oil in rheumatoid arthritis. Arthritis Rheum 1992; 35: S201.

96. Kremer J. Clinical studies of ω-3 fatty acid supplementation in patients with rheumatoid arthritis. Rheum Dis Clin North Am 1992; 17: 391–402.

97. Skoldstam L, Borjesson O, Kjallman A et al. Effects of six month fish oil supplementation in stable rheumatoid arthritis: a double blind, controlled study. Scand J Rheumatol 1992; 21: 178–185.

98. Kremer J, Lawrence D, Petrillo G et al. Effects of high dose fish oil on rheumatoid arthritis after stopping non-steroidal anti-inflammatory drugs: clinical and immune correlates. Arthritis Rheum 1995; 38: 1107–1114.

99. Lau C, Morely K, Belch J. Effects of fish oil supplementation on the non-steroidal anti-inflammatory drug requirements in patients with mild rheumatic arthritis: a double blind placebo controlled study. Br J Rheumatol 1993; 32: 982–989.

100. Belch J, Ansell D, Madhok R et al. Effects of altering dietary essential fatty acids on requirements for non-steroidal anti-inflammatory drugs in patients with rheumatoid arthritis: a double blind-placebo controlled study. Ann Rheum Dis 1988; 47: 96–104.

101. Cleland L, James M. Fish oil and rheumatoid arthritis: anti-inflammatory and collateral health benefits. J Rheumatol 2000; 27: 2305–2307.

102. Simopoulos A. Essential fatty acids in health and chronic disease. Am J Clin Nutr 1999; 70(suppl 3): 560s–569s.

103. Zurier RB, Rossetti RG, Jacobson EW et al. gamma-Linolenic acid treatment of rheumatoid arthritis. A randomized, placebo-controlled trial. Arthritis Rheum 1996; 39: 1808–1817.

104. Fisher P. Research into the homeopathic treatment of rheumatological disease: why and how? In: Lewith GT, Aldridge D, eds. Clinical research methodology for complementary therapies. London: Hodder & Stoughton, 1993.

105. Linde K, Clausius N, Ramirez G et al. Are the clinical effects of homeopathy placebo effects? A meta-analysis of placebo-controlled trials. Lancet 1997; 350: 834–843.

106. Gibson RG, Gibson SL, MacNeill AD, Buchanan WW. Homoeopathic therapy in rheumatoid arthritis: evaluation by double-blind clinical therapeutic trial. Br J Clin Pharmacol 1980; 9: 453–459.

107. Fisher P, Greenwood A, Huskisson EC et al. Effect of homeopathic treatment on fibrositis (primary fibromyalgia). Br Med J 1989; 299: 365–366.

108. Goleman D, Gurin J, eds. Mind body medicine: how to use your mind for better health. New York: Consumer Reports Books; 1993.

109. Astin JA, Harkness E, Ernst E. The efficacy of 'distant healing': a systematic review of randomized trials. Ann Intern Med 2000; 132: 903–910.

110. Superio-Cabuslay E, Ward MM, Lorig KR. Patient education interventions in osteoarthritis and rheumatoid arthritis: a meta-analytic comparison with nonsteroidal antiinflammatory drug treatment. Arthritis Care Res 1996; 9: 292–301.

111. Lorig K, Laurin J, Gines GE. Arthritis self-management. A five-year history of a patient education program. Nurs Clin North Am 1984; 19: 637–645.

112. Lorig K, Holman H. Arthritis self-management studies: a twelve-year review. Health Educ Q 1993; 20: 17–28.

113. Astin JA, Beckner W, Soeken K *et al*. Psychological interventions for rheumatoid arthritis: a meta-analysis of randomized controlled trials. Arthritis Rheum 2002; 47: 291–302.

114. Van Tulder MW, Ostelo R, Vlaeyen JW *et al*. Behavioral treatment for chronic low back pain: a systematic review within the framework of the Cochrane Back Review Group. Spine 2000; 25: 2688–2699.

115. Hadhazy VA, Ezzo J, Creamer P, Berman BM. Mind–body therapies for the treatment of fibromyalgia. A systematic review. J Rheumatol 2000; 27: 2911–2918.

116. Morley S, Eccleston C, Williams A. Systematic review and meta-analysis of randomized controlled trials of cognitive behaviour therapy and behaviour therapy for chronic pain in adults, excluding headache. Pain 1999; 80: 1–13.

117. Kruger JM, Helmick CG, Callahan LF, Haddix AC. Cost-effectiveness of the arthritis self-help course. Arch Intern Med 1998; 158: 1245–1249.

118. Hellman CJ, Budd M, Borysenko J *et al*. A study of the effectiveness of two group behavioral medicine interventions for patients with psychosomatic complaints. Behav Med 1990; 16: 165–173.

119. Kennell J, Klaus M, McGrath S *et al*. Continuous emotional support during labor in a US hospital. A randomized controlled trial. JAMA 1991; 265: 2197–2201.

120. Caudill M, Schnable R, Zuttermeister P *et al*. Decreased clinic use by chronic pain patients: response to behavioral medicine intervention. Clin J Pain 1991; 7: 305–310.

121. Eisenberg DM. Advising patients who seek alternative medical therapies. Ann Intern Med 1997; 127: 61–69.

REGIONAL AND WIDESPREAD PAIN

13 Neck pain

Les Barnsley

Definition

- A common regional pain syndrome usually arising from undefined mechanical or musculoskeletal disturbance
- Occurs acutely with marked hypomobility
- Chronic symptoms are poorly understood

Clinical features

- May rarely be a feature of serious underlying malignant, infective or inflammatory disorder
- Can occur in association with neurologic involvement – myelopathy and radiculopathy
- No examination or imaging findings are known that reliably identify the source of pain
- May be investigated with techniques targeting the pain, e.g. cervical zygapophyseal joint blocks and discography

INTRODUCTION

The neck provides a link of great flexibility between the sensory platform of the head and the trunk. Simultaneously it provides vital conduits for neural and vascular tissue between the brain and the rest of the body. These conflicting priorities are achieved through the structure of the cervical spine, which combines strength with an extraordinary range of movement. The strength is achieved through a bony tube made up of the individual vertebrae. The range of movement is achieved through a complex articular system involving ligamentous intervertebral discs and paired posterior zygapophyseal joints in the lower neck, and loosely constrained synovial joints at the upper levels. The discs fissure posteriorly as part of the normal aging process[1], permitting rotatory movements through an oblique axis[2]. The posterior, zygapophyseal joints have no bony constraint and facilitate a broad range of movement through having flat surfaces that glide in concert to permit flexion and extension and in opposite directions to produce rotation. This complex is the subject of almost constant activity, with the neck being reported to move over 600 times per hour or once every 6 seconds[1].

Pain perceived in the region of the neck arises as a result of noxious stimulation of any of the structures innervated by the cervical spinal nerves. These encompass local sources of pain among the intrinsic structures of the cervical spine and distant sources that refer pain to the neck by virtue of being supplied by nerves that arise in the neck but leave the cervical region and enter the head or thoracic region. The majority of neck pain is acute and self-limiting and can be attributed to mechanical problems but a small percentage of neck pain becomes chronic, and it is these patients that are the focus of this chapter. Upon investigation, most instances of chronic neck pain will prove to be musculoskeletal in origin and are usually recognizable as such, but it is incumbent upon the physician assessing neck pain to exclude other serious and potentially treatable pathology. Fortunately, this rarely presents a dilemma as the history and physical examination typically permit ready differentiation of musculoskeletal causes from other causes of neck pain. Once non-mechanical conditions have been excluded the second responsibility is to provide a diagnosis as to the structure and pathology producing the neck pain. Only with a sound anatomic diagnosis can therapy be targeted and rational.

Frequently discussed in association with neck pain, but really a separate problem, is the question of cervical nerve root or cervical cord compression. These problems warrant assessment on their own merits, independent of any associated neck pain, and are considered later.

EPIDEMIOLOGY

Although less common than low back pain, neck pain represents a common human experience: its universality and unpleasantness is reflected by the colloquial use of the term 'pain in the neck' to describe a particularly disagreeable circumstance or individual. Population-based Finnish studies attest to a lifetime prevalence of chronic neck pain (pain lasting for more than 3 months) of 71%, with 41% of those surveyed reporting episodes of neck pain in the most recent month. The point prevalence was 9.5% for males and 13.5% for females[3]. A survey in Saskatchewan province in Canada revealed a rate of disabling neck pain of over 4%[4]. The incidence of acute, self-limiting neck pain and stiffness is not known but the general clinical impression is that it represents a common problem; the prevalence was 18% in a randomly sampled population[5]. The determinants of chronic, mechanical neck pain are still incompletely studied. There is no doubt that trauma, particularly whiplash injury, is an important cause of chronic neck pain, with approximately 25% of those with acute neck pain following whiplash injury suffering chronic pain[6]. A clear relationship has been demonstrated between the nature of occupation and neck pain, with manual workers having higher frequencies of neck pain than those with sedentary jobs[7]. Other positive associations with neck pain include self-reported heavy workload, level of education[8] (probably a confounding factor with heavy workload) and depression[9]. Although often touted as a cause of neck pain, 'poor posture' has not been proved to be causally related to neck pain, largely because of difficulty in establishing a universal definition of what constitutes poor posture. It has been shown, however, that prolonged extreme flexion of the neck will precipitate neck pain, most probably through strain of the posterior zygapophyseal joint capsules[10]. It is unclear to what extent this can be extrapolated to less extreme postures. Neck pain is also more common with increasing age[11], so that neck pain in a young adult without a history of trauma should prompt a search for non-mechanical causes. The relationship of neck pain to body habitus has not been studied. Where neck pain is part of a systemic disease, its epidemiology will follow that of the underlying problem.

CLINICAL FEATURES

Neck pain may be classified as being referred from distant (non-cervical structures), arising through involvement of cervical structures by

TABLE 13.1 NON-MUSCULOSKELETAL SOURCES OF NECK PAIN

Structure	Condition
Pharynx	Pharyngitis
Larynx	Laryngitis
	Carcinoma
Trachea	Tracheitis
Thyroid	Thyroiditis
Lymph nodes	Lymphadenitis
Carotid arteries	Carotidynia
	Dissection
	Inflammation
Aorta	Aneurysm
	Dissection
Heart	Angina
	Infarction
Pericardium	Pericarditis
Diaphragm	Inflammation by blood, infection

Structures and examples of conditions that may refer pain to the neck.

TABLE 13.3 FEATURES OF PAIN TO BE ELICITED FROM THE CLINICAL HISTORY

- Mode and time of onset
- Site of pain
- Quality of pain
- Radiation of pain
- Frequency and duration of episodes of pain
- Pattern of episodes
- If periodic, mode of onset and time of onset
- Aggravating factors
- Relieving factors
- Associated features

neoplastic, inflammatory or infectious disease, or as being mechanical or musculoskeletal in origin. Diseases that may refer pain to the neck are outlined in Table 13.1. Fortunately, these conditions are usually readily recognized through their other clinical characteristics such as exertion-induced pain in angina, but the need for a complete history, including features other than those symptoms referable to the neck, is highlighted. A cross tabulation of those conditions that can affect the components of the cervical spine is shown in Table 13.2. This approach, considering each structure and then the processes that may affect it, is more readily recalled than an exhaustive list of all candidate problems. The clinical history should cover those characteristics of the pain outlined in Table 13.3. Each category reveals features that enable serious and distinctive conditions to be identified or, at least, strongly suspected.

Onset of pain

The setting in which the complaint of pain starts is most helpful in raising the suspicion of a diagnosis of non-mechanical neck pain. The patient's age and a past history of malignancy, particularly of the lung, breast, prostrate, thyroid or kidney, should raise the possibility of metastatic bone disease. Previous surgery, immunosuppression and past infections increase the risk of hematogenous osteomyelitis or septic arthritis. Inflammatory conditions such as ankylosing spondylitis, rheumatoid arthritis and polymyalgia rheumatica are suggested by involvement of areas other than

the cervical spine, a history of pain and stiffness on first rising and after immobility ('gelling') and systemic features such as weight loss or sweats. Polymyositis and dermatomyositis may affect the neck muscles but the myalgias are widespread, are always associated with weakness and hence do not present a diagnostic problem in terms of neck pain.

Musculoskeletal pain typically arises following trauma or unaccustomed activity[12]. Acceleration and/or deceleration (whiplash) injuries in motor vehicle accidents are probably the most common cause of traumatic neck pain (see below), although sports injuries and industrial accidents lead to similar symptoms. Occasionally, musculoskeletal pain can occur in the absence of a history of trauma, indicating that intrinsic disease processes, such as osteoarthritis, may be responsible for the development of pain.

Details of any trauma should be carefully documented so that the direction and magnitude of the forces that were applied to the neck can be estimated. Flexion imparts compressive forces to the vertebral bodies and discs and distractive forces on posterior spinal elements such as the zygapophyseal joint capsules and posterior neck muscles. Conversely, extension injuries compress posterior cervical structures such as the articular pillars and zygapophyseal joints while distracting anterior components such as the anterior anulus fibrosus of the disc, the vertebral endplates and anterior longitudinal ligament[6]. It has been noted that extension injuries appear to carry a worse prognosis for the development of chronic pain than flexion or lateral flexion injuries[13].

Quality of pain

The pain of mechanical, musculoskeletal derangement is typically dull, deep and aching. Exacerbations are usually short-lived, sharp pains superimposed on the chronic symptoms. Pain that does not follow this pattern, for instance pain that is shooting or electrical, should raise suspicion that neural structures are involved. Deep, unremitting pain with no periods of relief is a sinister sign implying ongoing distention, defor-

TABLE 13.2 MUSCULOSKELETAL STRUCTURES AND PATHOLOGIC PROCESSES

	Muscles	Joints	Discs	Bone	Dura	Ligament	Other
Infectious		Septic arthritis	Discitis	Osteomyelitis	Abscess Meningitis		Epidural abscess
Neoplastic				Primary Secondary	Neurofibroma Meningioma		Spinal cord tumor
Inflammatory	PM/DM, PMR	RA	Discitis? AS				
Metabolic				Paget's disease Osteoporosis Osteomalacia			

The table lists the musculoskeletal structures of the neck and potentially pathologic processes that may affect them. AS, ankylosing spondylitis; PM/DM, polymyositis/dermatomyositis; PMR, polymyalgia rheumatica; RA, rheumatoid arthritis.

mation or invasion of pain-sensitive structures, which may occur in malignancy.

Frequency and duration of episodes of pain

Mechanical or non-inflammatory musculoskeletal pain is typically experienced in episodes that are related to movement and exertion. This is particularly true in post-traumatic neck pain[14]. The pain is made worse by particular postures or exercises and is characteristically improved by rest and immobility. Pain that does not follow this pattern, that is not altered by movement and that worsens spontaneously, suggests a more sinister underlying cause.

Site and radiation of pain

Musculoskeletal pain is typically perceived over the posterior aspect of the neck and rarely radiates past the anterior border of the sternomastoid muscle. Pain in the anterior part of the neck usually indicates disease of one of the anterior structures (Table 13.1). Intrinsic neck pain can radiate into the head and down on to the shoulders. Headache is particularly common in those patients with upper cervical pathology, particularly at C3 and above. Pain from structures at these levels is often perceived in the distribution of the first division of the trigeminal nerve or the back of the head and neck, and is most probably mediated through the trigeminocervical nucleus in the upper spinal cord[15]. Pain from lower cervical levels can be referred to the shoulder girdle, arm, interscapular region and chest wall[16]. It has been observed that the more severe the pain, the larger the area of referral.

Significance of site and radiation of neck pain

In considering musculoskeletal or mechanical neck pain, the key issue is to determine the site of origin of the pain. However, there are no means by which a single structure such as the dura, cervical zygapophyseal joints or intervertebral discs can be singled out as the source on the basis of clinical history and examination. Studies of normal individuals have demonstrated the patterns of pain referral stemming from the noxious stimulation of cervical structures. The intervertebral discs were studied by Cloward, who showed that probing the anterior part of the cervical discs produced pain in the posterior neck, several segments below the level stimulated (Fig. 13.1a)[17]. Classic studies by Feinstein *et al.* in the 1950s revealed that injections of hypertonic saline into deep cervical muscles produced distinct patterns of pain, again over the posterior neck (Fig. 13.1b)[18]. More recent studies have concentrated on the synovial joints of the cervical spine. Dwyer *et al.* distended the capsules of the cervical zygapophyseal joints (C2/3–C6/7) of normal volunteers[19]. Each joint had a reproducible and characteristic pattern of pain referral (Fig. 13.1c). The lowermost joint, C6/7, had a sclerotome that involved the posterior lower neck extending well across the scapula, so that it is conceivable that pain arising from this joint could be mistakenly considered to be arising from the shoulder. Moving cephalad, C5/6 stimulation resulted in pain over the crook of the neck, but above the spine of the scapula and C4/5 and C3/4 referred pain to the mid-neck with biases to the lower and upper neck respectively. The uppermost joint assessed in this series was C2/3. Pain from C2/3 was located in the suboccipital region, extending up on to the occipital part of the skull and down to the upper half of the neck. Similar methodology was used by Dreyfus *et al.* to investigate referral patterns of pain from the atlantoaxial and atlanto-occipital joints[20]. They injected and distended these joints in normal volunteers and found that this produced pain in the suboccipital region (Fig. 13.1d). It is important to note that there is extensive overlap between different structures, so that 'disc pain' may occur in an identical distribution to zygapophyseal joint pain or deep muscle pain. Moreover, adjacent structures have extensive overlap in the area to which they refer pain. In particular, the upper cervical zygapophyseal joints and the atlantoaxial and atlanto-occipital joints all refer pain to the suboccipital region.

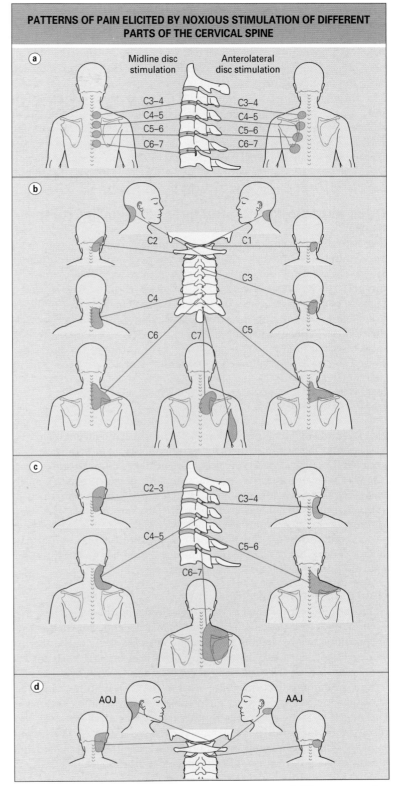

PATTERNS OF PAIN ELICITED BY NOXIOUS STIMULATION OF DIFFERENT PARTS OF THE CERVICAL SPINE

Fig. 13.1 Patterns of pain elicited by noxious stimulation of different parts of the cervical spine. The black dot represents the site stimulated to produce the pain pattern represented by the shaded area. (a) Intervertebral discs – probing of the discs in the midline anteriorly and lateral to the midline anteriorly. (Modified from Cloward[17].) (b) Deep musculoligamentous tissue – site of pain consistently produced by the injection of 6% saline into the interspinous region, just to the right of the midline, at cervical levels from C1 to C8. (Modified from Feinstein *et al.*[18]) (c) Zygapophyseal joints – sites of pain consistently produced by distention of the cervical zygapophyseal joints from C2/3–C6/7 through intra-articular injections of contrast medium. (Modified from Dwyer *et al.*[19]) (d) Upper cervical synovial joints – sites of pain consistently produced by distention of the atlantooccipital (AOJ) and atlantoaxial (AAJ) joints through intra-articular injections of contrast medium. (Modified from Dreyfus *et al.*[20])

The clinical consequence of this information is that it is impossible to determine the site of origin of neck pain on the basis of the site of pain alone. At best, the approximate level of involvement may be determined, but in practice this may be up to two or even three segments out and may reflect pain from a number of different structures. To complicate the issue further, a single source of pain may produce pain over a wide area through enhanced receptive fields of spinal neurons, so that pain may appear diffuse and unfocused. It is incumbent upon the physician to carefully assess the core of such pain when considering where to start further investigation. This can be facilitated by asking the patient to identify the most consistent pain, the core of the pain or where the pain seems to start. Pain maps and diagrams of the affected body part completed by the patient may be useful in this regard.

Other musculoskeletal structures referring pain to the neck

Somatic referred pain is typically referred distally, such as hip pain to the knee, shoulder pain to the upper arm and neck pain to the shoulder. However, two structures have been shown to refer pain proximally to the neck, potentially drawing attention away from the true source of pain. In similar experiments on normal volunteers, injection of hypertonic saline solution into the acromioclavicular joint[21] and sternoclavicular joints[22] frequently produced pain in the neck, sometimes with little local discomfort over the target joint. This information requires that these structures be evaluated as potential sources of neck pain in individual patients.

Associated features

Infections are typically accompanied by fevers and malaise as well as specific features reflecting the tissues involved. Pain arising from malignant disease may be accompanied by paraneoplastic conditions such as peripheral neuropathy, hypercalcemia or features of metastatic disease elsewhere. Symptoms that may accompany primary neck pain are dizziness and visual disturbances, which may be unaccompanied by abnormalities on conventional neurologic examination. The exact pathophysiologic basis for these symptoms has not been elucidated but a variety of hypotheses and increasing volumes of experimental data suggest an organic basis[6]. These symptoms should not be interpreted as indicating a neurotic basis for the neck pain.

Neurologic abnormalities

Neurologic symptoms such as paresthesia and subjective weakness may occur in neck pain patients. Their significance depends on whether they are accompanied by definite neurologic signs. Weakness in the absence of neurologic signs may seem to suggest a non-organic basis for the complaints but a variety of experimental studies have shown that pain has an inhibitory effect on motor neuron pools, resulting in a greater demand for effort and a consequent subjective sensation of weakness[23]. Paresthesia suggestive of nerve root irritation may arise, however, as a result of thoracic outlet syndrome caused by spasm of the scalene muscle[24]. This spasm seems to compress the lower trunk of the brachial plexus, causing the patient to experience paresthesia in the absence of clinical and imaging evidence of nerve root compression.

Hard neurologic signs are an uncommon finding in patients whose primary complaint is of neck pain but if neurologic impairment is detected the thrust of investigation should be to determine the site and nature of the lesion. Coexistent neck pain and neurologic deficit may be due to intrinsic disease of the cord, dura or nerve roots by neoplasia or infection (Table 13.2), or by compression of neural tissue by bone or discs that are themselves intrinsic sources of pain. The clinical assessment should establish whether the spinal cord, nerve roots or both are affected. The unexplained onset of, or presence of, impaired sphincter function, lower limb weakness and a sensory level are indicative of cord compression and demand urgent assessment by myelography (with or without computed tomography (CT) scan) or magnetic resonance imaging (MRI). These imaging modalities should determine whether a reversible cause of cord compression is present and allow the planning of any decompressive procedures.

Signs suggestive of a nerve root disorder, such as loss of a reflex or reflexes, dermatomal sensory loss or myotomic motor weakness (Fig. 13.2) may require confirmation by nerve conduction studies. Subsequent imaging of the course and origin of the nerve root(s) by myelography, CT or MRI often demonstrates the site and nature of the lesion and helps to ascertain whether the problem is intrinsic disease of the nerve or external compression. In the absence of neurologic signs, where neck pain alone is the clinical problem, there is little justification for nerve conduction studies, CT scans or MRI scans. However, there is experimental evidence to suggest that nerve root irritation can produce radiating, non-dermatomal patterns of pain[25].

CERVICAL NERVE ROOT COMPRESSION

Pain arising from overt compression or disease of the nerve root typically follows the appropriate dermatome and is therefore felt in the arm and not the neck. This pain will typically be radicular in quality, in other words, pain that is perceived in a narrow band on the skin of the arm and that has electrical, radiating or shooting properties. However more somatic pain (i.e. deep, diffuse aching) in proximal structures can be produced by nerve root compression[25]. However, pain that is perceived in the forearm or hand is unlikely to be somatic referred pain and is more likely to be radicular in origin.

Depending upon the severity of nerve root involvement, such pain may be accompanied by neurologic symptoms such as numbness, paresthesia, altered sensation and motor weakness. Pain may be perceived across the top of the shoulder from C4, and the face and head from lesions affecting C2 and C3[26]. However, these are uncommon levels to be affected, so much so that isolated lesions at these levels should prompt a systematic search for sinister space-occupying pathology. The overwhelming majority of cervical root lesions occur at the lower levels, C6, C7 and C8, which all tend to produce symptoms referable to the forearm and hand and which have distinctive clinical features (Fig. 13.2). Because of the extensive overlap of dermatomes in the arm and the complex central representation of the upper limb, the pain referred to the arm through root irritation may be far more diffuse than the traditional diagrams of dermatomes would suggest. The usual etiology of cervical nerve root pain is compromise of the exiting nerve root by so called 'spondylitic change'. This is a broad term, the use of which should be discouraged. In general it is taken to mean degenerative changes that take place with increasing age in the cervical spine affecting the cervical vertebrae, the intervertebral discs, the uncinate processes and the zygapophyseal joints. Unlike in the lumbar spine, disc prolapse itself is not the predominant cause of cervical nerve root irritation. This is because the nerve root in the lower cervical spine lies in the lower part of the foramen, at or below the level of the disc[27]. More typically, this part of the foramen is compromised by osteophytic involvement from the adjacent uncinate process or through hypertrophic changes in the adjacent zygapophyseal joint[1]. Where disc lesions do occur, the pathology is different from that affecting the lumbar spine. The discs fissure posteriorly as part of the normal aging process, so that there is no intact posterior anulus to 'bulge' in the manner described in the lumbar spine. Rather, disc contributions to neural encroachment are more likely to be discrete fragments of the disc that herniate into the foramen to cause neural compromise, either through direct pressure or through inciting a local inflammatory response. This has been demonstrated in a surgical study of radicular pain after whiplash injury, which found that all patients with persistent neurologic features had disc fragments that had been misdiagnosed as prolapses on MRI[28].

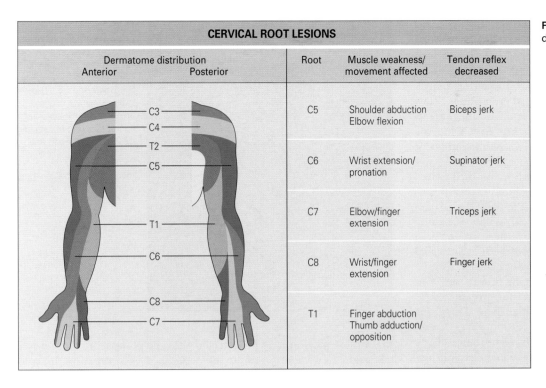

CERVICAL ROOT LESIONS			
Dermatome distribution Anterior Posterior	Root	Muscle weakness/ movement affected	Tendon reflex decreased
	C5	Shoulder abduction Elbow flexion	Biceps jerk
	C6	Wrist extension/ pronation	Supinator jerk
	C7	Elbow/finger extension	Triceps jerk
	C8	Wrist/finger extension	Finger jerk
	T1	Finger abduction Thumb adduction/ opposition	

Fig. 13.2 Cervical root lesions. Sensory and motor distribution of the cervical roots.

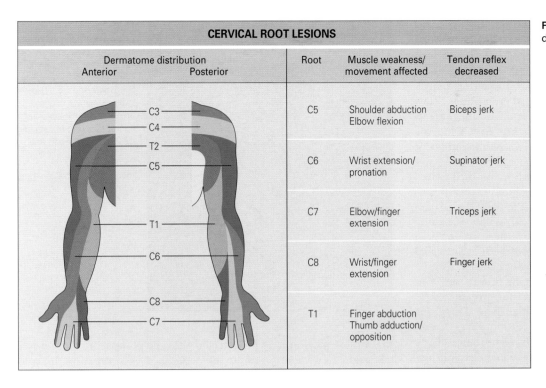

CLINICAL EXAMINATION

It is a time-honored belief that a careful clinical examination is an important and useful means of arriving at a diagnosis. For neck pain, this is only partly true. The principal role of the clinical examination is to exclude other conditions that may be present and contributing to the pain, such as infection, malignancy or inflammatory arthropathy, or to exclude neurologic involvement. Once these issues have been dealt with, and the diagnosis is that of isolated or mechanical neck pain, the diagnostic utility of clinical examination of the neck is extremely limited.

General examination

The general examination is performed to exclude non-mechanical causes of neck pain. This should be particularly focused on any system(s) where abnormalities have been suggested by the history. In addition, examination of the temperature, skin, joints, lymph nodes, abdomen and breasts should be performed. The yield from such assessment in the setting of neck pain is not known and is probably low but the serious consequences of missing a potentially treatable systemic illness, malignancy or infection make the performance of such an examination mandatory.

Neurologic examination

The aims of a neurologic examination in the presence of neck pain are to exclude cervical nerve root lesions or spinal cord lesions. The former requires a detailed examination of the arms. The muscles should be examined for wasting and fasciculation indicative of lower motor neuron lesions. Tone and power should then be assessed, before testing the biceps (C5/6), triceps (C6/7), supinator (C5/6) and finger (C8) jerks. Sensation to light touch and pain (pin prick) should then be checked, looking particularly for any dermatomal sensory loss. The lower limbs should be similarly examined, with the principal aim being the exclusion of any upper motor neuron signs indicative of cord compression due to the painful lesion in the neck. It is important to examine first the gait and then the lower limbs for spasticity, clonus, upgoing toes (Babinski's sign), hyper-reflexia and weakness. The trunk and lower limbs should be assessed for evidence of a sensory level.

Local examination

The neck examination again requires that non-mechanical causes, such as local infection, bruising, lymphadenitis, etc., are excluded. This is readily accomplished with routine inspection and palpation. The other cervical structures, such as the larynx, thyroid, lymph nodes and carotid arteries, should be carefully palpated for evidence of swelling or tenderness. However, in the absence of suggestive history, the yield from such examination is likely to be small. The neck should be examined for tenderness. This is best achieved by exerting pressure first on a control area such as the occipital protuberance. This pressure should then be applied along the spinous processes and then the articular pillars as well as the trapezii. This at least provides some standardization of the stimulus and permits some grading of response, e.g. tender, very tender, exquisitely tender. Unfortunately, the localization of tenderness contributes little in the way of diagnostic information. There has been no demonstrated correlation between tenderness in a particular area and a specific anatomic diagnosis. At most, examination for tenderness permits the approximate level of any causative pathology to be estimated. Tenderness is also a subjective finding, so that it is subject to reporting biases from patients keen to either exaggerate or diminish their problems.

Neck movement

Examination of the neck for mechanical problems traditionally incorporates the documentation of active and passive ranges of movement. The obsession with ranges of movement stems from a vain desire to provide a functional assessment of the patient and is no doubt fueled in part by the fact that most medicolegal assessments require a detailed range of movement estimation to enable percentage impairment to be calculated. However, basic research casts grave doubts on the diagnostic utility and reliability of such assessments. Detailed cineradiographic techniques employed by Van Mameren et al. to assess flexion and extension have revealed that even normal individuals display marked variation in the pattern and amplitude of both segmental and total ranges of neck movement[29]. They concluded that, at least in the sagittal plane, range of movement was unsuitable as a parameter of cervical spine mobility. Such variability in controlled laboratory situations is likely to translate to a much larger error in clinical situations with the added variability of many observers and different measurement environments. Therefore, only gross abnormalities of range of motion, such as reproducible asymmetry of movement, are likely to be assessed reliably. Notwithstanding any concerns over the reliability of measurements of neck movement, their clinical utility is open to serious question. Biomechanical studies have shown that 50% of cervical rotation takes place at the atlantoaxial joints[30]. The remaining rotation occurs in approximately equal proportions below C2, so that each segment contributes less than 7° of movement. Therefore, even complete fusion of a segment below C1–C2 may be clinically undetectable and will most probably fall within measurement error.

At the same time, it is conceivable that a painful lesion of the neck below C1–C2 may produce marked loss of movement, in excess of 50% of range, because of reflex inhibition of muscles due to pain, fear of pain being produced or local muscle spasm due to pain. This is readily appreciated in patients with acute hypomobility, whose site of pain (typically in the lower neck) would be inconsistent with atlantoaxial joint pain but whose range of movement is markedly reduced. Despite these observations, some have advocated that reduction of range of movement in the neck of greater than 50% is a 'non-organic' sign, suggestive of abnormal illness behavior[31], a potentially dangerous assumption.

An even more fundamental issue is the diagnostic significance of any observed motion restriction. No correlations have been established between motion abnormalities and any specific anatomic diagnoses. Therefore, the measurement of ranges of motion in the neck provides no reliable or discriminatory diagnostic information. At best, restriction of movement in the neck indicates that there is one or more of:

- disturbance of the neuromuscular control of the neck
- a painful lesion aggravated by movement
- a mechanical restriction anywhere in the complex articular arrangements between two or more vertebrae.

Similar concerns pertain to the observation of pain at extremes of range of movement.

Test for nerve root entrapment

A number of special maneuvers and tests have been proposed for the identification of nerve root compression. The most specific of these has been found to be the compression test. The patient's neck is moved passively into extension and rotated to the symptomatic side. Axial pressure is then applied to the neck by the examiner. This series of movements has been shown to narrow the intervertebral foramina. If the patient's radicular symptoms are reproduced, then the test is positive[32]. This test has good inter-rater reliability and is highly specific, but relatively insensitive. The combination of a positive compression test and abnormal neurologic signs in the arm is strongly predictive of nerve root compression on CT myelography.

INVESTIGATIONS

Radiographs

Plain radiographs of the cervical spine are ordered almost universally for patients presenting with neck pain. This may be appropriate where there is a history suggestive of severe trauma likely to produce fracture or severe subluxation, or where major instability is suspected. The most useful views in these circumstances are lateral flexion and extension views, open mouth views and to a lesser extent the anteroposterior view. To assess for subluxation, lines linking the anterior vertebral bodies, posterior vertebral bodies and posterior border of the intervertebral canal in a lateral projection are constructed. These should describe a smooth arc (Fig. 13.3). The presence of a 'step' in this arc is a sign of subluxation, either through retrolisthesis or spondylolisthesis. Gross abnor-

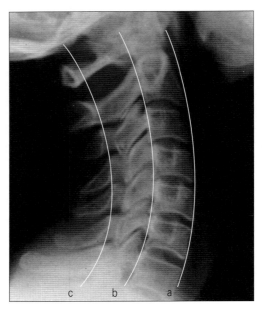

Fig. 13.3 Plain lateral radiograph of a normal cervical spine. Lines joining the anterior part of the vertebral body (a), the posterior aspect of the vertebral body (b), and the anterior border of the laminae (c), should describe a smooth arc.

malities of motion may be detected through comparing flexion and extension views, and instability demonstrated by comparing the construction lines described above on flexion and extension views.

Of particular note is the issue of atlantoaxial instability. This occurs almost exclusively in rheumatoid arthritis but can occur in the presence of other destructive lesions affecting the odontoid peg or transverse or alar ligament complex. This is assessed by comparing the gap between the anterior part of the odontoid peg and the posterior margin of the anterior arch of the atlas as seen on lateral flexion and extension views. This should normally be less than 2.5 mm in women and 4 mm in men.

Plain radiographs may also be useful in excluding primary bone disorders such as Paget's disease, significant sclerotic malignant infiltration of bone and destructive lesions such as osteomyelitis. However, standard views of the cervical spine are complex pictures with many structures being superimposed on all views, in contrast to a radiograph of a long bone. This means that radiographs tend to be insensitive in the detection of small abnormalities, such as purely lytic lesions without significant cortical bone destruction. Where such lesions are suspected but not detected on plain films, further imaging with CT, MRI or nuclear medicine techniques is desirable.

Congenital lesions, such as hypoplastic vertebral bodies or fusion of segments (most typically between C2 and C3) are also detectable on plain films. It is not known what the true relationship of many of these abnormalities is to symptoms, but it would be tempting to argue that a fused segment places increased mechanical stress on the adjacent segment, which may in turn lead to pain. A more detailed description of these abnormalities can be found in Resnick's excellent monograph[33]. Rheumatic disorders affecting the spine, such as diffuse idiopathic skeletal hyperostosis and ankylosing spondylitis, have characteristic radiographic appearances. The former causes large osteophytic linking between adjacent vertebrae but is more common in the lower thoracic spine. Ankylosing spondylitis is considered in detail in Chapter 21.

For those patients with mechanical pain, the value of plain radiographs is much more limited. It is commonly stated that neck pain is due to cervical spondylosis, which is a radiologic diagnosis. However, it has been repeatedly demonstrated that the presence of degenerative or spondylitic changes in the spine does not correlate with symptoms of neck pain. In seminal work conducted over 30 years ago, Freidenburg and Miller studied 92 pairs of age- and sex-matched patients with and without neck pain[34]. Plain cervical films were obtained for all patients. The incidence of degenerative changes rose with age, was most common at the C5/6 level, both at the intervertebral disc and the zygapophyseal joints, but bore no relationship to the presence of neck pain. This finding was ratified by Heller *et al.*, who failed to find any relationship between symptoms of neck pain and the presence of degenerative changes identified on lateral views of the cervical spine in patients undergoing barium swallows[35]. Therefore, the finding of degenerative or spondylitic changes on plain radiographs of the cervical spine has no discriminatory or diagnostic value: it is a sign of increasing age and provides no help for the physician seeking to explain a patient's neck pain.

Computed tomography

The principal value of CT in the assessment of cervical lesions is the visualization and measurement of the bony conduits through which the neural tissue must pass. This ability can be enhanced by the introduction of radio-opaque contrast medium into the thecal sac (CT myelography), which permits direct visualization of the nerve roots and sheaths and the spinal cord itself. CT is of less value in assessing soft tissues. The selection of these investigations would therefore be dictated by the clinical suspicion of a neurologic abnormality, either cervical myelopathy, cord compression or cervical nerve root compression. For neck pain alone, without neurologic symptoms or signs and without clinical or plain radiographic evidence of non-mechanical disorder, the role of CT remains to be determined. There are no extant studies relating CT abnormalities to symptoms in patients with neck pain. Therefore, in the presence of clinically benign neck pain, CT should only be obtained where there is a desire to clarify an abnormality detected on plain films or to assess neural compression or compromise.

Magnetic resonance imaging

Similar comments pertain to the use of MRI, which is highly specific and sensitive for disc herniations when compared to surgical findings and has results comparable to CT myelography (Fig. 13.4)[36]. Magnetic resonance imaging is particularly helpful in visualizing intracord pathology in the cervical region (such as demyelination, intra-axial tumors and spinal cord infarction) and enables accurate appraisal of developmental defects such as the Arnold–Chiari malformation. It has high sensitivity (92%) and specificity (96%) for the detection of osteomyelitis, including that affecting the spine[37].

However, for the assessment of neck pain of mechanical origin, MRI, like CT, has not been validated. It has been shown that nearly one-fifth of all asymptomatic patients had abnormalities on MRI scans, with 60% of older patients having abnormalities of their intervertebral discs[38].

Intradiscal lesions occurring in the anterior anulus have been found on MRI scans in patients with neck pain following whiplash injury[39] and would appear to match pathologic lesions reported in patients dying in motor vehicle accidents[40]. However, it has not yet been established that these 'rim lesions' seen on MRI are a source of pain. Surface coil MR images of isolated cervical spines have revealed that, even with optimal imaging parameters, the soft tissue components of the zygapophyseal joints are seen poorly, if at all[41]. Therefore, it is unlikely that MRI will provide useful data in the assessment of subtle but painful injuries or other pathologic processes affecting these structures. This technique should be reserved for those patients in whom there is a clinical suspicion of intraspinal pathology, neural compromise or other neurologic disorder. It should not be a routine investigation in patients with a clinical history of uncomplicated mechanical neck pain.

Isotope scans

The most commonly used nuclear medicine technique in the assessment of neck pain is bone scanning using technetium-99m-labeled methylene diphosphonate (^{99m}Tc-MDP). This technique is highly sensitive for the detection of bony pathology with the notable exception of those lesions that have a purely lytic pathology, particularly multiple myeloma (Fig. 13.5). However, for the tumors that most commonly metastasize to bone – lung, breast, prostate, thyroid and kidney – the technique is the investigation of choice for the early detection of metastases. Bone scanning may also be useful in the detection of infection; it will often show avid uptake in the affected region. Using an early, angiographic assessment during the injection of the radiopharmaceutical and a blood pool image a short time later, increased vascularity can be assessed which can help differentiate infection or inflammation from degenerative change. Areas of increased radiopharmaceutical uptake in the cervical spine must be assessed with knowledge of the usual pattern of uptake. Notable in the cervical spine is the normal, physiologic increase in uptake over the C2 spinous process compared with lower cervical vertebrae[42]. Only one study of the utility of bone scanning for a specific cause of neck pain has been undertaken[43]. This study assessed the sensitivity and specificity of single photon emission CT (SPECT) and planar bone scans against a criterion standard of cervical zygapophyseal joint pain established by diagnostic blocks (see below). The study revealed bone scans to have negligible accuracy in the diagnosis of cervical zygapophysial joint pain after whiplash injury.

Bone scans have an important role in the assessment of patients where tumor or infection are suspected but plain radiographs are normal or

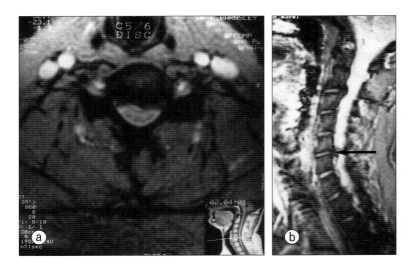

Fig. 13.4 Disc herniation on MRI. Axial (a) and sagittal (b) MRI scans of a 47-year-old man with neck pain and decreased left biceps jerk with numbness over his thumb following a motor vehicle accident. The scans demonstrate a significant left posterolateral disc protrusion (arrow) at C5/6, which significantly compromises the exiting C6 nerve root.

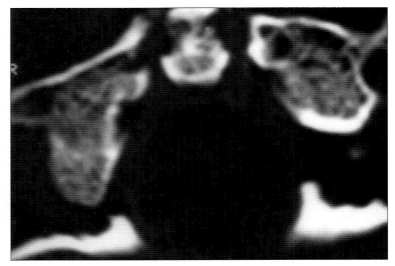

Fig. 13.5 Detection of myeloma. CT scan of a 63-year-old man with known multiple myeloma who developed neck pain. Plain radiographs and bone scan failed to demonstrate the osteolytic lesions affecting the odontoid peg.

equivocal. In this setting their superior sensitivity to early disturbances in osteoblastic activity may reveal important pathology well before plain radiographic changes emerge. A difficult area is differentiating increased uptake from degenerative changes in the neck from other, more sinister, pathologies. This may require further imaging of the region of interest with CT or MRI where significant doubt exists. However, in the cervical spine, degenerative changes typically affect the intervertebral joints so that increased uptake in these regions should arouse less suspicion than uptake localized to, say, the vertebral body.

The role of other nuclear medicine techniques, such as tumor thallium, indium-labeled white cell and gallium studies, is in the pursuit of specific diagnoses suggested on history, examination, plain radiographs, other imaging modalities or routine blood tests. They should not be used for screening patients with clinically benign neck pain.

Blood tests

Blood tests have no role in the assessment of pain that is mechanical on the basis of history and clinical examination. Where other problems such as tumor or infection are suspected they may provide supportive evidence. The most useful investigations would be complete blood count (CBC), erythrocyte sedimentation rate (ESR) and/or C reactive protein, and serum alkaline phosphatase. Infection and tumor are typically associated with an elevated ESR, infection with an elevated white cell count and Paget's disease with an increased alkaline phosphatase. It should be emphasized that these investigations have no role in the routine screening of patients where there are no historical or physical findings to suggest anything other than mechanical pain.

Myelography

Myelography is the introduction of radiographic contrast medium into the cerebrospinal fluid in the subarachnoid space with images then being collected as the contrast spreads or is guided to the area of interest. The primary value of myelography is not the elucidation of a source of neck pain but the demonstration of the outline of the subarachnoid space, in particular the spinal cord and nerve root sheaths. This is of value in revealing intrusions upon the cervical spinal canal and intervertebral foramina and compression of the cord or nerve roots by discs and disc fragments, infection or tumors. It may also reveal narrowing of the cervical spinal canal in patients with cervical myelopathy. Intraspinal lesions may be detected through the demonstration of expansion of the cord itself. However, all these lesions would need to be suspected on the basis of neurologic symptoms and signs and would rarely, if ever, present with neck pain alone.

Investigations targeting pain

In the absence of reliable morphologic correlates of mechanical neck pain on imaging, it is necessary to target the pain itself to identify the painful structure. This can be accomplished either by stimulating a potentially painful structure and determining whether pain is produced or by anesthetizing a structure and determining whether pain is relieved, thereby implicating that structure as a source of pain.

Zygapophyseal joint blocks

The techniques for the diagnosis of cervical zygapophyseal joint pain rely on the simple principle that, if a given joint is a source of pain, anesthetizing that joint will relieve the pain. There are two techniques by which the cervical zygapophyseal joints can be anesthetized. Local anesthetic can be injected into the joint or, alternatively, the nerves that convey pain from the joint can be anesthetized.

Intra-articular joint blocks

Intra-articular blocks of the cervical zygapophyseal joints are performed under fluoroscopic control. The procedure has been described using either a posterior or a lateral approach. In either case, a narrow-gauge

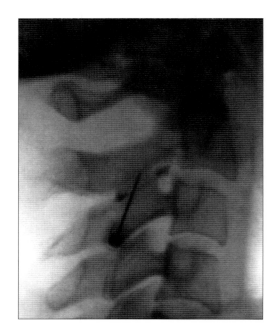

Fig. 13.6 Arthrogram of the C2/3 zygapophyseal joint. A needle has been placed into the center of the joint and injected contrast medium has filled the loose inferior and posterior recesses.

spinal needle is directed towards the center of the target joint. Once the needle is felt to have pierced the joint capsule, a minimal volume of contrast medium must be injected to confirm intra-articular placement (Fig. 13.6). Thereafter, 0.7–1.0ml of local anesthetic can be injected to anesthetize the joint.

The total injected volume should not exceed the joint capacity (generally accepted to be 1.0ml), since distention beyond this volume may cause capsular rupture. Nevertheless, even when smaller volumes have been employed, extra-articular leakage has been observed in up to 17% of cases[44]. The direction of spread after extra-articular leakage has been reliably described. Epidural spread has been reported but is believed to be rare and has only been reported when more than 1.0ml of injectant was used.

Theoretically, extra-articular spread may compromise the specificity of an intra-articular block by anesthetizing structures other than the target joint. The risk of this is minimized by using minimal volumes to infiltrate the joint and by monitoring the spread of the contrast medium used to confirm intra-articular placement of the needle. Any significant spread to the epidural space or spinal nerve would result in numbness or other neurologic signs. A postprocedural neurologic examination should be performed to detect any such inadvertent effects.

Medial branch blocks

Cervical medial branch blocks are a more expedient way to anesthetize a cervical zygapophyseal joint. They are easier to perform, are less painful to the patient and appear to provide the same diagnostic information[45]. They are performed under fluoroscopic control using either a posterior or a lateral approach. These blocks take advantage of the anatomy of the nerve supply to the cervical zygapophyseal joints.

Innervation of the cervical zygapophyseal joints

The cervical zygapophyseal joints are innervated by articular branches derived from the medial branches of the cervical dorsal rami. The C4–C8 dorsal rami arise from their respective spinal nerves just outside the intervertebral foramina and pass dorsally over the roots of the transverse processes. Lateral branches of the dorsal rami enter the lateral and superficial posterior neck muscles (splenius, iliocostalis and longissimus).

The medial branches of the typical cervical dorsal rami course posteriorly, hugging the waists of their ipsisegmental articular pillars. They are covered by the tendinous slips of origin of the semispinalis capitis

CERVICAL ZYGAPOPHYSEAL JOINT INNERVATION

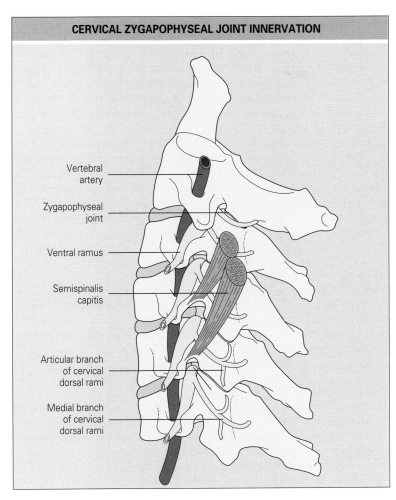

Vertebral artery

Zygapophyseal joint

Ventral ramus

Semispinalis capitis

Articular branch of cervical dorsal rami

Medial branch of cervical dorsal rami

Fig. 13.7 Cervical zygapophyseal joint innervation. A posterolateral view of the cervical spine illustrating the course of the medial branches of the cervical dorsal rami. All muscles except the origins of the semispinalis capitis at C4 and C5 have been removed. The medial branches of the cervical dorsal rami are seen to course across the waist of the articular pillars. At C4 and C5, they are shown covered by the tendinous origins of the semispinalis capitis. Articular branches arise from each medial branch, on the posterior aspect of the articular pillar, to innervate the zygapophyseal joints above and below. The medial branches are well away from the ventral rami of the spinal nerves and the vertebral artery.

(Fig. 13.7). Articular branches arise as the nerve approaches the posterior aspect of the articular pillar. An ascending branch innervates the zygapophyseal joint above and a descending branch innervates the joint below (Fig. 13.7). Consequently, each typical cervical zygapophyseal joint receives a dual innervation, from the medial branch above and from the medial branch below its location. Beyond the zygapophyseal joints the medial branches of the cervical dorsal rami supply the semispinalis and multifidus muscles.

The medial branches of the C3 dorsal ramus comprise a deep medial branch that passes around the waist of the C3 articular pillar, as described above, and participates in the innervation of the C3/4 zygapophyseal joint. The superficial medial branch of C3 is larger and is known as the third occipital nerve. It winds around the lateral aspect and then the posterior aspect of the C2/3 zygapophyseal joint. As it does so, it furnishes from its deep aspect articular branches to the C2/3 zygapophyseal joint[46]. Articular branches may also arise from a communicating loop which crosses the back of the joint between the third occipital nerve and the C2 dorsal ramus. Beyond the C2/3 zygapophyseal joint, the third occipital nerve furnishes muscle branches to the semispinalis capitis and becomes cutaneous over the suboccipital region. In

this respect the C3 dorsal ramus is the only cervical dorsal ramus below C2 that regularly has a cutaneous distribution. The dorsal rami of C4 and C5 may have cutaneous branches, whereas those from C6–C8 rarely do.

The cervical medial branches below the third occipital nerve, i.e. those supplying C3/4–C6/7, can be anesthetized by placing a small amount

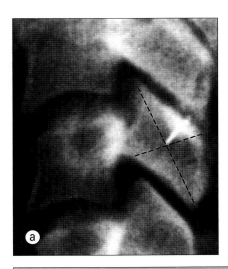

(a)

CERVICAL MEDIAL BRANCH BLOCK

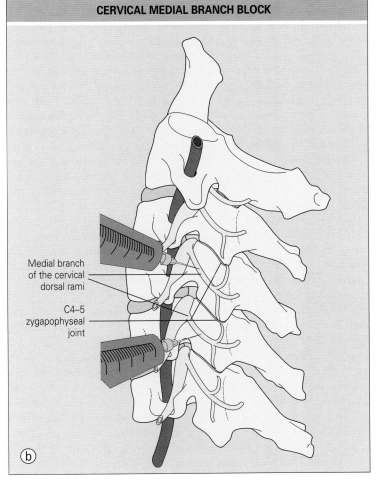

Medial branch of the cervical dorsal rami

C4–5 zygapophyseal joint

(b)

Fig. 13.8 Cervical medial branch block. (a) Radiograph illustrating a needle correctly placed for an injection on to the medial branch of the C5 dorsal ramus. The target point is the centrode of the articular pillar as seen on a true lateral view. (b) A schematic diagram of medial branch blocks of the C4 and C5 dorsal rami to anesthetize the C4/5 zygapophyseal joint. Needles inserted from a lateral approach are positioned for infiltration of the medial branches of the cervical dorsal rami of C4 and C5. Note that the needle tips are proximal to the origins of the ascending and descending articular branches.

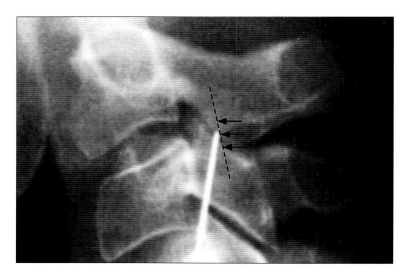

Fig. 13.9 Injecting the third occipital nerve. Lateral radiograph of the cervical spine with arrows indicating the target points for injections to anesthetize the third occipital nerve and thus the C2/3 zygapophyseal joint. The points lie along a line that vertically bisects the articular pillar of C3 seen on a lateral projection. The middle point lies over the joint line, the upper point over the subchondral plate of the C2 inferior articular surface and the lower over the subchondral plate of the superior articular surface of C3.

(0.5ml) of local anesthetic on to the nerve as it passes across the waist of the articular pillar. This is accomplished by placing a needle under image intensifier guidance on to the centrode of the articular pillar, usually from a lateral approach (Fig. 13.8). It has been shown that injections so placed do not spread laterally, posteriorly or inferiorly to affect any other diagnostically important structure; they remain constrained against the articular pillar and hence the nerve, by the medial aspect of the semispinalis capitis tendon and muscle[47]. The third occipital nerve is anesthetized by placing local anesthetic on to the nerve as it passes across the C2/3 joint, which it ultimately innervates. Because of the more variable course of this nerve, lying on the convex aspect of the joint rather than the concavity at the waist of the lower articular pillars, three injections are placed to bracket its less consistent course (Fig. 13.9).

To fully anesthetize a given zygapophyseal joint at typical cervical levels, both medial branches that supply it must be blocked. Thus, in the case of a C5/6 zygapophyseal joint, the medial branches of C5 and C6 must be anesthetized. In the case of the C2/3 zygapophyseal joint, the third occipital nerve must be blocked. Adequate blockade of this nerve is indicated by the onset of numbness in its cutaneous territory.

Notwithstanding the correct technical execution of these blocks, their value as a diagnostic tool hangs on the correct interpretation of the patient's responses. This involves both the patient's reporting and the physician's interpretation of that report, which are necessarily subjective. Formal appraisal of the value of single blocks finds them wanting in accuracy, with a 27% false-positive rate[48]. To circumvent this, two blocks should be used, administered on different occasions, using anesthetics with different durations of action, in random order under double-blind conditions. The veracity of the patient's response is then adjudicated through their report of the duration of pain relief afforded by the anesthetic given. Since the medial branches below the third occipital nerve do not have reliable cutaneous representation, the only way that a patient can tell which anesthetic was used is through the duration of pain relief. It is therefore axiomatic that only a patient with pain can correctly identify the longer-acting local anesthetic. This approach has been formally tested, and found to be a valid means of identifying cervical zygapophyseal joint pain[49].

A further refinement to this process is the addition of a third, placebo injection using normal saline as the injectant. A standard criterion of failure to respond to a double-blind administered placebo and any positive response to the local anesthetics reveals that simply using the two anesthetics results in high specificity but poor sensitivity[50]. Whichever approach is adopted depends on the aim of the investigation. Where aggressive neurolytic therapy is being considered, the extra accuracy afforded by triple, saline-controlled blocks may be warranted. Other situations, where less invasive therapy is being considered, may require only double blocks.

In summary, medial branch blocks are an exciting new tool for the diagnosis of cervical zygapophyseal joint pain. They are valid techniques that, when correctly and thoughtfully applied, provide a syndromic, anatomic diagnosis in many patients with otherwise undiagnosable neck pain. Studies using these techniques attest to a prevalence of cervical zygapophyseal joint pain of 54% in patients with chronic neck pain (whiplash) after motor vehicle accidents[51] and a lower prevalence of 36% in less selected patients[52].

Other anesthetic blocks

Anesthetic blocks of other structures, such as the greater occipital nerve and ventral rami of the spinal nerves, can occasionally be useful in confirming or eliminating structures in their territories as causes of pain but in contrast to zygapophyseal joint blocks these procedures do not have documented reliability and specificity and do not currently have a place in the routine assessment of the neck pain patient.

Provocation discography

The only regularly used provocative test in the neck is provocation cervical discography, in which a disc is punctured by a needle and distended by injecting contrast media. A positive discogram occurs when the procedure reproduces the patient's usual pain and implicates that disc as the source of pain[53]. The response can occasionally be confirmed by injecting local anesthetic in order to try to abolish the pain[54]. In practice the procedure itself can be quite painful and it is often difficult for the patient to judge whether it is their usual pain that is being reproduced.

The reliability of discography has been called into question by the observation that, in a significant proportion of patients, pain reproduced by discography can be completely eliminated by subsequent zygapophyseal joint blocks at that level[55]. Since zygapophyseal joint blocks do not have any effect on pain perception from the disc, these observations must indicate that discograms are liable to false-positive interpretations, wrongly incriminating the disc as a cause of pain when the true problem resides in the zygapophyseal joint. Furthermore, if zygapophyseal joint pain can be reproduced by stressing the disc at that segment, other structures with the same segmental nerve supply or mechanical relationships to the disc may be being falsely incriminated by seemingly positive discograms. On the basis of current evidence, discograms should only be considered as true positives if zygapophyseal joint blocks at that level are negative (i.e. no pain relief). The side effects of discography have been assessed in a audit study in a single practice, which revealed the rate of discitis to be 0.16% per injection[56].

PATHOGENESIS OF NECK PAIN

The exact cause of most mechanical neck pain remains elusive. As it is not a life-threatening problem, there is a paucity of pertinent pathological data and, as the previous section suggests, currently available imaging modalities provide morphologic information that does not necessarily correlate with pain. In the case of acute neck pain, it has been suggested that the pain and hypomobility may stem from entrapment of the intra-articular menisci of the cervical zygapophyseal joint in the large capsular recesses of these joints, with inflammation, pain and stiffness ensuing before the meniscus is 'reduced'[57]. This may account for the rapid response of such acute hypomobility to mobilizing therapy. The source of more chronic neck pain remains arcane. The pathologic data concerning necks focuses on those problems that lead to neurologic compromise. Where pain alone is the clinical problem, there is little more than theory and deduction, a poor substitute for data. However, the use of techniques such as zygapophyseal joint blocks and discography enables the anatomic source of pain at least to be identified in a number of cases. In the case of the disc, anular tears extending into the innervated outer third of the disc may well be the source of pain[58] but why normal age-related changes, including extensive posterolateral fissuring, fail to cause pain in a significant proportion of patients is not understood[59].

A variety of lesions resulting from trauma to the neck could affect the cervical zygapophyseal joints (see below). Many of these could result in premature osteoarthritic change which can be expected to be painful. Alternatively, intra-articular adhesions, capsulitis (analogous to frozen shoulder) or ongoing synovitis may be responsible for chronic zygapophyseal joint pain. For those patients without discogenic or zygapophyseal joint pain, the other candidate structures include the dura. However, studies of rat dura suggest that, below the tentorium, the dura is endowed with few nociceptive nerves[60]. A broader view of neck pain should also incorporate the possibility that some chronic neck pain is mediated within the spinal cord through 'wind up' of neuronal networks, principally in the posterior horn. The presence of these so called 'vicious circuits' has long been suspected but is still to be definitively demonstrated.

There are views that chronic neck pain may be a multifactorial problem, representing a complex interplay between biological, psychological and social factors – the so called 'biopsychosocial' model. Pain is recognized as a phenomenon arising from nociceptive excitation perceived in a psychological and social milieu. It is generally accepted that pain, particularly chronic pain, is frequently associated with impaired social functioning and psychological distress. It is therefore difficult to separate causative from incidental relationships. Some light has been thrown on this issue by the observation that, when chronic neck pain has been fully relieved, evidence of psychological distress disappears[61]. This would suggest that the psychological distress was a consequence rather than cause of the chronic pain.

TREATMENT

The treatment of neck pain due to infection, tumor or inflammatory disease such as rheumatoid arthritis is necessarily the treatment of the underlying disorder, and is not further considered in this chapter. The treatment of mechanical neck pain can be divided into those treatments that are not targeted at any particular structure, and are therefore non-specific, and those that are targeted at a particular painful structure within the neck. The aim of treatment is to relieve pain and thereby improve function.

Non-specific treatments
Analgesics
The most commonly used non-specific treatments for neck pain are simple analgesics such as acetaminophen (paracetamol). These have an important role in acute neck pain and can also be used safely over long periods of time in more chronic problems where other treatment is ineffective. In patients with more severe pain, synthetic and non-synthetic opioids such as dextropropoxyphene or codeine can be used but the potential for abuse and dependency needs to be considered before they are prescribed. These concerns should not prevent the physician from treating severe, refractory and incapacitating pain appropriately. Tricyclic antidepressants, in doses considerably less than those used in depression, can be used as co-analgesics. They are particularly useful where nocturnal sedation is desirable and where depression is present. Other newer agents such as tramadol and gabapentin have not yet been formally studied for neck pain.

Exercises
In common with many treatments of neck pain, there are no extant studies dealing with exercise as a single treatment modality compared to placebo. Neck exercises have two principal aims. The first is to restore a normal range of motion. The second is to strengthen the neck musculature. Application of the latter approach may be useful in patients with recurrent episodes of acute pain with hypomobility. It has been suggested that these episodes are related to entrapment of the intra-articular menisci of the cervical zygapophyseal joints[57] and it seems reasonable to expect that stronger supportive musculature may help to prevent these episodes. Analogous to articular problems elsewhere in the body, there would be logic in preserving range of movement in the neck joints to prevent contracture and loss of range of motion.

Whether the complexity of the cervical articular system permits individual joints to be actively mobilized by a patient is uncertain. However, the benign nature of the intervention and the potential benefits favor the inclusion of exercise in the treatment program for neck pain patients. This suggestion is supported by observations from a recent study that compared exercise therapy (simple exercise or MedX-enhanced) to manipulative therapy. It concluded that, for chronic neck pain, the use of strengthening exercise, whether in combination with spinal manipulation or in the form of a high-technology MedX program, appears to be more beneficial to patients with chronic neck pain than the use of spinal manipulation alone[62].

Physical therapy
Physical therapy incorporates a number of potentially therapeutic modalities such as heat, cold, interferential, ultrasound, traction, massage, passive and active range of motion exercises and muscle strengthening techniques. Systematic reviews of the physical therapy literature have concluded that there is little evidence for the efficacy of these modalities and call for further studies[63,64]. The undoubted fact that some patients report modest and temporary benefit from these approaches should encourage more formal appraisals but whether any single modality or combination of modalities is definitely efficacious remains unknown. Current evidence suggests no benefit of non-manipulative physical therapy over standard medical care[65].

Manual therapy/manipulation
A variety of 'hands on' techniques have been described in the treatment of neck pain. The best studied and most widely practiced are short-lever high-velocity 'adjustments', usually described as manipulations and used principally by chiropractors, the aim of which is to correct so-called vertebral subluxations. The other leading technique is known as mobilization and involves oscillatory movements through both the physiologic and accessory movements of spinal joints. The aim is to stretch tight joint capsules of symptomatic joints. The pathophysiologic basis for either of these approaches remains to be clearly demonstrated. Key issues of inter- and intrarater reliability for the diagnosis of vertebral subluxation or tight joints have yet to be resolved. Studies to date have therefore lumped together all patients with neck pain, and have also often included lumbar pain. At best, these studies show small benefit, of uncertain clinical significance, for manual techniques over conventional physical therapy modalities and best medical care[65].

A comprehensive meta-analysis of manual techniques for cervical pain and headache has concluded that mobilization was probably of benefit for acute neck pain and that manipulation is slightly better than mobilization or physical therapy for chronic neck pain[66]. However, the most important message was that much more quality research is required before decisions on using manual techniques can be considered truly evidence-based. The same article attempted to quantify the risks of cervical manipulation and concluded on the basis of a number of assumptions that the risk of death or serious injury was in the order of less than 1/500 000–1 000 000 manipulations. However, the serious nature of the complications, such as cerebrovascular accident from carotid and vertebral artery dissection, requires that this treatment should not be considered benign.

Manipulation under anesthetic

The principle behind manipulation under anesthetic is that stiff and possibly painful joints are 'freed up' or intra-articular adhesions broken by passive manipulation of the neck unhindered by voluntary or involuntary muscle contraction. A single quality study has considered this treatment in which 21 patients were randomly assigned to receive manipulation and an amnesic dose of diazepam or the diazepam alone. The blinding was well maintained and no differences in postprocedural pain levels were observed between the control and treatment groups[67]. With the small but finite risks of anesthesia, this form of therapy cannot be recommended on the basis of available evidence.

Pillows and posture correction

There is a paucity of reliable data to show that either 'posture correction' or the use of variously profiled pillows helps patients with chronic neck pain. However, these are benign interventions and in the absence of proven efficacious treatment their use may be justified.

Although again lacking empiric clinical trial evidence, the modification of workplace environments and practices to decrease extreme movements of the neck and decrease the amount of time that a fixed cervical posture is maintained are sensible adjuncts to other therapy and have some basis in that extreme cervical postures have been shown to be associated with neck pain in normal individuals.

Specific treatments

Zygapophyseal joints

When a definitive diagnosis of cervical zygapophyseal joint pain has been made, therapy can be targeted at the specific joint. Injection of these joints with corticosteroids has been advocated on the basis of open studies but a randomized controlled trial of corticosteroid injected into painful cervical zygapophyseal joints after whiplash injury has shown no benefit over injections of local anesthetic, with neither group obtaining useful relief[68]. It is not known whether patients whose pain arises spontaneously also fail to respond to intra-articular corticosteroids.

The other treatment modality proposed for cervical zygapophyseal joint pain is denervation of the joint, typically through percutaneous radiofrequency neurotomy of the medial branches of the cervical dorsal rami. Open studies have indicated that such techniques, when correctly performed, result in prolonged pain relief in around 70% of patients whose painful joint is below C2/3 and about 50% of patients with a painful C2/3 joint[69]. These results have been confirmed in a randomized controlled trial that demonstrated prolonged relief of zygapophyseal joint pain following percutaneous radiofrequency neurotomy. The active treatment group had a median duration of pain relief of 263 days, compared with 8 days in the control group[70]. Similar results have been reproduced by other groups[71].

The long-term effects of denervating a cervical zygapophyseal joint are not known but clinical experience on limited numbers of patients has indicated no lasting adverse effects, with the procedure being safely repeated at such time as the pain recurs over periods up to 3 years. Surgical intervention for proven cervical zygapophyseal joint pain has not yet been described.

Discs

The treatment options for proven disc pain are limited. By virtue of their diffuse innervation, they cannot be denervated to control pain in a manner analogous to that for the cervical zygapophyseal joints. Moreover, the exact site of pain production within a painful disc cannot yet be determined so that sclerosing or excising particular disc components is not currently a viable option. The current practice for the treatment of sus-

pected or proven cervical disc pain is cervical disc excision, usually with fusion, carried out from an anterior approach. The rationale for this approach is simple – remove the part that hurts – but empirical efficacy studies on the effects of cervical spine surgery on neck pain are not available. The only studies available are open, non-randomized and constitute retrospective reviews of individual practitioners' experiences[72,73]. Randomized, controlled studies of this operation on patients with proven disc pain are needed. For the time being, physicians contemplating such invasive intervention should ensure that the diagnosis of cervical disc pain is sound and that the patient is made aware of the potential risks of such operations, as well as the uncertainty of response.

Treatment of cervical nerve root compression

Natural history

Fundamental to any consideration of treatment of cervical nerve root irritation is a clear understanding of the natural history. This has recently been reviewed in detail[74]. The majority of patients with cervical radicular pain will have resolution of their pain over a few weeks or months. Over prolonged periods of observation, less than 10% of patients have persisting moderate or severe disablity[75].

Treatment modalities

There are very few interventions that have been shown, unequivocally, to be any better than others in the treatment of cervical nerve root pain. In particular, a three-armed, randomized study failed to show any long-term differences between a cervical collar, physiotherapy or surgery[76]. However, it would appear that any reasonable treatment is better than no intervention, with patients in the treated arms of trials reporting better satisfaction than those in placebo arms. Typical treatments that can be expected to increase patients' perceptions of improvement include physiotherapy, traction, transcutaneous electrical nerve stimulation (TENS), analgesics and isometric exercises. These types of intervention can be applied with the understanding that there is a generally favorable natural history and that there is no evidence for the superiority of any one intervention over any other. The choice therefore hinges upon minimizing harm.

Corticosteroid injections

Corticosteroid injections into the epidural space, either through an interlaminar route or into the root sleeve, have been advocated for radicular pain. No quality data exist but patient series suggested useful responses[74]. However, unpublished and published reports of serious or fatal complications from such procedures suggests that they cannot be advocated at this point in time[77].

Surgery

Surgery has the potential to relieve the compression on the affected nerve root and should therefore be able to 'cure' cervical radiculopathy and pain from cervical nerve root entrapment. However, this does not seem always to be the case. Marshaling the available empirical evidence suggests that, in the acute setting, surgery is likely to improve symptoms faster than conservative measures, without making any long-term difference when compared to conservative treatment. In the chronic arena, surgery is likely to improve symptoms in the majority of patients but is unlikely to effect a 'cure'[74]. In the absence of serious underlying cause of radiculopathy (e.g. tumor, infection), reasonable indications for surgery would include progressive neurological deficit or refractory and disabling pain.

WHIPLASH

Whiplash injuries warrant particular mention in any discussion of neck pain. Whereas there is no doubt that whiplash injuries are a common cause of acute neck pain, there remains vigorous debate about the frequency with which they cause chronic pain.

Biomechanics

Biomechanical studies have demonstrated that the traditional view of hyperextension as the primary event in whiplash is an incomplete and simplistic explanation for the behavior of the cervical spine in rear-end accidents. In particular, it has been found that axial compression and unnatural double curvatures of the cervical spine are important and potentially damaging components of the cervical spine's response to inertial loading. Cadaver experiments have demonstrated that, after rear-end impact, the lower cervical spine is thrust upwards and forwards[78]. The neck is, therefore, compressed from below. The lower cervical segments are extended while the upper segments are relatively flexed. As a result, the cervical spine assumes an S shape during the first 50–75ms. Thereafter, all segments are progressively extended until the head is thrown forwards into extension. Similar observations were reported in experiments in which normal volunteers were studied using high-speed cineradiography during simulated collisions of approximately 5kph[79]. The authors again emphasized the compression imparted to the cervical spine.

A more detailed cineradiographic study of normal volunteers described the motion of individual cervical segments during the extension phase of whiplash[80]. In this study, an individual was subjected to an 8kph impact, which resulted in a 4g acceleration. Again, the initial movement drove the C6 vertebra upwards. As it moved, the C6 vertebra extended underneath the rest of the cervical spine, causing the higher segments to undergo a small initial flexion, of some 2–5° in amplitude, before undergoing extension. The net result of these movements was that the cervical spine assumed an S shape at about 100ms, as lower segments commenced extension while higher segments were still undergoing initial flexion (Fig. 13.10). These movements took place around abnormal axes of rotation, with the pathological axes being higher than normal. As a result, the anterior end of the vertebra separated from the vertebral body below, and posteriorly to the tip of the inferior articular process chiseled into the supporting superior articular process. Subsequently, the cervical spine underwent extension, as described in the classical model. These observations provide a biomechanical substrate for injuries to several structures in the spine, most notably the cervical zygapophysial joints, which seem to be particularly susceptible to damage through uncontrolled rotation through abnormal axes[82].

Pathology

Our understanding of the pathology of whiplash has languished behind that of other spheres of rheumatology, primarily because of the paucity

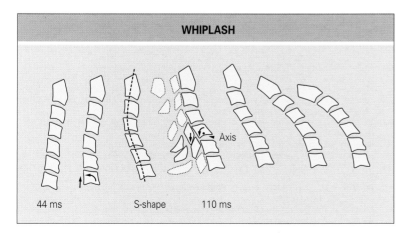

Fig. 13.10 Whiplash. The appearance of sequential radiographs of the cervical spine during the extension phase of whiplash. At 110ms the C5 vertebra rotates about an abnormally high axis of rotation, causing the vertebral body to separate anteriorly from C6 (arrowhead), and the inferior articular process of C5 to chisel into the superior articular process of C6 (arrow). (Redrawn from Barnsley et al.[6], based on Kaneoka et al.[81])

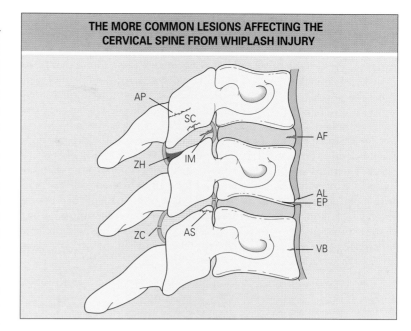

Fig. 13.11 The more common lesions affecting the cervical spine from whiplash injury. AP, articular pillar fracture; AF, tear of the anulus fibrosus of the intervertebral disc; AL, tear of the anterior longitudinal ligament; AS, fracture involving the articular surface; EP, endplate avulsion and/or fracture; IM, contusion of the intra-articular meniscus of the zygapophyseal joint; SC, fracture of the subchondral plate; VB, vertebral body fracture; ZC, rupture of tear of the zygapophyseal joint capsule; ZH, hemarthrosis of the zygapophyseal joint. (Adapted from Barnsley et al.[6])

of pathological material and the generally benign nature of the condition. Simply put, very few people die of whiplash. However, there are a number of pathological entities whose existence has been determined through clinical, animal, cadaveric and postmortem studies[6]. These are summarized in Figure 13.11. Notwithstanding the extent and variety of lesions possible after whiplash, plain radiographs have been shown to be profoundly insensitive to the detection of all but the most severe bony injuries of the cervical spine. A total of 22 cervical spines were harvested from patients who had died of head injuries[83]. The specimens were X-rayed under optimal conditions and the films studied by specialist orthopedic radiologists. They were then sectioned in submillimeter slices and photographed. This revealed 245 injuries to various structures. Only four were detected on plain X-rays, even on a second look.

Natural history

The natural history of whiplash is, for the most part, benign. Most patients recover within a few weeks of injury and have no residual symptoms. It has been argued that apparent differences in the rates of chronicity in whiplash in different countries are evidence that chronic whiplash is a socially programmed phenomenon pivoting on the presence of a compensation system[84]. However, a careful analysis of the data reveals that many of the studies proffered to support this view were compromised by small sample size, poor study design and inappropriate endpoints such as insurance claims rather than clinical information[85,86]. Moreover, competent follow-up studies have revealed that a significant proportion of patients develop chronic symptoms. A series of follow-up studies of an inception cohort of patients assembled in the UK in the early 1980s has been most revealing. They demonstrate that most patients destined to improve do so within a few months, with very little improvement after 2 years. The frequency of chronic symptoms classified as intrusive or severe at 15 years (presumably well after the settlement of any compensation claim) was in the order of 25%[87].

Treatment of acute whiplash injury

Treatment in the acute phase of whiplash is aimed at preventing chronicity, minimizing symptoms and improving function. A recent review of the conservative treatment of acute whiplash found that treatments such as cervical collars, rest and passive physical modalities were generally inferior to programs involving activation, multimodal interventions emphasizing improved function and simple reassurance and encouragement to resume normal activities[88]. A single randomized trial has investigated the use of high-dose intravenous methylprednisolone for the acute management of whiplash injury[89]. Based on the beneficial effect of steroids on spinal cord injury, this study compared the effects of high-dose intravenous methylprednisolone administered over 24 hours with a placebo infusion in 40 patients. Most of the patients had neurological signs and probably represented a more severely injured group than is commonly reported. At 6 months, there was a highly significant difference in the number of sick days taken between the two groups in favor of the treatment group.

Treatment of chronic whiplash

There are very few controlled studies of the treatment of chronic neck pain after whiplash injury. The single most promising avenue has been that of percutaneous radiofrequency neurotomy for chronic cervical zygapophyseal joint pain, described above[70]. This remains a palliative treatment but one that can be highly valuable for patients with constant and debilitating pain. Otherwise, the rather unsatisfactory options for the management of any chronic neck pain, as discussed above, can be applied.

SUMMARY

Neck pain is a common and usually self-limiting disorder but it is important to exclude serious underlying illness and neurological involvement. Future progress in the field of chronic and refractory pain will depend upon reliably identifying the source of pain, typically through invasive analgesic or provocation techniques. Many current treatments are not supported by properly constructed trials.

REFERENCES

1. Bland JH, Boushey DR. Anatomy and physiology of the cervical spine. Semin Arthritis Rheum 1990; 20: 1–20.
2. Penning L. Normal movements of the cervical spine. AJR 1978; 130: 317–326.
3. Makela M, Heliovaara M, Sievers K et al. Prevalence, determinants, and consequences of chronic neck pain in Finland. Am J Epidemiol 1991; 134: 1356–1367.
4. Cote P, Cassidy JD, Carroll L. The Saskatchewan Health and Back Pain Survey. The prevalence of neck pain and related disability in Saskatchewan adults. Spine 1998; 23: 1689–1698.
5. Westerling D, Jonnson BG. Pain from the neck shoulder region and sick leave. Scand J Soc Med 1980; 8: 131.
6. Barnsley L, Lord SM, Bogduk N. The pathophysiology of whiplash. In: Teasell RW, Shapiro A, eds. Spine state of the art reviews. Cervical flexion–extension/whiplash injuries 12: 2. Philadelphia: Hanley & Belfus; 1998: 209–242.
7. Holt L. Frequency of symptoms for different age groups and professions. In: Hirsch C, Zotterman Y, eds. Cervical pain. New York: Pergamon Press; 1971: 17–20.
8. Jacobsson L, Lindgarde F, Manthorpe R, Ohlsson K. Effect of education, occupation and some lifestyle factors on common rheumatic complaints in a Swedish group aged 50–70 years. Ann Rheum Dis 1992; 751: 835–843.
9. Leino P, Magni G. Depressive and distress symptoms as predictors of low back pain, neck-shoulder pain, and other musculoskeletal morbidity: a 10-year follow-up of metal industry employees. Pain 1993; 53: 89–94.
10. Harms Ringdahl K, Ekholm J. Intensity and character of pain and muscular activity levels elicited by maintained extreme flexion position of the lower-cervical–upper-thoracic spine. Scand J Rehabil Med 1986; 18: 117–126.
11. Lawrence JS. Disc degeneration: its frequency and relationship to symptoms. Ann Rheum Dis 1969; 28: 121–138.
12. Frykholm R. The clinical picture. In: Hirsch C, Zotterman Y, eds. Cervical pain. Oxford: Pergamon Press; 1972: 5–16.
13. Macnab I. Whiplash injuries of the neck. Manitoba Med Rev 1966; 46: 172–174.
14. Bring G, Westman G. Chronic posttraumatic syndrome after whiplash injury. A pilot study of 22 patients. Scand J Prim Health Care 1991; 9: 135–141.
15. Bogduk N. Cervical causes of headache and dizziness. In: Grieve G, ed. Modern manual therapy of the vertebral column. Edinburgh: Churchill Livingstone; 1986: 289–302.
16. Bogduk N. Innervation and pain patterns in the cervical spine. Clin Phys Ther 1988; 17: 1–13.
17. Cloward RB. Cervical diskography: a contribution to the etiology and mechanism of neck, shoulder and arm pain. Ann Surg 1959; 150: 1052–1064.
18. Feinstein B, Langton NJK, Jameson RM, Schiller F. Experiments on pain referred from deep somatic tissues. J Bone Joint Surg 1954; 36A: 981–997.
19. Dwyer A, Aprill C, Bogduk N. Cervical zygapophyseal joint pain patterns. I: a study in normal volunteers. Spine 1990; 15: 453–457.
20. Dreyfuss P, Michaelsen M, Fletcher D. Atlanto-occipital and atlantoaxial joint pain patterns. Spine 1994; 19: 1125–1131.
21. Gerber C, Galantay RV, Hersche O. The pattern of pain produced by irritation of the acromioclavicular joint and the subacromial space. J Shoulder Elbow Surg 1998; 7: 352–355.
22. Hassett G, Barnsley L. Pain referral from the sternoclavicular joint: a study in normal volunteers. Rheumatology (Oxford) 2001; 40: 859–862.
23. Stokes M, Young A. The contribution of reflex inhibition to arthrogenous muscle weakness. Clin Sci 1984; 67: 7–14.
24. Capistrant TD. Thoracic outlet syndrome in whiplash injury. Ann Surg 1977; 185: 175–178.
25. Slipman CW, Plastaras CT, Palmitier RA et al. Symptom provocation of fluoroscopically guided cervical nerve root stimulation. Are dynatomal maps identical to dermatomal maps? Spine 1998; 23: 2235–2242.
26. Poletti CE. C2 and C3 radiculopathies: anatomy, patterns of cephalic pain and pathology. APS J 1992; 1: 272–275.
27. Pech P, Daniels DL, Williams AL, Haughton VM. The cervical neural foramina: correlation of microtomy and CT anatomy. Radiology 1985; 155: 143–146.
28. Jónsson H Jr, Cesarini K, Sahlstedt B, Rauschning W. Findings and outcome in whiplash-type neck distortions. Spine 1994; 19: 2733–2743.
29. Van Mameren H, Drukker J, Sanches H, Beursgens J. Cervical spine motion in the sagittal plane (I) range of motion of actually performed movements, an X-ray cinematographic study. Eur J Morphol 1990; 28: 47–68.
30. Penning L, Wilmink JT. Rotation of the cervical spine. A CT study in normal subjects. Spine 1987; 12: 732–738.
31. Sobel JB, Sollenberger P, Robinson R et al. Cervical nonorganic signs: a new clinical tool to assess abnormal illness behaviour in neck pain patients: a pilot study. Arch Phys Med Rehabil 2000; 81: 170–175.
32. Viikari Juntura E, Porras M, Laasonen EM. Validity of clinical tests in the diagnosis of root compression in cervical disc disease. Spine 1989; 14: 253–257.
33. Resnick D. Additional congenital or heritable anomalies and syndromes. In: Resnick D, ed. Diagnosis of bone and joint disorders. Philadelphia: WB Saunders; 1995: 4269–4308.
34. Friedenberg ZB, Miller WT. Degenerative disc disease of the cervical spine a comparative study of symptomatic and asymptomatic patients. J Bone Joint Surg 1963; 45A: 1171–1178.
35. Heller CA, Stanley P, Lewis-Jones B, Heller RF. Value of X-ray examinations of the cervical spine. Br Med J 1983; 287: 1276–1278.
36. Mobic MT, Masyrak TJ, Mulopulos GP et al. Cervical radiculopathy: prospective evaluation with surface coil MR imaging, CT with metrizamide and metrizamide myelography. Radiology 1986; 161: 753–759.
37. Unger E, Moldofsky P, Gatenby R et al. Diagnosis of osteomyelitis by MR imaging. AJR 1988; 150: 605–610.
38. Boden SD, McCowin PR, Davis DO et al. Abnormal magnetic-resonance scans of the cervical spine in asymptomatic subjects. J Bone Joint Surg 1990; 72A: 1178–1184.
39. Davis SJ, Teresi LM, Bradley WGJ et al. Cervical spine hyperextension injuries: MR findings. Radiology 1991; 180: 245–251.
40. Taylor JR, Twomey LT. Acute injuries to cervical joints: an autopsy study of neck sprain. Spine 1993; 9: 1115–1122.
41. Fletcher G, Haughton VM, Khang-Cheng Ho, Shiwei Yu. Age-related changes in the cervical facet joints: studies with cryomicrotomy, MR, and CT. Am J Neuroradiol 1990; 11: 27–30.
42. Murray IP, Frater CJ. Prominence of the C2 vertebra on SPECT. A normal variant. Clin Nucl Med 1994; 19: 855–859.
43. Barnsley L, Lord SM, Thomas P et al. SPECT bone scans for the diagnosis of symptomatic cervical zygapophysial joints. Br J Rheumatol 1993; 32(suppl 2): 52.
44. Dory MA. Arthrography of the cervical facet joints. Radiology 1983; 148: 379–382.
45. Bogduk N, Marsland A. The cervical zygapophyseal joints as a source of neck pain. Spine 1988; 13: 610–617.
46. Bogduk N. The clinical anatomy of the cervical dorsal rami. Spine 1982; 7: 319–330.
47. Barnsley L, Bogduk N. Medial branch blocks are specific for the diagnosis of cervical zygapophyseal joint pain. Regional Anesth 1993; 18: 343–350.
48. Barnsley L, Lord SM, Wallis BJ, Bogduk N. False-positive rates of cervical zygapophyseal joint blocks. Clin J Pain 1993; 9: 124–130.
49. Barnsley L, Lord SM, Bogduk N. Comparative local anaesthetic blocks in the diagnosis of cervical zygapophyseal joint pain. Pain 1993; 55: 99–106.
50. Lord SM, Barnsley L, Bogduk N. The utility of comparative local anaesthetic blocks versus placebo-controlled blocks for the diagnosis of cervical zygapophyseal joint pain. Clin J Pain 1995; 11: 208–213.

51. Barnsley L, Lord SM, Wallis BJ, Bogduk N. The prevalence of chronic cervical zygapophyseal joint pain after whiplash. Spine 1995; 20: 20–26.
52. Speldewinde GC, Bashford GM, Davidson IR. Diagnostic cervical zygapophyseal joint blocks for chronic cervical pain. Med J Aust 2001; 174: 174–176.
53. Simmons EH, Segil CM. An evaluation of discography in the localization of symptomatic levels in discogenic disease of the spine. Clin Orthop 1975; 108: 57–69.
54. Roth DA. Cervical analgesic discography: a new test for the definitive diagnosis of the painful-disk syndrome. JAMA 1976; 235: 1713–1714.
55. Bogduk N, Aprill C. On the nature of neck pain, discography, and cervical zygapophyseal joint blocks. Pain 1993; 54: 213–217.
56. Zeidman SM, Thompson K, Ducker TB. Complications of cervical discography: analysis of 4400 diagnostic disc injections. Neurosurgery 1995; 37: 414–417.
57. Mercer S, Bogduk N. Intra-articular inclusions of the cervical synovial joints. Br J Rheumatol 1993; 32: 705–710.
58. Bogduk N, Windsor M, Inglis A. The innervation of the cervical intervertebral discs. Spine 1988; 13: 2–8.
59. Ohnmeiss DD, Guyer RD, Mason SL. The relation between cervical discographic pain responses and radiographic images. Clin J Pain 2000; 16: 1–5.
60. Kumar R, Berger RJ, Dunsker SB, Keller JT. Innervation of the spinal dura. Myth or reality? Spine 1996; 21: 18–26.
61. Wallis BJ, Lord SM, Bogduk N. Resolution of psychological distress of whiplash patients following treatment by radiofrequency neurotomy: a randomised double-blind placebo controlled trial. Pain 1997; 73: 15–22.
62. Bronfort G, Evans R, Nelson B et al. A randomized clinical trial of exercise and spinal manipulation for patients with chronic neck pain. Spine 2001; 26: 788–799.
63. Tan JC, Nordin M. Role of physical therapy in the treatment of cervical disk disease. Orthop Clin North Am 1992; 23: 435–449.
64. Gross AR, Aker PD, Goldsmith CH, Peloso P. Physical medicine modalities for mechanical neck pain disorders (Cochrane review). In: The Cochrane Library. Oxford: Update Software; 2001.
65. Koes BW, Bouter LM, Van Mameren H et al. Randomised clinical trial of manipulative therapy and physiotherapy for persistent back and neck complaints: results of one year follow up. Br Med J 1992; 304: 601–605.
66. Hurwitz EL, Aker PD, Adams AH et al. Manipulation and mobilization of the cervical spine: a systematic review of the literature. Spine 1996; 21: 1746–1760.
67. Sloop PR, Smith DS, Goldenberg E, Dore C. Manipulation for chronic neck pain: a double-blind controlled study. Spine 1982; 7: 532–535.
68. Barnsley L, Lord SM, Wallis BJ, Bogduk N. Lack of effect of intra-articular corticosteroids for chronic cervical zygapophyseal joint pain. N Engl J Med 1994; 330: 1047–1050.
69. Lord SM, Barnsley L, Bogduk N. Percutaneous radiofrequency neurotomy in the treatment of cervical zygapophyseal joint pain: a caution. Neurosurgery 1995; 36: 732–739.
70. Lord SM, Barnsley L, Wallis BJ et al. Percutaneous radio-frequency neurotomy for chronic cervical zygapophyseal-joint pain. N Engl J Med 1996; 335: 1721–1726.
71. Sapir DA, Gorup JM. Radiofrequency medial branch neurotomy in litigant and nonlitigant patients with cervical whiplash: a prospective study. Spine 2001; 26: E268–E273.
72. Whitecloud TS, Seago RA. Cervical discogenic syndrome. Results of operative intervention in patients with positive discography. Spine 1987; 12: 313–316.
73. Pawl RT. Headache, cervical spondylosis, and anterior cervical fusion. In: Nyhus LM, ed. Surgery annual. New York: Appleton-Century-Crofts; 1977: 391–408.
74. Bogduk N. Medical management of acute cervical radicular pain: an evidence based approach. Newcastle: Newcastle Bone and Joint Institute; 1999.
75. Radhakrishnan K, Litchy WJ, O'Fallon WM, Kurland LT. Epidemiology of cervical radiculopathy. A population-based study from Rochester, Minnesota, 1976 through 1990. Brain 1994; 117: 325–335.
76. Persson LC, Carlsson CA, Carlsson JY. Long-lasting cervical radicular pain managed with surgery, physiotherapy, or a cervical collar. A prospective, randomized study. Spine 1997; 22: 751–758.
77. Brouwers PJ, Kottink EJ, Simon MA, Prevo RL. A cervical anterior spinal artery syndrome after diagnostic blockade of the right C6-nerve root. Pain 2001; 91: 397–399.
78. Grauer JN, Panjabi MM, Cholewicki J et al. Whiplash produces an S-shaped curvature of the neck with hyperextension at lower levels. Spine 1997; 22: 2489–2494.
79. Matsushita T, Sato TB, Hirabyashi K et al. X-ray study of the human neck motion due to head inertia loading. Proceedings of the 38th Stapp Conference, 1994. Society for Automotive Engineers Paper no. 942208: 55–64
80. Human cervical spine kinematics during whiplash loading. Tokyo: 1997.
81. Kaneoka K, Ono L, Inaini S, Hayashi K. Abnormal segmental motion of the cervical spine during whiplash loading. J Jpn Orthop Assoc 1997; 71: S1680.
82. Cusick JF, Pintar FA, Yoganandan N. Whiplash syndrome: kinematic factors influencing pain patterns. Spine 2001; 26: 1252–1258.
83. Jónsson H Jr, Bring G, Rauschning W, Sahlstedt B. Hidden cervical spine injuries in traffic accident victims with skull fractures. J Spinal Disorders 1991; 4: 251–263.
84. Ferrari R, Russell AS. Epidemiology of whiplash: an international dilemma. Ann Rheum Dis 1999; 58: 1–5.
85. Merskey H. Commentary on 'Whiplash in Lithuania'. Pain Res Manag 1997; http://www.pulsus.com/Pain/02_01/mers_ed.htm.
86. Teasell RW, Merskey H. The Quebec Task Force on whiplash-associated disorders and the British Columbia Whiplash Initiative: a study of insurance company initiatives. Pain Res Manag 1999; 4: 141–149.
87. Squires B, Gargan MF, Bannister GC. Soft-tissue injuries of the cervical spine. 15-year follow-up. J Bone Joint Surg 1996; 78B: 955–957.
88. Peeters GG, Verhagen AP, De Bie RA, Oostendorp RA. The efficacy of conservative treatment in patients with whiplash injury: a systematic review of clinical trials. Spine 2001; 26: E64–E73.
89. Pettersson K, Toolanen G. High-dose methylprednisolone prevents extensive sick leave after whiplash injury. A prospective, randomized, double-blind study. Spine 1998; 23: 984–989.

14 Low back pain and lumbar spinal stenosis

David G Borenstein

- Low back pain represents one of the most common symptoms, being second only to the common cold
- The anatomic source of 'mechanical back pain', which accounts for more than 90% of low back pain episodes, cannot be differentiated precisely
- One of the most important roles of the physician is to recognize non-mechanical causes
- Investigations should be limited to the few patients with persistent or progressive pain and those in whom a non-mechanical cause is suspected

INTRODUCTION

Low back pain is a ubiquitous health problem. It represents the most frequent disorder of mankind after the common cold[1,2]. Between 65% and 80% of the world's population develop back pain at some point during their lives. A review of three time periods studied by the National Ambulatory Care Survey in the USA revealed mechanical low back pain as the fifth most common reason (2.8%) for physician office visits. Of these visits, non-specific low back pain was the most frequent diagnostic group at 56.8%[3]. Data from the US Health Interview Survey indicate that impairments of the back and spine are the chronic conditions that most frequently cause activity limitation among people aged 45 years or under and that they represent the third most common reason for impairment in people aged 45–64 years[4].

In some countries the surgical subspecialties of orthopedics and neurosurgery are most frequently associated with low back pain evaluation and treatment, despite the fact that the vast majority of patients do not require surgical intervention. Surgeons evaluate a large number of patients with non-surgical lesions in order to identify the relative few who require back surgery. In the USA, unlike Europe, rheumatologists have concentrated their efforts on the spondyloarthropathies and have shied away from patients with mechanical low back pain. Since they are experts in the conservative management of musculoskeletal disorders, rheumatologists are in many ways the most appropriate physicians to complete the initial and subsequent evaluation of patients with low back pain of any etiology and to plan a treatment program. They constantly use patient education, physical modalities and drug therapy, which are the cornerstones for treatment of back patients.

EPIDEMIOLOGY

Musculoskeletal impairment is the most prevalent impairment in people aged up to 65 years, with back and spine impairments the most frequently reported subcategory at 51.7%[5]. Back and spine impairments are more common in women (70.3 per 1000 population) than in men (57.3 per 1000 population). Caucasians have back pain more frequently than Blacks (68.7 per 1000 versus 38.7 per 1000) respectively. Increasing age is associated with a greater frequency of back pain, ranging from 75.9 to 93.6 per 1000 population in individuals 65 to more than 84 years of age.

Most episodes of back pain are not incapacitating. Over 50% of all patients with back pain improve after 1 week, while more than 90% are better at 8 weeks[6]. The remaining 7–10% continue to experience symptoms for longer than 6 months. However, as many as 75% of individuals who improve are at risk of having a relapse of back pain in the next 12 months[7]. The high costs associated with low back pain are related to these individuals with chronic pain. For example, the US estimated cost of industrial claims for low back pain in 1995 was US$8.8 billion despite a decrease in the number of claims[8]. Frymoyer has estimated that the direct cost of back pain in the USA in 1990 was over US$27.6 billion[9].

Many risk factors described for back pain involve occupational or psychologic characteristics. Occupational factors include jobs that require lifting beyond the worker's physical capabilities, or in an awkward position. Workers involved in heavy duty labor who are aged over 45 years have a 2.5 times greater risk of absence from work secondary to back pain than workers aged 24 years or younger[10]. Those individuals with an initial episode of back pain lasting 3 months or more have a risk for recurrence of 26.7% in the year following an initial pain episode versus 19.9% for an initial episode of 1 day's duration[11].

A number of psychologic conditions are associated with back pain. Neurosis, hysteria and conversion reaction are more frequently associated with acute back pain than depression[12]. Depression is a frequent complication of patients who develop chronic low back pain, although psychological distress predisposes to both a new episode and chronicity. Cigarette smoking is associated with an increased risk of back pain, although the data are inconsistent[13]. Although obesity is a minor factor in the causation of back pain, excessive weight facilitates perpetuation of episodes[14].

As many as 90% of patients with back pain have a 'mechanical' reason for their pain[15]. Mechanical low back pain implies that pain is secondary to overuse of a normal anatomic structure, to trauma or to deformity of an anatomic structure. Frequently, however, no such trauma or deformity can be identified with certainty. The remaining 10% of adults with back pain have the symptom as a manifestation of a systemic illness[16]. Over 70 non-mechanical illnesses may be associated with back pain[17]. Careful clinical evaluation helps separate patients with mechanical back pain from those with non-mechanical back pain.

CLINICAL EVALUATION

The evaluation of a patient with low back pain requires an organized and thoughtful approach that should be tailored to the specific complaints of the patient. In rare circumstances, a patient's symptoms and signs can be related to an identifiable pathologic process involving a specific anatomic structure. In these cases, specific therapy can be given. However, in most cases, the offending anatomic structure, be it bone, muscle, ligament, fascia or disc, cannot be identified as the specific source of back pain. Fortunately, the natural history of the symptom is resolution, frequently over a short period of time, so all interventions seem to work, whether it is limitation of activity, over-the-counter medications, temperature modalities or the therapies of alternative practitioners such as chiropractors. Although the diagnostic process is inexact for many patients, it nevertheless remains essential to identify a specific abnormality.

The physician plays an essential role in the evaluation and treatment of low back pain patients and their recovery. The very nature of the interaction of a person and a physician makes that individual view themselves as being sick. The physician may encourage this behavior by evaluating or treating an individual in too aggressive a manner. This may be a particular problem for individuals who have been injured at work. It is essential for the physician to downplay 'illness behavior' in these patients. Patients with low back pain need to be encouraged to resume normal activities as soon as possible and to be constantly reminded that the vast majority of individuals improve over a 2–3-week period.

HISTORY

The clinical history is an essential step in evaluating patients with low back pain. Certain disorders occur more commonly in younger individuals while others are associated with older patients (Fig. 14.1). The sex of the patient may also help select potential causes of low back pain (Table 14.1).

The duration and location of pain help inform the subsequent kinds of questions. Mechanical low back pain tends to have an onset associated with a physical task and is usually of short duration (days to weeks). Medical causes of low back pain tend to have a more gradual onset with no identifiable precipitating factor. These causes of low back pain are frequently present from weeks to months. Most back pain is limited to the lumbosacral area of the low back. Radiation of pain in the thighs or to the knees may be related to referred pain from elements of the spine (muscle, ligaments or apophyseal joints). Pain that radiates from the low back to below the knees is usually neurogenic in origin and suggests a pathologic process affecting spinal nerve roots.

Current episode

Most of the time spent in obtaining the clinical history is used to elucidate the factors that affect the pain. The history is directed towards understanding the chronological development of low back pain, its character and its response to therapy. The anatomic structures of the lumbosacral spine receive specific types of sensory innervation that are associated with distinct qualities of pain. The major categories of pain are superficial somatic, deep somatic (spondylogenic), radicular, neurogenic, visceral-referred and psychogenic (Table 14.2).

TABLE 14.1 SEX PREVALENCE OF LOW BACK PAIN CONDITIONS		
Male predominant	Spondyloarthropathies	
	Vertebral osteomyelitis	
	Benign and malignant neoplasms	
	Paget's disease	
	Retroperitoneal fibrosis	
	Peptic ulcer disease	
	Work-related mechanical disorders	
Female predominant		Polymyalgia rheumatica
		Fibromyalgia
		Osteoporosis
		Parathyroid disease
Equal frequency		Inflammatory bowel disease
		Pituitary disease
		Subacute bacterial endocarditis

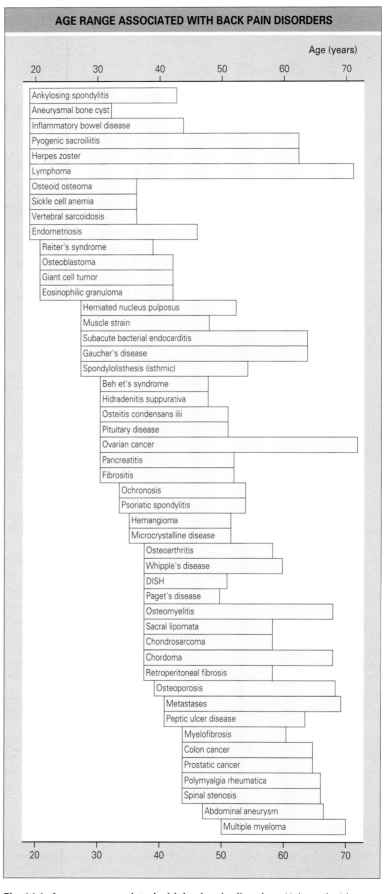

Fig. 14.1 **Age range associated with back pain disorders.** (Adapted with permission from Borenstein *et al.*[17]).

TABLE 14.2 CATEGORIES OF LOW BACK PAIN

Category	Source/pathologic entity	Quality
Superficial somatic	Skin, subcutaneous tissues (cellulitis)	Sharp, burning
Deep somatic	Muscles, fascia, periosteum, ligaments, joints, vessels, dura (arthritis)	Sharp, dull ache, boring
Radicular	Spinal nerves (herniated disc, spinal stenosis)	Radiating, shooting, tingling
Neurogenic	Mixed motor sensory nerves (femoral neuropathy)	Burning
Visceral-referred	Abdominal viscera, pelvic viscera, aorta (autonomic sensory nerves)	Boring, colicky, tearing
Psychogenic	Cerebral cortex (conversion reaction, malingering)	Variable

- **Superficial somatic pain** is associated with disorders that affect the skin and subcutaneous tissues. These tissues are well innervated by cutaneous A fibers that cover very small fields. Pathogenic processes in these tissues cause sharp or burning pain.
- **Deep somatic pain** has its source in the vertebral column, the surrounding muscles and the attaching tendons, ligaments and fascia. These structures are supplied by the sinuvertebral nerves and the unmyelinated pain fibers of the posterior primary rami of the spinal nerves. Deep somatic pain is characterized by a deep, dull ache that is maximal over the involved site and often radiates into the thighs but rarely below the knees. Acute injury to these tissues is associated with a sharp stab of pain at the moment of injury followed by a dull ache that may persist for weeks and may be associated with tenderness on palpation and reflex muscle spasm.
- **Radicular pain** is related to involvement of the proximal spinal nerves with inflammation, or any processes that decrease blood flow to the nerve. This type of pain is lancinating, shooting, burning, sharp and tender in quality and radiates from the low back to the lower extremity in the distribution of the compromised spinal nerve. In addition to the shooting pain, aching and spasm may be experienced in the thigh and calf muscles.
- **Neurogenic pain** results from involvement of the sensory portion of a peripheral nerve. Diabetic neuropathy is a good example. This type of pain is described as burning, tingling, crushing, gnawing or skin-crawling and tends to be sustained in most circumstances.
- **Visceral-referred pain** arises from abnormalities in organs that share segmental innervation with the lumbosacral spine. The back pain may be described as gripping, cramping, aching, squeezing, crushing, tearing, stabbing or burning, depending on the affected organ. The wider distribution of viscerogenic pain differs from the more precise localization of somatic pain.
- **Psychogenic pain** is perceived at the level of the cerebral cortex. It does not follow any dermatomal pattern and may be of any quality. The patient may describe the pain in terms of suffering or punishment. Terms used in this circumstance might include 'being hit' or 'being burned with a red hot poker'[18]. In most circumstances, psychogenic pain is resistant to all therapies. Patients who suffer from depression, hysteria or conversion reaction tend to exhibit psychogenic pain.

In addition to the quality of pain, elucidating factors that aggravate and alleviate pain is helpful in defining potential sources for the symptom. Typically, mechanical disorders worsen with activity, including prolonged sitting and standing, and improve with recumbency.

While some patients with medical disorders that affect the spine, such as compression, or pathologic fractures or acute infection, may also find relief of their pain with recumbency and even complete immobility, most find no association with body position. Exceptions include patients with a spondyloarthropathy, who classically report increased pain and stiffness when they remain in bed for a few hours; patients with tumors that involve the structures of the lumbar spine, who are worse with

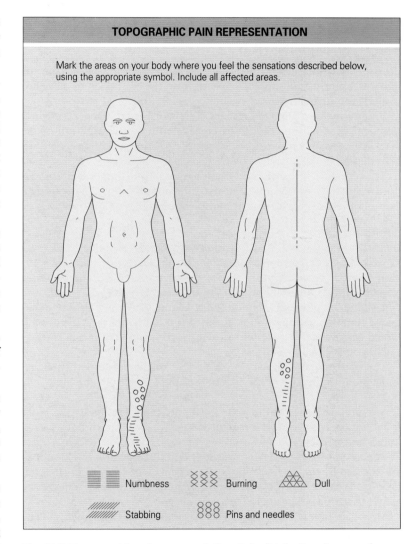

TOPOGRAPHIC PAIN REPRESENTATION

Mark the areas on your body where you feel the sensations described below, using the appropriate symbol. Include all affected areas.

Numbness   Burning   Dull

Stabbing   Pins and needles

Fig. 14.2 Topographic pain representation. Pain distribution diagram of a patient with radiculopathy secondary to a lumbar intervertebral disc herniation.

recumbency; and patients with viscerogenic pain, in whom moving around trying to achieve a comfortable position is characteristic.

The severity of pain may be measured by a number of means. Patients may fill in a diagram with the location, quality and severity of pain (Fig. 14.2). These diagrams are a way of documenting the extent of pain involvement and subsequent response to therapy.

Family and social history

Familial predisposition does occur in certain medical illnesses associated with back pain. Of particular importance is the group of illnesses that cause spondyloarthropathy.

Occupational and social history is important for identifying those patients at risk of developing mechanical low back pain. The association of work and the onset of pain is important in regard to compensation. The patient's opinion about the association of the pain and their work must be determined as well as their expectation of work-related sickness payments for injury and return to work[19].

Past medical history

In most circumstances, past medical history and a review of systems add little additional information. Previous history of malignancy, arthritis or metabolic bone disease may be significant. The review of systems may identify the patient who has a systemic disorder causing back pain but does not realize the association between the two (skin rash and spondyloarthropathy).

PHYSICAL EXAMINATION

In patients with a history suggestive of mechanical low back pain, the physical examination should concentrate on the evaluation of musculo-skeletal and neural tissues of the lumbosacral spine.

When a medical cause of low back pain is suspected, a general medical physical examination should be completed before evaluation of the back. Changes in various organ systems (e.g. skin, ocular, gastrointestinal) may be noted in patients with medical low back pain.

The objective of the physical examination of the lumbosacral spine is to demonstrate those static and dynamic abnormalities that can help sort out the disease entities that may be responsible for low back pain.

Standing

The patient stands undressed, facing away from the examiner. The spine is viewed for curvatures and postural deformities. A list is present if the first thoracic vertebra is not centered over the sacrum. The posterior superior iliac spines should be of equal height. The gluteal folds and knee joints should be at identical levels. Laterally, hyperlordosis or a flattened lumbosacral curve may be identified, while marked kyphosis is noted best from this position. Anteriorly, the shoulders and iliac wings should be of equal height.

The patient should squat in place. This maneuver tests the general strength and integrity of the function of the joints from the hip to the toes.

The muscle power of the lower extremity can be tested by toe raises standing on both feet. The patient is asked to rise up on both feet 10 times followed by a further 10 times on each foot independently. This test measures first sacral root function. Fifth lumbar root function may be assessed by the Trendelenburg test. The patient is asked to stand on one leg. Weakness of hip abduction is highlighted by the sagging of the pelvis to the side opposite to the affected leg.

Spinal motion is important in terms of symmetry and rhythm. The patient is asked to flex, extend and laterally bend the lumbosacral spine. As the patient bends forwards, it is important to observe the quality of spinal flexion in terms of the smooth reversal of the normal lumbar lordosis as the spine flexes forwards. Patients with localized mechanical disorders maintain the lordosis while bending from the hips when asked to flex forwards. Patients with injuries in musculoskeletal structures at the L4/5 and L5/S1 interspaces will experience abnormal motion secondary to protective muscle contraction.

After full flexion, it is helpful to observe how the patient regains the erect posture. Patients with back lesions return to the erect position utilizing a fixed lordosis and rotating the pelvis with the help of knee and hip flexion. Pain that increases with forward flexion suggests an abnormality in the anterior elements of the spine, including discogenic disease.

The patient should then be asked to extend the spine while limiting movement of the hip or knee. Pain that is increased by extension sug-gests disease in the posterior elements of the spinal column, including the apophyseal joints.

The exact source of pain with lateral bending is difficult to determine. Pain that is elicited on the same side as the bending motion suggests an apophyseal joint origin for the discomfort. Pain that is produced in a paraspinous location on the side opposite to the lateral bending motion may be of muscular, ligamentous or fascial origin. Spinal rotation is best examined when the patient is seated.

Bending forward over a table

Palpation of the spine and surrounding tissues with the back supported by the arms is possible with the patient bent forwards over a table. Palpation detects local tenderness, increased muscle tone or bony defects over the spinous processes. Sacroiliac tenderness may be elicited with direct percussion over these joints.

Kneeling

The ankle reflex is best determined in the kneeling position. It may also be elicited with the patient seated on the examining table.

Seated on a chair

Dorsiflexion power of the foot, a fifth lumbar nerve root function, is best tested by seating the patient on a chair and pushing down on the patient's foot with the heel on the floor. The maneuver should be continued for a minute to allow for detection of weakness in the muscle. Patients who feign weakness may either resist pressure for a few seconds and then release the muscle suddenly or in a manner resulting in a 'cogwheel' effect. Function of the L5 nerve root may also be tested by asking the patient to dorsiflex the large toe of the foot.

Seated on the examining table

Reflexes may be elicited when the patient is seated on the examining table. The knee reflex reflects the integrity of the L4 nerve root. Asymmetry of the reflexes should only be accepted if the abnormality persists on repeated testing.

In the seated position, the plantar response may be tested by lifting the straight leg and stroking the lateral aspect of the foot. Patients with radicular abnormalities will experience pain down the leg below the knee to the ankle or foot. Patients will also lean backwards to minimize the traction on neural elements (tripod sign). Patients with hamstring tightness will experience thigh pain but no pain radiation below the knee. A Babinski reflex (extension of the large toe and spreading of the other toes) should be plantar, since the spinal cord conus is situated at L1/2 level.

Hip flexor strength is tested by asking the patient to lift the thigh off the examining table. Downwards pressure by the examiner helps distinguish differences in strength from side to side.

Lying supine

The supine position is excellent for testing the status of the nerve roots, peripheral nerves and hip joints. A neurologic abnormality will give objectivity to a patient's subjective complaints. Any compression or traction on the dura surrounding a nerve will compress its contents and encroach upon the nerve and its blood supply. With inflammation of the nerve, pain is produced along the course of the peripheral nerve causing dysesthesias, motor weakness and decreased reflex function associated with the affected nerve root. Of the possible neurologic abnormalities, persistent muscle weakness is the most reliable indicator of persistent nerve compression with loss of nerve conduction[20]. Sensory findings are less reliable since they are affected by the state of fatigue and emotional state of the patient. Reflex changes are also not as reliable as motor function. Previous episodes of nerve compression may cause a loss of reflexes, which may not return even with recovery of motor and sensory function[21]. Older individuals may lose reflex function, particu-

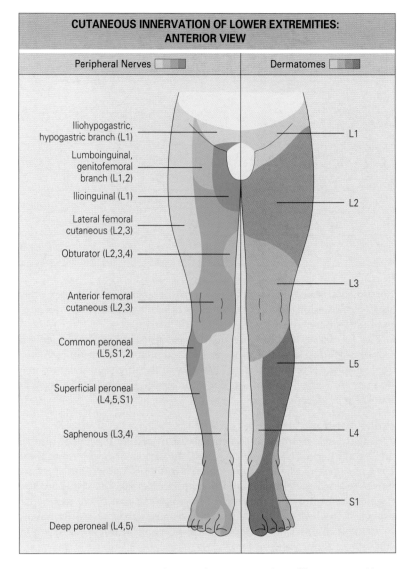

CUTANEOUS INNERVATION OF LOWER EXTREMITIES: ANTERIOR VIEW

Peripheral Nerves | Dermatomes

Iliohypogastric, hypogastric branch (L1)
Lumboinguinal, genitofemoral branch (L1,2)
Ilioinguinal (L1)
Lateral femoral cutaneous (L2,3)
Obturator (L2,3,4)
Anterior femoral cutaneous (L2,3)
Common peroneal (L5,S1,2)
Superficial peroneal (L4,5,S1)
Saphenous (L3,4)
Deep peroneal (L4,5)

L1
L2
L3
L5
L4
S1

Fig. 14.3 Cutaneous sensory innervation. Anterior view of lower extremities illustrating skin areas supplied by nerve roots (right) and peripheral nerves (left).

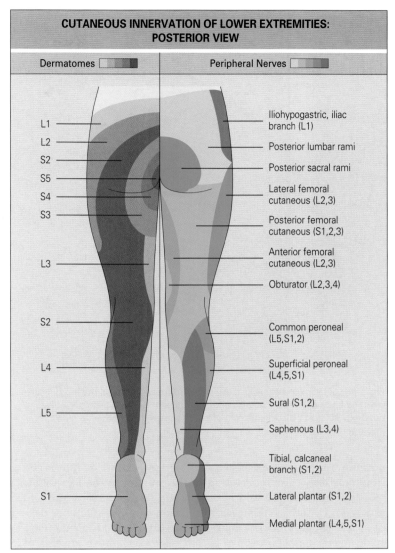

CUTANEOUS INNERVATION OF LOWER EXTREMITIES: POSTERIOR VIEW

Dermatomes | Peripheral Nerves

L1
L2
S2
S5
S4
S3
L3
S2
L4
L5
S1

Iliohypogastric, iliac branch (L1)
Posterior lumbar rami
Posterior sacral rami
Lateral femoral cutaneous (L2,3)
Posterior femoral cutaneous (S1,2,3)
Anterior femoral cutaneous (L2,3)
Obturator (L2,3,4)
Common peroneal (L5,S1,2)
Superficial peroneal (L4,5,S1)
Sural (S1,2)
Saphenous (L3,4)
Tibial, calcaneal branch (S1,2)
Lateral plantar (S1,2)
Medial plantar (L4,5,S1)

Fig. 14.4 Cutaneous sensory innervation. Posterior view of lower extremities illustrating skin areas supplied by nerve roots (left) and peripheral nerves (right).

larly in the ankles. The loss of reflexes is then symmetric. Patients who lose reflex function in both lower extremities acutely on the basis of compression have impingement of the cauda equina.

Upper motor neuron and peripheral nerve abnormalities may also cause neurologic dysfunction. Patients with upper motor neuron dysfunction develop muscle spasticity, hyper-reflexia and a Babinski reflex. Sensory and motor abnormalities associated with peripheral nerve injuries depend on the location of the damaged nerve. An injury to a single nerve root may have little effect on motor or cutaneous function if the area is supplied by nerves from multiple levels. However, if a peripheral nerve is injured, a specific muscle may become paralyzed or specific skin areas become anesthetic (Figs 14.3 & 14.4) The distinction between upper motor, nerve root and peripheral nerve lesions is essential for the differential diagnosis of back pain. Different disease processes preferentially affect upper motor (multiple sclerosis), nerve root (disc herniation) or peripheral nerve (diabetes).

The straight-leg-raising test detects irritation of the sciatic nerve (L4, L5, S1). The passive raising of the leg by the foot with the knee extended stretches the sciatic nerve, its nerve roots and dural attachments (Fig. 14.5). When the dura is inflamed and stretched, the patient will experience pain along its anatomic course to the lower leg, ankle and foot. Dural movement starts at 30° of elevation. Pain of dural origin

should not be felt below that degree of elevation. Pain is maximum between 30° and 70° of elevation. Symptoms at greater degrees of elevation may be of nerve root origin but may also be related to mechanical low back pain secondary to muscle strain or joint disease[22]. Dorsiflexion of the foot will exacerbate the radicular pain. Pain may also be experienced in the leg below the knee when the contralateral normal leg is raised. The presence of contralateral pain suggests a large central lesion in the spinal canal causing traction on the opposite nerve root when the normal leg is raised. The crossed straight-leg-raising test is insensitive but highly specific[23].

In the supine position, leg lengths should be measured to document discrepancies. The hip joints should be moved through their range of motion. Differentiation of hip pain from sacroiliac joint pain may be determined by the Patrick or 'faber' (**f**lexion, **ab**duction, **e**xternal **r**otation) test.

Neurologic function may be tested with the patient in the supine position. The sensory, motor and reflex functions of the lumbar spine and lower extremities should be assessed.

It is useful to measure muscle strength on a five-point scale for: extension and flexion (knee); abduction and adduction (hip); and eversion and inversion and dorsiflexion and plantar flexion (foot). When testing muscle power, the intervening joints should be in a neutral position. Pressure is applied by the examiner to a non-articular structure for a

SCIATIC STRETCH TEST

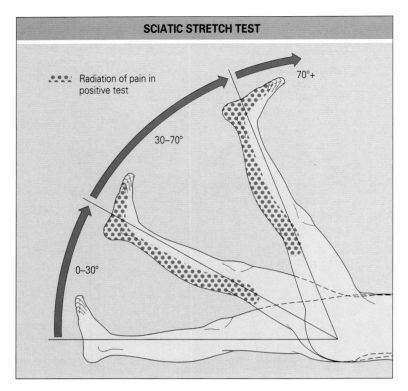

Fig. 14.5 Sciatic stretch test. In the straight-leg-raising test, the leg is lifted with the knee extended. Sciatic roots are tightened over a herniated disc between 30° and 70°. Dorsiflexion of the foot increases pain with nerve impingement

minimum of 5 seconds. When feasible, both sides should be tested simultaneously. The innervation of the muscles to the legs follows a sequential pattern. L2 and L3 supply hip flexion and L4 and L5 hip extension; L3 and L4 supply knee extension and L5 and S1 knee flexion; L4 and L5 supply ankle dorsiflexion and S1 and S2 ankle plantar flexion; ankle inversion is a function of L4 and ankle eversion is a function of L5 and S1 (Table 14.3).

Tender motor points are important diagnostically and prognostically. Motor points represent the main neuromuscular junctions for the involved muscle groups and are constant for an individual patient. Patients with tender motor points remain symptomatic for longer than do those without[24].

Function of the three most commonly affected nerve roots should be tested in both the supine and prone positions (Table 14.4). When S1 is compressed, the gastrocnemius becomes weak. The Achilles reflex (ankle jerk) is diminished or absent, and atrophy of the calf is present if the nerve compression is chronic. The posterior calf and lateral side of the foot may have decreased sensation (S1 distribution).

Compression of L5 leads to weakness in the extension of the large toe and, less completely, in the everters and dorsiflexors of the foot. The sensory deficit associated with L5 is noted over the anterior tibia and the

TABLE 14.3 MOTOR INNERVATION OF THE LOWER EXTREMITIES

Region	Backward	Forward
Hip	L4, L5 extension	Flexion L2, L3
Knee	L5, S1 flexion	Extension L3, L4
Ankle	S1, L2 plantarflexion	Inversion L4 Dorsiflexion L4, L5 Eversion L5, S1

TABLE 14.4 LUMBAR ROOT LESIONS

Root	Muscle weakness/movement affected	Tendon reflex decreased
L2	Hip flexion/adduction	
L3	Hip adduction Knee extension	Knee jerk
L4	Knee extension Foot inversion/dorsiflexion	Knee jerk
L5	Hip extension/abduction Knee flexion Foot/toe dorsiflexion	
S1	Knee flexion Foot/toe plantar flexion Foot eversion	Ankle jerk
Cutaneous, motor and reflex functions of the lower extremity.		

dorsomedial aspect of the foot down to the great toe. No reflex other than the posterior tibial reflex, which is difficult to obtain, is associated with the L5 nerve root.

The L4 nerve supplies the quadriceps muscles of the upper leg. Quadriceps muscle weakness, demonstrated in knee extension, is associated with L4 nerve compression. Atrophy of the thigh musculature may be marked. Sensory loss affects the anteromedial aspect of the leg. The patellar tendon reflex is lost.

Prone position

The neurologic examination is completed by testing for higher lumbar and sacral nerve root function. Dural irritation of nerve roots from L2–L4 are tested by the femoral stretch test (Fig. 14.6). With the knee bent, the thigh is elevated from the examining table. The test is positive if pain is reproduced in the front of the thigh (L2 and L3) or the medial aspect of the leg (L4). Gluteus maximus strength is tested by having the patient contract the buttocks. Asymmetry of contraction or atrophy suggests an abnormality of S1.

Upper and lower sacral roots are tested by sensory examination of the skin over the lower legs, buttocks and perineum. If a patient has saddle anesthesia, a positive straight-leg-raising test in both legs and abnormal sphincter tone, a cauda equina compression syndrome should be suspected.

FEMORAL LEG STRETCH

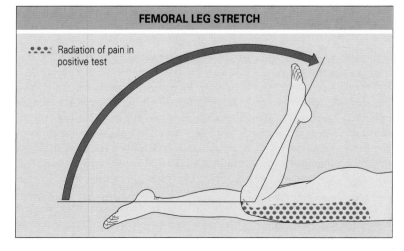

Fig. 14.6 Femoral leg stretch. In the femoral stretch test, the knee is flexed and lifted superiorly. Sharp pain generated in the anterior thigh is considered to constitute a positive test.

Other systems

The final part of the evaluation involves the genital and rectal examinations. This part of the examination is completed in patients who have symptoms and signs suggestive of medical low back pain. These examinations are helpful in detecting patients with prostatic abnormalities, rectal cancer or endometriosis.

A number of ancillary physical examination tests may be used to confirm abnormalities discovered during the routine examination. These tests are listed in Table 14.5.

Non-organic physical signs

Patients who are involved with litigation or claims for work-related sickness payment occasionally exaggerate their symptoms. In these patients,

the objective findings do not match the subjective complaints[25]. Waddell has described five tests that identify individuals with 'functional' or 'exaggerated' symptoms (Table 14.6)[26]. A finding of three or more of the five signs is clinically significant. Isolated positive signs are ignored.

Value of results

Although the physical examination adds essential information for the evaluation of patients with low back pain, problems exist in the reproducibility and significance of abnormal findings. Part of the difficulty in the evaluation of low back pain is the lack of definition for physical signs. McCombe et al. evaluated the reproducibility between three observers of 54 physical signs used for back pain evaluation[27]. The signs that were adequately reproducible included:

- measurements of lordosis (by tape measure from the maximum kyphosis of the thoracic spine to that of the sacrum)
- flexion range (Schober test)
- determination of pain location on flexion and lateral bend
- straight-leg-raising test (pendulum goniometer measurement of the angle at which pain was first experienced and angle of maximum tolerance)
- determination of pain location in the thigh and legs
- sensory changes in the legs.

Nerve root tension signs were reliable if the location of pain was described. Reproducibility of bone tenderness over the sacroiliac joints, spinous processes and iliac crests was greater than that associated with soft tissue structures.

The question of the predictive validity of disturbed sensory and motor function was tested prospectively by Jensen in 52 patients with lumbar disc herniations confirmed at surgery[28]. The positive predictive value of disturbed sensation in the L5 dermatome and weakness of foot dorsiflexion was 76% for herniation from the fourth lumbar disc. The positive predictive value of altered sensation in the S1 dermatome was only 50%.

TABLE 14.5 ANCILLARY TESTS FOR EVALUATION OF LOW BACK PAIN	
Schober test	Lumbosacral motion
Contralateral straight-leg-raising test	Nerve root compression
Bow string sign	Nerve root compression
Hoover test	Patient effort

TABLE 14.6 WADDELL TESTS FOR FUNCTIONAL LOW BACK PAIN	
Tenderness to superficial touch	
Simulation tests	Axial loading
	Spinal rotation in one plane
Distraction tests	Inconsistent results on confirmatory testing
Regional disturbances	Abnormalities not following neuroanatomic structures
Overreaction	Disproportionate verbalization

TABLE 14.7 CLASSIFICATION OF ACTIVITY-RELATED SPINAL DISORDER		
Classification	Symptoms	Working status at time of evaluation
1	Pain without radiation	W (working) I (idle)
2	Pain + radiation to extremity, proximally	
3	Pain + radiation to extremity, distally*	
4	Pain + radiation to lower limb, neurologic signs	
5	Presumptive compression of a spinal nerve root on a simple radiograph (i.e. spinal instability or fracture)	
6	Compression of a spinal nerve root confirmed by: • Specific imaging techniques (CT, myelography or MRI) • Other diagnostic techniques (e.g. electromyography, venography)	
7	Spinal stenosis	
8	Postsurgical status, 1–6 months after intervention	
9	Postsurgical status, >6 months after intervention	
	9.1 Asymptomatic; 9.2 Symptomatic	
10	Chronic pain syndrome	W (working) I (idle)
11	Other diagnosis	

* Not applicable to the thoracic segment.
(Modified from Spitzer et al.[29])

Since it is impossible in most patients to identify the precise anatomic source of the pain, the Quebec Task Force on Spinal Disorders has suggested abandoning non-validated diagnostic terms such as lumbar sprain, lumbar strain, discopathy, facet syndrome and ligamentitis. Instead, they have proposed a simple classification of activity-related spinal disorders in 11 categories, based on history, clinical and paraclinical examinations and response to treatment[29] (Table 14.7).

Most patients with mechanical low back pain may be treated without any specific investigation during the initial visit. On the other hand, patients in whom the history and physical examination suggest a medical cause for their pain will require further diagnostic tests[30].

INVESTIGATIONS

Plain radiographs

A plain radiograph of the lumbar spine is not a necessary part of the initial evaluation of patients with back pain unless they have a history of major trauma, or acute constitutional symptoms. The Quebec Task Force on Spinal Disorders suggested that, without neurologic dysfunction, plain radiographs should not be done during the first week of an acute episode of back pain[30].

Plain radiographs are associated with a number of drawbacks. Patients with back pain of a mechanical origin frequently have radiographs that are normal. In adults under the age of 50, the yield of unexpected findings can be as low as 1 in 2500[15]. In addition, many individuals with radiographic abnormalities may be entirely asymptomatic[31]. Thus, congenital abnormalities, including spina bifida, transitional vertebrae, Schmorl's nodes and mild scoliosis, are only rarely causes of back pain[32]. In those over 50 the prevalence in the normal population of radiographic change is very high: 67% of normal individuals have evidence of intervertebral disc degeneration, of whom two-thirds are asymptomatic. In addition osteoarthritis of apophyseal joints noted on radiographs is not closely correlated with symptoms[33]. Conversely, abnormalities confirmed at operation are not identified by plain radiographs. In one study, plain radiographs failed to identify two-thirds of those who at surgery were found to have disc protrusion[34].

When abnormalities are found, radiologists may disagree over the clinical significance of the findings[35]. It is perhaps not surprising that in a review of 35 studies there is a wide reported range in the strength of associations between non-specific low back pain and radiographic abnormalities on plain X-ray, degeneration, in the form of disc space narrowing, sclerosis and osteophytes[36]. The findings of spondylolysis, spondylolisthesis and spina bifida were not associated with back pain. Plain radiographs deliver a significant amount of radiation to the skin and lumbar spine and add a significant cost to the initial evaluation of patients[37].

When lumbar radiographs are obtained, a single lateral film may be adequate (Fig. 14.7). Padley et al. reviewed lumbosacral spine radiographs of 200 patients with back pain and no neurologic signs[38]. The single lateral film was as satisfactory diagnostically as a three-film series. The single projection had the added benefit of reduced cost and exposure of the patient to radiation. Others have suggested that anteroposterior and lateral views are adequate for evaluation[39,40]. The coned lateral view of the lumbosacral junction and oblique views do not identify therapeutically important lesions that cannot be seen on the other views[41].

Plain radiographs may be recommended for patients who have a systemic medical illness such as an inflammatory arthropathy, infection, tumor or significant fractures. The clinical practice guidelines issued in the USA for the Agency for Health Care Policy and Research (AHCPR) for acute low back pain have recommended that criteria for obtaining plain films include older age, recent significant trauma, history of prolonged steroid use, prior cancer, recent infection, fever, drug abuse, unexplained weight loss or pain with recumbency[42]. In a review of these guidelines, Suarez-Almazor et al. reported that the recommendation for X-ray based upon older age alone may be insufficiently specific resulting in excessive use of radiographs during the initial visit. The use of criteria of failure to respond to therapy and signs of systemic illness is more cost-effective[43].

Radionuclide bone scintigraphy

Bone scintigraphy is of limited utility in low back pain patients. Bone scintigraphy detects increased bone turnover of any etiology. Mechanical and non-mechanical lesions associated with increased bone metabolism will result in a positive scan. Therefore, bone scintigraphy should be used selectively.

Technetium-99m diphosphonate scans are useful in screening for infection, tumors, inflammatory arthritis and fractures[44,45]. The sensitivity of bone scan is generally equal to magnetic resonance imaging (90% versus 96%), but is less specific, for example, in detecting vertebral osteomyelitis (78% versus 92%)[46]. Gallium and indium scans increase the specificity when used with a technetium scan but are less sensitive when used alone[47]. Bone scintigraphy is better than magnetic resonance imaging (MRI) when evaluation of the whole skeleton is required[47]. Patients with metastatic disease may be unaware of bone lesions in other parts of the skeleton (Fig. 14.8). Increased activity in appendicular joints

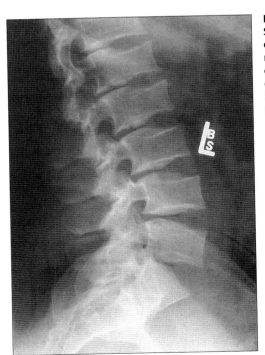

Fig. 14.7
Spondyloepiphyseal dysplasia. Plain radiograph, lateral view, demonstrating elongation of vertebral bodies at multiple levels of the spine.

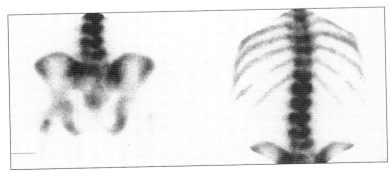

Fig. 14.8 Technetium bone scan. Increased tracer activity throughout the axial skeleton secondary to metastatic prostate cancer.

as well as in axial joints is suggestive of polyarthritis, usually associated with a spondyloarthropathy.

Bone scan is best reserved for the patient with one of the following:

- constitutional symptoms of fever and/or weight loss
- pain with recumbency
- failure to respond to conservative therapy
- abnormal laboratory tests including elevated sedimentation rate or anemia.

Computed tomography

Computed tomography (CT) is useful for evaluating abnormalities of the lumbosacral spine, where the spatial anatomy is complex[48]. CT creates cross-sectional images of the internal structure of the spine at various levels and, with reformatting, can formulate sagittal and coronal images. The CT scan is the best technique for assessing the bony architecture of the spinal column, including the sacroiliac joints, before changes are noted on plain radiographs[49]. In addition, the structural relationships of soft tissues (ligaments, nerve roots, fat, intervertebral discs) can be evaluated as they relate to their bony environment. CT is an excellent technique for identifying mechanical disorders, including spinal stenosis, spondylosis, spondylolisthesis, trauma and congenital anomalies (Fig. 14.9)[50–53]. CT can visualize cortical bone destruction, calcified tumor matrix and soft tissue extension of tumors affecting the spine and is superior to MRI in this regard (Fig. 14.10)[54]. CT can also be used in an outpatient setting for percutaneous needle biopsy guidance of bony lesions[55].

The clinical significance of CT abnormalities must be evaluated in the setting of the patient's clinical findings. In a study of 53 asymptomatic patients with lumbar CT scans, abnormal findings were described in 34.5% of individuals[56]. In patients aged less than 40, 19.5% had a CT diagnosis of an intervertebral disc herniation. In patients aged over 40, 50% had abnormal findings, including disc herniation, spinal stenosis and apophyseal joint degeneration. In addition, there was agreement among the three neuroradiologists in only 11% of the cases. The implication of the study is that a patient with no historical or physical findings indicative of spinal pathology has a one in three chance of having an abnormal CT scan. Surgical intervention cannot be based upon anatomic abnormalities without clinical symptoms and physical signs that correlate with radiographic findings. CT should be used as a confirmatory, not diagnostic, test.

Myelography

Once the only means to identify spinal cord and nerve root compression, myelography has fallen out of favor as a radiographic technique, as

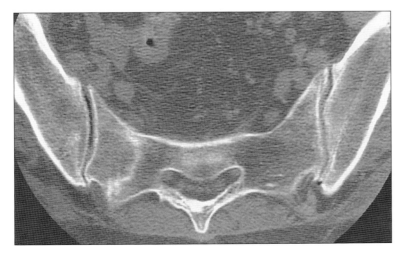

Fig. 14.9 Fracture. CT study of sacral spine demonstrating sacral fracture not visualized with plain radiographs.

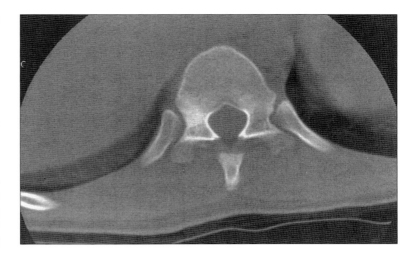

Fig. 14.10 Osteoid osteoma. CT study of thoracic spine demonstrating increased sclerosis associated with an osteoid osteoma.

it is associated with a number of drawbacks. Myelography is an invasive procedure requiring the injection of contrast media through a spinal needle. The procedure requires hospitalization for some patients. All the complications associated with a lumbar puncture may occur with a myelogram (headache, hematoma, infection, back pain and seizures)[57]. However, in combination with CT, myelography is helpful in detecting cord compression caused by fracture and soft tissue impingement associated with tumors. The use of a water-soluble contrast agent, metrizamide, also provides information about the dynamic movement of cerebrospinal fluid. A complete block on myelography conclusively demonstrates pressure on neural elements. Cerebrospinal fluid may be removed for laboratory evaluation[58]. CT enhanced with contrast (CT myelogram) improves the accuracy of postoperative assessment of epidural fibrosis versus recurrent disc[59]. Arachnoiditis may also be evaluated by CT myelography. CT myelography is most helpful for these conditions when patients are unable to undergo MRI evaluation[60].

Like the CT scan, the myelogram should be employed as a confirmatory study. An abnormal myelogram without associated clinical abnormalities is not significant. An abnormal iophendylate myelogram may be identified in 24% of individuals without back pain[61]. The myelogram should be reserved for the preoperative situation to confirm the presence of a damaged disc, a congenitally anomalous nerve root or an unsuspected tumor. Myelography is not as accurate as CT or MRI for the diagnosis of herniated nucleus pulposus that is corroborated at time of discectomy[62].

Magnetic resonance imaging

Magnetic resonance imaging has revolutionized the radiographic evaluation of the lumbosacral spine. MRI has a number of advantages compared to other radiographic techniques. The procedure is non-invasive and uses magnetism and radio waves instead of ionizing radiation to generate its image. It is well tolerated by most patients except for claustrophobic individuals, who may require sedation to remain in the limited confines of the machine. The entire length of the spinal cord and canal may be evaluated in multiple planes. MRI is able to define bony and soft tissue structures without intrathecal contrast. Patients who are not candidates for MRI evaluation include those on life support systems and those who have a cardiac pacemaker, or ferromagnetic clips in the abdomen or on blood vessels. Pacemakers may revert to a fixed rate mode. Metal clips may migrate. Although non-ferromagnetic appliances are not attracted to the magnets, the metal degrades the MRI image.

Many radiologists believe that MRI has become the primary imaging modality for the study of the spine[63]. It is an excellent technique to view

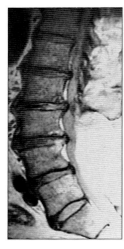

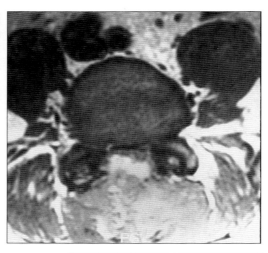

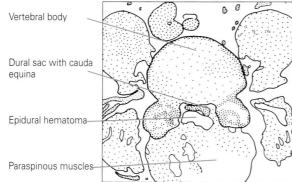

Vertebral body

Dural sac with cauda equina

Epidural hematoma

Paraspinous muscles

Fig. 14.11 Epidural hematoma. Postoperative sagittal and axial MRI studies showing an epidural hematoma compressing the cauda equina.

the spinal cord. It identifies syringomyelia, atrophy, cord infarction, cord injury, multiple sclerosis and intramedullary tumors (Fig. 14.11)[64]. The development of contrast media (gadopentetate dimeglumine) for MRI has improved the characterization of spinal cord tumors[65,66].

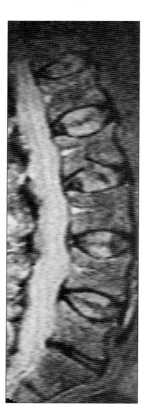

Fig. 14.12 Spinal cord tumor. Lumbar spine MRI study of a multiple myeloma patient with abnormal bone marrow signal throughout the vertebral bodies, associated with remodeling and pathologic fractures.

Contrast-enhanced MRI is able to identify spinal cord pial metastases not visible by other radiographic techniques[67]. MRI delineates the extent of extradural tumor invasion of the spinal canal and compression or displacement of the spinal cord. It can identify the vertebral bodies in which bone marrow has been replaced with tumor (Fig. 14.12)[68,69].

Magnetic resonance imaging is an excellent technique for detecting infection of the spine, including discitis, osteomyelitis, epidural abscess, paraspinal abscess and myelitis[70]. It is more sensitive in the detection of vertebral osteomyelitis than plain radiographs or CT[71]. Changes in the vertebral bodies and adjacent intervertebral disc spaces are visualized on T1-weighted images as areas of low signal intensity. On T2-weighted images, high signal intensity is seen crossing the involved bone and disc space.

Magnetic resonance imaging is also a useful technique for evaluating mechanical disorders of the lumbosacral spine. Disorders of the intervertebral disc are readily detected. Herniations can be identified in the sagittal plane and confirmed on the axial images[72]. Early degenerative changes are revealed by the loss of water, indicated by the darkening of the disc on the T2-weighted image. MRI is also useful in the assessment of traumatic and non-traumatic fractures of vertebral bodies[73].

As with CT and myelography, MRI findings are only significant in patients with correlating clinical symptoms and signs. Boden *et al.* reported on a total of 104 MRI scans of 67 asymptomatic and 37 symptomatic individuals interpreted by three neuroradiologists for abnormalities[74]. The radiologists read 19 of 67 (28%) of the asymptomatic people as having substantial abnormalities. Herniated discs (24%) and spinal stenosis (4%) were the most common findings. Older persons (aged 60–80 years) had the majority of the abnormal findings. Therefore, the finding of an abnormal disc is more reliable in a symptomatic individual less than 60 years of age. Jensen *et al.* completed a MRI study on 98 asymptomatic individuals[75]. Only 36% of these individuals (mean age 42.3 years) had normal results. Some 52% had a disk bulge at one level, 27% had a protrusion and 1% had an extrusion. An abnormality at two levels or more was noted in 38%[75]. Other investigators have reported similar results in different asymptomatic populations[76,77].

Many questions remain over the optimal sequence of radiographic tests for the evaluation of the lumbosacral spine. A consensus agrees that MRI is the most useful technique for lumbar spine imaging. In the diagnosis of herniated discs and spinal stenosis, MRI has a sensitivity equal to or greater than that of CT or myelography[78]. In a study comparing MRI with contrast CT for the diagnosis of herniated disc confirmed at surgery, MRI was associated with 90.3% accuracy while CT had an accuracy rate of only 77.4%[79]. MRI had greater sensitivity (88% accuracy) than myelography (75%) for the diagnosis of herniated discs[80]. It is also accurate in the diagnosis of spinal stenosis. A 96.6% agreement between MRI and contrast CT was identified for 41 patients evaluated for spinal stenosis in the central canal, lateral recess and foramens[81]. In addition, MRI was able to identify disc degeneration in 74 of 123 interspaces while CT identified only 27. Currently, MRI is the technique of choice for investigation of spinal stenosis and disc degeneration. The major limitation on MRI is the cost, which varies, ranging from US$800 to US$1600 if contrast is required.

Other radiographic techniques

A number of other radiographic techniques are available for the evaluation of the lumbosacral spine. They are used infrequently compared to the techniques already discussed.

Spinal angiography permits the identification of the arterial origins and the venous drainage of vascular lesions of the spinal cord and column[82]. Arteriovenous malformations are characterized by arteriovenous communication without an intervening capillary network.

Abnormalities of disc integrity may be missed on plain radiographs and CT scans. Lumbar discography is a procedure associated with the injection

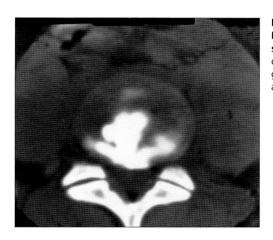

Fig. 14.13 Postdiscography CT scan. A scan demonstrating a painful grade 4 disruption of an anulus fibrosus.

of contrast material through a percutaneous needle into the nucleus pulposus suspected of causing back pain. The reproduction of the patient's pain is considered a positive test (Fig. 14.13). The test is used for patients with a degenerative disc who may be considered for spinal fusion because of persistent pain[83]. Its clinical significance remains controversial[84]. The prevalence and significance of discographic abnormalities continue to be investigated[85]. MRI is equally sensitive in detecting disc degeneration by identifying high intensity zones in an intervertebral disc (Fig. 14.14).[86] However, MRI is unable to reproduce patient symptoms. The role of discography will be decided on its relevance to patient symptoms and the development of better, non-surgical, therapies.

Thermography is a non-invasive procedure that records infrared radiation emitted from body surfaces. Thermographers believe that a close correlation exists between abnormal thermograms and surgically proven herniated discs[87]. However, meta-analysis of 28 studies evaluating the role of thermography in the evaluation of radiculopathy revealed significant methodologic flaws in 27. The one high-quality study found no discriminant value for liquid-crystal thermography[88]. At present thermograms are not recommended for use in the routine decision-making for diagnosis of low back pain patients.

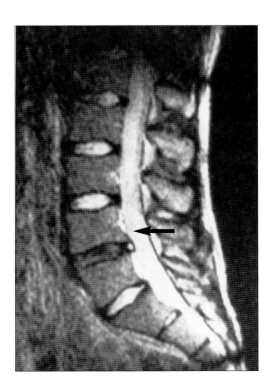

Fig. 14.14 Disc degeneration. MRI demonstrating a high intensity zone lesion (arrow) in the L4/5 intervertebral disc.

CLINICAL LABORATORY TESTS

The vast majority of individuals with low back pain do not require laboratory studies with their initial evaluation. However, patients who are elderly, who have constitutional symptoms or who have failed conservative therapy may benefit from a laboratory evaluation. The most useful test in helping to differentiate medical from mechanical low back pain is measurement of the erythrocyte sedimentation rate (ESR). An elevated ESR suggests the presence of inflammation in the body and, in the appropriate setting, should result in a more thorough evaluation of a patient for a systemic inflammatory disorder. In one study, an ESR of over 25mm/h had a false-positive rate of only 6%[89].

Abnormalities in the complete blood count (hematocrit, leukocyte or platelet count) may be indicative of an inflammatory disorder including neoplasms. Alterations of calcium concentration and alkaline phosphatase activity suggest diffuse bone disease. Elevated acid phosphatase activity may mirror the extent of metastases from prostatic cancer. An urinalysis can identify the individual with renal abnormalities (nephrolithiasis). Detection of occult blood in the stool is a screening test for ulcers or gastrointestinal tumors.

ELECTRODIAGNOSTIC STUDIES

Electrodiagnostic studies are extensions of the neurologic examination and provide a means to identify nerve and muscle damage. These tests can confirm the clinical suspicion of nerve root compression, define the distribution and severity of involvement and document or exclude other illnesses of nerves or muscles that contribute to the patient's symptoms and signs.

Electrodiagnostic tests are most helpful in documenting, objectively, neurophysiologic abnormalities in a patient where clinical examination (pain radiation, sensory changes, muscular weakness) does not necessarily indicate nerve root dysfunction[90]. Neurophysiologic tests can also document normal function where radiographic techniques have revealed anatomic abnormalities.

Electromyography (EMG) is the test most commonly ordered to document the presence of a radiculopathy[91]. Electromyography measures the action potentials of muscle fibers. As the nerve supplying a muscle becomes compressed, fibers to that muscle are lost and are eventually replaced with regenerated fibers. This process of denervation and reinnervation occurs over time (Fig. 14.15). Electromyography may not be able to document abnormalities until 3–4 weeks after the initial insult. Abnormalities associated with radiculopathy can include increased motor unit potentials, fibrillations and prolonged insertional activity. In a partially denervated muscle (the usual occurrence with herniated discs), the remaining axons from unaffected nerve roots grow to innervate more of the muscle fibers. The increase in the number of motor fibers per unit results in an asynchronous and prolonged muscle fiber depolarization. The result is a motor unit potential of longer duration and increased amplitude.

Fibrillations are action potentials that arise from small clusters of denervated healthy muscle fibers awaiting reinnervation. Once present, fibrillations may persist for months. Nerve fibers are damaged when entered by the EMG needle. This damage results in the production of electrical current, referred to as insertional activity. In normal fibers, insertional activity ceases once the needle electrode comes to rest. In radiculopathies, the insertional activity persists for seconds.

As opposed to EMG, nerve conduction tests become abnormal as soon as nerve damage occurs[92]. Nerve conduction tests include evaluation of H-reflex, F-response and somatosensory-evoked responses. The H-reflex is the electrical equivalent of a tendon reflex. It consists of a sensorimotor monosynaptic reflex arc that is measured over the gastrocnemius on stimulation of the posterior tibial nerve in the popliteal fossa. The H-reflex is commonly used for evaluation of S1 radiculopathy and is

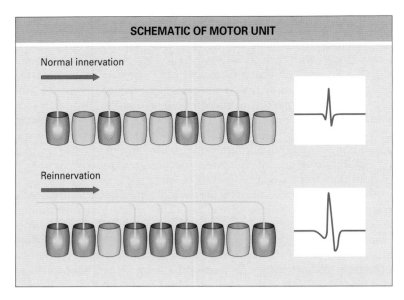

Fig. 14.15 Schematic of motor unit. A normal motor unit with four innervated muscle fibers and, below, reinnervation by terminal sprouting of an undamaged nerve fiber of fibers in a muscle partially denervated. Following reinnervation, corresponding action potentials (shown on the right) have greater duration and amplitude as a result of the increased number of innervated muscle fibers.

associated with a high degree of accuracy[93]. The time latency is standardized for age and the length of the limb. The time difference between the lower extremities should be 2ms or less.

An F-response exclusively measures motor nerve pathways between the point of stimulation and anterior horn cells in the spinal cord. It is not a reflex since no sensory nerves are involved. F-responses may be entirely normal in pure sensory radiculopathies. Unlike the H-reflex, the F-response is variable in latency and must be repeated to average the responses. In addition, many F-responses evaluate nerve roots of multiple levels. Single level radiculopathies may have normal F-responses[94]. F-response is reported as the minimal response or latency time; 2ms is the maximally allowed difference between the extremities.

Somatosensory-evoked responses measure the sensory pathways between the point of stimulation, the spinal cord and the scalp. The most commonly used means of eliciting the response for radiculopathies is stimulation of specific nerves, such as the sural nerve (S1) or superficial peroneal nerve (L5). By standardizing the latency in normal individuals of the same height and leg length, disturbances in nerve conduction can be assessed. Abnormal dermatomal and small sensory nerve responses are correlated with the presence of a radiculopathy[95].

The limitations of electrodiagnostic studies must be considered when evaluating patients with low back pain. These studies do not determine a specific diagnosis. An abnormal EMG is corroborative evidence of organic disease and helps the physician determine who is a potential candidate for surgical intervention. Electromyography changes may recede with resolution of the nerve impingement. However, patients with a good operative decompression with relief of symptoms may have EMG abnormalities persist 1 year after surgery[96]. In patients without neurologic dysfunction, EMG and nerve conduction tests are normal.

DIFFERENTIAL DIAGNOSIS

Most patients with low back pain will improve and will not require additional diagnostic testing. In times of increasing medical financial costs, diagnostic tests must be obtained in a thoughtful and time-efficient manner.

The primary objective for the physician is to return the patient with acute low back pain to regular activity as quickly as possible. Patients who continue with low back pain for 6 months or longer are unlikely to have resolution of pain and rarely return to their usual employment. The effort required to evaluate and treat patients effectively to prevent the evolution into a chronic pain syndrome is worthwhile. In achieving this goal, the physician must be concerned with making efficient and precise use of diagnostic studies, avoiding ineffectual surgery and making therapy available at a reasonable cost.

SYSTEMATIC APPROACH TO LOW BACK PAIN

Most patients with low back pain have a mechanical cause for their symptoms and do not require any diagnostic tests (Table 14.8). Individuals who must be evaluated more intensively are those with life-threatening disorders, such as cauda equina compression or expanding abdominal aneurysms (Fig. 14.16).

Patients with cauda equina compression have a symptom complex that may include low back pain, bilateral sciatica, saddle anesthesia or bladder and bowel incontinence. The most common mechanical causes of cauda equina compression are central herniations of intervertebral discs, while epidural abscesses, epidural hematomas and tumor masses constitute the most frequent non-mechanical causes. Once the diagnosis is suspected, the patient should undergo a radiographic procedure to visualize the affected anatomic area of the lumbosacral spine. MRI is the most sensitive radiographic technique for detecting these lesions. Patients are treated appropriately for their underlying abnormalities. Patients with cauda equina syndrome have the best opportunity for return of neurologic function if the cause of the compression can be eliminated within 48 hours[97].

TABLE 14.8 MECHANICAL LOW BACK PAIN					
	Muscle strain	**Spondylolisthesis**	**Herniated disc**	**Osteoarthritis**	**Spinal stenosis**
Age (years)	20–40	20–30	30–50	Over 50	Over 60
Pain pattern					
Initial location	Back	Back	Back	Back	Leg
Onset	Acute	Insidious	Acute	Insidious	Insidious
Standing	+	+	–	+	+
Sitting	–	–	+	–	–
Flexion	+	–	+	–	–
Extension	–	+	–	+	+
Straight leg-raising	–	–	+	–	+ (stress)
Plain radiograph	–	+	–	+	+

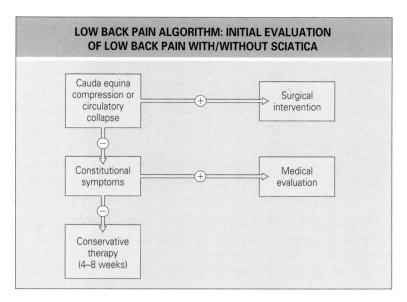

LOW BACK PAIN ALGORITHM: INITIAL EVALUATION OF LOW BACK PAIN WITH/WITHOUT SCIATICA

Fig. 14.16 Low back pain algorithm: initial evaluation of low back pain with/without sciatica.

A patient with tearing or throbbing back pain who has experienced acute dizziness may have an expanding abdominal aneurysm. Any change in the frequency, intensity or location of the pain suggests expansion in the size of the aneurysm. Patients with an abdominal aneurysm are usually older individuals who have had a history of lower extremity claudication. If patients complain of syncope or are hypotensive, they must be evaluated for an aneurysm on an emergency basis. Physical examination of the abdomen may reveal a pulsatile mass, abdominal bruits and decreased pulsations in the lower extremities. Patients with expanding aneurysms may be evaluated with CT or ultrasonography, depending on the patient's hemodynamic status. Patients with an expanding aneurysm require surgical correction of the aneurysmal defect.

Other patients with low back pain who need to be identified before therapy is initiated are those with medical low back pain. They usually present with one of the following:

- fever and/or weight loss
- increased pain on recumbency (sleeping in a chair)
- morning stiffness lasting hours
- acute, localized lumbosacral bone pain
- visceral pain associated with alterations in gastrointestinal or genito-urinary function.

Patients with any of these symptoms should be evaluated thoroughly.

Those without cauda equina syndrome or a medical illness may be started on conservative therapy without a laboratory or radiographic evaluation. One exception to this guideline is older individuals (aged over 50 years) with new-onset back pain. These patients may benefit from a plain radiograph of the lumbar spine and ESR measurement to detect neoplastic or infectious disorders[42].

Conservative management for acute low back pain includes patient education, controlled physical activity, non-steroidal anti-inflammatory drugs (NSAIDs), muscle relaxants or physical therapy. Any or all of these components of conservative management may be used in an individual patient.

The physician should decide on a course of therapy and continue it for a 4–6-week trial. The determination of a specific diagnosis, whether it be a muscular strain of the paraspinous muscles of the lumbar spine or a herniated intervertebral disc, is not important at this stage of the evaluation. The entire population of individuals with low back pain is treated in a similar manner. Some of these may require more elaborate diagnostic tests or more invasive therapy. However, conservative therapy and time is so effective (90% or more recovered at 2 months) that most patients do not require expensive tests or therapies. The opportunity to treat patients in this manner results from the fact that the vast majority of patients have non-radiating low back pain or back strain. The etiology of the pain associated with back strain is unclear. Possibilities include injury to muscle bundles, ligamentous or fascial attachments, mechanical stress associated with poor posture, or tears of the anulus fibrosus, among others. Patients complain of pain with an acute onset, frequently related to some traumatic event that involved excess effort in an awkward position or a contusion. The pain is localized to areas lateral to the midline near the lumbosacral junction. On occasion the pain may radiate across the midline or into the buttocks. On physical examination, patients demonstrate a decreased range of lumbar spine motion, tenderness to palpation over the involved muscle and increased muscle contraction. Laboratory and radiographic evaluations of these patients are normal. Any variation from normal should result in an evaluation for alternative diagnoses.

After 4–6 weeks have passed, patients in whom the initial treatment regimen fails are sorted into four groups, based upon the location and radiation of the residual pain. These groups include those with localized low back pain, leg pain below the knee (sciatica), anterior thigh pain and posterior thigh pain.

Localized low back pain

Patients with localized low back pain make up the largest group with residual pain (Fig. 14.17). Evaluation with plain radiographs of the lumbar spine is indicated, with flexion and extension views if spinal instability is suspected. Spondylolysis, with or without spondylolisthesis, is the most common structural abnormality to cause significant low back pain. Spondylolysis is a break in the pars interarticularis. If the defect permits displacement of one vertebra on another, it is termed a spondylolisthesis (Fig. 14.18). Individuals may have this abnormality without symptoms. Most patients with symptomatic spondylolisthesis

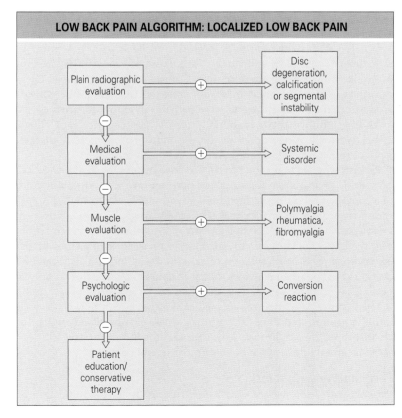

LOW BACK PAIN ALGORITHM: LOCALIZED LOW BACK PAIN

Fig. 14.17 Low back pain algorithm: localized low back pain.

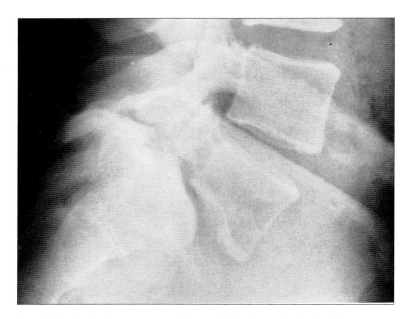

Fig. 14.18 Grade II developmental spondylolisthesis. At the L5–S1 level.

complain of pain when their spine is placed in extension (increased displacement) as opposed to flexion (which tends to normalize vertebral body position). Most patients have a good response to non-operative measures, including patient education, flexion exercises and a flexion back support. A small group will fail conservative management and require a fusion of the unstable segment. The development of progressive intervertebral disc degeneration associated with vacuum phenomenon and vertebral osteophytes at the olisthetic level in the third decade of life coincides with the development of increasing back pain. These individuals are likely to benefit from spinal fusion[98].

Localized low back pain may also be associated with disorders of the intervertebral discs and related apophyseal joints. Abnormalities may be noted on plain radiographic evaluation of the lumbar spine. Decreased disc height and apophyseal joint sclerosis may not cause low back pain. However, articular degeneration with apophyseal joint sclerosis may be associated with decreased back motion and back pain[99]. A point to remember is that older individuals who develop osteoarthritis are also more likely to develop more ominous causes of low back pain. These disorders (e.g. malignancy, infection, osteoporosis) should be considered before the physician ascribes the patient's pain to osteoarthritis.

Another abnormality occasionally seen is disc calcification. This is associated with ochronosis, calcium pyrophosphate dihydrate disease, hemochromatosis, hyperparathyroidism and acromegaly.

Patients who fail to respond to conservative management and who have no specific radiographic abnormalities may improve with a local injection of a combination of an anesthetic and a semisoluble corticosteroid preparation into the area of maximal tenderness. Many patients with local muscle strain experience complete relief of symptoms with the injection. This therapy should be given to individuals who will be compliant with the instructions regarding limitation of activity. These individuals should be cautioned to limit their activities for 24–48 hours to be sure that additional healing has occurred so that usual activities can be resumed.

The histories of patients with medical low back pain may be divided into five groups according to symptoms. These groups include individuals with fever or weight loss, pain with recumbency, morning stiffness, acute localized lumbosacral bone pain or visceral pain.

Fever and/or weight loss

Patients with fever and/or weight loss frequently have an infection or tumor as a cause of their pain. Neoplastic lesions also cause pain with recumbency and will be discussed in the following section.

TABLE 14.9 INFECTIOUS DISORDERS AFFECTING THE LUMBOSACRAL SPINE	
Vertebral osteomyelitis	Bacterial
	Tuberculous
	Fungal
	Spirochetal
	Parasitic
Discitis	
Pyogenic sacroiliitis	
All these may cause localized low back pain	

The clinical presentation of the patient with a spinal infection depends on the infecting organism (Table 14.9). Bacterial infections cause acute, toxic symptoms while tuberculous and fungal infections are indolent. The pain in bacterial infections is persistent, present at rest and exacerbated by motion. Pain radiating to the abdomen or both legs and the presence of abdominal discomfort may confuse the diagnosis. Paraplegia is more closely associated with lesions in the cervical or thoracic spine, but can occur with lumbar infections. Physical findings include decreased range of motion, muscle spasm and percussion tenderness over the involved bone. Plain radiographs may reveal localized areas of osteopenia. If radiographs are normal, technetium bone scintigraphy is indicated. MRI is a sensitive technique with which to investigate the entire lumbosacral spine for the presence of local infection. MRI also detects soft tissue extension of lesions beyond the bony confines of the vertebral column. CT should take place after MRI evaluation to delineate the bony architecture of lesions not visualized adequately by MRI (Fig. 14.19).

Vertebral osteomyelitis follows hematogenous spread from an extraosseous source and can be identified in 40% of patients[100]. Organisms may enter bone from nutrient arteries, or from the venous plexus of Batson, a valveless system of veins that supplies the spinal column. Organisms that cause osteomyelitis include bacteria, mycobacteria, fungi, spirochetes and parasites. The primary sources for spinal infections include the genitourinary tract, respiratory tract and skin. The most frequently encountered organism causing infection in 60% of cases is *Staphylococcus aureus*[101]. Gram-negative organisms are often grown from samples from the elderly and from parenteral drug abusers

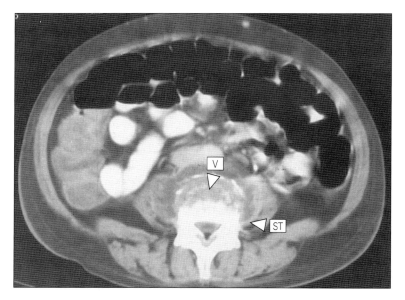

Fig. 14.19 Vertebral osteomyelitis. CT scan, axial view, demonstrating destruction of vertebral body (V) with soft tissue extension (ST) into the paravertebral space.

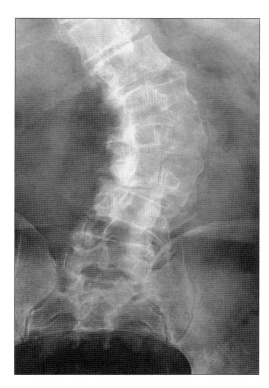

Fig. 14.20 Lumbosacral spine involvement. Pott's disease affecting the lumbosacral spine at L3, resulting in rotatory scoliosis and lateral calcification.

The definitive diagnosis of infection is based on the recovery and identification of the causative organism from blood cultures, or from aspirated material or biopsy of the lesion. Antibiotic therapy is adequate to cure most spinal infections. Surgical intervention for drainage is needed if neurologic dysfunction has occurred secondary to the infection.

Other infections that affect the lumbosacral spine include discitis and pyogenic sacroiliitis. Spondylodiscitis occurs in the setting of concurrent extraspinal infection[106]. Infection of the intervertebral disc space in adults is also associated with lumbar disc surgery. Approximately 3% of lumbar disc surgery patients develop disc space infections[107]. The ESR is almost universally elevated in the case of established disc space infections, often exceeding 100mm/h along with a leukocytosis[108]. Plain radiographs may be normal at the onset of infection but will demonstrate increasing destruction with prolonged duration of infection (Fig 14.21). Radiographic evidence of established disc infection includes:

- symmetric destruction of adjacent end plate surfaces of two vertebrae
- loss of disc height
- reactive new bone formation
- sclerosis of bone endplates, with or without evidence of bone destruction or bone formation
- soft tissue abscesses
- kyphosis or subluxations after there has been significant bone destruction.

On CT, changes in disc space and vertebral endplates can be seen, as can soft tissue abscesses (Fig. 14.22) Diagnosis is confirmed by identifying the causative organism from blood cultures or aspirated disc material. Six weeks of parenteral antibiotics and possibly additional oral antibiotic therapy usually provides adequate treatment for patients with radiologic evidence of disc space infection and a positive culture. During the acute phase a short course of bed rest is also indicated and patients who have severe muscle spasm or pain may benefit from the use of a light corset. The ESR provides a method of assessing the efficacy of therapy in these patients.

Surgical intervention, including drainage and debridement of spinal infections, is indicated in patients who develop paraparesis or paraplegia. The following factors appear to increase the risk of neurologic deficits:

- older age
- cervical or thoracic infection

(*Escherichia coli* and *Pseudomonas aeruginosa*[102] respectively). In patients who have undergone surgery or trauma to the spine, non-pathogenic organisms (diphtheroids, *Staphylococcus epidermidis*) may be associated with an indolent infection of the vertebral column[103]. Workers in the meat-processing industry may acquire a brucellosis infection[104]. Tuberculous and fungal infections of the vertebral column occur most often in the elderly and other immunocompromised individuals. Some 50–60% of individuals with skeletal tuberculosis have axial skeletal disease. The clinical presentation of a patient with tuberculous spondylitis is pain over the involved vertebrae, low-grade fever and weight loss. The process is indolent and may be present for years before diagnosis (Fig. 14.20)[105].

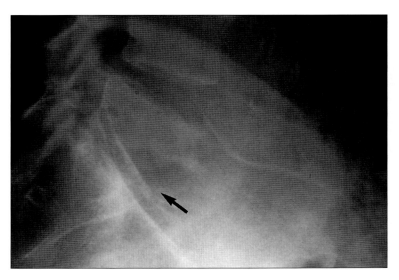

Fig. 14.21 Infection of the intervertebral disc space. Plain lateral radiograph of the lumbar spine showing narrowing of the L5/S1 disc space with new bone formation at the L5 endplate (arrow) and a soft tissue mass pushing the great vessels anteriorly. This finding of narrowing of the disc space and new bone formation with displacement of the great vessels strongly suggests the diagnosis of spinal infection with a soft tissue abscess.

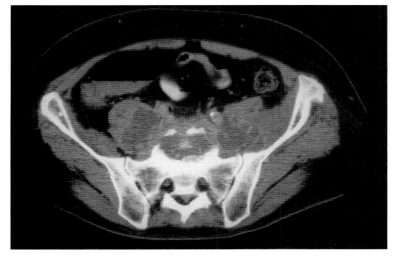

Fig. 14.22 Spinal infection imaged by CT of the lumbar spine. At the L5/S1 level lucent areas in both psoas muscles and destructive changes in the intervertebral disc space suggest the presence of spinal infection with bilateral abscesses.

- staphylococcal infection as opposed to other organisms
- coexisting diabetes or rheumatoid arthritis.

When surgical treatment is selected, controversy exists involving the use of bone grafts to achieve bony fusion. The experience of the spinal surgeon at the time of surgical debridement can help to determine the appropriate course of action.

Pyogenic sacroiliitis is an unusual form of septic arthritis[109]. The disease is associated with acute symptoms, severe sacroiliac joint pain and fever. Diagnosis of the causative organism may be obtained by blood cultures, fluoroscopic fine needle aspiration or open biopsy. Antibiotic therapy for 6 weeks is usually adequate to heal the infection without the need for surgical drainage.

Nocturnal pain/pain with recumbency

Tumors of the spinal column or spinal cord cause pain at night or with recumbency. Both benign and malignant neoplasms cause these symptoms. Nocturnal pain may be caused by swelling of neoplastic tissues associated with inactivity in the supine position or by stretching the neural tissues over the neoplastic mass.

A number of benign and malignant tumors are associated with involvement of the lumbosacral spine (Table 14.10). Benign lesions tend to cause local pain and involve the posterior elements of vertebrae. Malignant lesions cause more diffuse pain and systemic symptoms, and involve the anterior elements of vertebrae.

Patients with malignancies have pain that is gradual in onset but persistent in character and increasing in intensity. Physical examination shows localized tenderness over the lesion along with neurologic dysfunction if neural elements are compressed. Radiographic evaluation is very useful in detecting the location and characteristics of the neoplastic lesion.

An example of a benign tumor of bone that affects the lumbar spine is an osteoid osteoma. The tumor is most frequently found in young adults aged 20–30 years. Approximately 7% of osteoid osteomas occur in the spine, most frequently in the lumbar area[110]. The pain associated with this lesion is intermittent and vague initially, but with time becomes constant and aching, with a boring quality. The pain is not relieved with rest or application of heat. The pain is frequently exacerbated at night and disturbs sleep. In the spine, osteoid osteomas are associated with non-structural scoliosis. The appearance of marked paravertebral muscle spasm and the sudden onset of scoliosis in a young adult requires an evaluation for the presence of this lesion. The lesion is on the concave side of the scoliosis. The symptoms of osteoid osteoma may be present for a considerable time before plain radiographic findings become evident. The pain is relieved by low doses of NSAIDs.

Physical examination reveals local tenderness. Scoliosis is reversible early in the course of the lesion. With prolonged spasm, muscle atrophy may occur. Vertebral deformity may occur in young individuals who are growing. Hyperemia of the tumor may cause swelling and erythema of the skin if the lesion is superficial in location.

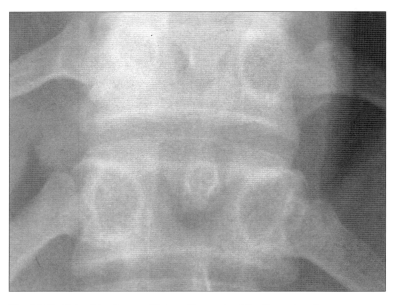

Fig. 14.23 Osteoid osteoma. Plain radiograph of the thoracic spine demonstrating sclerosis affecting the right pedicle of T11.

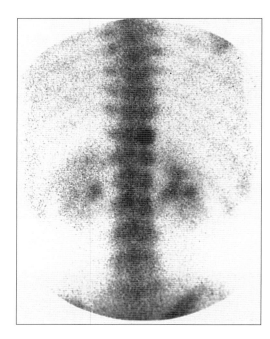

Fig. 14.24 Osteoid osteoma. Bone scintigraphy (posterior view) demonstrating increased uptake in T11. There is no other area of increased uptake in the skeleton.

The radiographic finding of a lucent nidus with a diameter of 1.5cm and a surrounding well-defined area of dense sclerotic bone is virtually pathognomonic of osteoid osteoma. The lesions are in the neural arch in 75% of affected vertebrae, articular facets in 18% and 7% in vertebral bodies (Fig. 14.23). Bone scans or CT scans should be employed if an osteoma is suspected and not found on plain radiographs (Fig. 14.24)[111,112].

The treatment for an osteoid osteoma is simple excision of the nidus and surrounding sclerotic bone. If the nidus is not entirely removed, recurrence of the lesion is possible and symptoms may persist. On occasion, osteoid osteomas may undergo spontaneous healing.

Multiple myeloma is the most common primary malignancy of bone in adults (27% of biopsied bone tumors)[113]. Patients range in age from 50 to 70 years, with only a rare patient below the age of 40. Low back pain is the initial complaint in 35% of patients. The pain is aching and intermittent at onset, aggravated by weight-bearing and improved with bed rest. Some patients may have radicular symptoms that mimic those of sciatica and arthritis[114]. Significant neurologic dysfunction, including paraplegia,

TABLE 14.10 NEOPLASTIC LESIONS OF THE LUMBOSACRAL SPINE		
Benign	**Malignant**	**Spinal cord tumors**
Osteoid osteoma	Multiple myeloma	Extradural metastases
Osteoblastoma	Chondrosarcoma	Intradural–extramedullary
Osteochondroma	Chordoma	Neurofibroma
Giant cell tumor	Lymphoma	Meningioma
Aneurysmal bone cyst	Skeletal metastases	Intramedullary
Hemangioma		Ependymoma
Eosinophilic granuloma		Astrocytoma
Sacroiliac lipoma		
All these may cause localized low back pain.		

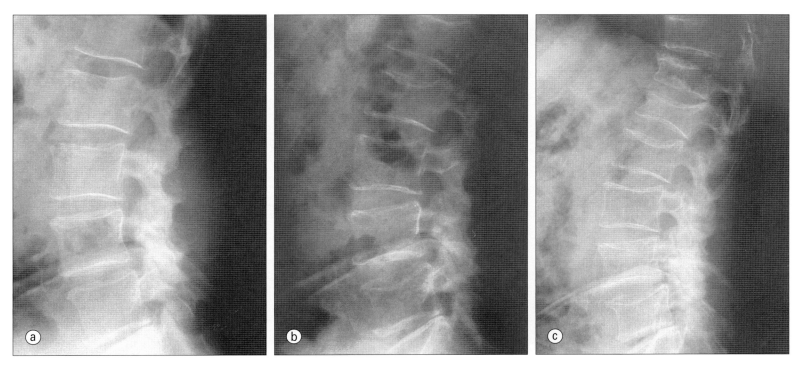

Fig. 14.25 Multiple myeloma. A series of plain radiographs taken over a 3-month period. Progressive osteopenia and pathologic compression fractures are noted. (a) Initial evaluation; (b) at 12 weeks; (c) at 14 weeks. Diagnosis was made at 12 weeks after initial presentation

occurs more commonly with solitary plasmacytoma than with multiple myeloma[115].

Physical examination may demonstrate diffuse bone tenderness, fever, pallor and purpura in the later stages of the illness. Signs of spinal cord compression are present if vertebral body collapse has progressed to a significant degree.

Laboratory testing reflects the systemic nature of this malignancy. Included in the abnormal findings may be anemia, leukocytosis, thrombocytopenia, elevated ESR, hypercalcemia, hyperuricemia, elevated creatinine and a positive Coombs test. An increase in serum proteins is secondary to the presence of abnormal immunoglobulins of any of the five classes. Urinalysis may detect Bence Jones protein formed by the production of excess immunoglobulin light chains. Bone marrow aspirate or biopsy reveals an excess number of plasma cells of varied histologic grades.

Plain radiographs demonstrate osteolysis without reactive sclerosis and sparing of the posterior elements of the spine (Fig. 14.25)[116]. Solitary plasmacytomas in the spine have variable radiographic appearances. They may be expansile, with or without reactive bone. They may invade an intervertebral disc space and mimic discitis. Bone scintigraphy does not detect myeloma since there is no reactive component of osteoblasts to the myeloma cells. MRI and CT are better techniques for identifying the presence and extent of myeloma lesions in the bone and soft tissues. MRI is able to detect spinal bone marrow involvement in asymptomatic myeloma patients[117].

The diagnosis of multiple myeloma is based upon clinical data, along with the detection of abnormal plasma cells on biopsy. Myeloma is treated with the use of chemotherapeutic agents to control the growth of the malignant plasma cells. In patients with cord compression, decompression laminectomy with or without local radiotherapy is indicated.

Skeletal metastases are 25 times more common than primary tumors as the cause of neoplastic lesions in the spine. Patients who are aged over 50 years are at greatest risk of developing metastatic disease. Autopsy results demonstrate that 70% of patients with primary tumors develop metastases to the thoracolumbar spine[118]. The common primary sources for skeletal metastases include tumors of the breast, prostate, lung, kidney, thyroid, colon, uterine cervix and bladder.

Lumbar pain is of gradual onset and increasing intensity. The symptoms are increased with motion, sneezing or coughing. The pain is local at the onset but may become radicular in character. Neurologic abnormalities may occur abruptly over a 4–6-month period.

Physical examination may demonstrate pain on palpation over the affected bone. Muscle spasm and limitation of motion are associated findings. Neurologic abnormalities are indicative of nerve root or spinal cord impingement.

Laboratory findings may include anemia, elevated ESR, abnormal urinalysis, increased alkaline phosphatase and, in metastatic prostate cancer, increased prostatic acid phosphatase. Histologic features of biopsy specimens may suggest the identity of the primary tumor but some lesions are too undifferentiated for identification.

Radiographic abnormalities depend on the character of the underlying malignancy. Kidney and thyroid metastases are typically osteolytic while colon lesions are osteoblastic. Mixed lytic and blastic lesions are noted with breast, lung, prostate or bladder tumors (Fig. 14.26). Plain radiographs may not show any abnormalities until 30–50% of bone calcium is lost[119]. Bone scans are positive in over 85% of patients with metastases. MRI is able to show tumor in the spinal cord, extraosseous extension and bone marrow replacement, while CT is more helpful for detecting cortical bone involvement and bone mineralization[120].

Neoplastic lesions may also occur inside the spinal canal. These intraspinal neoplasms may be extradural, between bone and the outermost covering of the spinal cord (the dura); intradural–extramedullary, between the dura and the spinal cord; and intramedullary, in the spinal cord proper. Extradural tumors are most commonly metastatic in origin. Intradural–extramedullary tumors are primarily meningiomas, neurofibromas or lipomas (Fig. 14.27). Intramedullary tumors are ependymomas or gliomas. The neurologic abnormalities associated with these unusual neoplasms are dependent on their location in the spinal cord and cauda equina. MRI, by its ability to define the exact location,

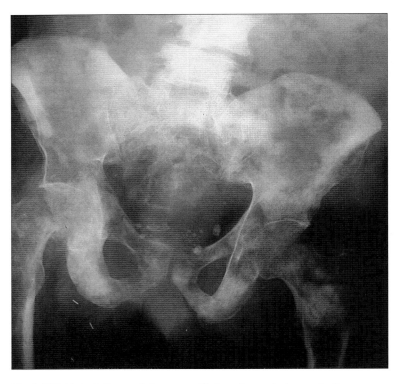

Fig. 14.26 Metastatic prostate cancer. Plain radiograph demonstrating osteoblastic lesions replacing lower lumbar vertebral bodies and most of the bony pelvis.

TABLE 14.11 RHEUMATIC DISORDERS AFFECTING THE LUMBOSACRAL SPINE	
Spondyloarthropathies	Ankylosing spondylitis Reactive arthritis Psoriatic arthritis Enteropathic arthritis
Behçet's syndrome	
Familial Mediterranean fever	
Whipple's disease	
Diffuse idiopathic skeletal hyperostosis	
All these may cause localized low back pain.	

size and character of the lesions, has revolutionized the visualization of intraspinal lesions[65].

Treatment of metastatic disease of the spine is directed towards pain palliation. A cure is rarely possible since most metastatic lesions are rarely solitary. Radiotherapy is useful to control spinal pain. Decompressive laminectomy is recommended for patients who have recently developed neurologic dysfunction.

Morning stiffness

Morning stiffness of the lumbosacral spine is a frequent symptom in patients with inflammatory arthropathies that affect the axial skeleton (Table 14.11). While morning stiffness of mechanical origin may last an hour or less, stiffness associated with the spondyloarthropathies typically lasts for hours. The spondyloarthropathies include a group of arthritides that inflame the sacroiliac joints and the axial skeleton. Patients with ankylosing spondylitis or enteropathic spondylitis have sacroiliitis initially and subsequently develop spondylitis. On rare occasions, patients have pain that is primarily in the lumbar spine and spares the sacroiliac joints (reactive arthritis, psoriatic spondylitis). They may also awaken during the night because of back pain.

Physical examination of the musculoskeletal system may demonstrate decreased mobility in the axial skeleton (i.e. Schober test, chest expansion). The general physical examination may discover physical findings unsuspected by the patient that help diagnose the specific spondyloarthropathy (oral ulcers, psoriatic skin lesions).

Laboratory tests may show a mild anemia and elevated ESR. Histocompatibility testing for the HLA-B27 haplotype is confirmatory but not diagnostic. Approximately, 8% of the Caucasian population is HLA-B27-positive but is unaffected by a spondyloarthropathy.

Plain radiographs of the sacroiliac joints represent the initial investigation of choice in patients suspected of having an inflammatory arthropathy of the axial skeleton (Fig. 14.28). Lumbar radiographs may show loss of lumbar lordosis and squaring of the vertebral bodies (Fig. 14.29). If plain radiographs are normal, tilting the radiography tube by 30° results in an image taken with the sacroiliac joint in one plane (Ferguson view). This view is helpful in detecting early changes of sacroiliitis. Bone scintigraphy can detect increased uptake in the sacroiliac joints but false-positive results frequently occur. CT scanning is the most sensitive test and may show early involvement of the sacroiliac joint when plain radiographs are normal or equivocal[121].

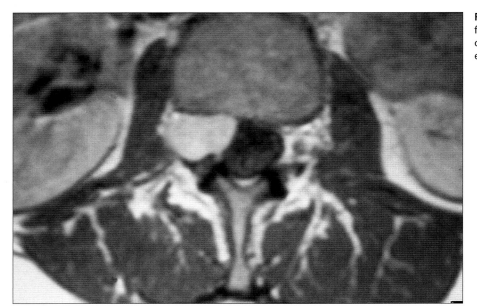

Fig. 14.27 Caudal neurofibroma. Transverse T1-weighted MRI following intravenous gadolinium shows an enhancing mass occluding the right neural foramen of L2. Note how local bone erosion has widened the neural foramen.

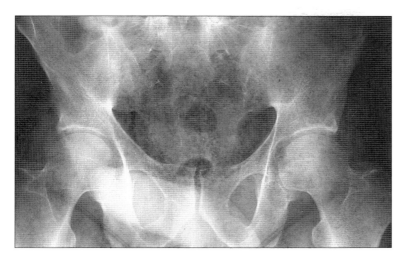

Fig. 14.28 Ankylosing spondylitis. Plain radiograph of the pelvis demonstrating bilateral sacroiliitis with fusion of the sacroiliac joints.

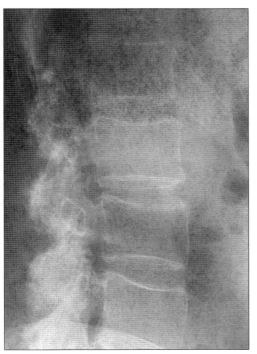

Fig. 14.29 Ankylosing spondylitis. Lateral view of lumbar spine demonstrating squaring of vertebral bodies, thin syndesmophytes, disc calcification and diffuse osteopenia.

Acute localized bone pain

Pain localized to the midline is frequently associated with disorders that affect osseous structures of the lumbar spine. Acute localized bone pain is usually caused by a fracture or expansion of bone. Any systemic process that increases mineral loss from bone, causes bone necrosis or replaces bone cells with inflammatory or neoplastic cells will weaken vertebral bone to the point where fracture may occur spontaneously or with minimal trauma (Table 14.12). Patients with acute fractures experience sudden onset of pain localized to the affected bone. Bone pain may be the initial manifestation of disease or may occur in the setting of associated symptoms. A medical history, including the review of systems, may elicit responses that suggest the underlying cause of the patient's back pain (kidney stones – hyperparathyroidism, chronic cough – sarcoidosis).

Physical examination shows localized tenderness with palpation of the affected areas of the spine. Muscle spasm may surround the area of bony tenderness.

Laboratory evaluation of patients with acute localized bone pain may be quite extensive. Therefore, screening tests should suit the most likely causes of the patient's symptoms. Anemia or an increased ESR should raise the suspicion of an inflammatory process. Serum chemistry may detect abnormalities of calcium metabolism associated with vitamin D deficiency (osteomalacia) or elevated parathormone level (hyper-

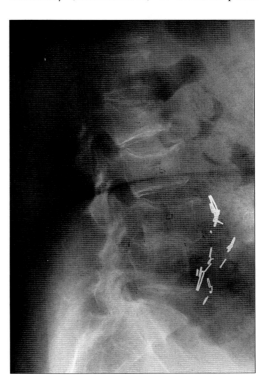

Fig. 14.30 Osteoporosis. Plain radiograph, lateral view, demonstrating diffuse osteopenia and multiple compression fractures.

parathyroidism). Elevations in alkaline phosphatase may suggest increased bone activity associated with neoplasms or Paget's disease.

Radiographic evaluation concentrates on the tender area noted with physical examination. Plain radiographs may show osteopenia if more than 30–50% of the bone calcium has been lost (Fig. 14.30). Areas of sclerosis related to healed fractures or Paget's disease may be identified (Fig. 14.31). Microfractures cause significant pain and may not be detected with plain films. Bone scintigraphy is useful in this context for detection of increased bone activity associated with fractures. CT scans may identify the location of a fracture or an area of bone that has been replaced by inflammatory tissue. MR scan is able to detect abnormalities of bone marrow that are associated with alterations in bone mineral density (Figs 14.32 & 14.33)[123].

Therapy for patients with acute localized bone pain must be tailored to the specific disease process causing their illness. In the instance of

TABLE 14.12 ENDOCRINOLOGIC, HEMATOLOGIC AND MISCELLANEOUS DISORDERS AFFECTING THE LUMBOSACRAL SPINE	
Endocrinologic/metabolic	Osteoporosis
	Osteomalacia
	Hyperparathyroidism
Hematologic	Hemoglobinopathy
	Myelofibrosis
	Mastocytosis
Miscellaneous	Paget's disease
	Subacute endocarditis
	Sarcoidosis
	Retroperitoneal fibrosis
All these may cause acute localized bone pain.	

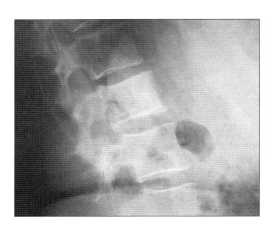

Fig. 14.31 Paget's disease. Plain radiograph demonstrating osteosclerotic alterations of bony trabeculae in L2 vertebral body. The body is slightly increased in size. This patient had elevation of serum alkaline phosphatase

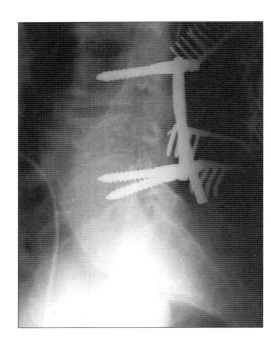

Fig. 14.34 Plasmacytoma. Postoperative plain radiograph, lateral view, demonstrating placement of rods to stabilize the spine and prevent neurologic damage.

severe bony compromise, stabilization of the spine may require bone graft and/or rod placement (Fig. 14.34). Vertebroplasty is a treatment for vertebral compression fractures that are matured over 6 weeks in duration that remain painful[123]. Methylmethacrylate is injected through a cannula into the collapsed vertebral body. The cement stabilizes the fracture and results in pain relief. In rare circumstances the cement will escape from the vertebral body if injection pressure is too great. A limitation of vertebroplasty is the inability of the procedure to reverse spinal kyphosis associated with fractures. Kyphoplasty uses an inflatable bone tamp to reverse kyphosis in fractures that are less than 6 weeks old[124].

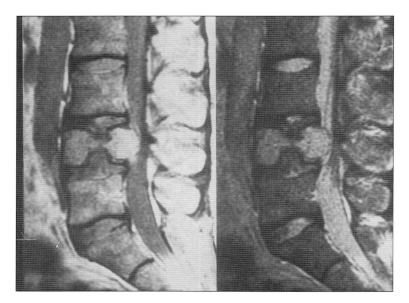

Fig. 14.32 Plasmacytoma. MRI scan, sagittal view, demonstrating replacement of the vertebral body with a mass lesion extending into the spinal canal.

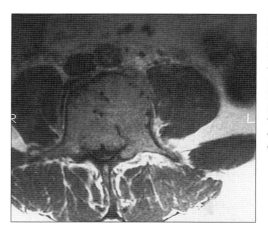

Fig. 14.33 Plasmacytoma. MRI scan, axial view, revealing replacement of the vertebral body and pedicles with a homogeneous mass. The mass has extended into the spinal canal, compressing the cauda equina.

This procedure is associated with rapid relief of spinal pain in individuals with acute fractures.

Visceral pain

Disorders of the vascular, genitourinary and gastrointestinal systems can cause stimulation of sensory nerves that results in the perception of pain both in the damaged area and in superficial tissues supplied by the same segments of the spinal cord (Table 14.13). The duration and sequence of visceral pain follows the periodicity of the involved organ. Colicky pain occurs in peristaltic waves and is associated with a hollow viscus, such as the ureter, uterus, gall bladder or colon. Throbbing pain is associated with vascular structures.

Back pain is rarely the only symptom of visceral disease. Vascular lesions cause dull, steady abdominal pain that is unrelated to activity. Back pain is usually associated with epigastric discomfort and may radiate to the hips or thighs if retroperitoneal structures are irritated. Rupture or acute expansion of the aneurysm is associated with tearing pain and circulatory collapse. Kidney pain is felt in the costovertebral angle. Ureteral pain from nephrolithiasis may cause dull flank pain with chronic distention or colic if obstruction occurs at the ureteropelvic junction. Patients with bladder infections may develop diffuse low back pain centered near the sacrum. Pain from genital organs may occur locally or in a referred pattern. Pain may be related to pancreatitis, peptic ulcer disease or colon or rectal disorders. Examination of the abdomen may be able to identify the maximum source of pain.

Patients who do not have constitutional symptoms should be asked specifically about muscle pain and stiffness. Patients aged over 50 years may have proximal stiffness around the hips and shoulders. These

TABLE 14.13 VISCEROGENIC PAIN REFERRED TO THE LUMBAR SPINE	
Vascular	Expanding aortic aneurysm
Genitourinary	Endometriosis Tubal pregnancy Kidney stone Prostatitis
Gastrointestinal	Pancreatitis Peptic ulcers Colonic cancer
All these disorders can cause referred pain to the lower back.	

patients may present with low back pain as well. Polymyalgia rheumatica must be considered in these older individuals. In younger individuals with more localized areas of pain, fibromyalgia may be the cause of low back pain[125]. Tender points are found in characteristic locations throughout the musculoskeletal system. Some patients may not even be aware of the tender points until they are pressed by the examiner.

The diagnosis of these disorders is a clinical one. Polymyalgia rheumatica is associated with an elevated ESR. Fibromyalgia usually has a normal ESR. The therapy for these illnesses is very different. Polymyalgia is treated with low-dose corticosteroids (prednisone, 10–20mg/day). Fibromyalgia is treated with mild aerobic exercise and moderate doses of tricyclic antidepressants.

If the medical evaluation remains unrevealing, the patient should be evaluated for any psychosocial difficulties. Drug habituation, depression, alcoholism and hysteria may be associated with low back pain. These patients will benefit from therapy directed at controlling their addiction or psychiatric difficulties.

Those patients who do not show any evidence of systemic medical illness or psychiatric difficulties should be educated about their back problem individually by the physician or in a back school. Back school reviews proper and efficient use of the body in work and recreation. Patients are given methods for dealing with the stresses of chronic pain. Many individuals are able to be more functional once they realize that their pain is not related to an acute illness. These individuals concentrate on maximizing their physical function in their daily activities as opposed to concentrating on the presence of pain.

Leg pain below the knee (sciatica)

Herniated disc

Sciatica is a frequent cause of continuing musculoskeletal pain despite a 4–6-week course of conservative management. Herniated disc with nerve impingement is associated with leg pain exacerbated with flexion of the lumbar spine or with prolonged sitting. Individuals may experience sensory or motor deficits corresponding to the degree of nerve compression. Bed rest does not accelerate recovery[126]. Further diagnostic tests are indicated to document the anatomic abnormalities associated with the patient's symptoms when pain persists (Fig. 14.35). Depending on the circumstances, the patient should undergo MRI or CT evaluation (Figs 14.36 & 14.37). Once the abnormality is identified (herniated disc) and medical disorders have been ruled out as possible causes of the patient's pain, additional therapy in the form of epidural corticosteroid injections may be given[127]. Long-acting corticosteroid is injected into the epidural space close to the location of nerve root compression. The procedure can be done in the outpatient setting. Although well-designed

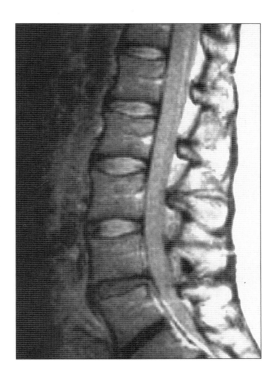

Fig. 14.36 Herniated intervertebral lumbar disc. Sagittal MRI demonstrates a herniated disc with caudal migration of the disc at the L4/5 interspace.

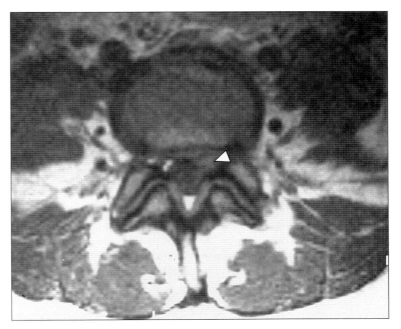

Fig. 14.37 Herniated intervertebral lumbar disc. Axial MRI demonstrates a herniated disc (arrow) blocking the left neural foramen.

controlled studies are needed to prove the efficacy of this therapy, over 90% of patients with sciatica have described improvement in rest and walking pain over a 1-month period[128]. The maximum benefit is noted after 4 weeks. The injection may be given as a series of three over a 3–6-week period. The injections are discontinued once leg pain is resolved.

If epidural steroids are effective in alleviating the patient's leg pain, the patient should be encouraged to increase physical activity, although limiting activities that increase intradiscal pressure, such as heavy lifting or sitting for long periods of time. Patients with a disc herniation should be on restricted work for a 3-month period before resuming more typical physical activities.

If the epidural corticosteroid therapy has not been effective and the patient is considering surgical intervention, the individual must be

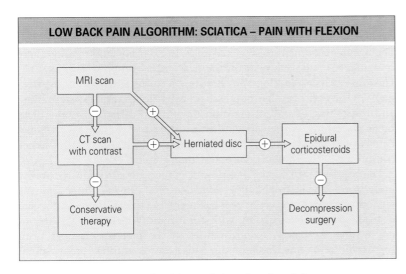

LOW BACK PAIN ALGORITHM: SCIATICA – PAIN WITH FLEXION

Fig. 14.35 Low back pain algorithm: sciatica – herniated disc.

re-evaluated for the persistence of a neurologic deficit and a positive tension sign. Electrodiagnostic tests may be obtained to confirm the presence of a radiculopathy and its level in the spinal cord. Preliminary studies report that sequestrated intervertebral discs that are highlighted by the contrast material gadolinium are more likely to resorb spontaneously than protruded discs that do not absorb contrast[129].

The choice of surgical procedure (laminectomy with discectomy versus microdiscectomy) is beyond the scope of this chapter. Discectomy produces better pain relief than non-surgical treatment over a 4-year period but may not persist at 10-year followup[130]. Needless to say, the success of any of these surgical procedures is dependent on choosing the patient who requires surgery. Surgery for sciatica is helpful in relieving leg pain. It should not be done to improve back pain.

Lumbar spinal stenosis

The second group of patients whose symptoms are based upon mechanical pressure on the neural elements are those with spinal stenosis. These individuals experience leg pain with standing or walking (neurogenic claudication) (Fig. 14.38). Spinal stenosis can be defined as narrowing of the spinal canal secondary to degenerative changes that occur in the spinal canal with time (Fig. 14.39). Other forms of spinal stenosis occur secondary to congenital abnormalities, traumatic, postsurgical, or metabolic disorders.

Epidemiology

The prevalence of narrowing of the lumbar spinal canal increases with the age of the population. The definition of stenosis has an affect on the prevalence of the condition. A midsagittal narrowing to less than 10.0mm is unequivocally pathologic[131]. Clinical recognition of the syndrome is very much age-related, with few cases diagnosed under the age of 50 years.

Myelographic[132], computed tomographic[56] and magnetic resonance imaging studies[74] of living patients have all shown that 20–25% of asymptomatic populations older than 40 years have marked narrowing of the lumbar spinal canal. These *in vivo* measurements support the conclusion drawn from postmortem morphometry studies that many cases of 'morphologic' lumbar spinal stenosis have no recognizable clinical expression.

Etiology and pathogenesis

The lumbar spinal canal is bounded anteriorly by lumbar discs, vertebral bodies and the posterior longitudinal ligament, laterally by the laminae and facet joints and posteriorly by the ligamentum flavum (Fig. 14.40).

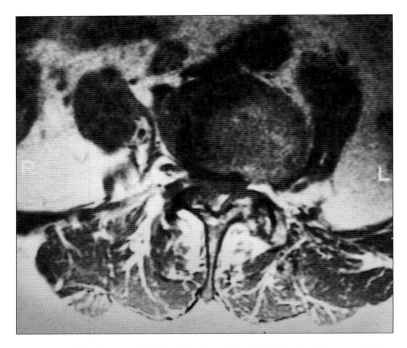

Fig. 14.39 Spinal stenosis. MRI, axial view, of the L3/4 disc level demonstrating osteophytic overgrowth, disc degeneration and ligamentous hypertrophy. The cauda equina is compressed in the central area of the canal.

The nerve root canals through which spinal nerves exit the spinal canal are bounded anteriorly by the posterior surface of discs and vertebral body, posteriorly by facet joints and pars interarticularis and medially by the central vertebral canal[133]. Stenosis develops when there is a relative narrowing of the dimensions of the lumbar spinal canal due to either congenital or acquired factors. The midsagittal diameter of the spinal canal is narrowest at the bodies of the second, third and fourth lumbar vertebrae and widens at the level of the fifth lumbar vertebra.

Congenital spinal abnormalities tend to produce interpedicular narrowing such as that observed in achondroplasia, while acquired lumbar spinal stenosis is usually the result of spondylotic change and tends to cause midsagittal narrowing. Most cases of lumbar spinal stenosis syndrome are the result of both congenital and acquired narrowing of the lumbar spinal canal, thus limiting the utility of any rigid etiologic classification[134].

Pathologic studies of the lumbar nerve root canal show that lumbar spondylosis is associated with reduction in the vertical dimension due to disk space narrowing, posterior bulging of the intervertebral discs, retropulsion of anulus fibrosus remnants and the formation of sclerotic ridges around the vertebral endplates (Fig. 14.40). Osteoarthritic facet joints project osteophytes anteriorly from the superior articular processes, and there are often synovial effusions, hemarthroses and derangements of meniscal synovial folds. In extension and rotation there is significant encroachment on the nerve root complex (Fig. 14.40)[135]. Flexion–extension myelography has shown consistent anterior displacement of the entire lumbar dural sac on extension, caused by shortening and thickening of the ligamentum flavum[136]. Furthermore, the discs bulge posteriorly, particularly at the L3/4 and L4/5 levels, and with spinal extension there is also facet joint subluxation anteriorly, further compromising the dimensions of the lumbar spinal canal.

The precise mechanisms that produce pseudoclaudication are poorly understood. The neuropathology of patients has shown chronic segmental compression of nerves at regular intervals corresponding to the site of myelographic obstruction, with confirmatory histologic features of nerve fiber damage[137]. Abnormalities of the pial vessels have been reported[138] and some patients have high cauda equina cerebrospinal fluid pressures[139]. Any or all of these factors may play a role in the genesis of pseudoclaudication.

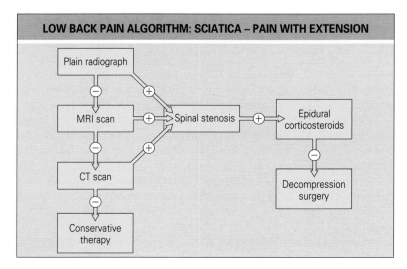

LOW BACK PAIN ALGORITHM: SCIATICA – PAIN WITH EXTENSION

Fig. 14.38 Low back pain algorithm: sciatica – spinal stenosis.

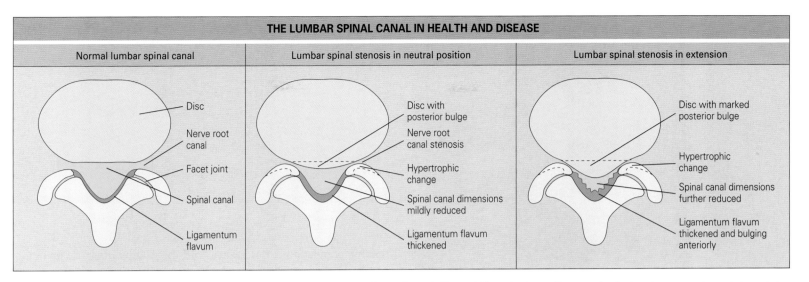

THE LUMBAR SPINAL CANAL IN HEALTH AND DISEASE

| Normal lumbar spinal canal | Lumbar spinal stenosis in neutral position | Lumbar spinal stenosis in extension |

Disc
Nerve root canal
Facet joint
Spinal canal
Ligamentum flavum

Disc with posterior bulge
Nerve root canal stenosis
Hypertrophic change
Spinal canal dimensions mildly reduced
Ligamentum flavum thickened

Disc with marked posterior bulge
Hypertrophic change
Spinal canal dimensions further reduced
Ligamentum flavum thickened and bulging anteriorly

Fig. 14.40 The lumbar spinal canal in health and disease. (Left) The normal spinal canal. (Center) The spinal canal in central spinal and nerve root canal stenosis in the neutral position. (Right) The effect of lumbar extension on the spinal canal.

Clinical features

The most characteristic symptom is pseudoclaudication, defined as any discomfort that occurs in the buttock, thigh or leg on standing or walking that is relieved by rest and is not produced by peripheral vascular insufficiency. At times, similar symptoms can occur while lying down and are relieved only by walking around. Such discomfort is generally described as pain but is occasionally appreciated as numbness or weakness, with many patients experiencing various combinations of these symptoms[137].

Pseudoclaudication is generally relieved by lying down or sitting and adopting a posture of flexion at the waist. In daily life, such relief is achieved by, for example, leaning forwards on a shopping cart, leaning on a church pew or adopting a bent forwards position while walking (simian stance). Such pseudoclaudication typically affects multiple dermatomes and is difficult to ascribe to a single nerve root lesion. Some 40% of cases have bilateral symptoms[137].

Sciatica due to lumbar spinal stenosis is distinct from the sciatica that typically follows herniation of the nucleus pulposus. Objective neurologic signs are frequently absent. Restriction of straight leg-raising (Lasègue's sign) is present in only 10% of cases of sciatica due to lumbar spinal stenosis. Ankle jerks are absent in 40%, knee jerks are absent in 10% and a small percentage have sensory loss or weakness[137,140]. A condition identical to meralgia paraesthetica can be produced by stenosis at the upper lumbar levels[141].

Bowel and bladder sphincter disturbance can develop but are relatively uncommon. Their presence constitutes an absolute indication for surgery to stabilize the deficit and allow some potential for recovery of bladder function[142]. Rarely, intermittent priapism has been reported as a manifestation of lumbar spinal stenosis[143]. Men have been described who are unable to void in the standing position but are able to do so while sitting, a cauda equina equivalent of pseudoclaudication.

Restriction of lumbar spinal motion is common in this condition since most cases have significant and often severe spondylotic changes. It has been estimated that 65% of patients who undergo lumbar spinal surgery for lumbar spinal stenosis have significant mechanical lumbar pain[137]. This probably represents a substantial underestimate of the extent of lumbar pain in this context since the more mechanical lumbar pain a patient has the less likely they are to be offered lumbar spinal surgery.

Investigations

The purpose of investigation is to confirm the diagnosis in patients with a clinically defined lumbar stenosis syndrome and, if necessary, to exclude other diseases. Imaging techniques and neurophysiologic investigations allow demonstration of the defined anatomy so that appropriate therapy can be planned. The imaging techniques are complementary and in most cases a combination of techniques is necessary.

Plain films usually show abnormalities in lumbar spinal stenosis, although they are not diagnostic of spinal canal narrowing. However, it is unusual to demonstrate absolutely normal lumbar plain films in this condition. Plain film changes that may be associated with stenosis include narrowing of disc spaces, apophyseal joint osteoarthritis and degenerative spondylolisthesis, particularly at L4/5[137]. These features are common in asymptomatic older individuals and their predictive value is limited. Measurement of interpedicular diameter and midsagittal measurements are of questionable clinical significance. Spondylolysis with spondylolisthesis frequently causes distortion of the nerve root exit foramen, which may lead to compromise of the exiting nerve but only rarely causes stenosis of the central lumbar canal.

Computed tomograms visualize structures localized to a single spinal level and can demonstrate articular facet hypertrophy, enlargement of laminae, hyperplasia and ossification of the ligamentum flavum, and disc prolapse (Fig. 14.41). The technique allows definition of the osseous margins and shape of the lumbar spinal canal. CT scanning provides better visualization of the lateral recesses and nerve root exit canals than does myelography and allows visualization of the spinal canal below the level of a myelographic block. Although abnormal dimensions are described, the clinical correlations with these are poor. A trefoil shape of the lumbar canal is typical of severe lumbar spinal stenosis. The presence of normal epidural fat makes significant mechanical nerve root compromise unlikely.

Contrast myelography remains valuable in defining the extent of lumbar spinal stenosis and the degree of nerve root entrapment, although it is better suited to definition of stenosis of the central lumbar canal than stenosis isolated to the lateral recesses. Demonstration of obstruction to dye flow can be dependent on posture, with compression of the dural sac by the ligamentum flavum and disc being more severe in extension (Fig. 14.42). Myelography can also be extended to allow demonstration of the conus medullaris and the lower thoracic levels. The combination of contrast myelography and CT directed at specific levels can demonstrate lateral recess and/or nerve root canal with greater definition than CT or myelography alone.

Magnetic resonance imaging reveals changes of stenosis in 21% of asymptomatic subjects over the age of 60 years[75]. MRI and contrast CT are comparable in demonstrating spinal stenosis at any one segment[143].

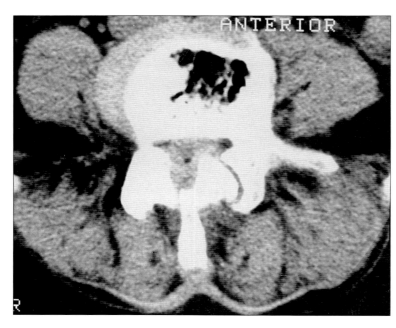

Fig. 14.41 Lumbar spine stenosis. CT showing thickened ligamentum flavum, facet joint hypertrophy and posterior disc bulging. Note absence of epidural fat with trefoil deformity of lumbar spinal canal.

TABLE 14.14 DIFFERENTIAL DIAGNOSIS OF LUMBAR SPINAL STENOSIS SYNDROME
• Lumbar spondylosis without spinal stenosis
• Herniated nucleus pulposus
• Atherosclerotic occlusive peripheral vascular disease
• Spinal tumors
• Restless leg syndrome
• Peripheral nerve entrapment
• Cervical and thoracic spinal stenosis
• Peripheral neuropathy
• Anterior tibial compartment syndrome

tomatic population is not known, and this complicates interpretation. Much of the usefulness of electromyography lies in excluding peripheral neuropathy and peripheral nerve entrapment syndromes[147]. Cortical somatosensory-evoked potentials provide a sensitive test of neurologic compromise and have been used in assessing the adequacy of neural decompression intraoperatively[148]. The specificity of this test is uncertain, and it is expensive; it is currently more of a research tool than a routine clinical procedure.

Differential diagnosis

A number of conditions must be distinguished from lumbar spinal stenosis syndrome (Table 14.14). Peripheral vascular disease can be distinguished by a careful history and physical examination. Vascular laboratory studies and vascular surgical consultation are helpful in individuals who demonstrate findings suggestive of both disorders[149]. The possibility of a herniated nucleus pulposus causing sciatica is associated with abrupt onset. Peripheral nerve entrapment may produce radicular complaints indistinguishable from spinal nerve compression. Electromyography with nerve conduction studies is usually required for their diagnosis[147]. Lumbar spinal stenosis may be associated with stenosis in the cervical and thoracic areas. Some cases of thoracic spinal stenosis produce a pure pseudoclaudication syndrome[150]. Furthermore, myelopathy due to more rostral narrowing of the spinal canal will result in difficulty in walking and sphincter disturbance, symptoms that can easily be confused with those due to lumbar neurologic compromise[151].

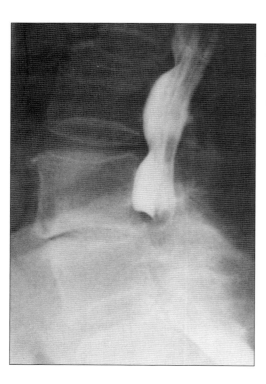

Fig. 14.42 Lumbar spine stenosis: myelogram in extension. Note increased block with marked posterior indentation due to the ligamentum flavum.

There are few adequate studies comparing these various imaging modalities[144]. On balance, MRI and CT myelography are comparable in establishing the radiologic (in contrast to clinical) diagnosis of lumbar spinal stenosis[145].

Electromyography is frequently abnormal if performed exhaustively. Of 37 patients with surgically proven lumbar spinal stenosis, 34 had an abnormality on electromyogram with evidence of one or more radiculopathies[137]. These abnormalities can be difficult to interpret, with one study demonstrating that 11 of 36 patients with stenosis had electromyographic abnormalities at levels higher than those expected based on myelography[146]. The frequency of similar positive findings in an asymp-

Anterior thigh pain

A small group of individuals develop anterior thigh pain in conjunction with back pain. Such pain has a number of possible sources (Fig. 14.43). Pain in the anterior thigh is related either to hip disease, a hernia, kidney disorders, femoral neuropathy or retroperitoneal process (anterior). Hip arthritis causes pain that is primarily in the groin. However, the peripheral nerves that supply the hip joint also innervate muscles in the low back and anterior thigh. Hip disease may present as lateral low back and anterior thigh pain. A careful physical examination, including range of motion of the hips, will identify those individuals with decreased hip motion. The patient's pain should be recreated by putting tension on the hip joint. Plain films of the hips should document the presence of joint disease (Fig. 14.44).

An inguinal hernia can cause anterior thigh pain. Occasionally, the pain radiates into the lateral low back. Physical examination will identify patients with direct and indirect hernias.

Patients with kidney disease may present with anterior thigh pain. Nephrolithiasis will cause pain that radiates from the back into the genitalia or anterior thigh. A simple urinalysis may identify hematuria or pyuria suggesting a renal source for the pain. An intravenous pyelogram may be obtained to evaluate more fully the urinary system.

LOW BACK PAIN ALGORITHM: SCIATICA – ANTERIOR THIGH PAIN

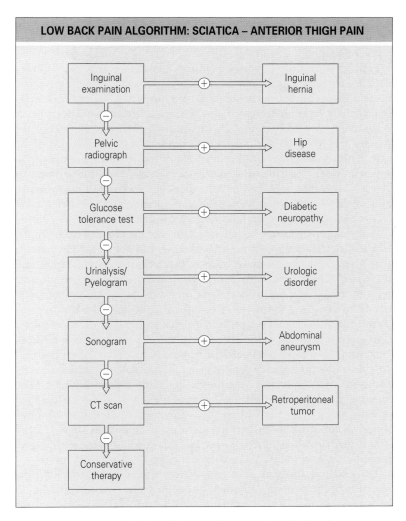

Fig. 14.43 **Low back pain algorithm: sciatica – anterior thigh pain.**

Disorders of the femoral nerve may be associated with anterior thigh pain. The anterior femoral cutaneous nerve (L2, L3) supplies the anterior thigh. Peripheral neuropathies, particularly due to diabetes, may affect the femoral nerve.

Any retroperitoneal process may refer pain to the anterior thigh. Retroperitoneal structures that may cause pain include the aorta and

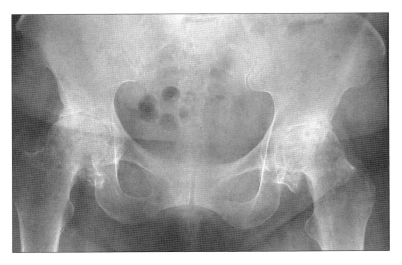

Fig. 14.44 **Hip arthritis.** Plain radiograph of pelvis demonstrating severe osteoarthritis of both hips. The patient had presented with back and knee pain. Hip examination revealed no motion of the joint. Back pain was reduced with joint replacement.

LOW BACK PAIN ALGORITHM: POSTERIOR THIGH PAIN

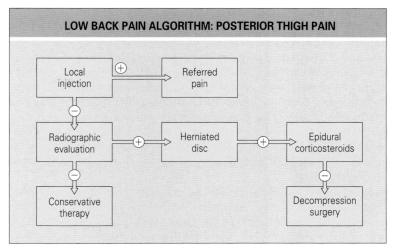

Fig. 14.45 **Low back pain algorithm: sciatica – posterior thigh pain.**

kidneys. Tumor or infiltrative processes that involve the retroperitoneum may also cause back and anterior thigh pain. If a retroperitoneal process is suspected, CT evaluation is appropriate to determine the status of the aorta, kidney and lymph nodes.

Posterior thigh pain

The fourth group of patients will complain of pain that radiates from the low back into the posterior thigh. These patients may have referred or radicular pain (Fig. 14.45). Patients with referred pain have it on the basis of injury to the bony, ligamentous and muscular components of the lumbar spine. The muscles of the posterior thigh and buttocks have the same embryologic origin as those of the lumbar spine. An injury to these structures in the lumbar spine may be referred to the posterior thigh. These patients may respond to a local injection of corticosteroid and anesthetic into the maximum point of tenderness in the lumbar spine. Patients with referred pain do not improve with surgical intervention.

Patients with lesions compressing the L2 and L3 nerve roots may experience pain on the medial and lateral portions of the posterior thigh. These areas are supplied with cutaneous nerves that have their origin at the L2 and L3 spinal cord levels. Occasionally, L4 lesions may also cause similar symptoms and signs. MRI evaluation can identify causes of nerve impingement at higher levels of the spinal cord. Electrophysiologic studies can corroborate the presence of a radiculopathy. Surgical intervention should only be contemplated when the clinical and laboratory data document a radiculopathy and conservative therapy has been ineffective.

MANAGEMENT

No single form of therapy is effective for all forms of back pain. Patients with systemic causes for back pain must be treated with specific therapies effective for their underlying disease. Antibiotics are effective for osteomyelitis while chemotherapeutic agents are effective in slowing the growth of malignant plasma cells in multiple myeloma.

The vast majority of patients have low back pain on a mechanical basis. In most circumstances, the mechanical disorder causing the symptoms cannot be identified. Despite the inability to identify the specific source of the patient's pain, the physician is faced with treating the patient to decrease their symptoms. Ideally, therapy would decrease symptoms without any toxicities. This circumstance does not exist, and even conservative therapy has its potential risks. The risks associated with NSAIDs, muscle relaxants and injection therapy must be compared to the possibilities of infection, paralysis and death associated with surgical intervention. It is the role of the physician to maximize medical therapy so that surgical intervention is considered in the appropriate clinical setting. Only 1–2% of patients with low back pain will undergo lumbar spine surgery[42].

A panel of spine experts recently reviewed the medical literature concerning the efficacy of the components of therapy for low back pain[42]. In general, most components of back pain therapy were found to be without adequate studies demonstrating efficacy. The therapeutic recommendations of the panel include the following.

- Bed rest for more than 4 days is not helpful and may debilitate the patient. During the acute phase, patients are encouraged to ambulate as tolerated.
- Relief of pain may be accomplished most safely with non-prescription analgesics or non-steroidal medication. Spinal manipulation is helpful during the first 4 weeks in patients without radiculopathy.
- Low-stress aerobic activities can be safely started in the first 2 weeks of symptoms. Trunk muscle exercises should be delayed at least 2 weeks.
- Patients should be encouraged to return to usual activities, both vocational and recreational, as soon as possible.

The guidelines take into account the natural history of low back pain, which is associated with symptom improvement in the vast majority of patients within 2 months of the onset of symptoms. Patients who have persistent or progressive pain or who have radicular pain may require additional interventions.

Frequently the ability of the patients to cope with their symptoms can be helped by careful explanation of the cause of the symptoms. Not all patients with the clinical syndrome require surgical intervention. The key to conservative management lies in the patient's acceptance of mild disability, since most continue to be symptomatic in the longer term. Some patients improve spontaneously, presumably because of resolution of an acute disc prolapse in an already compromised canal. In one series of 32 untreated spinal stenosis patients followed for 4 years, only 15% worsened, with the remainder unchanged or improved[152].

Controlled physical activity

Components of a conservative management program for low back pain patients include patient education, 'controlled physical' activity, bed rest, exercise and drug therapy in the form of NSAIDs and muscle relaxants. Of all the therapies, controlled physical activity is employed most frequently. Many patients spontaneously go to bed to assume a supine position when they develop mechanical back pain. The duration of bed rest should be kept to a minimum. Scientific data supports regular activity as being as effective a therapy as a short course of bed rest[153–155].

The biomechanical rationale for bed rest is that intradiscal pressures are lower in the supine position. However, rolling over in bed may result in increased intradiscal pressure. In addition, the number of patients with herniated discs compared to muscle strain is small. The exact mechanism that causes improvement in pain associated with muscle and ligament injury is unknown.

Bed rest is not benign if it is continued for too long. Muscles become deconditioned. Cardiovascular function diminishes. Individuals lose time from work and, with continuing bed rest, start to view themselves as ill[99].

Busy patients rarely stay in bed unless their back pain is severe. Most patients strictly limit their recreational activities and minimize the time lost at their job. The best outcome for low back pain is associated with those individuals who resume normal activity as opposed to extension exercises or bed rest. Resumption of normal activity is to be encouraged to improve the resolution of back pain[154].

Physical modalities

Physical modalities may be used to diminish symptoms for short periods of time. These counterirritant forms of therapy include ice massage, hot packs, diathermy, ultrasound and transcutaneous electrical nerve stimulation (TENS). These therapies may be applied by the patient themselves or by a therapist.

Patients with acute low back pain may experience analgesia with ice massage or cold packs. Cold temperatures decrease swelling, pain and muscle spasm during the acute phase of an injury. Cold reduces metabolic activity locally, decreases muscle spindle activity and slows nerve conduction. A cold pack may be placed in a towel and applied to the painful area of the back if the patient cannot tolerate the stroking of the skin with ice massage. Cold relieves pain and spasm for longer than superficial heat. Patients who experience increased α motor neuron discharges with cold application will experience increased muscle spasm and cannot tolerate this form of therapy. Patients may experience at least 33% reduction in pain following ice massage[156].

Heat is another form of counterirritant therapy that has utility in the treatment of low back pain patients. Heat should not be used in patients with back pain secondary to trauma. Heat causes vasodilatation and increased blood flow. This can cause increased damage to an area recently traumatized. However, heat increases the elastic properties of connective tissues and may be of particular utility in patients who complain of stiffness associated with their back pain. Heat also decreases γ fiber activity, muscle spindle excitability and resting muscle tension. Heat may be applied to superficial or deep structures. Superficial heat penetrates to the subcutaneous tissues. Hydrocollator packs, heating pads, infrared heat and whirlpools generate superficial heat. The maximal safe exposure for these forms of therapy is 30 minutes applied directly to the skin at 45°C. Deep heat generated by diathermy or ultrasound penetrates to structures below the subcutaneous tissues. Deep heat is given in 20-minute sessions. Heat has been shown to be helpful for reducing pain in hospitalized patients with low back discomfort[157].

The practical application of temperature modalities depends on the response of the patient. Although, physiologically, cold therapy should be used in patients with acute pain, and heat in patients with chronic pain, these modalities may have the opposite effect. The recommendation should be cold for acute pain and heat for chronic pain initially. If the patient does not respond, or has an exacerbation of symptoms, the opposite temperature modality should be tried.

Transcutaneous electrical nerve stimulation therapy is based upon the gate control theory of pain, which suggests that counterstimulation of the sensory system will modify pain perception in the cerebral cortex. TENS preferentially stimulates low-threshold αA fibers. The stimulation of these fibers is thought to inhibit the nociceptive impulses of the small C unmyelinated and αD fibers. The effect of TENS on pain is not mediated through opiate receptors. The electrical stimulation is produced by an electrical pulse generator, which delivers current that can be varied in form, intensity and frequency to superficial electrodes. The optimal placement of the electrodes is proximal to the painful area. The average time for the onset of analgesia is approximately 20 minutes. Therapy should be given for at least 30 minutes. The pain relief from TENS may be present only during stimulation or may last for a considerable period of time. TENS is not indicated for patients with acute low back pain[42]. TENS has been shown to be superior to massage and equivalent to cold therapy[158]. However, a large, randomized, placebo-controlled study found no benefit of TENS for chronic low back pain[159]. The role of TENS in the therapy of low back pain is in question and it should not be considered usual therapy.

Drug therapy

A variety of drugs is widely used in the therapy of patients with acute and chronic low back pain. The types of medication used have included analgesics, NSAIDs, muscle relaxants and antidepressants. Medications should be used for a limited period and monitored constantly. Additional analgesics or non-steroidal medications should be tried if the initial drugs are ineffective. The potential toxicities of the agents must also be considered when choosing an agent for a patient.

Analgesics

Non-narcotic (acetaminophen) and narcotic (codeine, oxycodone, meperidine) analgesics have been used for low back pain. Patients who are intolerant of NSAIDs may benefit from acetaminophen (paracetamol), in doses of 500–650mg every 4 hours. A slow-release form of the drug may allow for a more prolonged analgesic effect in back pain patients. The drug has a synergistic effect with the NSAIDs and may be used in combination to increase analgesia without increasing toxicity.

Tramadol, a non-narcotic analgesic, is a useful agent that can be given independently or in combination with non-steroidal drugs for the relief of chronic low back pain. This agent is most helpful for individuals with back pain who are unable to tolerate non-steroidal anti-inflammatory agents and narcotic analgesics.

Narcotic analgesia should be reserved for patients with severe pain associated with a herniated disc. Codeine in doses of 30–60mg every 4–6 hours, in combination with an NSAID or acetaminophen, is an effective analgesic. This form of therapy may be used in an outpatient setting along with controlled physical activity and temperature modalities. However, codeine does have the potential to cause constipation, which may exacerbate low back pain. Patients should be told to increase fiber in their diets and consume increased amounts of liquids to decrease the potential for this side effect. Stronger narcotic analgesia should be reserved for patients who are unable to perform activities of daily living because of persistent pain. The continuation of narcotic analgesics in the outpatient setting should be discouraged unless the patient is committed to maximizing physical function through increased activity. Dependence and tolerance frequently result from the continued use of narcotics. Their use in chronic low back pain should be strictly limited[160].

Non-steroidal anti-inflammatory drugs

Non-steroidal anti-inflammatory drugs have analgesic properties in low doses and anti-inflammatory properties at higher doses. Different NSAIDs have greater potentials as analgesics or as anti-inflammatory agents. Some NSAIDs combine both characteristics. The onset of action of the agents is also an important characteristic. In acute back pain, a rapid onset of action is important to control symptoms quickly. In chronic pain, the onset of action is not as important as efficacy and safety over extended periods of time.

Non-steroidal anti-inflammatory drugs have been studied in patients with acute and chronic back pain. Naproxen, piroxicam and diflunisal have been reported to be more effective than placebo in relieving low back pain[161,162]. From a practical viewpoint, NSAIDs as a class of agents are effective in low back pain therapy[163]. The problem that remains is that there is no specific selection criteria for the choice of a single agent for a specific patient with pain. The patient is given an NSAID with characteristics that fit the patient's symptoms and complicating medical problems (renal failure, gastric ulcer). The drug is given for a period of 2–4 weeks as a therapeutic trial and is continued if it is efficacious and well tolerated. The drug is changed if the initial agent is ineffective or associated with serious toxicity. In that circumstance, an NSAID from a different chemical group is selected in the hope that it will be efficacious. The process is continued until an effective NSAID is identified. Cyclo-oxygenase (COX)-2-selective inhibitors are indicated for low back pain treatment in individuals with a history of peptic ulcer disease or gastrointestinal intolerance to dual COX-I/COX-II inhibitors.

The NSAID is continued while the patient increases physical activity and regains confidence. It is discontinued once the individual resumes their normal daily activities in work and recreation. Patients with chronic low back pain may require NSAIDs for extended periods of time. NSAIDs are not used so much to relieve pain as to support the patient's efforts to be physically active. Patients with chronic pain may not achieve a total resolution of pain but should be encouraged to engage in as much physical activity as can be tolerated. NSAIDs help support the patient in this endeavor.

Muscle relaxants

Muscle relaxants are a group of drugs used to decrease muscle contraction present in patients with low back pain. The use of muscle relaxants in low back pain remains controversial[164]. The muscle relaxants used for low back pain patients work centrally to affect the activity of muscle stretch reflexes. Despite the skepticism concerning the pathophysiology of muscle spasm and the mechanism of action of these drugs, the muscle relaxants have been found to be effective for muscle contraction in the lumbar spine in scientific studies. Drugs including cyclobenzaprine, carisoprodol and chlorzoxazone have been shown to be more effective than placebo in treating patients with muscle spasm[165]. Of interest is the lack of efficacy of diazepam, a benzodiazepine, as a muscle relaxant for low back pain. In appropriately selected patients with acute muscle spasm, the combination of an NSAID and a muscle relaxant is more effective than the same NSAID alone[166]. The combination of a NSAID and a muscle relaxant offers significant relief of pain compared to other combinations of therapies, including those with narcotics[167]. The major toxicity of muscle relaxants is drowsiness. Also noted are headache, dizziness and dry mouth. Muscle relaxants should be used only during the time the spasm is palpable. Once the spasm has subsided, the drug should be discontinued.

Antidepressants

Tricyclic antidepressants have been used for the treatment of chronic pain for patients with or without depression. A number of mechanisms have been suggested to explain the pain relief associated with the tricyclics. One theory suggests that tricyclic antidepressants increase serotonin (5-hydroxytryptamine) levels in the pain inhibitory pathway in the central nervous system. Double-blind studies have documented the role of tricyclics for relieving chronic pain. Low doses in the range of 10–25mg may be needed to control symptoms[168]. Rare patients may require up to 150mg per day. The drug does not work immediately and may need to be continued for a number of weeks before decreased symptoms are noted. Newer antidepressants (sertraline, fluoxetine) are not as effective as tricyclics for chronic pain relief[169].

Injection therapy

Local or regional anesthesia given by injection is part of the therapeutic regimen for some patients with low back pain. By blocking peripheral pain input, the local area of pain can be eased as well as areas of referred pain and increased muscle tension. Patients who describe localized areas of muscle or ligamentous tenderness are candidates for local anesthetic therapy. The area injected may be an area of local trauma or a myofascial trigger point[170]. Trigger points are areas of the muscle that are painful at rest, prevent full lengthening of the muscle, weaken the muscle, refer pain in the muscle group on direct palpation and cause a local contraction when palpated. Trigger points may be found in the paraspinous muscles, the quadratus lumborum and the gluteal muscles. The point of maximum tenderness is injected with a combination of 1% lidocaine (lignocaine) and a depository form of corticosteroid[171]. A study by Garvey et al. suggests that needling the area with or without medication may have a beneficial effect[172]. Injections may be given on a weekly basis for 3–4 additional weeks. Controlled studies designed to evaluate the efficacy of this treatment modality have yet to be carried out.

Epidural corticosteroid injections are used for patients with nerve root compression who do not respond to conservative management. Corticosteroids are injected directly into the epidural space with the intention of increasing the anti-inflammatory effect in comparison to oral corticosteroids. The injections may be given on an outpatient basis. The course of therapy includes three injections given at variable intervals (days to weeks with herniated discs and over months for spinal stenosis). The efficacy of these injections for the therapy of herniated discs and spinal stenosis with radiculopathy has been questioned. Epidural injections have been found to be effective in some patients[173]. The benefits may include decreased pain and more rapid return of sensory function[174]. In patients who have radiculopathy secondary to compression and are poor candidates for surgical intervention, epidural corticosteroids may be considered.

Patients who have apophyseal joint disease may develop pain on a referred basis that simulates radicular pain. In this circumstance, patients have received injections of anesthetic and corticosteroid to decrease pain[175]. The injections are done under fluoroscopic control to document the appropriate placement of the needle into the facet joint. Facets both at and above the level of the involved joint must be blocked in order to obtain adequate analgesia since each facet joint receives sensory innervation from two spinal levels. Injections are given every 2–4 weeks for three sessions. The efficacy of these injections has been questioned[176]. Even in studies reporting a good response, the mean pain relief is only 30%. No specific historical or physical factors identify those patients with zygapophyseal joint disease who may benefit from injection[177]. With the results of these studies, the use of facet joint blocks must be limited.

Calcitonin dispensed by injections or nasal spray is useful in cases of lumbar spinal stenosis associated with Paget's disease[178]. Open studies have suggested that calcitonin may be effective in treating patients with neurogenic claudication without Paget's disease. A subsequent double blind study yielded less impressive results[179] and further studies indicate that such treatment is helpful but unlikely to be effective in severe neurogenic claudication with walking distances of less than 200 metres[180].

Exercise

Physical therapy, particularly in the form of therapeutic exercises, may be particularly helpful in controlling mechanical low back pain[181]. A number of different exercise programs are available for patients with low back pain. These include flexion exercises, extension exercises, stretching regimens and aerobic conditioning. As a generalization, patients with mechanical disorders of the discs prefer extension exercises, while those with posterior component disease prefer flexion exercises. In most circumstances patients eventually take part in a combination of both forms of exercise.

A recent study suggests that, with an exercise program, patients may feel worse before they feel better[182]. In this study, 2 months were required in patients with chronic low back pain before benefit was noted. The treating physician should find a physical therapist who is interested in taking care of back patients and communicate his/her concerns about patients to the therapist. The therapist can then try various exercise programs and modify them according to the patient's response. The time spent in encouraging the patient to participate in exercises and becoming physically fit is well worth the effort.

Exercises may also play a significant role in preventing back pain in asymptomatic individuals. In a comparison with educational strategies, mechanical supports and risk modification, exercises that strengthen back and abdominal muscles were the only intervention associated with decreased frequency and duration of low back pain[183].

Complementary therapies

Complementary therapies are used for a variety of medical problems, including low back pain[184]. Therapies promoted for the treatment of low back pain include spinal manipulation, massage, acupuncture and magnets.

Spinal manipulation is recommended by the AHCPR guidelines. However, the guidelines do not specifically recommend that manipulation be done by a chiropractor. Experienced physical therapists have similar skills to mobilize the lumbar spine. Patient satisfaction with chiropractors is related to the chiropractor's willingness to listen to a patient's concerns. In a study of 215 patients who visited a physician and 242 who visited a chiropractor, overall satisfaction with care was three times greater with the chiropractors than with the physicians[185]. Patients had greater satisfaction with the information imparted by the chiropractors, which included graphic descriptions of the causes of pain and instructions on physical measures to improve back pain. Physicians were perceived as being less concerned about the patient's condition and pain and were less confident about the underlying cause of the patient's discomfort. Chiropractic care is associated with the greatest number of visits per episode and the highest outpatient cost compared to other health-care providers[186]. Osteopaths are health-care professionals who also offer manipulation as a therapy for low back pain. The number of osteopaths who offer manipulation therapy is limited.

Therapeutic massage has benefit for individuals with chronic low back pain. This therapy given once a week over 10 weeks has demonstrated benefit months after the last treatment. The efficacy of this form of treatment is limited to the availability of massage therapists[187]. This same study failed to identify significant benefit of acupuncture in chronic low back pain. Acupuncture techniques vary and this may have an effect on the outcome of a clinical trial.

A double-blind placebo-controlled trial was reported of magnets for back pain in individuals with chronic pain. This study demonstrated no significant difference between the study groups. Magnets did not decrease back pain in this trial[188].

Surgical treatment

A small percentage of individuals with low back pain require surgical intervention to improve their condition. Indications for surgery vary according to the patient characteristics but include sphincter and sexual dysfunction due to compression of the conus medullaris or cauda equina, severe radicular symptoms, particularly if there are progressive neurologic motor deficits, and radicular symptoms failing to respond to conservative management. The operative procedure is determined by the characteristics of the lesions and the skill of the surgeon with the specific technique.

With spinal stenosis, the success of surgical approaches depends on adequate decompression of areas of absolute stenosis and good judgment with respect to adequacy of decompression of areas of relative stenosis. Preoperative assessment and planning using multiple imaging techniques is essential. Prior to surgery there must be demonstration of compression of spinal nerve structures that correspond to the patient's clinical symptoms and signs. Surgery should not be carried out for clinically asymptomatic spinal stenosis.

Most patients require multiple level procedures and in one study 72% of patients had three or more laminae removed. In the follow-up of those patients 4 years after surgery, 64% reported that surgery had yielded good to excellent results but 36% still had more than half of their preoperative disability[137]. Similar results are reported for population-based series and from pooled series[189,190].

An analysis of laminectomy failure in 45 stenosis patients found that only half had the clinical picture of neurogenic claudication and only 10 had radiologic evidence of severe lumbar canal stenosis. The most common technical problem was inadequate neural decompression[191]. Comorbidities, including hip arthritis, osteoporosis and cardiovascular disease, are associated with persistent pain after surgical correction[192]. In summary, the more the clinical picture is one of pseudoclaudication with convincing radiology of neural compromise and the less it is mechanical low back pain the greater the chance of success with surgical intervention.

Some patients with lumbar spinal stenosis are left with persisting significant neurologic deficit, for example foot drop, despite maximal therapy, and such patients should have appropriate rehabilitation and orthoses to improve their functional status. Unfortunately, in spite of adequate conservative and operative management, some patients are left with ongoing severe back pain and limitation. Multidisciplinary pain management and functional restoration techniques should be considered for these patients, and the management involves both physical and psychologic assessment and treatment[193].

REFERENCES

1. Kelsey JL, White AA III. Epidemiology and impact of low back pain. Spine 1980; 5: 133–142.
2. Frymoyer JW, Pope MH, Costanza MC et al. Epidemiology studies of low back pain. Spine 1980; 5: 419–423.
3. Hart LG, Deyo RA, Cherkin DC. Physician office visits for low back pain: frequency, clinical evaluation, and treatment patterns from a U.S. national survey. Spine 1995; 20: 11–19.
4. National Center for Health Statistics. Limitation of activity due to chronic conditions, United States 1969–1970. Vital and Health Statistics Series 10, No. 80. Washington, DAC: National Center for Health Statistics.; 1973.
5. Andersson GBJ. Epidemiological features of chronic low-back pain. Lancet 1999; 354: 581–585.
6. Dixon A StJ. Progress and problems in back pain research. Rheumatol Rehabil 1973; 12: 165–175.
7. Van den Hoogen HJM, Koes BW, van Eijk JTM, Bouter LM. The prognosis of low back pain in general practice. Spine 1997; 22: 1515–1521.
8. Murphy PL, Volinn E. Is occupational low back pain on the rise? Spine 1999; 24: 691–697.
9. Frymoyer JW, Cats-Baril WL. An overview of the incidences and costs of low back pain. Orthop Clin North Am 1991; 22: 263–271.
10. Rossignol M, Suissa S, Abenhaim L. Working disability due to occupational back pain: three year follow-up of 2,300 compensated workers in Quebec. J Occup Med 1988; 30: 502–505.
11. Rossignol M, Suissa S, Abenhaim L. The evolution of compensated occupational spinal injuries: a three-year follow-up study. Spine 1992; 17: 1043–1047.
12. Merskey H. The characteristics of persistent pain in psychological illness. J Psychosom Res 1965; 9: 291–298.
13. Deyo RA, Bass JE. Lifestyle and low back pain: the influence of smoking and obesity. Spine 1989; 14: 501–506.
14. Leboeuf-Yde C, Kyvik KO, Bruun NH. Low back pain and lifestyle. Part II – Obesity: information from a population-based sample of 29,424 twin subjects. Spine 1999; 24: 779–784.
15. Nachemson A. The lumbar spine: an orthopaedic challenge. Spine 1976; 1: 59–71.
16. Deyo RA, Weinstein JN. Low back pain. N Engl J Med 2001; 344: 363–370.
17. Borenstein DG, Wiesel SW, Boden SD. Low back pain: medical diagnosis and comprehensive management. 2E. Philadelphia: WB Saunders; 1995: 181–589.
18. Klein RF, Brown W. Pain descriptions in medical patients. J Psychosom Res 1967; 10: 367–372.
19. Atlas SJ, Chang Y, Kammann E et al. Long-term disability and return to work among patients who have a herniated lumbar disc: the effect of disability compensation. J Bone Joint Surg 2000; 82A: 4–15.
20. Spengler DM, Freeman CW. Patient selection for lumbar discectomy. Spine 1979; 4: 129–134.
21. Blower PW. Neurologic patterns in unilateral sciatica. A prospective study of 100 new cases. Spine 1981; 6: 175–179.
22. Fahrni WH. Observation on straight leg raising with special reference to nerve root adhesions. Can J Surg 1966; 9: 44–48.
23. Vroomen PC, de Krom MC, Knottnerus JA. Diagnostic value of history and physical examination in patients suspected of sciatica due to disc herniation: a systematic review. J Neurol 1999; 246: 899–906.
24. Gunn CC, Chir B, Milbrandt WE. Tenderness at motor points: a diagnostic and prognostic aid to low back pain injury. J Bone Joint Surg 1976; 58A: 815–825.
25. Vallfors B. Acute, subacute, and chronic low back pain: clinical symptoms, absenteeism, and working environment. Scand J Rehabil Med 1985; 11(suppl): 1–98.
26. Waddell G, McCullogh JA, Kummel E, Venner RM. Non-organic physical signs in low back pain. Spine 1980; 5: 117–215.
27. McCombe PF, Fairbank JCT, Cockersole BC, Pynsent PB. Reproducibility of physical signs in low back pain. Spine 1989; 14: 908–918.
28. Jensen OH. The level-diagnosis of a lower lumbar disc herniation: the value of sensitivity and motor testing. Clin Rheumatol 1987; 6: 564–569.
29. Spitzer WO, LeBlanc FE, Dupier M. Scientific approach to the assessment and management of activity-related spinal disorders: a monograph for clinicians. Report of the Quebec Task Force on Spinal Disorders. Spine 1987; 12: S16–S21.
30. Deyo RA, Rainville J, Kent DL. What can the history and physical examination tell us about low back pain? JAMA 1992; 268: 760–765.
31. Witt I, Vestergaard A, Rosenklint A. A comparative analysis of X-ray findings of the lumbar spine in patients with and without lumbar pain. Spine 1984; 9: 298–300.
32. Deyo RA, Bigos SJ, Maravilla KR. Diagnostic imaging procedures for the lumbar spine. Ann Intern Med 1989; 111: 865–867.
33. Lawrence JS, Bremmer JM, Bier F. Osteo-arthrosis. Prevalence in the population and relationship between symptoms and x-ray changes. Ann Rheum Dis 1966; 25: 1–24.
34. Hakelius A, Hindmarsh J. The comparative reliability of preoperative diagnostic methods in lumbar disc surgery. Acta Orthop Scand 1972; 43: 234–238.
35. Deyo RA, McNeish LM, Cone RO III. Observer variability in the interpretation of lumbar spine radiographs. Arthritis Rheum 1985; 28: 1066–1070.
36. Van Tulder MW, Assendelft WJJ, Koes BW et al. Spinal radiographic findings and non-specific low back pain: a systematic review of observational studies. Spine 1997; 22: 427–434.
37. Liang M, Komaroff AL. Roentgenograms in primary care patients with acute low back pain. A cost-effective analysis. Arch Intern Med 1982; 142: 1108–1112.
38. Padley S, Gleeson F, Chisholm R, Baldwin J. Assessment of a single spine radiograph in low back pain. Br J Radiol 1990; 63: 535–536.
39. Eisenberg RL, Hedgcock MW, Williams EA et al. Optimum radiographic examination for consideration of compensation awards. II. Cervical and lumbar spines. AJR 1980; 135: 1071–1074.
40. Gehweiler JA Jr, Daffner RH. Low back pain: the controversy of radiologic evaluation. AJR 1983; 140: 109–112.
41. Scavone JG, Latshaw RF, Weidner WA. Anteroposterior and lateral radiographs: an adequate lumbar spine examination. AJR 1981; 136: 715–717.
42. Bigos S, Bowyer O, Braen G et al. Acute low back problems in adults. Clinical Practice Guideline No. 14. AHCPR Publication No. 95-0642. Rockville, MD: Agency for Health Care Policy and Research, Public Health Service, US Department of Health and Human Services; 1994.
43. Suarez-Almazor ME, Beleseck E, Russell AAS et al. Use of lumbar radiographs for the early diagnosis of low back pain: proposed guidelines would increase utilization. JAMA 1997; 277: 1782–1786.
44. Tumeh SS, Tohmeh AG. Nuclear medicine techniques in septic arthritis and osteomyelitis. Rheum Dis Clin North Am 1991; 17: 559–584.
45. Pomeranz SJ, Pretorius HT, Ramsingh PS. Bone scintigraphy and multimodality imaging in bone neoplasia: strategies for imaging in the new health care climate. Semin Nucl Med 1994; 24: 188–207.
46. Modic MT, Feiglin DH, Piraino DW. Vertebral osteomyelitis. Assessment using MR. Radiology 1985; 157: 157–166.
47. Adatepe MH, Powell DM, Issacs GH et al. Hematogenous pyogenic vertebral osteomyelitis. Diagnostic value of radionuclide bone imaging. J Nucl Med 1986; 27: 168–185.
48. Rosenthal DI, Mankin HJ, Bauman RA. Musculoskeletal application for computed tomography. Bull Rheum Dis 1983; 33: 1–4.
49. Golimbu C, Firooznia H, Rafii M. CT of osteomyelitis of the spine. AJR 1984; 142: 156–163.
50. Epstein BS, Epstein JA, Jones MD. Lumbar spinal stenosis. Radiol Clin North Am 1977; 15: 227–239.
51. Faerber EN, Wolpert SM, Scott RM et al. Computed tomography of spinal fractures. J Comput Assist Tomogr 1979; 3: 657–661.
52. Wang A, Wesolowski DP, Farak J. Evaluation of posterior spinal structures by computed tomography. Spine: State Art Rev 1988; 2: 439–465.
53. Carrera GF, Haughton VM, Syverstein A, Williams AL. Computed tomography of the lumbar facet joints. Radiology 1980; 134: 145–148.
54. Beltran J, Noto AM, Chakeres DW, Christofordis AJ. Tumors of the osseous spine: staging with MR imaging versus CT. Radiology 1987; 162: 565–569.
55. Herkowitz HN, Wesolowski DP. Percutaneous biopsy of the spine. Indications, techniques, results and complications. Update Spinal Disord 1980; 1: 3–9.
56. Wiesel SW, Tsourmas N, Feffer HL et al. A study of computer-assisted tomography. I. The incidence of positive CAT scans in an asymptomatic group of patients. Spine 1984; 9: 549–551.
57. Baker RA, Hillman BJ, McLennan JE et al. Sequelae of metrizamide myelography in 200 examinations. AJR 1978; 130: 499–502.
58. Weinstein JN. Differential diagnosis and surgical treatment of primary benign and malignant neoplasms. In: Frymoyer JW, ed. The adult spine: principles and practice. Raven Press: New York; 1991: 832.
59. Braun IF, Hoffman JC, Davis PC et al. Contrast enhancement in CT differentiation between recurrent disc herniation and post-operative scar. Am J Neuroradiol 1985; 6: 607–612.
60. Byrd SE, Cohn ML, Biggers SL et al. The radiographic evaluation of symptomatic post-operative lumbar spine patient. Spine 1985; 10: 652–661.
61. Hitselberger WE, Witten RM. Abnormal myelograms in asymptomatic patients. J Neurosurg 1969; 28: 204–206.
62. Albeck MJ, Hilden J, Kjaer L et al. A controlled comparison of myelography, computed tomography, and magnetic resonance imaging in clinically suspected lumbar disc herniation. Spine 1995; 20: 443–448.
63. Erly WK, Carmody RF. MRI of the spine. Crit Rev Diagn Imaging 1994; 35: 313–377.
64. Paushter DM, Modic MT, Masaryk TJ. Magnetic resonance imaging of the spine: applications and limitations. Radiol Clin North Am 1985; 23: 551–562.
65. Sze G, Stimac GK, Bartlett C et al. Multicenter study of gadopentetate dimeglumine as an MR contrast agent: evaluation in patients with spinal tumors. Am J Neuroradiol 1990; 11: 967–974.
66. Parizel PM, Baleriaux D, Rodesch G et al. Gd-DTPA-enhanced MR imaging of spinal tumors. Am J Neuroradiol 1989; 10: 249–258.
67. Lim V, Sobel DF, Zyroff J. Spinal cord pial metastases: MR imaging with gadopentetate dimeglumine. Am J Neuroradiol 1990; 11: 975–82.

68. Olson DO, Shields AF, Scheurich CJ et al. Magnetic resonance imaging of the bone marrow in patients with leukemia, aplastic anemia, and lymphoma. Invest Radiol 1986; 21: 540–546.

69. Traill Z, Richards MA, Moore NR. Magnetic resonance imaging of metastatic bone disease. Clin Orthop 1995; 312: 76–88.

70. Post MJD, Brown BC, Sze G. Magnetic resonance imaging of spinal infection. Rheum Dis Clin North Am 1991; 17: 773–794.

71. Sharif HS, Morgan JL, al-Shahed MS et al. Role of CT and MR in the management of tuberculous spondylitis. Radiol Clin North Am 1995; 33: 787–804.

72. Jensen MC, Kelly AP, Brant-Zawadzki MN. MRI of degenerative disease of the lumbar spine. Magn Reson Q 1994; 10: 173–190.

73. Kaplan PA, Orton DF, Russell JA. Osteoporosis with vertebral compression fracture, retropulsed fragments, and neurologic compromise. Radiology 1987; 165: 533–535.

74. Boden SD, Davis DO, Dina TS et al. Abnormal magnetic resonance scans of the lumbar spine in asymptomatic subjects: a prospective investigation. J Bone Joint Surg 1990; 72A: 403–408.

75. Jensen MC, Brant-Zawadzki MN, Obuchowski N et al. Magnetic resonance imaging of the lumbar spine in people without back pain. N Engl J Med 1994; 331: 69–73.

76. Weishaupt D, Zanetti M, Hodler J et al. MR imaging of the lumbar spine: prevalence of intervertebral disk extrusion and sequestration, nerve root compression, end plate abnormalities, and osteoarthritis of the facet joints in asymptomatic volunteers. Radiology 1998; 209: 661–666.

77. Stadnik TW, Lee RR, Coen HL et al. Annular tears and disk herniation: prevalence and contrast enhancement on MR images in the absence of low back pain or sciatica. Radiology 1998; 206: 49–55.

78. Kent DL, Larson EB. Magnetic resonance imaging of the brain and spine. Is clinical efficacy established after the first decade? Ann Intern Med 1988; 108: 402–424.

79. Fornistall RM, Marsh HO, Pay NT. Magnetic resonance imaging and contrast CT of the lumbar spine: comparison of diagnostic methods and correlations with surgical findings. Spine 1988; 13: 1049–1054.

80. Szypryt EP, Twining P, Wilde GP et al. Diagnosis of lumbar disc protrusion: a comparison between magnetic resonance imaging and radiculopathy. J Bone Joint Surg 1988; 70B: 717–722.

81. Schnebel B, Kingston S, Watkins R, Dillin W. Comparison of MRI to contrast CT in the diagnosis of spinal stenosis. Spine 1989; 14: 332–337.

82. Le Bras F, Wallman J, Barth MO, Gaston A. Spinal angiography. Spine: State Art Rev 1988; 2: 379–394.

83. Troisier G, Cypel D. Discography: an element of decision: surgery versus chemonucleolysis. Clin Orthop 1986; 206: 70–78.

84. Walsh TR, Weinstein JN, Spratt KF et al. Lumbar discography in normal subjects. A controlled, prospective study. J Bone Joint Surg 1990; 72A: 1081–1088.

85. Schwarzer AC, April CN, Derby R et al. The prevalence and clinical features of internal disc disruption in patients with chronic low back pain. Spine 1995; 20: 1878–1883.

86. April C, Bogduk N. High intensity zone: a pathognomonic sign of painful lumbar disc on MRI. Br J Radiol 1992; 65: 361–369.

87. Edeiken J, Wallace JD, Curley RF, Lee S. Thermography and herniated lumbar disks. AJR 1968; 102: 790–796.

88. Hoffman RM, Kent DL, Deyo RA. Diagnostic accuracy and clinical utility of thermography for lumbar radiculopathy: a meta-analysis. Spine 1991; 16: 623–628.

89. Waddell G. An approach to backache. Br J Hosp Med 1982; 28: 187–194.

90. Eisen A. Electrodiagnosis of radiculopathies. Neurol Clin 1985; 3: 495–510.

91. Haldeman S. The electrodiagnostic evaluation of nerve root function. Spine 1984; 9: 42–48.

92. Tonzola RF, Ackil AA, Shakani BT, Young RR. Usefulness of electrophysiological studies in the diagnosis of lumbosacral root disease. Ann Neurol 1981; 9: 305–308.

93. Baylan SP, Yu J, Grant AE. H-reflex latency in relation to ankle jerk electromyographic, myelographic, and surgical findings in back pain patients. Electromyogr Clin Neurophysiol 1981; 21: 201–206.

94. Fisher MA, Shivde AJ, Teixera C, Grainer LS. The F-response – a clinically useful physiological parameter for the evaluation of radicular injury. Electromyogr Clin Neurophysiol 1979; 19: 65–75.

95. Scarff TB, Ballmann DE, Toleikis JR. Dermatomal somatosensory evoked potential in the diagnosis of lumbar root entrapment. Surg Forum 1981; 32: 489–491.

96. Tullberg T, Svanborg E, Issacsson J et al. A preoperative and postoperative study of the accuracy and value of electrodiagnosis in patients with lumbosacral disc herniation. Spine 1993; 18: 837–842.

97. Shapiro S. Medical realities of cauda equina syndrome secondary to lumbar disc herniation. Spine 2000; 25: 348–352.

98. Floman Y. Progression of lumbosacral isthmic spondylolisthesis in adults. Spine 2000; 25; 342–347.

99. Borenstein DG, Burton JR. Lumbar spine disease in the elderly. J Am Geriatr Soc 1993; 41: 167–175.

100. Ross PM, Flemming JL. Vertebral body osteomyelitis: spectrum and natural history: A retrospective analysis of 37 cases. Clin Orthop 1976; 118: 190–198.

101. Digby JM, Kersley JB. Pyogenic non-tuberculous spinal infection: an analysis of thirty cases. J Bone Joint Surg 1979; 61B: 47–55.

102. Kido D, Bryan D, Halpern M. Hematogenous osteomyelitis in drug addicts. AJR 1973; 118: 356–363.

103. Schofferman L, Schofferman J, Zuckerman J et al. Occult infection causing persistent low back pain. Spine 1989; 14: 417–419.

104. Young EJ. Human brucellosis. Rev Infect Dis 1983; 5: 821–842.

105. Gorse GJ, Pais MJ, Kusske JA, Cesario TC. Tuberculous spondylitis: a report of six cases and a review of the literature. Medicine 1983; 62: 178–193.

106. Hadjipavlou AG, Mader JT, Necessary JT et al. Hematogenous pyogenic spinal infections and their surgical management. Spine 2000; 25: 1668–1679.

107. Pilgaard S. Discitis following removal of lumbar intervertebral disc. J Bone Joint Surg 1969; 51A: 713–716.

108. Perrone C, Saba J, Behloul Z et al. Pyogenic and tuberculous spondylodiskitis (vertebral osteomyelitis) in 80 adult patients. Clin Infect Dis 1994; 19: 746–750.

109. Vyskocil JJ, McIlroy MA, Brennan TA, Wilson FM. Pyogenic infection of the sacroiliac joint: case reports and review of the literature. Medicine 1991; 70: 188–197.

110. Cohen MD, Hanington DM, Ginsburg WW. Osteoid osteoma: 95 cases and a review of the literature. Semin Arthritis Rheum 1983; 12: 265–281.

111. Winter PF, Johnson PM, Hilal SK, Feldman F. Scintigraphic detection of osteoid osteoma. Radiology 1977; 122: 177–178.

112. Wedge HJ, Tchang S, MacFadyen DJ. Computed tomography in localization of spinal osteoid osteomas. Spine 1981; 6: 423–427.

113. Dahlin DC, Unni KK. Bone tumors: general aspects and data on 8,542 cases, 4th ed. Springfield, IL: Charles C Thomas; 1986: 193–207.

114. Bayrd ED, Heck FJ. Multiple myeloma: a review of 83 proved cases. JAMA 1947; 133: 147–157.

115. Valderrama JAF, Bullough PG. Solitary myeloma of the spine. J Bone Joint Surg 1968; 50B: 82–90.

116. Jacobson HG, Poppel MH, Shapiro JH, Grossberger S. The vertebral pedicle sign: a roentgenographic finding to differentiate metastatic carcinoma from multiple myeloma. AJR 1958; 80: 817–821.

117. Moulopoulos LA, Dimopoulos MA, Smith TL et al. Prognostic significance of magnetic resonance imaging in patients with asymptomatic multiple myeloma. J Clin Oncol 1995; 13: 251–256.

118. Fornasier VL, Horne JG. Metastases to the vertebral column. Cancer 1975; 36: 590–594.

119. Edelstyn GA, Gillespie PG, Grebbel FS. The radiological demonstration of skeletal metastases: experimental observations. Clin Radiol 1967; 18: 158–162.

120. Galasko CSB. Diagnosis of skeletal metastases and assessment of response to treatment. Clin Orthop 1995; 312: 64–75.

121. Kozin F, Camera GF, Ryan LM et al. Computed tomography in diagnosis of sacroiliitis. Arthritis Rheum 1981; 24: 1479–1485.

122. Steiner RM, Mitchell DG, Rao VS et al. Magnetic imaging of bone marrow. Diagnostic value in diffuse hematologic disorders. Magn Reson Q 1990; 6: 17–34.

123. Jensen ME, Dion JE. Percutaneous vertebroplasty in the treatment of osteoporotic compression fractures. Neuroimag Clin North Am 2000; 10: 547–568.

124. Watts NB, Harris ST, Genant HK. Treatment of painful osteoporotic vertebral fractures with percutaneous vertebroplasty or kyphoplasty. Osteoporosis Int 2001; 12: 429–437.

125. Borenstein D. Prevalence and treatment outcome of primary and secondary fibromyalgia in patients with spinal pain. Spine 1995; 20: 1055–1060.

126. Vroomen PCAJ, de Krom MCTFM, Wilminik JT et al. Lack of effectiveness of bed rest for sciatica. N Engl J Med 1999; 340: 418–423.

127. Carette S, Leclaire R, Marcoux S et al. Epidural corticosteroid injections for sciatica due to herniated nucleus pulposus. N Engl J Med 1997; 336: 1634–1640.

128. Bush K, Hillier S. A controlled study of caudal epidural injections of triamcinolone plus procaine for the management of intractable sciatica. Spine 1991; 16: 572–575.

129. Komori H, Okawa A, Haro H et al. Contrast-enhanced magnetic resonance imaging in conservative management of lumbar disc herniation. Spine 1998; 22: 67–73.

130. Gibson JNA, Grant IC, Waddell G. The Cochrane review of surgery for lumbar disc prolapse and degenerative lumbar spondylosis. Spine 1999; 24: 1829–1832.

131. Eisenstein S. Lumbar vertebral canal morphometry for computerized tomography in spinal stenosis. Spine 1983; 8: 187–191.

132. Hitselberger WE, Witten RM. Abnormal myelograms in asymptomatic patients. J Neurosurg 4 1968; 28: 204–206.

133. Lee CY, Rauschning W, Glenn W. Lateral lumbar spinal canal stenosis: classification, pathologic anatomy and surgical decompression. Spine 1988; 13: 313–320.

134. Arnoldi CC, Brodsky AE, Cauchoix J et al. Lumbar spinal stenosis and nerve root entrapment syndromes: definition and classification. Clin Orthop 1976; 115: 4–5.

135. Rauschning W. Normal and pathologic anatomy of the lumbar root canals. Spine 1987; 12: 1008–1019.

136. Penning L, Wilmink JT. Biomechanics of lumbosacral dural sac: a study of flexion–extension myelography. Spine 1981; 6: 398–408.

137. Hall S, Bartleson JD, Onofrio BM et al. Lumbar spinal stenosis: Clinical features, diagnostic procedures and results of treatment in 68 patients. Ann Intern Med 1985; 103: 271–275.

138. Watanabe R, Parke WW. Vascular and neural pathology of lumbosacral spinal stenosis. J Neurosurg 1986; 64: 64–70.

139. Magnaes B. Clinical recording of pressure on the spinal cord and cauda equina. J Neurosurg 1982; 57: 57–63.

140. Jonsson B, Stromqvist B. Symptoms and signs in degeneration of the lumbar spine. A prospective consecutive study of 300 operated patients. J Bone Joint Surg 1993; 75B: 381–385.

141. Guo-Xiang J, Wei-Dong X, Ai-Haow. Spinal stenosis with meralgia paraesthetica. J Bone Joint Surg 1988; 70B: 272–273.

142. Deen HG, Zimmerman RS, Swanson SK, Larson TR. Assessment of bladder function after lumbar decompressive surgery for spinal stenosis: a prospective study. J Neurosurg 1994; 80: 971–974.

143. Ram Z, Findler G, Spiegelman R et al. Intermittent priapism in spinal canal stenosis. Spine 1987; 12: 377–378.

144. Kent DL, Haynor DR, Larson EB, Deyo RA. Diagnosis of lumbar spinal stenosis in adults: A meta-analysis of the accuracy of CT, MR, and myelography. AJR 1992; 158: 1135–1144.

145. Bischoff RJ, Rodriguez RP, Gupta K et al. A comparison of computed tomography–myelography, magnetic resonance imaging and myelography in the diagnosis of herniated nucleus pulposus and spinal stenosis. J Spinal Dis 1993; 6: 289–295.

146. Seppalainen AM, Alaranta H, Soini J. Electromyography in the diagnosis of lumbar spinal stenosis. Electromyogr Clin Neurophysiol 1981; 21: 55–66.

147. Saal JA, Dillingham MF, Gamburd RS, Fanton GS. The pseudoradicular syndrome. Lower extremity peripheral nerve entrapment masquerading as lumbar radiculopathy. Spine 1988; 13: 926–930.

148. Herron LD, Trippi AC, Gonyeau M. Intraoperative use of dermatomal somatosensory-evoked potentials in lumbar stenosis surgery. Spine 1987; 12: 379–383.

149. Dodge LD, Bohlman HH, Rhodes RS. Concurrent lumbar spinal stenosis and peripheral vascular disease. Clin Orthop 1988; 230: 141–148.

150. Yamamoto I, Matsumae M, Ikeda A et al. Thoracic spinal stenosis: experience with 7 cases. J Neurosurg 1988; 68: 37–40.

151. Dagi TF, Tarkington MA, Leech JJ. Tandem lumbar and cervical spinal stenosis. J Neurosurg 1988; 66: 842–849.

152. Johnsson KE, Rosen I, Uden A. The natural course of lumbar spinal stenosis. Clin Orthop 1992; 27: 82–86.

153. Deyo RA, Diehl AK, Rosenthal M. How many days of bed rest for acute low back pain? A randomized clinical trial. N Engl J Med 1986; 315: 1064–1070.

154. Malmivaara A, Hakkinen U, Aro T et al. The treatment of acute low back pain – bed rest, exercises, or ordinary activity? N Engl J Med 1995; 332: 351–355.

155. Waddell G, Feder G, Lewis M. Systematic reviews of bed rest and advice to stay active for acute low back pain. Br J Gen Pract 1997; 47: 647–652.

156. Melzack R, Jeans ME, Stratford JG, Monks RC. Ice massage and transcutaneous electrical stimulation: comparison of treatment of low back pain. Pain 1980; 9: 209–217.

157. Landon BR. Heat or cold for the relief of low back pain? Phys Ther 1967; 47: 126–130.

158. Melzack R, Vetere P, Finch L. Transcutaneous electrical nerve stimulation for low back pain. A comparison of TENS and massage for pain and range of motion. Phys Ther 1983; 63: 489–493.

159. Deyo RA, Walsh N, Martin D et al. A controlled trial of transcutaneous electrical nerve stimulation (TENS) and exercise for chronic low back pain. N Engl J Med 1990; 322: 1627–1634.

160. Jamison RN, Raymond SA, Slawsby EA et al. Opioid therapy for chronic noncancer back pain: a randomized prospective study. Spine 1998; 23: 2591–2600.

161. Berry H, Bloom B, Hamilton EBD, Swinson DR. Naproxen sodium, diflunisal, and placebo in the treatment of chronic back pain. Ann Rheum Dis 1982; 41: 129–132.

162. Videman T, Osterman K. Double-blind parallel study of piroxicam versus indomethacin in the treatment of low back pain. Ann Clin Res 1984; 16: 156–160.

163. Koes BW, Scholten RJPM, Mens JMA et al. Efficacy of nonsteroidal anti-inflammatory drugs for low back pain: a systematic review of randomized clinical trials. Ann Rheum Dis 1997; 56: 214–223.

164. Johnson EW. The myth of skeletal muscle spasm. Am J Phys Med Rehabil 1989; 68: 1.

165. Elenbaas JK. Centrally acting oral skeletal muscle relaxants. Am J Hosp Pharm 1980; 37: 1313–1322.

166. Borenstein DG, Lacks S, Wiesel SW. Cyclobenzaprine and naproxen versus naproxen alone in the treatment of acute low back pain. Clin Ther 1990; 12: 125–131.

167. Cherkin DC, Wheeler KJ, Barlow W et al. Medication use for low back pain in primary care. Spine 1998; 607–614.

168. Hameroff SR, Crago BR, Cork RC et al. Doxepin effects on chronic pain, depression and serum opioids. Anesth Analg 1982; 61: 187.

169. Atkinson JH, Slater MA, Williams RA et al. Effects of nonadrenergic and serotonergic antidepressants on chronic low back pain intensity. Pain 1999; 83: 137–145.

170. Travell JG, Simons DG. Myofascial pain and dysfunction: the trigger point manual. Baltimore: Williams & Wilkins; 1983.

171. Swezey RL, Clements PJ. Conservative treatment of back pain. In: Jayson MIV, ed. The lumbar spine and back pain, 3rd ed. Edinburgh: Churchill Livingstone; 1987: 299–314.

172. Garvey TA, Marks MR, Wiesel SW. A prospective, randomized, double-blind evaluation of trigger point injection. Spine 1989; 14: 962–964.

173. Dilke TFW, Burry HC, Grahame R. Extradural corticosteroid injection management of lumbar nerve root compression. Br Med J 1973; 2: 635–637.

174. Carette S, LeClaire R, Marcoux S et al. Epidural corticosteroid injections for sciatica due to herniated nucleus pulposus. N Engl J Med 1997; 336: 1634–1640.

175. Jackson RP, Jacobs RR, Montesano PX. Facet joint injection in low back pain: a prospective statistical study. Spine 1988; 13: 966–971.

176. Carette S, Marcoux S, Truchon R et al. A controlled trial of corticosteroid injections into facet joints for chronic low back pain. N Engl J Med 1991; 325: 1002–1007.

177. Schwarzer AC, Wang S, Bogduk N et al. Prevalence and clinical features of lumbar zygapophyseal joint pain: a study in an Australian population with chronic low back pain. Ann Rheum Dis 1995; 54: 100–106.

178. Herzberg L, Bayliss D. Spinal cord syndrome due to non-compressive Paget's disease of bone: a spinal artery steal phenomenon reversible with calcitonin. Lancet 1980; 2: 13–15.

179. Porter W, Miller CG. Neurogenic claudication and root claudication treated with calcitonin. A double-blind trial. Spine 1988; 13: 1061–1063.

180. Eskola A, Pohjolainen T, Alaranta H et al. Calcitonin treatment in lumbar spinal stenosis: a randomized placebo-controlled, double-blind, cross-over study with one-year follow-up. Calcif Tissue Int 1992; 50: 400–403.

181. Jackson CP, Brown MD. Is there a role for exercise in the treatment of patients with low back pain? Clin Orthop 1983; 179: 39–45.

182. Manniche C, Hesselsoe G, Bentzen L et al. Clinical trial of intense muscle training for chronic low back pain. Lancet 1988; 2: 1473–1476.

183. Lahad A, Malter AD, Berg AO et al. The effectiveness of four interventions for the prevention of low back pain. JAMA 1994; 272: 1286–1291.

184. Borenstein D. Complementary therapies. In: Borenstein D. Back in control! A conventional and complementary prescription for eliminating back pain. New York: M Evans; 2001: 124–144.

185. Cherkin DC, MacCormack FA. Patient evaluations of low back pain care from family physicians and chiropractors. West J Med 1989; 150: 351–355.

186. Shekelle PG, Markovich M, Louie R. Comparing the costs between provider types of episodes of back pain care. Spine 1995; 20: 221–227.

187. Cherkin DC, Eisenberg D, Sherman KJ et al. Randomized trials comparing traditional Chinese medical acupuncture, therapeutic massage, and self-care education for chronic low back pain. Arch Intern Med 2001; 1081–1088.

188. Collacott EA, Zimmerman JT, White DW et al. Bipolar permanent magnets for the treatment of chronic low back pain: a pilot study. JAMA 2000; 283: 1322–1328.

189. Atlas SJ, Keller RB, Robson D et al. Surgical and nonsurgical management of lumbar spinal stenosis: four-year outcomes from the Maine Lumbar Spine Study. Spine 2000; 25: 556–562.

190. Amundsen T, Weber H, Nordal HU et al. Lumbar spinal stenosis: conservative or surgical management? A prospective 10-year study. Spine 2000; 25: 1424–1436.

191. Deen HG, Zimmerman RS, Lyons MK et al. Analysis of early failures after lumbar decompressive laminectomy for spinal stenosis. Mayo Clin Proc 1995; 70: 33–36.

192. Katz JN, Stucki G, Lipson SJ et al. Predictors of surgical outcome in degenerative lumbar spinal stenosis. Spine 1999; 24; 2229–2233.

193. Mayer TG, Gatchel RJ, Kishino N et al. Objective assessment of spine function following industrial injury. A prospective study with comparison group and one year follow-up. Spine 1985; 10: 482–493.

REGIONAL AND WIDESPREAD PAIN

15 The shoulder

Seamus E Dalton

- Shoulder motion involves four articulations: the glenohumeral, acromioclavicular, sternoclavicular and scapulothoracic
- The stability of the shoulder is provided by ligaments and the rotator cuff muscles
- Common shoulder disorders include rotator cuff tendinitis, rotator cuff tears, capsulitis (frozen shoulder), glenohumeral arthritis and acromioclavicular syndromes
- Most shoulder conditions can be diagnosed clinically by a careful history and physical examination. In tendon conditions, there is pain on active and resisted motion but passive range of motion tends to be normal. In capsulitis and glenohumeral arthritis, active and passive motions are painful, there is no pain on resisted motion and passive motion is decreased

FUNCTIONAL ANATOMY

The clavicle, scapula and humerus make up the bony skeleton of the shoulder girdle. The relationship of these bones with the axial skeleton is maintained largely through muscular attachments and also through the articulation of the clavicle with the thoracic cage at the sternoclavicular joint. Shoulder movement occurs through many planes and is achieved through motion at four articulations: the glenohumeral, acromioclavicular, sternoclavicular and scapulothoracic. Some constraint is also afforded to the head of the humerus through the subacromial joint by the overlying acromion and coracoacromial ligament. The glenohumeral joint is a multiaxial joint that allows the greatest freedom of movement of any joint of the body, although this is at the expense of stability. The bones of the shoulder girdle combine to provide a mobile framework upon which glenohumeral motion can take place. Ligamentous support is important in maintaining the stability of the joints of the shoulder and allowing synchronous movements to take place. Muscles act as prime movers at the shoulder as well as providing some dynamic stability to the glenohumeral joint.

Glenohumeral joint

The glenohumeral joint is not a true ball and socket joint and allows a certain amount of gliding movement, which is increased when there is laxity of the musculoligamentous support to the joint. Inherent bony stability is poor because of the shallow glenoid fossa and larger humeral head. The glenoid labrum is a rim of fibrocartilage at the periphery of the glenoid that effectively deepens the glenoid fossa and increases its diameter and contact with the humeral head, thereby affording some increased stability (Fig. 15.1). The joint capsule is lax, especially inferiorly, which allows rotation and elevation. In conditions where the capsule contracts there is restriction of glenohumeral motion. Restriction in this capsule posteriorly can aggravate or even give rise to secondary subacromial impingement. The joint capsule is thickened anteriorly to form separate components known as the glenohumeral ligaments,

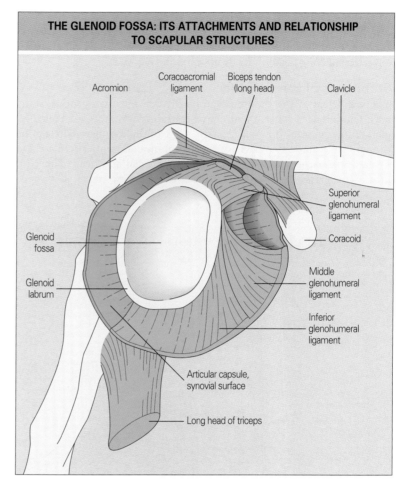

THE GLENOID FOSSA: ITS ATTACHMENTS AND RELATIONSHIP TO SCAPULAR STRUCTURES

Fig. 15.1 The glenoid fossa: Its attachments and relationship to scapular structures.

which act to strengthen the anterior and inferior capsule. The superior glenohumeral ligament runs from the anterosuperior aspect of the glenoid to the proximal edge of the lesser tuberosity of the humerus, with the middle glenohumeral ligament running just below this. The inferior glenohumeral ligament runs from the anteromedial aspect of the glenoid to the distal edge of the lesser tuberosity and proximal shaft of the humerus and has three components[1]. It is important in the provision of anteroinferior stability to the joint, particularly with the arm in abduction and external rotation, and has also been shown to provide some posterior stability[2].

Deficiencies in this ligament complex are important in the development of instability. Several studies have described a number of anatomic variations in the glenohumeral ligaments and capsulolabral attachments that need to be differentiated from truly pathological conditions[3,4]. With the advent of magnetic resonance imaging (MRI) and arthroscopy, these variants have been demonstrated in the normal and symptomatic population. An example is the variable development of the middle glenohumeral ligament and anterosuperior labrum, with normal variants such as the Buford complex (absent anterior superior labrum and cord-like middle glenohumeral ligament) and sublabral hole (or window), often being mistakenly identified as a pathological lesion, i.e. Bankart defect (isolated tear in the anterior inferior glenoid labrum).

The coracohumeral ligament runs from the coracoid process to the greater tuberosity and capsule and has a minor role to play in stabilizing the humeral head. The coracoacromial ligament extends from the undersurface of the medial acromion to the superolateral border of the coracoid process. Therefore, along with the acromion, it acts as a roof over the subacromial space under which the rotator cuff tendons slide, with the subacromial bursa lying between. This structure has been implicated in the pathology of impingement of the shoulder[5]. The transverse humeral ligament runs between the greater and lesser tuberosities, covering the long head of the biceps tendon (Fig. 15.2).

Stabilizers of the shoulder

The stabilizers of the shoulder can be divided into two groups: static and dynamic (i.e. passive and active restraints). The capsule, labrum, glenohumeral and, to a lesser extent, coracohumeral ligaments can be thought of as static stabilizers of the glenohumeral joint. There are two sleeves of muscles about the shoulder; superficial and deep. The deep group comprises the rotator cuff muscles – supraspinatus, subscapu-

laris, infraspinatus and teres minor – and the tendon of the long head of biceps. This layer acts dynamically to stabilize the humeral head in the glenoid fossa during shoulder movement, while simultaneously providing rotation (through subscapularis, teres minor and infraspinatus) and abduction (through supraspinatus).

The rotator cuff has also been shown to provide some passive restraint to glenohumeral joint translation, especially posteriorly[6]. During the initiation of shoulder abduction or elevation, the larger, more powerful deltoid muscle, if unopposed, would pull the humeral head superiorly towards the acromion. The rotator cuff muscles and the biceps tendon act as humeral head depressors to prevent this translational movement superiorly. This is known as the 'force-couple'. The subscapularis also acts to resist the tendency of the humeral head to sublux anteriorly in the upper ranges of abduction, although its role is less important than was previously thought[7,8]. Dysfunction of the rotator cuff muscles, either through weakness or a tear, results in diminished stabilization of the humeral head. This leads to weakness of the arm in elevation as well as superior migration of the humeral head, increasing the likelihood of subacromial compression or impingement (Fig. 15.3)[9]. Therefore, the four tendons of the rotator cuff grip the humeral head and act as guy-ropes to stabilize it during shoulder movement, resisting this sliding tendency within the joint.

Furthermore, there is a gap, or thinning of the cuff, between the supraspinatus and subscapularis tendons known as the 'rotator interval', which is composed of the coracohumeral ligament, the superior glenohumeral ligament and part of the joint capsule[10]. The rotator interval is of variable size, has a role in the prevention of inferior translation of the humeral head and may be implicated in some patients with anterior glenohumeral instability. Two functionally different parts of the rotator cuff have been identified and it has been reported that the coracohumeral ligament is an important structure in the rotator interval that

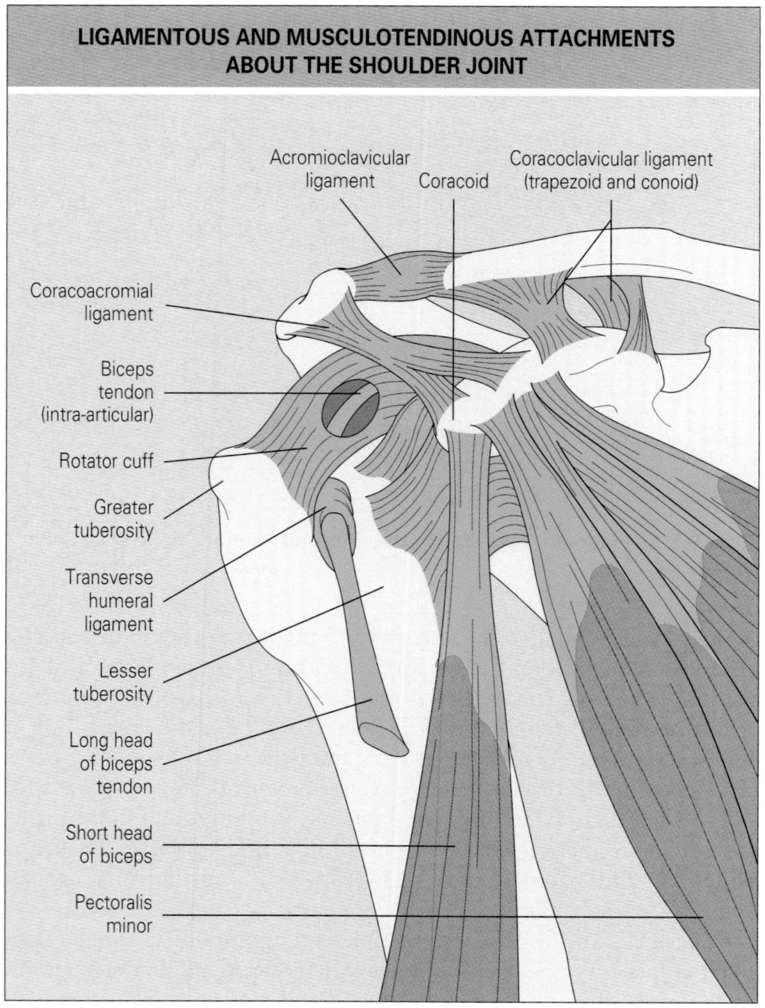

LIGAMENTOUS AND MUSCULOTENDINOUS ATTACHMENTS ABOUT THE SHOULDER JOINT

Acromioclavicular ligament
Coracoid
Coracoclavicular ligament (trapezoid and conoid)

Coracoacromial ligament

Biceps tendon (intra-articular)

Rotator cuff

Greater tuberosity

Transverse humeral ligament

Lesser tuberosity

Long head of biceps tendon

Short head of biceps

Pectoralis minor

Fig. 15.2 Ligamentous and musculotendinous attachments about the shoulder joint.

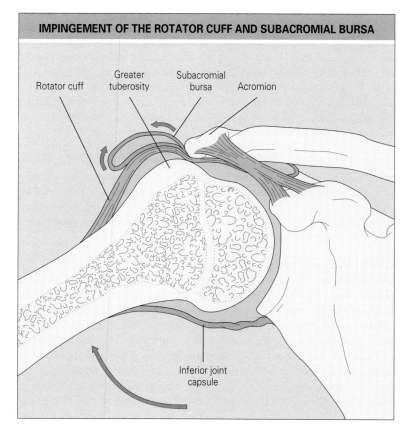

IMPINGEMENT OF THE ROTATOR CUFF AND SUBACROMIAL BURSA

Rotator cuff
Greater tuberosity
Subacromial bursa
Acromion

Inferior joint capsule

Fig. 15.3 Impingement of the rotator cuff and subacromial bursa.
Mechanism of impingement of the rotator cuff and subacromial bursa between the humeral head and overlying coracoacromial arch.

appears to have a role in the control of external rotation as well as inferior translation.

The biceps tendon arises from the superior labrum or directly from the supraglenoid tubercle, although a number of variations in this attachment have been reported. The long head of biceps acts as a humeral head depressor in full abduction and has also been shown to contribute to anterior stability of the shoulder[11]. However a recent study suggests that its role as a stabilizer of the glenohumeral joint is either a passive one or dependent on tension associated with elbow and forearm activity[12].

The outer sleeve of muscles comprises the deltoid, teres major, pectoralis major, latissimus dorsi and trapezius muscles. They act as prime movers of the humerus, although the trapezius acts through movement of the scapula and clavicle. The combination of these large muscles (which provide abduction, flexion, extension, adduction and a degree of rotation) with the deep layer of rotator cuff muscles (which provide more rotation of the humeral head and act as a stabilizing force) allows the expansive movement of the arm in actions such as reaching behind one's back or behind the head.

The deltoid muscle has three bellies; anterior, middle and posterior, producing respectively flexion, abduction and extension of the shoulder. All three muscles converge to an insertion on the deltoid tubercle on the lateral aspect of the humeral shaft. The rotator cuff muscles originate from the scapula and attach to the greater (supraspinatus, infraspinatus and teres minor) and lesser (subscapularis) tuberosities of the humerus.

Nerve supply to the glenohumeral joint is provided by those peripheral nerves supplying muscles acting upon the joint: the axillary, suprascapular, subscapular and musculocutaneous nerves. Innervation is via the fifth, sixth and seventh cervical roots, and the brachial plexus passes anterior and inferior to the glenohumeral joint.

Acromioclavicular joint

A fibrous disc separates the non-congruous surfaces of the distal end of the clavicle and the acromion and allows movement at this joint. During abduction and elevation the clavicle rotates through 30–40° and this largely occurs at the sternoclavicular joint[13]. There is a small amount of movement at the acromioclavicular joint and compressive force is applied to the joint in full elevation and horizontal adduction, which is the basis of stress tests applied to this joint. The joint is stabilized posteriorly by the posterior transverse ligament and inferiorly by the inferior ligament, and the deltoid and trapezius muscles act to provide some anterior and superior stability through their fascial layer. Of particular importance are the conoid and trapezoid, or coracoclavicular, ligaments, which maintain the close relationship between the scapula and clavicle during shoulder movement.

Scapulothoracic joint

The scapula lies against the posterolateral aspect of the thoracic wall, rotating and sliding laterally in abduction, elevation and flexion. It provides the origin for the rotator cuff muscles as well as the deltoid muscle and the trapezius inserts along its superior aspect. The scapulothoracic joint represents that articulation between the scapula and thoracic cage, and motion here is important for normal functioning of the shoulder.

Scapulohumeral rhythm

Elevation and abduction of the arm involves synchronous motion at the glenohumeral and scapulothoracic joints. As elevation increases above 90°, so does the proportion of scapulothoracic motion relative to glenohumeral motion. Scapulohumeral rhythm is representative of the ratio between movement at these two joints and is important in several shoulder disorders. Disturbance of the normal scapulohumeral rhythm affects the biomechanics of the shoulder joint and may result in secondary impingement or tendinitis of the shoulder. This is well demonstrated in elite swimmers or participants in overhead sports, in whom muscle imbalances such as serratus anterior fatigue can give rise to tendinitis or

impingement in this manner. Several muscles (levator scapulae, serratus anterior, trapezius, rhomboids) act to stabilize and control movement of the scapula, and the balance between scapula elevators, rotators, depressors, retractors and protractors provides scapular control and determines scapulothoracic movement. Scapular control by these muscles is becoming better understood as an important factor in glenohumeral instability and rotator cuff dysfunction. Muscle imbalance about the scapula can also lead to fatigue and overactivity in the levator and upper trapezius muscles particularly.

Sternoclavicular joint

Like the acromioclavicular joint, the sternoclavicular joint contains an intra-articular fibrous disc, which allows rotation of the clavicle during abduction and elevation. Strong ligaments stabilize this joint anteriorly and posteriorly.

Bursae

Significant variation exists in regard to the number and extent of bursae around the shoulder. The subacromial bursa lies between the rotator cuff (mainly supraspinatus tendon) and overlying acromion. This bursa does not consist of a distinct sac and its synovial layers blend in with and are firmly attached to the acromion and rotator cuff. In subacromial impingement and rotator cuff tendinitis there is reactive inflammation of this bursa. The subscapularis bursa communicates with the synovial joint cavity between the superior and middle glenohumeral ligaments, and the synovial membrane of the joint invests the tendon of the long head of biceps. Other bursae include the subdeltoid, coracoid, infraserratus and bursae at the insertion of the tendon of trapezius and at the tendon insertions on the humerus.

HISTORY AND PHYSICAL EXAMINATION

History

Shoulder pain may be seen in association with several medical conditions and may be referred from cervical, thoracic or abdominal sources. Any history suggestive of such a secondary cause, for example diabetes or Raynaud's phenomenon, may be crucial in diagnosis. Similarly, the mechanism of any precipitating injury is of value. A fall on an outstretched arm can give rise to instability in the younger patient or a rotator cuff tear in the elderly. A fall on the point of the shoulder may result in injury to the rotator cuff or acromioclavicular joint. Throwing injuries tend to stress the capsulolabral complex and ligament attachments of the glenohumeral joint and can also give rise to rotator cuff or bicipital tendinitis.

A thorough history is essential, since the location and type of pain varies between conditions. Pain referred from the cervical spine is often maximal over the suprascapular region with associated paresthesia or pain referred into the upper limb. Acromioclavicular and sternoclavicular pain is usually well localized to the involved joint. Pain from rotator cuff pathology is usually felt at the outer aspect of the upper arm or deltoid region. Adhesive capsulitis tends to give rise to an intense aching deep in the shoulder, although features similar to rotator cuff pathology are common in the early stages. Radiating pain into the arm may indicate cervical pathology, thoracic outlet syndrome, compressive neuropathy, brachial neuritis or reflex sympathetic dystrophy. Night pain tends to be of two main types: either sharp pain associated with movement, indicative of a rotator cuff tendinitis or acromioclavicular pathology; or pain of a deep, constant aching nature more suggestive of capsulitis or a chronic tear of the rotator cuff.

Inspection

This should be carried out from anterior, posterior and lateral aspects. The patient's ability to undress should be observed, as difficulty may indicate functional limitations. Areas of erythema and bruising should be noted. Although uncommon, swelling of the shoulder joint may be seen anteriorly in the projection of the subscapularis bursa. Deformity of the shoulder girdle exists with acromioclavicular joint separation or fractures of the clavicle or humerus. It is important to look for positioning of the shoulder such as asymmetric elevation or overprotraction. Neck positioning should also be recorded. Rupture of the long head of biceps tendon is readily seen with anterior bulging in the upper arm. Muscle wasting may be present in cases of cervical or brachial neuropathy (e.g. suprascapular nerve entrapment) but is also seen with chronic rotator cuff pathology in the supraspinatus and infraspinatus muscle bellies. Scapulohumeral and scapulothoracic rhythm during elevation should be assessed and any asymmetry noted. Winging of the scapula, demonstrated by asking the patient to do a push-up against the wall, is indicative of serratus anterior weakness (as in long thoracic nerve palsy) but can also occur with muscular dysfunction. Excessive depression of the scapula ('dumping') that is maintained through a range of abduction of the shoulder often indicates weakness of the upper trapezius and can lead to shoulder pain and symptoms of brachialgia and thoracic outlet syndrome.

Palpation

This should assess the presence of tenderness, swelling and instability of the acromioclavicular, sternoclavicular and glenohumeral joints. Tenderness over the tendon of the long head of biceps and the bicipital groove is common in bicipital tendinitis but comparison with the normal shoulder is necessary as this tendon is normally sensitive to touch. There may be tenderness over the rotator cuff insertions to the greater and lesser tuberosities but this is not always present in rotator cuff tendinitis. Acute calcific tendinitis is exquisitely tender over the involved tendon. The lateral margin of the subacromial joint can be palpated for swelling and tenderness and the glenohumeral joint itself may be tender in chronic or acute instability or capsulitis. An effusion of the glenohumeral joint should be differentiated from subacromial swelling, although communication between the two may exist in degenerative conditions where there is a full-thickness tear of the rotator cuff. Osteophytes can also be palpated at the margins of these joints, as can crepitus, if present.

Instability of the acromioclavicular and sternoclavicular joints is readily demonstrable but glenohumeral instability requires a more detailed examination combining assessment of laxity in anterior, posterior and inferior directions with stress and apprehension tests to determine the presence of symptomatic instability. This assessment needs to be carried out in the young adult presenting with shoulder pain, since underlying instability is a frequent cause of tendinitis around the shoulder. Muscles of the shoulder girdle and neck region should be palpated for trigger points and tender points, typically present with myofascial syndromes and fibromyalgia respectively.

Mobilization

Active and passive ranges of motion of both shoulders should be assessed in the planes of abduction, forward flexion and external rotation, both with the arm by the side and at 90° abduction. Internal rotation is frequently assessed as a combined maneuver with extension in bringing the arm up behind the back. This is limited in many periarticular conditions and a better assessment of true glenohumeral joint restriction is done by measuring true internal rotation with the arm by the side and the elbow extended, using the epicondyles as markers for comparison with the other shoulder. Any limitation of movement should be noted as well as any discrepancy between active and passive motion. Glenohumeral joint pathology is unlikely in the presence of a normal range of passive motion.

Further assessment should include passive adduction of the flexed and internally rotated shoulder to look for tightness of the posterior structures, namely the posterior capsule and external rotator cuff muscles, as this is often seen in chronic cuff pathology. Resisted shoulder movements are performed to assess involvement of muscles and tendons. The patient is asked to resist a specific movement in order to elicit an isolated, isometric contraction in the particular muscle group. The supraspinatus is tested with the arm abducted to 90°, flexed to 30° and internally rotated (i.e. thumb downwards). The examiner then resists abduction from this position. However in symptomatic cases this is often very painful and resisted flexion (at 30° flexion) with the arm internally rotated is often a sensitive and less aggravating test of rotator cuff (particularly supraspinatus) function. Resisted internal rotation tests the subscapularis and resisted external rotation tests the infraspinatus and teres minor. Resisted abduction should also be carried out with the arm by the side. Biceps function can also be tested by resisting shoulder flexion with the elbow extended (Speed's test) or resisting supination with the elbow flexed to 90° (Yergason's test), although the validity and specificity of these tests is questionable. Any assessment must include an examination of the cervical spine to assess range of motion and the presence of any referred upper limb pain (see Chapter 13).

Special movements

Specific examination techniques can be employed to further localize the source of pain in the shoulder region. Various tests for impingement have been described. In one of these the arm is flexed to 90°, adducted and then forcefully internally rotated and slightly elevated by the examiner, with the scapula stabilized by the examiner's other hand (Fig. 15.4a). In another variation the arm is placed in the adducted, flexed, internally rotated position and the patient is asked to externally rotate the arm against resistance (Fig. 15.4b). A further impingement test is carried out by passively forcing the arm into full forward flexion while the examiner stabilizes the top of the scapula with the other hand (Fig. 15.4c). In all situations a positive test is recorded if pain is felt as the subacromial bursa and the rotator cuff are forced against the

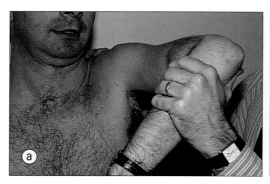
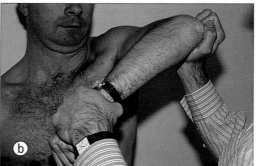
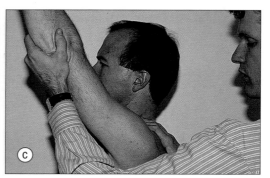

Fig. 15.4 Impingement tests. (a) Forced passive internal rotation. (b) Resisted external rotation. (c) Forced passive full forward flexion.

undersurface of the acromion, although it appears likely that these tests also provoke contact between anatomical structures associated with internal impingement.

Apart from Speed's and Yergason's tests, a further bicipital provocation test can be performed by asking the patient to abduct the arm to 90° with the palm upwards. The arm is then slowly adducted (with the elbow extended) across the midline and the chest against resistance[14]. In cases of bicipital tendon involvement a catching pain is felt in the region of the bicipital groove as the arm crosses in front of the shoulder joint (Fig. 15.5). O'Brien's test has been described as a provocation test for superior labral and biceps anchor pathology (SLAP lesions) but it also elicits pain in acromioclavicular joint disorders.

Pain at the acromioclavicular joint can be localized by performing various stress tests. In one the arm is held with the elbow and shoulder extended and then passively adducted across behind the back (Fig. 15.6). In another, less specific maneuver the arm is abducted to 90° and then

adducted across the patient's chest under the chin. In both tests pain is felt over an inflamed acromioclavicular joint at the limits of these movements. Assessment for a thoracic outlet syndrome is always difficult and several maneuvers are described that may provoke the symptoms of neurovascular compression. A number of upper limb neural tension tests have also been described and are useful when assessing the etiology of diffuse or non-specific upper limb pain.

The patient should be assessed for the presence of joint hypermobility. Laxity of the glenohumeral joint in anterior and posterior directions is determined by carrying out drawer tests in which the humeral head is gripped firmly and moved backwards and forwards in the glenoid fossa. This is best carried out with the patient lying supine and the abducted arm supported by the examiner's hand (Fig. 15.7). Inferior laxity is assessed by applying distal retraction to the arm while palpating the gap between the humeral head and acromion. Presence of a distinct gap can be felt and even seen, and is referred to as a positive sulcus sign. If

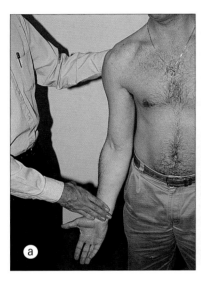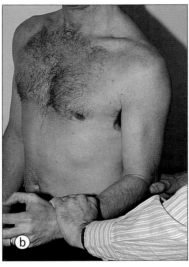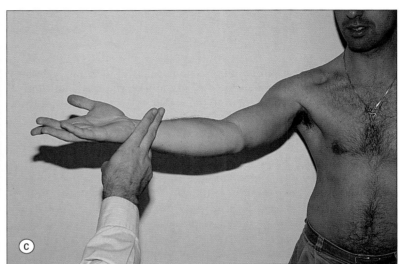

Fig. 15.5 Clinical tests for bicipital tendinitis. (a) Speed's test. (b) Yergason's test. (c) Bicipital provocation test.

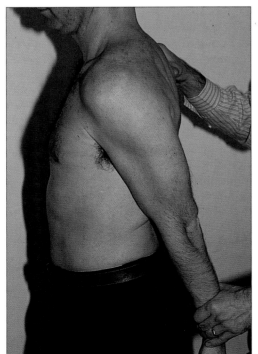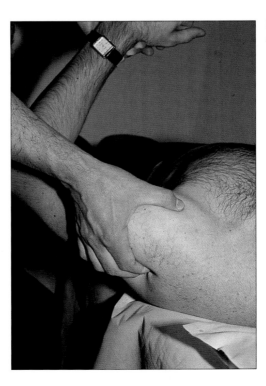

Fig. 15.6 An adduction stress test of the acromioclavicular joint.

Fig. 15.7 The anterior drawer test.

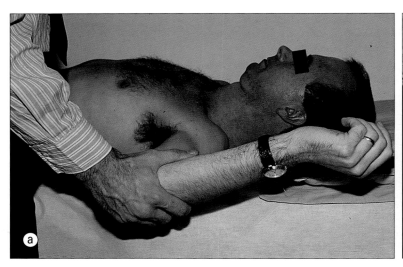
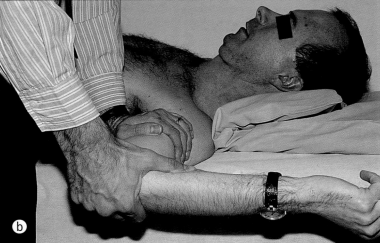

Fig. 15.8 A stress test for anterior glenohumeral instability. (a) The examiner slowly extends and externally rotates the abducted arm. (b) Containment sign: applying pressure anteriorly relieves the symptoms and allows further external rotation.

present this is indicative of multidirectional laxity of the joint. Anterior apprehension and stress tests are carried out with the examiner slowly extending and externally rotating the abducted arm with the patient supine. A positive test occurs when the patient experiences pain or apprehension during this maneuver and is confirmed when these symptoms disappear as the examiner's free hand applies a downward, i.e. stabilizing, force to the anterior aspect of the upper humerus. This often allows further external rotation of the arm (Fig. 15.8). Symptoms return as this stabilizing force is slowly withdrawn. It is important to differentiate between a positive test eliciting pain alone, as opposed to apprehension, as this may simply indicate internal impingement as opposed to true instability. The posterior stress test is carried out by applying gentle axial pressure to the humerus with the arm in the forward flexed, internally rotated and slightly adducted position, again in an attempt to reproduce pain and apprehension.

DIFFERENTIAL DIAGNOSIS OF SHOULDER PAIN

The glenohumeral joint may be affected as part of widespread joint disease, i.e. a polyarthropathy such as rheumatoid arthritis, crystal arthropathy or other inflammatory arthropathies. Septic arthritis, neuropathic (Charcot's) arthritis, osteonecrosis and idiopathic destructive arthritis are all conditions that can affect the shoulder joint in isolation. In articular disorders of the shoulder there may be swelling, and invariably there is an effect on passive and active motion of the glenohumeral joint with pain, restriction of motion and often crepitus.

Periarticular conditions affecting the shoulder can be loosely grouped into those with and without capsulitis. If there is no capsular involvement then passive joint motion is largely unaffected, whereas active movement may be limited by pain and/or weakness (e.g. rotator cuff disorders). With capsulitis there is multidirectional restriction of passive motion, and differentiation from articular conditions of the shoulder is made on clinical and radiologic grounds.

Referred pain to the shoulder can occur with cervical disorders, Pancoast's tumor of the lung, subphrenic pathology, entrapment neuropathies and brachial neuritis. In these conditions passive and often active movements of the shoulder are largely unaffected and there is usually little or no pain when testing rotator cuff function. However cervicobrachial pain is often associated with painful restriction of passive and active shoulder motion and may be confused with adhesive capsulitis. Again, differentiation from disorders of the shoulder is possible with an adequate history and examination (Table 15.1).

ROTATOR CUFF DISORDERS

The spectrum of disorders affecting the rotator cuff ranges from the mild transient tendinitis that follows an episode of glenohumeral instability in the young patient to a complete tear in the degenerative rotator cuff of the older patient. The anatomic configuration of the shoulder joint is such that the cuff is subjected to stresses when the arm is in the elevated position. Impingement can occur as the supraspinatus tendon is compressed between the humeral head and the overlying anterior acromion, coracoacromial ligament and even the inferior border of the acromioclavicular joint[5,15]. Impingement may be structural due to the presence of an acromial spur or degenerative acromioclavicular joint but it may also be functional, due to superior migration of the humeral head during abduction and elevation[9]. Mechanical impingement by the coracoid process on the rotator cuff or rotator interval has also been recognized as a clinical entity, although the diagnosis can only be confidently confirmed at the time of surgery[16]. Underlying glenohumeral instability is a frequent cause of rotator cuff tendinitis, particularly in the younger patient, as is eccentric overload in the throwing athlete, where the rotator cuff muscles act as decelerators of the throwing arm.

As the rotator cuff becomes inflamed, thinned or torn, its function as a humeral head depressor is compromised and superior migration of the humeral head can occur through the unopposed action of the deltoid, giving rise to further impingement. In the degenerative cuff with a complete tear this can eventually result in a cuff arthropathy with osteoarthritis at the subacromial and glenohumeral joints. The subacromial bursa lies between the rotator cuff tendons and the overlying coracoacromial arch and becomes inflamed with this impingement. This is a reactive process and is usually a secondary phenomenon, although primary subacromial bursitis can result from trauma.

Rotator cuff tendinitis
Clinical presentation and features
Presentation depends to a degree on the age of the patient and the likely etiology. Tendinitis resulting from eccentric overload or glenohumeral instability in the young adult usually presents acutely following an activity such as throwing. In the middle-aged individual, onset may be more gradual, reflecting the underlying chronic changes seen in the involved tendon. The patient may present with aching and discomfort in the shoulder, pain on movement and a history of repetitive or strenuous upper limb activity. The elderly patient may present with no history of antecedent trauma or repetitive activity and there is usually a gradual

TABLE 15.1 DIFFERENTIAL DIAGNOSIS OF SHOULDER PAIN: CLINICAL AND RADIOGRAPHIC FEATURES OF COMMON CAUSES OF SHOULDER PAIN

Diagnosis	Age	Type of onset	Location of pain	Night pain	Active range of motion	Passive range of motion	Impingement signs	Radiation of pain	Paras-thesia	Weakness	Instability	Radiographic changes	Special features
Rotator cuff tendinitis	Any	Acute or chronic	Deltoid region	+	↓↓ guarding	Normal	+++	–	–	Only due to pain	Look for	In chronic cases	Painful arc of abduction
Rotator cuff tears (chronic)	Over 40 years	Often chronic	Deltoid region	++	↓↓↓	Normal (may ↓ later)	++	–	–	++	–	+	Wasting of cuff muscles
Bicipital tendinitis	Any	Overuse	Anterior	–	↓ guarding	Normal	+	Occasionally into biceps	–	Only due to pain	Look for	None	Special examination tests
Calcific tendinitis	30–60 years	Acute	Point of shoulder	++	↓↓↓ guarding	Normal except for pain	+++	–	–	Only due to pain	–	++	Tenderness ++
Capsulitis ëfrozen shoulderí	Over 40 years	Insidious	Deep in shoulder	++	↓↓	↓↓	+	–	–	–	–	–	Global range of motion ↓
Acromioclavicular joint	Any	Acute or chronic	Over joint	Lying on side	↓ full elevation	Normal	–	–	–	–	–	In chronic cases	Local tenderness
Osteoarthrosis of glenohumeral joint	Over 40 years	Insidious	Deep in shoulder	++	↓↓	↓↓	–	–	–	May have mild	–	+++	Crepitus
Glenohumeral instability	Usually <25 years	Episodic	Anterior or posterior	–	Only appre-hension	Only appre-hension	Possible	–	+ with acute episodes	+ with acute episodes	+++	Often	Stress tests
Cervical spondylosis	Over 40 years	Insidious	Supra-scapular	Often	Normal	Normal	–	++	+++	+	–	In cervical spine	Pain with neck movement
Thoracic outlet syndrome	Any	Usually with activity	Neck shoulder arm	–	Normal	Normal	–	++	++	++	–	–	Special examination tests

onset of increasing shoulder discomfort, night pain, pain with movement and weakness if a degenerative tear is present. Except in the young patient with a history of explosive arm activity or trauma, onset tends to be gradual and aggravated by movements such as abduction and elevation or sustained overhead activity, which are commonly sports- or occupation-related. Patients frequently complain that they have difficulty reaching up behind their back when dressing. The pain at night usually occurs when rolling on to the affected side and is typically felt in the deltoid region rather than the point of the shoulder, although this can occur. Active movements may be restricted by pain and in the more severe or chronic cases a secondary capsulitis can develop, further restricting movement at the shoulder.

Findings on examination include a painful arc of abduction usually occurring between 70° and 120°. When lowering from full abduction there is often a 'catch' of pain, usually at midrange as impingement occurs, particularly when there is associated scapular dyskinesia. Passive motion tends to be full and pain-free if adequate muscle relaxation can be achieved. Point tenderness over the greater tuberosity and distal rotator cuff can occur but is not always present. The diagnosis is confirmed by reproducing pain when resisting movement of the affected tendon and with impingement testing. In the older patient, acromioclavicular joint arthritis is often present and there may be early joint stiffness.

Pathology
Impingement has been shown to occur in forward flexion when the anterior margin of the acromion impinges on the supraspinatus tendon[5,17]. Vascular studies have demonstrated that there is a constant area of avascularity or 'critical zone' extending from a point approximately 1cm proximal to the point of insertion of the tendon into the

greater tuberosity, and this compromise in microvascularity is seen with the arm in the adducted (neutral) position[18]. However, studies by Iannotti et al. have detected substantial blood flow in this critical zone using a laser Doppler[19]. It has long been supposed that this region of relative hypovascularity is compromised in elevation and abduction, thereby producing an inflammatory response and subsequent tendinitis. The pathology of this impingement syndrome has been classified by Neer into three stages:

● stage I: edema and hemorrhage of the tendon
● stage II: fibrosis of the subacromial bursa and tendinitis of the rotator cuff
● stage III: tendon degeneration, bony changes at the acromion and humeral head and eventual tendon rupture.

The bicipital tendon is frequently involved as part of this condition but is not usually the primary pathology. Generally, stage I is the pathology found in those under 25 years, stage II occurs in patients aged 25–40 years and stage III in those aged over 40 years of age. However in recent years our understanding of rotator cuff pathology has improved. Neer's initial proposal that rotator cuff tendinopathy resulted from subacromial impingement has been questioned and found to be an oversimplification of the pathogenesis of rotator cuff disease. There appear to be both extrinsic and intrinsic mechanisms involved[20].

Histological studies have shown that degenerative changes are more prominent on the articular surface of the rotator cuff insertions[21] and a number of radiological studies have confirmed the relative incidence of bursal, articular surface, intrasubstance and lamination tears of the rotator cuff.

There appears to be progressive tendon failure leading to cuff rupture with the prevalence of cuff tears increasing with age in the asymptomatic population[22–24]. Full-thickness tears have been reported in 20–30% and partial thickness tears have been found in a further 20–30% of people aged over 60 years of age, with the prevalence of full-thickness tears rising to 50% in those aged over 70. Possible etiological factors include trauma, attrition, ischemia and impingement. Recent work has looked at biochemical changes within the tendon matrix that may predispose to tendon rupture[25–27].

Investigations

Plain radiographs may show evidence of calcification in the rotator cuff tendons in chronic cases, and in long-standing cases there are changes suggestive of rotator cuff degeneration, i.e. cystic and sclerotic changes at the greater tuberosity insertion. Ultrasonography and MRI can be used to identify changes of rotator cuff tendinitis and partial tears but in the case of ultrasonography interpretation is fairly observer-dependent. Dynamic ultrasonography can also demonstrate thickening of the subacromial bursa and impingement[28].

Diagnostic pitfalls

Pain felt in the deltoid may suggest referred cervical pain, although this is more likely to present with suprascapular pain referring down into the arm. Pain on active arm movement and impingement testing will assist in differentiation, and preservation of passive range of movement will differentiate a capsulitis from rotator cuff tendinitis. In cases of tendinitis due to underlying instability – and this must be suspected in patients under 25 years of age – examination should confirm symptomatic instability.

Management

The treatment of rotator cuff tendinitis is often difficult and usually made impossible by continued participation in aggravating activities. Rest and activity modification are necessary to prevent the problem becoming chronic. Initial treatment should be directed at reducing inflammation by means of physical modalities and non-steroidal anti-inflammatory drugs (NSAIDs) if required. When there is failure to settle symptoms by these means, a subacromial injection of corticosteroid can be used taking care not to inject the rotator cuff directly[29]. As well as reducing pain, treatment should be directed at restoring range of motion and the normal biomechanics of shoulder movement, paying particular attention to scapular control and scapulohumeral rhythm. This is especially important in cases where such a disturbance in biomechanics has aggravated or even precipitated the problem. Proprioceptive taping can be used to assess the role of scapular dyskinesia in the genesis of dynamic subacromial impingement and is a useful tool in the early rehabilitation of shoulder dysfunction. Once the pain has reduced and normal shoulder movement patterns have been restored, a strengthening program should be instituted concentrating on rotator cuff exercises in order to restore its function as a humeral head stabilizer and depressor, thereby reducing the likelihood of further injury.

The younger patient with instability needs a full stabilization rehabilitation program and rarely requires injection to the shoulder. The older patient with a degenerative rotator cuff and associated acromioclavicular joint pathology may be resistant to conservative treatment.

Indications for surgery vary according to the age of the patient, stage of impingement or tendinitis, and the symptoms. The major indication for surgical intervention is pain and, in the presence of an intact rotator cuff, failure to respond to a conservative program within 1 year is a reasonable indication for surgery[30,31]. This involves subacromial decompression and may consist of an anterior acromioplasty and resection of the coracoacromial ligament, both of which can be carried out arthroscopically. Any impingement due to acromioclavicular joint pathology must also be addressed at operation. The results of subacromial decompression have generally been reported as good or excellent. However, there is a significant body of opinion that impingement usually results from a disturbance of normal glenohumeral kinematics attributable to capsular tightness, glenohumeral instability, scapulohumeral dysfunction or loss of rotator cuff function as a humeral head stabilizer. Therefore an accurate clinical diagnosis and evidence of subacromial impingement at surgery is important in determining outcome following subacromial decompression[32]. In some patients a capsular release or stabilization procedure may be more appropriate. In other words, subacromial impingement is frequently the result rather than the cause of shoulder dysfunction.

Prevention

In the young patient or athlete, attention to proper preparation for exercise and correct technique is important. Many athletes develop muscular imbalances about the shoulder, either through tightness or weakness, and secondary impingement and tendinitis can result if these are not corrected. In the older patient avoidance of sustained above-shoulder activities or explosive lifting will help prevent this condition from deteriorating or perhaps even developing.

Rotator cuff tears

Clinical presentation and features

Rotator cuff tears may be acute or chronic, partial or full-thickness. Partial tears may occur in any age group following trauma, but the full-thickness (or complete) tear is unusual in the patient under 40 years of age. In the young adult a partial tear can result from a fall or explosive shoulder movement and presents very much as a rotator cuff tendinitis, although onset is acute. Also, full active range of motion may be preserved. The acute complete rupture after trauma should be readily diagnosed. The mechanism of injury is usually a fall onto the outstretched arm, a hyperabduction injury or a fall onto the side of the shoulder. Bruising is often delayed and occurs in the upper arm, and there is usually an immediate loss of active abduction with weakness of abduction and external rotation. There is a close association between dislocation of the shoulder in the patient over 40 years of age and partial or complete tears of the rotator cuff. In one review of 40 patients the prevalence of full-thickness tears was 90%[33,34].

Chronic full-thickness tears are found in 7–27%[35,36] of patients at autopsy, and many patients with a documented complete tear of the supraspinatus tendon have full active abduction, often in the absence of pain, even in the presence of abnormal glenohumeral kinematics and superior humeral head migration[37]. There may be no history of trauma and symptoms frequently become apparent with increased activity, although the clinical expression of rotator cuff tears is variable[38]. The usual picture is one of pain on abduction and flexion with varying degrees of loss of active movement depending on the size of the tear. The patient may complain of weakness of abduction, flexion and internal or external rotation depending on the tendon involved.

Night pain is common and often severe. Examination reveals many of the features of rotator cuff tendinitis but there is often an inability to maintain the arm in abduction when lowering from the elevated position, i.e. a positive 'drop-off' sign. Subacromial crepitus and pain on impingement testing are present. A common clinical finding is wasting of the infraspinatus and, to a lesser extent, supraspinatus muscle bellies, together with weakness of abduction, but more often weakness of external rotation reflects the size of the tear. Rupture of the long head of the biceps tendon is frequently associated with chronic rotator cuff pathology.

Pathology

The incidence of degenerative cuff tears increases with age, as does the size of the tear[39,40]. Superior migration of the humeral head against the undersurface of the acromion occurs as the incompetent rotator cuff fails to stabilize and depress the humeral head and therefore counteract the pull of the deltoid. This leads to degenerative change both at the subacromial joint and secondarily at the glenohumeral joint, known as rotator cuff arthropathy. Management is difficult because of the combination of cuff deficiency and arthritic change. Neer estimates that 4% of cuff tears ultimately progress to a cuff arthropathy[41].

Investigation

Features of chronic rotator cuff degeneration can be seen on plain radiography with sclerosis and cystic changes at the greater tuberosity. Osteophyte formation may be present along the anterior inferior acromion, with possible acromioclavicular joint osteoarthritis. With a complete tear there may be superior migration of the humeral head and narrowing of the subacromial space (less than 6mm indicates a tear). This finding is seen in cuff arthropathy where there is degenerative change in the subacromial compartment and glenohumeral joint.

Full-thickness tears are readily demonstrated with single- or double-contrast arthrography, and sensitivity approaches 90%. Partial tears can occasionally be seen (Fig. 15.9). Estimation of the size of the defect using this technique is unreliable. Ultrasonography can identify tears, both full and to a lesser extent partial thickness[42] (Fig. 15.10). MRI compares favorably with arthrography in the diagnosis of complete tears (Fig. 15.11) but is less consistent in the assessment of partial tears, and interpretation is difficult[43] (Fig. 15.12). Arthroscopy may be used to establish the diagnosis in the patient with shoulder pain who requires further assessment. It is particularly useful in the assessment of instability while at the same time allowing visualization of the rotator cuff, subacromial bursa, intra-articular bicipital tendon and glenoid labrum. It also has a role in the estimation of the size of a cuff tear prior to more definitive surgery.

Management

Initially, partial rotator cuff tears should all be managed conservatively, as for rotator cuff tendinitis, although corticosteroid injection is not

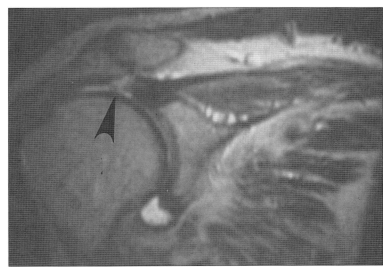

Fig. 15.11 MRI of complete rotator-cuff tear. T2-weighted MR image of the shoulder shows discontinuity of the supraspinatus tendon indicative of complete tear (arrow). The proximal tendon margin is frayed and retracted 1.5cm. Focal swelling and increased signal in opposing articular cartilages of the glenohumeral joint are evidence of early degenerative disease.

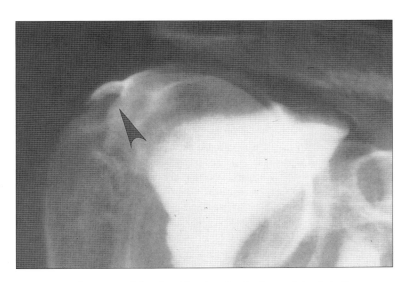

Fig. 15.9 Arthrogram of the shoulder showing leakage of dye into the supraspinatus tendon confirming a partial tear (arrow). This investigation is more accurate in the assessment of full-thickness tears of the rotator cuff.

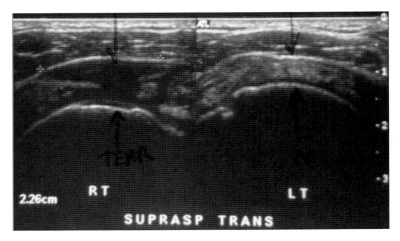

Fig. 15.10 Ultrasound of acute full-thickness rotator cuff tear.

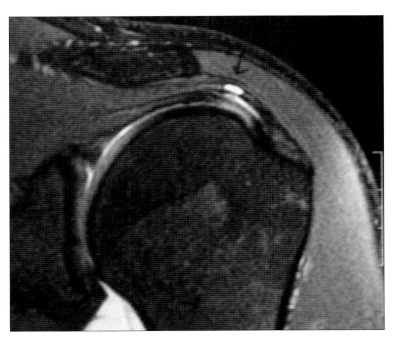

Fig. 15.12 MRI of complex rotator cuff pathology. The image shows a partial articular surface rotator cuff tear along with a laminar defect and small cyst in the distal supraspinatus tendon.

advisable within 4–6 weeks of an acute injury. The surgical management of complete tears is somewhat controversial. Acute ruptures in the young or active patient should be managed surgically earlier rather than later. In the older or less active patient it is reasonable to have a trial of conservative management but if there is no substantial improvement within 3 months then subacromial decompression and repair is advisable[44].

Chronic complete tears should all be treated with an adequate conservative program in the first instance. Failure to achieve pain relief is a major indication for surgical intervention. Any operative procedure should be directed primarily at relief of impingement, debridement of the cuff tear and usually, but not always, repair of the defect[45]. Surgery should also be considered where there is an associated rupture of the biceps tendon as these cases appear more likely to develop a cuff arthropathy.

The results of surgical repair of rotator cuff tears are usually good but depend on the age of the patient and on the size and age of the tear. Pain relief is usually achieved but recovery of strength is less predictable and restoration of joint motion may depend on the amount of postoperative stiffness that develops. A major predictor of outcome following cuff repair is the degree of rotator cuff muscle atrophy and fatty infiltration present, which can be assessed preoperatively with computed tomography or MRI[46]. Therefore a number of factors must be taken into account when deciding whether to proceed to surgery. These include the patient's age and occupation, the size and type of tear (repair of lamination and complex tears can be difficult) and the presence of tendon retraction and muscle atrophy. Surgery should be delayed if there is an associated capsulitis, and a capsular release may be required beforehand. Full-thickness tears of the subscapularis are best repaired early, as delayed closure may not be possible once the torn tendon has retracted. In large retracted tears a latissimus dorsi or pectoralis major muscle transfer may be required to close the defect and improve function.

BICIPITAL TENDINITIS

Clinical presentation and features
Although frequently diagnosed, bicipital tendinitis is not often seen in isolation and usually occurs in association with rotator cuff tendinitis or impingement, or with glenohumeral instability[47]. Primary involvement of the tendon is seen as an overuse injury in sports such as weightlifting where there is a repetitive stress placed upon the tendon, or after prolonged and repetitive carrying (e.g. of small children). The bicipital tendon acts as a secondary stabilizer of the humeral head and the translational movement seen with glenohumeral laxity can place increased stress upon the tendon, leading to tendinitis. As with rotator cuff tendinitis, the young patient with bicipital tendinitis should be assessed for instability. With chronic impingement or rotator cuff degeneration the biceps tendon may become fibrotic and attenuated and eventually rupture. Acute ruptures are also seen in young power-lifters and the diagnosis is made easily in the acute presentation.

Pain is usually felt over the anterior aspect of the shoulder, often radiating into the biceps muscle, with well localized tenderness over the tendon as it runs in the bicipital groove. Pain is felt with overhead activities and often with shoulder extension and elbow flexion. Examination may reveal features of impingement, rotator cuff tendinitis and instability, all of which are important in determining the etiology of bicipital tendinitis. Pain may be reproduced with resisted elbow flexion, supination and shoulder flexion and various provocation tests are described, although none appear to be consistently positive. Passive shoulder extension stretches the biceps and may be painful. Rupture of the tendon is evident when there is the characteristic deformity of the upper arm with bunching up of the lateral muscle belly of the biceps, best seen with resisted elbow flexion and supination.

Acute rupture of the transverse humeral ligament can result in subluxation or dislocation of the tendon. This can present with symptoms similar to bicipital tendinitis but often a more specific complaint is made of catching and a clicking sensation at the shoulder. Clinical examination may demonstrate subluxation of the tendon, which is felt as the arm is passively moved through internal and external rotation while in the 90° abducted position. Medial dislocation of the tendon is often found in association with tears of the subscapularis tendon.

Pathology
The tendon of the long head of biceps may be involved at several sites: its attachment to the superior glenoid labrum, which may be injured in a fall or throwing action ('SLAP' lesion[48]); as it runs across the glenohumeral joint (intra-articular); or as it runs in the bicipital groove (extra-articular). The transverse humeral ligament stabilizes the tendon in the bicipital groove and if this mechanism is disrupted subluxation or dislocation of the tendon can result. This tends to occur as the arm is rotated in the abducted position. The tendon can become inflamed, thickened and fibrotic in chronic cases and it has been shown that bicipital groove anatomy correlates with biceps tendon disease[49]. In the older patient there may be attenuation and thinning of the tendon and eventual rupture. This latter presentation is almost always indicative of underlying rotator cuff degeneration as the bicipital tendon appears to become stressed in its attempt to act as a humeral head depressor in cases of rotator cuff incompetence. Also, the presence of a complete rotator cuff tear exposes the intra-articular portion of the bicipital tendon to the overlying acromion and further impingement.

Investigation
Special radiographic views demonstrate the bicipital groove, allowing assessment of its depth and the presence of any hypertrophic spurring. Filling of the synovial extension around the tendon is seen on arthrography and may be reduced in cases of chronic fibrosis. The tendon and any surrounding fluid can be seen well with ultrasonography (Fig. 15.13), and this assists in the diagnosis of tears, both partial and complete, as well as tendinitis. It can also be used to demonstrate subluxation/dislocation of the tendon. MRI or arthroscopy allows visualization of the intra-articular portion of the tendon and its labral attachment (Fig. 15.14).

Management
It is necessary to establish whether the tendinitis is primary or secondary, since a failure to address any underlying rotator cuff pathology or

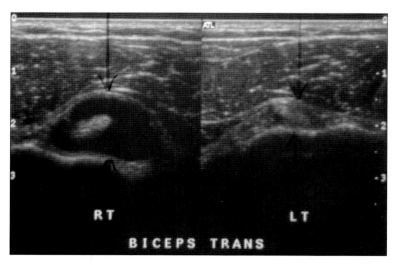

Fig. 15.13 Ultrasound of bicipital tendinitis. Transverse image showing large effusion in the long head of biceps tendon sheath.

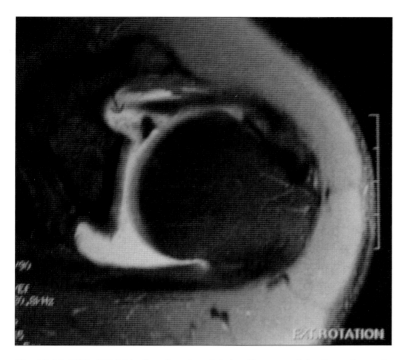

Fig. 15.14 MRI of SLAP lesion showing debris adjacent to labral tear (arrow).

instability will lead to a recurrence of symptoms. The principles of management are rest, physical modalities and NSAIDs as required. Low-power laser therapy has been reported to have a beneficial effect, although this has been disputed[50,51]. Corticosteroid injection is helpful in chronic cases but care should be taken not to inject the tendon itself. An intra-articular injection or injection to the bicipital groove may be given but both are best done under ultrasound guidance. Since most cases of bicipital tendinitis are secondary, they usually settle as the primary condition is treated. The primary cases due to lifting or other activities respond to rest and simple anti-inflammatory measures. Surgery can be considered in chronic resistant cases; this may involve subacromial decompression in cases of impingement, or tenodesis when there is chronic thickening of the tendon in the groove. Rupture of the tendon is normally treated conservatively except in the occasional young patient where upper arm strength is critical to their sport or profession. Usually, weakness following this injury is not significant. Subluxation of the tendon is usually treated conservatively, although occasionally surgery is necessary and medial subluxation/dislocation of the tendon out of the groove frequently indicates the presence of a tear in the subscapularis tendon which may not be apparent with ultrasonography. Any conservative program must include range of motion exercises, stretches and, once symptoms have settled, a graduated eccentric and concentric biceps and rotator cuff strengthening program.

SUBACROMIAL BURSITIS

The close relationship between the subacromial bursa and the rotator cuff, specifically the supraspinatus tendon, is such that the term subacromial bursitis is frequently used when describing the pathology of impingement. In most cases inflammation of the bursa arises as part of the impingement process and coexists with an underlying rotator cuff tendinitis. This bursitis is therefore a reactive phenomenon. In chronic cases the bursa becomes thickened and fibrotic and surgical excision or debridement may be necessary. Treatment of rotator cuff tendinitis is directed at reducing the inflammation in the subacromial space or bursa as well as reducing the impingement.

Acute traumatic bursitis in the form of hemorrhage and edema can occur as a result of a fall or a direct blow to the point of the shoulder. Pain on abduction is present but differentiation from rotator cuff tendinitis is possible on the basis of increased tenderness and fluid at the subacromial space. A period of rest combined with simple measures, such as ice, usually allows resumption of normal activities, but occasionally persistent impingement develops, requiring further treatment.

CAPSULITIS

Introduction

Capsulitis of the shoulder remains a condition both difficult to define and universally awkward to manage. Many labels have been given to the situation where there is a painful restriction of shoulder movement apparently of soft tissue origin. These include frozen shoulder, periarthritis or pericapsulitis of the shoulder, adhesive capsulitis and adherent or obliterative bursitis. There has been an attempt to classify patients with a painful stiff shoulder according to the presence or absence of capsular joint restriction as seen at arthrography[52]. Perhaps incorrectly, the term 'frozen shoulder' is applied to many conditions where restriction of movement is largely due to pain from an underlying condition, such as rotator cuff tendinitis, rather than to the classic global restriction of glenohumeral joint motion seen with a true adhesive capsulitis.

Primary capsulitis of the shoulder can be defined as a condition of unknown etiology in which there is a painful restriction of glenohumeral movement in all planes of motion, both active and passive, in the absence of joint degeneration sufficient to explain this restriction. A similar condition, known as secondary capsulitis, exists when the condition is associated with a clearly defined clinical disorder or precipitating event. Underlying diseases associated with this condition are diabetes mellitus, thyroid disease, hyperlipidemia, pulmonary disorders such as tuberculosis or carcinoma, and cardiac disease or surgery. Myocardial infarct, cerebrovascular accident or shoulder trauma may precipitate the development of a shoulder capsulitis. Dupuytren's disease is often seen in association with adhesive capsulitis and it has been suggested that the two conditions may have similar biochemical and histological characteristics[53]. Following traction or hyperabduction injuries to the shoulder a mixed clinical picture of capsulitis and cervicobrachialgia may develop, further complicating diagnosis and treatment.

Clinical presentation and features

Estimation of the prevalence of adhesive capsulitis is difficult due to variation in populations studied and diagnostic criteria used but it appears to be approximately 2–3% in non-diabetics[54–56]. Onset under the age of 40 years is rare, with the mean age of onset being in the sixth decade. Women are affected more often than men. Involvement of the contralateral shoulder occurs in 6–17% of patients over the subsequent 5 years[57]. It is commonly stated that recurrence in the same shoulder does not occur, although there has been a recent case report[58]. There is a frequent history of minor shoulder strain or injury prior to the onset of symptoms but whether this represents a true strain of the shoulder or simply the earliest awareness of pain is unclear. The natural history of this condition has been assessed by various authors and it appears that there are three phases in its development and progression. The shoulder moves from being simply painful to being painful and stiff and eventually to being less painful but profoundly stiff. This last stage appears to be self-limiting and recovery is gradual and spontaneous. These stages have been termed painful, adhesive and resolution. The duration of each stage in the overall condition varies considerably but approximate durations are 3–8 months for the painful phase, 4–6 months for the adhesive phase and 1–3 years for the resolution phase. The extent of recovery is variable, with quoted figures of 33–61% of patients having a clinically detectable limitation of shoulder movement and, although many remain asymptomatic, 7–15% of patients may have a persisting functional disability[59–63]. The extent to which the duration of the painful and adhesive phases determines the degree of residual disability remains controversial.

Painful phase

This is characterized by the insidious onset of symptoms, usually in the form of pain on shoulder movement and background ache in the shoulder region, often in the upper trapezius muscle. As the condition becomes established there is the development of increasing pain at rest and at night, the latter becoming quite disturbing and frequently waking the patient in the absence of a history of precipitative movement. Muscle spasm may develop, further limiting shoulder movement, which becomes restricted with the increase in pain and stiffness at the shoulder. Towards the end of this phase stiffness becomes a major complaint.

Adhesive phase

Usually after several months the character of pain alters and becomes less severe. There is a reduction in pain at rest and at night but discomfort and a more severe pain at the limits of movement persist. Shoulder movement becomes more restricted during this phase and this can lead to periscapular pain due to the increase in scapulothoracic motion.

Resolution phase

The pain is less evident and the dominant symptom is restriction of shoulder movement, which often appears less distressing for the patient now that the pain has eased. There is a slow and gradual improvement in range of motion, although this is frequently incomplete. The onset and rate of recovery are variable and unpredictable.

Clinical examination

The physical signs alter to a degree as the condition progresses, with pain, often severe, present in the earlier stages. Differentiation from rotator cuff tendinitis is possible on the basis of a global restriction of passive movement rather than simply the loss of abduction and flexion that is seen with chronic rotator cuff conditions. A useful early clinical indicator of developing capsulitis is pain at the limit of passive external rotation of the shoulder with the arm by the side. In the painful phase there is painful restriction of active and passive motion (often mild in the earlier stages). There may be pain on impingement testing and resisted movement, although this is less common than in rotator cuff tendinitis. Associated findings are tenderness in the upper trapezius muscle and early scapula hitching in elevation. In the latter phases the important finding is significant restriction of glenohumeral movement with a compensatory increase in scapulothoracic motion during flexion and abduction. Pain may be present but there is less discrepancy between active and passive ranges. Disuse atrophy of the rotator cuff and deltoid muscles may exist. Joint line tenderness is common in the painful phase.

Pathophysiology

The etiology of adhesive capsulitis is not known and the evidence for its association with the aforementioned conditions or trauma is unconvincing. Capsulitis is more prevalent in diabetics (prevalence 10–20%), usually occurring at a younger age and often associated with prolonged duration of the diabetes, insulin dependence, the development of limited joint mobility syndrome and widespread microvascular disease. Bilateral involvement is also more common in diabetes[54–55]. The links between diabetes and capsulitis may revolve around microvascular disease, abnormalities of collagen repair or predisposition to infection[64]. An association between capsulitis and thyroid disease and pulmonary conditions has been noted but provides little information regarding its pathogenesis[65–68]. Histologic studies have failed to demonstrate the presence of inflammatory cell infiltrates, granulomas or vasculitis in the joint capsule or synovium. Also, there is nothing to implicate infection, crystal arthropathy or trauma.

Histologic studies of the joint capsule early in the disease are difficult to perform and the heterogeneity of patients loosely labeled as having capsulitis makes study of this condition difficult. However, Lundberg[54] noted an increase in fibrous tissue, fibroblast numbers and vascularity with no change in the synovial lining and no inflammatory cell infiltrate. Bunker has reported that fibroblasts and myofibroblasts lay down a dense type III collagen matrix in the shoulder joint capsule, leading to joint contracture[69]. Cytokine, matrix metalloproteinase (MMP) and MMP inhibitor abnormalities have been reported. Several studies have looked at a variety of immunologic factors, and no immunologic disturbance has been demonstrated[70].

Investigation

Diagnosis is made largely on clinical grounds since there are few abnormalities found on investigation. Elevations of erythrocyte sedimentation rate (ESR), acute phase reactants and globulin levels are not usually seen, and calcium metabolism appears normal on testing. Plain radiographs are not helpful in making the diagnosis except to exclude widespread osteoarthritic changes, calcific tendinitis or neoplasm. In the younger patient presenting with clinical features of adhesive capsulitis, avascular necrosis should be suspected and must be excluded before considering intraarticular corticosteroid injection.

Classic features at arthrography are limitation of joint volume with a loss of the normal dependent axillary fold or pouch and irregularity of the capsular insertion to the anatomic neck of the humerus. Some authors insist that these changes must be present in order to make a diagnosis of adhesive capsulitis. Between 10% and 30% of patients who undergo arthrography have a demonstrable complete tear of the rotator cuff[52,62]. Other studies have suggested that a significant number of patients with a clinical diagnosis of adhesive capsulitis have normal findings at arthrography[62]. Arthroscopy allows further evaluation of these patients and different stages of synovitis and contracture have been described[52].

Bone scintigraphy may demonstrate increased isotope uptake in the affected shoulder region but this appears to have no predictive value in terms of outcome or response to treatment and is therefore of limited diagnostic value[71]. An average reduction in bone mineral content of 50% in the affected humeral head has been demonstrated, although again this is of little diagnostic or therapeutic value[54]. Ultrasonography has been used and typical findings are a biceps sheath effusion, restriction of movement and subacromial impingement resulting from the capsular contracture, but these features are not diagnostic and patients are often mistakenly treated for impingement tendinitis.

Management

Many therapies have been tried in an attempt to modify the natural history of capsulitis, and clinical studies of the efficacy of various treatment methods have been compromised by difficulties with patient selection, diagnostic criteria and the variability in the natural resolution of the condition. The emphasis of treatment in the early stages should be on pain reduction and minimization of joint restriction. Analgesics and anti-inflammatory drugs provide limited relief of pain but do little to alter the course of the disorder. Physiotherapy utilizes physical modalities to modify pain and reduce protective muscle spasm while attempting to encourage range of motion exercises early on in order to maintain joint mobility. Shoulder immobilization should be discouraged if at all possible, although in the painful phase the patient tends to minimize shoulder movement.

Few treatments have been shown to consistently affect rate of recovery or limit restriction of movement. Intra-articular corticosteroid injections have been shown to improve pain and range of movement to a degree, although no long-term benefit has been demonstrated[72–75]. Intra-articular injection is best done under ultrasound guidance or fluoroscopy and failure to do so in previous studies may account for the variable response to corticosteroid injection in the past. It still remains a useful and often effective means of relieving pain and hastening recovery. Oral corticosteroids have also been shown to improve pain but not to affect the rate of recovery[76]. Careful utilization of analgesic or anti-inflammatory drugs with physiotherapy may be of benefit, although this may be due to a reduction in the protective spasm seen in the untreated patient.

Hydrodistention of the joint capsule has been used as a treatment in various stages of this condition but no consensus has been reached with regard to its benefits. Manipulation under anesthetic has been used to restore joint motion but may involve rupture of the inferior capsule and possibly the subscapularis tendon at its insertion. Care should be taken when carrying out this procedure, especially in the elderly patient, in order to avoid humeral fracture, shoulder dislocation or a significant rotator cuff rupture. Aggressive early rehabilitation in the immediate postmanipulation period is needed in order to maintain joint mobility, and patient co-operation with and tolerance of this treatment is essential. Manipulation during the painful phase is not recommended since painful recontraction of the capsule may occur and this treatment method is usually reserved for the adhesive phase once the pain has settled.

Arthroscopic capsulotomy can be used to treat recalcitrant cases of frozen shoulder. Some authors do not restrict the use of this treatment to those patients who no longer have significant pain and advocate arthroscopic capsular release over manipulation, given that it allows direct visualization of the joint capsule and therefore less risk of tendon rupture[77–79]. For many patients, however, once the painful phase of their condition has subsided the prospect of this painful procedure is not appealing. Improvement in range of movement following manipulation or capsulotomy is variable and is perhaps dependent upon patient selection. Long-term recovery appears unchanged, although resolution may be accelerated immediately following manipulation[52,61,63].

ACROMIOCLAVICULAR SYNDROMES

Introduction
Pain localized to the acromioclavicular joint is commonly seen as either an acute or a chronic condition. In the younger patient this joint is frequently subjected to trauma as a result of falls or contact sport. This may result in an acute injury and may also predispose the joint to further problems, such as instability or secondary osteoarthritis. Infection of this joint is rare but septic arthritis has been described[80].

Trauma
Disruption of the acromioclavicular joint may be seen in association with fractures of the outer end of the clavicle and often leads to the development of secondary osteoarthritis. More common are injuries to the joint itself, which are graded according to the degree of disruption of the joint capsule and supporting ligaments. Grade I injury involves minor sprain to the joint capsule without ligament disruption. Grade II injury involves subluxation of the joint with downward displacement of the acromion relative to the distal end of the clavicle. There is stretching of the inferior acromioclavicular ligaments, and stretching and possibly a partial tear, but not complete rupture, of the coracoclavicular ligaments. In a grade III injury complete dislocation of the joint occurs through rupture of the coracoclavicular ligaments. Grade III injuries can be further classified (often as grades IV, V and VI) according to the extent (and direction) of disruption or perforation of the overlying deltotrapezius fascial or muscle layer by the displaced outer end of the clavicle.

Clinical presentation and features on physical examination
The mechanism of injury usually involves a fall directly on to the point of the shoulder. Pain is localized to the top of the shoulder in the region of the involved joint, which is tender and often swollen to palpation. Abduction is often limited, both actively and passively, according to the degree of joint disruption. With a minor injury where there is good preservation of movement, acromioclavicular joint stress tests can be carried out to localize symptoms. In complete dislocation of the joint a visible step deformity is seen and examination will determine whether or not this dislocation can be reduced. This is important in the determination of the extent of any grade III injury. The patient often describes a feeling of the shoulder having dropped, due to the downward displacement of the acromion.

Management
For the grade I or grade II injury, treatment is largely symptomatic, with analgesics and provision of a sling for days to weeks depending on the symptoms. Shoulder movements should be encouraged as pain settles, and functional recovery is excellent.

Controversy exists over the management of grade III injuries. Provided perforation of the overlying muscle or fascial layer has not occurred, most patients settle with conservative treatment over a period of 6–10 weeks. Strapping of the joint has no effect on long-term stability and is not indicated in these patients[81]. Although effective, surgical stabilization by means of internal fixation is usually unnecessary; it is associated with a significant complication and failure rate and long-term results are not demonstrably better than for non-operative treatment. Recent surgical advances have lowered the complication rate and therefore the threshold for considering surgical repair or reconstruction of the acromioclavicular joint, particularly in manual workers or people dependent on overhead function. However surgery is usually reserved for severe grade III disruptions or where an individual's occupation may be compromised by persistent deformity or instability at that joint.

Late sequelae
Patients may present with persistent pain at the acromioclavicular joint. This represents low-grade joint inflammation and may be associated with an underlying instability, early development of secondary osteoarthritis or osteolysis of the distal end of the clavicle. Persistent pain following joint injury may also result from damage to the intra-articular fibrocartilage sustained at the time of injury. Treatment is symptomatic, with anti-inflammatory medication or injection of intra-articular corticosteroid for resistant cases. Delayed surgical stabilization may be carried out in cases of gross instability and tears of the fibrocartilage can be debrided arthroscopically. Long-term treatment is as for osteoarthritis of the joint.

Osteolysis of the clavicle
Osteolysis of the distal clavicle is a condition that may follow an acute injury or repetitive stress to the shoulder[82].

Symptoms are usually similar to those of acromioclavicular inflammation, with aching and pain at the limits of flexion and abduction. Radiographic changes typically show resorption of the distal clavicle, often with osteophyte formation, osteoporosis or tapering (Fig. 15.15). Response to activity modification and conservative treatment is usually satisfactory but excision of the distal clavicle may be necessary. There may even be reconstitution of the distal clavicle with rest[83].

Osteoarthritis
Acromioclavicular joint morphology appears to be associated with the development of osteoarthritis[84]. A previous history of joint injury is common when osteoarthritis of this joint occurs in isolation, but the joint may also be involved as part of generalized osteoarthritis.

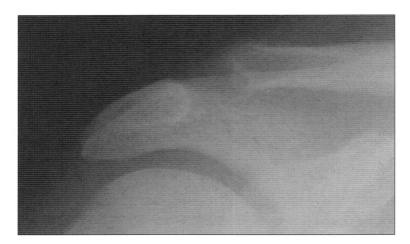

Fig. 15.15 Radiographic changes of osteolysis of the clavicle.

Clinical features

Pain and tenderness are localized to the joint, which is often prominent because of osteophyte formation. Pain exists on full abduction or horizontal adduction and can also be reproduced with adduction of the extended arm. Crepitus is frequently localized to the joint. It is important to note that osteoarthritis of the joint is often seen in association with rotator cuff degeneration, and inferior osteophytes at the acromioclavicular joint may contribute to the development of a rotator cuff tear. Clinical features of both conditions frequently coexist, especially in the older patient.

Investigation

Osteoarthritis can be diagnosed on plain radiography and an arthrogram may reveal the presence of a complete tear of the rotator cuff. Traction or weight-bearing views can be taken in order to demonstrate joint instability.

Management

Initial management consists of local modalities and the use of analgesic or anti-inflammatory drugs. A suitable exercise program should be provided in order to restore normal scapulohumeral rhythm, glenohumeral range of motion, and deltoid and rotator cuff strength once symptoms have settled. Intra-articular corticosteroid injection usually provides good symptom relief but often needs to be repeated. Cases resistant to conservative treatment may require surgery, which usually consists of excision arthroplasty of the joint while ensuring that instability is minimized. Careful assessment of rotator cuff function is important and, in the presence of a significant tear, rotator cuff repair or an acromioplasty may be indicated. Excision arthroplasty may also be indicated in the younger patient with chronic symptoms, whether due to degenerative change, osteolysis or instability.

CALCIFIC TENDINITIS

The prevalence of radiologically detectable calcification in the rotator cuff tendons is reported to be 2.7–7.5%, occurring in both symptomatic and asymptomatic shoulders[85,86]. It often involves the supraspinatus tendon and has been reported as being more common in women, housewives and sedentary individuals. Bosworth[87] estimated that 35–45% of individuals with calcification seen on radiography developed symptoms. Frequently bilateral, it usually occurs between the ages of 40 and 60 years but can present as an acute condition in the younger patient. Patients may present with chronic symptoms of catching pain with movement due to impingement.

Acute calcific tendinitis has a quite different presentation with acute severe pain limiting passive or active shoulder movement almost com-

pletely, with exquisite point tenderness and occasionally erythema over the involved tendon. The onset of symptoms can be rapid with no history of injury or overuse and this occurs during the resorptive phase of calcification.

Patients can therefore be divided into two groups: first, those patients with an acute onset of severe pain and limitation of movement, often in the absence of any previous shoulder symptoms; second, patients who have a more chronic catching pain associated with movement presenting as an impingement problem.

Pathophysiology

It has been argued by various authors that calcification occurs as part of a degenerative process involving the rotator cuff tendons, largely because it is rarely seen in people before the fourth decade[88]. Also, complete cuff tears have been found in 21% of patients with calcific tendinitis[89]. Histologic studies have confirmed that calcification follows on from tendon fibrosis and subsequent necrosis[89,90]. Uhthoff and colleagues[91,92] have proposed a model for the pathogenesis of calcific tendinitis based on its clinical presentation as a self-healing condition in which the calcific process is actively mediated by cells in a viable environment. They classify the disease in three stages: precalcific, calcific and postcalcific. In the precalcific stage it is thought that there is fibrocartilaginous transformation in the avascular or 'critical' zone of the supraspinatus tendon. In the calcific stage calcium crystals are deposited in matrix vehicles to form large deposits (known as the formative phase). After a variable period of inactivity (resting period) there is spontaneous resorption of the calcium by means of peripheral vascularization and phagocytosis of the deposit (resorptive phase). Following removal of the calcium the space is filled with granulation tissue (postcalcific stage). Occasionally a deposit can rupture into the overlying subacromial bursa. There has been a reported association between this condition and HLA-A1[93].

Investigation

A plain radiograph will identify and localize the calcific deposit to a particular tendon, usually the supraspinatus. In the formative phase of calcification the deposit is well defined and homogenously dense. In the resorptive phase, usually presenting as the acute condition, the deposit is less well defined, irregular and has a fluffy, less dense appearance (Fig. 15.16). Degenerative rotator cuff disease and arthropathy may have radiologically detectable calcification but this is usually associated with other features of these conditions and the areas of calcification are usually small, stippled and close to the tendon insertion at the greater tuberosity.

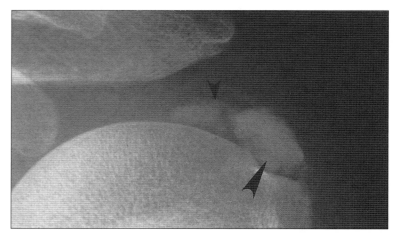

Fig. 15.16 Calcific tendinitis: formative phase (large arrow) and resorptive phase (small arrow).

Laboratory investigation usually does not reveal any abnormality of calcium or phosphate metabolism. There is no associated leukocytosis, raised ESR or change in serum alkaline phosphatase activity.

Management

Asymptomatic patients require no specific treatment. In patients with chronic symptoms conservative management should consist of mobility and strengthening exercises about the glenohumeral joint, physical modalities and NSAIDs for symptom relief if required. An injection of corticosteroid should only be given if there are clear-cut features of impingement and subacromial inflammation and should only be repeated with caution. In the acute stages treatment should include resting the arm in a sling, analgesics, anti-inflammatory medication and local application of ice. Injection of corticosteroid should be avoided as this may inhibit the resorption of calcium; occasionally, needling and aspiration of the deposit under ultrasound control may result in a subsequent reduction in pain. Injection of subacromial lidocaine should also be given for temporary relief of pain. Some authors advocate corticosteroid injection in the acute phase[92].

Surgical intervention is indicated when conservative management of the chronic condition has failed and there are persistent features of impingement. The deposit can be removed arthroscopically or at an open procedure and may be followed up by resection of the coracoacromial ligament and anterior acromioplasty, although there is some evidence that these additional procedures are unnecessary and in some cases associated with a poorer outcome.

SCAPULOTHORACIC BURSITIS

Scapulothoracic crepitus should by no means always be considered a pathologic symptom since it is frequently found in the normal population[94]. Rarely, it may represent changes in the bony structure of the deep surface of the scapula or underlying ribs, such as an osteochondroma of the scapula or a rib exostosis. These lesions tend to give rise to a more pronounced snapping sound and may result in deviation of the scapula away from the chest wall. Soft tissue causes are more common, and frequently a diagnosis of scapulothoracic bursitis is made, although the exact pathology if present is difficult to define. Crepitus is frequently found in association with muscular complaints and probably represents a frictional sound as the scapula glides across the underlying muscle layers. Treatment is probably best directed at relief of symptoms and postural exercises, although subscapular injections have been given with variable results and at considerable risk of pneumothorax. Arthroscopic debridement has also been described.

GLENOHUMERAL INSTABILITY

Glenohumeral instability is becoming better understood as a major cause of symptoms and pathology around the shoulder joint. The more traditional orthopedic model of shoulder dislocation, whether acute or recurrent, has been expanded to encompass the more subtle but equally important subluxations and occult instabilities that can play an important role in the development of shoulder pain, especially in a young active population. Glenohumeral instability can be classified according to the etiology, direction, type and circumstance of the instability, although in reality this represents a spectrum of disorders ranging from traumatic unidirectional dislocation with a Bankart lesion to the atraumatic multidirectional instability resulting from bilateral glenohumeral laxity[95]. Symptomatic subluxation or instability often presents as a painful shoulder with all the signs and features of a rotator cuff or bicipital tendinitis, but a careful history and examination coupled with a high index of suspicion in the young adult should confirm the presence of instability.

In throwing athletes with occult instability the increased glenohumeral rotation, angulation and anterior translation of the humeral head causes the posterior aspect of the rotator cuff to be pinched between the humeral head and posterosuperior glenoid rim. This is known as 'internal impingement'[96]. A number of potential pathological sites of pain exist and differentiation between internal impingement and symptoms of instability can be difficult[97–99]. It is, however, important to distinguish between internal as opposed to external (subacromial) impingement as the etiology, treatment and rehabilitation differs considerably in the two conditions.

Management of tendinitis in the young patient with instability should be directed at the resolution of symptoms, restoration of normal flexibility and scapular control, correction of faulty technique in athletes and then a suitable strengthening program for the dynamic stabilizers of the shoulder joint, notably the rotator cuff muscles. Also, correction of any muscle imbalance about the shoulder girdle is important. Arthroscopy allows closer evaluation of shoulder pathology and has an important role in the treatment of symptomatic instability, even to the extent of carrying out stabilization procedures to the biceps anchor or glenoid labrum as well as formal reconstruction.

REFERENCES

1. Turkel SJ, Panio MW, Marshall JL, Girgis FG. Stabilizing mechanisms preventing anterior dislocation of the glenohumeral joint. J Bone Joint Surg 1981; 63A: 1208–1217.
2. O'Brien SJ, Neves MC, Arnoczky SP et al. The anatomy and histology of the inferior glenohumeral ligament complex of the shoulder. Am J Sports Med 1990; 18: 449–456.
3. Gohlke F, Essigkrug B, Schmiz F. The pattern of the collagen fiber bundles of the capsule of the glenohumeral joint. J Shoulder Elbow Surg 1994; 3: 111–128.
4. Williams MM, Snyder SJ, Buford D Jr. The Buford complex, the cord-like middle glenohumeral ligament and absent anterosuperior labrum complex: a normal anatomic capsulolabral variant. Arthroscopy 1994; 10: 2417.
5. Neer CS. Anterior acromioplasty for the chronic impingement syndrome in the shoulder: a preliminary report. J Bone Joint Surg 1972; 54A: 41–50.
6. Debski RE, Sakane M, Woo SL-Y et al. Contribution of the passive properties of the rotator cuff to glenohumeral stability during anterior-posterior loading. J Shoulder Elbow Surg 1999; 8: 324–329.
7. Itoi E, Newman SR, Kuechle DK et al. Dynamic anterior stabilizers of the shoulder with the arm in abduction. J Bone Joint Surg Br 1994; 76: 834–836.
8. Alpert SW, Pink MM, Jobe FW et al. Electromyographic analysis of deltoid and rotator cuff function under varying loads and speeds. J Shoulder Elbow Surg 2000; 9: 47–58.
9. Chen S-K, Simonian PT, Wickiewicz TL et al. Radiographic evaluation of glenohumeral kinematics: a muscle fatigue model. J Shoulder Elbow Surg 1999; 8: 49–52.
10. Jost B, Koch PP, Gerber C. Anatomy and functional aspects of the rotator interval. J Shoulder Elbow Surg 2000; 9: 336–341.
11. Rodosky MW, Harner CD, Fu FH. The role of the long head of the biceps muscle and superior glenoid labrum in anterior stability of the shoulder. Am J Sports Med 1994; 22: 121–130.
12. Levy AS, Kelly BT, Lintner SA et al. Function of the long head of the biceps at the shoulder: electromyographic analysis. J Shoulder Elbow Surg 2001; 10: 250–255.
13. Inman VT, Saunders JB de CM, Abbott LC. Observations on the function of the shoulder joint. J Bone Joint Surg 1944; 26: 1–30.
14. Dalton SE. Clinical examination of the painful shoulder. In: Hazleman BL, Dieppe PA, eds. The shoulder joint. Baillière's Clinical rheumatology. London: Baillière Tindall; 1989: 453–474.
15. Wuelker N, Plitz W, Roetman B. Biomechanical data concerning the shoulder impingement syndrome. Clin Orthop 1994; 303: 242–249.
16. Dumontier C, Sautet A, Gagey O, Apoil A. Rotator interval lesions and their relation to coracoid impingement syndrome. J Shoulder Elbow Surg 1999; 8: 130–135.
17. Sigholm G, Styf J, Korner L, Herberts P. Pressure recording in the subacromial bursa. J Orthop Res 1988; 6: 123–128.
18. Rathbun JB, MacNab I. The microvascular pattern of the rotator cuff. J Bone Joint Surg 1970; 52B: 540–553.
19. Iannotti JP, Swiontkowski M, Esterhafi J, Boulas HJ. Intraoperative assessment of rotator cuff vascularity using laser Doppler flowmetry. Abstract presented to AAOS Meeting, Las Vegas, NV, 1989.
20. Soslowsky LJ, Thomopoulos S, Tun S et al. Overuse activity injures the supraspinatus tendon in an animal model: a histologic and biomechanical study. J Shoulder Elbow Surg 2000; 9: 79–84.

21. Sano H, Ishii H, Trudel G, Uhthoff HK. Histologic evidence of degeneration at the insertion of 3 rotator cuff tendons: a comparative study with human cadaveric shoulders. J Shoulder Elbow Surg 1999; 8: 574–579.

22. Fukuda H, Mikasa M, Yamanaka K. Incomplete thickness rotator cuff tears diagnosed by subacromial bursography. Clin Orthop 1987; 223: 51–58.

23. Yamanaka K, Fukuda H, Hamada K, Mikasa M. Incomplete thickness tears of the rotator cuff. Orthop Traumatol Surg (Tokyo) 1983; 26: 713.

24. Tempelhof S, Rupp S, Seil R. Age-related prevalence of rotator cuff tears in asymptomatic shoulders. J Shoulder Elbow Surg 1999; 8: 296–299.

25. Riley GP, Harrall RL, Constant CR et al. Tendon degeneration and chronic shoulder pain: changes in the collagen composition of the human rotator cuff tendons in rotator cuff tendinitis. Ann Rheum Dis 1994; 53: 359–366.

26. Riley GP, Harrall RL, Constant CR et al. Glycosaminoglycans of human rotator cuff tendons: changes with age and in chronic rotator cuff tendinitis. Ann Rheum Dis 1994; 53: 367–376.

27. Dalton S, Cawston TE, Riley GP et al. Human shoulder tendon biopsy samples in organ culture produce procollagenase and tissue inhibitor of metalloproteinases. Ann Rheum Dis 1995; 54: 571–577.

28. Farin PU, Jaroma H, Harju A, Soimakallio S. Shoulder impingement syndrome: sonographic evaluation. Radiology 1990; 176: 845–849.

29. Tillander B, Franzen LE, Karlsson MH, Norlin R. Effect of steroid injections on the rotator cuff: an experimental study in rats. J Shoulder Elbow Surg 1999; 8: 271–274.

30. Nielsen KD, Wester JU, Lorensten A. The shoulder impingement syndrome: the results of surgical decompression. J Shoulder Elbow Surg 1994; 3: 12–16.

31. Brox JI, Gjengedal E, Uppheim G et al. Arthroscopic surgery versus supervised exercises in patients with rotator cuff disease (stage II impingement syndrome): a prospective, randomized, controlled study in 125 patients with a 2.5-year follow-up. J Shoulder Elbow Surg 1999; 8: 102–111.

32. Patel VR, Singh D, Calvert PT, Bayley JIL. Arthroscopic subacromial decompression: results and factors affecting outcome. J Shoulder Elbow Surg 1999; 8: 231–237.

33. Berbig R, Weishaupt D, Prim J, Shahin O. Primary anterior shoulder dislocation and rotator cuff tears. J Shoulder Elbow Surg 1999; 8: 220–225.

34. Hawkins RJ, Bell RH, Hawkins RH, Koppert GJ. Anterior dislocation of the shoulder in the older patient. Clin Orthop 1986; 206: 192–198.

35. Grant JCB, Smith CG. Age incidence of rupture of the supraspinatus tendon. Anat Rec 1948; 100: 666.

36. Hazlett JW. Tears of the rotator cuff. J Bone Joint Surg 1971; 53B: 772.

37. Yamaguchi K, Sher JS, Andersen WK et al. Glenohumeral motion in patients with rotator cuff tears: a comparison of asymptomatic and symptomatic shoulders. J Shoulder Elbow Surg 2000; 9: 6–11.

38. Duckworth DG, Smith KL, Campbell B, Matsen FA. Self-assessment questionnaires document substantial variability in the clinical expression of rotator cuff tears. J Shoulder Elbow Surg 1999; 8: 330–333.

39. Hijioka A, Suzuki K, Nakamura T, Hojo T. Degenerative change and rotator cuff tears: an anatomical study in 160 shoulders of 80 cadavers. Arch Orthop Trauma Surg 1993; 112: 61–64.

40. Sher JS, Uribe JW, Posada A et al. Abnormal findings on magnetic resonance images of asymptomatic shoulders. J Bone Joint Surg 1995; 77A: 10–15.

41. Neer CS. Rotator cuff arthropathy. J Bone Joint Surg 1983; 65A: 1232–1244.

42. Read JW, Perko M. Shoulder ultrasound: diagnostic accuracy for impingement syndrome, rotator cuff tear and biceps tendon pathology. J Shoulder Elbow Surg 1998; 7: 264–271.

43. Stiles RG, Otte MT. Imaging of the shoulder. Radiology 1993; 188: 603–613.

44. Hawkins RJ, Misamore GW, Hobeika PE. Surgery for full-thickness rotator cuff tears. J Bone Joint Surg 1985; 67A: 1349–1355.

45. Hoe-Hansen CE, Palm L, Norlin R. The influence of cuff pathology on shoulder function after arthroscopic subacromial decompression: a 3- and 6-year follow-up study. J Shoulder Elbow Surg 1999; 8: 585–589.

46. Fuchs B, Weishaupt D, Zanetti M et al. Fatty degeneration of the muscles of the rotator cuff: assessment by computed tomography versus magnetic resonance imaging. J Shoulder Elbow Surg 1999; 8: 599–605.

47. Sethi N, Wright R, Yamaguchi K. Disorders of the long head of the biceps tendon. J Shoulder Elbow Surg 1999; 8: 644–654.

48. Snyder SJ, Karzel RP, Del Pizzo W. SLAP lesions of the shoulder. Arthroscopy 1990; 6: 274–279.

49. Pfahler M, Branner S, Refior HJ. The role of the bicipital groove in tendopathy of the long biceps tendon. J Shoulder Elbow Surg 1999; 8: 419–424.

50. England S, Farrell AJ, Coppock JS et al. Low power laser therapy of shoulder tendonitis. Scand J Rheumatol 1989; 18: 427–431.

51. Gam AN, Thorsen H, Lonnberg F. The effect of low-level laser therapy on musculoskeletal pain: a meta-analysis. Pain 1993; 52: 63–66.

52. Neviaser RJ, Neviaser TJ. The frozen shoulder. Diagnosis and management. Clin Orthop 1987; 223: 59–64.

53. Smith SP, Devaraj WS, Bunker TD. The association between frozen shoulder and Dupuytren's disease. J Shoulder Elbow Surg 2001; 10: 149–151.

54. Lundberg BJ. The frozen shoulder. Acta Orthop Scand 1969; 119(suppl): 1–59.

55. Bridgman JF. Periarthritis of the shoulder and diabetes mellitus. Ann Rheum Dis 1972; 31: 69–71.

56. Satter MA, Luqman WA. Periarthritis: another duration-related complication of diabetes mellitus. Diabetes Care 1985; 8: 507–510.

57. Rizk TE, Pinals RS. Frozen shoulder. Semin Arthritis Rheum 1982; 11: 440–452.

58. Cameron RI, McMillan J, Kelly IG. Recurrence of a 'primary frozen shoulder': a case report. J Shoulder Elbow Surg 2000; 9: 65–67.

59. Shaffer B, Tibone JE, Kerlan RK. Frozen shoulder. A long-term follow-up. J Bone Joint Surg 1992; 74A: 738–746.

60. Lloyd-Roberts GC, French PR. Periarthritis of the shoulder. A study of the disease and its treatment. Br Med J 1959; 1: 1569–1571.

61. Reeves B. The natural history of the frozen shoulder syndrome. Scand J Rheumatol 1976; 4: 193–196.

62. Binder A, Bulgen DY, Hazleman BL, Roberts S. Frozen shoulder: a long-term prospective study. Ann Rheum Dis 1984; 43: 361–364.

63. Hazleman BL. The painful stiff shoulder. Rheumatol Rehabil 1972; 11: 413–421.

64. Nash P, Hazleman BL. Frozen shoulder. In: Hazleman BL, Dieppe PA, eds. The shoulder joint. Baillière's clinical rheumatology. London: Baillière Tindall; 1989: 551–566.

65. Wohlgethan JR. Frozen shoulder in hyperthyroidism. Arthritis Rheum 1987; 30: 936–939.

66. Bowman C, Jeffcoate W, Patrick M, Doherty M. Bilateral adhesive capsulitis, oligoarthritis and proximal myopathy as a presentation of hypothyroidism. Br J Rheum 1988; 27: 62–64.

67. Johnson JTH. Frozen shoulder syndrome in patients with pulmonary tuberculosis. J Bone Joint Surg 1959; 41A: 877–882.

68. Saha ND. Painful shoulder in patients with chronic bronchitis and emphysema. Am Rev Respir Dis 1966; 94: 455–456.

69. Bunker TD, Anthony PP. The pathology of frozen shoulder. J Bone Joint Surg Br 1995; 77: 677–683.

70. Bulgen DY, Binder A, Hazleman BL, Park JP. Immunological studies in frozen shoulder. J Rheumatol 1982; 9: 893–898.

71. Binder A, Bulgen DY, Hazleman BL. Frozen shoulder: an arthrographic and radionuclear scan assessment. Ann Rheum Dis 1984; 43: 365–369.

72. Bulgen DY, Binder A, Hazleman BL. Frozen shoulder: prospective clinical study with an evaluation of three treatment regimens. Ann Rheum Dis 1984; 43: 353–360.

73. Lee PN, Lee M, Haq AM et al. Periarthritis of the shoulder: trial of treatments investigated by multivariate analysis. Ann Rheum Dis 1974; 33: 116–119.

74. Richardson AT. The painful shoulder. Proc R Soc Med 1975; 8: 731–736.

75. Rizk TE, Pinals RS, Talaiver AS. Corticosteroid injections in adhesive capsulitis: investigation of their value and site. Arch Phys Med Rehabil 1991; 72: 20–22.

76. Binder A, Hazleman BL, Parr G, Roberts S. A controlled study of oral prednisolone in frozen shoulder. Br J Rheum 1986; 25: 288–292.

77. Pollock RG, Duralde XA, Flatow EL, Bigliani LU. The use of arthroscopy in the treatment of resistant frozen shoulder. Clin Orthop 1994; 304: 30–36.

78. Watson L, Dalziel R, Story I. Frozen shoulder: a 12-month clinical outcome trial. J Shoulder Elbow Surg 2000; 9: 16–22.

79. Omari A, Bunker TD. Open surgical release for frozen shoulder: surgical findings and results of the release. J Shoulder Elbow Surg 2001; 10: 353–357.

80. Griffith PH III, Boyadjis TA. Acute pyoarthrosis of the acromioclavicular joint: a case report. Orthopedics 1984; 7: 1727–1728.

81. Rockwood CA, Young DC. Disorders of the acromioclavicular joint. In: Rockwood CA, Matsen FA, eds. The shoulder, vol 2. Philadelphia, PA: WB Saunders; 1990: 413–476.

82. Cahill BR. Osteolysis of the distal part of the clavicle in male athletes. J Bone Joint Surg 1982; 64A: 1053–1058.

83. Levine AH, Pais MJ, Schwartz EE. Post traumatic osteolysis of the distal clavicle with emphasis on early radiologic changes. Am J Rheumatol 1976; 127: 781–784.

84. De Palma AF. Surgery of the shoulder, 2nd ed. Philadelphia, PA: JB Lippincott; 1973.

85. Bosworth BM. Calcium deposits in the shoulder and subacromial bursitis: a survey of 12 122 shoulders. JAMA 1941; 116: 2477–2482.

86. Welfling J, Kahn MF, Desroy M et al. Les calcifications de l'epaule. II: La maladie des calcifications tendineuses multiples. Rev Rhum 1965; 32: 325–334.

87. Bosworth BM. Examination of the shoulder for calcium deposits. J Bone Joint Surg 1941; 23: 567–577.

88. McLaughlin HL. Lesions of the musculotendinous cuff of the shoulder. III: Observations on the pathology, course and treatment of calcific deposits. Ann Surg 1946; 124: 354–362.

89. Hsu HC, Wu JJ, Jim YF et al. Calcific tendinitis and rotator cuff tearing: a clinical and radiographic study. J Shoulder Elbow Surg 1994; 3: 159–164.

90. MacNab I. Rotator cuff tendinitis. Ann R Coll Surg Engl 1973; 53: 271–287.

91. Uhthoff HK. Calcifying tendinitis: An active cell-mediated calcification. Virchows Arch [A] 1975; 366: 51–58.

92. Uhthoff HK, Sarkar K. Calcifying tendinitis. In: Hazleman BL, Dieppe PA, eds. The shoulder joint. Baillière's clinical rheumatology. London: Baillière Tindall; 1989: 567–581.

93. Sengar DPS, McKendry RJ, Uthoff HK. Increased frequency of HLA-AI in calcifying tendinitis. Tissue Antigens 1987; 29: 173–174.

94. Milch H. Snapping scapula. Clin Orthop 1961; 20: 139–150.

95. Dalton SE, Snyder SJ. Glenohumeral instability. In: Hazleman BL, Dieppe PA, eds. The shoulder joint. Baillière's Clinical Rheumatology. London: Baillière Tindall; 1989: 511–354.

96. Walch G, Boileau P, Noel E, Donell ST. Impingement of the deep surface of the supraspinatus tendon on the posterosuperior glenoid rim: an arthroscopic study. J Shoulder Elbow Surg 1992; 1: 238–245.

97. Davidson PA, Elattrache NS, Jobe CM, Jobe FW. Rotator cuff and posterior-superior glenoid labrum injury associated with incrossed glenohumeral motion: a new site of impingement. J Shoulder Elbow Surg 1995; 4: 384–390.

98. McFarland EG, Hsu C-Y, Neira C, O'Neil O. Internal impingement of the shoulder: a clinical and arthroscopic analysis. J Shoulder Elbow Surg 1999; 8: 458–460.

99. Edelson G, Teitz C. Internal impingement in the shoulder. J Shoulder Elbow Surg 2000; 9: 308–315.

REGIONAL AND WIDESPREAD PAIN

16

The elbow

Michael D Chard

- The elbow is a complex hinge joint essential for the positioning and full use of the hand
- Relevant anatomy includes the radiohumeral and ulnohumeral hinge, the connecting proximal radioulnar joint, the radial head, the medial and lateral epicondyles, the ulnar nerve groove, the muscles spanning the elbow and the olecranon bursa
- Soft tissue lesions such as lateral epicondylitis and olecranon bursitis are far more frequent than many common joint diseases
- Diagnosis of elbow conditions is largely based on pain characteristics, location of swelling, presence of point tenderness and the results of passive, active and resisted motion

FUNCTIONAL ANATOMY

Bony joint structure

The elbow is considered to be a hinge joint but is more accurately a hinged joint about a trochlea or pulley. This allows for the motions of pronation and supination of the forearm. The combination of flexion and rotation at the elbow enables the hands to be brought into view and provides a steady

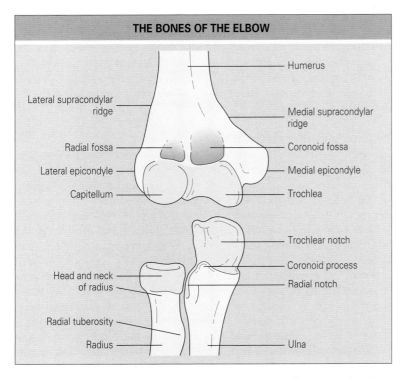

THE BONES OF THE ELBOW

- Humerus
- Lateral supracondylar ridge
- Medial supracondylar ridge
- Radial fossa
- Coronoid fossa
- Lateral epicondyle
- Medial epicondyle
- Capitellum
- Trochlea
- Trochlear notch
- Coronoid process
- Head and neck of radius
- Radial notch
- Radial tuberosity
- Radius
- Ulna

Fig. 16.1 The bones of the elbow. Expanded view of the elbow joint showing the bony features.

but adjustable base for the hands to make best use of the highly mobile fingers and opposable thumb. It is a compound synovial joint since it is composed of articulation between the ulnar notch and trochlea of the humerus, and between the radial head and humeral capitellum (Fig. 16.1). In continuity with these is the proximal radioulnar joint[1].

At its distal end the humerus is expanded to form a modified condyle, widest transversely, and consists of articular and non-articular parts. The capitellum on the lateral aspect is curved, forms less than half a sphere and contributes anterior and inferior surfaces. A shallow groove separates the capitellum from the medial trochlea, which has anterior, inferior and posterior surfaces. Its medial margin projects inferiorly and the edge is the main determinant of the angulation between the long axis of the radius and ulna in an extended supinated position. Medial and lateral bony projections of the lower humerus form the epicondyles which, along with olecranon, coronoid and radial fossas, make up the non-articular part of the condyle. The fossas accept the relevant parts of the ulna and radius during extremes of extension and flexion movements. Above the larger medial and less prominent lateral epicondyle formed by the flaring of the distal humerus are the supracondylar ridges. The medial epicondyle provides a groove for the ulnar nerve as it crosses the elbow to enter the forearm.

At its proximal end the radius has a head, neck and tuberosity. The head is discoid, with a proximal shallow cup for the humeral capitellum and an articular periphery that is deepest medially where it contacts the ulnar radial notch. Distal to this is the constriction of the neck, which leads on medially to the bony prominence of the tuberosity. The large proximal ulna has large olecranon and coronoid processes, with a large trochlear and smaller radial notches to articulate with humerus and radius. The deep trochlear notch articulating with the humeral trochlea is a major contributor in making the elbow joint one of the most congruous and inherently stable. Together, the ulnohumeral and radiohumeral joints provide approximately 50% of the joint stability, the rest being due to soft tissue constraint.

Ligaments, capsule and synovium

Varus–valgus stability of the elbow is largely due to the collateral ligaments (Fig. 16.2)[2]. The medial (ulnar) collateral ligament has anterior, posterior and inferior (oblique) parts. It forms a triangular band with its apex attached around the medial epicondyle and extending in a fan-shaped fashion to insert into a proximal tubercle on the medial coronoid margin (anteriorly) and the medial margin of olecranon (posteriorly). The anterior portion is the most important elbow stabilizer. The lateral (radial) collateral ligament is attached low on the lateral epicondyle and extends to the annular ligament. Its superficial fibers are blended with those of the attachment of supinator and extensor carpi radialis brevis.

The annular ligament is a strong band that encircles the radial head, holding it against the radial notch of the ulna. It attaches to the edge of the notch anteriorly and on a ridge at, or just behind, the edge posteriorly. The proximal annular border is continuous with the cubital capsule, except posteriorly where the capsule passes deep to it at the

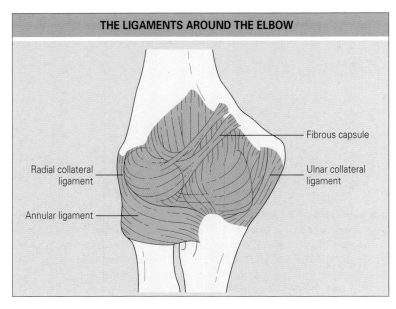

THE LIGAMENTS AROUND THE ELBOW

Fig. 16.2 The ligaments around the elbow. Anterior view of the elbow joint showing the ligaments and capsule.

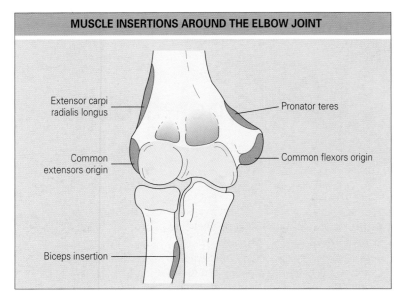

MUSCLE INSERTIONS AROUND THE ELBOW JOINT

Fig. 16.3 Muscle insertions around the elbow joint. Anterior view of the elbow joint showing the muscle insertions.

radial notch. The distal annular border attaches loosely to the radial neck after passing over a synovial reflection. Posterior to the ligament are the anconeus and the interosseus recurrent artery. Where the ligament internally is in contact with the radial head, it is lined with a thin layer of cartilage, but distally it is covered by a reflected fold of synovium on the radial neck.

The articular capsule of the elbow joint is a thin structure. Anteriorly it is broad, attaching proximally to the front of the humerus, medial epicondyle (above the coronoid) and radial fossa (in continuity on its sides with the collateral ligaments) and distally attaching to the edge of the ulna, coronoid process and annular ligament. It receives fibers from the brachialis. Posteriorly it attaches to the humerus behind the capitellum, around the olecranon fossa (except inferiorly) and the back of the medial epicondyle, and extends to the superior and lateral margins of the olecranon. Laterally it is continuous with the superior radioulnar joint capsule deep to the annular ligament. The anconeus and triceps are related to it posteriorly.

There is sometimes irregularity of the synovial lining of the joint in the coronoid process on flexion, usually occurring adjacent to the medial collateral ligament, but otherwise it is smooth. There are four fat pads between synovium and capsule; one in the synovial fold, which partly divides the joint into humeroradial and humeroulnar parts, and the others in relation to the fossas of the lower end of the humerus.

Muscles and bursae

Muscles that are related to the elbow joint are the brachialis (in front) the triceps and anconeus (behind), the supinator and common extensor tendon (laterally) and the common flexor tendon and flexor carpi ulnaris (medially) (Fig. 16.3). Anterior to the brachialis, the biceps tendon passes on its way to insertion into the radial tuberosity. The common superficial flexor tendon is attached to the medial epicondyle and the common superficial extensor tendon to the lateral epicondyle, both exterior to the joint capsule. The anconeus attaches to the posterior aspect of the lateral epicondyle. Above the medial epicondyle on the supracondylar ridge is attached the humeral head of the pronator teres, while the lateral supracondylar ridge gives attachment to the extensor carpi radialis longus. The triceps passes posteriorly over the elbow joint to insert into the olecranon. Numerous bursal structures have been reported but the main bursa around the elbow is the super-

ficial olecranon bursa, which separates the olecranon from the overlying skin. This forms in late childhood[3]. A small bicipitoradial bursa is found close to where the biceps tendon inserts into the posterior aspect of the radial tuberosity. Superficial epicondylar and radiohumeral bursae are sometimes found.

Movement

Consideration of movement at the elbow functionally includes the cubital joint itself and the proximal radioulnar joint. The cubital hinge joint traverses an area of flexion of around 150°. Pronation of 75–80° and supination of 85–90° are achievable but require an intact distal radioulnar joint as well as the proximal one[4]. The combination leads to the large variety of movements possible at this articulation. Because of the shape of the trochlea, extension results in valgus positioning of the forearm to the arm of 10–15° (more in women), the 'carrying angle'. In flexion, a similar degree of varus positioning helps when bringing the hand in close proximity to the mouth. Flexion at the elbow is carried out by the brachialis and biceps, the latter also acting as a supinator of the forearm. The brachioradialis muscle assists their action. Extension is carried out by the triceps aided by the anconeus.

Neurovascular relationships

The elbow joint receives articular arteries from numerous periarticular anastomoses that are supplied mainly by the brachial artery. Articular nerves are derived principally from the radial and musculocutaneous nerves but the median, ulnar and sometimes the anterior interosseous nerves contribute. These nerves follow the supply of blood vessel and probably contain vasomotor fibers as well as pain and proprioception afferents. The neurovascular structures of the arm have an intimate relationship with the joint capsule. The brachial artery traverses the joint anteriorly, just medial to the biceps tendon in the antecubital space. The musculocutaneous nerve innervates the biceps and brachialis above the level of the elbow and terminates distally to form the lateral cutaneous nerve of the forearm. The course of the median nerve takes it anterior to the joint capsule and medial to the biceps tendon and brachial artery. The radial nerve passes anterior to the lateral epicondyle, descending beneath brachialis and brachioradialis muscles. The ulnar nerve traverses the elbow in the ulnar groove behind the medial epicondyle.

CLINICAL EXAMINATION

Introduction

The examination of the elbow must be preceded by a precise history to allow emphasis to be placed on particular areas. Complaints usually consist of pain, loss of movement, weakness, clicking or locking. There may be sharply localized pain, typical of extra-articular pathology, deep joint pain or the poorly localized pain of ulnar neuropathy with or without typical paresthesia extending to the hand. The functional interplay between elbow, shoulder and wrist means that examination of all these joints may be necessary. Referred pain in the elbow, especially from the neck or shoulder, is usually diffuse. Examination must include comparison of right and left arms (Table 16.1).

Inspection

Inspection is very important since much of the elbow joint is subcutaneous and so alterations in soft tissue or bony anatomy are easily seen. Anteriorly viewing the elbow in the extended, supinated position allows assessment of the carrying angle. It is increased in certain congenital conditions, such as Turner's syndrome, and may be altered by fractures around the elbow. Synovial proliferation and effusion are each detected as a fullness in the region of the lateral infracondylar recess. The swelling may be obliterated by pressure in the case of effusion. A hard bony swelling is detected where there is radial head pathology, such as previous fracture. Posteriorly, swelling of the subcutaneous olecranon bursa may be detected, and in rheumatoid arthritis nodules often occur extending distally along the border of the ulna. Occasionally ulnar neuritis may result in enlargement of the ulnar nerve, which is seen medially.

Palpation

Palpation of the subcutaneous lateral and medial epicondyles and olecranon tip is easily undertaken. Tenderness over the lateral epicondyle is typical of lateral epicondylitis. The radial head is palpated by gentle pressure over the radiocapitellar joint and assessed during pronation and supination movements. Loose bodies may be detected in the infracondylar recess. Medially the ulnar nerve may be palpated to detect thickening, and assessment with the elbow in flexion and extension detects ulnar nerve subluxation. The nerve may displace anteriorly during flexion, sometimes with an obvious snap, and be associated with ulnar nerve paresthesia. Posteriorly, the tip of the olecranon and the olecranon fossa above can be felt if the elbow is not in full extension. Flexion to around 15° also enables assessment of the collateral ligaments. These may be palpated. Varus stress with the humerus in full internal rotation, and valgus stress in full external rotation, test for lateral and medial instability respectively but abnormality is often subtle and requires experience to detect[5].

Movement

Active and passive ranges of movement should be measured, including flexion, extension and rotation. Most frequently, a reduced range of movement is due to pain. After injury, elbow joint extension is both the first movement to be lost and the last to recover. The normal range of flexion–extension, 0–150°, is in excess of that needed for everyday activity, which is of the order of 30–130°. Forcibly moving the joint beyond the pain-free range helps to identify the predominant cause of the restriction. In extension, posterior pain indicates a posterior impingement problem, whereas anterior pain indicates tightness of the anterior capsule. The reverse is true for loss of flexion. Early in arthritis flexion and extension are limited but rotational movements are often spared. Motion is best assessed with the elbow flexed to 90° and held to the side of the body, with supination often greater than 85° and a little less for pronation.

Pain should be sought on resisted active movements, particularly where there is no major intra-articular pathology. These are carried out with the elbow held at 90°. Flexion and supination strength is normally greater than extension and pronation. Passive, but not resisted, movements producing pain indicate intra-articular pathology, whereas pain on resisted movement alone indicates a musculotendinous pathology associated with that movement. To complete the assessment of muscles around the elbow, resisted flexion and extension of the wrist must be performed[6]. Neurologic examination must not be omitted, with particular attention paid to structures supplied by the C5, C6 and C7 nerve roots. Biceps jerk (C5), brachioradialis reflex (C6) and triceps jerk (C7) should also be assessed.

DIFFERENTIAL DIAGNOSIS OF ELBOW PAIN

Pain felt at the elbow may be due to either local pathology or referred pain (Table 16.2). As indicated above, shoulder and cervical problems frequently produce pain referred to the elbow. In the case of cervical spine lesions the pain is often associated with frank neurologic symptoms. Although referred pain is usually part of more generalized arm pain symptoms, it may be localized. Examination of the neck and shoulder is therefore important in the assessment of elbow pain. Intrathoracic pathology can give rise to arm pain but is rarely localized to the elbow.

True elbow pain may be related to joint disease but is more commonly due to lesions of the soft periarticular tissues. These causes can usually be distinguished by history and appropriate examination. Primary osteoarthritis is not common but elbow involvement frequently occurs in more generalized inflammatory arthritis. The joint can be inflamed in gout or affected by septic arthritis. Traumatic effusions occur and the joint may be involved by a fracture of the bones, minor fractures sometimes being missed and only presenting as an effusion. A traumatic/overuse form of osteochondritis of the radial head can occur in some throwing sports, especially in the teenage child. The joint may be affected by loose bodies and synovial osteochondromatosis. Traumatic partial subluxation of the radial head through the annular ligament occurs in children, especially if they have a hypermobile tendency.

TABLE 16.1 EXAMINATION OF THE ELBOW		
Inspection	Swelling	Joint
		Bursa
	Deformity	
	Carrying angle	
Palpation	Synovial	
	Joint line epicondyles/soft tissues	
	Ulnar nerve	
Movement	Active	
	Passive	
	Resisted	
Other	Upper limb neurologic examination	
	Neck and shoulder	

TABLE 16.2 DIFFERENTIAL DIAGNOSIS OF ELBOW PAIN		
Local	Articular	Arthritis, osteochondritis, loose bodies, subluxation
	Periarticular	Lateral and medial epicondylitis, olecranon bursitis, ligamentous lesions, entrapment neuropathy
Referred		Cervical and shoulder disease

Plain anteroposterior and lateral radiographs are useful in assessing joint pathology. Further investigation of the joint is best carried out by arthroscopy[7] rather than tomography or arthrography, although magnetic resonance imaging, where available, is a better non-invasive alternative[8–10]. High-resolution ultrasound (sonography) is a further less costly alternative but is very dependent on operator skill[11]. These techniques also allow assessment of the periarticular soft tissues.

SOFT TISSUE ELBOW LESIONS

Introduction

Apart from lateral epicondylitis ('tennis elbow'), medial epicondylitis ('golfer's elbow') and olecranon bursitis, soft tissue lesions at the elbow are relatively rare. Biceps tendinitis is characterized by local pain and tenderness in the region of the bicipital tuberosity of the radius, with pain on resisted flexion and supination. Pain on resisted flexion alone indicates the rarer brachialis muscle lesion, with pain and tenderness that is less well localized and is found behind the biceps tendon. Although uncommon, such a tear is particularly prone to develop

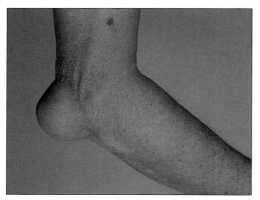

Fig. 16.4 A case of olecranon bursitis in early rheumatoid arthritis.

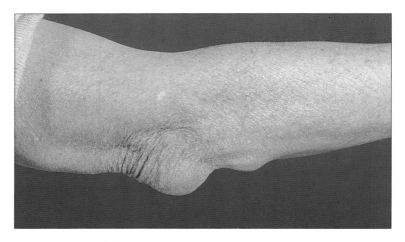

Fig. 16.5 A case of olecranon bursitis in later rheumatoid arthritis; a rheumatoid nodule is also shown.

myositis ossificans, which in the early phases produces a warm, firm mass that can be mistaken for tumor[6]. Pain on resisted supination alone is said to indicate a supinator lesion, but this very rarely if ever occurs and pain would be felt further down the forearm. It is unusual to have a lesion at the site of triceps insertion into the olecranon (triceps tendinitis) but instead these occur higher in the arm at the musculotendinous junction. Ligamentous lesions do not usually occur in isolation, most often being associated with traumatic joint synovitis or effusion, if not frank joint derangement or fracture. Medially, a ligamentous lesion may form at least part of the elbow injury caused by some throwing sports, such as javelin.

Olecranon bursitis

Bursal inflammation around the elbow can occur and principally affects the olecranon bursa. Both epicondylar and radiohumeral bursitis have been reported but are rare, producing vague symptoms around the elbow with swelling. They have in the past been suggested as causes of

	Traumatic (idiopathic) non-inflammatory	**Aseptic inflammatory**			**Septic inflammatory**
		Rheumatoid arthritis	**Crystalline**	**Uremia**	
Clinical symptoms					
Trauma	+++	+	+	0/+	+++
Tenderness	+	+	++	+	+++
Skin breakage	+	0	0	0	+++
Clinical signs					
Fever	0	0	0	0	++
Warmth	+	+	++	+	+++
Erythema	+	+	++	+	+++
Cellulitis	0	0	+	+	+++
Lymphadenopathy	0	0/+	0/+	0	++
Edema	0/+	0/+	0/+	0	++
Bursal fluid					
Color	C, S, H	C, S	S, H	S	S, H, P
White blood cells per mm³	50–10 000 (mean 1100)	1000–60 000 (mean 3000)	1000–20 000 (mean 2900)	1200	350–450 000 (mean 75 000)
Gram stain	Negative	Negative	Negative	Negative	Positive (70%)
Crystals	Negative	Rare cholesterol	Monosodium urate or pyrophosphate	Rare	Negative
Culture	Negative	Negative	Negative	Negative	Positive

TABLE 16.3 DIFFERENTIAL DIAGNOSIS OF OLECRANON BURSITIS

Differential diagnosis: 0, usually absent; +, rare; + +, occasional; +++, common. Bursal fluid color: C, clear; H, hemorrhagic; P, purulent; S, serosanguineous.

tennis elbow but rarely, if ever, have the same clinical features. The olecranon bursa is a subcutaneous synovial pouch located on the extensor aspect of the elbow. It allows the skin to glide freely over the olecranon process, preventing tissue tears. Because of its superficial position over the olecranon, with little soft tissue padding, the olecranon bursa is vulnerable to trauma by friction or a blow and to infection through abrasions, puncture wounds or cellulitis. Olecranon bursitis occurs when the bursa swells because of trauma, inflammation or infection (Fig. 16.4). Such swelling occurs easily and is readily visible. The swelling may be the result of fluid accumulation but may be due to synovial tissue hypertrophy or fibrosis. In addition to trauma, the bursa may also be involved in crystal arthropathies (gout or rarely calcium pyrophosphate arthritis) or in generalized inflammatory arthritis, especially rheumatoid arthritis. Swelling of the olecranon bursa may be seen in association with rheumatoid nodules on the ulnar border of the forearm (Fig. 16.5). Rheumatoid nodules may form within the bursa but intrabursal nodules may also form as a consequence of traumatic fibrosis or gouty tophi and result in bursal swelling.

Olecranon bursitis is fairly frequently seen in outpatients (approximately 3 in 1000 rheumatology outpatient visits) and when septic may occasionally require hospitalization (about 1 in 1000 hospitalizations). The condition is most commonly seen in younger men as a consequence of recurrent elbow trauma either due to work (e.g. automobile mechanics, miners) or related to leisure activities (playing darts, gymnastics, gardening). There is often no obvious precipitating cause of olecranon bursitis. It rarely occurs in childhood for developmental reasons[3].

Olecranon bursitis can be classified clinically into three general categories (Table 16.3):

- traumatic (or idiopathic) non-inflammatory
- aseptic inflammatory
- septic inflammatory.

Appropriate therapy depends on the bursitis category. Therefore, it is important for the cause to be defined as soon as possible through history, examination and where appropriate, bursal aspiration. The main diagnostic challenge is to distinguish septic and non-septic olecranon bursitis as the septic form has the greatest potential for morbidity and must be diagnosed as soon as possible. A clinician must also be aware there is a potential for a rapid change in the cause of the bursitis, i.e. a change from non-septic to septic. This should be considered at each follow-up visit.

Questions regarding occupation, duration of symptoms and possible trauma or skin injury are important aspects of the history. Information on other causes of bursitis such as rheumatoid arthritis, gout or uremia should be sought. Diabetes or conditions associated with immunosuppression can increase the risk of sepsis. During the physical examination the size and turgor of the bursa should be noted (and size change at follow-up visits). Warmth and erythema of the bursa or skin along with the presence of nodules or lymphadenopathy provide important clues. An effusion in the adjacent elbow joint may occur, especially with inflammatory arthritis. Evidence of trauma, particularly with skin breakage, should be sought. General physical status should be assessed, particularly looking for fever.

In traumatic or idiopathic olecranon bursitis, pain is usually localized and typically does not occur on passive or resisted movement. It is usually provoked by leaning on the elbow or flexion with a constriction around the elbow such as a coat sleeve. Tenderness should be sought about the tip of the olecranon and will be present, sometimes with palpable thickening of the bursal wall, even in the absence of significant effusion; it is generally very sensitive to pressure. Septic olecranon bursitis occurs less frequently (around 25% of hospital cases) but it is important and should not be missed. Usually it occurs following an abrasion or

may be associated with an initial cellulitis of the skin. Septic olecranon bursitis usually causes pain with elbow flexion and sometimes with resisted extension but it is different from acute arthritis as gentle passive extension is unimpaired[12].

Patients with asymptomatic or obviously traumatic bursitis may be symptomatically treated and observed. Where inflammation or infection is suspected, percutaneous diagnostic aspiration of the bursa is indicated. Aspiration of the bursa both reduces symptoms and allows assessment of the fluid (see Chapter 6 for technical aspects). Along with gross visualization of blood staining, or turbidity of the fluid, white cell count and differential, and Gram stain with culture of the fluid should be undertaken to exclude infection. Polarized light microscopy should be performed to reveal any crystals. Elbow radiographs are rarely necessary and should only be used to exclude traumatic fracture or pre-existing joint injury. Diagnostic elements are summarized in Table 16.3.

Therapeutic options

Non-inflammatory, traumatic (or idiopathic) bursitis usually responds to simple conservative therapy including rest, elbow protection and anti-inflammatory drug treatment. Padded elbow support may help to prevent further trauma and skin abrasion. Percutaneous needle aspiration should be considered for patients having significant symptoms. The aspiration itself reduces symptoms and in addition a compressive elastic bandage may be used to prevent recurrence of swelling. If infection has been satisfactorily excluded by culture, local corticosteroid injection may be performed, which is effective in speeding recovery[13]. However, this can lead to complications (infection, skin atrophy, chronic pain) and should only be used sparingly for traumatic bursitis. In inflammatory olecranon bursitis, related to rheumatoid arthritis or crystalline arthropathy, intrabursal corticosteroid injection is useful. In such cases it should be proceeded by aspiration and investigation to exclude infection. An injection of 20mg of methylprednisolone acetate usually leads to rapid recovery.

The finding of infection requires appropriate antibiotic therapy and reaspiration of pus as necessary. *Staphylococcus aureus* is the most frequently found organism although a group A β-hemolytic streptococcus or *Streptococcus epidermidis* is less commonly found[12,14]. Rarely *Haemophilus influenzae* and *Pseudomonas* species may be the cause. In immunocompromised patients (malignancy, human immunodeficiency virus (HIV)-positive status or systemic corticosteroid therapy), special cultures for mycobacteria, fungi or anaerobic bacteria may be necessary.

Patients who fail to respond to outpatient therapy or who at the outset have more severe initial infection need to be hospitalized for intravenous antibiotic therapy. This includes patients with high fever, chills, prolonged duration of symptoms and cellulitis. Hospitalization also needs to be considered for those with complicating medical conditions (diabetes, uremia, rheumatoid arthritis) and immunosuppression.

Repeated aspiration of the infected bursa is essential and may initially need to be carried out on a daily basis. This can be done percutaneously or if necessary with the placement of a suction-irrigation system. Measuring the cell counts and repeated culture should be used to monitor the response to therapy. Patients requiring initial intravenous antibiotic therapy can be switched to oral medication as soon as signs and symptoms show consistent improvement. In general, antibiotic therapy should be continued for 10–14 days, although there is evidence that patients commencing treatment within a week of onset actually require only half this duration to sterilize the bursa.

Surgical drainage or bursectomy is occasionally required in the management of olecranon bursitis. If repeated traumatic bursitis occurs then surgical removal of the bursa should be considered, either arthroscopically or by open resection. Persistent aseptic inflammatory bursitis may require open resection. Bursectomy may be required for septic bursitis if the acute infection fails to resolve or if after repeated infection, a fibrotic, chronically inflamed bursa is left[15].

Lateral epicondylitis

Used synonymously with the term 'tennis elbow', this condition is one of the most common lesions of the arm. The first description is attributed to Runge in 1873[16] but the name 'tennis elbow' is derived from Morris's description of 'lawn tennis arm' in *The Lancet* in 1882[17]. Around 1–3% of the population are affected by it[18,19], mostly those aged between 40 and 60 years, the dominant arm being affected most frequently. Some 40–50% of tennis players suffer with it, mainly older players[20,21], but in clinical practice fewer than 5% of cases are due to the game[22]. It is found most often in non-athletes and the majority are not manual workers. Many cannot describe any specific precipitating factors[23].

Etiopathology

There have been more than 25 suggested causes of the condition[24], and this reflects the use of the diagnosis non-specifically for lateral elbow pain. Pathologic material for study is relatively rare as most cases do not come to surgery. Reported operative findings in relatively few chronic cases have included periostitis[16], infection[24], radiohumeral joint disease[25], radial nerve entrapment[26] and a lesion of the orbicular (annular) ligament[27]. It is believed, however, that the majority of cases are due to a musculotendinous lesion of the common extensor tendon at the attachment to the lateral epicondyle or nearby, especially that portion derived from extensor carpi radialis brevis[6,22].

Macroscopic tears in the common extensor tendon are sometimes found at operation[22] but repeated high-dose local corticosteroid injections may have affected findings. Microfractures, cystic and fibrinoid degeneration and round cell infiltrations, immature fibrous tissue, hyaline degeneration and vascular plus fibroblastic proliferation ('angiofibroblastic tendinosis'; Fig. 16.6), sometimes with calcific debris, and attempts at repair have been described[21,22,28–30]. Some cases show a chronic traction effect. Histologic evidence of inflammation has not been found. The changes seen are similar to those seen in the rotator cuff with advancing age, where tendon vascular factors are believed to be important[31]. The relationship of such findings to the acute lesion is uncertain. Ischemic stress may be important because the tenoperiosteal junction (enthesis) and nearby tendon are relatively avascular, since the blood supply is a watershed of that derived from muscle and bone and working muscle takes up the blood supply at the expense of tendon.

Age is an important factor, since lateral epicondylitis rarely occurs before the age of 30 years. Adult maturity is associated with alterations in the enthesis, including changes in collagen content, reduction in cells and ground substance and increase in lipids, which then probably predispose it to injury[32]. Other possible changes that may be important, including those due to tendon elasticity, have yet to be elucidated. The onset of symptoms may be brought on by overuse and hence lateral epicondylitis is more often seen in the active middle-aged than the less active elderly. In manual workers relative overuse of wrist and finger extensors may precipitate the condition, which most often affects the dominant arm. Sometimes there may be bilateral involvement, either due to increased stress placed on the unaffected arm or resulting from a general tendency to soft tissue lesions that occurs in some individuals[22,23].

Clinical findings

Lateral epicondylitis usually arises slowly and apparently spontaneously; a blow or acute traumatic strain is relatively rarely remembered. Pain is localized to the lateral epicondyle but may spread up and down the upper limb. Grip is impaired because of pain, and this may result in restricted daily activities. Tenderness over the epicondyle is usual, although maximum tenderness is sometimes found at nearby sites[6,27]. The other cardinal sign is increase in pain on resisting wrist dorsiflexion with the elbow in extension (Fig. 16.7). Symptoms may also be precipitated by extending the elbow with the wrist flexed (Fig. 16.8) and by resisted middle finger extension. Resisted supination may also be painful. The range of movement of the elbow is usually normal but a few degrees of extension may be lost in some severe and chronic cases. It is important to exclude other conditions producing elbow pain, especially that referred from the cervical spine or shoulder, as well as arthritis of the elbow, although this is usually obvious.

A nerve entrapment around the elbow may produce diagnostic confusion. Radial tunnel syndrome or compression of the posterior interosseous nerve[26] can produce lateral elbow and upper forearm pain.

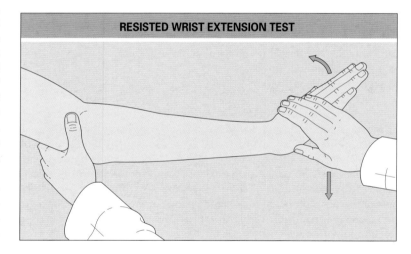

Fig. 16.7 **Resisted wrist extension test.**

RESISTED WRIST EXTENSION TEST

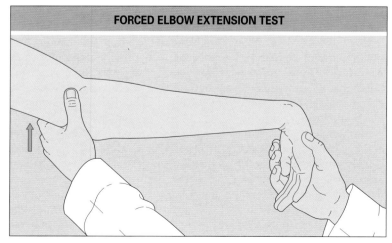

FORCED ELBOW EXTENSION TEST

Fig. 16.8 **Forced elbow extension test.**

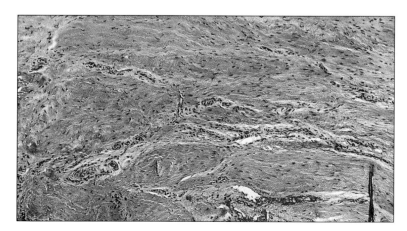

Fig. 16.6 **Angiofibroblastic hyperplasia.**

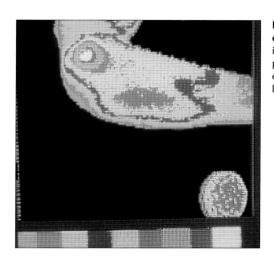

Fig. 16.9 Lateral epicondylitis. An infrared thermographic pattern in lateral epicondylitis showing localized 'hot spot'.

It can be the cause of apparent lateral epicondylitis that is unresponsive to conservative treatment but is believed to be a rare cause of resistant cases[33]. These entrapments have been found to be due to compressive lesions caused by abnormal fibrous bands in front of the radial head, a sharp tendinous origin of extensor carpi radialis brevis or a radial recurrent fan of vessels. More rarely, a lipoma or ganglion has been found to be the cause. Compression of the posterior interosseous nerve may occur where it passes through the supinator muscle just below the elbow joint. A well-defined arcade of Frohse is present in 30% of subjects[34] and makes a compression neuropathy more likely. Diffuse pain, symptoms distal to the lateral epicondyle and the presence of muscle weakness may be useful distinguishing features.

Investigations

Investigations are not usually required but radiographs of the elbow may be helpful in excluding joint disease and may occasionally show lateral soft tissue calcification. Electromyography may be helpful in excluding a nerve entrapment. Quantitative assessment of severity and response to treatment is difficult but grading pain, tenderness and pain on resisted wrist extension can be helpful and lifting graded weights and grip strength measurement aid objectivity[35]. A truly objective measurement is that of infrared thermography of the affected elbow, which shows a discrete localized area of increased heat near the lateral epicondyle in 98% of affected elbows (Fig. 16.9). Analysis of the gradient across the abnormal area reveals a correlation with clinical severity[35]. Lack of general availability of this technique means it is mainly a research tool. Magnetic resonance imaging has been used to identify tissue abnormalities prior to surgery in chronic cases[36]. High-resolution ultrasound may also be of use[11].

Management

Over 40 treatment regimens for lateral epicondylitis have been described in the literature, ranging from the extremes of 'prolonged observation' to X-ray therapy. Reduced activity may result in resolution of symptoms in a few patients and may be effective in early cases especially with some

form of splinting (Table 16.4). A simple sling can be used but is unlikely to be effective as the forearm is usually held in position with the wrist flexed. A plaster cast or brace may be helpful but, since 4–6 weeks of immobility are required, these risk a long-term fixed flexion deformity. However, a hinged brace may be tried, which has a reduced risk of residual flexion deformity. A cock-up wrist splint reducing tension on forearm extensors is an alternative. Oral non-steroidal anti-inflammatory drugs (NSAIDs) are often used, but evidence for their efficacy is tenuous[37]. NSAID gels may be as useful and a trial of treatment in early or mild cases would be appropriate.

Numerous physical modalities of treatment have been used to treat lateral epicondylitis but the efficacy of most of them remains unproven. Ultrasound, by its ability to cross myofascial planes and concentrate near bone, has theoretical advantages. A double-blind controlled trial has confirmed an advantage for pulsed therapeutic ultrasound. A total of 63% of patients improved and the technique had the merit of being non-painful with a relapse rate lower than that after corticosteroid injection[38]. Medical laser light therapy has been used as treatment in recent years but published placebo controlled trials have not confirmed efficacy using varying techniques[39,40]. Extracorporeal shock wave therapy has recently been advocated for persistent cases but further placebo-controlled trial confirmation is awaited[41]. Acupuncture has also been used in treatment[42].

Local injections of corticosteroids have been widely used and have been shown to be superior to saline and local anesthetics[43]. There is a rapid response with corticosteroids; however, this may not produce a better outcome at 6 months after injection than lidocaine (lignocaine) alone or affect long-term outcome[37,44]. The newer corticosteroid preparations may produce a quicker response but they may also lead to loss of subcutaneous fat, with dimpling and depigmentation, especially with repeated injection. Local corticosteroid injections (see Chapter 6) are both efficacious and cost-effective, with around 90% of subjects responding. But the injection may cause increased pain for up to 72 hours afterwards and a significant number of patients relapse[23]. The injection may be repeated after 2–4 weeks, in the event of either failure to respond or relapse, but should not be repeated more than twice as it is unlikely then to be effective, increases risk of side effects and predisposes to chronic pain[45].

Role of surgery

Surgical intervention is considered for the 10% of cases failing to respond to conservative treatments. The value of manipulation as a means of avoiding surgery is controversial. It may be effective when performed under general anesthetic by an experienced practitioner, particularly using the method of Mills in conjunction with a local corticosteroid injection[46]. Approaches to surgical management have attempted to correct the presumed pathology. Excision of tissues around the epicondyle, removal of the synovial fringe of the radiohumeral joint or partial removal of the annular ligament have all been advocated. Denervation of the lateral epicondyle has been used to relieve symptoms in a few cases. Most commonly either repair of tears[22] and removal of abnormal tendon is undertaken[29] or a procedure to lengthen the muscle tendon complex is carried out. Such lengthening has been achieved either by the less favored distal tenotomy[47] or by a 'lateral release' procedure involving division of the origin of the common extensor tendon[48–50].

Advocates of removal of abnormal tendon and repair claim a better response and are concerned about weakness caused by a 'lateral release'. Others believe the 'lateral release' gives as good long-term results of around 90%, using a simpler procedure that may even be carried out under local anesthetic. The good results from a procedure that can be carried out as day-case surgery have led to an assertion that extensor origin release should be considered earlier in the course of the condition

TABLE 16.4 MANAGEMENT OF LATERAL EPICONDYLITIS	
Early/mild	Rest, splinting, NSAID
Established	Local corticosteroid injection
	Ultrasound
Resistant	Manipulation?
	Surgery – lateral release

after failure of initial conservative treatment[50]. It has been suggested that endoscopic direct vision release could improve responses and identify other associated lesions but it is technically challenging and time-consuming[51]. There is general agreement that extensive lateral release with resection of the proximal third of the annular ligament is best avoided because of the risk of subsequent elbow instability[52].

It must be admitted that most described treatments for lateral epicondylitis, conservative or operative, are not supported by robust scientific evidence. Until there is greater proof, clinicians have to be guided by the available evidence, a pragmatic, if subjective, viewpoint and clinical experience[53].

Prognosis

Lateral epicondylitis has been considered to be a self-limiting disorder with patients improving with or without treatment within 1 year[6]. This good prognosis contrasts with reported relapse rates of between 18% and 50% 6 months after conservative treatment[54,55]. In one study, 40% of patients had prolonged minor discomfort, which in some persisted for 5 years. Manual workers, especially mechanics, builders and domestic workers, are most susceptible to recurrence on resumption of the activity that induced the initial pain[23]. Early treatment may improve prognosis. Firm strapping of the forearm muscles just distal to the elbow joint, or the use of one of the commercial elbow splints, may be helpful. Patients should be instructed to avoid straining the arm for at least 3 months. Although emphasis is on rest, graded exercises to strengthen forearm muscles may be prescribed, especially in the rehabilitation back to sport. In a few cases, persistence of lateral elbow pain despite local treatment is due to a cervical lesion that was not originally clinically apparent, and re-examination may be necessary. Up to 10% of patients fail to respond to physical therapy and injections[46].

Medial epicondylitis

Otherwise known as 'golfer's elbow', this condition is around 15 times less commonly seen than lateral epicondylitis[22]. It is a lesion of the common flexor tendon at the medial epicondyle. As with 'tennis elbow', a sporting cause is relatively rare. The condition is usually milder and often pain and tenderness are less well localized to the medial epicondyle, being felt a little distal to the flexor origin. Pain on resisted wrist flexion with the elbow in extension is the most reliable sign (Fig. 16.10), although rarely flexion of the fingers rather than of the wrist best elicits symptoms. The pathology and management are essentially the same as those for lateral epicondylitis.

SUMMARY

The elbow is a hinged joint to which is added the pronation and supination motion of the forearm, producing a steady adjustable base to make best use of the hands. Elbow pain is due either to joint disease or more commonly to a lesion of the soft periarticular tissues. Referred pain from the neck and shoulder can give rise to diagnostic confusion and must be excluded by appropriate examination. Nerve entrapment about the elbow can mimic the pain of a soft tissue lesion. Lateral epicondylitis is the most frequent periarticular lesion, affecting 1–3% of the population, mainly in middle life, but despite its common name of 'tennis elbow' it is rarely due to the sport. Medial epicondylitis and olecranon bursitis are the other common periarticular lesions. Diagnosis is clinical and straightforward, based on relevant history and examination. Olecranon bursitis and some elbow joint conditions may be effectively treated by aspiration and local corticosteroid injection but the possibility of an underlying infection must be considered and examination of synovial fluid is necessary before injection.

Epicondylitis can be successfully treated in 90% of cases by local corticosteroid injection into the tender tendon origin at the humeral epicondyle (see Chapter 6). The injection is not infrequently painful initially and relapse may occur requiring further injection. No more than two repeat injections should be given and the arm should not be strained for at least 3 months afterwards. Pulsed therapeutic ultrasound, when used optimally, can be an effective alternative that is non-painful but is less frequently successful. Other modalities of treatment are of uncertain or unconfirmed benefit. For the 10% of resistant cases, manipulation under general anesthetic may be tried but in general a surgical lateral release procedure should be considered.

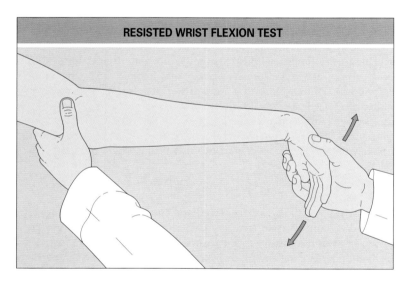

RESISTED WRIST FLEXION TEST

Fig. 16.10 Resisted wrist flexion test.

REFERENCES

1. Williams PL, Bannister LH, Berry MM *et al.*, eds. Gray's anatomy, 38th ed. Edinburgh: Churchill Livingstone; 1995.
2. Morrey BF, An KN. Articular and ligamentous contributions to stability of the elbow joint. Am J Sports Med 1983; 11: 315–319.
3. Chen J, Alk D, Eventov I, Wientroub S. Development of the olecranon bursa: an anatomic cadaveric study. Acta Orthop Scand 1987; 58: 408–409.
4. Boone DC, Azen SP. Normal range of motion of joints in male subjects. J Bone Joint Surg 1979; 61A: 756–759.
5. Yocum LA. The diagnosis and non-operative treatment of elbow problems in the athlete. Clin Sports Med 1989; 8: 439–451.
6. Cyriax J H. Diagnosis of soft tissue lesions. II: Treatment by manipulation, massage and injection. In: Textbook of orthopaedic medicine. London: Baillière Tindall; 1982.
7. Baker CL, Brooks AA. Arthroscopy of the elbow. Clin Sports Med 1996: 15: 261–281.
8. Miller TT. Imaging of elbow disorders. Orthop Clin N Am 1999; 30: 21–36.
9. Schweitzer M, Morison WB. Arthropathies and inflammatory conditions of the elbow. Magn Reson Imaging Clin North Am 1997; 5: 503–517.
10. Fritz RC, Steinbach LS, Tirman PF, Martinez S. MR imaging of the elbow. An update. Rad Clin North Am 1997; 35: 117–144.
11. Connel D, Burke F, Coombes P *et al*. Sonographic examination of lateral epicondylitis. AJR 2001; 176: 777–782.
12. Canoso JJ, Barza M. Soft tissue infections. Clin Rheum Dis 1993; 19: 293–309.
13. Smith DL, McAfee JH, Lucas LM *et al*. Treatment of nonseptic olecranon bursitis. A controlled blinded prospective trial. Arch Intern Med 1989; 149: 2527–2530.
14. Ho G, Su EY. Antibiotic therapy of septic bursitis: its implication in the treatment of septic arthritis. Arthritis Rheum 1981; 24: 905–910.
15. Stewart NJ, Manzanares JB, Morrey BF. Surgical treatment of a septic olecranon bursitis. J Shoulder Elbow Surg 1997; 6: 49–54.
16. Runge F. Zur Genese und Behandlung des Schreiberkrampfes. Berl Klin Wschr 1873; 10: 245–248.
17. Morris H. Rider's sprain. Lancet. 1882; 2: 557.
18. Allander E. Prevalence, incidence and remission rates of some common rheumatic diseases and syndromes. Scand J Rheumatol 1974; 3: 145–153.

19. Kivi P. The aetiology and conservative treatment of humeral epicondylitis. Scand J Rehabil Med 1982; 15: 37–41.
20. Gruchow HW, Pelletier BS. An epidemiologic study of tennis elbow. Am J Sports Med 1979; 7: 234–238.
21. Nirschl RP, Pettrone FA. Tennis elbow. J Bone Joint Surg 1973; 61A: 832–839.
22. Coonrad RW, Hooper WR. Tennis elbow: course, natural history, conservative and surgical management. J Bone Joint Surg 1973; 55A: 1177–1187.
23. Binder AI, Hazleman BL. Lateral humeral epicondylitis – a study of natural history and the effect of conservative therapy. Br J Rheumatol 1983; 22: 73–76.
24. Cyriax JH. The pathology and treatment of tennis elbow. J Bone Joint Surg 1936; 18: 921–940.
25. Newman JH, Goodfellow JW. Fibrillation of the radial head as one cause for tennis elbow. Br Med J 1975; 2: 328–330.
26. Roles NC, Maudsley RH. Radial tunnel syndrome: resistant tennis elbow as a nerve entrapment. J Bone Joint Surg 1972; 54B: 499–508.
27. Bosworth DM. The role of the orbicular ligament in tennis elbow. J Bone Joint Surg 1955; 37A: 527–533.
28. Sarkar K, Uhthoff HK. Ultrastructure of the common extensor tendon origin in tennis elbow. Virchows Arch A 1980; 386: 317–330.
29. Nirschl RP, Pettrone FA. Tennis elbow: the surgical treatment of lateral epicondylitis. J Bone Joint Surg 1979; 61A: 832–839.
30. Regan W, Lester E, Coonrad R, Morrey BF. Microscopic histopathology of chronic refractory lateral epicondylitis. Am J Sports Med 1992; 20: 746–749.
31. Chard MD, Cawston TE, Riley GP et al. Rotator cuff degeneration and lateral epicondylitis: a comparative histological study. Ann Rheum Dis 1994; 53: 30–34.
32. Neipal GA, Sitaj S. Enthesopathy. Clin Rheum Dis 1979; 5: 857–862.
33. Van Rossum J, Buruma OJS, Kamphrisen HAC, Onvlee GJ. Tennis elbow – a radial tunnel syndrome? J Bone Joint Surg 1978; 60A: 197–208.
34. Spinner H. The arcade of Frohse and its relationship to posterior interosseous nerve paralysis. J Bone Joint Surg 1968; 50A: 809–812.
35. Binder A, Parr G, Page Thomas P, Hazleman B. A clinical and thermographic study of lateral epicondylitis. Br J Rheumatol 1983; 22: 77–81.
36. Potter HG, Hannefin JA, Morwessel RM et al. Lateral epicondylitis: correlation of MR imaging, surgical and histopathological findings. Radiology 1995; 196: 43–46.
37. Hay EM, Paterson SM, Lewis M et al. Pragmatic randomised controlled trial of local corticosteroid injection and naproxen for treatment of lateral epicondylitis in primary care. Br Med J 1999; 319: 964–968.
38. Binder A, Hodge G, Greenwood AM et al. Is therapeutic ultrasound effective in treating soft tissue lesions? Br Med J 1985; 292: 512–514.
39. Lundberg T, Haker E, Thomas M. The effect of laser versus placebo in tennis elbow. Scand J Rehab Med 1987: 135–138.
40. Krasheninnkoff M, Ellitsgaard N, Rogvi-Hansen B et al. No effect of low power laser in lateral epicondylitis. Scand J Rheumatol 1994; 23: 260–263.
41. Rompe JD, Hopf C, Kullmerk et al. Analgesic effect of extracorporeal shock wave therapy on chronic tennis elbow. J Bone Joint Surg 1996; 78B: 233–237.
42. Brattberg G. Acupuncture therapy for tennis elbow. Pain 1983; 16: 285–288.
43. Day BH, Gordindasamy N, Patnaik R. Corticosteroid injection in the treatment of tennis elbow. Practitioner 1978; 220: 459–462.
44. Price R, Sinclair H, Heinrich I, Gibson T. Local injection treatment of tennis elbow – hydrocortisone, triamcinolone and lignocaine compared. Br J Rheumatol 1991; 30: 39–44.
45. Coonrad RW. Tendinopathies of the elbow. Instructional course lectures of the American Academy of Orthopaedic Surgeons 1991; 40: 25–32.
46. Wadsworth TG. Tennis elbow: conservative, surgical and manipulative treatment. Br Med J 1987; 294: 621–624.
47. Garden RS. Tennis elbow. J Bone Joint Surg 1961; 43: 100–106.
48. Calvert PT, Macpherson IS, Allum RL, Bentley G. Simple lateral release in treatment of tennis elbow. J R Soc Med 1985; 78: 912–915.
49. Verhaar J, Walenkamp G, van Mameren H, van der Linden T. Lateral extensor release for tennis elbow. A prospective long term follow-up study. J Bone Joint Surg 1993; 75A: 1034–1043.
50. Bankes MJK, Jessop JH. Day-case simple extensor origin release for tennis elbow. Arch Orthop Trauma Surg 1998; 117: 250–251.
51. Kuklo TR, Taylor KF, Murphy KP et al. Arthroscopic release for lateral epicondylitis: a cadaveric model. Arthroscopy 1999; 15: 265–268.
52. O'Neil J, Sarkar K, Uhthoff HK. A retrospective study of surgically treated cases of tennis elbow. Acta Orthop Belg 1980; 46: 189–190.
53. Boyer M I, Hastings H II. Lateral tennis elbow 'Is there any science out there?' J Shoulder Elbow Surg 1999; 8: 481–941.
54. Clarke AK, Woodland J. Comparison of two steroid preparations used to treat tennis elbow, using the hypospray. Rheumatol Rehabil 1975; 14: 47–49.
55. Nevelos AB. The treatment of tennis elbow with triamcinolone acetonide. Curr Med Res Opin 1980; 6: 507–509.

REGIONAL AND WIDESPREAD PAIN

17 The wrist and hand

Adel G Fam

■ Pain in the wrist and hand may have its origin in the bones and joints, periarticular soft tissues (cutaneous and subcutaneous tissues, palmar fascia, tendon sheaths), nerve roots and peripheral nerves, and vascular structures or be referred from the cervical spine, thoracic outlet, shoulder or elbow.

■ Precise diagnosis rests upon a meticulous history, a thorough examination and a few rationally selected diagnostic studies.

INTRODUCTION

The hand is the chief sensory organ of touch and is uniquely adapted for grasping. The radial side of the hand performs pinch grip between the fingers and thumb, while the ulnar side performs power grip between the fingers and palm.

FUNCTIONAL ANATOMY

The bones of the hand are divided into a central fixed unit for stability, and three mobile units for dexterity and power[1]. The fixed unit comprises the eight carpal bones tightly bound to the second and third metacarpals (Fig. 17.1). The three mobile units projecting from the fixed unit are:

● the thumb, the first carpometacarpal (CMC) joint, which permits extension, flexion, abduction and adduction, for powerful pinch and grasp and fine manipulations
● the index finger, endowed with independent extrinsic extensors and flexors and powerful intrinsic muscles, for precise movements alone or with the thumb
● the middle, ring and little fingers for power grip, a function enhanced by slight movements of the fourth and fifth metacarpals at their CMC articulations.

The axis of the wrist and hand is an extension of the longitudinal axis of the radius and the third metacarpal, with the wrist in the neutral position and the dorsal surface of the hand in the same plane as that of the distal radius[2].

Wrist (radiocarpal) joint

This is an ellipsoid joint between the distal radius and articular disc proximally and the scaphoid, lunate and triquetrum distally[1–3] (Fig. 17.1). The articular capsule is strengthened by the radiocarpal (dorsal and palmar) and collateral (radial and ulnar) ligaments. The articular disc, or triangular fibrocartilage of the wrist, joins the radius to the ulna. Its base is attached to the ulnar border of the distal radius and its apex to the root of the ulnar styloid process. The synovial cavity of the distal radioulnar joint is L-shaped and extends distally beneath the triangular fibrocartilage but is usually separated from the radiocarpal joint.

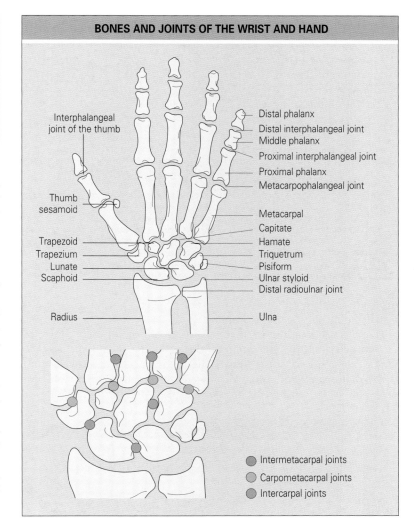

BONES AND JOINTS OF THE WRIST AND HAND

Interphalangeal joint of the thumb
Distal phalanx
Distal interphalangeal joint
Middle phalanx
Proximal interphalangeal joint
Proximal phalanx
Metacarpophalangeal joint
Thumb sesamoid
Metacarpal
Capitate
Hamate
Trapezoid
Trapezium
Triquetrum
Lunate
Pisiform
Scaphoid
Ulnar styloid
Distal radioulnar joint
Radius
Ulna

● Intermetacarpal joints
● Carpometacarpal joints
● Intercarpal joints

Fig. 17.1 Bones and joints of the wrist and hand.

The radiocarpal, intercarpal, midcarpal (located between the proximal and distal rows of the carpal bones), CMC and intermetacarpal joints often intercommunicate through a common synovial cavity (Fig. 17.1).

The carpal bones form a volar concave arch or carpal tunnel, with the pisiform and hook of the hamate on the ulnar side and the scaphoid tubercle and crest of the trapezium on the radial side[1–3]. The four bony prominences are joined by the flexor retinaculum (transverse carpal ligament), which forms the roof of the carpal tunnel. The palmaris longus (absent in 10–15% of the population) partly inserts into the flexor retinaculum and partly fans out into the palm, forming the palmar aponeurosis (fascia). The aponeurosis broadens distally and divides into four digital slips which attach to the finger flexor tendon sheath,

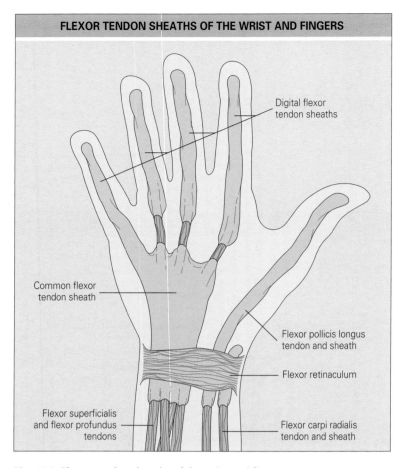

FLEXOR TENDON SHEATHS OF THE WRIST AND FINGERS

Digital flexor
tendon sheaths

Common flexor
tendon sheath

Flexor pollicis longus
tendon and sheath

Flexor retinaculum

Flexor superficialis
and flexor profundus
tendons

Flexor carpi radialis
tendon and sheath

Fig. 17.2 Flexor tendon sheaths of the wrist and fingers.

metacarpophalangeal joint capsules and proximal phalanges. There is usually no digital slip to the thumb.

Tendons crossing the wrist are enclosed for part of their course in tenosynovial sheaths. The common flexor tendon sheath encloses the long flexor tendons of the fingers (flexor digitorum superficialis and flexor digitorum profundus) and extends from approximately 2.5cm proximal to the wrist crease to the mid-palm. It runs with the flexor

pollicis longus tendon sheath and the median nerve through the carpal tunnel (Fig. 17.2). The tendon sheath of the little finger is usually continuous with the common flexor sheath. The flexor pollicis longus tendon to the thumb runs through a separate tenosynovial sheath but may join the common flexor sheath. The flexor carpi radialis is invested in a short tendon sheath as it crosses the volar aspect of the wrist between the split radial attachment of the flexor retinaculum. The flexor retinaculum straps down the flexor tendons as they cross at the wrist. The ulnar nerve, artery and vein cross over the retinaculum but are sometimes covered by a fibrous band – the superficial part of the transverse carpal ligament – to form the ulnar tunnel, or Guyon's canal.

On the dorsum of the wrist, the extensor tendons pass through six tenosynovial, fibro-osseous tunnels beneath the extensor retinaculum (dorsal carpal ligament): abductor pollicis longus and extensor pollicis brevis are usually in a single sheath (first extensor compartment, most radial), extensor carpi radialis longus and brevis, extensor pollicis longus, extensor digitorum communis and extensor indicis proprius, extensor digiti minimi and extensor carpi ulnaris (sixth extensor compartment, most ulnar; Fig 17.3). Each tenosynovial sheath extends about 2.5cm proximally and distally from the retinaculum. The extensor retinaculum, by its deep attachments to the distal radius and ulna, binds down and prevents bowstringing of the extensor tendons as they cross the wrist. The anatomic snuffbox corresponds to the depression between the extensor pollicis longus tendon and the tendons of the abductor pollicis longus and extensor pollicis brevis.

Movements of the wrist include palmar flexion, dorsiflexion (extension), ulnar deviation, radial deviation and circumduction. The intercarpal joints, particularly the lunate-capitate joint, contribute to wrist dorsiflexion and palmar flexion[4]. Prime wrist palmar flexors are the flexor carpi radialis, flexor carpi ulnaris and palmaris longus. The prime dorsiflexors are the extensor carpi radialis longus and brevis and the extensor carpi ulnaris.

Pronation (palm of the hand turned backward) to 90° and supination (palm turned forward) to 90° of the hand and forearm occur at the proximal and distal radioulnar joints.

The carpometacarpal joints

The first CMC joint is a saddle-shaped, very mobile joint between the trapezium and the base of the first metacarpal[1,5]. It allows 40–50° of

Fig. 17.3 Extensor tendons and tendon sheaths of the wrist.

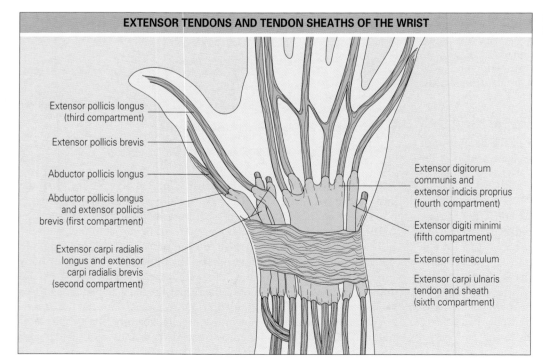

EXTENSOR TENDONS AND TENDON SHEATHS OF THE WRIST

Extensor pollicis longus
(third compartment)

Extensor pollicis brevis

Abductor pollicis longus

Abductor pollicis longus
and extensor pollicis
brevis (first compartment)

Extensor carpi radialis
longus and extensor
carpi radialis brevis
(second compartment)

Extensor digitorum
communis and
extensor indicis proprius
(fourth compartment)

Extensor digiti minimi
(fifth compartment)

Extensor retinaculum

Extensor carpi ulnaris
tendon and sheath
(sixth compartment)

thumb flexion–extension (parallel to the plane of the palm) and 40–70° of adduction–abduction (perpendicular to the plane of the palm). These movements are important in bringing the thumb into opposition with the fingers. The second and third CMC joints are relatively fixed but the fourth and fifth are mobile, allowing the fourth and fifth metacarpals to flex forward (15–30°) toward the thumb during power grip.

The metacarpophalangeal joints

The metacarpophalangeal (MCP) joints are modified hinge joints that lie about 1cm distal to the knuckles (metacarpal heads)[1,5,6] (Fig. 17.1). Their capsule is strengthened by the radial and ulnar collateral ligaments on the sides and by the palmar (volar) plate on the volar surface. The collateral ligaments are loose in the neutral position, allowing radial and ulnar deviations, but become tight in the flexed position, preventing side-to-side motion (referred to as sagittal cam effect). The deep transverse metacarpal ligament joins the volar plates of the second to fifth MCP joints. The MCP joint of the thumb is large and has two sesamoid bones overlying its volar surface.

When the long extensor tendon of the digit reaches the metacarpal head, it is joined by the tendons of the interossei and lumbrical and expands over the dorsum of the MCP joint and digit forming the extensor hood or expansion (Fig. 17.4). The expansion divides over the dorsum of the proximal phalanx into an intermediate slip, which is inserted principally into the base of the middle phalanx, and two collateral slips, which are inserted into the base of the distal phalanx.

The first MCP joint permits 50–70° palmar flexion and 10–30° dorsiflexion. Radial and ulnar deviations are limited to less than 10–20°. The other MCP joints allow 90° palmar flexion, 30° dorsiflexion, and 35° of radial and ulnar movements. The extensor pollicis brevis, extensor indicis proprius, extensor digitorum communis and extensor digiti minimi dorsiflex the MCP joints. The palmar flexors are the flexor pollicis brevis, lumbricals, interossei and flexor digiti minimi brevis assisted by the long flexors. Radial and ulnar movements at the second to fifth MCP joints are a function of the intrinsic muscles.

The interphalangeal joints

The proximal and distal interphalangeal (PIP and DIP) joints of the fingers and the interphalangeal (IP) joint of the thumb are hinge joints[1,5,6]. Their capsules are strengthened by the collateral ligaments on the sides and by the volar plates on the palmar surface, which serve to limit hyperextension, particularly at the PIP joints. Unlike the MCP joints, the radial and ulnar collateral ligaments remain taut in all positions, providing side-to-side stability throughout the range of movement.

The flexor tendon sheaths for the fingers enclose the tendons of flexor digitorum superficialis and profundus to their insertions on the middle and distal phalanges respectively. The sheaths extend from just proximal to the MCP joints to the bases of the distal phalanges (Fig. 17.2). The thumb flexor pollicis longus tendon sheath extends proximally to the carpal tunnel.

The flexor sheath of the little finger is often continuous with the wrist common flexor tendon sheath. Segmental condensations, or annular pulleys, in the digital flexor sheaths prevent bowstringing of the tendons and are mechanically critical for full digital flexion[1,5,7].

The PIP joints do not normally hyperextend. They allow 100–120° palmar flexion. The DIP joints permit 50–80° palmar flexion and 5–10° dorsiflexion. The IP joint of the thumb allows 80–90° palmar flexion and 20–35° dorsiflexion. The flexor digitorum superficialis flexes the PIP joints and the flexor digitorum profundus flexes the DIP joints of the fingers. The prime dorsiflexors are the interossei and lumbrical muscles. The flexor pollicis longus flexes the IP joint of the thumb and the extensor pollicis longus dorsiflexes the joint.

PHYSICAL EXAMINATION

Inspection

The wrist and hand are inspected for any swelling or deformity[2,5,6]. Arthritis of the radiocarpal joint produces a diffuse swelling distal to the radius and ulna. Extensor wrist tenosynovitis, by contrast, presents as a linear or oval-shaped dorsal swelling localized to the distribution of the tendon sheath. When the fingers are actively extended, the distal margin of the swelling moves proximally and folds in, like a sheet being tucked under a mattress (tuck sign)[2]. Tenosynovitis of the common flexor tendon sheath presents as a swelling over the volar aspect of the wrist just proximal to the carpal tunnel (volar hot dog sign). The wrist is a common site for ganglia (Fig. 17.5). A ganglion is a cystic swelling arising from a joint capsule or from a tendon sheath. It is synovium-lined and contains a clear, thick, jelly-like fluid.

Wrist deformities are common in rheumatoid arthritis (RA) and other chronic inflammatory arthritides. They include volar subluxation of the

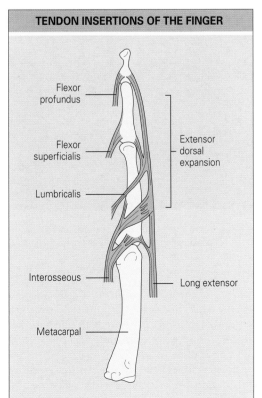

Fig. 17.4 Tendon insertions of the finger.

TENDON INSERTIONS OF THE FINGER

Flexor profundus

Flexor superficialis

Lumbricalis

Interosseous

Metacarpal

Extensor dorsal expansion

Long extensor

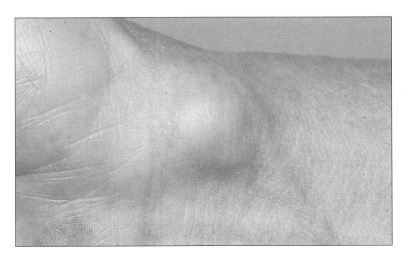

Fig. 17.5 A ganglion on the volar aspect of the wrist

carpus with a visible step opposite the radiocarpal joint, carpal collapse (loss of carpal height to less than half the length of the third metacarpal, with inability to admit the tips of the patient's index and middle fingers), and radial posturing of the carpus (radial deviation of the carpus from the axis of the wrist and hand). Chronic arthritis of the distal radioulnar joint results in instability and dorsal subluxation of the ulnar head with a 'piano key' movement on downward pressure.

Entrapment of the median nerve in the carpal tunnel (carpal tunnel syndrome) can lead to atrophy of the thenar muscles. In RA, rupture at the wrist of an extensor tendon to the little or ring finger is associated with inability to actively dorsiflex the digit at the MCP joint.

Deformities of the fingers and thumb are common in RA. The fingers are inspected for swelling of the MCP, PIP or DIP joints, deformities, clubbing, subcutaneous nodules, gouty tophi, Heberden's or Bouchard's nodes, sclerodactyly, telangiectasia, ischemic digital ulcers, pitted scars, nailfold infarcts, periungual erythema or psoriatic skin/nail lesions[5]. MCP synovitis produces a diffuse swelling of the joint that may obscure the valleys between the knuckles. Swelling of a PIP joint produces a fusiform or spindle-shaped finger. Digital flexor tenosynovitis produces a diffuse tender swelling over the volar aspect of the finger (sausage finger). MCP joint deformities include ulnar drift, volar subluxation (often visible as a step) and flexion deformities. Boutonnière deformity describes a finger with flexion of the PIP joint and hyperextension of the DIP joint (Fig. 17.6). A swan-neck deformity describes the appearance of a finger in which there is hyperextension of the PIP joint and flexion of the DIP joint (Fig. 17.6). A Z-shaped deformity of the thumb is flexion of the MCP joint and hyperextension of the IP joint (Fig. 17.6). Telescoped shortening of the digits, produced by partial resorption of the phalanges secondary to psoriatic arthritis, RA or other destructive arthritis, is often associated with concentric wrinkling of the skin (opera-glass hand).

Thickening and contracture of the palmar aponeurosis (Dupuytren's contracture) often produces flexion deformities of the ring and, less commonly, the little and middle fingers.

Palpation

The wrist is palpated with the joint in slight palmar flexion[2,3]. The margins of a swollen synovium are detected most reliably by the thumbs firmly palpating the dorsal surface of the wrist while the fingers of both

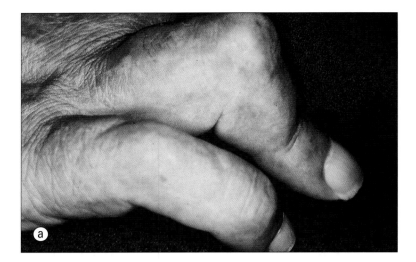

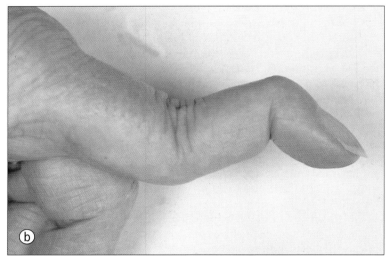

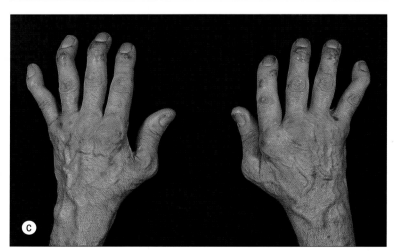

Fig. 17.6 Deformities of the fingers and thumb. (a) Boutonnière and (b) swan-neck deformity of the fingers; (c) 'Z'-shaped deformity of the thumb.

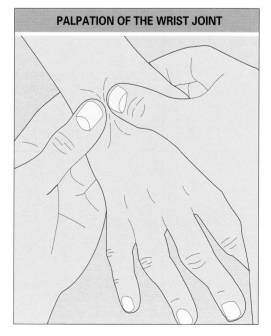

PALPATION OF THE WRIST JOINT

Fig. 17.7 Palpation of the wrist joint.

hands support the joint (Fig. 17.7). The joint is difficult to palpate from the volar surface because of the overlying flexor tendons. The presence of fluctuance indicates a large wrist effusion: pressure with one hand on one side of the joint produces a fluid wave transmitted to the second hand placed on the opposite side of the wrist.

Wrist tenosynovitis produces a superficial, linear, tender swelling extending beyond the joint margins. A crepitus may be palpable and movements of the involved tendon often produce pain.

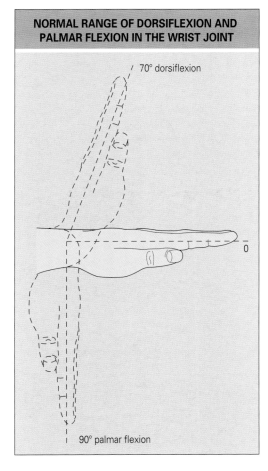

NORMAL RANGE OF DORSIFLEXION AND PALMAR FLEXION IN THE WRIST JOINT

70° dorsiflexion

0

90° palmar flexion

Fig. 17.8 Normal range of dorsiflexion and palmar flexion in the wrist joint.

The normal range of movement at the wrist comprises 80–90° palmar flexion, 70–80° dorsiflexion, 40–50° ulnar deviation and 15–20° radial deviation (Fig. 17.8).

The first CMC joint is palpated for tenderness, swelling or crepitus. Osteoarthritis is associated with crepitus and 'squaring' of the joint.

Synovitis of the MCP joint is detected most reliably by palpating firmly with the thumbs over the dorsal surface of the joint on each side of the extensor tendon, while the forefingers support the joint over the volar aspect (Fig. 17.9).

The joint is difficult to palpate from the volar aspect because of the thickened skin of the palm, overlaying fat pad and intervening flexor tendon sheath.

The PIP and DIP joints are palpated for tenderness, synovial thickening, or effusion using the thumbs and forefingers of both hands placed on opposite sides of the joint[3] (Fig. 17.10). To detect an effusion, compression of the joint by one hand produces ballooning or a hydraulic lift sensed by the other hand (balloon sign). Unlike PIP synovitis, dorsal knuckle pads produce a non-tender thickening of the skin localized to the dorsal surface of the PIP joints.

Finger tenosynovitis produces linear tenderness, volar swelling, thickening, nodules and/or crepitus of the flexor tendon sheath. Tendon nodules usually occur at the level of the metacarpal heads opposite the proximal annular pulley of the sheath. These can be palpated in the palm while the patient slowly flexes and extends the affected finger.

The range of movements at the MCP, PIP and DIP joints is assessed by asking the patient to extend the fingers, make a fist, then flex the fingers so that the fingertips touch the palm opposite the MCP joints. To test for stability of the MCP joint, the joint is palmar flexed to 90° to tighten the radial and ulnar collateral ligaments, and the corresponding metacarpal is then held in one hand while the other hand moves the finger from side to side to test the integrity of the collateral ligaments. The stability of the radial and ulnar collateral ligaments of the PIP and DIP joints can be assessed by applying side strain with the joint in the neutral position.

Special maneuvers

In carpal tunnel syndrome, percussion of the median nerve at the flexor retinaculum (just radial to the palmaris longus tendon at the distal wrist crease) produces paresthesia in the median nerve distribution: thumb, index and middle fingers and the radial half of the ring finger (Tinel's

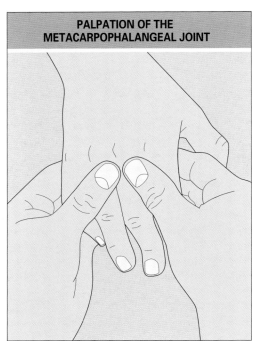

PALPATION OF THE METACARPOPHALANGEAL JOINT

Fig. 17.9 Palpation of the metacarpophalangeal joint.

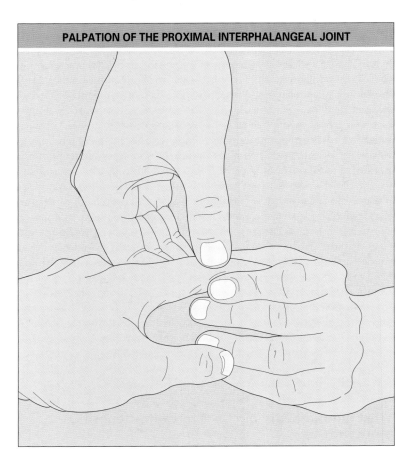

PALPATION OF THE PROXIMAL INTERPHALANGEAL JOINT

Fig. 17.10 Palpation of the proximal interphalangeal joint.

sign)[2,3]. Sustained palmar flexion of the wrist for 30–60 seconds may induce finger paresthesia (Phalen's wrist flexion sign). If the wrist cannot be flexed because of arthritis, pressure over the median nerve for 30 seconds often produces the same effect.

In de Quervain's stenosing tenosynovitis of the abductor pollicis longus and extensor pollicis brevis (see below), Finkelstein's test is a useful diagnostic maneuver. Passive ulnar deviation of the wrist with the fingers flexed over the thumb placed in the palm stretches the tendons and reproduces the pain over the distal radius and the radial side of the wrist[2].

In vascular disorders of the hand, the patency of the radial and ulnar arteries can be assessed by Allen's test[1]. The patient elevates the hand and makes a fist while the examiner occludes both the radial and the ulnar arteries at the wrist. The patient then extends the fingers and repeats the maneuver until blanching of the hand is seen. Each artery is then released and the color of the hand returns to normal. If either artery is occluded, the hand remains blanched when this artery alone is released.

In swan-neck finger deformity, tightness and shortening of the intrinsic muscles (interossei and lumbricals) results in restriction of PIP flexion when the MCP joint is dorsiflexed. Thus, with the MCP joint dorsiflexed, the range of PIP flexion is less than that when the MCP joint is palmar flexed (positive Bunnell's test)[5].

DIFFERENTIAL DIAGNOSIS OF WRIST AND HAND PAIN

Pain in the wrist and hand is a relatively common symptom of diverse causes[8–10]. It may have its origin in the bones and joints of the wrist and hand, periarticular soft tissues (cutaneous and subcutaneous tissues, palmar fascia, tendon sheaths), nerve roots and peripheral nerves or vascular structures, or be referred from the musculoskeletal structures of the cervical spine, thoracic outlet, shoulder or elbow. Table 17.1 provides a classification of painful disorders of the wrist and hand based upon the site of origin of pain and its predominant location. Precise diagnosis rests upon a meticulous history, a thorough examination of the joints, periarticular structures, cervical spine, nerve and blood supplies to the hand, and a few rationally selected diagnostic studies.

As with any other clinical problem, assessment begins with a complete history, which should take account of the onset, location, character, duration and modulating factors of pain. The onset of hand musculoskeletal disorders is often insidious. A history of unaccustomed, repetitive or excessive hand activity is particularly important in the diagnosis of wrist, thumb, or finger tenosynovitis due to an overuse syndrome. A detailed occupational history is important for determining whether the hand tendinitis is work-related, either as a cumulative trauma disorder, or an acute injury. Abnormal tensile stresses, exceeding the elastic limits of tendons, can lead to cumulative microfailure of the molecular links between tendon fibrils; a phenomenon referred to as 'fibrillar creep'. With aging, tendons become less flexible and less elastic, rendering them more susceptible to injury. A shortened musculotendinous unit, from lack of regular stretching exercises, is more prone to cumulative trauma disorder. Initial diagnostic studies include a complete blood count, erythrocyte sedimentation rate, hand radiographs, synovial fluid analysis (when available), and if indicated, serum uric acid, rheumatoid factor, and antinuclear antibody test. Additional studies are sometimes required and include skeletal scintigraphy, ultrasonography, nerve conduction studies, noninvasive vascular (Doppler) studies, arteriography, computed tomography (CT), magnetic resonance imaging (MRI), arthrography and synovial biopsy.

SPECIFIC DISORDERS OF THE WRIST AND HAND

Wrist tenosynovitis and De Quervain's stenosing tenosynovitis

A total of 22 extrinsic tendons cross the wrist, providing a unique combination of power and dexterity to the hand. Each tendon passes

TABLE 17.1 DIFFERENTIAL DIAGNOSIS OF WRIST AND HAND PAIN	
Articular	
Arthritis of wrist, MCP, PIP and/or DIP due to	Trauma, hypermobility, sprain RA (wrist, MCP, PIP joints) Osteoarthritis (first CMC, PIP and DIP joints) Other forms of arthritis: gout, psoriatic arthritis, infection Joint neoplasms
Periarticular	
Subcutaneous	RA nodules, gouty tophi, painful subcutaneous calcific nodules in scleroderma, glomus tumor of nail bed
Palmar fascia	Dupuytren's contracture
Tendon sheath	Wrist extensor tenosynovitis, including de Quervain's tenosynovitis and extensor carpi radialis tenosynovitis Wrist volar flexor tenosynovitis (including carpal tunnel syndrome) Thumb flexor tenosynovitis (trigger or snapping thumb) Finger flexor tenosynovitis (trigger finger) Pigmented villonodular tenosynovitis (giant cell tumor of the tendon sheath)
Acute calcific periarthritis Ganglion	Wrist, MCP, and rarely PIP and DIP
Osseous	
Bone lesions	Fractures, neoplasms, infection, osteonecrosis including Kienböck's disease (lunate) and Preiser's disease (scaphoid)
Neurologic	
Nerve entrapment syndromes Median nerve	Carpal tunnel syndrome (at wrist) Pronator teres syndrome (at pronator teres) Anterior interosseous nerve syndrome
Ulnar nerve	Cubital tunnel syndrome (at elbow) Guyon's canal (at wrist)
Posterior interosseous nerve syndrome	Radial nerve palsy (spiral groove syndrome)
Lower brachial plexus	Thoracic outlet syndrome, Pancoast's tumor
Cervical nerve roots *Spinal cord lesion* Spinal tumors, syringomyelia	Herniated cervical disc, tumors
Vascular	
Vasospastic disorders with Raynaud's phenomenon	Scleroderma, occupational vibration syndrome, etc.
Small- or large-vessel vasculitis	With digital ischemia, ischemic ulcers, e.g. systemic lupus erythematosus, RA and Takayasu's arteritis
Referred pain	
Cervical spine disorders Reflex sympathetic dystrophy syndrome (RSDS)	Shoulder–hand syndrome and causalgia
Cardiac	Angina pectoris

through a narrow fibro-osseous canal lined by a tubular synovial sheath. A wrist or finger tendon sheath is lined by an inner or visceral synovial layer that adheres closely to the tendon and an outer or parietal synovium that covers the inside of the fibrous tendon sheath. The visceral and parietal synovial tubes are united longitudinally by the mesotendon, a synovial fold that transmits vessels and nerves to the tendon. The mesotendon may disappear partially in some tendon sheaths, and be represented by threads or vinculae[11].

Excessive loads or repetitive movements of a tendon through its tendon sheath can cause chronic reactive or stenosing tenosynovitis with inflammation, fibrosis and thickening of the sheath, and 'fibrillar creep' of the tendon with swelling, edema and bunching of the fibres[9,11,12]. This results in an impediment to smooth gliding of the tendon through its sheath and ultimately 'catching', 'triggering' or 'locking' on either side of the retinacular ligament or annular pulley. Less frequently, tenosynovitis may result from an isolated traumatic event.

Clinically, tenosynovitis is characterized by local pain, swelling and stiffness. There is linear tenderness and crepitus over the affected tendon sheath, and the pain is made worse by placing the tendon under tension, either by muscular contraction or by passive stretching.

De Quervain's stenosing tenosynovitis of the abductor pollicis longus and extensor pollicis brevis, trigger finger or thumb, and wrist common flexor tenosynovitis, are often due to 'primary' tenosynovitis caused by occupation- or avocation-related cumulative microtrauma. Primary 'overuse' stenosing tenosynovitis affecting other wrist tendon sheaths is less frequent. Secondary causes of tenosynovitis are less common and include rheumatoid arthritis, systemic lupus erythematosus, scleroderma, psoriatic arthritis, reactive arthritis, infection (bacterial, mycobacterial, fungal and viral), microcrystalline (gouty, pyrophosphate and hydroxyapatite or calcific tenosynovitis), amyloid deposition, sarcoidosis and pigmented villonodular tenosynovitis.

De Quervain's tenosynovitis

De Quervain's stenosing tenosynovitis is most common in women between 30 and 50 years of age[9,11–14]. Repetitive activity, involving pinching with the thumb while moving the wrist in radial and ulnar directions, results in frictional inflammation with thickening and stenosis of the fibrous tendon sheath as it passes over the distal radius beneath the extensor retinaculum[15].

De Quervain's tenosynovitis may also occur in association with RA[16], psoriatic arthritis, other inflammatory synovitis, direct trauma, pregnancy and during the postpartum period[17].

Most patients report several weeks or months of pain on the radial aspect of the wrist and at the thumb base during pinch grip, grasping, and other

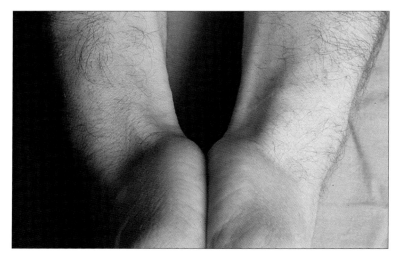

Fig. 17.11 De Quervain's tenosynovitis of the wrist.

thumb and wrist movements. The affected tendon sheath is tender and often swollen 1–2cm proximal to the radial styloid (Fig. 17.11). Finkelstein's test is positive and a tendon crepitus may be palpable[9,11–14]. Patients may have other forms of tenosynovitis such as carpal tunnel syndrome or trigger finger or thumb.

The diagnosis of de Quervain's tenosynovitis is often confused with osteoarthritis of the first CMC joint and with the intersection syndrome. The latter is due to tenosynovitis of the second extensor compartment (extensor carpi radialis longus and brevis) at its intersection with the tendons of the first extensor compartment (abductor pollicis longus and extensor pollicis brevis)[12,18]. This syndrome, which results from frequent repetitive wrist movements particularly in athletes (rowers, canoeists, weight lifters), is associated with pain, tenderness, swelling and sometimes crepitus over the dorsoradial aspect of distal forearm, about 4cm proximal to the wrist joint[12,18]. This differentiates the intersection syndrome from the more distal de Quervain's tenosynovitis.

Treatment of de Quervain's tenosynovitis consists of local heat therapy, nonsteroidal anti-inflammatory drugs (NSAIDs), and wrist and thumb splinting[9,11–14,16,17]. A radial-gutter light support splint immobilizes the wrist in slight extension and radial deviation and the first MCP joint in slight extension. The IP joint of the thumb is left unrestricted. Modification of hand activities, avoiding inciting tasks that require repetitive thumb movements or pinch grasping, is important. These measures are usually effective in alleviating symptoms. In patients with more severe or persistent pain, one or more local corticosteroid injections into the affected tendon sheath are often beneficial, giving complete and lasting relief in about 70% of patients[19–22]. This can be done through a dorsoradial approach. A 27-gauge needle is inserted tangentially into the distal end of the abductor pollicis longus and extensor pollicis brevis tendon sheath 1cm proximal to the radial styloid. If correctly placed, injection of a local anesthetic distends the sheath, producing a swelling proximal to the extensor retinaculum. Methylprednisolone acetate 5–7.5mg is then instilled into the sheath. Surgical decompression of the first extensor compartment, with or without tenosynovectomy, is indicated in those with persistent or recurrent symptoms for more than 6 months[12–14,19,21,23]. A septated tendon sheath, with separate compartments for the abductor pollicis longus and extensor pollicis brevis, can lead to recurrence due to incomplete release of the tendon sheath[12,19,23].

Trigger finger or thumb (stenosing digital tenosynovitis)

Trigger finger or thumb, also known as stenosing digital tenosynovitis or snapping finger or thumb, is the most common repetitive strain injury of the hand[11,12,14]. The anatomic lesion is a tenosynovitis of the flexor tendons of the finger or thumb, which results in fibrosis, constriction and occasionally fibrocartilaginous metaplasia localized to the first annular pulley that overlies the MCP joint[9,11,14,24–26]. A nodular thickening of the tendon often develops at the site of stenosis.

The nodule and/or tendon sheath constriction interfere mechanically with normal tendon gliding, resulting in pain over the area of the pulley and 'snapping', 'triggering' or 'catching' movement of the finger or thumb. Pain along the course of the sheath with active or resisted flexion, and pain on stretching the tendon passively in extension, are common. Intermittent locking of the digit in flexion may also develop, particularly upon arising in the morning. Passive extension of the PIP joint of the finger or IP joint of the thumb may produce crepitus and a popping sensation as the digit is straightened. Examination reveals tenderness over the area of the proximal pulley often associated with linear tenderness and swelling of the flexor tendon sheath, tendon crepitus and limitation of digital flexion and extension. A nodular tendon swelling can often be palpated in the palm just proximal to the MCP joint as it moves during finger or thumb flexion and extension. Over time, guarding on the part of the patient to fully range the digit, can lead to a fixed flexion deformity of the PIP joint.

The most common cause of trigger finger or thumb is overuse trauma of the hands from repetitive gripping activities with increased pull and friction on the flexor tendons[9,11,14,24–26]. The disorder is characteristically restricted to one digit, usually the thumb, middle, ring, little or index fingers in this order. Other causes of flexor digital tenosynovitis include RA[16], psoriatic arthritis, diabetes mellitus[27], amyloidosis, hypothyroidism, sarcoidosis, pigmented villonodular tenosynovitis and infections, including tuberculosis and sporotrichosis A[9].

Management consists of modification of hand activities, local heat treatment, gentle exercises and NSAIDs as required[11,12,14,25]. Extension splinting of the affected digit at night prevents painful flexion during sleep. Trigger finger or thumb, including childhood trigger thumb[28], may resolve spontaneously. One or more corticosteroid injections of the affected flexor tendon sheath are effective and often curative in the majority of patients[9,11,12,24,25,29–31]. A 27-gauge needle is inserted tangentially into the flexor tendon sheath proximal to the first annular pulley, opposite the volar surface of the metacarpal head. The needle is advanced until gentle passive movements of the finger (or thumb) makes a crepitant sensation, indicating that the needle-tip is rubbing against the surface of the tendon. The needle is then withdrawn 0.5–1.0 mm before injecting 5–7.5 mg methylprednisolone acetate into the sheath. Surgical release with transaction of the fibrous annular pulley of the finger or thumb flexor sheath is required rarely for those with chronic symptoms not responding to medical treatment[11,12,23–25,31]. Favorable results have been reported with 'closed' percutaneous trigger finger release, using a hypodermic needle to section the first annular pulley[26,32].

Dupuytren's contracture

This is a relatively common condition characterized by nodular thickening and contraction of the palmar fascia drawing one or more fingers into flexion at the MCP joints[33–36]. In most patients, Dupuytren's contracture affects the ulnar side of both hands. The fourth finger is usually affected earliest, followed by the fifth, third, and second fingers in decreasing order of frequency. Fibrous nodules, resulting from contraction of proliferating fibroblasts and myofibroblasts in the superficial layers of the palmar fascia, are the earliest abnormality. The dermis is invaded by fibroblastic cells, resulting in puckering, dimpling and tethering of the overlying skin (Fig. 17.12). There is usually little pain initially and if no further progression occurs the hand function is preserved and no treatment is required. However, after a variable period of months or years, the aponeurotic thickening may extend distally to involve the digits. The fingers become flexed at the MCP joints by taut fibrous bands or 'cords' radiating from the palmar fascia, and the hand cannot be placed flat on a table (positive table-top test)[10,33–36]. Although there is no direct involvement of the joints or tendons, progressive flexion deformity of the fingers can lead to severe functional impairment.

The etiology of Dupuytren's contracture is poorly understood[33–40]. The disorder occurs most frequently in Caucasians of Celtic or Scandinavian origin. It is rare in non-Caucasians. Its incidence rises with increasing age, and the sex ratio is predominantly male (7:1). Familial predisposition is frequent, suggesting an autosomal dominant pattern with variable penetrance. Cytogenetic studies of Dupuytren's nodules have shown non-specific chromosomal abnormalities, including clonal numerical changes involving trisomies of chromosomes 7 and 8[40]. A pathogenetic role for local repetitive injury and occupational trauma remains unproven[33–41]. Dupuytren's contracture has been observed in association with idiopathic epilepsy, alcohol abuse, tobacco smoking, diabetes mellitus, chronic pulmonary disease, human immunodeficiency virus infection and reflex sympathetic dystrophy syndrome[33–36]. The disorder has also been reported following treatment with a matrix metalloproteinase inhibitor[42]. Patients with Dupuytren's disease are at risk of developing other localized fibroses, including nodular plantar fibromatosis, nodular fasciitis of popliteal fascia, Peyronie's disease and knuckle pads[33,43]. The cause of these fibrosing diseases is unknown but seems to be determined by a dominant gene with high penetrance in males, usually middle-aged white men of Celtic ancestry[33].

Pathologically, the early lesion of Dupuytren's disease is characterized by marked fibroblastic proliferation, vascular hyperplasia and clusters of macrophages and T lymphocytes. This is followed by dense, disorderly collagen deposition with thickening of the palmar fascia and nodule formation[33–36,44]. The abnormal fascia demonstrates elevated total amounts of collagen with increased content of reducible cross links and hydroxylysine[45]. About 25% of the collagen is type III, which is normally present in small amounts in the palmar fascia. Ultrastructurally, contractile, smooth-muscle-like fibroblasts or myofibroblasts surrounded by bundles of disarrayed collagenous fibrils and completely or partially occluded capillaries are present in the fibrotic nodules and cords[44]. Although myofibroblasts are not specific to Dupuytren's contracture, they are believed to be responsible for contraction of the palmar fascia and finger deformities. The finding of isolated foci of fibroblasts positive for smooth muscle α-actin (an antibody marker for myofibroblasts) dispersed in the dermis remote from the main Dupuytren's tissue may explain the high recurrence rate of Dupuytren's disease after fasciectomy[46]. Both interleukin-1α and IL-1β, tumor necrosis factor-α, the vasoactive prostaglandins PGE_2 and $PGF_{2\alpha}$, and fibronectin, are present in increased concentrations in Dupuytren's nodules and are thought to influence myofibroblast contractility and contribute to the formation of the contracture[37,39,45]. Increased expression of growth factors, such as transforming growth factor-β, platelet-derived growth factor, basic fibroblast growth factor and epidermal growth factor, in Dupuytren's fascial lesions suggests that these polypeptides may play a role in fibroblastic proliferation[34,39,45]. Adhesion molecules, which enhance transendothelial migration of inflammatory cells, are also expressed in Dupuytren's lesions: integrin VLA4 on macrophages and lymphocytes, and vascular cell adhesion molecule-1 on endothelial cells[37].

Production of oxygen-derived free radicals may also be an important feature of the pathogenesis of Dupuytren's and other fibrotic conditions. Excessive formation of superoxide, hydrogen peroxide and hydroxyl radicals, resulting from microvascular occlusion and relative ischemia of the palmar fascia, can lead to tissue damage and enhanced fibroblastic proliferation[39,45]. Flow cytometry of inflammatory cells from Dupuytren's lesions has demonstrated predominance of CD3-positive T lymphocytes, macrophages and increased expression of major histocompatibility complex (MHC) class II proteins[47]. An association between Dupuytren's contracture, HLA-DR3 and autoantibodies to type I–IV collagen has also been demonstrated[39,48]. Factor XIIIa-positive dermal dendrocytes of macrophage lineage, are present in and around

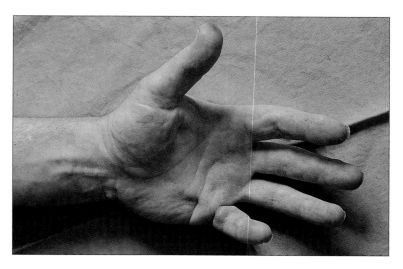

Fig. 17.12 Dupuytren's contracture of the palmar fascia.

Dupuytren's nodules[39,49]. These cells may be an important local source of fibrogenic cytokines[39,49]. These observations suggest that Dupuytren's disease may represent a T-cell-mediated autoimmune disorder[47–49]. In late stages of the disease, the lesions become less cellular and more fibrotic.

Dupuytren's contracture runs a variable course. Some patients show little change or incapacity over a period of many years, while in others fascial contraction progresses rapidly, with severe deformity and impairment of hand function.

Treatment depends on the rate of progression and severity of the lesions. Recent observations suggest that MRI may be useful in assessing the extent and degree of cellularity, and hence 'activity' of the lesion[50]. In patients with mild disease, local heat, stretching exercises and use of protective padded gloves during heavy manual grasping tasks are often helpful[33–37,51]. Many patients learn the benign nature of the contracture and adapt to the disorder. In more severe lesions with pain and inability to straighten the fingers, intralesional corticosteroid injections may be beneficial[33–37,51]. Local injections of collagenase, an enzyme that breaks collagen, and intralesional infiltrations of interferon-γ, a cytokine produced by T-helper lymphocytes that inhibits fibroblastic proliferation and collagen formation, are promising but untested new treatments[51]. In those with advanced disease with progressive digital contracture of more than 30°, a positive table-top test and functional impairment, limited or total palmar fasciectomy with or without skin graft replacement, is indicated[33–37,52]. The risk of recurrence is increased in young patients with active bilateral disease and cellular nodules and in those with a strong family history and/or other ectopic fibrotic lesions[52,53].

Ganglions of the wrist and hand

A ganglion is a mucin-filled, thin-walled, uni- or multilocular cyst attached to an adjacent joint capsule, tendon or tendon sheath[9,10,54,55]. A ganglion is the most common soft tissue tumour of the hand, accounting for 50–75% of all masses. Ganglions occur most frequently in women between the ages of 20 and 40 years.

A dorsal wrist ganglion, arising from and attached to the capsule of the scapholunate joint, is the most common site (60–70%)[54]. A volar wrist ganglion attached to the capsule of the radiocarpal joint is the second most frequent location (20%). Other ganglia include flexor digital tendon sheath ganglion arising from the proximal annular ligament of the sheath (10%), mucous cysts or ganglia of the distal and proximal interphalangeal joints, in association with osteoarthritic Heberden's and Bouchard's nodes respectively[55], ganglia of the extensor and flexor tendons of the wrist, a ganglion arising from the triquetrohamate joint within the ulnar canal (Guyon's canal)[56] and intraosseous ganglia.

The typical ganglion presents insidiously as a relatively painless, nontender, smooth cystic nodular swelling over the dorsum of the wrist. Ganglia can be soft, firm or feel so tense that they may be mistaken for a bony swelling[54,57]. Patients seek advice because of swelling and rarely pain and limitation of movements. Impairment of function may result from pressure of the ganglion on a peripheral nerve, e.g. the ulnar nerve in the canal of Guyon[56] or the median nerve in the carpal tunnel[58].

Radiographs of the affected region are often unrevealing except for a soft tissue swelling. Ultrasonography, CT and MRI may be required in patients with deep-seated ganglia. MRI is particularly suited to delineating the contiguity of ganglia with the outer fibres of joint capsules or tendon sheaths[56,59].

Microscopically, the wall of the ganglion is made up of compressed collagen fibres incompletely lined with fibroblast-like cells, simulating synovium[56]. There are few or no inflammatory cells. The capsular attachment of the cyst contains numerous mucin-filled clefts that intercommunicate via a small, often tortuous duct, with an adjacent joint or tendon sheath. A ganglion cyst is filled with clear, thick, highly viscous, sticky, jelly-like mucinous fluid containing a high concentration of hyaluronic acid in addition to glucosamine, albumin and globulin. The fluid is thicker and more viscous than normal synovial fluid.

The pathogenesis of ganglia is poorly understood. An association with trauma has been postulated but the link is rarely proven; only about 10% of patients report a specific antecedent trauma. Minor cumulative trauma has also been implicated but there is no obvious correlation with patient's occupation. Trauma, by stretching the joint capsule or tendon sheath, can cause joint fluid to burrow through minute ducts in the capsule or tendon sheath to form a tortuous duct leading to the subcutaneous ganglion cyst[55,60]. Communication between the adjacent joint (usually the wrist) and the cyst has been demonstrated with arthrography but not with a ganglion cystogram[60]. This suggests that the tortuous duct acts as a one-way valve connecting the joint to the cyst. This valve mechanism explains many of the features of ganglia – their aggravation by joint movements and relief by rest, their tendency to ramify into tendons, nerves and even bone, and the high recurrence rate from simple excision without removal of the valve mechanism and capsular attachment[55,60].

Ganglia may subside with resting the affected joint, enlarge with activity and may rupture or disappear spontaneously. Patient reassurance about the benign nature of ganglia is often the only treatment required. Historically, the classical treatment of slamming the cyst with a mallet or a family Bible is rarely successful. Non-operative treatment is associated with a high recurrence rate and includes rupture of the ganglion by direct digital pressure, simple needle aspiration[61], needle puncture[62] and injections of hyaluronidase or a sclerosing solution[55]. Aspiration of the ganglion and instillation of a corticosteroid (e.g. 5mg methylprednisolone acetate) may reduce the size of the mass and alleviate symptoms for a varying period of time[54,55]. Incision of the ganglion capsule with a tenotomy knife, and expression of the contents subcutaneously is sometimes effective.

Surgical excision is indicated in patients with symptomatic ganglia not responding to more conservative methods[54,55]. The likelihood of recurrence is low if the ganglion and its attachment to the adjacent joint capsule and tendon sheath are completely excised.

REFERENCES

1. Markison RE, Kilgore ES. Hand. In: Davis JH, ed. Clinical surgery. St Louis: CV Mosby; 1987: 2292–2353.
2. McMurtry RY, Little AH. The wrist. In: Little AH, ed. The rheumatological physical examination. Orlando, FL: Grune & Stratton; 1986: 83–89.
3. Kauer JMG. Functional anatomy of the wrist. Clin Orthop 1980; 149: 9–20.
4. Ferris BD, Stanton J, Zamora J. Kinematics of the wrist. Evidence for two types of movements. J Bone Joint Surg 2000; 82B: 242–245.
5. McMurtry RY. The hand. In: Little AH, ed. The rheumatological physical examination. Orlando, FL: Grune & Stratton; 1986: 91–100.
6. Williams PL, Warwick R, Dyson M, Bannister LH. Joints of the upper limb. In: Williams JL, Warwick, R, Dyson M et al., eds. Gray's anatomy, 37th ed. Edinburgh: Churchill Livingstone; 1989: 499–516.
7. Strauch B, de Moura W. Digital flexor tendon sheath: an anatomic study. J Hand Surg 1985; 10: 785–810.
8. Bluestone R. A practical approach to hand pain. J Musculoskel Med 1989; 6: 75–85.
9. Canoso JJ. Bursitis, tenosynovitis, ganglions, and painful lesions of the wrist, elbow and hand. Curr Opin Rheumatol 1990; 2: 276–821.
10. Fam AG. The wrist and hand. In: Klippel JH, Dieppe PA, eds. Rheumatology, 2nd ed. St Louis: Mosby; 1997: section 4, 9.1–9.8.
11. Fam AG. Bursitis and tendinitis: a practical approach to diagnosis. Geriatrics 1992; 8: 35–42.
12. Thorson E, Szabo RM. Common tendinitis problems in the hand and forearm. Orthop Clin North Am 1992; 23: 65–74.
13. Field JH. De Quervain's disease. Am Fam Physician 1979; 20: 103–104.

14. Thompson JS, Phelps TH. Repetitive strain injuries. How to deal with 'the epidemic of the 1990s'. Postgrad Med 1990; 88: 143–149.
15. Clarke MT, Lyall HA, Grant JW, Matthewson MH. The histopathology of De Quervain's disease. J Hand Surg 1998; 23B: 732–734.
16. Gray RG, Gottlieb NL. Hand flexor tenosynovitis in rheumatoid arthritis. Prevalence, distribution, and associated rheumatic features. Arthritis Rheum 1977; 20: 1003–1008.
17. Nygaard IE, Saltzman CL, Whitehouse MB, Hankin FM. Hand problems in pregnancy. Am Fam Physician 1989; 39: 123–126.
18. Grundberg AB, Keagan DS. Pathologic anatomy of the forearm: intersection syndrome. J Hand Surg 1985; 10A: 299–302.
19. Harvey FJ, Harvey PM, Horsley MW. De Quervain's disease: surgical or nonsurgical treatment. J Hand Surg 1990; 15A: 83–7.
20. Witt J, Pess G, Gelberman RH. Treatment of de Quervain's tenosynovitis: a prospective study of the results of injection of steroids and immobilization in a splint. J Bone Joint Surg 1991; 73A: 219–222.
21. Weiss A-PC, Akelman E, Tabatabai M. Treatment of De Quervain's disease. J Hand Surg 1994; 19A: 595–598.
22. Zingas C, Failla JM, Van Holsbeeck M. Injection accuracy and clinical relief of De Quervain's tendinitis. J Hand Surg 1998; 23A: 89–96.
23. Sampson SP, Wisch D, Badalamente MA. Complications of conservative and surgical treatment of de Quervain's disease and trigger fingers. Hand Clin 1994; 10: 73–82.
24. Freiberg A, Mulholland RS, Levine R. Nonoperative treatment of trigger fingers and thumbs. J Hand Surg 1989; 14A: 553–558.
25. Kraemer BA, Young VL, Arfken C. Stenosing flexor tenosynovitis. South Med J 1990; 83: 806–811.
26. Sampson SP, Badalamente MA, Hurst LC, Seidman J. Pathobiology of the human A1 pulley in trigger finger. J Hand Surg 1991; 16A: 714–721.
27. Yosipovitch G, Yosipovitch Z, Karp M, Mukamel M. Trigger finger in young patients with insulin dependent diabetes. J Rheumatol 1990; 17: 951–952.
28. Dunsmuir RA, Sherlock DA. The outcome of treatment of trigger thumb in children. J Bone Joint Surg 2000; 82B: 736–738.
29. Rhoades CE, Gelberman RH, Manjarris JF. Stenosing tenosynovitis of the fingers and thumb. Results of a prospective trial of steroid injection and splinting. Clin Orthop 1984; 190: 236–238.
30. Anderson B, Kaye S. Treatment of flexor tenosynovitis of the hand 'trigger finger' with corticosteroids. A prospective study of the response to local injection. Arch Intern Med 1991; 151: 153–156.
31. Patel MR, Bassini L. Trigger fingers and thumb: when to splint, inject or operate. J Hand Surg 1992; 17A: 110–113.
32. Pope DF, Wolfe SW. Safety and efficacy of percutaneous trigger finger release. J Hand Surg 1995; 1995 20A: 280–283.
33. Wooldridge WE. Four related fibrosing diseases. When you find one, look for another. Postgrad Med 1988; 84: 269–274.
34. Benson LS, Williams CS, Kahle M. Dupuytren's contracture. J Am Acad Orthop Surg 1998; 6: 24–35.
35. Rayan GM. Clinical presentations and types of Dupuytren's disease. Hand Clinics 1999; 15: 87–96.
36. Saar JD, Grothaus PC. Dupuytren's disease: an overview. Plast Reconstruct Surg 2000; 106: 125–134.
37. Meek RMD, McLellan S, Crossan JF. Dupuytren's disease. A model for the mechanism of fibrosis and its modulation by steroids. J Bone Joint Surg 1999; 81B: 732–738.
38. Kloen P. New insights in the development of Dupuytren's contracture: a review. Br J Plastic Surg 1999; 52: 629–635.
39. Yi IS, Johnson G, Moneim MS. Etiology of Dupuytren's disease. Hand Clinics 1999; 15: 43–51.
40. Dal Cin P, De Smet L, Sciot R et al. Trisomy 7 and trisomy 8 in dividing and non-dividing tumour cells in Dupuytren's disease. Cancer Genet Cytogenet 1999; 108: 137–140.
41. Liss G, Stock S. Can Dupuytren's contracture be work-related? Review the evidence. Am J Ind Med 1996; 29: 521–532.
42. Hutchison JW, Tierney GM, Parsons SL, Davis TRC. Dupuytren's disease and frozen shoulder induced by treatment with a matrix metalloproteinase inhibitor. J Bone Surg 1998; 80B: 907–908.
43. Connelly TJ. Development of Peyronie's and Dupuytren's diseases in an individual after single episodes of trauma: a case report and review of the literature. J Am Acad Dermatol 1999; 41: 106–108.
44. Murrell GAC, Francis MJO, Howlett CR. Dupuytren's contracture. Fine structure in relation to aetiology. J Bone Joint Surg 1989; 71B: 367–373.
45. Badalamente MA, Hurst LC. The biochemistry of Dupuytren's disease. Hand Clin 1999; 15: 35–42.
46. McCann BG, Logan A, Belcher H et al. The presence of myofibroblasts in the dermis of patients with Dupuytren's contracture. A possible source for recurrence. J Hand Surg 1993; 18B: 656–661.
47. Baird KS, Alwan WH, Crossan JF, Wojciak B. T-cell-mediated response in Dupuytren's disease. Lancet 1993; 341: 1622–1623.
48. Neumuller J, Menzel J, Millesi H. Prevalence of HLA-DR3 and auto-antibodies to connective tissue components in Dupuytren's contracture. Clin Immunol Immunopathol 1994; 71: 142–148.
49. Sugden P, Andrew JG, Andrew SM, Freemont AJ. Dermal dendrocytes in Dupuytren's disease: a link between the skin and pathogenesis? J Hand Surg 1993; 18B: 662–666.
50. Yacoe ME, Bergman AG, Ladd AL, Hellman BH. Dupuytren's contracture: MR imaging findings and correlation between MR signal intensity and cellularity of lesions. AJR 1993; 160: 813–817.
51. Hurst LC, Badalamente MA. Non-operative treatment of Dupuytren's disease. Hand Clin 1999; 15: 97–107.
52. Armstrong JR, Hurren JS, Logan AM. Dermofasciectomy in the management of Dupuytren's disease. J Bone Joint Surg 2000; 82B: 90–94.
53. Rombouts J-J, Noël H, Legrain Y, Munting E. Prediction of recurrence in the treatment of Dupuytren's disease: evaluation of a histologic classification. J Hand Surg 1989; 14A: 644–652.
54. Nelson CL, Sawmiller S, Phalen GS. Ganglions of the wrist and hand. J Bone Joint Surg 1972; 54A: 1459–1464.
55. Angelides AC. Ganglions of the hand and wrist. In: Green DP, Hotchkiss RN, Pederson WC, eds. Green's operative surgery, 4th ed. New York: Churchill Livingstone; 1999: 2171–2183.
56. Subin GD, Mallon WJ, Urbaniak JR. Diagnosis of ganglion in Guyon's canal by magnetic resonance imaging. J Hand Surg 1989; 14A: 640–643.
57. Kleinert HE, Kutz JE, Fishman JH. Etiology and treatment of the so-called mucous cyst of the finger. J Bone Joint Surg 1972; 54A: 1455–1458.
58. Kerrigan JJ, Bertoni JM, Jaeger SH. Ganglion cysts and carpal tunnel syndrome. J Hand Surg 1988; 13A: 763–765.
59. Feldman F, Singson RD, Staron RB. Magnetic resonance imaging of para-articular and ectopic ganglia. Skeletal Radiol 1989; 18: 353–358.
60. Andreu L, Eiken O. Arthrographic studies of wrist ganglions. J Bone Joint Surg 1971; 53A: 299–302.
61. Zubowicz VN, Ishii CH. Management of ganglion cysts of the hand by simple aspiration. J Hand Surg 1987; 12A: 618–620.
62. Richman JA, Gelberman RH, Engber WD et al. Ganglions of the wrist and digits: results of treatment by aspiration and cyst wall puncture. J Hand Surg 1987; 12A: 1041–1043.

18 The hip

Bernard Mazières

- The hip joint is the best example in the human body of a ball-and-socket synovial joint. It is an exceptionally strong and stable articulation which also exhibits a wide range of multiaxial movements
- These apparently contradictory properties of the hip joint allow a person to stand erect while also permitting complex activities such as walking, running, squatting and dancing
- Degenerative and inflammatory diseases of the hip are common and can lead to severe functional disability. Prosthetic replacement has changed the prognosis of this disability, but fracture of the femoral neck is still the source of nearly 20% of deaths within a year of the trauma

FUNCTIONAL ANATOMY

The hip joint is formed by the rounded head of the femur which joins the cup-shaped cavity of the acetabulum (Figs 18.1 & 18.2). The femoral head forms about two thirds of a sphere and is entirely covered with hyaline cartilage, except for the fovea, to which the ligamentum teres is attached. The head is mounted on the 8–10cm neck which forms an angle of about 125–140° with the shaft of the femur. When the angle decreases below this range, either because of congenital or acquired disorders, this is referred to as coxa vara. When it is increased above this range, this is referred to as coxa valga (Fig. 18.3). Two bony prominences project from the femoral neck: the greater trochanter, situated laterally, onto which are inserted several of the gluteal muscles; and the lesser trochanter, situated medially, onto which are inserted the hip flexors. Both trochanters are united anteriorly by a roughened ridge, called the intertrochanteric line, and posteriorly by a smoother crest, the intertrochanteric crest.

The acetabulum is formed by the union of the ilium, ischium and pubis. It faces laterally, downwards and slightly forwards to accommodate the femoral head. In contrast to the shallow glenoid fossa of the scapula, the acetabulum is deeper and therefore provides some intrinsic stability to the joint. In addition, its rim is reinforced by a strong lip of fibrocartilage, the acetabular labrum, which deepens the socket and forms a tight collar around the femoral head, adding significantly to the stability of the joint. The articular area of the acetabulum has the outline of a horseshoe (Fig. 18.2). The center of the cavity or acetabular fossa is occupied by a fat pad which is covered with synovial membrane. The lower margin of the acetabulum, or acetabular notch, allows passage to the ligamentum teres which contains a small branch from the obturator artery that supplies blood to the region of the fovea. The inferior margin of the acetabulum is closed in by the transverse acetabular ligament.

The thickness of the hyaline cartilage covering the femoral head varies significantly from one area to the other. It is thickest on the superior and posterior aspects of the head (3mm) and thins down to 0.5mm at the peripheral margin. Similarly, the acetabular cartilage ranges from 2–2.5mm in its posterosuperior segment to 1mm peripherally (Fig. 18.4).

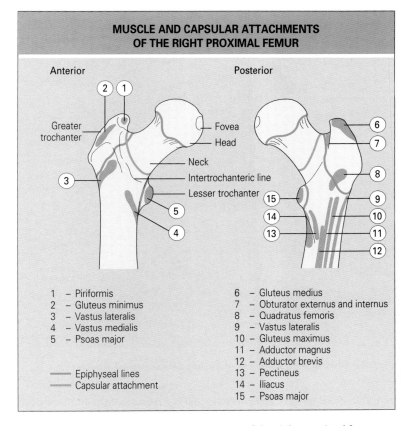

MUSCLE AND CAPSULAR ATTACHMENTS OF THE RIGHT PROXIMAL FEMUR

Anterior — Posterior

Greater trochanter — Fovea — Head — Neck — Intertrochanteric line — Lesser trochanter

1 – Piriformis
2 – Gluteus minimus
3 – Vastus lateralis
4 – Vastus medialis
5 – Psoas major

Epiphyseal lines
Capsular attachment

6 – Gluteus medius
7 – Obturator externus and internus
8 – Quadratus femoris
9 – Vastus lateralis
10 – Gluteus maximus
11 – Adductor magnus
12 – Adductor brevis
13 – Pectineus
14 – Iliacus
15 – Psoas major

Fig. 18.1 Muscular and capsular attachments of the right proximal femur. Anterior and posterior aspects of the proximal right femur, showing the attachments of the muscles and hip capsule.

The fibrous articular capsule of the hip is attached proximally to the margin of the acetabulum and labrum and to the transverse acetabular ligament. Distally, it surrounds the head and neck of the femur and is attached anteriorly to the intertrochanteric line and posteriorly to the neck, slightly proximal to the intertrochanteric crest. The inner surface of the capsule is lined with the synovial membrane while its outer aspect is reinforced by three strong ligaments: the iliofemoral, ischiofemoral and pubofemoral ligaments (Fig. 18.5). Of these, the thick iliofemoral is the strongest and most important. It covers the anterior aspect of the joint. It has a Y-shaped appearance and is attached proximally to the acetabular margin and the anterior inferior iliac spine, and distally to the intertrochanteric line. The ligament is relaxed in flexion and tense in extension, thus preventing excessive extension of the hip and helping to maintain erect posture. The weaker ischiofemoral and pubofemoral ligaments strengthen the capsule posteriorly and inferiorly, respectively.

In the majority of individuals, the medial femoral circumflex artery, which is a branch of the common femoral artery, supplies most of the blood to the head and neck of the femur, even if the true vascularization

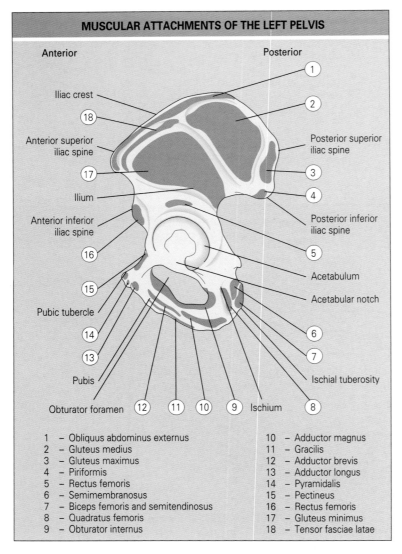

MUSCULAR ATTACHMENTS OF THE LEFT PELVIS

Anterior   Posterior

Iliac crest

18

Anterior superior
iliac spine

17

Ilium

Anterior inferior
iliac spine

16

15

Pubic tubercle

14

13

Pubis

Obturator foramen   12   11   10   9   Ischium   8

1

2

Posterior superior
iliac spine

3

4

Posterior inferior
iliac spine

5

Acetabulum

Acetabular notch

6

7

Ischial tuberosity

1	– Obliquus abdominus externus	10	– Adductor magnus
2	– Gluteus medius	11	– Gracilis
3	– Gluteus maximus	12	– Adductor brevis
4	– Piriformis	13	– Adductor longus
5	– Rectus femoris	14	– Pyramidalis
6	– Semimembranosus	15	– Pectineus
7	– Biceps femoris and semitendinosus	16	– Rectus femoris
8	– Quadratus femoris	17	– Gluteus minimus
9	– Obturator internus	18	– Tensor fasciae latae

Fig. 18.2 Muscular attachments of the left pelvis – lateral aspect.

of the femoral head is still controversial[1,2]. Fracture of the femoral neck may therefore disrupt the blood supply to the femoral head and lead to osteonecrosis. In some patients, anastomoses with the small vessels of the ligamentum teres may prevent this from occurring[3].

The origin and insertion of the muscles of the hip region are shown in Figures 18.1 and 18.2. The main flexor of the thigh at the hip joint is the iliopsoas muscle. The chief extensors are the gluteus maximus and the hamstrings. The chief abductors are the gluteus medius and the gluteus minimus, while the chief adductors are the adductor longus, brevis and magnus. The main medial rotators are the tensor fasciae lata, gluteus medius and gluteus minimus and the main lateral rotators are the obturator muscles, gemelli and quadratus femoris.

Several bursae are found in the hip region. The three most important clinically include: the trochanteric bursa, which lies between the gluteus maximus muscle and the posterolateral aspect of the greater trochanter; the iliopsoas bursa, which is located between the psoas tendon and the hip capsule, just lateral to the femoral vessels; and the ischiogluteal bursa, which lies between the gluteus maximus muscle and the ischial tuberosity.

HISTORY AND PHYSICAL EXAMINATION

History

Hip pain is a common symptom with diverse etiologies. In the majority of instances, a diagnosis can be made with reasonable certainty by a careful history and physical examination.

● One of the most important aspects of the history is asking the patient to locate precisely the site of the pain. Typically, hip disease manifests itself with pain in the groin which may radiate to the anterior, lateral or medial thigh, sometimes as far as the knee. However, not unusually, the pain may localize laterally to the greater trochanter, medially to the adductors, or posteriorly to the buttock. When these locations are associated with pain in the groin, it is usually easy to evoke hip pathology. The other etiologies of pain in the groin and anterior thigh area include iliopsoas bursitis, adductor tendinitis, hernias and pain from retroperitoneal structures.

● Trochanteric bursitis is by far the most common cause of lateral trochanteric pain, although hip disease, as mentioned previously, and thoracolumbar pathology may also refer pain into this area. Buttock pain can be caused by referred back and sacroiliac pain, hip disease, ischiogluteal bursitis or vascular insufficiency.

● Characterizing some of the alleviating and aggravating factors can help to differentiate certain disorders. For example, pain in the trochanteric area aggravated by lying in the lateral decubitus position is highly suggestive of trochanteric bursitis, while pain in the ischiogluteal area aggravated by the sitting position should suggest an ischiogluteal bursitis. Groin pain aggravated by walking and relieved by rest is suggestive of a degenerative hip arthropathy, while pain in the same location, when associated with morning stiffness lasting more than 30 minutes and relieved by activity, is typical of an inflammatory arthropathy. Vascular insufficiency tends to present with buttock pain aggravated by walking and relieved within minutes by rest.

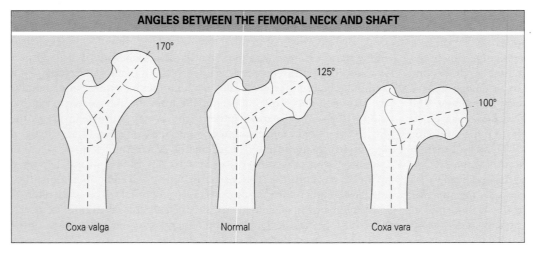

ANGLES BETWEEN THE FEMORAL NECK AND SHAFT

170°

125°

100°

Coxa valga   Normal   Coxa vara

Fig. 18.3 Angles between the femoral neck and shaft in adults.

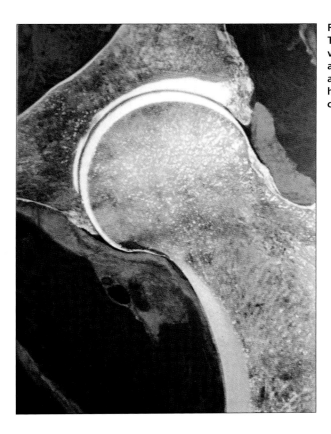

Fig. 18.4
Thickness
variations of
acetabular
and femoral
head
cartilages.

be noted. An exaggerated lumbar lordosis, especially if associated with a slight flexion of the knee, should alert the examiner to the possibility of a flexion deformity of the hip.

- Pelvic tilting should also be noted. Tilting of the pelvis can be due to leg length discrepancy, scoliosis or hip disease. In the presence of leg length discrepancy, pelvic elevation will be present on the side of the longer leg when the patient stands with both legs parallel and the feet flat on the floor. The skin folds of the gluteal and popliteal regions will be higher on the longer leg. Hip disease may result in adduction or abduction deformities. An adduction deformity will be compensated by an upward tilt of the pelvis on the side of the adducted thigh, in order to allow the legs to be parallel during walking (Fig. 18.6). In contrast, an abduction deformity will be compensated by an elevation of the uninvolved side. In both cases, measurement of the actual length of the legs will be equal.
- Rotational deformities of the hip are best evaluated with the patient facing the examiner. A vertical line drawn from the mid inguinal area should cross the middle of the patella and the middle of the ankle. Any deviation from this line defines a rotational deformity.
- Particular attention should be paid to the patient's gait. There are two phases to the normal walking cycle: the stance phase, which begins with the heel strike and ends with the toe-off, and the swing phase, which begins with the toe-off and ends with the heel strike. During the stance phase, the hip joint loads three times the body weight. Pain in the hip may cause a patient to walk with an antalgic gait: in this case, the stance phase on the painful extremity is shorter than on the uninvolved side as the patient attempts to hurry off the painful limb as quickly as possible. Weakness of the gluteus medius will produce a Trendelenburg (abductor) gait: in this instance, the upper part of the body is thrown towards the weak limb during the stance phase in order to maintain balance because the abductors are unable to hold the pelvis level. Bilateral weakness of the gluteus medius will result in a

Inspection

The hip region should be inspected with the patient in both the standing and supine positions. In the standing position, the patient should be observed from the anterior, posterior and lateral aspects. Standing behind the patient, the presence of abnormal spinal curvatures should

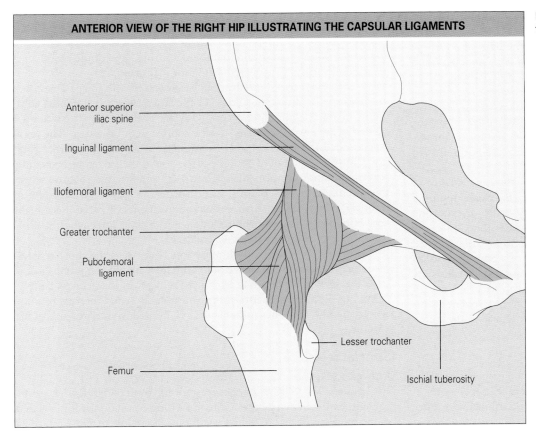

Fig. 18.5 Anterior view of the right hip illustrating the capsular ligaments.

ANTERIOR VIEW OF THE RIGHT HIP ILLUSTRATING THE CAPSULAR LIGAMENTS

- Anterior superior iliac spine
- Inguinal ligament
- Iliofemoral ligament
- Greater trochanter
- Pubofemoral ligament
- Lesser trochanter
- Femur
- Ischial tuberosity

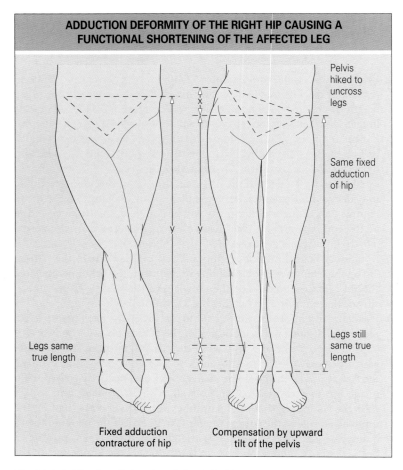

ADDUCTION DEFORMITY OF THE RIGHT HIP CAUSING A FUNCTIONAL SHORTENING OF THE AFFECTED LEG

Pelvis hiked to uncross legs

Same fixed adduction of hip

Legs still same true length

Legs same true length

Fixed adduction contracture of hip

Compensation by upward tilt of the pelvis

Fig. 18.6 Adduction deformity of the right hip causing a functional shortening of the affected leg.

waddling gait: the patient's upper body shifts laterally from side-to-side during the stance phase. Often, patients with a painful hip have components of both an antalgic and a Trendelenburg gait: the stance phase is shorter on the involved extremity and the upper part of the body is thrown towards the painful limb during the stance phase in order to avoid contraction of the gluteus medius, which might produce painful spasms.

● With the patient lying supine, the examiner should observe the position of the lower extremities. Advanced hip diseases often cause the affected extremity to be held in flexion, abduction and external rotation, since this position relaxes the articular capsule and tends to lessen pain by reducing pressure in the joint.

● Finally, the inguinal region should be inspected for any evidence of swelling. Enlargement of the iliopsoas bursa can cause inguinal swelling by one of two mechanisms: a localized bursitis, or extension of hip synovitis in the few individuals (15%) in whom the joint cavity communicates with the bursa. Such swelling has to be differentiated from adenopathies and hernias. In the absence of a communication with the iliopsoas bursa, synovitis of the hip will not usually cause any visible swelling or erythema, since the joint lies too deep to the skin surface. Similarly, trochanteric bursitis is only rarely associated with visible swelling in the greater trochanter region because of the thickness of the muscles and fat pad overlying the bursa.

Palpation

Because of its deep location, the hip joint cannot be palpated directly. However, in the presence of hip disease, percussion of the heel or simultaneous firm compression of both trochanters may occasionally produce pain in the inguinal region. The bony landmarks and soft tissues of the hip

area should be palpated systematically while noting any evidence of tenderness or swelling. With the patient in the supine position, these include:

● the anterior superior iliac spine
● the contents of the inguinal area (from outside to inside: iliopsoas bursa, femoral nerve, artery and vein, lymph nodes, pubic tubercle and symphysis pubis)
● the muscles of the anterior thigh and the adductor muscles.

With the patient lying on one side, the greater trochanter and the iliotibial tract should be palpated. The ischial tuberosity is best examined in this position after passively flexing the hip and knee. Finally, with the patient in the prone position, the examiner will palpate the iliac crest, posterior superior iliac spine, sacroiliac joint, sciatic nerve and gluteus muscles.

Mobility

The hip joint is capable of movements in three planes: sagittal (flexion and extension), frontal (abduction and adduction) and horizontal (internal and external rotations). Similarly to the shoulder, the hip is capable of circumduction. With the exception of extension, all these movements are best assessed passively with the patient lying in the supine position on a firm table. Throughout the examination, the pelvis must be stabilized by the hand of the examiner in order to avoid including pelvic motion in the measurements. Inter-observer errors in the measurements are in the order of 5–10%, while intra-observer errors are somewhat less (1–5%). To measure the ranges of motion with an acceptable level of consistency and accuracy, certain procedural principles must be followed in a systematic fashion and the measurement of joints with multiple axes may require different positions for different motions[4].

With the knee flexed to 90°, the hip can be flexed to about 135°. However, when the knee is extended, hip flexion is limited to only 90°.

The hip can be abducted to 45–50°. By placing the hand on the opposite anterior superior iliac spine, the examiner can easily feel the pelvis beginning to move at the end point of hip abduction. The intermalleolar distance between full abduction of both hips is occasionally used as a quantitative measure of hip abduction, but it is a poorly reproducible measure.

Adduction of the hip is limited to 30–40° and is assessed similarly to abduction with the exception that the stabilizing hand of the examiner is placed on the ipsilateral anterior superior iliac crest.

External and internal rotation can be measured with the patient either in the prone or supine positions. In the latter, which is the most commonly used in practice, the knee and hip are flexed to 90°. The examiner holds the knee with one hand and the ankle with the other. The leg is then rotated inwards (external rotation) and outwards (internal rotation). Movements should be stopped as soon as the pelvis starts moving. External rotation is normally limited to 45° and internal rotation to 35°. In patients with very painful hip disorders (often in the context of trauma), it may be easier to evaluate movements of rotation with the legs extended by simply rolling one leg at a time internally (internal rotation) and externally (external rotation).

Hip extension is normally limited to 20–30°. It is the most difficult movement to measure. It can be done with the patient lying prone or sideways. Again, it is important to fix the pelvis to get an adequate measure.

Among all the movements of the hip, abduction and internal rotation are usually the first ones to be painful or limited in the presence of hip pathology.

Special tests
Patrick's test

Patrick's test is used as a screening test for hip joint pathology. The test is sometimes designated by the acronym FABER, based on the initial letters of the movements that it evaluates (flexion, abduction, external rotation).

PATRICK'S TEST (FABER TEST)

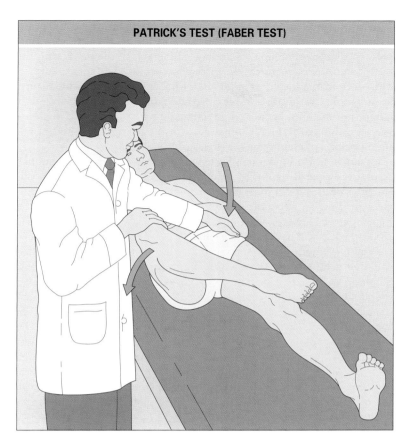

Fig. 18.7 Patrick's test (FABER test). The contralateral iliac crest is stabilized with downward pressure while lowering the ipsilateral flexed, abducted and rotated leg. Rapid lowering tests the sacroiliac joint, while slow lowering tests the hip joint.

THE TRENDELENBURG SIGN

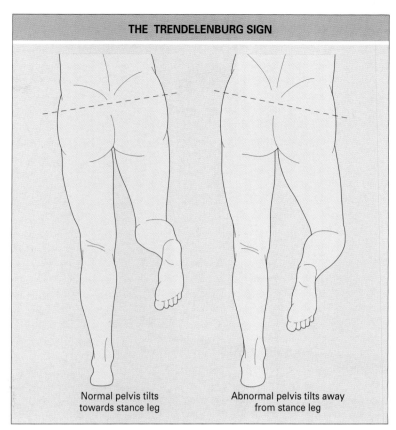

Normal pelvis tilts towards stance leg

Abnormal pelvis tilts away from stance leg

Fig. 18.8 The Trendelenburg sign. In a negative test, the pelvis tilts towards the stance leg because of adequate abductor contraction. In a positive test, the pelvis tilts away from the stance leg.

With the patient lying supine, the knee and hip are flexed to 90° and the foot of the examined extremity is placed on top of the opposite knee. The thigh is then slowly fully abducted and externally rotated towards the examining table (Fig. 18.7). The presence of groin pain, spasm or limitation of movement is suggestive of hip pathology. Patrick's test can also be used to stress the sacroiliac joints. To do so, one hand is placed on the abducted knee and the other on the opposite anterior superior iliac spine. Pain localized to the back when sudden pressure is applied simultaneously on each of these points, suggests sacroiliac pathology (see Chapter 28).

Trendelenburg's test

Trendelenburg's test is designed to evaluate the strength of the gluteus medius muscle. Normally, when a patient stands on one extremity, the abductor muscles on the weight-bearing side contract in order to maintain balance. This contraction causes the pelvis on the opposite side to rise slightly. In the presence of weak abductors or any condition which interferes with gluteus medius action (such as that caused by dislocation of the hip, coxa vara or arthritis), the pelvis on the contralateral side will not rise and may actually drop (Fig. 18.8). Patients with this sign will exhibit a Trendelenburg gait.

Thomas test

The Thomas test is designed to evaluate the presence of a flexion contracture of the hip. With the patient lying supine, the thigh opposite the side to be tested is fully flexed on the abdomen in order to correct for any compensatory lumbar lordosis. Failure of the hip tested to lie flat on the examining table indicates the presence of a flexion contracture of that hip (Fig. 18.9).

THE THOMAS TEST

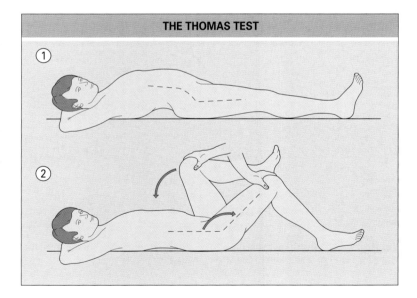

Fig. 18.9 The Thomas test. A flexion deformity of the hip is masked by an increased lumbar lordosis (1). Flexion of the contralateral hip flattens the lordosis and reveals the flexion deformity of the hip (2).

Ober's test

Ober's test is designed to evaluate the presence of contracture of the iliotibial band. With the patient lying on one side, the lower knee and hip are flexed in order to eliminate lumbar lordosis, the upper leg is extended and abducted and then slowly lowered. Failure of the extremity to fall on the table when the supporting hand is withdrawn suggests the presence of contracture of the iliotibial band (Fig. 18.10).

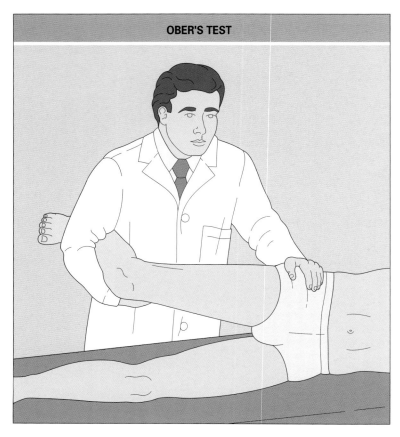

OBER'S TEST

Fig. 18.10 Ober's test. In the presence of contraction of the iliotibial band, the uppermost hip remains abducted and does not drop back towards the table when the leg is released.

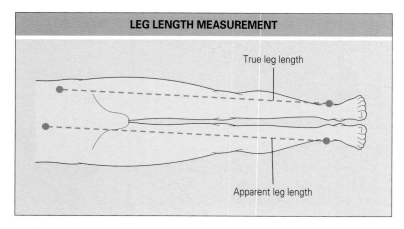

LEG LENGTH MEASUREMENT

True leg length

Apparent leg length

Fig. 18.11 Leg length measurement. The measurement is best made from the anterior superior iliac spine to the lateral malleolus.

Leg length measurement

Measurements of leg length are best performed with the patient lying supine with the legs fully extended and placed 15–20cm apart. Measurements are made from the anterior superior iliac spine to the middle of the lateral malleolus (Fig. 18.11). It is preferable to use the lateral malleolus as a landmark rather than the middle malleolus, in order to avoid measurement errors due to muscle wasting or obesity. A difference in length between the two legs of 1cm or less is not clinically significant.

Various radiologic techniques have been proposed to alleviate the lack of precision observed with clinical measurements of leg length. The simplest consists of obtaining a standing radiograph of the pelvis with the feet positioned 15–20cm apart[5]. In the absence of joint contractures, a difference in the height of the femoral heads indicates leg inequality. Scanography is a more complex method which requires taking radiographs of the hips, knees and upper ankles with the patient lying on a special calibrated frame[6]. Compared with the previous method, it has the advantage of identifying the bones which are shorter.

An apparent (or functional) leg length discrepancy on inspection may result from a pelvic tilt due to a scoliosis or abduction or adduction contractures of the hip. In these situations, measurements from the umbilicus will show an apparent shortening of the leg on the side with the higher pelvis. However, when measured from the anterior superior iliac spine, the legs will have the same length.

True leg length discrepancy can be due to various congenital or acquired disorders, many of which occur during childhood. The most common of these include: congenital dislocation of the hip; acetabular dysplasia; Legg–Perthes disease; slipped capital femoral epiphysis; and congenital coxa vara. Leg length discrepancy is associated with an increased incidence of trochanteric bursitis on the longer side. The longer leg is typically held in adduction under a tilted pelvis. This results in decreased acetabular covering of the femoral head. The increased localized stress on the remaining weight-bearing area of the femoral head may contribute to the development of osteoarthritis[7]. Indeed, an increased incidence of osteoarthritis of the hip on the side of the longer leg has been reported.

DIFFERENTIAL DIAGNOSIS OF HIP PAIN

Pain in the hip region may arise from the hip joint itself, adjacent bones or periarticular soft tissues (cutaneous and subcutaneous tissues, muscles, tendons and bursae). In addition, thoracolumbar spine disorders, intra-abdominal pathologies and peripheral vascular diseases can present with referred pain in this region and should therefore be considered in the differential diagnosis. A classification of hip pain, based upon the tissues primarily involved, is outlined in Table 18.1. Of these, osteoarthritis of the hip, trochanteric bursitis and spinal disorders account for the vast majority of conditions seen in clinical practice. A detailed history and careful physical examination of the joints (hip, pubis and sacroiliac), periarticular soft tissues, nerve and blood supply, abdomen and thoracolumbar spine are essential for a precise diagnosis.

Lumbar spine disorders

Pain in the posterior aspect of the hip area is most often referred from the lumbar spine. The history and physical examination usually allow the examiner to separate hip disease from a low back disorder. Most patients with lumbar and/or buttock pain have a mechanical cause for their symptoms[8]. The value of imaging techniques is extremely limited in these patients[9], the great majority of whom fortunately improve with simple conservative measures[10].

Mechanical disorders of the thoracolumbar junction (T12 and L1) may refer pain to the greater trochanter area and thus may mimic trochanteric bursitis. Such pain referral is due to the fact that the skin overlying the greater trochanter is innervated by a cutaneous branch originating from the dorsal rami of T12–L1[11] (Fig. 18.12). Pain on palpation and mobilization of the spinous processes of the lower thoracic and upper lumbar vertebrae may orient the examiner towards the correct origin.

Nerve root compression from L2 to L4 may mimic hip disease by causing referred pain in the inguinal area and the anterior aspect of the thigh. In these cases, neurologic deficits and a positive femoral stretch

TABLE 18.1 DIFFERENTIAL DIAGNOSIS OF HIP PAIN	
Articular	**Periarticular**

Inflammatory joint diseases
  Rheumatoid arthritis
  Spondyloarthropathies
  Polymyalgia rheumatica
	Bursitis
	  Trochanteric
	  Iliopsoas
	  Ischiogluteal

Degenerative joint diseases
  Primary osteoarthritis
  Secondary osteoarthritis
	Tendinitis
	  Trochanteric
	  Adductor

Metabolic joint diseases
  Gout
  Pseudogout
  Ochronosis
  Hemochromatosis
  Wilson's disease
  Acromegaly
	Acute calcific periarthritis
	Heterotopic calcifications

	Osseous

Infections	Bone lesions
	  Fractures, neoplasms, infection, osteonecrosis of
	  the femoral head, metabolic bone disease (Paget's
	  disease of bone, stress fractures, osteomalacia,
	  hyperparathyroidism, renal osteodystrophy), reflex
	  sympathetic dystrophy (transient migratory
	  osteoporosis)

Tumors
  Benign
    Pigmented villonodular
    synovitis
    Osteochondromatosis
  Malignant
    Synovial sarcoma
    Synovial metastasis
	In children
	  Congenital dislocation of the hip ⎤
	  Acetabular dysplasia ⎟ Usually not
	  Coxa vara ⎟ painful
	  Slipped capital femoral epiphysis ⎦
	  Legg–Perthes disease
	  Rickets

Hemarthrosis	

In children
  Transient ētoxicí synovitis
  Juvenile chronic arthritis
	Neurologic

	Entrapment neuropathies
	  Lateral femoral cutaneous nerve
	  (meralgia paresthetica)
	Lumbar nerve root compression
	  L2, L3 and L4

Referred pain	
	Vascular
Thoracolumbar spine Intra-abdominal structures Retroperitoneal structures	
	Atherosclerosis of aorta iliac vessels

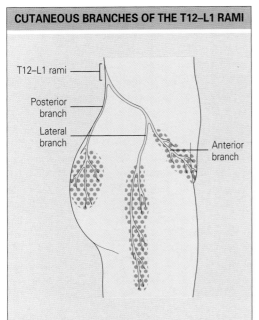

CUTANEOUS BRANCHES OF THE T12–L1 RAMI

T12–L1 rami

Posterior branch

Lateral branch

Anterior branch

Fig. 18.12 Cutaneous branches of the T12–L1 rami. Cutaneous branches originating from these rami innervate the skin overlying the iliac crest, the inguinal region and the greater trochanter area.

test in the absence of pain or limitation of motion of the hip should evoke the diagnosis. Meralgia paresthetica defines the clinical picture produced by entrapment of the lateral femoral cutaneous nerve as it passes under the inguinal ligament. This condition, which has to be differentiated from L2 to L4 nerve root compression, is discussed in more detail in Chapter 14.

Sacroiliac disorders can also cause buttock pain. When the patients present with an insidious onset of pain associated with severe morning stiffness that is relieved by activity, the diagnosis of sacroiliitis is usually considered. However, when these characteristics are lacking, the diagnosis may be missed, especially since the bedside techniques for sacroiliac joint examination are unreliable[12].

Intra-abdominal pathologies

Various intra-abdominal and retroperitoneal conditions can refer pain to the hip region (the inguinal and anterior thigh areas especially). Chief among these are inflammatory processes about the iliopsoas muscle, such as retroperitoneal appendicitis, tuberculous abscess or pelvic inflammatory disease. Irritation of the psoas often causes the patient to flex the hip or hold it rigidly extended. Flexion of the joint against resistance aggravates the pain (positive iliopsoas test). Hernias (inguinal or femoral) can usually be easily detected on physical examination if the examiner specifically looks for them. Ureteral stones are among the other conditions that can typically refer pain to the hip area. The history is usually characteristic.

Peripheral vascular diseases

Thrombosis or aneurysm formation of branches of the aorta or iliac vessels may give rise to buttock, thigh or leg pain that may be confused with hip pain. The aggravation of pain with activity and rapid relief with rest, together with the presence of decreased or absent peripheral pulses or bruits on physical examination, should orient the clinician to the correct diagnosis.

Hip diseases

In practice, there are three levels of difficulty in the diagnosis of hip disease. When symptoms are long-standing, radiographs will usually show characteristic changes and the diagnosis should pose no difficulty. For instance, it is easy to diagnose Paget's disease involving the femur and hip joint. Similarly, primary hip osteoarthritis is readily diagnosed in the presence of subchondral sclerosis, marginal osteophytes and superolateral joint space narrowing. The same applies to late stages of osteonecrosis when flattening of the femoral head has occurred or to chondrocalcinosis when calcific deposits are visible in the hyaline cartilage and/or acetabular labrum.

In other more difficult cases, radiographs are abnormal but are not characteristic of a specific disorder. For example, localized or diffuse osteopenia or sclerosis of the femoral head, and/or neck and/or acetabulum may be observed, suggesting bone pathology. Similarly, one may notice minimal joint space narrowing, sometimes with subchondral erosions and/or osteopenia, but without osteophytes or sclerosis. In these cases an inflammatory arthritis may be suspected. Radiographs are useful in confirming that the hip is affected but other investigations are usually needed to establish a definite diagnosis. In each circumstance, diagnostic modalities should be guided by the history and other physical findings. A clinical suspicion of early osteonecrosis may require magnetic resonance imaging for confirmation. An arthrogram may be helpful in documenting chondromatosis, synovial tumors, labrum tears or local thinning of the cartilage in the weight-bearing areas of an early osteoarthritic joint. The suspicion of a chronic septic or crystal-induced synovitis would require joint aspiration for synovial fluid analysis.

The most difficult diagnostic situation occurs when the patient presents with hip pain and a normal radiograph. All the conditions listed in Table 18.1 must be considered. A careful history and physical examination become even more important in this situation. The presence of pain at the extremes of abduction and internal rotation suggest early hip disease caused by arthritis or osteonecrosis. Limitation of hip movements in all directions in a diabetic patient suggests an adhesive capsulitis of the hip joint. The presence of systemic symptoms, such as fatigue, fever, weight loss or worsening of pain at night, suggests infection or malignancy. Baseline laboratory tests and other imaging techniques including radionuclide bone scan and magnetic resonance imaging may be especially useful when the plain radiograph is normal.

SOME SPECIFIC NON-ARTHRITIC HIP DISORDERS

Transient osteoporosis

Transient osteoporosis of the hip is a rare condition that affects children and young and middle-aged adults of both sexes[13]. In pregnant women, typically the left hip is affected (Fig. 18.13), but involvement of the right hip has also been described[14]. Patients present with groin pain, sometimes referred to the anterior knee on weight bearing. The ESR is occasionally raised, but this may be difficult to distinguish from the normal elevation seen in pregnancy. There may be an associated effusion; in this case, synovial fluid is pale yellow, clear, with normal viscosity and the aspirate contains less than 1000 cells/mm^3, with a majority of mononuclear cells, no crystal and is sterile. Synovial biopsies tend to be normal but occasionally show a non-specific, mild, chronic inflammatory change.

Isotope scans may be positive much earlier than radiographic evidence of demineralization of the femoral head. Computed tomography (CT) can be used to demonstrate demineralization in idiopathic cases.

The cause of transient osteoporosis is unknown, but theories have implicated both endocrine changes and local compression of vessels or nerves resulting in a transient algodystrophy. These theories are unlikely to be correct, as these changes have also been seen in early pregnancy and non-pregnant states. Complete recovery in 2–6 months is the rule.

Conservative management is usually the rule unless otherwise clinically indicated[14]. Radiographs should be avoided if possible. Ultrasound may reveal an effusion, which can be aspirated in order to provide therapeutic effect and allow microscopic and microbiological investigation. Investigations in most cases, unless clinically indicated, can usually be delayed until after delivery. Non-steroidal anti-inflammatory agents (NSAIDs) should be avoided, particularly around the third trimester, because of the potential effects on the fetal circulation. Acetaminophen (paracetamol) crosses the placenta easily, but with no effects on the fetus. Codeine and propoxyphene are also safe, but large amounts may result in fetal withdrawal symptoms.

Osteitis pubis

Osteitis pubis is a sterile symmetric condition without evidence of true osteomyelitis of the os pubis[15]. Onset often follows a urogenital surgical procedure and it is more common than osteomyelitis. Erosive symmetric osteitis pubis may often be associated with seronegative spondyloarthropathy but is less painful and disabling than in postsurgical cases. Traumatic osteitis pubis occurs in athletes undertaking running and kicking sports and an avulsion stress fracture at the origin of the gracilis muscle near the symphysis pubis has occasionally been implicated. Chondrocalcinosis of the symphysis pubis is a well-known radiologic finding in, for example, primary hyperparathyroidism but acute symphysitis in this context has not been reported.

The typical symptom of osteitis pubis is pain in both groins exacerbated by walking and partially relieved by rest. On examination, there is marked tenderness over the symphysis pubis and over the inferior pubic rami, painful and decreased bilateral hip joint abduction, painful hip joint adduction with muscle spasms and pain on lateral compression of the pelvis. Evidence of urogenital infection, e.g. prostatitis, epididymo-orchitis or sepsis elsewhere, may give a high probability of true osteomyelitis but may be misleading[16]. Pyrexia may occur in both infective and non-infective cases.

The ESR is raised in all cases. Plain radiographs may be normal for several weeks after onset of pain. Rarefaction and erosion of the os pubis then occurs with widening of the joint space (Fig. 18.14). Healing with sclerotic changes and bone apposition then follows, usually within 6 months. Simple degenerative changes are also common, especially in women after childbirth. Bone scintigraphy is always positive and probably the single most useful test (Fig. 18.15). It does not distinguish infective cases but a positive indium-labeled leukocyte scan would strongly indicate osteomyelitis. Thorough investigation for bacterial infection is essential. Aspiration needle biopsy may be helpful and sometimes open biopsy to obtain adequate tissue samples for culture and histology may be indicated. Various organisms have been implicated in infective cases, e.g. *Staphylococcus aureus*, *Pseudomonas aeruginosa* and *Escherichia coli*. Histology reveals thickened bone trabeculae, fibrous replacement of marrow by a non-specific chronic inflammatory infiltrate of lymphocytes and plasma cells, an absence of acute inflammatory changes and typically negative cultures.

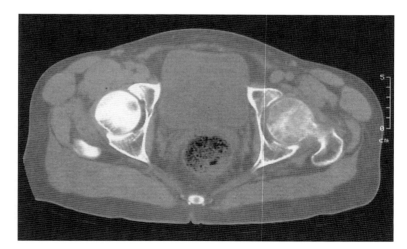

Fig. 18.13 Marked osteoporosis of the head of the left femur in a case of transient painful osteoporosis of the hip.

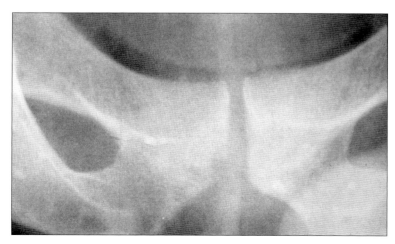

Fig. 18.14 Osteitis pubis. This anteroposterior radiograph of the pelvis shows widening of the symphysis pubis and erosion of bone in the inferior part of the right pubic ramus.

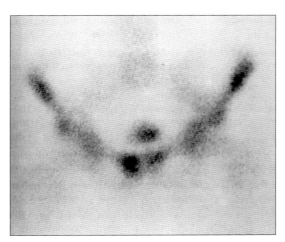

Fig. 18.15 Osteitis pubis. On this bone scan, taken 3 hours after injection of 99mTc-labeled diphosphonate, increased retention of isotope is seen at the symphysis pubis.

Most cases are self-limiting and settle with conservative therapy using, for example, NSAIDs, analgesics and physical therapy. Therapeutic trials of broad-spectrum antibiotics in the deteriorating patient may also be used even in the absence of proven infection. Osteitis pubis associated with osteomyelitis requires 6–12 weeks of appropriate antibiotics, e.g. ofloxacin, ciprofloxacin or flucloxacillin.

If severe pain continues for more than 6 months, and all conservative measures have been exhausted, it is worth considering a generous wedge resection of the symphysis pubis, which only rarely leads to pelvic instability as body weight is transmitted mainly through posterior pelvic structures[17].

The pathophysiology of osteitis pubis without osteomyelitis remains obscure. The posterior structures of the symphysis pubis drain into the veins of the lower urinary tract and incompetence of venous valves has been demonstrated. Retrograde venous flow in the retropubic area associated with urogenital infection or trauma might recur. This may lead to bone hyperemia and demineralization. Transient osteonecrosis is another possibility. Perhaps more convincingly, osteitis pubis with pain and reversible bone loss following trauma may be an example of algo-dystrophy (reflex sympathetic dystrophy).

Periarticular soft tissue problems
Several problems of the hip are related to the soft tissue structures around the joint and its surrounding muscles. Although relatively common, many of these problems are poorly defined, misdiagnosed or both[18]. Numerous bursae are found in the hip region. Since they are lined with synovial tissue, they may be affected by all the inflammatory diseases affecting the hip joint, such as rheumatoid arthritis, and infectious or crystal-induced synovitis. Most commonly however, bursitis and tendinitis around the hip are induced by trauma or repetitive microtrauma.

Trochanteric bursitis
Trochanteric bursitis is the most common cause of pain about the hip region. The soft tissues that cross the bony posterior portion of the greater trochanter are protected from it by the three trochanteric bursae. The gluteus maximus bursa, which separates the fibers of gluteus maximus from the greater trochanter, is the most important of these bursae. It is not palpable unless it is distended or inflamed. Patients with trochanteric bursitis present with a deep, aching pain sometimes associated with a burning sensation on the lateral aspect of the hip and thigh. The pain increases with activities such as walking, squatting and climbing stairs, and is associated with a limp in 15% of patients[19]. Typically the pain decreases at rest, although it is frequently worse at night, especially when the patient is lying on the affected side. Tenderness can be elicited on palpation of the area around the greater trochanter which

may feel boggy, at least in thin patients. Resisted abduction of the hip when the patient is lying on the opposite side may accentuate the discomfort. The movements of the hip are normal, but in severe cases discomfort can limit motion. Trochanteric bursitis is more common in women. It can occur as an isolated condition but is more frequently seen in association with damage to the ipsilateral hip joint, mechanical back strain and obesity[20]. The alteration in gait secondary to these conditions is often accompanied by a limitation of internal rotation of the hip and reflex tightening of the external rotators. These factors may increase the tension of gluteus maximus on the iliotibial band, and potentiate bursal inflammation[21]. Potential precipitating factors include local trauma, leg length inequalities, jogging and other athletic and stressful activities.

Slight irregularities of the greater trochanter or peritrochanteric calcifications of the bursa are sometimes seen on plain radiographs. Bone scintigraphy may show local increased uptake[20]. The differential diagnosis of increased radio-uptake in this region includes stress fractures, local infection and bone and soft tissue tumors. Clinically, however, hip disease and referred thoracolumbar pain are the two conditions that mimic trochanteric bursitis most commonly. The course of trochanteric bursitis is varied: an acute phase may last several days, followed by the gradual abatement of symptoms. However, in many patients, low-grade discomfort may persist for weeks or months.

Treatment includes continuous rest. Patients engaged in sports should be advised to reduce their level of activity, especially running and standing for prolonged periods on the affected limb. NSAIDs can be used but results are often disappointing[19]. Ultrasound is useful only in a minority of patients. The efficacy of massages has not been studied. In uncontrolled series, infiltration of a local anesthetic and of a long-acting corticosteroid preparation in the trochanteric bursa has been shown to be helpful in confirming the diagnosis and bringing long-term relief[18–21]. It is considered by many to be the most effective treatment modality.

Failure of trochanteric bursitis to respond to conservative treatment may be due to tightness of the iliotibial band, as evidenced by a positive Ober's test. Referral to physiotherapy for exercises to stretch out the fascia lata femoris in these patients may be worthwhile. In patients with true leg length discrepancy, trochanteric bursitis tends to occur on the longer leg because of the increased stress imposed on the abductors. In these patients, a heel lift may be indicated. Various surgical procedures have been proposed for refractory cases of trochanteric bursitis but these are rarely, if ever, necessary[22,23].

Iliopsoas bursitis
Iliopsoas bursitis has been described in association with a variety of hip disorders, including osteoarthritis, rheumatoid arthritis, synovial chondromatosis, pigmented villonodular synovitis, osteonecrosis and septic arthritis[24]. While the bursa communicates with the hip cavity in only 15% of adults, a communication has been documented in most reported cases of bursitis. Several theories may explain this finding: hip synovitis with excessive synovial fluid accumulation may cause enlargement of the iliopsoas bursa via a pre-existing communication; a weakened inflamed hip capsule may rupture into the adjacent bursa, creating a new communication; or the bursa itself may be enlarged by the inflammatory process[25].

The direction and degree of bursal enlargement are the most important factors in clinical presentation. The majority of patients are asymptomatic or present with a painful inguinal mass[26,27]. Others may present with leg swelling or varicosities secondary to femoral vein compression[28] or femoral nerve compression[29], thus making the diagnosis more difficult. Several cases of bladder and bowel compression have also been reported. Computed tomography has been proposed as the best diagnostic test to document iliopsoas bursitis (Fig. 18.16). Arthrography followed by the instillation of corticosteroids is also an effective diagnostic and therapeutic modality. Surgical excision of the bursa is occasionally necessary.

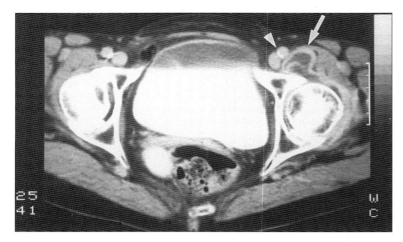

Fig. 18.16 CT scan of a patient with rheumatoid arthritis. The scan shows an enlarged fluid-filled iliopsoas bursa (arrow) communicating with the hip joint and displacing the neurovascular bundle (arrowhead). (With permission from Letourneau *et al.*[28])

Ischiogluteal bursitis

Ischiogluteal bursitis is most commonly seen in patients engaged in jobs which favor repeated friction of the ischial bursae[29]. In the standing position, the gluteus maximus forms a thick pad over the ischial tuberosity. When the thigh is flexed, as in the sitting position, the distal border of the gluteus maximus moves superiorly, leaving the ischial tuberosity subcutaneous. Weavers repeatedly extend one limb and then the other in the practice of their craft. The repeated friction on the ischial bursa may lead to inflammation of the bursae or 'weaver's bottom'. Patients with ischiogluteal bursitis complain of exquisite pain over the ischia, which is aggravated by sitting and lying. Local tenderness on palpation of the ischia is always found. Enthesitis, such as seen in ankylosing spondylitis and other spondyloarthropathies, can give rise to a similar clinical picture. Symptoms may be alleviated by using an 8–10cm rubber cushion with holes cut for the ischial prominences. Trunk and knee-to-chest stretching exercises while lying on the cushion should be encouraged. A local injection of corticosteroid may be used in refractory cases. Care should be taken not to inject the sciatic nerve which passes just laterally to the bursa.

Adductor tendinitis

Adductor tendinitis tends to occur in patients engaged in sports activities involving straddling, such as horseback riding, gymnastics and dancing, as well as in enthusiasts of aerobic exercise classes, especially in those individuals with an inadequate or insufficient warming-up period. The pain is typically felt in the groin and inner aspect of the thigh and is increased by passive abduction of the thighs and active adduction against resistance. Tenderness may also be elicited by local palpation of the adductor muscles, especially near their insertion on the front of the pubis. The differential diagnosis of adductor tendinitis include hernias, genitourinary afflictions (prostatitis, epididymitis, urethritis, hydrocele, etc.), osteitis pubis and arthritis of the hip. Treatment consists of rest and ice during the acute phase. NSAIDs, ultrasound and progressive stretching exercises are used in the subacute phase. Local corticosteroid injections are reserved for patients resistant to these conservative modalities.

'Snapping hip syndrome'

Some patients complain of pain in the hip region associated with an audible and palpable snapping sensation, usually felt in the lateral trochanteric area[30]. This is an uncommon entity reported most frequently in young individuals. Symptoms typically occur in activities such as climbing or walking upstairs during which a taut iliotibial band slips over the greater trochanter. On examination, the patient can usually reproduce the snapping sensation by flexing and internally rotating the thigh, and the examiner can sometimes feel the snapping sensation by applying a palm to the greater trochanter area. Treatment consists essentially of exercises to stretch the iliotibial band. Cases of snapping hip caused by slipping of the iliopsoas tendon over an osseous ridge on the lesser trochanter have been reported[30].

REFERENCES

1. Gautier E, Ganz K, Krügel N et al. Anatomy of the medial femoral artery and its surgical implications. J Bone Joint Surg 2000; 82B: 679–683.
2. Crock HV. Anatomy of the medial femoral artery and its surgical implications (letter). J Bone Joint Surg 2001; 83B: 149–150.
3. Sevitt S. Avascular necrosis and revascularization of the femoral head after intracapsular fracture: a combined arteriographic and histological study. J Bone Joint Surg 1964; 46B: 270–296.
4. Lea RD, Gerhardt JJ. Range-of-motion measurements. J Bone Joint Surg 1995; 77A: 784–798.
5. Clarke GR. Unequal leg length: an accurate method of detection and some clinical results. Rheum Phys Med 1982; 11: 385–390.
6. Morscher E, Figner G. Measurement of leg length. In: Hungerford DS, ed. Progress in orthopedic surgery, volume 1, Leg length discrepancy: the injured knee. New York: Springer-Verlag; 1977: 21–27.
7. Bjerkreim I. Secondary dysplasia and osteoarthritis of the hip joint in functional and in fixed obliquity of the pelvis. Acta Orthop Scan 1974; 45: 873–882.
8. Spitzer WO, Leblanc FE, Dupier M. Scientific approach to the assessment and management of activity-related spinal disorders: a monograph for clinicians. Report of the Quebec Task Force on Spinal Disorders. Spine 1987; 12: S1–S59.
9. Witt I, Vestergaard A, Rosenklint A. A comparative analysis of x-ray findings of the lumbar spine in patients with and without lumbar pain. Spine 1984; 9: 198–299.
10. Berquist-Ullman M, Larsson U. Acute low back pain in industry. A controlled prospective study with reference to therapy and confounding factors. Acta Orthop Scand 1977; 170: S1–S17.
11. Maigne R. Low back pain of thoracolumbar origin. Arch Phys Med Rehabil 1980; 61: 389–395.
12. Russell AS, Maksymowych W, LeClercq S. Clinical examination of the sacroiliac joints: a prospective study. Arthritis Rheum 1981; 24: 1575–1577.
13. Schapira D. Transient osteoporosis of the hip. Semin Arthritis Rheum 1992; 22: 98–105.
14. Bradwell JD, Burns JE, Kingbury GH. Transient osteoporosis of the hip in pregnancy. J Bone Joint Surg 1989; 71: 1252–1257.
15. Coventry MB, Mitchell WC. Osteitis pubis. J Am Med Assoc 1961; 178: 898–905.
16. Sexton DJ, Heskestad L, Lambeth WR et al. Postoperative pubic osteomyelitis misdiagnosed as osteitis pubis: report of 4 cases and review. Clin Infect Dis 1993; 17: 695–700.
17. Grace JN, Sim FH, Shives TC et al. Wedge resection of the symphysis pubis for the treatment of osteitis pubis. J Bone Joint Surg 1989; 71A: 358–364.
18. Lotke PA. Soft tissue afflictions. In: Steinberg ME, ed. The hip and its disorders. Philadelphia: Saunders; 1991: 669–682.
19. Schapira D, Nahir M, Scharf Y. Trochanteric bursitis: a common clinical problem. Arch Phys Med Rehabil 1986; 67: 815–817.
20. Little H. Trochanteric bursitis: a common cause of pelvic girdle pain. Can Med Assoc J 1979; 120: 456–458.
21. Swezey RL. Pseudo-radiculopathy in subacute trochanteric bursitis of subgluteus maximus bursa. Arch Phys Med Rehabil 1976; 57: 387–390.
22. Gordon EJ. Trochanteric bursitis and tendinitis. Clin Orthop 1961; 20: 193–202.
23. Zoltan DJ, Clancy WG, Keene JS. A new operative approach to snapping hip and refractory trochanteric bursitis in athletes. Am J Sports Med 1986; 14: 201–204.
24. Toohey AK, LaSalle TL, Martinez S, Polisson RP. Iliopsoas bursitis: clinical features, radiographic findings, and disease associations. Semin Arthritis Rheum 1990; 10: 41–47.
25. Melamed A, Bauer CA, Howard Johnson J. Iliopsoas bursal extension of arthritic disease of the hip. Radiology 1967; 89: 54–58.
26. Underwood PL, McLeod RA, Ginsburg WW. The varied manifestations of iliopsoas bursitis. J Rheumatol 1988; 15: 1683–1685.
27. Helfgott SM. Unusual features of iliopsoas bursitis. Arthritis Rheum 1988; 31: 1331–1333.
28. Letourneau L, Dessureault M, Carette S. Rheumatoid iliopsoas bursitis presenting as unilateral femoral nerve palsy. J Rheumatol 1991; 18: 462–463.
29. Swartout R, Compere EL. Ischio-gluteal bursitis. J Am Med Assoc 1974; 227: 551–552.
30. Schaberg JE, Harper MC, Allen WC. The snapping hip syndrome. Am J Sports Med 1984; 12: 361–365.

19 The knee

John A Fairclough and Geoffrey P Graham

- The knee, the largest human joint, is comprised of two joints, the patellofemoral and the tibiofemoral

- Knee stability is provided by four major ligaments, the anterior and posterior cruciate and medial and lateral collateral ligaments, which, along with the bony anatomy, provide dynamic stability to the joint

- The prepatellar and the pretendinous bursae are subcutaneous sacs independent from the joint. When distended, the gastrocnemius–semimembranosus bursa, which communicates with the joint in 50% of adults, causes a Baker's cyst

- Knee pain may arise from the joint itself, from periarticular tissues such as tendons and bursae, or from distant sites such as the hip or femur

- An accurate diagnosis of knee conditions can usually be made on the basis of the history and physical examination. Standard investigations include synovial fluid analysis, conventional radiography (X-ray), magnetic resonance imaging and arthroscopy

FUNCTIONAL ANATOMY

Skeletal

The knee is a highly modified hinge joint consisting of two separate articulations, the tibiofemoral and the patellofemoral, which share a common synovial cavity (Fig. 19.1).

The shape of the articular surfaces contributes significantly to the articular mechanics of the rotation of the knee throughout its range of movements.

The distal femur is bicondylar; the medial femoral condyle is larger and projects further posteriorly and distally than the lateral condyle, with the lateral femoral condyle projecting further anteriorly despite its smaller anteroposterior diameter (Fig. 19.2).

The anterior posterior axis is not straight, as the medial femoral condyle diverges from the sagittal midline, resulting in a divergence of the condyles that in flexion is approximately 28°. The difference in size of the condyles in addition to the divergence explains the 'screw home mechanism.' As the knee extends, the medial side has further to travel and hence the tibia continues to rotate externally, taking with it the tibial tubercle.

The proximal tibia consists of two articular areas or condyles, which are separated by the tibial eminence (Fig. 19.3). The medial condyle is concave and longer in the anteroposterior plane than the lateral, which is smaller and mildly convex. Both condylar surfaces rise to a bony intercondylar eminence, which acts as a reference point for the insertion of the cruciate ligaments.

The second major joint of the knee is the patellofemoral joint. This is highly specialized in shape and function, having the body's greatest thickness of hyaline cartilage, which reaches a thickness of up to 5mm in the midline to resist the large pressures that are exerted upon it. The patella itself is a sesamoid bone within the quadriceps tendon that includes three lateral and four medial facets[1] (Fig. 19.4). The fourth or 'odd' facet only articulates with the femur toward the full extent of flexion with some contact with the medial condyle. There is no true separation of the patellofemoral and tibiofemoral condylar articulation in the human, although the lateral femoral condyle has a small sulcus indicating the line of separation. The shape of the medial and lateral condyles form the trochlear groove of the patellofemoral joint, which measures approximately 140°, along which the patella travels during knee movement (Fig. 19.2). As the knee starts to flex from full extension, first the distal part of the patella surface is contacted and subsequently the zone of contact passes proximally on the patella while the femoral contact zone moves distally; the excursion of movement on the lateral tibial plateau is less than on the medial condyle. In full extension, the patella lies just above the trochlea and centralizes within the trochlea during the first 30° of flexion.

The femoral and tibial condyles are covered with thick hyaline cartilage and articulate with each other, with the crescent shaped fibrocartilaginous menisci interposed. The triangular cross-section of a meniscus has an upper surface that is convex from side to side and is flattened on its tibial surface. The thickened posterior border is attached to the capsule and the sharpened free edge lies in the joint. The menisci are not covered with synovium and are divided into two zones. The peripheral parameniscal area is vascular and covers approximately the outer third of the meniscus with the central zone being fibrocartilage. The lateral meniscus is nearly circular and the medial meniscus is semicircular (Fig. 19.5). Their ends are attached to the intercondylar area of the tibia with attachments at the circumference to the meniscotibial and meniscofemoral ligaments, which are part of the capsule of the joint[2]. The lateral meniscus is attached to the femur posteriorly by the inconstant meniscofemoral ligaments of Wrisberg and Humphrey. The popliteus tendon enters the joint through a deficiency in the capsule adjacent to the lateral meniscus and may be attached to it[3,4]. The menisci transmit approximately 60% of the force through the normal tibiofemoral joint and play a role in lubrication. They alter shape in order to maintain congruity of the joint as the knee flexes and extends. The peripheral 10–30% of the meniscus and the anterior and posterior horns receive a blood supply from the geniculate vessels and have the potential for repair[5]. The rest of the meniscus is avascular and is nourished from the synovial fluid, so there is little potential for healing in this area.

Ligamentous

There are four major ligaments in the knee, the anterior and posterior cruciate and medial and lateral collateral ligaments with capsular thickenings that contribute greatly to the rotatory stability of the knee.

The medial collateral ligament is a broad ligament whose superficial layer arises from the medial epicondyle and fans out over the medial side of the tibia where its posterior border blends with the capsule of the knee joint[6,7]. The deep layer originates with the superficial layer but, just above the joint line, inserts into the medial meniscus, acting as a stabilizer to the fibrocartilage. The deep layer then proceeds distally to blend

SAGITTAL SECTION OF THE KNEE JOINT

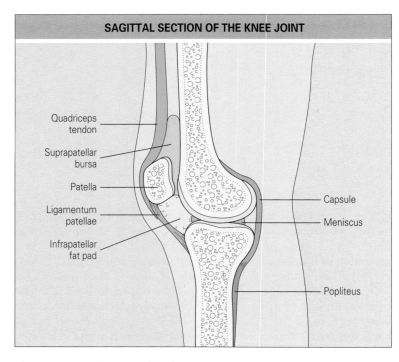

Quadriceps tendon

Suprapatellar bursa

Patella

Ligamentum patellae

Infrapatellar fat pad

Capsule

Meniscus

Popliteus

Fig. 19.1 Sagittal section of the knee joint, showing the components.

THE PATELLOFEMORAL JOINT

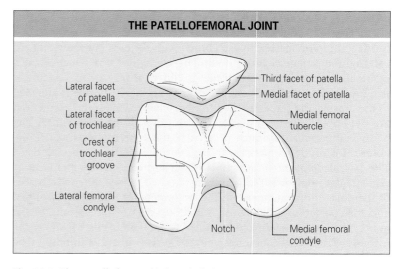

Lateral facet of patella

Lateral facet of trochlear

Crest of trochlear groove

Lateral femoral condyle

Third facet of patella

Medial facet of patella

Medial femoral tubercle

Notch

Medial femoral condyle

Fig. 19.2 The patellofemoral joint – inferior view.

TIBIAL PLATEAU

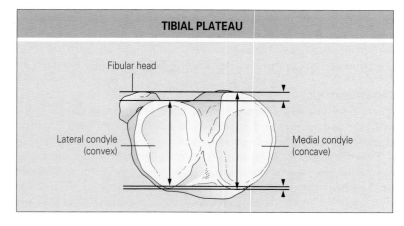

Fibular head

Lateral condyle (convex)

Medial condyle (concave)

Fig. 19.3 Tibial plateau – superior view.

FACETS OF THE PATELLA

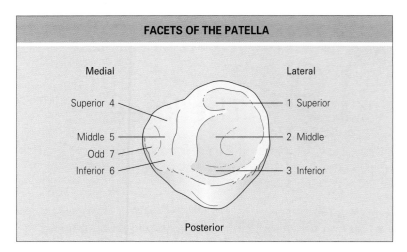

Medial

Superior 4

Middle 5

Odd 7

Inferior 6

Lateral

1 Superior

2 Middle

3 Inferior

Posterior

Fig. 19.4 Facets of the patella. The figure shows the intra-articular surface of the patella, demonstrating the position of the facets.

again with the superficial layer as it inserts in an oblique manner into the tibia approximately 10cm below the joint line. The lateral collateral ligament is smaller and shorter, arising from the lateral femoral condyle and inserting into the posterior aspect of the fibular head. The popliteus tendon is a fundamental part of the lateral stabilizing structures in the knee and passes from the posterior surface of the tibia through a hiatus in the lateral meniscus before inserting just anterior and inferior to the lateral collateral ligament.

The anterior cruciate ligament (ACL) is comprised of two main bundles and, although intra-articular, is extrasynovial. It has two bands: an anteromedial, which is taut when the knee is flexed, and a postero-lateral, which is taut when the knee is extended[8]. The posterolateral bundle is inserted into the lateral aspect of the tibial origin, is the largest and strongest of the bundles and has its origin from the most posterior part of the femoral attachment. The anteromedial bundle originates from the anterior femoral origin and inserts into the medial side of the tibial insertion. The bundles spiral around each other, allowing a constant tension throughout knee movement. The ACL lies flat at 90° of flexion and more vertically in extension.

The posterior cruciate ligament (PCL) is also extrasynovial, arises in front of the medial femoral condyle, spirals inferiorly and flattens into a large insertion just lateral to the midline on the posterior aspect of the tibia (Fig. 19.6).

The capsular structures on the posteromedial side are thickened in a band running obliquely, the posterior oblique ligament. The semimem-branosus muscle has five major bands inserting on the posteromedial side of the tibia reinforcing the posteromedial capsule.

The posterolateral aspect of the knee is complex and damage to it causes major instability. There are three main layers, the deepest of which is the posterior capsule, which encloses the lateral collateral liga-ment (Fig. 19.7). A thickening of the capsule arising from the fibular head is known as the arcuate ligament. Further thickenings of the capsule contributing to the stability of the posterolateral back corner are the fabellofibular ligament and the popliteofibular ligament, extending from the fibular head to the popliteus tendon. The latter provides support for resisting a posterior translation, external rotation and varus angulation.

Knee movement

The movements that occur are complex and involve both rolling and gliding and rotation of the femur on the tibia. The axis of rotation alters as the knee is flexed and extended. The normal motion of the knee is controlled by the shape of the articular surfaces and menisci and by the

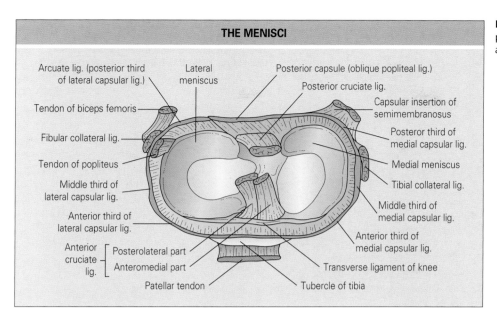

THE MENISCI

Arcuate lig. (posterior third of lateral capsular lig.)

Lateral meniscus

Posterior capsule (oblique popliteal lig.)

Posterior cruciate lig.

Tendon of biceps femoris

Capsular insertion of semimembranosus

Fibular collateral lig.

Posteror third of medial capsular lig.

Tendon of popliteus

Medial meniscus

Middle third of lateral capsular lig.

Tibial collateral lig.

Anterior third of lateral capsular lig.

Middle third of medial capsular lig.

Anterior cruciate lig. — Posterolateral part / Anteromedial part

Anterior third of medial capsular lig.

Patellar tendon

Transverse ligament of knee

Tubercle of tibia

Fig. 19.5 The menisci. The superior surface of the tibial plateau, demonstrating the anatomical position, size and attachments of the menisci.

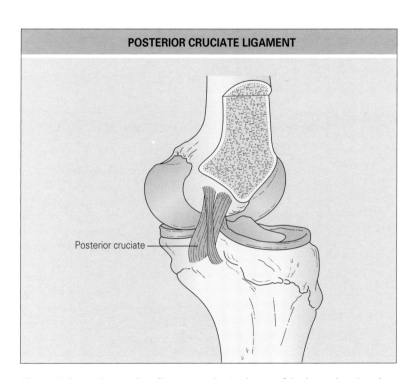

POSTERIOR CRUCIATE LIGAMENT

Posterior cruciate

Fig. 19.6 Posterior cruciate ligament – Sagittal view of the knee showing the origin and attachments of the posterior cruciate ligament.

tension in the ligaments and capsule. Alteration in the configuration of any of these structures due to injury or disease can cause abnormal motion to occur.

The passive motion of the knee averages 0–135° and, because of the asymmetry, the first 30° of flexion is accompanied by the rolling of the lateral femoral condyle posteriorly more than the medial condyle. This allows the femur and tibia to unlock from full extension and occurs independent of any dynamic muscle action.

In health the center of the hip, the center of the knee and the center of the ankle lie in a straight line. Because of the medial inclination of the femur, the long axes of the femur and tibia form a valgus angle of approximately 7°. Disease or an abnormality of growth may alter this: genu valgum represents an increase and genu varum a decrease in the angle (Fig. 19.8).

Patellofemoral movement

The patella articulates with the trochlear groove of the femur and its function is to increase the mechanical advantage of the quadriceps. In full extension only the lower part of the patella is in contact with the articular cartilage of the femur. As the knee is flexed the patella enters the trochlear groove and sits centrally in it. A line drawn from the anterior superior iliac spine to the center of the patella represents the line of pull of the quadriceps, which is lateral to the long axis of the femur. The angle formed by this line and a line drawn from the center of the patella to the tibial tubercle is called the Q angle (Fig. 19.9)[10]. The larger the Q angle, the larger is the force vector tending to pull the patella laterally. In a normal knee the Q angle measures approximately 15°; an angle exceeding 20° is abnormal. Genu valgum, persistent femoral anteversion and external tibial torsion increase this angle and therefore increase the tendency for the patella to dislocate. The factors acting against dislocation are the lower fibers of the vastus medialis, the shape of the patellofemoral joint and the fact that the lateral condyle is higher than the medial. The medial collateral ligament runs forward and down from the medial femoral condyle to a broad insertion on the subcutaneous border of the tibia, deep to the pes anserinus.

The quadriceps muscle consists of the rectus femoris and the three vasti: intermedius, medialis and lateralis. It is the main extensor of the knee and inserts into the patella via the quadriceps tendon into the tibial tuberosity. Fibrous expansions from the vastus medialis and lateralis run obliquely to insert into the sides of the patella, the patellar tendon and the tibia to form the medial and lateral patellar retinacula[7,11]. The iliotibial band is a thickening of the fascia lata on the lateral aspect of the thigh[12]. Proximally, the tensor fascia lata muscle inserts into it. Its distal insertion is into Gerdy's tubercle on the tibia and more proximally by oblique fibers that blend with the lateral patellar retinacula. It helps to stabilize the lateral side of the joint and acts as an extensor when the knee is already near full extension. As the knee is flexed the iliotibial band moves backwards behind the center of rotation of the knee and acts as a flexor. The hamstrings are the main flexors of the knee, helped by the gastrocnemius, sartorius and gracilis. Medial rotation of the flexed knee is controlled by the medial hamstrings (semimembranosus and semitendinosus), popliteus, sartorius and gracilis. Lateral rotation is controlled by the biceps femoris alone.

There are a number of bursae around the knee joint, all of which may become inflamed. The bursae in front of the knee are the prepatellar bursa, which is subcutaneous and lies over the lower half of the patella,

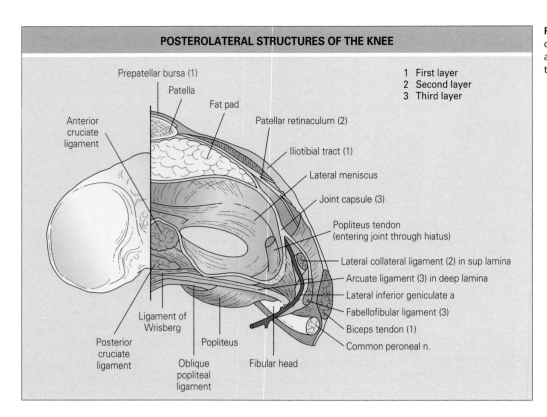

POSTEROLATERAL STRUCTURES OF THE KNEE

Prepatellar bursa (1)
Patella
Fat pad
Anterior cruciate ligament
Patellar retinaculum (2)
Iliotibial tract (1)
Lateral meniscus
Joint capsule (3)
Popliteus tendon (entering joint through hiatus)
Lateral collateral ligament (2) in sup lamina
Arcuate ligament (3) in deep lamina
Lateral inferior geniculate a
Fabellofibular ligament (3)
Biceps tendon (1)
Common peroneal n.
Ligament of Wrisberg
Posterior cruciate ligament
Popliteus
Oblique popliteal ligament
Fibular head

1 First layer
2 Second layer
3 Third layer

Fig. 19.7 Posterolateral structures of the knee. The drawing shows the complexity of the layers and attachments controlling the posterior rotation of the tibial plateau. Redrawn from Seebacher et al.[9]

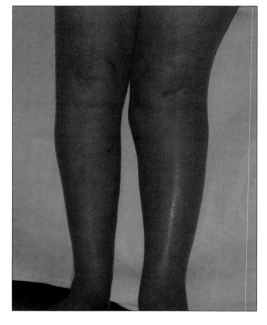

Fig. 19.8 Standing picture demonstrating a valgus left knee with a mild varus angulation of the right knee.

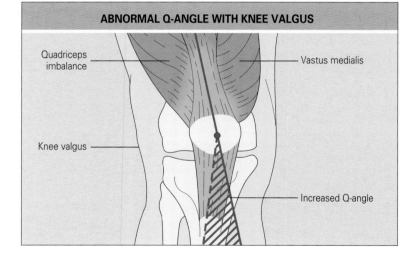

ABNORMAL Q-ANGLE WITH KNEE VALGUS

Quadriceps imbalance
Vastus medialis
Knee valgus
Increased Q-angle

Fig. 19.9 Abnormal Q angle with knee valgus.

the infrapatellar bursa, which lies over the patellar tendon and tibial tubercle, and the deep infrapatellar bursa, which separates the patellar tendon from the upper tibia. On the medial side the anserine bursa is superficial to the medial collateral ligament and separates it from the tendons of sartorius, gracilis and semitendinosus. The common insertion of these three tendons lies superficial to the medial collateral ligament over the upper tibia and is called the pes anserinus. Other smaller bursae may be present deep to the medial collateral ligament[6,13]. Bursae lie deep to the semimembranosus and medial head of the gastrocnemius and may enlarge to form a swelling in the popliteal fossa[14]. On the lateral side, bursae may lie deep to the lateral head of gastrocnemius, between the lateral collateral ligament and the biceps femoris, and around the popliteus, separating it from the lateral femoral condyle and the lateral ligament.

HISTORY AND EXAMINATION

The clinical history remains the cornerstone of diagnosis in knee pathology[15]. The pattern of disease changes with age and mechanism of any injury.

Certain pathologies, such as Osgood–Schlatter disease, occur only in the adolescent, while chondrocalcinosis and degenerative hyaline cartilage problems are conditions seen predominantly in older adults. Non-traumatic swelling in the knee may also be associated with concomitant medical disease, such as gout or infection, and, as with any other aspect in medicine, arriving at an accurate diagnosis is dependent on obtaining a detailed and thorough history. The mechanism of any traumatic incident should be detailed with particular note of the presence of any audible 'pop' and the timing of any swelling in the knee. Swelling occurring within the first few minutes after any injury indicates a hemarthrosis and a popping noise is associated with a rupture of the ACL in over a third of cases. Normally, the history will suggest a diagnosis and a physical examination is then performed to confirm this suspicion.

The tests described below should be relevant for the particular history and individual in question. The approach needs to consider the patient's age, the pattern of injury and the patient's general condition. There is however significant overlap between the various diagnostic groups.

Inspection

It is important that the whole lower limb is exposed The patient should be asked to stand with the feet a few inches apart. The alignment of the knees and the presence of varus or valgus deformity on weight-bearing should be noted. The normal knee is aligned at approximately 7° of valgus and, although variations of the degree of varus or valgus alignment may be constitutional, such findings can indicate underlying knee pathology. The degree of clinical varus is the distance between the knees with the feet together and the degree of valgus is the distance between the medial malleoli with the knees together. Hip, ankle and foot problems can affect the knee joint biomechanics and lead to secondary symptoms in the knee. Variations in the proximal femur, such as femoral anteversion or a contracture of the hip, will lead to internal rotation of the femur and the patella being inwardly facing or 'squinting'.

Likewise, the knee should be viewed from the side to note the degree of genu recurvatum or the presence of a flexion contracture. A recurvatum deformity is usually obvious on standing and persistent femoral anteversion causes 'squinting' of the patella (Fig. 19.10).

The degree of tibial rotation compared with the position of the patella is indicated by the position of the malleoli and foot in relation to the patella. Any suspicion of excessive tibial torsion is confirmed from the angle that the foot makes to the thigh in the prone examination. Abnormalities of the foot and ankle, especially those related to hindfoot

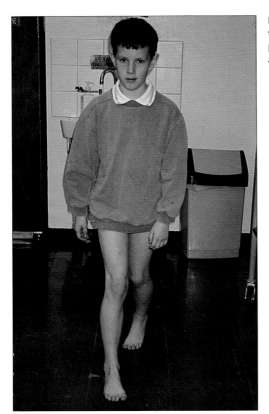

Fig. 19.10 Squinting of the patella caused by persistent femoral anteversion.

valgus, can produce torsion of the tibia and abnormalities of the patellofemoral complex leading to anterior knee pain.

Palpation

Any swelling within the synovial cavity is seen above and on either side of the patella and patellar tendon (Fig. 19.11). A swelling that does not extend above the patella suggests local injury or an enlarged bursa. Inflammation of the pre- or infrapatellar bursae causes a characteristic swelling over the front of the knee. There may be scars from previous surgery, injury or infection. More subtle changes of smaller effusions, however, can be detected by milking fluid out of the suprapatellar pouch with one hand while gently squeezing the sulci on either side of the patellar tendon.

A thickening of the synovium, as in synovitis, may be difficult to distinguish from an intra-articular effusion but is in general identified by a firmer, spongy feeling of the swelling, which cannot easily be compressed, rather than the more easily compressed synovial effusion.

Extra-articular soft tissue swellings are normally localized and more superficial; prepatellar and infrapatellar bursitis, Osgood–Schlatter disease and infrapatellar jumper's knee all have specific anatomical sites.

The size, shape and length of the patella in relation to the patellar ligament should be sought. Palpation of the knee joint is performed, identifying the structures around the knee beginning with the quadriceps tendon and continuing distally over the patella, the patellar tendon, tibial tubercle and soft tissues, noting any specific area of thickening, defect or tenderness. Lateral and posterior palpation should include the lateral femoral condyle, epicondyle, collateral ligament, head of femur, iliotibial track and, specifically, the peroneal nerve.

Change in the contour of these areas or any specific swelling may indicate a specific diagnosis. A small swelling on the joint line on the lateral side of the knee, for example, is almost certainly a meniscal cyst (Fig. 19.12).

Palpation of the hamstrings and the popliteal fossa may identify the presence of a popliteal or 'Baker's' cyst. Not all swellings in the popliteal fossa are Baker's cysts and the nature of the swelling should be closely noted. In rare circumstances a popliteal aneurysm may present as knee pain, being easily differentiated by its pulsatile nature and normally the presence of a bruit. Palpation is continued medially, including the joint line, the medial collateral ligament and pes anserinus area. Signs of bruising over the medial collateral ligament may indicate an injury to that structure and bruising in the calf may indicate rupture of the joint capsule. A swelling over the tibial tubercle in children indicates possible Osgood–Schlatter disease. Tumors around the knee may present as a swelling, particularly in children. Dilated veins over a swelling is an ominous sign, often indicating a neoplastic process.

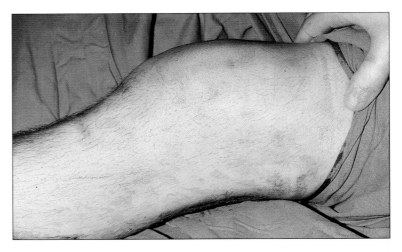

Fig. 19.11 Swelling within the synovial cavity.

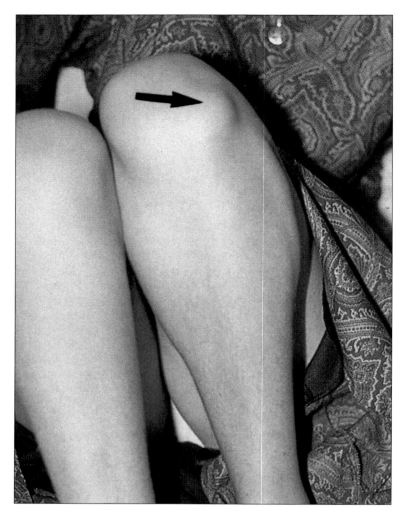

Fig. 19.12 Lateral meniscal cyst, visible on the lateral joint, associated with a horizontal cleavage tear of the lateral meniscus.

The temperature of the joint should be compared first to the ipsilateral pretibial area and then to the contralateral knee; an increase in temperature suggests an inflammatory process.

Tenderness over the insertions or course of the medial collateral ligament after injury is suggestive of a medial collateral ligament sprain, particularly if associated with localized bruising. The lateral collateral ligament may be palpated in the flexed knee when a varus stress is

applied. Swelling and tenderness over its course is suggestive of a sprain.

Motion

Both passive and active motion need to be assessed. The normal passive range is from 0–135°, although considerable variation occurs. Hyperextension in individuals may be normal and indicate a higher risk of certain diagnoses. Individuals with hyperextension of the knee may be at increased risk of ACL tears.

The degree of internal and external rotation of the tibia is noted with the knees flexed to 90° and the hip–foot angle recorded. The 'screw home mechanism' is assessed during active extension. At 90° of flexion the tibial tubercle is normally directly below the patella, whereas in full extension it moves laterally. Any degree of concern about the possible lack of full extension can be more easily seen by placing the patient in the prone position and assessing heel height. Any obvious muscle wasting can be noted. The specific measurements of quadriceps girth, however, is of only marginal use subject to marked areas of measurement.

The measurement of Q angle should be undertaken with the patient in the supine position. The angle is formed by the intersection of a line drawn from the anterior-superior iliac spine to the center of the patella and a second line running from the central patella to the tibial tubercle (Fig. 19.9). Any angle above 15° should be regarded with caution and over 20° as being abnormal.

Patellofemoral joint evaluation

Finally, attention is devoted to the patellofemoral joint. The movements of the patella are assessed when the knee is flexed and extended and palpation of the joint during movement should be undertaken. Occasionally, bands of tissue, mainly on the medial parapatellar region, can be palpated and click as the knee moves. These bands are known as plica and may be the source of anterior knee pain. The patellar apprehension test is performed in the relaxed patient with the knee flexed to 30° (Fig. 19.13). A lateral force is applied to the medial board of the patella. As the patella moves laterally, the patient feels an incipient subluxation of the knee and resists further movements and may withdraw from the examiner, which indicates a patellar instability complex.

A further test for evaluation of the stability, especially of the lateral retinaculum, is the patella tilt test. With the patient supine, and the knee fully extended, the examiner gently lifts the edge of the patella away from the lateral femoral condyle and any degree of tilting is noted. At this point any specific tenderness over the medial and lateral facets of the patella can be noted.

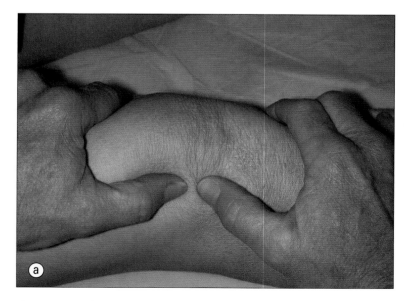
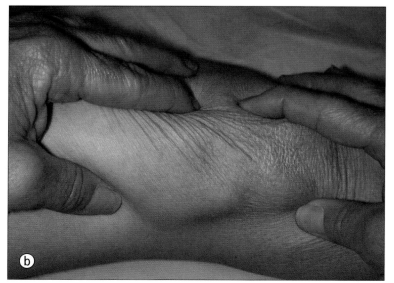

Fig. 19.13 Patellar apprehension test showing lateral force being applied to the patella as the knee is in the early range of flexion.

Finally, patellofemoral mechanics may be affected by the presence of a tight iliotibial band. The Ober's test is useful in evaluating the contractures of the latter band. In this test the patient is rotated onto the non-affected side and the limb maximally abducted. With the knee flexed to 90° the abducted limb is then gently released and any degree of persistent adduction may indicate a contraction of the iliotibial band (Fig. 19.14).

Gait

The majority of symptoms related to knee function are dynamic in origin and hence it is important to assess the function of the knee in its

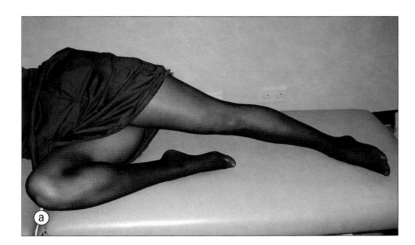

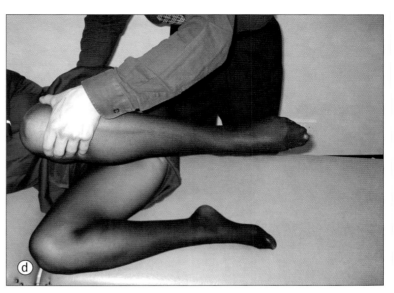

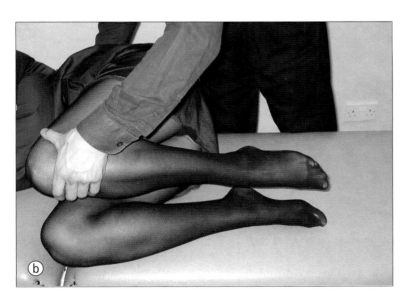

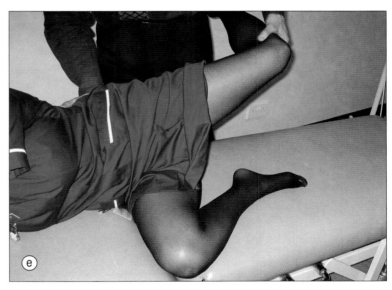

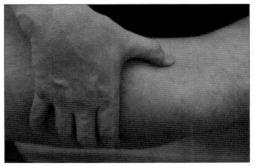

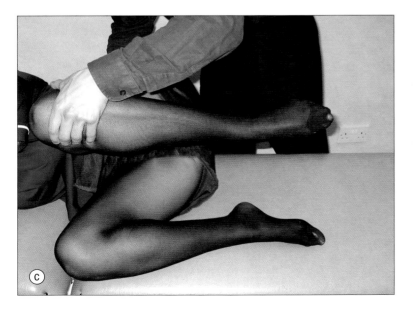

Fig. 19.14 Ober's test to evaluate iliotibial band flexibility and symptomatology. (a) The test is performed with the patient lying on the side opposite to that being tested, with the lower hip flexed. (b) Flex the hip on the side being tested. (c) While the hip is flexed, maximally abduct the hip. (d) With the hip now in maximal abduction, extend the hip. It is important to maintain stabilization of the pelvis to keep it perpendicular and maintain the neutral rotation of the femur. (e) Allow the thigh to abduct. Note stabilizing position of hand. (inset) As the thigh is allowed to adduct, the lateral tibial band is palpated, often reproducing the patient's symptoms.

normal gait pattern. The normal gait is smooth and rhythmic. Frequently a minor degree of varus or lateral thrust is emphasized in the gait pattern, as in severe osteoarthritis.

Minor degrees of flexion contracture lead to an alteration in the weight-bearing pattern with poor heel strike and rotation of the hips, and are much more apparent in the dynamic assessment of gait than in the static position.

SPECIFIC DISORDERS OF THE KNEE

The remainder of this chapter will focus on specific knee disorders. Clinically, most patients present with knee pain and the major causes of this symptom in each of the major periods of life are considered separately (Table 19.1). Secondly, the knee is subject to some very specific injuries, including meniscal tears and cruciate rupture. The second half of this chapter separately reviews these and other consequences of injury.

KNEE PAIN

Children

Pain in the infant or early adolescent is uncommon but is always significant. The limping child must always be treated with a degree of urgency and a cause for the symptoms must be confirmed. In the toddler or young child the cause of knee pain may frequently be referred from the hip; thus Perthes disease or a missed dislocated hip frequently present with knee pain.

Transient synovitis of the hip or an irritable hip in childhood can frequently present with knee pain and a similar condition of non-specific inflammation can be seen in the young infant. The presence of any effusion in a young child should likewise be dealt with with a degree of urgency, to rule out the presence of a bacterial infection.

Septic arthritis and osteomyelitis

Septic arthritis of the knee in children is not uncommon. The infection is usually blood-borne but may occur after a puncture wound. The patient complains of severe pain on even the slightest movement and is generally unwell with a tensely swollen knee and a fever. Joint aspiration should be immediately performed for synovial fluid cell count and differential, Gram stain and culture. Thorough arthroscopic washout should be commenced as soon as the diagnosis is suspected. This is more efficient than arthrotomy and may need to be repeated. Arthrotomy is required if loculi have formed that cannot be broken down arthroscopically. Antibiotics should only be started after fluid has been sent for culture and sensitivity. The differential diagnosis includes other inflammatory processes such as juvenile chronic arthritis and non-specific synovitis.

Acute hematogenous osteomyelitis commonly affects the lower femoral and upper tibial metaphyses. The diagnosis is clinical, with tenderness over the area, and is supported by an increased white cell count and erythrocyte sedimentation rate (ESR). Radiographic changes may take a number of days to appear. A sympathetic effusion may be present in the knee joint.

Other causes

In the child under 10 years, internal derangement of the knee is very uncommon. Mechanical symptoms of pain, clicking and giving way may be reported, however, indicating a tear to a discoid meniscus. The lateral meniscus occasionally will not differentiate into its normal shape and lies as a thick band of fibrocartilaginous tissue, which may tear and produce symptoms akin to the bucket-handle tear locking seen in later age-groups.

The treatment of this is by arthroscopically removing the medial fragment of the meniscus, leaving a more anatomical meniscal shape.

Although tumors are rare in children, Ewing's osteosarcoma or forms of leukemia may occasionally present with atypical joint pain. Any finding of tenderness or systemic symptoms should be thoroughly investigated, which should include anterior and posterior radiograph of the hip and knee.

Inflammatory joint conditions such as juvenile ankylosing spondylitis and juvenile idiopathic arthritis may present as a single joint problem in the knee.

Early adolescence

In this age group, between 10 years and skeletal maturity, the knee is subject to more adult forces and activity levels. As a result of this, overuse injuries become more prominent and specific conditions of adolescence such as osteochondritis dissecans and slipped upper femoral

	Cause		
Age group	**Intra-articular**	**Periarticular**	**Referred**
Childhood (2–10 years)	Juvenile chronic arthritis Osteochondritis dissecans Septic arthritis Torn discoid lateral meniscus	Osteomyelitis	Perthes disease Transient synovitis of the hip
Adolescence (10–18 years)	Osteochondritis dissecans Torn meniscus Anterior knee pain syndrome Patellar malalignment	Osgood–Schlatter disease Sinding-Larsen–Johansson syndrome Osteomyelitis Tumors	Slipped upper femoral epiphysis
Early adulthood (18–30 years)	Torn meniscus Instability Anterior knee pain syndrome Inflammatory conditions	Overuse syndromes Bursitis	Rare
Adulthood (30–50 years)	Degenerate meniscal tears Early degeneration following injury or meniscectomy Inflammatory arthropathies	Bursitis Tendinitis	Degenerative hip disease secondary to hip dysplasia or injury
Older age (>50 years)	Osteoarthritis Inflammatory arthropathies	Bursitis Tendinitis	Osteoarthritis of the hip

TABLE 19.1 COMMON CAUSES OF KNEE PAIN IN DIFFERENT AGE GROUPS

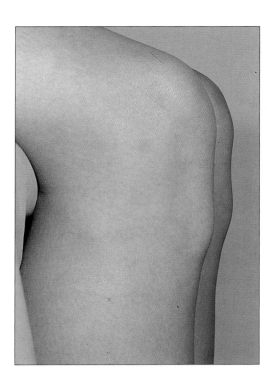

Fig. 19.15
Osgood–Schlatter disease. Enlarged tibial tuberosity.

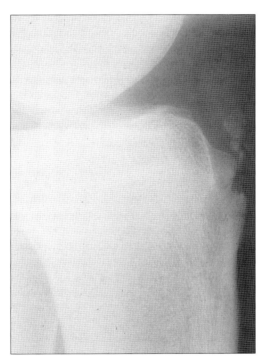

Fig. 19.16
Osgood–Schlatter disease. Loose ossicles in the patellar tendon.

epiphysis need to be considered. It is common, however, for a child to present with a mild limp and aching pain and discomfort in the knee and be examined on several occasions and to be found to have a normal knee examination, but still limp.

Examination of the hip, however, can reveal the presence of a slipped upper femoral epiphysis. In this child, there will be a reduction of flexion of the hip, internal rotation and abduction, which may not produce any hip pain but may cause minor discomfort in the ipsilateral knee. It is essential in this age group to be aware of this condition and take appropriate pelvic X-rays.

Osgood–Schlatter disease

Osgood–Schlatter disease is a traction apophysitis of the tibial tuberosity[16]. It occurs most commonly in those aged 10–14 years and is associated with overuse. The patients present complaining of pain over the tibial tuberosity, particularly on activity[17]. The clinical findings are of tenderness over the tibial tuberosity, which is often enlarged (Fig. 19.15).

Resisted extension can provoke the symptoms. The condition is frequently bilateral, although one side may be significantly more affected than the other with a swelling, occasionally the size of a small egg, present on the tibial tubercle. It is, however, a benign condition and can be treated with advice. There is no indication to prohibit the child from performing sporting activity and the exclusion of a child from sport may well be detrimental. The concept of resting in plaster for a period of time is unnecessary and the condition resolves at skeletal maturity.

Occasionally, the fragmentation of the apophysis with the production of small ossicles, as shown in Figure 19.16, may cause some discomfort in the adult and removal of the ossicles may be necessary in rare circumstances.

Sinding-Larsen–Johansson syndrome

This is a condition similar to Osgood–Schlatter disease occurring at the distal pole of the patella. It is a traction apophysitis and is related to overuse[18]. The patient complains of pain at the distal pole of the patella on activity. This area is tender and radiographs show fragmentation (Fig. 19.17). In this particular group it is important to assess the overall gait of the individual as there is a frequent association with a gait abnormality – for example, related to external rotation of the tibia from a pes planar valgus foot. The condition responds to rest but may persist into adolescence as jumper's knee.

Osteochondritis dissecans

Osteochondritis dissecans occurs most commonly in the knee joint. A fragment of cartilage with its underlying subchondral bone becomes detached and may become loose in the joint. Boys are affected more commonly than girls. The second decade is the usual time for presentation but it may occur earlier.

The symptoms are usually of an aching pain during and after activity. Clicking and giving way may occur. An antalgic gait may be present. There is often a mild effusion and tenderness over the site of the lesion. Wasting of the quadriceps is an early sign. If the fragment separates, symptoms of locking occur and a loose body may be palpable, usually in the suprapatellar pouch. Wilson's sign may be positive. The test involves straightening the internally rotated knee from a flexed position – pain at

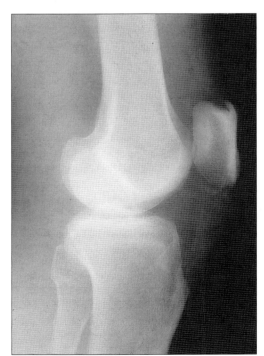

Fig. 19.17 **Sinding-Larsen–Johansson syndrome.** Radiograph showing fragmentation of the lower pole of the patella.

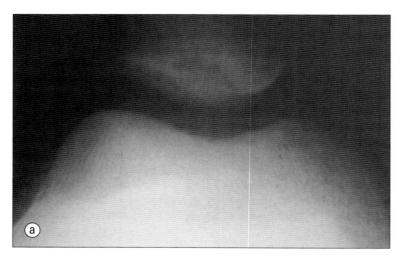

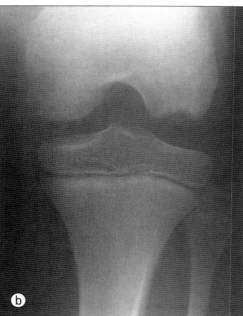

Fig. 19.18 Radiographic appearances of osteochondritic lesions of (a) the patella and (b) the lateral femoral condyle.

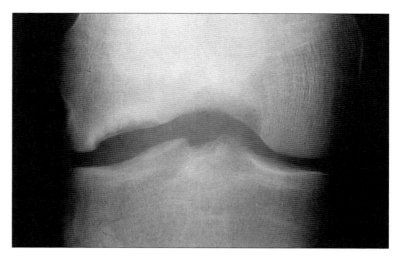

Fig. 19.19 Radiograph of a notch view. The radiographs shows an osteochondral defect in a 17-year-old with a defect over the weight-bearing area of the lateral femoral condyle.

30° of flexion that is relieved by externally rotating the tibia is said to be diagnostic of osteochondritis dissecans[19].

The lesions occur most commonly on the lateral aspect of the medial femoral condyle but may also affect the posterior aspect of the lateral condyle, the trochlea and the patella. Abnormalities of ossification also occur in these sites and may be mistaken for osteochondritis dissecans.

Osteochondritic lesions of the condyles can often be seen on antero-posterior and lateral radiographs but are best seen on a tunnel view. The radiographic appearance is diagnostic, showing a well-circumscribed fragment of subchondral bone (Fig. 19.18). If the fragment has become detached, an irregularity is seen at the site (Fig. 19.19). Computed tomography (CT) scanning and magnetic resonance imaging (MRI) are useful to confirm the diagnosis and to define the extent of the lesion. In cases of doubt, a bone scan may be useful to differentiate osteochondritis dissecans from abnormalities of ossification. A hot spot around the lesion confirms active disease; the uptake decreases with healing of the lesion[20].

Treatment of the undisplaced fragment in the younger child has historically involved rest and avoidance of activities that might injure the knee until the lesion is healed. The etiology of the condition, however, is incompletely understood and there is little evidence that prolonged rest alters the prognosis of the condition; long-term immobilization should be avoided[21,22]. There is no evidence that immobilization is effective and a symptomatic approach to return to normal activity is optimal. The prognosis is better in younger patients before skeletal maturity in whom the fragment does not separate.

Treatment of the older child follows the same lines but, if the symptoms persist and if the fragment generally does not separate, arthroscopic assessment should be undertaken and the fragment should be debrided and drilled if necessary. Loose fragments should be fixed if they are large. This procedure may be performed open or arthroscopically using fine K-wires or Herbert screws. Smaller fragments loose in the joint should be removed arthroscopically. The defect that is left should be debrided and will fill with fibrocartilage. The long-term consequences of such a defect are incompletely understood. In certain defects the hyaline cartilage loss may cover a large part of the articular surface and would suggest a greater risk of degenerate osteoarthritis in the future than is observed in the long term.

Concern over the prognosis of large defects has led to their treatment by a variety of surgical procedures to attempt to reproduce the hyaline cartilage surface (Fig. 19.20). The long-term result of such surgical intervention is not known but methods involve either the transfer of plugs of hyaline cartilage from another part of the knee to the defect (osteochondral transfer, OCT) or an attempt to grow hyaline cartilage by culturing autologous chondrocytes and implanting them into the defect under a periosteal graft (autologous cartilage implantation, ACI). Occasionally, the first indication that an individual has suffered from osteochondritis dissecans is when s/he presents with mechanical locking and radiological investigation shows a detached loose body from an old lesion (Fig. 19.21).

Late teens/early adulthood

In the age group from early skeletal maturity to early adulthood the most common causes of swelling and discomfort in the knee are related to trauma. Direct blows to the knee may produce an effusion with no intra-articular damage, but effusions that do not settle must be investigated thoroughly.

Anterior knee pain

Anterior knee pain of adolescence is one of the most frequent presentations in this age group. It encompasses a wide variety of pathologies and may produce considerable emotional and physical disability, while proving a major diagnostic challenge to the clinician[23]. Despite many advances in the understanding and investigation of knee pathology, anterior knee pain remains a diagnostic enigma. Frequently the patients are unable to identify specific causation and report only activities of daily living, such as stair climbing, squatting or getting out of chairs as a cause of their problems.

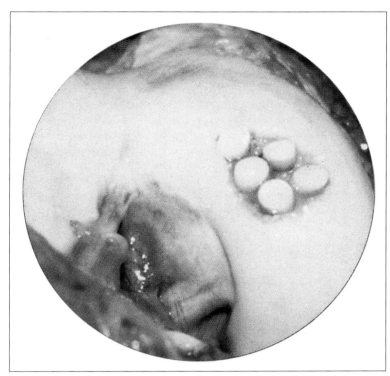

Fig. 19.20 Osteochondral transfer: multiple osteochondral plugs. A large defect in the weight-bearing area of the medial femoral condyle has been filled with cylinders of hyaline cartilage and underlying cancellous bone harvested from donor sites on the ipsilateral knee, either from the lateral parapatellar region or the intercondylar notch.

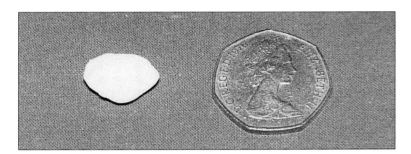

Fig. 19.21 Osteochondral loose body. Loose body removed arthroscopically from a teenage boy presenting with an acute locked knee. Investigation showed the fragment to have originated from previously asymptomatic osteochondritis of the femoral condyle.

The clinical examination should be designed to determine the anatomical site of pain and to assess when the anterior knee pain is maximal. Specific areas of tenderness lead to specific diagnoses, such as infrapatellar tendonitis, synovitis or parapatellar strain. The presence of a marked tender area over the medial or lateral side to the knee associated with the band may indicate a plica syndrome.

Radiological investigation of anterior knee pain should include a standard anteroposterior and lateral radiograph and a skyline view of the patella, which may show, especially in individuals with patellar subluxation, alteration to the shape of the femoral condyles.

The increasing use of MRI has led to the ability to be able to statically assess the shape and degree of health of the hyaline cartilage of the patellofemoral joint, and also to get dynamic sequences that indicate the overall function of the patellofemoral joint.

Once other forms of pathological causes of knee pain have been excluded, including that of patellofemoral subluxation, a group of patients will be left who have aching pain and discomfort in the knee, which can be frequently debilitating, with no obvious cause.

Two main factors have historically been felt to be causal in the etiology of anterior knee pain; firstly, the presence of so-called chondromalacia patellae or hyaline cartilage change; and secondly, malalignment of the patellofemoral joint.

Chondromalacia patellae

A diagnosis of chondromalacia patellae or softening of the articular cartilage of the patella can only be made at arthroscopy or arthrotomy. It is a pathologic diagnosis and should not be used to describe the clinical syndrome of pain arising from the anterior knee joint. However, patients with anterior knee pain may be found to have chondromalacia patellae. It may be associated with patellar malalignment, in which case it is probably due to impact loading and shearing of the articular cartilage as the patella is compressed against the lateral femoral condyle. Articular cartilage is poor at resisting shear forces and repetitive impact loading and shear may both be shown to produce cartilage softening. The majority of cases associated with malalignment respond to correction of the underlying abnormality, provided cartilage loss has not occurred. Idiopathic chondromalacia patellae usually responds to the conservative measures of isometric quadriceps exercises and hamstring stretching.

Bipartite patella

Bipartite patella occurs when the ossification centers of the patella fail to fuse. The defect is seen as a lucent line, usually at the superolateral corner of the patella, where it may be mistaken for a fracture. Occasionally, the synchondrosis may fracture as a result of repetitive stress and cause pain and tenderness. Rest in a padded knee splint is usually curative.

Plica syndrome

Embryologically, the knee is divided into three synovial compartments, which break down in the fourth intrauterine month. Failure of complete breakdown leaves synovial shelves or plicae. Pain arising from these is termed the plica syndrome. The infrapatellar plica (ligamentum mucosum) is the most common but does not usually become inflamed or cause pain. The suprapatellar plica is a remnant of the membrane that separates the suprapatellar pouch from the rest of the knee. This may be virtually complete, with only a small foramen, or it may be seen as a crescentic fold[24]. It occasionally causes symptoms if it becomes inflamed. The medial patellar plica runs along the medial wall of the joint from the suprapatellar pouch to the infrapatellar fold. It is the most frequently symptomatic, becoming inflamed as a result of impingement as it passes over the medial femoral condyle. Occasionally it may be large and cover the medial femoral condyle. The medial patellar plica is the great imitator of symptoms in the knee and can be a diagnostic problem. It may present with pain, typically over the medial femoral condyle, but this may be generalized. A snapping sensation or giving way are also common. The diagnosis may be made clinically by palpating a tender thickened band over the medial femoral condyle. Commonly it is made at arthroscopy, when a plica may be seen to impinge on the medial femoral condyle and there may be an associated impingement lesion. Treatment is initially rest, but the plica may need to be resected arthroscopically if symptoms persist[25].

Malalignment

Historically, measurements of the normal biomechanical access and relationship of indicators of malalignment such as a high Q angle or patellofemoral tilting were suggested as being pathologic. It is now more common to use a combination of Merchant's views, congruence angles and tibial sulcus angle (Fig. 19.22). Patients who have bilateral radiological signs with similar patellofemoral tilt or congruence angles may only have unilateral symptoms.

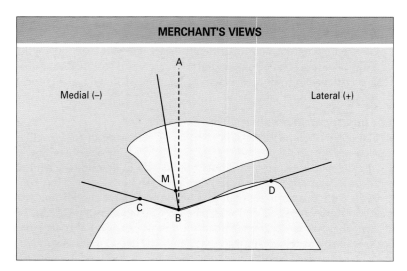

Fig. 19.22 Merchant's views. The congruence angle is determined by firstly bisecting the sulcus angle CBD angle with a line AB. A line joining the median patella ridge M is constructed to join the base of the sulcus at point B. The congruence angle MBA is noted as positive if medial to AB and negative if lateral. (Adapted from Merchant AC, Mercer RL, Jacobsen RH, Cool CR. Roentgenographic analysis of patello-femoral congruence. J Bone Joint Surg 1974; 56A: 1391–1396)

Initially, avoidance of aggravating the symptomatology of the knee is important, whether this be by modification of the patient's activity level or by the use of taping of the patellofemoral joint (McConnell taping) to reduce the load across the joint and reduce the patient's symptomatology (Fig. 19.23)[26]. Rehabilitation, however, requires that muscles are used and the patellofemoral taping and muscle strengthening exercises are essential in regaining normal knee function.

It is inappropriate to force patients to try and strengthen the quadriceps mechanism (e.g. by using unchained quadriceps extension) which may aggravate what is clearly an already uncomfortable joint.

ADULTHOOD

Bursitis

Inflammation of the bursae around the knee is common and on occasion may cause diagnostic difficulty. An accurate knowledge of the anatomic sites of the bursae is helpful.

Prepatellar bursitis is common. The condition is related to recurrent trauma and is seen most often in people who spend a lot of time kneeling, such as carpet-fitters and, in earlier times, housemaids (hence the eponym, 'housemaid's knee'). Diagnosis is usually obvious, with a hot, red, well-circumscribed and fluctuant swelling over the front of the patella. The skin in the area is often thickened. Although the bursa may look infected, in most cases it is not. The inflammation may be caused by trauma or gout. Aspiration is necessary to prove infection and gout. Traumatic cases settle with rest and avoidance of kneeling. Gout responds to non-steroidal anti-inflammatory drugs (NSAIDs). Septic bursitis is treated with rest, preferably with a posterior plaster splint, serial aspirations and parenteral followed by oral antibiotics. Surgical drainage is necessary in loculated or otherwise unimproved cases. Recurrent episodes of inflammation or infection may require surgical excision of the bursa.

Infrapatellar bursitis. The common term for this condition is 'parson's knee'. The presentation and treatment are the same as for prepatellar bursitis.

Anserine bursitis. This term tends to be used loosely to describe pain over the medial aspect of the upper tibia in the region of the anserine bursa. While inflammation of the bursa may be the origin of the pain, it may also arise from the medial collateral ligament or pes anserinus insertion, and the exact anatomic site may be impossible to identify. The conditions of anserine bursitis, medial ligament syndrome and pes anserinus tendonitis may therefore be impossible to separate. Treatment is initially by rest and NSAIDs. In persistent cases injection of a small amount of corticosteroid into the painful area is usually curative.

Bursae on the lateral side of the knee deep to the iliotibial band and the lateral ligament may occasionally become inflamed and cause symptoms.

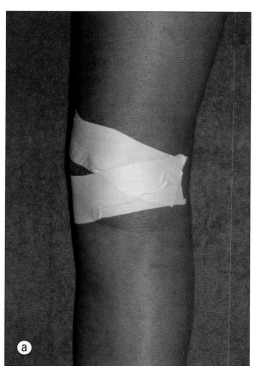

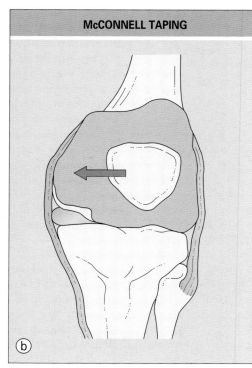

Fig. 19.23 McConnell taping. (a) Left knee showing a form of McConnell taping used to treat anterior knee pain in a middle-aged woman with lateral patellar pain. (b) The direction in which it is intended to pull the patella by the taping method to affect patellar tracking. Arrow indicates the direction of force applied by the patella taping.

Tendinitis and ligament syndromes

Although many tendons cross and are inserted in and around the knee joint, surprisingly few are associated with pathology or debilitating conditions. The major tendinous problem that occurs in and around the knee is associated with the patellar tendon, which is in a unique position, being part of the patellofemoral complex and under immense strain during flexion and extension.

Patellar tendinitis (jumper's knee)[27] is a condition that most commonly affects young sportsmen but may also affect older patients. The symptoms are of pain at the inferior pole of the patella that is brought on by activity, particularly climbing stairs, running and jumping. The condition is a subject of conjecture as to the etiology of pain and the method of treatment. In certain individuals mucoid degeneration of the patellar tendon at its insertion into the inferior pole of the patella can be noted while in others no specific abnormality can be determined. The majority of cases respond to rest, modification of training activities and NSAIDs. For those that do not, injection of a small amount of corticosteroid (<40mg) into the tender area may be of benefit. As with most tendinopathies there is a potential risk with repeated injection of corticosteroids around tendons of softening or rupture. Occasionally, operative treatment to excise the involved portion of tendon is necessary. The role of the intra-articular fat pad in the prognosis of knee pain associated with the infrapatellar region is incompletely understood; however, occasionally arthroscopic removal of the inferior pole of the patella and/or portions of the fat pad may be of assistance if conservative methods have failed.

Pes anserinus tendinitis. The pes anserinus insertion may become inflamed but this may be indistinguishable clinically from anserine bursitis and the medial ligament syndrome. In cases of overuse, rest is usually curative but in persistent cases a small amount of corticosteroid may be injected into the point of maximum tenderness.

Popliteus tendinitis is also an overuse injury, which causes pain over the lateral aspect of the joint. It is caused by inflammation of the popliteus tendon as it passes beneath the arcuate ligament complex. Symptoms usually settle with rest and NSAIDs.

Iliotibial band friction syndrome (runner's knee) occurs in runners and is due to overuse[28]. It tends to occur in patients with genu varum and planus feet. The symptoms are of pain over the lateral epicondyle of the femur during running and are thought to be due to friction between the iliotibial band and the femur and may be due to an inflamed bursa. Tenderness is found over the lateral epicondyle. The symptoms usually settle with rest but in resistant cases a corticosteroid injection into the tender site may help.

Medial ligament syndrome is an ill-defined syndrome in which the patient complains of pain at the site of insertion of the medial ligament. Examination reveals tenderness over the insertion of the ligament, and valgus stress may exacerbate the pain. It is more common in women than in men and is associated with valgus knees and the pain amplification syndrome. As stated previously, it may be difficult to differentiate from anserine bursitis and pes anserinus tendonitis. The etiology is obscure but in some cases an inflammatory arthropathy, such as ankylosing spondylitis, is present. Treatment is initially conservative with rest and heat. Persistent symptoms usually settle following injection of a small amount of corticosteroid into the painful area.

Pellegrini–Stieda disease. Following an injury to the medial collateral ligament, the patient presents with pain over the femoral insertion, particularly on activity. The area is tender to palpation and pain is elicited on stressing the ligament. Radiographs reveal characteristic calcification at the ligament insertion[29] (Fig. 19.24). The condition is most probably due to calcification of a hematoma following injury to the femoral insertion of the medial collateral ligament. Treatment consists of rest and NSAIDs, since the condition is usually self-limiting.

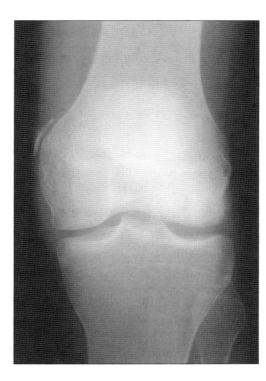

Fig. 19.24 Pellegrini–Stieda disease. Radiograph showing calcification of the insertion of the medial collateral ligament.

Occasionally, a small amount of corticosteroid injected into the area will help to resolve a persistent case.

Popliteal cysts and swelling

Swellings occurring in the popliteal region are common and should be called popliteal cysts regardless of where they originate[14]. They may occur at any age from childhood onwards. The frequency of a communication between the knee joint and the gastrocnemius–semimembranosus bursa increases with age[30,31]. The communication occurs where the tendon of the medial head of gastrocnemius leaves the joint capsule. With increasing age, degeneration and loss of elasticity occurs in the capsule, allowing a tear into the bursa to occur when the knee is extended. Fluid in the knee joint may then flow into the bursa, causing it to distend.

The presenting complaint is usually of a swelling at the back of the knee. The swelling may be associated with aching and is more prominent when the knee is extended. In children there is usually no other abnormality found on examination of the knee but in adults the cysts are most commonly associated with rheumatoid arthritis and osteoarthritis. Plain radiographs may show a soft tissue swelling, and double-contrast arthrography will confirm the diagnosis in those that communicate with the joint. Ultrasound is a reliable method of differentiating cysts from aneurysms and solid swellings. CT scanning and MRI are useful, particularly where the diagnosis is in doubt and for preoperative planning. The differential diagnosis includes popliteal artery aneurysm, ganglia, nerve sheath tumors and sarcoma.

Popliteal cysts may become very large as the result of a valve effect probably caused by inspissated debris, particularly in rheumatoid arthritis. If they burst they may simulate a deep vein thrombosis (pseudothrombophlebitis syndrome). The signs in the calf are similar but differentiation can usually be made due to a history of swelling in the popliteal fossa and the sudden onset of pain, often with a sensation of water running down the leg. Ultrasound in the early stages usually differentiates between the two. A venogram may be needed to conclusively rule out deep vein thrombosis.

Treatment in children should be conservative, as the cysts commonly decrease in size spontaneously and those which are operated on have a high recurrence rate. Treatment in adults should be aimed at the underlying pathology[32]. Knee aspiration and corticosteroid injection may be performed. Arthroscopic knee synovectomy often leads to spontaneous resorption of the cyst.

Synovial chondromatosis

Synovial chondromatosis is a rare condition of unknown etiology in which multiple metaplastic foci of cartilage develop in joints, tendon sheaths and bursae. It occurs as a result of metaplasia in the subsynovial connective tissue. The cartilaginous bodies may become pedunculated or loose in the joint (Fig. 19.25). The knee is by far the most common joint affected by both intra-articular and extra-articular disease. Milgram[33] classified the disease into three phases: early, with active intrasynovial disease but no loose bodies; transitional, with active intrasynovial disease and loose bodies; and late, with multiple loose bodies but no synovial disease.

The condition tends to occur in middle age but may present as early as the late teens[34]. Pain is the usual presenting feature, commonly associated with swelling. Locking may be a feature when the lesions are loose or pedunculated. Examination reveals a swollen knee with thickened synovium, crepitus on movement and palpable loose bodies. In the later stages the range of motion may be decreased.

Radiographs in the early stages may show multiple, stippled cartilaginous bodies. Double-contrast arthrography is useful. In the later stages of the disease when the lesions have calcified they become more obvious on plain radiographs. Treatment of symptomatic disease involves arthroscopy or arthrotomy and removal of symptomatic loose bodies. In the first and second phases of disease the active synovium should be excised. Total synovectomy is impractical and unnecessary. Recurrence is only likely with generalized active disease, in which case a second arthrotomy may be necessary. The condition tends to resolve with time.

Pigmented villonodular synovitis

This condition, which tends to affect young adults, is characterized by a proliferative synovial reaction. The synovium becomes nodular and brown in color. The etiology of the condition is unknown. The knee joint is the most commonly affected joint.

The presenting complaint is usually of pain and swelling. Locking may occur if the proliferative synovium becomes trapped between the joint surfaces. Examination reveals a swollen joint with thickened synovium and limitation of movement. Radiographs show lytic bone lesions and soft tissue swelling. Double contrast arthrography shows multiple filling defects in the synovium, which are diagnostic. MRI shows bone and synovial changes that are highly suggestive of the condition. Aspiration of brown synovial fluid in the absence of recent trauma is characteristic and may often be the first indication of the disease. On arthroscopy, thickened nodular synovium which is reddish brown in color is seen. Histological examination shows a stroma of reticulum and collagen fibers with multi-nucleated giant cells, foam cells and hemosiderin deposits.

Treatment is by synovectomy, preferably arthroscopic. This may need to be repeated, as the disease is liable to recur. Marked bone destruction can occur and may require radiation therapy in extreme cases[35].

KNEE INJURIES

The knee remains the most common joint to be injured in sporting activity. The structures traumatized most commonly are the soft tissues and ligaments surrounding the knee and less frequently the intra-articular structures, the menisci, and cruciate ligaments.

Meniscal injuries

The meniscus in the young is a resilient fibrocartilaginous structure. With age and degenerative change it loses this resilience and becomes stiffer. Thus, different types of meniscal injury are seen in different age groups.

Meniscal injuries are common in young adults, usually occurring secondary to sport injuries and often in combination with ligamentous injury (particularly rupture of the ACL). Meniscal injuries are also associated with chronic instability. The mechanism of the injury is usually a twisting force applied to the weight-bearing knee, causing entrapment of the meniscus between the tibial and femoral condyles. The resulting tear is usually longitudinal. If the tear is extensive the inner portion may displace into the joint causing the knee to lock (a bucket handle tear; Fig. 19.26). This locking may be intermittent as the torn portion flips in and out of the joint. A tear may extend to the inner margin of the meniscus, forming a 'parrot beak' tear. The flap formed can displace into the joint, causing intermittent locking. Peripheral meniscal detachment may also occur.

In the older age group, where the meniscus is less elastic, degenerative tears can occur[36]. These tears are usually horizontal cleavage tears or radial tears running into the substance of the meniscus.

The history of an acute meniscal tear in a young adult is often characteristic. A twisting injury occurs, causing immediate severe pain. The patient is unable to weight-bear and may be unable to fully extend the knee if a bucket handle tear has lodged in the joint. The knee swells within several hours. If a cruciate ligament rupture is also present, a hemarthrosis will accumulate within an hour. The patient complains of pain well localized to the joint line. Examination reveals a painful knee

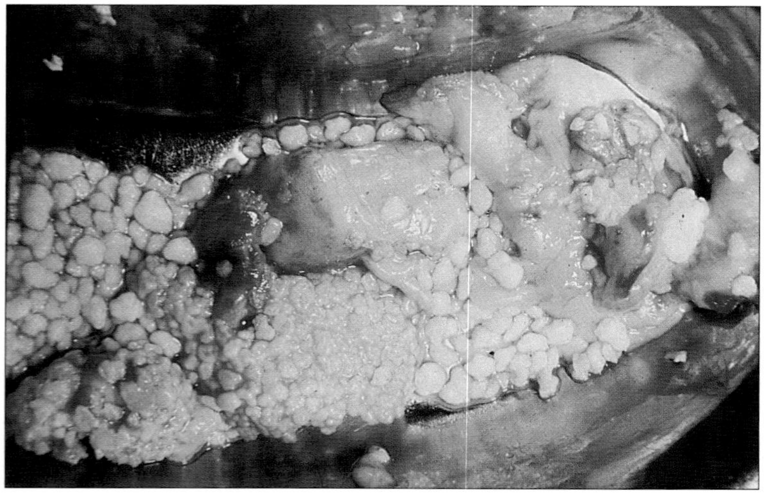

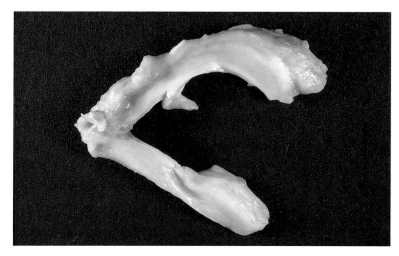

Fig. 19.25 Synovial chondromatosis. Cartilaginous bodies in the joint.

Fig. 19.26 Bucket-handle tear of the meniscus. (With permission from Bullough PG. Orthopaedic pathology, 3rd ed. London: Mosby-Wolfe; 1997.)

with tenderness over the joint line adjacent to the tear. An effusion is virtually always present and, if the torn portion has displaced into the joint, a springy block to full extension is felt.

In a chronic tear the patient may complain of pain over the joint line and a feeling of 'catching'. Joint line tenderness is usually present. True locking occurs when the torn portion of the meniscus displaces into the joint, causing loss of full extension. Locking due to a meniscal tear always occurs with the knee flexed, although not necessarily weight-bearing. Examination of a knee locked due to a meniscal tear reveals a springy block to extension; forced extension is painful. Flexion is usually full or only mildly reduced due to pain. Patients often confuse locking with stiffness and it is important to distinguish between the two. If the knee unlocks with a click or a clunk it is suggestive of a meniscal tear.

McMurray's test[37] is widely used to diagnose meniscal tears. The test involves flexing and extending the knee while the tibia is first internally rotated and then externally rotated, with the thumb and fingers over the joint line. Pain and an associated click are said to be diagnostic of a meniscal tear. Apley's grinding test[38] is performed with the patient prone and the knee flexed. Downward pressure is exerted on the tibia while it is internally and externally rotated. Pain or a clicking sensation are said to be suggestive of a meniscal tear. However, these tests are not specific.

While the majority of acute and chronic meniscal injuries can be diagnosed on the history and examination, confirmation may be obtained by arthrography, MRI or arthroscopy (Fig. 19.27). Although MRI is accurate, if the tear is symptomatic, arthroscopy is preferable, as the tear can be excised at the same time.

The treatment of a symptomatic meniscal tear in a young adult depends on the site of the tear. If the tear is peripheral, in the outer one-third, there is potential for healing and surgical repair should be considered. If the tear involves the avascular inner two thirds, arthroscopic partial meniscectomy is the treatment of choice. The recovery following this is much quicker than following arthrotomy and total meniscectomy.

It is well recognized that total meniscectomy increases the risk of degenerative change[39]. Jackson found a 21% incidence of degeneration following total meniscectomy compared with a 5% incidence on the other side[40]. The effect of partial meniscectomy has not been determined but it is likely that the rate of degeneration will be less than with total meniscectomy. As much of the meniscus as possible should be retained to leave a 'balanced' stable rim.

In older patients with degenerative tears, an initiating injury may not be remembered. Patients usually complain of acute, well-localized joint line pain, which may wake them from sleep. Examination usually reveals joint line tenderness and a small effusion, although this is not a constant feature. Plain radiographs may reveal mild degenerative change, and arthrography or MRI will confirm the diagnosis. Symptoms often settle

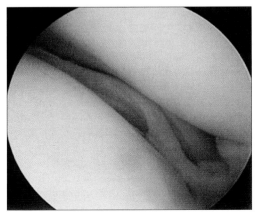

Fig. 19.27 Arthroscopic view of meniscal tear.

with conservative treatment but arthroscopic resection of the torn portion of the meniscus may be required.

Ligamentous injuries

Ligamentous injuries are common in young athletes. The diagnosis and treatment of knee ligament injuries has improved over the past 15 years. The recognition of rotatory instability as a result of ligamentous injury and its effect on knee function has been an important advance. Arthroscopy has enabled accurate diagnosis of intra-articular pathology and recognition of the association between instability, meniscal tears and degeneration. Most of the ligaments of the knee have dual roles; the loss of one ligament may initially be masked by the secondary restraining structures. Over a period of time these secondary restraints may stretch and the instability become evident.

A ligament sprain is an injury in which the fibers are torn. In a first-degree sprain there are torn fibers but unimpaired function. In a second degree sprain more fibers are torn, with stretching of the ligament, causing abnormal joint movement. A third-degree sprain implies complete tearing and loss of function with marked abnormal motion. This is used synonymously with the term 'rupture'[41]. The degree of instability following a ligament injury is described by the amount of abnormal tibial movement that occurs in relation to the femur during testing. Hence 1+ laxity is up to 5mm; 2+ is 5–10mm; and 3+ is 10–15mm. The pivot shift phenomenon is also scored on a 0–3 scale.

Examination of the unstable knee varies depending on the time from injury. In the acute phase, examination may be difficult because of pain and swelling. The knee should be examined for localized swelling, bruising and effusion or hemarthrosis; 70% are associated with an ACL tear. Examination and arthroscopy under general anesthetic may be necessary to define the extent of the damage if pain precludes an adequate clinical assessment. Radiographs should always be obtained to rule out associated fractures.

Tests for collateral ligament rupture

The integrity of the medial collateral ligament is tested by applying a valgus stress with the knee held in 30° of flexion. Opening of the joint compared to the other side suggests laxity or rupture of the medial collateral ligament and posteromedial capsule. The test should be repeated with the knee in full extension. If laxity is present it suggests a tear of the medial collateral ligament, medial capsule, posteromedial corner and the PCL[42]. This is because in full extension all these structures act as a check to valgus movement. The same test should be repeated using a varus stress with the knee in 30° of flexion to test the lateral collateral ligament and posterolateral capsule. The test should be repeated in full extension to test these and the PCL[43].

Test for cruciate ligament laxity

With the knees flexed to 90° the profile of each knee should be examined. In PCL rupture the tibia sags back compared to the normal side, and when the tibia is pushed posteriorly no solid end point is felt. If this posterior sag is not recognized, a PCL rupture may be mistaken for an ACL rupture as the tibia is reduced from its subluxated position during the anterior drawer test (Fig. 19.28). In ACL rupture the knee may be seen to hyperextend slightly, as the ACL helps to limit extension. The anterior drawer test is performed with the knee flexed to 90° and the hamstrings relaxed. The tibia is pulled forwards on the femur. An increase in anterior translation of the tibia on the femur compared to the other side is suggestive of an ACL tear. If the PCL is intact, on internal rotation of the foot the amount of anterior drawer will be reduced. This is due to the PCL tightening and drawing the tibia onto the femur. With the foot in external rotation the anterior translation is often increased due to unwinding of the PCL.

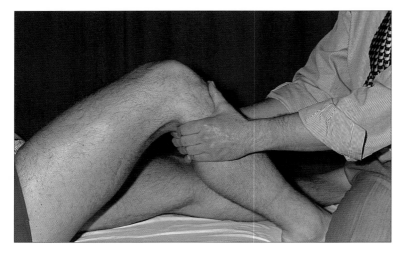

Fig. 19.28 The anterior drawer test. The test is performed with the knee in 90° of flexion and should be repeated with the tibia in internal and external rotation.

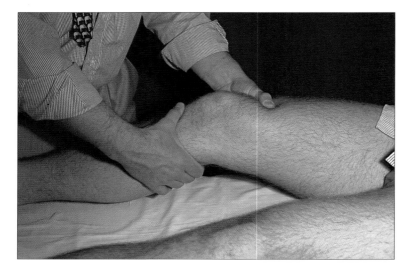

Fig. 19.29 Lachman test for tears of the cruciate ligaments.

The Lachman test is similar to the anterior drawer test but the knee is held in 20° of flexion and the tibia is pulled forward on the femur[44]. An increase in this anterior translation suggests an ACL tear (Fig. 19.29). If the examiner's hands are small or the patient has a large leg, it often helps to rest the patient's knee on the examiner's thigh.

Rotatory instability

Anterolateral rotatory instability is the most common type to occur with ACL rupture. The ACL is the primary restraint to anterior translation and internal rotation of the tibia on the femur. When it is ruptured the tibia is able to move forwards and internally rotate on the femur. This subluxation of the lateral tibial condyle occurs at between 15° and 20° of knee flexion, causing the pivot shift phenomenon[45]. The pivot shift is simply the term used to describe the phenomenon of subluxation or reduction of the tibia on the femur in a knee with anterolateral rotatory instability. This subluxation is what the patient describes as the knee 'giving way'. The secondary restraints of capsule, collateral ligaments and muscles may prevent subluxation during activity but, if they have been damaged or become lax due to excessive loading and subsequent stretching, functional instability can occur.

A variety of tests have been described for the pivot shift phenomenon. The jerk test for anterolateral instability is performed with the examiner's upper hand over the tibia and the thumb behind the head of the

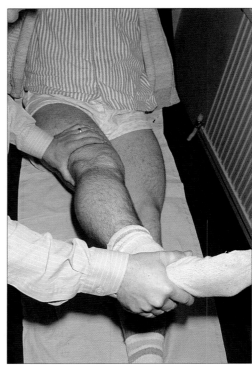

Fig. 19.30 The pivot shift test. Anterolateral tibial subluxation is created by applying an internal rotation and valgus force to the tibia while holding the knee in full extension. As the knee is flexed the tibia will suddenly reduce, often accompanied by a click.

fibula exerting a valgus force on the knee. The examiner's other hand internally rotates the foot (Fig. 19.30). As the knee is extended the lateral tibial condyle subluxates forwards, usually with a clunk, which the patient may recognize as the sensation experienced when the knee gives way. If the knee is then extended the tibial condyle will reduce again, often with a second clunk.

Anteromedial instability may also occur when the ACL is damaged in association with a lax medial collateral ligament and capsule. In this case the medial tibial condyle subluxates forwards. Anteromedial and anterolateral instability may coexist.

The reverse pivot shift is the opposite of the pivot shift phenomenon and is due to posterior subluxation of the lateral tibial condyle because of an injury to the posterolateral corner of the knee, and often the PCL as well[46]. The reverse pivot shift test is essentially the reverse of the jerk test. The foot is held externally rotated while the upper hand applies a valgus force to the knee. As the knee is extended the lateral tibial condyle reduces at approximately 20° of flexion with a clunk.

Anterior cruciate ligament injuries

The ACL is often injured with surprisingly little force. An acute tear is usually associated with a hemarthrosis[47]. A pitfall occurs when an ACL tear is associated with capsular disruption when a tense hemarthrosis does not accumulate as the blood leaks out into the calf. Bruising and swelling in the calf is often an indication of serious knee disruption. The injury is usually a twisting injury. Two main mechanisms are recognized: a valgus external rotation injury to a flexed knee associated with damage to other structures; and a hyperextension internal rotation injury resulting in an isolated ACL tear. The patient usually feels the knee go out of joint and may hear a 'pop'. The ACL injury may be missed in the acute phase if other more obvious structures, such as the medial collateral ligament, are damaged. The Lachman test is a reliable indicator of ACL rupture and may be performed on an acutely injured knee without causing too much discomfort. In children, avulsion of the tibial spines tends to occur rather than a mid-substance tear.

Radiographs should be taken to look for avulsion injuries of the tibial spines and other associated fractures. A small flake of bone may be seen to be avulsed from the lateral aspect of the tibial condyle just above the fibula[48]. This is called a Segond fracture (Fig. 19.31) and if present

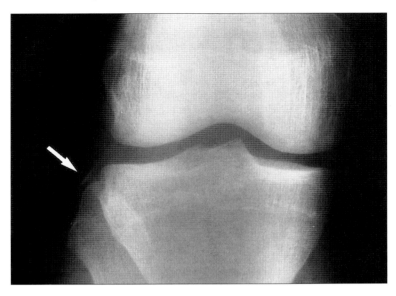

Fig. 19.31 Segond fracture. The figure demonstrates the flake of bone (arrowed), showing the avulsion of the anterolateral capsule in the region of Gerdy's tubercle, frequently associated with ACR.

indicates a 60–70% chance of an ACL injury. If there is doubt about the diagnosis an examination under anesthesia and arthroscopy should be performed.

Approximately 60% of patients with an ACL rupture will have an associated meniscal tear and 20% will have an osteochondral fracture.

The symptoms of an ACL-deficient knee are giving way, swelling and pain. The patient experiences symptoms with twisting or jumping maneuvers. The symptoms are due to rotational instability rather than loss of anteroposterior stability. Symptoms of locking may occur but these are usually due to a coexisting meniscal tear rather than to the ACL rupture itself. The incidence of meniscal tears in knees with functional anterolateral instability increases with time[49].

Treatment for acute ACL tears is controversial and beyond the scope of this chapter. Most cases can be treated conservatively and any subsequent functional instability treated later. In athletes with ACL and associated ligamentous and meniscal damage, acute surgery is indicated.

Symptomatic chronic tears of the ACL in young patients that have not responded to conservative measures may be treated by intra-articular replacement of the ACL with autogenous tissue, such as patellar or semitendinosus tendon. In older patients extra-articular repair may control the instability[46,50].

Posterior cruciate ligament injury

This is much less common than ACL tears and usually occurs as a result of a road traffic accident, when a blow to the anterior aspect of the tibia in a flexed knee forces the tibia posteriorly, rupturing the PCL. Unless other structures have also been damaged, the function of the knee following PCL rupture is usually good and reconstruction is not necessary[51]. Conservative treatment consists of a plaster cast for 6 weeks with the knee in 20° of flexion, followed by rehabilitation in a knee brace.

Medial collateral ligament injuries

The medial collateral ligament is usually injured as a result of a valgus force, often associated with external rotation of the tibia. The classic example is a skiing injury where the ski moves laterally, causing a valgus external rotation force on the knee. In the acute phase the findings are of swelling and bruising over the course of the ligament with tenderness over the joint line or femoral insertion. Loss of full extension may be present in an incomplete tear due to pain as the ligament comes under

tension in the last 20° of extension. Such injuries may be associated with meniscal or ACL injury necessitating an examination under anesthetic and arthroscopy. Treatment for isolated medial collateral ligament tears is conservative, consisting of 4 weeks in a cast brace with the range of motion set between 40° and 60° and then a further 4–6 weeks in a light brace to protect the ligament during rehabilitation[52].

Lateral collateral ligament injuries

The lateral collateral ligament is rarely injured in isolation but is usually torn in association with damage to the posterolateral ligament complex (lateral capsule, arcuate ligament and popliteus tendon). The cruciate ligaments may also be damaged. The mechanism of injury is usually a varus force on a flexed knee. The ligament usually ruptures at its fibular insertion or it may avulse the fibular styloid. A peroneal nerve palsy may be associated with a lateral collateral ligament tear and should be looked for at the time of the injury. Little functional instability arises from an isolated tear of the lateral collateral ligament, which may therefore be treated conservatively in a similar manner to the medial collateral ligament. Lesions of the lateral collateral ligament associated with capsular or cruciate ligament damage should be repaired acutely in active young athletes.

Patellofemoral injuries

Injuries of the patellofemoral joint are common in children and adolescents.

Congenital dislocation

Congenital dislocation occurs in infancy and involves irreducible lateral displacement of the patella[53]. It is associated with genu valgum, a small patella, hypoplasia of the lateral femoral condyle and tethering of the lateral capsule. Treatment is surgical, to release the tight lateral structures and realign the patella.

Habitual dislocation

In habitual dislocation lateral displacement of the patella occurs every time the knee is flexed. It is due to contracture of the vastus lateralis and iliotibial band with an abnormal insertion of the iliotibial band into the patella[54]. Because of this lateral contracture the patella must dislocate to allow the knee to flex. The constant physical sign is an inability to flex the knee when the patella is held reduced. Treatment is usually surgical and involves proximal realignment of the quadriceps mechanism by releasing the contracted lateral structures and, if necessary, lengthening the rectus femoris.

Recurrent dislocation and subluxation

Recurrent dislocation and subluxation of the patella are conditions in which intermittent episodes of dislocation or subluxation occur, and may be grouped together under the heading of patellar instability. This is common in adolescence, particularly in girls, but may also occur in younger children. It is associated with a variety of developmental abnormalities. These include generalized or localized joint laxity, patella alta and hypoplasia of the lateral femoral condyle. Genu valgum, external tibial torsion and persistent femoral anteversion increase the Q angle and predispose to patellar instability.

In adolescence, patellar instability may follow an acute traumatic dislocation or occur spontaneously[55]. In acute dislocation the patient describes the patella dislocating laterally and may reduce it by pushing it back. Examination in the acute phase reveals a painful swollen knee with obvious lateral dislocation of the patella. If the patella has already been reduced the chief findings are of tenderness over the torn medial retinaculum associated with knee swelling. Acute dislocation may be associated with an osteochondral fracture of the lateral femoral condyle. Treatment in the acute phase is by immobilization in a plaster cast for 4 weeks, which allows the torn retinacular fibers to heal, followed by an isometric exercise program to restore the power of the quadriceps, particularly the vastus medialis obliquus.

In the chronic phase the diagnosis of recurrent dislocation is straightforward. The patient is usually an adolescent girl describing episodes of lateral dislocation of the patella, which either reduce spontaneously or she pushes back. The episodes usually occur during activities that involve knee flexion but in severe cases may occur during everyday activities. Recurrent subluxation of the patella is more common than dislocation and is caused by the same factors, but the diagnosis may be more difficult to make. The patient often complains of a feeling of instability as the patella rides up on the lateral femoral condyle, and the knee may give way. Pain is due to compression of the lateral facet of the patella against the lateral femoral condyle. Pseudo-locking due to pain is common. The majority of cases are secondary to weakness of the vastus medialis obliquus associated with bony malalignment.

Examination may reveal any of the anatomic abnormalities mentioned above, and the patella may be found to track laterally on flexion of the knee. In the majority of adolescent girls with this condition there is poor muscle tone in the quadriceps, particularly the vastus medialis, and the Q angle may be increased as a result of the factors mentioned earlier[10]. Patellar tracking should be assessed clinically, as described in the section on examination. The apprehension test is usually positive in recurrent subluxation and dislocation. This is performed with the knee flexed to 30° and the examiner gently pushing the patella laterally. A positive test occurs when the patient feels as though the patella is going to dislocate; occasionally the patient will push the examiner's hand away. In some girls with a small, high patella it may be seen to sit laterally in full extension.

Lateral and anteroposterior views of the knee are useful to look for femorotibial malalignment, osteochondral fractures and patella alta (Fig. 19.32). Patella alta is recognized on the lateral view by comparing the length of the patella to the length of the patellar tendon. In normal knees the ratio is 1. In patella alta the patella is relatively short compared to the tendon and the ratio is less than 0.8[56]. Skyline views of the patella with the knee flexed at 30–40° may show it to be tilted laterally and to ride high on the lateral femoral condyle. A variety of special views and measurements have been described to quantify the degree of subluxation or tilting. The patella should sit centrally in the trochlea with an equal joint space medially and laterally. The skyline views may show it to be tilted laterally with a narrower joint space on the lateral

side. Occasionally, sclerosis may be seen in the subchondral bone of the lateral facet indicating increased stress through it. The angle formed by the lateral facet of the patella and a line drawn across the femoral condyles is called the lateral patellofemoral angle and should be open laterally. If the lines are parallel or the angle is open medially this suggests patellar malalignment[57]. CT scanning with the knee straight and flexed to 30° and 60° may show a laterally displaced patella and a deficient lateral femoral condyle. Unfortunately, radiographic findings such as these are common in the asymptomatic population and should only be taken as significant in conjunction with the clinical picture.

Recurrent dislocation or subluxation of the patella should initially be managed conservatively with isometric quadriceps and hamstring exercises[58]. Most patients will respond to conservative management provided they continue the exercises. Unfortunately many do not and the resultant weakening of the quadriceps may lead to recurrence. In the compliant patients who do not respond to conservative treatment, surgery is usually necessary as the condition can be disabling. An arthroscopic lateral release may be tried if there is a tight lateral tether but open surgery to realign the patella may be necessary.

Other injuries

The most common tendon injury around the knee occurs in the elderly and affects the extensor mechanism. Catching a foot against the edge of a pavement, or tripping, with contraction of the quadriceps may be enough to cause rupture or avulsion of an already degenerate patellar or quadriceps tendon. On examination the patient is unable to extend the knee and there may be a high-riding patella if the patellar tendon has ruptured. If the quadriceps tendon has been avulsed a gap may be palpable above the patella. Fracture of the patella may be secondary to quadriceps contraction or a fall. It is associated with bruising, swelling and tenderness over the patella, and radiographs will confirm the diagnosis.

A direct blow to the knee, particularly the patellofemoral joint, or a minor strain, is likely to produce an effusion in the joint, which develops over a period of 12 hours. The stiffness and discomfort in the knee increase during this period.

Limitation of function is generally slight and spontaneous recovery occurs over a period of 2–3 days, although aching pain may persist for up to 2 weeks. In more severe strains there is tenderness over the ligaments.

THE RELATIONSHIP OF INJURY TO DEGENERATION

The role of trauma in initiating a degenerative process in the knee is well recognized. Intra-articular fractures affect the congruence of the joint, leading to increased pressure loading across the hyaline cartilage, which is then subject to early degeneration.

The importance of accurate reduction of intra-articular fractures is therefore paramount, although the risk of degeneration persists to a minor degree even with full anatomical reconstruction.

Any injury that alters the biomechanics of the knee joint and leads to an alteration in the pressure occurring across the hyaline cartilage surfaces will lead to degeneration. It has been indicated that the removal of meniscal material is known to cause degenerative processes to occur in the knee. Although this takes many years to develop, the removal of the meniscus, especially on the lateral side, will inevitably lead to a narrowing of the joint space and collapse of the joint into a malaligned position.

Where total meniscectomy has been performed there is a high likelihood that the patient will need a knee replacement in later life. The rate of degeneration varies depending on concomitant ligamentous injuries and the age and function of the individual, but most individuals will have significant symptomatology related to the meniscal removal within 40 years.

The role of ligamentous injury in stimulating degenerate change in the knee is now well recognized. The ACL, when torn, produces an instab-

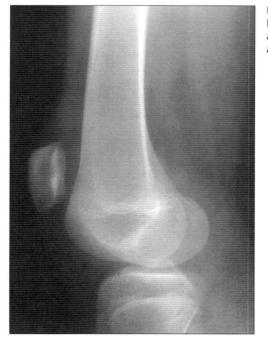

**Fig. 19.32
Radiographic appearance of patella alta.**

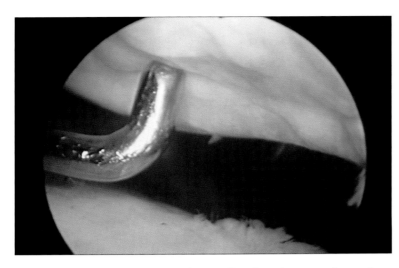

Fig. 19.33 Degeneration of the hyaline cartilage knee in an anterior cruciate deficient knee. Arthroscopic view of the loss of the hyaline cartilage from the medial femoral condyle in an anterior cruciate deficient knee.

ility pattern in the knee that, in both treated and untreated individuals, leads to an increased risk of degenerative change (Fig. 19.33). There is little historical evidence to support the suggestion that the stabilization of an individual with an ACL-deficient knee will reduce degenerative change[59].

There are encouraging short-term reports of a potential reduction in the rate of secondary meniscal tears and degeneration with modern reconstructive methods but no long-term prospective study has yet shown conclusive evidence of a reduction in the rate or extent of osteoarthritis. The multifactorial nature of knee ligament instability and the different activity levels of individuals both before and after surgery make long-term studies difficult to interpret. The present evidence suggests that, once an ACL is torn, the prognosis in terms of function of the knee and long-term risk of degenerate change is deleteriously affected.

Stabilization can reduce the symptomatology, reduce the risk of meniscal tears and increase short-term activity levels but is still associated with long-term morbidity.

The understanding of the mechanical function of the knee has progressed rapidly over the last two decades, as have the methods for determining the degeneration of hyaline cartilage in the osteoarthritic knee. The natural history of any single patient who has an osteoarthritic knee is multifactorial and there can be no certainty in suggesting a single method of management that will produce the optimum result for that individual.

INJECTION OF THE KNEE

Although the knee is a large joint that is readily accessible for both drainage of fluid and injection using a wide-bore needle, access to the joint cavity may prove to be difficult, especially in patients without an effusion and with large amounts of adipose tissue.

The capsule of the knee is large and expands almost a hand's breadth above the patella, but contains, in the non-inflamed patient, only a few milliliters of synovial fluid. In addition, the fat pad lies behind the patellofemoral joint and fits snugly against the condylar surface, filling the potential space in the anterior aspect of the knee.

The most reliable technique for accessing the knee approaches from the lateral side. With the patient lying supine the upper and lateral borders of the patella are noted. The patella is moved sideways in order to palpate the gap inferiorly between the patella and the lateral femoral condyle. Although local anesthetic need not be used universally, 2ml of 1% lidocaine inserted into the injection site in the subcutaneous tissue using a 22 gauge needle will enable the injection or aspiration of material from the knee to be accomplished painlessly. Having instilled the local anesthetic an 18 or 21 gauge needle is inserted under the patella at the superolateral aspect and the needle will be felt to meet initial resistance before entering the joint cavity. A free injection of fluid or aspiration of any effusion will be easily accomplished. The appropriate dose of corticosteroid for the knee joint is 40mg of methyl prednisolone.

The knee may also be approached from the anteromedial or anterolateral aspect with the knee held in 90° of flexion. Caution must be applied when using this technique as injection into the fat pad is easy and this may well stimulate pain and discomfort.

Degenerative disease is the most common cause of knee pain in those aged over 50 years. The knee is affected by osteoarthritis more commonly than any other joint (see Chapter 39). The pain is associated with stiffness and swelling, especially after activity. Loose bodies secondary to the degeneration may cause episodes of sharp pain associated with locking of the joint. Periarticular causes include bursitis and tendonitis. Referred pain in this age group is usually secondary to osteoarthritis of the hip.

REFERENCES

1. Goodfellow J, Hungerford DS, Zindel M. Patello-femoral mechanics and pathology: I. Functional anatomy of the patello-femoral joint. J Bone Joint Surg 1976; 58B: 287–290.
2. Price CT, Allen WC. Ligament repair in the knee with preservation of the meniscus. J Bone Joint Surg 1978; 60A: 61–65.
3. Last RJ. Some anatomical details of the knee joint. J Bone Joint Surg 1948; 30B: 683–688.
4. Last RJ. The popliteus muscle and the lateral meniscus. J Bone Joint Surg 1950; 32B: 93–99.
5. Arnoczky SP, Warren RF. Microvasculature of the human meniscus. Am J Sports Med 1982; 10: 90–95.
6. Brantigan OC, Voshell AF. The tibial collateral ligament: its function, its bursae and its relation to the medial meniscus. J Bone Joint Surg 1943; 25: 121–131.
7. Warren LF, Marshall JL, Girgis FG. The prime static stabiliser of the medial side of the knee. J Bone Joint Surg 1974; 56A: 665–674.
8. Girgis FG, Marshall JL, Al Monajem ARS. The cruciate ligaments of the knee joint. Clin Orthop 1975; 106: 216–231.
9. Seebacher JR, Ingilis AE, Marshal JL et al. The structure of the posterolateral aspect of the knee. J Bone Joint Surg 1982; 64A 536–541.
10. Aglietti P, Insall JN, Cerulli G. Patellar pain and incongruence I: measurements of incongruence. Clin Orthop 1983; 176: 217–224.
11. Fulkerson JP, Gossling HR. Anatomy of the knee joint lateral retinaculum. Clin Orthop 1980; 153: 183–188.
12. Kaplan EB. The iliotibial tract. Clinical and morphological significance. J Bone Joint Surg 1985; 40A: 817–832.
13. Henigan SP, Schneck CD, Mesgarzadeh M, Clancy M. The semimembranosus–tibial collateral ligament bursa. J Bone Joint Surg 1994: 76A: 1322–1327.
14. Burleson RJ, Bickel WH, Dahlin DC. Popliteal cyst. A clinico-pathological survey. J Bone Joint Surg 1956; 38A: 1265–1274.
15. Apley AG, Solomon L. The knee joint. In: Apley's system of orthopaedics and fractures, 6th ed. London: Butterworths; 1982: 277–305.
16. Osgood RB. Lesions of the tibial tubercle occurring during adolescence. Boston Med Surg J 1903; 148: 114.
17. Ogden JA, Southwick WO. Osgood–Schlatter's disease and tibial tuberosity development. Clin Orthop 1976; 116: 180–189.
18. Sinding-Larsen C. A hitherto unknown affection of the patella in children. Acta Radiol 1921; 1: 171.
19. Wilson JN. A diagnostic sign in osteochondritis dissecans of the knee. J Bone Joint Surg 1967; 49B: 440–447.
20. Cahill B. The treatment of juvenile osteochondritis dissecans and osteochondritis dissecans of the knee. Clin Sports Med 1985; 4: 367.
21. Hughston JC, Stone M, Andrews JR. The suprapatellar plica: its role in internal derangement of the knee. J Bone Joint Surg 1973; 55A: 1318.
22. Aichroth P. Osteochondritis dissecans of the knee. A clinical survey. J Bone Joint Surg 1971; 53B: 440–447.
23. Stanitski CL. Anterior knee pain syndromes in the adolescent. J Bone Joint Surg 1993; 75A: 1407–1416.
24. Johnson DP, Eastwood DM, Witherow PJ. Symptomatic synovial plicae of the knee. J Bone Joint Surg 1993; 75A: 1485–1496.

25. Patel D. Arthroscopy of the plicae: synovial folds and their significance. Am J Sports Med 1978; 6: 217.
26. McConnell J. The management of chondromalacia patellae: a long-term solution. Aust J Physiother 1986; 32: 215–223.
27. James SL. Running injuries to the knee. J Am Acad Orthop Surg 1995; 3: 309–318.
28. Renne JW. The iliotibial band friction syndrome. J Bone Joint Surg 1975; 57A: 1110–1111.
29. Nachlas IW, Olpp JL. Para-articular calcification (Pellegrini–Stieda) in affectations of the knee. Surg Gynecol Obstet 1945; 81: 206–212.
30. Lindgren PG, Willen R. Gastrocnemio-semimembranosus bursa and its relation to the knee joint. I. Anatomy and histology. Acta Radiol 1977; 18: 497–512.
31. Lindgren PG. Gastrocnemio-semimembranosus bursa and its relation to the knee joint. IV. Clinical considerations. Acta Radiol 1978; 19: 609–622.
32. Rauschning W, Lindgren PG. Popliteal cysts (Baker's cysts) in adults. I. Clinical and roentgenological results of operative excision. Acta Orthop Scand 1979; 50: 583–591.
33. Milgram JW. Synovial osteochondromatosis: a histo-pathological study of thirty cases. J Bone Joint Surg 1977; 59A: 792–801.
34. Maurice H, Crone M, Watt I. Synovial chondromatosis. J Bone Joint Surg 1988; 70B: 807–811.
35. Flandry F, Hughston JC. Pigmented villonodular synovitis. J Bone Joint Surg 1987; 69A: 942–949.
36. Noble J, Hamblen DL. The pathology of the degenerate meniscus lesions. J Bone Joint Surg 1975: 57B: 180–186.
37. McMurray TP. The semilunar cartilages. Br J Surg 1941; 29: 407.
38. Apley AG. The diagnosis of meniscus injuries. Some new clinical methods. J Bone Joint Surg 1947; 29: 78–84.
39. Fairbank TJ. Knee joint changes after meniscectomy. J Bone Joint Surg 1948; 30B: 664–670.
40. Jackson JP. Degenerative changes in the knee after meniscectomy. Br Med J 1968; 2: 525–527.
41. Noyes FR, Grood ES, Torzilli PA. The definitions of terms for motion and position of the knee and injuries of the ligaments. J Bone Joint Surg 1989; 71A: 465–471.
42. Hughston JC, Andrews JR, Cross MJ, Moschi A. Classification of knee ligament instabilities. Part 1. The medial compartment and cruciate ligaments. J Bone Joint Surg 1976; 58A: 159–172.
43. Hughston JC, Andrews JR, Cross MJ, Moschi A. Classification of knee ligament instabilities. Part 2. The lateral compartment. J Bone Joint Surg 1976; 58A: 173–179.
44. Torg JS, Conrad W, Kalen V. Clinical diagnosis of anterior cruciate ligament instability in the athlete. Am J Sports Med 1976; 4: 84–93.
45. Galway RD, Beaupre A, Macintosh DL. Pivot shift: a clinical sign of symptomatic anterior cruciate insufficiency. J Bone Joint Surg 1972; 54B: 763–4.
46. Jakob RP, Hassler H, Staeubli HU. Observations on rotatory instability in the lateral compartment of the knee. Acta Orthop Scand 1981; 191(Suppl): 1–32.
47. DeHaven KE. Diagnosis of acute knee injuries with hemarthrosis. Am J Sports Med 1980; 8: 9–14.
48. Fairclough JA, Graham GP, Dent CM. Radiological sign of chronic anterior cruciate ligament deficiency. Injury 190; 21: 401–2.
49. Indelicato PA, Bittar ES. A perspective of lesions associated with ACL insufficiency in the knee. A review of 100 cases. Clin Orthop 1985; 198: 77–80.
50. Ireland J, Trickey EL. Macintosh tenodesis for anterolateral instability of the knee. J Bone Joint Surg 1980; 62B: 340–345.
51. Cross MJ, Powell JF. The long term follow up of posterior cruciate ligament rupture: a study of 116 cases. Am J Sports Med 1984; 12: 292–297.
52. Indelicato PA. Non operative treatment of complete tears of the medial collateral ligament of the knee. J Bone Joint Surg 1983; 65A: 323–329.
53. Jones RD, Fisher RL, Curtis BH. Congenital dislocation of the patella. Clin Orthop 1976; 119: 177–183.
54. Williams PF. Quadriceps contracture. J Bone Joint Surg 1968; 50B: 278–284.
55. Fulkerson JP. Patellofemoral pain disorders: evaluation and management. J Am Acad Orthop Surg 1994; 2: 124–132.
56. Insall J, Salvati E. Patella position in the normal knee joint. Radiology 1971; 101: 101–104.
57. Laurin CA, Levesque HP, Dussault R et al. The abnormal lateral patellofemoral angle: a diagnostic roentgenographic sign of recurrent patellar subluxation. J Bone Joint Surg 1978; 60A: 55–60.
58. Hungerford DS, Lennox DW. Rehabilitation of the knee in disorders of the patellofemoral joint: relevant biomechanics. Orthop Clin North Am 1983; 14: 397–402.
59. Graham GP, Fairclough HA. Early osteoarthritis in young sportsmen with severe antero-lateral instability of the knee. Injury 1988; 19: 247–248.

20 Fibromyalgia and related syndromes

Don L Goldenberg

Clinical features

- A chronic musculoskeletal syndrome characterized by diffuse pain in the absence of synovitis or myositis
- Unremarkable musculoskeletal examination except for tenderness upon palpation of discrete anatomical locations termed tender points
- Associated symptoms include fatigue, sleep disturbances, headaches, irritable bowel syndrome, paresthesias, cognitive disturbances, depression and anxiety

HISTORY

Accurate accounts of fibromyalgia symptoms were reported in the mid-1800s. François Valleix described tender points in 1841 noting 'if, in the interval of the shooting pains, one asks a patient what is the seat of his pain, he replies then by designating limited points. It is only with the aid of pressure that one discovers exactly the extent of the painful points'[1]. Sir William Gowers coined the term 'fibrositis' in 1904, although he actually described regional pain syndromes[2]. He also reported the presence of fatigue and sleep disturbances. Kellgren, in the 1930s, provided eloquent descriptions of referred muscle pain after the injection of hypertonic saline into deep muscle tissue[3]. The distribution of pain referral patterns was uniform and differed from dermatomal patterns. During the next half century, fibrositis, as it was then called, was considered by some to be a common cause of muscular pain, by others to be a manifestation of 'tension' or 'psychogenic rheumatism', and by the rheumatology community in general to be a nonentity.

TABLE 20.1 DIAGNOSTIC FEATURES OF FIBROMYALGIA
Cardinal features*
Chronic, widespread pain Tender points on examination
Characteristic features
Fatigue Sleep disturbances Stiffness Paresthesias Headaches Irritable bowel syndrome Raynaudís-like symptoms Depression Anxiety
*For classification criteria, patients must have pain for at least 3 months involving the upper and lower body, right and left sides, as well as axial skeleton, and pain in at least 11 of 18 tender points on digital examination.

The current concept of fibromyalgia was ushered in by studies from Smythe and Moldofsky in the mid-1970s[4]. They characterized the most common tender points and also reported that patients with fibromyalgia had disturbances in deep and restorative sleep, and that selective stage 4 interruptions induced the symptoms of fibromyalgia. Yunus and others then reported on the major clinical manifestations of patients with fibromyalgia seen in rheumatology clinics[5].

DIAGNOSTIC CRITERIA

Diagnostic criteria for fibromyalgia were suggested, based on the presence of certain symptoms and tender points, together with the exclusion of rheumatic or systemic diseases. Different authors debated the optimal number of tender points, as well as the relevance of the concept of primary and secondary fibromyalgia. Subsequently, a North American multicenter study compared 293 patients with fibromyalgia and 265 control patients with rheumatic disorders that could be easily confused with fibromyalgia, such as 'possible' rheumatoid arthritis (RA) or neck and back pain syndromes. Based on these comparisons, criteria for the classification of fibromyalgia were recommended and adopted by the American College of Rheumatology (Table 20.1)[6]. The combination of widespread pain, defined as pain that was bilateral, above and below the waist, and included axial involvement, together with at least 11 of 18 specified tender points, yielded a sensitivity of 88% and a specificity of 81%. There were no significant differences between patients considered to have primary or secondary fibromyalgia, and for classification purposes such distinctions were to be discarded. No exclusions were made, irrespective of laboratory or radiographic findings.

Controversy persists as to whether fibromyalgia is a discrete entity[7–11]. There has also been concern that attaching an illness label to common symptoms reinforces exaggerated somatic concerns. Nevertheless, the concept of fibromyalgia as a clinical syndrome has been useful for epidemiological and therapeutic studies[7–10]. Furthermore, most physicians report that the fibromyalgia diagnostic label provides reassurance to patients that their symptoms are real, and that many other people have similar symptoms.

EPIDEMIOLOGY

Fibromyalgia is a very common rheumatic disorder, with a prevalence of 1–4% of the population[12–14]. The prevalence has varied as widely as 0–4% in men and 2.5–10.5% in women. Overall, about 75% of those with fibromyalgia are women[14]. The mean patient age at diagnosis is in the fifth decade, with prevalence increasing with age, reaching 7–8% in women of age 60–80 years[12–15]. The prevalence and clinical manifestations of fibromyalgia in children has varied from 1 to 7%[16].

Chronic widespread pain *per se* is more prevalent, occurring in 10–20% of the population[12,15]. Fibromyalgia represents one end of a continuum of pain and fatigue in the population at large[7–10,14,15]. Compared with other patients with chronic widespread pain, those with fibromyalgia have more severe pain and fatigue, more somatic symptoms and worse overall health[7,8,15]. Factors associated with fibromyalgia and also with chronic widespread pain include female sex, pain duration, four or more somatic symptoms, and depression[7–10,14–16]. A number of other disease states have been associated with fibromyalgia, including RA, systemic lupus erythematosus, osteoarthritis, Sjögren's syndrome, neck and back pain, hepatitis C infection and Lyme disease[7–10].

CLINICAL MANIFESTATIONS AND DIAGNOSIS

The cardinal symptom of fibromyalgia is diffuse, chronic pain. The pain often begins in one location, particularly the neck and shoulders, but then becomes more generalized[5,6,9,10,12]. Patients with fibromyalgia typically report that 'it hurts all over'. The muscle pain is often described as burning, radiating or gnawing, and the intensity of the pain as modest or severe. In most studies utilizing pain intensity surveys, such as the

TABLE 20.2 SYNDROMES THAT OVERLAP WITH FIBROMYALGIA

- Chronic fatigue syndrome
- Myofascial pain syndrome
- Irritable bowel syndrome
- Muscle, migraine headaches
- Irritable bladder, interstitial cystitis
- Gulf War syndrome

McGill Pain Questionnaire[17] and visual analog scales, the self-rating of pain intensity by patients with fibromyalgia has been greater than that of those with RA.

Most patients also report profound fatigue[9,10]. This is especially notable at the time of arising from sleep, but also is marked in the mid-

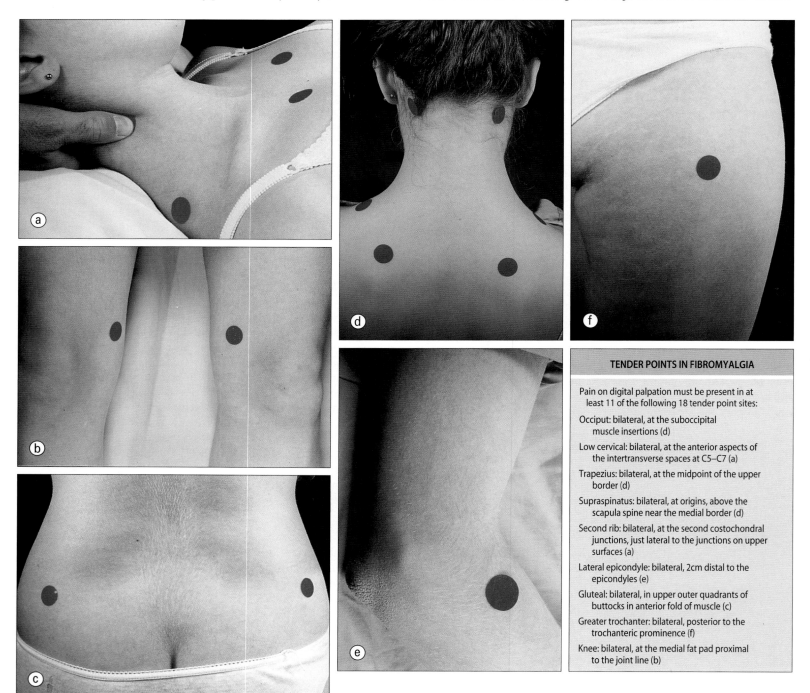

TENDER POINTS IN FIBROMYALGIA

Pain on digital palpation must be present in at least 11 of the following 18 tender point sites:

Occiput: bilateral, at the suboccipital muscle insertions (d)

Low cervical: bilateral, at the anterior aspects of the intertransverse spaces at C5–C7 (a)

Trapezius: bilateral, at the midpoint of the upper border (d)

Supraspinatus: bilateral, at origins, above the scapula spine near the medial border (d)

Second rib: bilateral, at the second costochondral junctions, just lateral to the junctions on upper surfaces (a)

Lateral epicondyle: bilateral, 2cm distal to the epicondyles (e)

Gluteal: bilateral, in upper outer quadrants of buttocks in anterior fold of muscle (c)

Greater trochanter: bilateral, posterior to the trochanteric prominence (f)

Knee: bilateral, at the medial fat pad proximal to the joint line (b)

Fig. 20.1 Locations of the nine pairs of tender points for diagnostic classification of fibromyalgia.

afternoon. Seemingly minor activities aggravate the pain and fatigue, although prolonged inactivity heightens their symptoms. Patients are stiff in the morning and wake unrefreshed, even if they have slept for 8–10 hours. Patients with fibromyalgia characteristically sleep 'lightly', waking frequently during early morning and having difficulty getting back to sleep.

Headaches are frequently present, in as many as 70% of patients; they are often described as muscular, but in one study migraine-type headaches were noted in 50% of patients[18,19]. Irritable bowel syndrome is present in more than 50% of patients[18,20–22]. Surveys have shown that 30% of patients with chronic undifferentiated headaches and irritable bowel syndrome have fibromyalgia[19–22]. Irritable bladder and interstitial cystitis have been commonly reported[23]. These common syndromes overlap with fibromyalgia clinically and physiologically (Table 20.2). Raynaud's phenomenon or excess sensitivity to cold, dizziness, difficulty concentrating, dry eyes and dry mouth, palpitations, and sensitivity to foods, medications and allergens are common[24].

On examination, patients usually appear well, with no obvious systemic illness or articular abnormalities. Many patients describe some joint or soft tissue swelling, but no obvious synovitis is present. As fibromyalgia may complicate any systemic arthritis, the presence of osteoarthritis or RA does not exclude coexistent fibromyalgia. Patients invariably complain of muscle weakness; however, formal muscle testing does not reveal objective weakness, provided the pain does not prevent the patient from achieving maximal effort. Numbness and tingling, especially in the extremities, are present in more than 75% of patients, yet a neurological examination usually does not demonstrate any significant abnormalities.

Thus the only reliable finding on examination is the presence of several tender points[9]. Although various sets of 'best' tender point discriminators in fibromyalgia have been proposed, the currently recommended nine pairs of tender points should be routinely examined, because they were chosen for classification criteria (Fig. 20.1). The examiner must gain experience with the technique and in locating these sites. The patient should be seated comfortably on the examination table and queried as to the presence of pain after the palpation of each bilateral anatomical site. Palpation should be done with the thumb or forefinger, applying pressure approximately equal to a force of 4kg[6]; excessive force may elicit pain in anyone. A systematic palpation of each site, beginning at the suboccipital muscle insertion at the posterior skull, progressing ultimately to the medial fat pad of the knee 2cm proximal to the joint line, should be followed (Fig. 20.1). 'Control' anatomical sites, such as over the thumbnail, midforearm and forehead, should also be palpated. These sites are not as painful on pressure as the selected anatomical sites, although most patients with fibromyalgia are more tender to palpation

TABLE 20.3 MANUAL AND DOLORIMETER TENDER POINT SCORES IN 293 FIBROMYALGIA PATIENTS AND 265 CONTROLS		
Manual tender points	Fibromyalgia	Controls
Mean tenderness (0–4 scale)	1.5	0.5
Number of sites (maximum=24)		
Mild or more than mild tenderness	19.7	8.0
Moderate or more than moderate	12.5	3.6
Severe	5.0	1.3
Mean dolorimeter scores (0–6.5kg/cm scale)		
'Active' 18 sites (9 pairs)	3.4	4.9
Control 6 sites (3 pairs)	5.0	5.8

at any soft tissue site, compared with normal controls. Patients are often not aware of the location of many of the tender points.

The diagnostic utility of a tender point evaluation has been objectively documented with the use of a dolorimeter or algometer – pressure loaded gauges that accurately measure force per area – and by manual palpation (Table 20.3)[6]. Such instruments are useful in controlled studies but, in the clinic, digital palpation is adequate. The nine pairs of tender points are by no means inclusive, but they are representative. The criterion of at least 11 of 18 tender points is recommended for classification purposes, but should not be considered essential to diagnosis in individual patients. Patients with fewer than 11 tender points certainly can be diagnosed with fibromyalgia, provided other symptoms and signs are present. Women with fibromyalgia have lower pain thresholds than men, resulting in greater tender point scores[25,26]. Other common findings on examination include muscle 'spasm' or taut bands of muscle – sometimes referred to by patients as nodules – skin sensitivity, in the form of skin roll tenderness, or dermatographism (Fig. 20.2). Purplish mottling of the skin is often noted, especially of the legs after exposure to the cold. This is sometimes believed to be livido reticularis, but more accurately probably represents cutis marmorata.

INVESTIGATIONS

Laboratory and radiological investigations in fibromyalgia are largely unrevealing, and primarily useful for excluding other conditions[9]. At an initial evaluation, minimal baseline blood tests probably should include

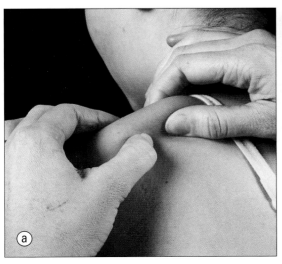
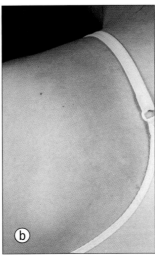

Fig. 20.2 Skin rolling tenderness (a) and reactive hyperemia (b) in fibromyalgia.

a complete blood count, an erythrocyte sedimentation rate, standard blood chemistry and thyroid function studies. These all are usually normal in fibromyalgia. Unless there is evidence of an associated arthritis or possible cervical or lumbar radiculopathy, plain radiographs, computed tomography scans, nuclear scans or magnetic resonance imaging are not generally necessary. Serological tests such as rheumatoid factor, antinuclear antibodies, or Lyme antibody assays are of dubious diagnostic utility. Unless there is a clinical suspicion of a systemic connective tissue disease or Lyme disease, routine ordering of such tests will yield a large proportion of 'false positive' values, because each of these tests may be positive in healthy individuals. Approximately 10% of patients with fibromyalgia will have a positive antinuclear antibody test[24].

Complaints of paresthesias and minor cognitive dysfunction often lead to costly and invasive neurological testing[27]. Unnecessary surgery, especially carpal tunnel release (which does not improve symptoms) or disc 'decompression', is common in patients with fibromyalgia. However, an informal or formal assessment of mood and functional impairment should be performed in all patients. Generally, this can be performed with simple self-administered questions, but formal evaluation by a mental health professional should be obtained from patients with obvious mood disturbances. Muscle biopsies should not be performed unless there is clinical evidence suggesting inflammatory or metabolic myopathy. A careful sleep history should be obtained, including questions regarding possible sleep apnea, which is more common in men than women with fibromyalgia.

DIFFERENTIAL DIAGNOSIS

The somewhat vague and nebulous symptoms of chronic, generalized pain and fatigue are present in many rheumatic and non-rheumatic diseases. Furthermore, fibromyalgia may occur concurrently with many chronic illnesses, including RA or systemic lupus erythematosus. In some reports, 10–30% of patients with RA, Sjögren's syndrome and systemic lupus erythematosus had fibromyalgia[28,29]. Certain rheumatic diseases such as RA, Sjögren's syndrome or systemic lupus erythematosus may present initially with diffuse pain and fatigue (Table 20.4). The characteristic synovitis and systemic features of connective tissue disorders are not features of fibromyalgia. Ankylosing spondylitis or other inflammatory back conditions may present with axial skeleton pain and stiffness, but the characteristic radiological features of spondylitis are diagnostic. Polymyalgia rheumatica may mimic fibromyalgia, although tender points have not been consistently reported. An increased erythrocyte sedimentation rate is present in the vast majority of patients with polymyalgia rheumatica and most respond extremely well to modest doses of corticosteroids. Inflammatory myositis and metabolic myopathies cause muscle weakness and muscle fatigue, but usually are not associated with diffuse pain. Furthermore, patients with fibromyalgia do not have significant muscle weakness, other than that related to pain or disuse, and they have normal muscle enzyme tests and normal or non-specific histopathological findings on muscle biopsy.

Certain non-rheumatic systemic illnesses such as hypothyroidism may mimic fibromyalgia (Table 20.4). However, there is no evidence that correcting the thyroid abnormality ameliorates the fibromyalgia, or that the majority of patients with fibromyalgia have a history of thyroid dysfunction. As noted above, peripheral neuropathies, entrapment syndromes (such as carpal tunnel syndrome) and neurological disorders (such as multiple sclerosis and myasthenia gravis) are sometimes considered in the differential diagnosis. However, the standard neurological examination, in addition to electromyography and nerve conduction velocities, are usually normal in fibromyalgia.

The most confusing conditions in the differential diagnosis include a group of poorly understood disorders that may be best considered as part of the fibromyalgia concept or to overlap with it (Table 20.2). Such conditions include chronic fatigue syndrome (CFS), myofascial pain syndrome, irritable bowel syndrome, migraine, interstitial cystitis and Gulf War syndrome. Chronic fatigue syndrome and myofascial pain syndrome are especially difficult to distinguish from fibromyalgia and are considered in detail below.

Chronic fatigue syndrome

The history of CFS bears a striking resemblance to that of fibromyalgia[30,31]. The term 'neurasthenia' was popularized by George Beard to account for patients with chronic unexplained fatigue[30]. The connection of chronic fatigue and infections, especially viral, was reported commonly during the polio epidemics of the 1930s and 1940s. Outbreaks of apparent postviral chronic fatigue were reported from Los Angeles County Hospital, the Royal Free Hospital in London, in Iceland, in Australia, and in many other locations. Some authors emphasized the chronic neuropsychiatric symptoms and the term 'benign myalgic encephalomyelitis' was used. Despite speculation that these conditions were related to a viral illness, extensive serological, virological and epidemiological studies did not demonstrate an infectious etiology.

During the mid-1980s, the concept of chronic Epstein–Barr virus infection as a cause of what is now termed CFS became popular. However, despite increased antibody titers to Epstein–Barr virus antigens in many patients, there was no evidence that Epstein–Barr virus was causally associated with the vast majority of cases of CFS. The working case definition for CFS, like that for fibromyalgia, is based on clinical symptoms and signs. The cardinal symptom is chronic, debilitating fatigue, and the evaluation discloses no other systemic illness. Fibromyalgia and major depression or anxiety do not exclude the diagnosis of CFS. In direct comparisons, 30–70% of patients with fibromyalgia have met the working case definition for CFS[32–34].

Demographic, clinical, biological and psychiatric studies have demonstrated overlap of CFS and fibromyalgia[31–37]. CFS has been most often reported in previously healthy, young and middle-aged females. There has been a predominance of white middle-class patients, although selection bias may account for this. Similar subtle neuroendocrine, psychiatric and neuroimaging findings have been demonstrated in CFS and in fibromyalgia, as discussed below. One of the most

---

TABLE 20.4 DIFFERENTIAL DIAGNOSIS AND SYSTEMIC ILLNESSES THAT ARE ASSOCIATED WITH FIBROMYALGIA

Condition	Helpful differential features	% with FM
Rheumatoid arthritis	Synovitis, serologic tests, increased erythrocyte sedimentation rate (ESR)	12
Systemic lupus erythematosus	Dermatitis, systemic vasculitis (renal, central nervous system, etc.)	22
Sjögren's syndrome	Lymphadenopathy, biopsy of salivary glands	11
Polymyalgia rheumatica	Increased ESR, elderly, response to steroids	?
Myositis	Increased muscle enzymes, weakness more than pain	?
Hypothyroidism	Abnormal thyroid function tests	?
Neuropathies	Clinical and electrophysiologic evidence of neuropathy	7

TABLE 20.5 COMPARISON OF FIBROMYALGIA AND MYOFASCIAL PAIN SYNDROMES		
Variable	Fibromyalgia	Myofascial pain
Examination	Tender points	Trigger points
Location	Generalized	Regional
Response to local therapy	Not sustained	'Curative'
Sex	Females:males, 10:1	(?) Equal
Systemic features	Characteristic	(?)

intriguing issues has been the relationship of a prior infection to fibromyalgia and CFS[38].

Regional myofascial pain syndromes (repetitive strain syndrome)

Myofascial pain syndromes encompass common regional pain disorders, including specific syndromes such as temporomandibular joint syndrome, in addition to the so-called repetitive strain syndrome (see below). Myofascial pain syndromes overlap with fibromyalgia (Table 20.5). Myofascial pain is defined by the presence of trigger points, which include a localized area of deep muscle tenderness, located in a taut band in the muscle, and a characteristic reference zone of perceived pain that is aggravated by palpation of the trigger point[39-41]. Some authors also insist on the presence of a local twitch response.

The relationship of *trigger* points to *tender* points is not clear. Although trigger points may be latent – that is, not associated with pain – they are usually very tender. The location of the trigger point is deep within the muscle belly. Trigger points are said to cause decreased muscle stretch and pain with contraction. A 'twitch response', believed to be pathognomonic of an active trigger point, is a visible or palpable contraction of the muscle produced by a rapid snap by the examining finger on the taut band of muscle. There is a characteristic pattern of referred pain (Fig. 20.3). Some investigators have questioned the reliability of the trigger point evaluation and have found little difference between the symptoms and tender point examination in patients with fibromyalgia and those with myofascial pain syndrome[39-41]. Clinical, electromyographic and outcome studies have suggested that myofascial pain is a localized form of fibromyalgia[39,40].

The terms 'repetitive strain syndrome' and 'chronic whiplash' are often used when myofascial pain occurs in the context of activities involving repetitious movement or postural constraint[41-44]. However, as with fibromyalgia, there is no evidence of persisting tissue damage or injury. The term repetitive strain syndrome has been used in conjunction with epidemics of unexplained musculoskeletal pain triggered by apparent injury or work-related activities. 'Writer's cramp' was first noted among mail clerks of the British Civil Service in the 1830s and attributed by the workforce to the introduction of the steel nib. In 1908, 'telegraphist's cramp' was added to the schedule of diseases that was covered by the British Workman's Compensation Act of 1906. In Australia in the 1980s, repetitive strain injury was diagnosed in up to 30% of workers. The condition affected both blue- and white-collar workers, had a female predominance, was more prevalent in non-Australian-born workers, and was not uniformly represented in workplaces, even in those with identical ergonomic and social backgrounds. Very few self-employed persons developed the problem. Media and political pressure fueled the expanding number of claims made for repetitive strain injury, until the causal nature of the symptoms was questioned. By the early 1990s, the condition had receded to a low endemic rate similar to that observed a decade earlier (Fig. 20.4)[41].

ETIOLOGY

The etiology of fibromyalgia has been debated for more than a century. It is unlikely that fibromyalgia, or for that matter any chronic pain condition, is 'caused' by a single factor. Many patients with fibromyalgia cannot identify any one event that precipitated their symptoms. The most common factors that patients do identify are a flu-like or 'viral' illness; minor or substantial physical trauma, such as a fall or a motor vehicle accident; emotional trauma; or changes in medication, especially withdrawing corticosteroids (Table 20.6)[20,41-47].

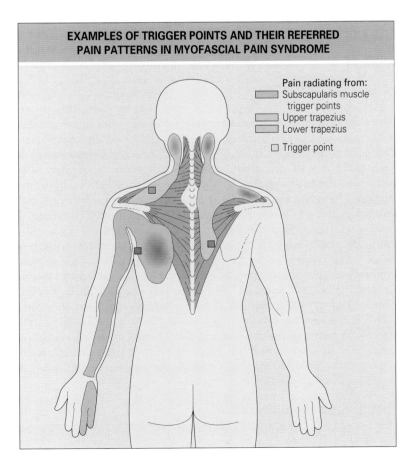

EXAMPLES OF TRIGGER POINTS AND THEIR REFERRED PAIN PATTERNS IN MYOFASCIAL PAIN SYNDROME

Pain radiating from:
- Subscapularis muscle trigger points
- Upper trapezius
- Lower trapezius
- □ Trigger point

Fig. 20.3 Examples of trigger points and their patterns of referred pain in myofascial pain syndrome.

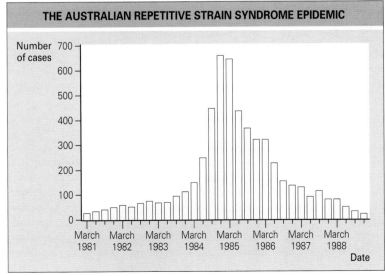

THE AUSTRALIAN REPETITIVE STRAIN SYNDROME EPIDEMIC

Fig. 20.4 The Australian repetitive strain syndrome epidemic.

TABLE 20.6 MOST COMMON PRECIPITATING FACTORS IN FIBROMYALGIA
Flu-like viral illness
Usually unspecified
Chronic fatigue syndrome
HIV infection
Lyme disease
Physical trauma
Emotional trauma
Medications, especially steroid withdrawal

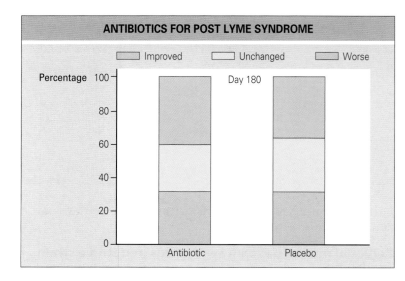

Fig. 20.5 Antibiotics for post Lyme syndrome. Results of a randomized trial of 6 months of antibiotic treatment for patients with chronic pain and fatigue after appropriately treated Lyme disease: overall SF-36 outcome, all patients. (Modified with permission from Klempner *et al.*[38])

Infection

Of particular interest has been the association of fibromyalgia and infections, also a topic of enormous debate in CFS[38,45,46]. Fibromyalgia has been noted to follow various viral diseases. Usually the specific infection is not known, although hepatitis C and human immunodeficiency virus infections have been associated with fibromyalgia[47]. It is common for patients to develop widespread pain during acute infectious mononucleosis and 20% of patients in one study met criteria for fibromyalgia[45]. However, only 1% met criteria for fibromyalgia 6 months after the viral illness. About 25–40% of patients with documented Lyme disease who were treated appropriately with antibiotics developed persistent pain and fatigue, consistent with fibromyalgia/chronic fatigue syndrome[47,48]. Although there has been no evidence of persistent Lyme infection, these chronic symptoms have often been treated with prolonged antimicrobial therapy. Randomized, controlled studies have demonstrated that such antibiotic treatment does not improve the chronic pain and fatigue of 'post Lyme syndrome' (Fig. 20.5)[38].

Trauma

There is evidence that trauma and structural musculoskeletal conditions may precipitate fibromyalgia[49,50]. A study in Israel found that fibromyalgia was 10 times more likely to develop after a neck injury than after a leg fracture[49]. The force of initial impact and the patient's psychiatric history before the collision were found to be inversely correlated with the diagnosis of post-traumatic fibromyalgia[51]. Both widespread pain and fibromyalgia have been associated with joint hypermobility[52].

PATHOGENESIS

Genetics

Preliminary reports suggest a possible familial basis for fibromyalgia[53,54]. Such reports have been strengthened by observations of associations with specific polymorphisms. Thus the S/S genotype of the promoter region of the serotonin transporter gene was present at a greater frequency among patients with fibromyalgia compared with controls[53]. The patients with the S/S genotype had higher levels of depression and psychological distress.

Muscle abnormality

There is decreased efficiency of the work performance and difficulty in relaxing the postural muscles in patients with fibromyalgia compared with pain-free controls[55,56]. Dynamic and isometric muscle strength are, however, similar to those in controls matched for the level of exercise[57]. Further, although intrinsic muscle abnormalities have been demonstrated in fibromyalgia, most investigators now believe they are secondary to inactivity and pain (Fig. 20.6). For example, no differences were noted in the concentrations of phosphocreatine, inorganic phosphate and intracellular pH of the upper trapezius and tibialis anterior muscles after exercise when 13 women with fibromyalgia were compared with 13 sedentary control females, using phosphorus magnetic resonance spectroscopy[58].

Autonomic and central nervous system abnormality

During the past decade, fibromyalgia research has focused on the autonomic and central nervous systems. Increased skin hyper-reactivity, cold sensitivity and orthostatic intolerance noted in fibromyalgia suggest alterations in the autonomic nervous system (Fig. 20.6). Autonomic dysfunction was demonstrated utilizing power spectral analysis to detect increased heart rate variability in women with fibromyalgia compared with healthy, age-matched controls[59]. The same investigators also demonstrated orthostatic intolerance in men with fibromyalgia characterized by sympathetic hyperactivity and concomitantly reduced parasympathetic activity[60].

Fibromyalgia is a disorder of abnormal pain processing (Fig. 20.6). There are profound differences between the sexes with respect to analgesic responses, across all animal species. This may help explain the decreased pain tolerance in women with fibromyalgia as compared with men. Pain signals are modulated by endogenous and exogenous processes. Patients with fibromyalgia have reduced pain tolerance to pressure, heat and electrical pulse, at both classic tender points and control points. The concentration of substance P in the cerebrospinal fluid was threefold greater in patients with fibromyalgia than in normal controls[61]. Substance P release may signal enhanced synthesis of nitrous oxide[62]. The regional cerebral blood flow, as detected by single photon emission computed tomography, has been found to be reduced in the left and right hemithalami, the right heads of the caudate nuclei and the pontine tegmentum in patients with fibromyalgia compared with controls[63,64]; these are important pain processing areas in the brain. Central nervous system sensitization is the working model proposed to explain heightened pain perception[65]. Patients with fibromyalgia demonstrated abnormal temporal summation of pain, called 'wind-up', after a series of repetitive thermal stimulations[66].

Psychological abnormality

It is not surprising that many authors have concluded that fibromyalgia is a psychiatric illness or a manifestation of psychophysiological abnormalities[10,18]. Patients look well, and there are no objective findings to account for the chronic symptoms on the basis of the physical examination, or laboratory or radiological findings. Furthermore, many patients do report depression, anxiety and high levels of stress. Thus fibromyalgia has often been considered to be a form of 'masked' depression or a somatization disorder.

Controlled studies using standard psychiatric instruments and applying validated operational diagnostic criteria have concluded the following[18,67-72]:

- There are greater psychological symptoms in patients with fibromyalgia than in controls, but increased scores on tests such as the Minnesota Multiphasic Personality Inventory may be related to pain and do not differentiate physical from psychological symptoms
- The majority of patients with fibromyalgia do not have an active psychiatric illness, although major depression is found in 20–30% of patients, and anxiety disorder in 10–20%
- There is a greater prevalence of a lifetime and family history of depression in patients with fibromyalgia compared with those with RA and with normal controls
- There is no evidence for a specific personality type, such as obsessive–compulsive disorder, and somatoform disorders are unusual
- Psychiatric illness is related to healthcare-seeking behavior, rather than to the fibromyalgia.

Investigators from the University of Alabama compared patients with fibromyalgia and people in the community who had symptoms of fibromyalgia but were not being followed for the condition – so-called non-patients – and healthy community controls[72]. The patients with fibromyalgia had a significantly greater number of lifetime psychiatric diagnoses than the non-patients, although the latter did not differ from controls (Fig. 20.7). The patients also had higher levels of psychological distress. This finding has also been noted in patients with irritable bowel syndrome.

Fibromyalgia, depression, anxiety disorders, migraine, CFS and irritable bowel syndrome have been termed 'affective spectrum disorders' or 'functional somatic syndromes'. Each is characterized by multiple, unexplained somatic symptoms and psychological distress[10,18,67,73]. The risk of chronic, widespread pain was significantly associated with indicators of somatization, especially with high scores on the Illness Behavior Scale[73]. A past history of increased physical and emotional trauma, including sexual abuse in childhood, has also been reported in fibromyalgia[73-76]. Such chronic stress also fits the hypothesis regarding various traumatic events being associated with fibromyalgia (Fig. 20.6)[77,78].

Sleep disturbance

Sleep disturbances[79-83] and cognitive disturbances also point to abnormalities of the central nervous system. Alpha intrusion during sleep can

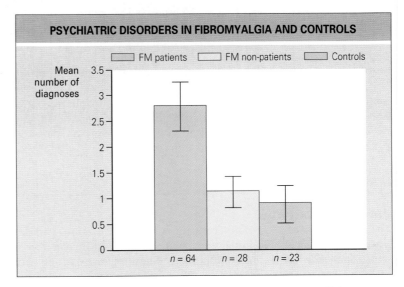

Fig. 20.7 Psychiatric disorders in fibromyalgia. Comparison of lifetime psychiatric diagnoses in patients with fibromyalgia (FM), fibromyalgia 'non-patients' and controls. (Modified from Aaron *et al.*[72] This material was used by permission of Wiley-Liss Inc., a subsidery of John Wiley & Sons Inc. © 1996.)

Fig. 20.6 A possible pathophysiologic model of fibromyalgia.

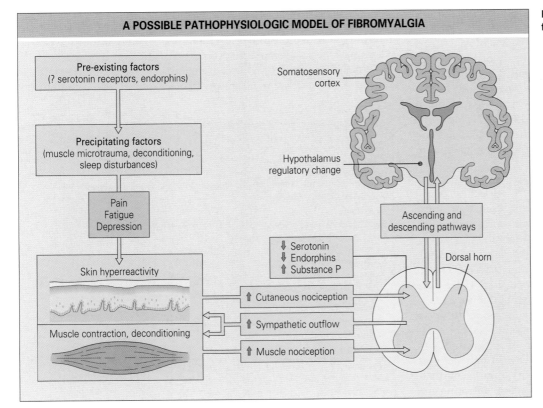

be of different patterns, and phasic alpha activity (simultaneous with delta activity) has been found to correlate best with symptoms of fibromyalgia[79]. Periodic limb movements and sleep apnea may also complicate the condition[80,81]. The initial reports of Moldofsky and coworkers[4] that slow-wave sleep disruption triggered symptoms of fibromyalgia have been recently reproduced[82]. Circadian rhythms of women with fibromyalgia did not differ from those of healthy controls[83].

Neuroendocrine abnormality

There is significant evidence for disturbances of the neurohormonal system in patients with fibromyalgia (Fig. 20.6)[85]. A number of studies have demonstrated reduced concentrations of growth hormone and prolactin, and altered serotoninergic pathways in some patients with fibromyalgia[86–89]. Most intriguing has been evidence for altered response of the central stress axis[85,90,91]. Corticotropin releasing hormone is an important regulator of the stress axis. Women with fibromyalgia displayed an impaired ability to activate the hypothalamic–pituitary portion of the stress axis and the sympathoadrenal system[90]. Infusion of interleukin 6, which stimulates release of corticotropin releasing hormone, caused an exaggerated norepinephrine and heart rate response and a delayed release of adrenocorticotropic hormone in patients with fibromyalgia compared with controls[91].

MANAGEMENT

Patient education

The cornerstone of successful treatment is patient education. Patients with fibromyalgia should initially be taught what the syndrome represents. They may have been told that there is nothing really wrong with them, or that it is 'all in their heads'. They need to understand that the illness is real, not imagined, but also that it is not likely to be caused by an infection or other illness over which the patient has no control. Patients must be told that this is not a deforming or deteriorating condition, and that it is never life threatening or a cosmetic problem. Analogies with conditions such as migraine can be useful. The complicated psychosocial and physiological interactive pathway (Fig. 20.6) should be discussed as a basis for treatment. At the initial visit, the role of sleep and mood disturbances should be reviewed.

There is no single approach to the optimal management of patients with fibromyalgia. Patients vary widely in the severity of their symptoms and in the prominence of individual symptoms. Therefore, treatment must be tailored to each individual and specifically to the symptoms that most impair each person. A stepwise approach guided by symptom severity and psychosocial issues works best (Table 20.7). Because, at present, there is no highly effective therapy, patients and their physicians must be flexible and willing to try various modalities of treatment.

Drug treatment

Drug treatment may be used for pain relief, to improve sleep, to treat the fatigue, or to relieve depression. Many of the medications used in the treatment of fibromyalgia affect each of those symptoms and it is impossible to tease out their mechanisms of action[90] (Table 20.7). In general, anti-inflammatory medications have not been better than placebo in clinical trials, and simple analgesics are usually tried first. There have been no controlled trials of selective cyclo-oxygenase-2 inhibitors.

The tricyclic antidepressants, such as amitriptyline, in addition to cyclobenzaprine, have been studied more than any other class of medication in fibromyalgia[93,94]. They clearly have been of some efficacy in decreasing pain and improving the overall well-being of patients with fibromyalgia. Even with low doses of the tricyclics, dry mouth, constipation, fluid retention, weight gain and difficulty concentrating are common. Initially, patients are generally prescribed very low doses, such

as amitriptyline or desipramine 5–10mg, 1–3h before bedtime. The dose may be increased after 2 weeks, with increases of 5mg at 2 week intervals. The final dose should be set by the patient, on the basis of efficacy and side effects, always keeping the dose as low as possible. The doses typically studied in randomized placebo controlled trials have been amitriptyline 25–50mg and cyclobenzapine 10–20mg, usually given as a single dose at bedtime. It is unlikely that the efficacy of tricyclic agents in fibromyalgia relates to their effect on depression, as the doses used have been 'subtherapeutic' for the treatment of depression, the improvement has been more rapid (usually within 2 weeks), and there has been no correlation of improvement with premorbid psychiatric disorders. Tricyclic antidepressants have an analgesic effect that may be related to their potentiation of endogenous opioids, and to their effect on brain serotonin and other neurogenic amines.

Three meta-analyses of the randomized placebo controlled trials of tricyclic antidepressants, serotonin reuptake inhibitors and S-adenosylmethionine demonstrated an odds ratio for improvement of 4.2[95–97]. However, the long-term use of these agents has not been well established. In general, the improvement with these drugs seems to fade over time. Serotonin reuptake inhibitors may also have some analgesic effect and help improve energy. The combination of fluoxetine hydrochloride and amitriptyline has been more effective than either medication alone or than placebo in decreasing pain and improving other symptoms of fibromyalgia (Fig. 20.8)[98]. Anecdotal reports have suggested that other selective serotonin reuptake inhibitors and venlafaxine may be useful in patients with fibromyalgia[99,100]. The tricyclic antidepressants may improve sleep disturbances, although clinical trials have not been able to correlate their efficacy with improved restorative sleep patterns. Clonazepam and L-dopa/carbidopa have been used to treat periodic limb movements.

Tramadol is a weak opioid agonist and also inhibits the reuptake of serotonin and norepinephrine at the level of the dorsal horn. It has recently been used with some efficacy in fibromyalgia[101]. Opioids have rarely been prescribed, because of the concern with addiction, although this is extremely rare in patients with chronic pain. Some rheumatologists have been comfortable utilizing opioids in unusual situations, whereas others typically refer such patients to a pain management unit. Ketamine, a dissociative anesthetic that blocks N-methyl-D-aspartate receptors, was demonstrated to relieve pain acutely in fibromyalgia[102]. There have been several recent clinical trials demonstrating some efficacy of the serotonin (5-hydroxytryptamine-3) receptor antagonists in fibromyalgia[103]. Other medications that have been advocated but not

---

TABLE 20.7 STEPWISE APPROACH TO FIBROMYALGIA TREATMENT

First-line treatment

Medications: simple analgesics, NSAIDs, low-dose tricyclic antidepressants* or serotonin receptor inhibitors
Education*
Exercise*: low impact, such as walking, water exercises
If mood disturbances, treat with appropriate medications

Second-line treatment

Medications: tramadol*, combinations of antidepressants* or other analgesics
Cognitive behavioral program*, stress management therapy*
Structured exercise program*
Physical medicine and rehabilitation program
Trigger point injections, acupuncture
Pain management program

* Evidence of efficacy in controlled clinical trials.
NSAIDs, non-steroidal anti-inflammatory drugs.

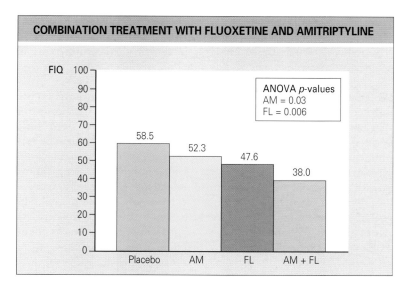

COMBINATION TREATMENT WITH FLUOXETINE AND AMITRIPTYLINE

Fig. 20.8 Combination treatment with fluoxetine and amitriptyline. Results of change in Fibromyalgia Impact Questionnaire (FIQ) comparing placebo, 25mg amitriptyline (AM), 20mg fluoxetine (FL) or both 25mg amitriptyline and 20mg fluoxetine (AM + FL). (Modified from Goldenberg et al.[93] This material is used by permission of Wiley-Liss Inc., a subsidiary of John Wiley & Sons Inc. © 1996.)

adequately tested include the benzodiazepines, intravenous and topical lidocaine hydrochloride, magnesium and malic acid, gabepentin, dextromethorphan and some of the newer antidepressants.

Non-drug treatment

Non-drug treatment of fibromyalgia includes exercise, physical therapy and related manual treatments, cognitive–behavioral treatments, education and multidisciplinary approaches (Table 20.7). During the past decade, a number of these therapeutic modalities have been tested in a controlled fashion. Generally, these treatments have been compared with wait-listed controls. More than 10 randomized clinical trials have focused on aerobic exercise[104–108]. Often, the aerobic exercise was accomplished by walking or bicycling, and the control consisted of stretching, or attention controls such as relaxation techniques. There was a high dropout rate in many of the studies. In general, the exercise group did better and were able to perform the conditioning exercise program. Some investigators reported no improvement in fibromyalgia symptoms[108]. Water exercise, especially in a warm-water pool, enhanced cardiovascular capacity and self-reported physical impairment, fatigue, pain and mood[106,107].

Unfortunately, despite reports demonstrating the beneficial effect of cardiovascular exercise, it is difficult to start and maintain patients with fibromyalgia in a structured cardiovascular exercise program. Patients generally perceive that their pain and fatigue worsen as they begin to exercise. The majority of patients are physically unfit. Therefore, it is important to instruct patients in the principles and methods of gradual incremental cardiovascular fitness programs. Low-impact aerobic activities such as fast walking, biking, swimming or water aerobics are most successful. However, the type and intensity of the program should be individualized, and physical therapists or exercise physiologists can provide helpful instruction.

Various forms of cognitive behavioral therapy have been evaluated in fibromyalgia[109,110]. These programs typically use multidisciplinary approaches, mind and body integration, and coping skills training, along with an educational component. Cognitive behavioral strategies have often focused on relaxation techniques and pain modification. Meditation, biofeedback and other types of relaxation training in addition to stress management have been promoted. Although placebo-controlled groups are not practical, the results of these programs have largely been positive. Other less well studied non-medical treatments include injections to tender

points, electromyographic biofeedback, hypnotherapy, transcutaneous electrical nerve stimulation, acupuncture and homeopathy[111,112].

Multidisciplinary pain management programs should be used in patients who have not responded to usual management[113–115]. Such programs should include pain management experts, an anesthesiologist, a physiatrist, a physical therapist and an occupational therapist, in addition to mental health professionals. Patients need to be followed at regular intervals until they have achieved some significant improvement and stability in their symptoms.

PROGNOSIS

In most longitudinal reports, fibromyalgia remains fairly constant over time[116]. By contrast, in the longest follow-up study from a single medical center, 14 years after the initial diagnosis of fibromyalgia, 67% of the patients felt better than when they were first diagnosed and 70% felt that their symptoms interfered little, if at all, with their daily activities or work[117]. Only 9% had to leave their job because of fibromyalgia. However, a multicenter study of more than 500 patients followed for 7 consecutive years also demonstrated little change in symptoms over time[118,119]. There was no significant change in health satisfaction, symptoms or functional disability, and more than 50% of the patients rated their health as fair or poor. Community based studies of patients with fibromyalgia suggest that the prognosis is better than that of patients from tertiary referral centers[120], and in one study 25% of patients had a complete remission of their symptoms 2 years after diagnosis[121].

Studies of healthcare utilization show that patients with fibromyalgia have an average of 10 outpatient medical visits each year and take an average of three medications per year for their fibromyalgia[119]. In 1996, the average yearly cost per patient was US$2274, similar to the cost of treating osteoarthritis.

Factors associated with improved outcome were a younger age and lower global and pain scores at the time of the initial diagnosis[122,123]. Pain is the most important determinant of 'global severity', but psychological status and functional disability contribute independently to severity. With regard to function in fibromyalgia, studies have reported varying disability rates, from 9 to 44%[117–124]. Disability has been most strongly associated with functional and work status, pain, mood disturbances, coping ability, depression, pending litigation and educational background. Patients in tertiary referral practices with a special interest in fibromyalgia may represent the 'tip of the iceberg' in terms of severity and functional disability; community based patients with fibromyalgia have fared much better in outcome.

The variable severity of fibromyalgia must be considered in any discussion of prognosis and outcome. The somewhat bleak outcome reported from tertiary referral clinics with a specialty interest in fibromyalgia may not be representative of the general community. Less problematic patients may often do well with simple reassurance, education and attention to physical fitness and ergonomic issues. Many patients respond well to very low doses of tricyclic antidepressants or other central nervous system medications and, particularly as their sleep improves, they cope well and find fibromyalgia to be no more than a nuisance condition. Nevertheless, most patients do continue to report chronic symptoms, and a complete and permanent remission is rather unusual.

MEDICOLEGAL ASPECTS

As might be expected from the disability numbers given above, fibromyalgia has become an important medicolegal issue[123,124]. Many patients with fibromyalgia and repetitive strain syndrome are involved in compensation, litigation or disability assessment. The issue of whether compensation is appropriate is one that has to be worked out by each individual and their healthcare providers, and the courts. However, in our litigious society, such issues have become common, and rheumatologists will by necessity have to render opinions in legal cases.

One simple way to deal with such questions is to state that fibromyalgia is never related to injury and is never disabling. Of course, such responses are contrary to what patients tell us, and physical trauma has been one of the most common precipitating factors in fibromyalgia. When physicians are asked to comment on whether fibromyalgia can cause disability, we can only respond by using subjective criteria such as the level of pain, exhaustion and distress that patients report.

In most studies, the ability of patients to work has been directly related to job satisfaction and the flexibility of their work. There is no evidence that compensation from workplace issues is helpful to illness outcome. Those patients who consider that physical trauma caused their symptoms tend to have a poorer outcome and more often seek disability compensation[125]. Patients should be encouraged to continue to work and be helped to modify their workplace and their life in general. If disability questions are raised:

- The diagnosis of fibromyalgia should be specified and confirmed according to current classification criteria. It is helpful to note that the locations of tender and control points are usually not known to patients, making it difficult to fake a tender point evaluation
- The prognosis is impossible to predict in any chronic condition. However, it should be stressed that the majority of patients are working full time
- The relationship of the 'injury' to fibromyalgia is best approached by using the terms 'precipitating factor' or temporal relationship of the 'injury' to the onset of symptoms. We do not know the 'cause' of fibromyalgia and it would be inappropriate to tackle issues of causation
- Reports do now describe significant work loss, work modifications and work disability in fibromyalgia. What is such disability related to, as there are no objective measures of physical impairment? Pain in fibromyalgia is more prominent than in many disabling conditions such as RA. Fatigue may also cause disability. However, according to

the social security guidelines of some countries, pain, without objective physical or laboratory abnormalities, is not a sufficient factor in disability determinations. Tender points might then be utilized as an objective measure of pain and dysfunction.

We should convince the patient that medicolegal issues may be a negative influence on the condition, and steer employers and lawyers to a course of rehabilitation rather than confrontation. A finite time away from work, devoted to a team approach to chronic pain rehabilitation, might be recommended. Formal evaluation of the patient by the rheumatologist, a physiatrist or physical therapist, and a mental health professional should provide a treatment plan. Evaluation of the patient's specific job and possible job modification, as well as workplace 'hardening', will be helpful. The goal of everyone must be to restore the patient's confidence and desire to return to work, with the knowledge that the team of professionals and the employer are 'on the patient's side' rather than being adversaries.

CONCLUSION

Fibromyalgia is a common condition that, despite being well described 150 years ago, is just beginning to be accepted as a discrete syndrome that can be readily distinguished from other causes of chronic musculoskeletal pain. It overlaps with other functional disorders such as CFS and irritable bowel syndrome. Controversy regarding the presence of inflammation, and confusion regarding terminology and overlap with other pain syndromes have resulted in a healthy skepticism about its existence[126–128].

Fibromyalgia is an appropriate diagnostic label when we encounter patients with chronic idiopathic musculoskeletal pain and fatigue[10,116]. Although rare individuals may exploit the diagnostic label for financial or psychosocial purposes, most patients will benefit by knowing that they are suffering from symptoms that affect a significant percentage of the population. Early diagnosis will decrease costly testing and healthcare utilization. Targeted therapeutic approaches based on an integrated mind and body model are being explored[109]. As fibromyalgia and related disorders are better understood, better treatment for these perplexing syndromes will become available.

REFERENCES

1. Reynolds MD. The development of the concept of fibrositis. J Hist Med Allied Sci 1983; 38: 5–35.
2. Gowers WR. Lumbago: its lessons and analogues. BMJ 1904; 1: 117–121.
3. Kellgren JH. Observations on referred pain arising from muscle. Clin Sci 1938; 3: 175–190.
4. Smythe HA, Moldofsky H. Two contributions to understanding the 'fibrositis syndrome'. Bull Rheum Dis 1978; 26: 928–931.
5. Yunus M, Masi AT, Calabro JJ et al. Primary fibromyalgia (fibrositis): clinical study of 50 patients with matched normal controls. Semin Arthritis Rheum 1981; 11: 151–171.
6. Wolfe F, Smythe HA, Yunus MB et al. The American College of Rheumatology 1990 criteria for the classification of fibromyalgia: Report of the Multicenter Criteria Committee. Arthritis Rheum 1990; 33: 160–172.
7. Croft P, Schollum J, Silman A. Population study of tender point counts and pain as evidence of fibromyalgia. BMJ 1994; 309: 696–699.
8. McBeth J, Macfarlane GJ, Benjamin S et al. Features of somatization predict the onset of chronic widespread pain: results of a large population-based study. Arthritis Rheum 2001; 44: 940–946.
9. Goldenberg DL. Fibromyalgia syndrome. An emerging but controversial condition. JAMA 1987; 257: 2782–2787.
10. Goldenberg DL. Fibromyalgia: why such controversy? Ann Rheum Dis 1995; 54: 3–5.
11. Rau CL, Russell IJ. Is fibromyalgia a distinct clinical syndrome? Curr Rev Pain 2000; 4: 287–294.
12. Wolfe F, Ross K, Anderson J et al. The prevalence and characteristics of fibromyalgia in the general population. Arthritis Rheum 1995; 38: 19–28.
13. Forseth KO, Gran JT, Husby G. A population study of the incidence of fibromyalgia among women aged 26–55 years. Br J Rheumatol 1997; 36: 1318–23.
14. White KP, Speechley M, Harth M et al. The London fibromyalgia epidemiology study: the prevalence of fibromyalgia syndrome in London, Ontario. J Rheumatol 1999; 26: 1570–1576.
15. White KP, Speechley M, Harth M et al. The London fibromyalgia epidemiology study: comparing the demographic and clinical characteristics in 100 random community cases of fibromyalgia versus controls. J Rheumatol 1999; 26: 1577–1585.
16. And AKK, Schanberg L. Juvenile fibromyalgia syndrome. Curr Rheumatol Rep 2001; 3: 165–171.
17. Melzack R. The short-form McGill pain questionnaire. Pain 1987; 30: 191–197.
18. Hudson JI, Goldenberg DL, Pope HG Jr et al. Comorbidity of fibromyalgia with medical and psychiatric disorders. Am J Med 1992; 92: 363–367.
19. Okifuji A, Turk DC, Marcus DA. Comparison of generalized and localized hyperalgesia in patients with recurrent headache and fibromyalgia. Psychosom Med 1999; 61: 771–180.
20. Sperber AD, Atzmon Y, Neumann L et al. Fibromyalgia in the irritable bowel syndrome: studies of prevalence and clinical implications. Am J Gastroenterol 1999; 94: 3541–3546.
21. Chun A, Desautels S, Slivka A et al. Visceral algesia in irritable bowel syndrome, fibromyalgia, and sphincter of Oddi dysfunction, type III. Dig Dis Sci 1999; 44: 631–636.
22. Chang L, Mayer EA, Johnson T et al. Differences in somatic perception in female patients with irritable bowel syndrome with and without fibromyalgia. Pain 2000; 84: 297–307.
23. Clauw DJ, Schmidt M, Radulovic D et al. The relationship between fibromyalgia and interstitial cystitis. J Psychiatr Res 1997; 31: 125–131.
24. Dinerman H, Goldenberg DL, Felson DT. A prospective evaluation of 118 patients with the fibromyalgia syndrome: prevalence of Raynaud's phenomenon, sicca symptoms, ANA, low complement, and Ig deposition at the dermal–epidermal junction. J Rheumatol 1986; 13: 368–373.
25. Yunus MB, Inanici F, Aldag JC, Mangold RF. Fibromyalgia in men: comparison of clinical features with women. J Rheumatol 2000; 27: 485–490.
26. Buskila D, Neumann L, Alhoashle A, Abu-Shakra M. Fibromyalgia syndrome in men. Semin Arthritis Rheum 2000; 30: 47–51.

27. Simms RW, Goldenberg DL. Symptoms mimicking neurologic disorders in fibromyalgia syndrome. J Rheumatol 1988; 15: 1271–1273.

28. Middleton GD, McFarlin JE, Lipsky PE. The prevalence and clinical impact of fibromyalgia in systemic lupus erythematosus. Arthritis Rheum 1994; 37: 1181–1188.

29. Bonafede RP, Downey DC, Bennett RM. An association of fibromyalgia with primary Sjögren's syndrome: A prospective study of 72 patients. J Rheumatol 1995; 22: 133–136.

30. Beard GM. Neurasthenia, or nervous exhaustion. Boston Med Surg J 1869; 3: 217–121.

31. Demitrack MA. Chronic fatigue syndrome and fibromyalgia. Psych Clinics N Am 1198; 21: 672–693.

32. Goldenberg DL, Simms RW, Geiger A, Komaroff AL. High frequency of fibromyalgia in patients with chronic fatigue seen in a primary care practice. Arthritis Rheum 1990; 33: 381–387.

33. White KP, Speechley M, Harth M et al. Co-existence of chronic fatigue syndrome with fibromyalgia syndrome in the general population. Scand J Rheumatol 2000; 29: 44–51.

34. Aaron LA, Buchwald D. A review of the overlap among unexplained clinical conditions. Ann Intern Med 2001; 134: 868–881.

35. Wessely S. Chronic fatigue: symptom and syndrome. Ann Intern Med 2001; 134: 838–843.

36. Skapinakis P, Lewis G, Meltzer H. Clarifying the relationship between unexplained chronic fatigue and psychiatric morbidity. Am J Psych 2000; 157: 1492–1498.

37. Kavelaars A, Kuis W, Knook L et al. Disturbed neuroendocrine–immune interactions in chronic fatigue syndrome. J Clin Endocrinol Metab 2000; 85: 692–696.

38. Klempner MS, Hu LT, Evans J et al. Two controlled trials of antibiotic treatment in patients with persistent symptoms and a history of Lyme disease. N Engl J Med 2001; 345: 85–92.

39. Wolfe F, Simons DG, Fricton J et al. The fibromyalgia and myofascial pain syndromes: a preliminary study of tender points and trigger points in persons with fibromyalgia, myofascial pain syndrome and no disease. J Rheumatol 1992; 19: 944–951.

40. Tunks E, McCain GA, Hart LE et al. The reliability of examination for tenderness in patients with myofascial pain, chronic fibromyalgia and controls. J Rheumatol 1995; 22: 944–952.

41. Littlejohn GO. Fibrositis/fibromyalgia syndrome in the workplace. Rheum Dis Clin N Am 1989; 15: 45–60.

42. Elert J, Kendall SA, Larsson B et al. Chronic pain and difficulty in relaxing postural muscles in patients with fibromyalgia and chronic whiplash associated disorders. J Rheumatol 2001; 28: 1361–1368.

43. Gallinaro AL, Feldman J, Natour J. An evaluation of the association between fibromyalgia and repetitive strain injuries in metalworkers of an industry in Guarulhos, Brazil. Joint Bone Spine 2001; 68: 59–64.

44. De Stefano R, Selvi E, Villanova M et al. Image analysis quantification of substance P immunoreactivity in the trapezius muscle of patients with fibromyalgia and myofascial pain syndrome. J Rheumatol 2000; 27: 2906–2910.

45. Rea T, Russo J, Katon W et al. A prospective study of tender points and fibromyalgia during and after an acute viral infection. J Rheumatol 1999; 159: 865–870.

46. Wittrup IH, Jensen B, Bliddal H et al. Comparison of viral antibodies in 2 groups of patients with fibromyalgia. J Rheumatol 2001; 28: 601–603.

47. Goldenberg DL. Do infections trigger fibromyalgia? Arthritis Rheum 1993; 36: 1489–1492.

48. Hsu VM, Patella SJ, Sigal LH. 'Chronic Lyme disease' as the incorrect diagnosis in patients with fibromyalgia. Arthritis Rheum 1993; 36: 1493–1500.

49. Buskila D, Neumann L, Vaisberg G et al. Increased rates of fibromyalgia following cervical spine injury. A controlled study of 161 cases of traumatic injury. Arthritis Rheum 1997; 40: 446–452.

50. White KP, Carette S, Harth M et al. Trauma and fibromyalgia: is there an association and what does it mean? Semin Arthritis Rheum 2000; 29: 200–216.

51. White KP, Ostbye T, Harth M et al. Perspectives on posttraumatic fibromyalgia: a random survey of Canadian general practitioners, orthopedists, physiatrists, and rheumatologists. J Rheumatol 2000; 27: 790–796.

52. Karaaslan Y, Haznedaroglu S, Ozturk M. Joint hypermobility and primary fibromyalgia: a clinical enigma. J Rheumatol 2000; 27: 1774–1746.

53. Offenbaecher M, Bondy B, de Jonge S et al. Possible association of fibromyalgia with a polymorphism in the serotonin transporter gene regulatory region. Arthritis Rheum 1999; 42: 2482–2488.

54. Yunus MB, Khan MA, Rawlings KK et al. Genetic linkage analysis of multicase families with fibromyalgia. J Rheumatol 1999; 26: 408–412.

55. Bansevicius D, Westgaard RH, Stiles T. EMG activity and pain development in fibromyalgia patients exposed to mental stress of long duration. Scand J Rheumatol 2001; 30: 92–98.

56. Elert J, Kendall SA, Larsson B et al. Chronic pain and difficulty in relaxing postural muscles in patients with fibromyalgia and chronic whiplash associated disorders. J Rheumatol 2001; 28: 1361–1368.

57. Hakkinen A, Hakkinen K, Hannonen P et al. Force production capacity and acute neuromuscular responses to fatiguing loading in women with fibromyalgia are not different from those of healthy women. J Rheumatol 2000; 27: 1277–1282.

58. Simms RW, Roy SH, Hrovat M et al. Lack of association between fibromyalgia syndrome and abnormalities in muscle energy metabolism. Arthritis Rheum 1994; 37: 794–800.

59. Cohen H, Neumann L, Shore M et al. Autonomic dysfunction in patients with fibromyalgia: application of power spectral analysis of heart rate variability. Semin Arthritis Rheum 2000; 29: 217–227.

60. Cohen H, Neumann L, Alhosshle A et al. Abnormal sympathovagal balance in men with fibromyalgia. J Rheumatol 2001; 28: 581–589.

61. Russell IJ, Orr MD, Littman B et al. Elevated cerebrospinal fluid levels of substance P in patients with the fibromyalgia syndrome. Arthritis Rheum 1994; 37: 1593–1601.

62. Larson AA, Giovengo SL, Russell IJ, Michalek JE. Changes in the concentrations of amino acids in the cerebrospinal fluid that correlate with pain in patients with fibromyalgia: implications for nitric oxide pathways. Pain 2000; 87: 201–211.

63. Mountz JM, Bradley LA, Modell JG et al. Fibromyalgia in women. Abnormalities of regional cerebral blood flow in the thalamus and the caudate nucleus are associated with low pain threshold levels. Arthritis Rheum 1995; 38: 926–938.

64. Kwiatek R, Barnden L, Tedman R et al. Regional cerebral blood flow in fibromyalgia: single-photon-emission computed tomography evidence of reduction in the pontine tegmentum and thalami. Arthritis Rheum 2000; 43: 2823–2833.

65. Bennett RM. Emerging concepts in the neurobiology of chronic pain: evidence of abnormal sensory processing in fibromyalgia. Mayo Clin Proc 1999; 74: 385–398.

66. Staud R, Vierck CJ, Cannon RL et al. Abnormal sensitization and temporal summation of second pain (wind-up) in patients with fibromyalgia syndrome. Pain 2001; 91: 165–175.

67. Hudson JI, Pope HG Jr. The relationship between fibromyalgia and major depressive disorder. Rheum Dis Clin N Am 1996; 22: 285–303.

68. McBeth J, Silman AJ. The role of psychiatric disorders in fibromyalgia. Curr Rheumatol Rep 2001; 3: 157–164.

69. Kurtze N, Gundersen KT, Svebak S. Quality of life, functional disability and lifestyle among subgroups of fibromyalgia patients: the significance of anxiety and depression. Br J Med Psychol 1999; 72: 471–484.

70. Okifuji A, Turk DC, Sherman JJ. Evaluation of the relationship between depression and fibromyalgia syndrome: why aren't all patients depressed? J Rheumatol 2000; 27: 212–219.

71. Nielson WR, Merskey H. Psychosocial aspects of fibromyalgia. Curr Pain Headache Rep 2001; 5: 330–337.

72. Aaron LA, Bradley LA, Alarcon GS et al. Psychiatric diagnoses in patients with fibromyalgia are related to health care-seeking behavior rather than to illness. Arthritis Rheum 1996; 39: 436–445.

73. McBeth J, Macfarlane GJ, Benjamin S et al. Features of somatization predict the onset of chronic widespread pain: results of a large population-based study. Arthritis Rheum 2001; 44: 940–946.

74. Van Houdenhove B, Neerinckx E, Lysens R et al. Victimization in chronic fatigue syndrome and fibromyalgia in tertiary care: a controlled study on prevalence and characteristics. Psychosomatics 2001; 42: 21–28.

75. Boisset-Pioro MH, Esdaile JM, Fitzcharles M-A. Sexual and physical abuse in women with fibromyalgia syndrome. Arthritis Rheum 1995; 38: 235–241.

76. Alexander RW, Bradley LA, Alarcon GS et al. Sexual and physical abuse in women with fibromyalgia: association with outpatient health care utillization and pain medication usage. Arthritis Care Res 1998; 11: 102–215.

77. Hassett AL, Cone JD, Patella SJ et al. The role of catastrophizing in the pain and depression of women with fibromyalgia syndrome. Arthritis Rheum 2000; 43: 2493–2500.

78. Sherman JJ, Turk DC, Okifuji A. Prevalence and impact of posttraumatic stress disorder-like symptoms on patients with fibromyalgia syndrome. Clin J Pain 2000; 16: 127–134.

79. Roizenblatt S, Moldofsky H, Benedito-Silva AA et al. Alpha sleep characteristics in fibromyalgia. Arthritis Rheum 2001; 44: 222–230.

80. Drewes AM. Pain and sleep disturbances with special reference to fibromyalgia and rheumatoid arthritis. Rheumatology (Oxford) 1999; 38: 1035–1038.

81. Tayag-Kier CE, Keenan GF, Scalzi LV et al. Sleep and periodic limb movement in sleep in juvenile fibromyalgia. Pediatrics 2000; 106: E70.

82. Lentz MJ, Landis CA, Rothermel J et al. Effects of selective slow wave sleep disruption on musculoskeletal pain and fatigue in middle aged women. J Rheumatol 1999; 26: 1586–1592.

83. Klerman EB, Goldenberg DL, Brown EN et al. Circadian rhythms of women with fibromyalgia. J Clin Endocrinol Metab 2001; 86: 1034–1039.

84. Glass JM, Park DC. Cognitive dysfunction in fibromyalgia. Curr Rheumatol Rep 2001; 3: 123–127.

85. Neeck G, Crofford LJ. Neuroendocrine perturbations in fibromyalgia and chronic fatigue syndrome. Rheum Dis Clin North Am 2000; 26: 989–1002.

86. Leal-Cerro A, Povedano J, Astorga R et al. The growth hormone (GH)-releasing hormone–GH–insulin-like growth factor-1 axis in patients with fibromyalgia syndrome. J Clin Endocrinol Metab 1999; 84: 3378–3381.

87. Dessein PH, Shipton EA, Joffe BI et al. Hyposecretion of adrenal androgens and the relation of serum adrenal steroids, serotonin and insulin-like growth factor-1 to clinical features in women with fibromyalgia. Pain 1999; 83: 313–319.

88. Landis CA, Lentz MJ, Rothermel J et al. Decreased nocturnal levels of prolactin and growth hormone in women with fibromyalgia. J Clin Endocrinol Metab 2001; 86: 1672–1678.

89. Maes M, Verkerk R, Delmeire L et al. Serotonergic markers and lowered plasma branched-chain-amino acid concentrations in fibromyalgia. Psychiatry Res 2000; 97: 11–20.

90. Adler GK, Kinsley BT, Hurwitz S et al. Reduced hypothalamic–pituitary and sympathoadrenal responses to hypoglycemia in women with fibromyalgia syndrome. Am J Med 1999; 106: 534–543.

91. Torpy DJ, Papanicolaou DA, Lotsikas AJ et al. Responses of the sympathetic nervous system and the hypothalamic–pituitary–adrenal axis to interleukin-6: a pilot study in fibromyalgia. Arthritis Rheum 2000; 43: 872–880.

92. Crofford LJ, Appleton BE. The treatment of fibromyalgia: a review of clinical trials. Curr Rheumatol Rep 2000; 2: 101–103.

93. Goldenberg DL, Felson DT, Dinerman H. A randomized, controlled trial of amitriptyline and naproxen in the treatment of patients with fibromyalgia. Arthritis Rheum 1986; 29: 1371–1377.

94. Carette J, Bell MJ, Reynolds WJ et al. Comparison of amitriptyline, cyclobenzaprine, and placebo in the treatment of fibromyalgia. A randomized, double-blind clinical trial. Arthritis Rheum 1994; 37: 32–40.
95. O'Malley PG, Balden E, Tomkins G et al. Treatment of fibromyalgia with antidepressants: a meta-analysis. J Gen Intern Med 2000; 15: 659–666.
96. Arnold LM, Keck PE Jr, Welge JA. Antidepressant treatment of fibromyalgia. A meta-analysis and review. Psychosomatics 2000; 41: 104–113.
97. Rossy LA, Buckelew SP, Dorr N et al. A meta-analysis of fibromyalgia treatment interventions. Ann Behav Med 1999; 21: 180–191.
98. Goldenberg DL, Mayskiy M, Mossey CJ et al. A randomized, double-blind crossover trial of fluoxetine and amitriptyline in the treatment of fibromyalgia. Arthritis Rheum 1996; 39: 1852–1859.
99. Anderberg UM, Marteinsdottir I, von Knorring L. Citalopram in patients with fibromyalgia – a randomized, double-blind, placebo-controlled study. Eur J Pain 2000; 4: 27–35.
100. Ninan PT. Use of venlafaxine in other psychiatric disorders. Depress Anxiety 2000; 12: 90–94.
101. Biasi G, Manca S, Manganelli, S et al. Tramadol in the fibromyalgia syndrome. Int J Clin Pharmacol Res 1998; 18: 13–19.
102. Graven-Nielsen T, Aspegren Kendall S, Henriksson KG et al. Ketamine reduces muscle pain, temporal summation, and referred pain in fibromyalgia patients. Pain 2000; 85: 483–491.
103. Stratz T, Muller W. The use of 5-HT3 receptor antagonists in various rheumatic diseases – a clue to the mechanism of action of these agents in fibromyalgia? Scand J Rheumatol Suppl 2000; 113: 66–71.
104. Gowans SE, deHueck A, Voss S et al. A randomized, controlled trial of exercise and education for individuals with fibromyalgia. Arthritis Care Res 1999; 12: 120–128.
105. Meiworm L, Jakob E, Walker UA et al. Patients with fibromyalgia benefit from aerobic endurance exercise. Clin Rheumatol 2000; 19: 253–257.
106. Mannerkorpi K, Nyberg B, Ahlmen M et al. Pool exercise combined with an education program for patients with fibromyalgia syndrome. A prospective, randomized study. J Rheumatol 2000; 27: 2473–2481.
107. Jentoft ES, Kvalvik AG, Mengshoel AM. Effects of pool-based and land-based aerobic exercise on women with fibromyalgia/chronic widespread muscle pain. Arthritis Rheum 2001; 45: 42–47.
108. Ramsay C, Moreland J, Ho M et al. An observer-blinded comparison of supervised and unsupervised aerobic exercise regimens in fibromyalgia. Rheumatology (Oxford) 2000; 39: 501–505.
109. Hadhazy VA, Ezzo J, Creamer P et al. Mind–body therapies for the treatment of fibromyalgia. A systematic review. J Rheumatol 2000; 27: 2911–2918.
110. Worrel LM, Krahn LE, Sletten CD et al. Treating fibromyalgia with a brief interdisciplinary program: initial outcomes and predictors of response. Mayo Clin Proc 2001; 76: 384–390.
111. Berman BM, Ezzo J, Hadhazy V et al. Is acupuncture effective in the treatment of fibromyalgia? J Fam Pract 1999; 48: 213–218.
112. Crofford LJ, Appleton BE. Complementary and alternative therapies for fibromyalgia. Curr Rheumatol Rep 2001; 3: 147–156.
113. Keel PJ, Bodoky C, Gerhard U et al. Comparison of integrated group therapy and group relaxation training for fibromyalgia. Clin J Pain 1998; 14: 232–238.
114. Bailey A, Starr L, Alderson M, Moreland J. A comparative evaluation of a fibromyalgia rehabilitation program. Arthritis Care Res 1999; 12: 336–340.
115. Turk DC, Okifuji A, Sinclair JD et al. Interdisciplinary treatment for fibromyalgia syndrome: clinical and statistical significance. Arthritis Care Res 1998; 11: 186–195.
116. Goldenberg DL. Fibromyalgia syndrome a decade later: what have we learned? Arch Intern Med 1999; 159: 777–785.
117. Kennedy M, Felson DT. A prospective long-term study of fibromyalgia syndrome. Arthritis Rheum 1996; 39: 682–685.
118. Wolfe F, Anderson J, Harkness D et al. Health status and disease severity in fibromyalgia: results of a six-center longitudinal study. Arthritis Rheum 1997; 40: 1571–1579.
119. Wolfe F, Anderson J, Harkness D et al. A prospective, longitudinal, multicenter study of service utilization and costs in fibromyalgia. Arthritis Rheum 1997; 40: 1560–1570.
120. MacFarlane GJ, Thomas E, Papageorgiou AC et al. The natural history of chronic pain in the community: a better prognosis than in the clinic? J Rheumatol 1996; 23: 1617–1620.
121. Granges G, Zilko P, Littlejohn GO. Fibromyalgia syndrome: assessment of the severity of the condition 2 years after diagnosis. J Rheumatol 1994; 21: 523–529.
122. Wolfe F, Anderson J, Harkness D et al. Work and disability status of persons with fibromyalgia. J Rheumatol 1997; 24: 1171–1178.
123. Wigers SH. Fibromyalgia outcome: the predictive values of symptom duration, physical activity, disability pension, and critical life events – a 4.5 year prospective study. J Psychosom Res 1996; 41: 235–243.
124. Bennett RM. Fibromyalgia and the disability dilemma. A new era in understanding a complex, multidimensional pain syndrome. Arthritis Rheum 1996; 39: 1627–1634.
125. Aaron LA, Bradley LA, Alarcon GS et al. Perceived physical and emotional trauma as precipitating events in fibromyalgia. Arthritis Rheum 1997; 40: 453–460.
126. Solomon DH, Liang MH. Fibromyalgia: scourge of humankind or bane of a rheumatologist's existence? Arthritis Rheum 1997; 40: 1553–1555.
127. Hadler NM. If you have to prove you are ill, you can't get well. The object lesson of fibromyalgia. Spine 1996; 21: 2397–2400.
128. Croft P, Burt J, Schollum J et al. More pain, more tender points: is fibromyalgia just one end of a continuous spectrum? Ann Rheum Dis 1996; 55: 482–485.

21 Sports medicine: the clinical spectrum of injury

J David Perry

- Sports medicine encompasses the science and medicine of exercise and sport
- Age, body habitus and anatomical variants contribute significantly to the risk of injury
- Immediate swelling of a joint implies hemarthrosis
- Hemarthrosis generally indicates significant intra-articular injury (fracture, ligamentous tears)
- Chronic overuse injuries affect mainly the soft tissues but about one-tenth of these injuries involve fatigue failure of bone (stress fractures)
- The characteristic pathology of chronic overuse conditions in Achilles and patellar tendons and rotator cuff is non-inflammatory tendinosis with neovascularization
- Stress fractures are suggested by 'crescendo' activity-related pain and localized tenderness; initial X-rays are often normal
- An underlying spondyloarthropathy should not be missed in a youngster with enthesitis or joint swelling without clear injury

INTRODUCTION

Sports medicine is the science and medicine of exercise and sport. Athletic endeavor, both elite and recreational, has advanced and expanded steadily, but medical practice has often been slow to respond to the changing needs of a more fitness-conscious society. However, there is now developing an increasing awareness of the benefits of active exercise in health promotion[1], so that physical exercise has become an important part of many people's daily routine. The Surgeon General's Report (1979) in the USA and the Health of the Nation (1992) strategy[2] in the UK highlighted the importance of regular exercise as a means of improving the general fitness of the population with the aim of reducing mortality rates from the cardiovascular diseases. Unfortunately, the increase in exercise consciousness has led to an epidemic of injury, much of it attributable to inappropriate or poorly advised activity.

The term 'athlete' is used loosely to describe any individual engaged in sport or regular exercise.

Scope of clinical problems

The purpose of this chapter is to highlight the mechanisms and risks of injury with particular reference to soft tissue problems. Some musculoskeletal problems are found almost exclusively in sportspeople but the common conditions covered in previous chapters occur frequently in this group as well, although their presentation, severity and management may differ. Chronic overuse injuries mainly affect soft tissues but about a tenth of these involve fatigue failure of bone. The nature of the injury is dependent on the type of sport and repetitive loading forces involved, the age and body habitus of the individual, and the training environment (e.g. properties of the training surface) and equipment, including footwear. All these factors must be taken into account, both in diagnosis and management, which should therefore aim to restore function and prevent reinjury by modifying training patterns and correcting biomechanics where feasible.

Major trauma causing fracture, ligamentous disruption or hemarthrosis requires immediate orthopedic opinion. Most of the patients presenting with acute traumatic hemarthrosis may have a significant intra-articular injury, such as anterior cruciate ligament (ACL) rupture, osteochondral fracture or meniscal tear. Frequently, however, because the significance of the presenting history is ignored, the diagnosis is not made until the patient presents with symptoms of instability or meniscal damage. Late diagnosis may therefore lead to increased risk of degenerative hyaline cartilage damage.

Inter-relationship between exercise, injury and musculoskeletal disease

It is equally important, when assessing patients with apparent injury through sport, to confirm that the 'injury' can be explained by the history of the forces or overuse described. Where it cannot, a primary rheumatologic disorder, possibly modified by the sporting activity, must be considered (Table 21.1). In adolescents and young adults, the most common inflammatory condition causing confusion is the enthesopathic or monoarticular presentation of the spondyloarthropathies. The predominantly lower limb involvement of the entheses by these

TABLE 21.1 THE SIMILARITIES BETWEEN SOFT TISSUE INJURY AND THE PERIPHERAL INVOLVEMENT OF SPONDYLOARTHROPATHY		Soft tissue involvement in spondyloarthritis
Common soft tissue injuries of the lower limb		
Hip girdle	Groin strains Adductor, hamstring Tendinitis Symphysis instability	Pelvic enthesopathies (especially adductor) Symphysitis
Knee	Sinding–Larsen–Johansson disease Patellar ligament tendinitis Osgood–Schlatter apophysitis	Enthesopathies of tibial tubercle and patellar poles

Hindfoot	Plantar fasciitis
	Achilles
	  Paratendinitis
	  Tendinosis
	  Deep tears
	Severís apophysitis (os calcis)
	Periosteal reaction due to stress fracture
		Plantar fasciitis
		Achilles
		  Tendinitis
		  Enthesopathy
		  Bursitis
		
		Periostitis at or close to enthesis

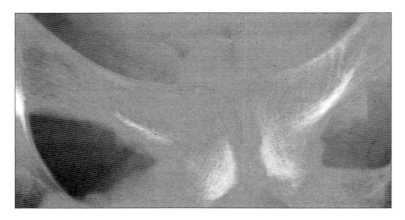

Fig. 21.1 Radiograph showing erosion of the symphysis pubis in a marathon runner.

conditions has many factors in common with the overuse injuries. Several studies[3,4] have shown that enthesitis is the most common initial presentation of seronegative spondyloarthritis and that children are frequently misdiagnosed and inappropriately investigated. Recognition of the importance of either a personal or a family history of associated problems is often crucial in separating this group from children with traumatic enthesopathy.

Furthermore, confusion may arise from the effects of injury on attachment sites, producing radiologic erosions indistinguishable from primary inflammatory involvement. An example of this is symphysitis or instability of the symphysis pubis through sport, with frank radiologic evidence of erosive change (Fig. 21.1). This is in keeping with the view that there are a limited number of ways in which a bone or joint can react to a variety of pathologic processes. It should be noted that these radiologic changes may be seen in asymptomatic sportspeople and must be interpreted with full consideration of the presenting history and physical examination.

Sport and exercise in society

Many factors, including labor-saving devices and motorized transport, have led to an overall decrease in the level of population fitness, in Western societies particularly. A simultaneous rise in the incidence of cardiovascular disease suggests that a change to a more sedentary lifestyle may be detrimental to the individual and potentially costly for society, although no clear cause-and-effect relationship has yet been shown. Nevertheless, epidemiologic evidence strongly supports the beneficial effect of physical exercise in reducing the morbidity and mortality levels due to the cardiovascular diseases, with active individuals also less likely to indulge in other potentially cardiotoxic pursuits, such as smoking. Physical activity can now also be considered a valuable component in the management of systemic hypertension, obesity and some forms of obstructive airway disease and musculoskeletal disease, such as osteoporosis.

The International Federation of Sports Medicine has recommended[5] in normal healthy individuals a regular program of three to five fairly vigorous aerobic exercise sessions each week, but with a prior screening examination by a doctor if the subject is over 35 years of age or has known 'risk' factors. Table 21.2 provides some indication of the epidemiology of the 'fitness craze'[9–12].

The physiologic effects of exercise

This is a complex subject beyond the scope of this chapter, but it is worth stressing that clinicians need to be aware, when examining patients for whatever reason, that some of the physiologic effects of exercise may cause apparent or real abnormalities of examination or investigation indices (Table 21.3). Evaluation of creatine kinase and

TABLE 21.2 FREQUENCY OF REGULAR EXERCISE IN THE GENERAL POPULATION

- 15% of Americans jog regularly
- 59% of American adults exercise regularly
- 16% of American adults exercise for more than 5 hours weekly
- 11% of American adults are joggers
- 50% of boys aged 8–16 years take part in competitive sport
- 25% of girls aged 8–16 years take part in competitive sport

TABLE 21.3 EFFECTS OF EXERCISE ON BLOOD PARAMETERS

Parameter	Effect	Reference
Hemoglobin Hematocrit	Chronic endurance training may increase plasma volume, diluting hemoglobin	9
MCH/MCHC	Progressive rise during marathon run probably due to loss of red cell water	9
WBC	Immediate leukocytosis during exercise, settling rapidly, delayed prolonged leukocytosis peaking some hours after exercise Immunomodulation through exercise	10 11
CPK	Chronic elevation in endurance exercise up to 19-fold increase, with peak 6–24 hours following a marathon	12
CRP	Peak elevation 24 hours after intense endurance exercise	13
Cortisol	Increase by high intensity aerobic and heavy resistance exercise and overtraining; less marked in well-conditioned athlete	14–16
Ferritin Antitrypsin	Marked rise after intense load in overtrained	17

CPK – creatine phosphokinase; CRP – C-reactive protein; MCH – mean corpuscular hemoglobin; MCHC – MCH concentration; WBC – white blood cells.

white cell count estimations must take account of recent exercise. Vigorous exercise leading to increased adrenocorticotropic hormone (ACTH) output and subsequent elevation of cortisol, as well as an endorphin response, particularly to anaerobic exercise, may modify the symptomatology of established inflammatory conditions such as ankylosing spondylitis[18]. It is important in any patient presenting with musculoskeletal symptoms, therefore, to assess the level of exercise that the individual maintains. Changes in activity level may affect symptomatology, including the duration of early morning stiffness.

THE EPIDEMIOLOGY OF INJURY

The frequency of injury is not always easy to assess because of the variability of reporting and attendance[19,20]. However, there is no doubt that the increased fitness awareness of Western society has led to a great increase in injuries (Table 21.4).

The issue of sport and osteoarthritis (OA) is a more complex relationship that has been extensively studied and is outside the scope of this chapter. There is, however, no consistent evidence of increased OA risk as a result of repetitive loading, unless there is significant biomechanical derangement or underlying traumatic or pre-existing hyaline cartilage change[27].

TABLE 21.4 THE EPIDEMIOLOGY OF INJURY		
Frequency (%)	Example	Reference
9	Casualty attendances in Finland due to sport	21
3	Casualty and routine outpatient attendances in Sweden due to sport	22
21	Childhood accidents seen in casualty sport-related	23
16	Sample of 50 men referred to a rheumatology clinic with back pain who appeared to have a sport-related problem	24
57	World class swimmers troubled by shoulder pain	25
30–50	Sports injuries of overuse type	26
	3.7 injuries occur per 1000 skier days	19
	9.4 injuries occur per 1000 player hours of ice hockey	20

Osteoporosis may be improved, both primarily and secondarily, by regular exercise[27]. However, it can also be caused by the amenorrhea induced by high-intensity training in some female athletes[28].

STRUCTURE AND FUNCTION

In discussing the mechanisms of overuse injury it is necessary to understand the structure and function of soft tissues[29,30].

Tendons and ligaments

Tendons comprise clusters of collagen fibrils interspersed with occasional fibrocytes. Larger tendons are made up of multiple fascicles separated by loose connective tissue, containing nerve fibers and blood vessels. Tendons passing through constricted areas or acting as a pulley across a sharp joint angle are invested with a tendon sheath, whereas the larger, heavily loaded tendons, such as the Achilles and patellar tendons, have a

paratendon. The enthesis is particularly susceptible to injury in young adolescents, tendons and ligaments effectively being stronger than bone at this age. If overloading to tendons and ligaments attaching to an epiphysis (apophysis) occurs, the resulting condition is an apophysitis, such as Osgood–Schlatter disease (Table 21.5). Paradoxically, adult tendons are more susceptible to intrasubstance tears, vascular insufficiency probably being a major factor in the localization of such injuries in the Achilles tendon at the watershed 4–6cm above the insertion. Structure therefore determines, in part, the type of response to injury, particularly as tendons must provide flexibility and resistance to tension. They allow concentration of force from a muscle, which may be large, to a relatively small attachment area. Others, for example in the hand, permit fine concentration of pull to provide precision.

In contrast, ligaments function passively, being superior for constant tension. They usually show a less regular orientation of collagen and contain elastin.

The collagen in tendons unaffected by injury is almost all type I, but in Achilles tendon rupture there may be an increase in type III, probably as part of repair of previous partial tear, rather than an intrinsic abnormality[31]. Nevertheless, this increase in type III collagen may lead to decreased resistance to tensile forces and therefore reinjury, supporting the view that Achilles tendon rupture frequently follows previous minor or asymptomatic degeneration[32].

Tendon loading

Tendon or ligament loading causes a brief alignment of fibers, as at rest they are slightly misaligned from parallel (crimping). Following this 'toe-in' period, there is linear extension to the limit of elasticity (according to Hooke's law of elasticity), at which point individual fiber failure and eventually complete rupture will occur (Fig. 21.2).

Healthy heavily loaded tendons such as the patellar tendon have been estimated as capable of coping with loads of up to four times the usual maximum load of everyday activity. Failure will, however, occur at lower loading if there is predisposing weakness due to:

- previous injury
- age changes
- abnormal collagen
- loss of strength due to inactivity.

TABLE 21.5 COMMON SITES OF TRACTION APOPHYSITIS			
Eponym	Site	Specific clinical features	Specific management features
Osgood–Schlatter disease	Tibial tubercle (patellar tendon)	Boys, esp. age 13–14 years Girls, esp. age 10–11 years Chronic condition may develop	Reduce activity initially Quadriceps strengthening and progressive stretching
Larsen–Johansson syndrome	Inferior patellar pole (patellar tendon)	Tender inferior patellar pole and radiographic evidence of small inferior patellar avulsion	If acute usually requires immobilization in cylinder cast
Severís	Os calcis (Achilles)	Relative increase in tightness of gastrocnemius/soleus, and weakness of dorsiflexors	Supervised flexibilty Dorsiflexion strengthening Orthotics if indicated
(Prominent) Accessory navicular syndrome	Navicular (at tibialis posterior attachment)	Due to apophyseal separation, often associated with pes planus and secondary pain due to irritation of soft tissues by prominent navicular	Orthotic Modify footwear
Thrower's elbow	Medial epicondyle, elbow	Medial epicondyle is last elbow growth plate to close Often due to poor technique in tennis players, and round arm throw in javelin	Modify technique

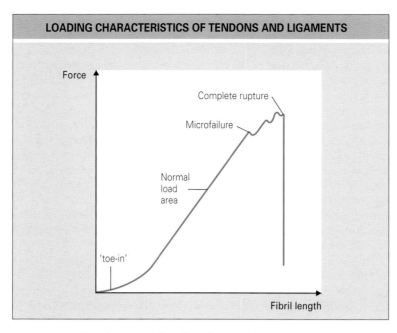

Fig. 21.2 Loading characteristics of tendons and ligaments.

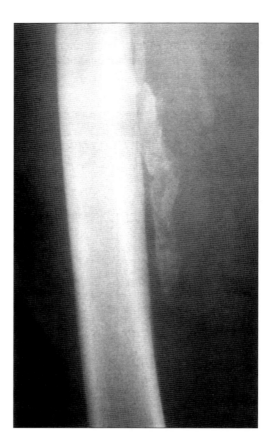

Fig. 21.3 Radiograph of the thigh showing myositis ossificans.

Immobilization particularly decreases the strength of the bone–ligament complex, with changes both in the ligament substance and attachment (enthesis). Noyes and colleagues demonstrated a 39% decrease in maximum failure load of primate ACL after 8 weeks' immobilization[33]. Histologically, there is ligament atrophy with increased collagen degradation and osteoclastic periosteal resorption around ligament insertion sites[34]. In the explosive loading of jumping or repetitive loading of endurance sports, there may therefore be microtearing of collagen fibers, followed by a cellular reaction with vascular proliferation, edema and increased tendon volume[35].

The other major factor in chronic soft tissue injury is the length of recovery time of tendon strength. Paratendinitis or tenosynovitis may further reduce tendon vascularization, because of increased diffusion distance. Healing is therefore often incomplete, leaving a weakened tendon subject to the risk of further tearing.

Muscle

Muscle injury

Muscles provide the power for movement, with a balanced control between agonists and antagonists, but injury is common in both trained and untrained individuals. Muscle contusions frequently result from direct blows to muscle. Partial and complete tears of the muscle tendon junctions occur primarily as a result of eccentric contractions, i.e. forceful contraction of the muscle as the muscle tendon unit is being lengthened. The muscle tendon junctions extend for a substantial length of muscle in the hamstrings and rectus femoris muscles, and these muscles are common sites of muscle tendon junction tears. The hamstrings cross two joints (the hip and the knee) and this may be one of the factors, as well as high loading, that make them so susceptible to tears.

Partial tears ('pulled muscle') can be deep (central) or superficial (peripheral), with the degree of tearing and bleeding influencing recovery. The latter can lead to major hematoma or, by later fibrosis, a deep intramuscular cyst.

Myositis ossificans

Myositis ossificans, the formation of bone within skeletal muscle, may also develop 6–8 weeks after muscle injury (Fig. 21.3). The exact mechanisms responsible for myositis ossificans are unknown. It is most commonly seen in the thigh but also may occur in the arm muscles.

Symptoms are continuing and excessive pain following injury, with loss of movement and muscular swelling with a deep woody feel. Active stretching and massage must be avoided as they aggravate the changes. Radiographic change may take 6 weeks to develop, with consolidation over the following months. Resorption may occur and surgery, which should only be considered if functional disability continues, must be delayed until active turnover (as judged by technetium scan) has stopped, usually over a year after injury.

Muscle soreness

More diffuse muscle symptoms after exercise are very common and can be broadly divided into three types:

- **Acute**, occurring during sustained isometric contractions at near tetanus levels
- **Delayed**, occurring 12–48 hours after exercise, particularly after eccentric work; this is probably due to ischemia during sustained contractions, with release of factors irritating pain receptors
- **Injury to muscle fibrils** can be caused by rapid repetitive movement with load, disturbing the normal control system of agonist and antagonist, with the risk of muscle and joint hyperextension; the rapid reversals of direction of stretch tax the elastic component of muscle.

Creatine phosphokinase (CPK) levels in plasma rise in individuals undergoing intensive training, and high levels are found for several days after marathon running, especially downhill running. Therefore these indices must be interpreted with great caution in athletes[12].

Muscular hypertrophy can cause compartmental syndrome (see below).

Chronic overuse and bone

Stress fractures

Stress fractures in bone occur in athletes as a result of fatigue failure in normal bone secondary to overloading through intensive exercise or biomechanically abnormal loading[36]. They should be considered as distinct from the fatigue failure in the bones of the elderly, where bone strength is either reduced through aging or markedly reduced because of osteoporosis. However, female amenorrheic athletes commonly suffer stress fractures due to osteoporosis[28,37].

The typical history is of localized increasing (crescendo) pain on exercise, easing with rest. With increasing severity, the pain occurs earlier on exercise and in some cases will eventually occur in everyday activities. Localized swelling may be seen, particularly in children and the elderly, with tenderness and, at some sites such as the fibula, pain on stressing by springing the bone at a more proximal site. Radiographs are frequently normal, although callus may become evident after about 6 weeks. Technetium scan will show localized increased uptake (Fig. 21.4). Pain induced by testing the site with high-frequency ultrasound can be helpful in supporting the diagnosis, before specific investigation. The most common site involved is the junction of the lower third of the medial tibia, followed by the tarsal bones, metatarsals, fibula and femur.

Early recognition and treatment is important as the athlete must not be advised to 'run it off', which, at a few sites, particularly the mid-tibia, risks complete fracture. Early immobilization, or surgery if severe, is advised by some in stress fractures of the mid-tibia, femoral neck and proximal diaphysis of the 5th metatarsal and navicular; but, in general, rest from the loading of sport is sufficient for other sites. It is important to maintain general fitness, and water training may be very helpful. Rest for 6 weeks is usually sufficient in mild cases but up to 12 weeks or longer may occasionally be necessary, and very graduated reloading is crucial thereafter. Biomechanical factors should be corrected.

Stress fracture of the pars interarticularis of one of the lower lumbar vertebrae can occur as a result of repetitive hyperextension stress, particularly in adolescent athletes in sports such as gymnastics and the high jump. Single photon emission computed tomography (SPECT) now appears to be the investigation of choice. If there is a spondylolysis on standard lateral or oblique spinal radiographs but no increased uptake on SPECT, the pars defect can be defined as long-standing, with no bony healing potential. If radiographs are normal but SPECT positive, computed tomography (CT) scan should be performed to grade the pars lesion.

Stress fracture of the tarsal navicular is often a chronic problem and is particularly seen in the running and jumping sports. In cases that do not settle rapidly, increased uptake on technetium bone scan (Fig. 21.4)

should be followed up by CT scan to assess the extent of fracture. In some series, recovery has been shown to take up to 6 months for undisplaced fractures. For the more serious displaced lesion, for which surgery is necessary, recovery times have been reported to be as long as 18–24 months.

It is vital that abnormal biomechanical factors are recognized and modified. Rigid pes cavus appears to increase the risk of metatarsal and femoral neck fracture. Excessive foot pronation increases tibial torsion and is found more commonly in stress fractures of the tibia and fibula. Female athletes should be screened for amenorrheic osteopenia.

Several other important etiological factors can be considered as part of the underlying cause of stress fractures. Muscle weakness reduces the shock absorption of the lower extremity and causes redistribution of forces to bone, increasing the stress at focal points. This probably is a factor in femoral neck stress fracture[28].

Stress fractures seen in non-weight-bearing bones of the upper extremity (e.g. the humerus in baseball pitchers) lend support to the view that muscle pull across a bone can produce sufficient repetitive force to produce fatigue failure. This is also likely to be the major component in lower medial tibial stress fractures, particularly where there is altered biomechanical loading through gait abnormalities, such as hyperpronation in the stance phase.

Compression stress fractures through direct loading force occur particularly in the calcaneum. Stress fractures can therefore be considered as focal structural weaknesses in bone that occur during remodeling (early osteoclastic resorption followed by osteoblastic activity) in response to the repeated application of subthreshold stresses. Increased uptake on technetium scanning at asymptomatic sites in athletes suggests that painless remodeling of bone is common in relation to stress – this can be considered as bone strain, representing a continuum of response to physical stress, similar to that seen with muscles, ligaments and tendons.

Individual sports are associated with quite specific stress fracture profiles, as summarized in Table 21.6.

Amenorrhea and reduced bone density

In female athletes, the beneficial effects of physical training may be offset by intensive exercise-induced amenorrhea. Although this change in

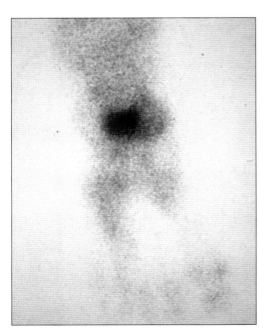

Fig. 21.4 Technetium scan showing localized uptake in navicular stress fracture.

Sport	Site of stress fracture
TABLE 21.6 PROFILE OF COMMON STRESS FRACTURES IN INDIVIDUAL SPORTS	
Basketball	Patella, calcaneum, hallux sesamoid femur and pubis
Cricket (fast bowlers)	Pars interarticularis, patella and tibia
Diving	Tibia
Fencing	Pelvis
Golf	Ribs (posterolateral, esp. 4th–6th)
Gymnastics	Upper limb and pars interarticularis
High jumping	Hallux sesamoid, patella and pars interarticularis (Fosbury flop)
Ice skating	Fibula
Javelin throwing	Olecranon or shaft of ulna
Long/triple jumping	Navicular, hallux sesamoid and pelvis
Rowing	Ribs
Running	Tibia, tarsal (especially navicular), metatarsal, femur, fibula and pelvis
Tennis	Humerus and ulna
Volleyball	Pisiform

reproductive physiology may appear to the athlete a 'pleasant convenience', secondary amenorrhea is known to be associated with reduced bone mass. Drinkwater showed decreased trabecular (spinal) density but normal cortical (radius) density, whereas Lindberg reported reduced cortical and trabecular density and a marked increase in stress fracture rate in amenorrheic athletes compared with a eumenorrheic group[37].

Intensive physical training before puberty can delay menarche and if commenced soon after menarche is associated with oligo- or amenorrhea and reduced levels of circulating estrogen. Since this can be seen in swimmers and gymnasts as well as runners, the type of physical activity appears unimportant, but the intensity is crucial. Marcus showed very low levels of body fat in amenorrheic athletes and Firsch suggested that a critical level of body fat is essential for normal estrogen status, although this is likely to be too simplistic a view[37].

In practical terms, physicians seeing amenorrheic female athletes should exclude an organic cause for the amenorrhea; the athlete should be counseled about the risk in terms of reduced bone strength and modified training schedules should be discussed.

Injury in relation to body habitus

Generalized joint laxity or hypermobility (Fig. 21.5) is usually inherited as a benign multisystem disorder of connective tissue or benign joint hypermobility syndrome (BJHS). More serious causes such as Ehlers–Danlos syndrome are rare, but even the benign condition is associated with an increased risk of soft tissue injuries and chronic pain[38,39]. Selection for some activities, such as gymnastics and dance, may favor the hypermobile but may result in a higher incidence of injury. However, it is worth noting that measures of hypermobility, such as the Beighton index[40], designed as an epidemiological tool, may miss important localized laxity, which may be a major factor in some joint injuries, such as those of the shoulder.

Injury factors in children

Children are included in the epidemic of overuse injuries, but several factors in the growing child modify the type of injury seen.

- Ligaments and tendons are comparatively stronger in relation to bone than in adult structures; injuries therefore most commonly occur at the attachment site (enthesis) (apophysis).
- Growth spurts may lead to rapid lengthening of bone with measurable increase in muscle–tendon tightness, causing loss of flexibility that adds to the risk of overuse injury.

- Growth cartilage is located not only at the epiphyses and joint surfaces but also at the apophyseal attachments of major muscle–tendon complexes. Apophysitis (e.g. Osgood–Schlatter disease) is an unfortunate term implying primary inflammation, whereas lesions of the apophyseal attachment in growing children are usually primarily traumatic in origin. They need, however, to be differentiated from the enthesitis of inflammatory arthritis (Table 21.1).
- Asymmetric traction loads or partial separation through sudden trauma to a growth plate (epiphysis), if not recognized, will lead to uneven growth, with risk of long bone asymmetry. This will alter the loading through joints, and the altered biomechanics carries the risk of premature OA in adult life.
- Excessive use of weight training can lead to marked asymmetry of muscle growth and joint laxity (e.g. 'tennis shoulder'). As a general rule, growing children should only use their own body weight for muscle strengthening.
- Osteochondritis dissecans (Fig. 21.6) is usually considered to be predominantly a condition of the immature skeleton, possibly related to trauma or ischemia or a combination of these factors.

Anatomic variants

Minor anatomic variants, which in the non-athlete may have no significance, may lead to specific injury problems when major stress or recurrent overuse affects these sites. Common examples are the os trigonum, leading to posterior impingement at the ankle, leg-length inequality and the offset anatomy of the patellar mechanism, although abnormalities in the latter are commonly associated with symptoms in non-athletic teenage girls as well.

Relationship of the patella to the femur and tibia (Q-angle)

The position of the patella is assessed by measurement of the Q-angle, between a line drawn from the anterior superior iliac spine to the center of the patella and the line of the patellar tendon to the tibial tubercle (Fig. 21.7; see also Chapter 19). The ratio of the patellar tendon length to patellar length should be less than 1.2:1. The patella tends to be displaced laterally during forced extension of the knee, but this is counteracted by the buttress of the prominent lateral surface of the lower femur and by the retaining action of the lower fibers of vastus medialis obliquus, which insert into the medial patellar border.

An increased Q-angle (Fig. 21.8) and/or hyperextension (genu recurvatum) increases the risk of patellar subluxation and anterior knee pain,

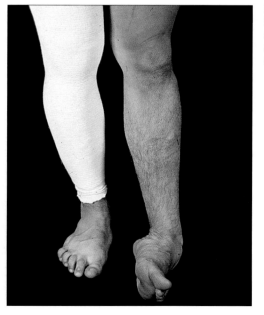

Fig. 21.5 Generalized hypermobility associated with anterior cruciate rupture of the right knee.

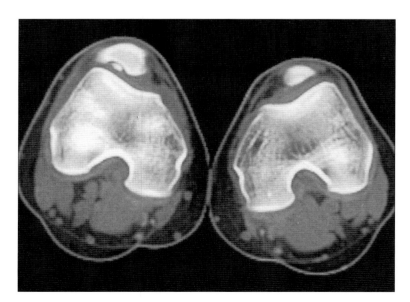

Fig. 21.6 Osteochondritis dissecans of the right patella, due to traumatic dislocation, demonstrated by CT scan.

THE PATELLAR Q-ANGLE

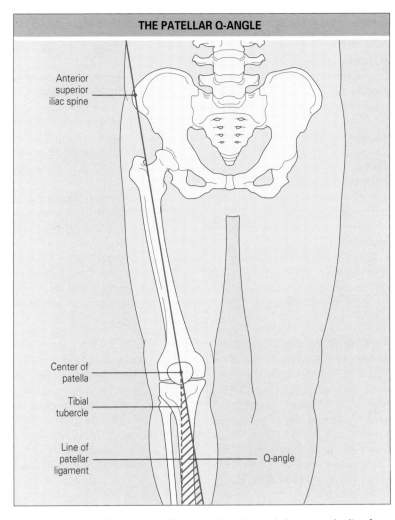

Anterior superior iliac spine

Center of patella

Tibial tubercle

Line of patellar ligament

Q-angle

Fig. 21.7 The patellar Q-angle. The Q-angle is the angle between the line from the anterior superior iliac spine through the center of the patella and the line of the patellar ligament (i.e. patellar center to tibial tubercle).

ABNORMAL Q-ANGLE WITH KNEE VALGUS

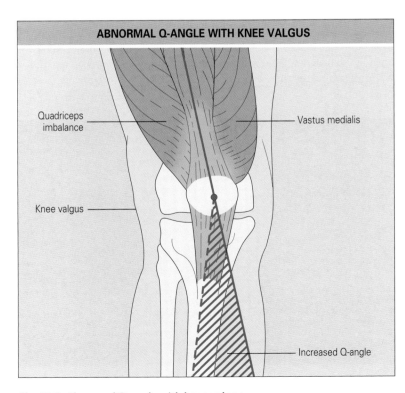

Quadriceps imbalance

Vastus medialis

Knee valgus

Increased Q-angle

Fig. 21.8 Abnormal Q-angle with knee valgus.

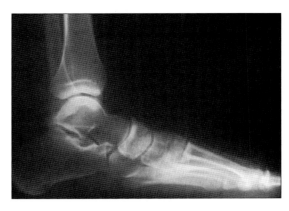

Fig. 21.9 Radiograph of large os trigonum associated with posterior heel pain in a runner.

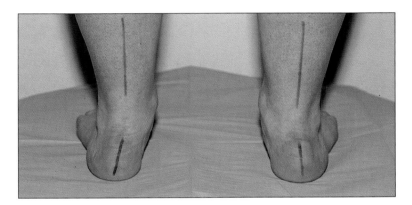

Fig. 21.10 Hyperpronation of the feet with hind foot valgus.

with or without true chondromalacia patellae found at arthroscopy. Patella alta with recurvatum increases the risk of anterior horn meniscal injury, medial collateral ligament injury and anterior or posterior ligament rupture. Such individuals should be counseled about the need to change to lower-risk non-contact sports.

Management of anterior knee pain must include a period of reduced activity, vastus medialis strengthening and correction of foot hyperpronation, if present, as this also effectively increases the Q-angle.

Os trigonum

The presence of an os trigonum (an unfused epiphysis of the posterior tubercle of the talus; Fig. 21.9) may lead to posterior heel pain, particularly in sports involving maximal plantar flexion, such as long jumping and dancing *en pointe*. The os trigonum impinges between the tibia and the calcaneum, as the foot plantar flexes. There may also be a pre-Achilles bursitis.

Abnormalities of gait

Walking and running are coordinated processes of extraordinary complexity, in which individual movements occur at many body sites simultaneously in three planes. The six major components of gait are pelvic rotation and tilt, lateral pelvic displacement, knee extension and flexion and ankle joint movement. If there is a fault in this co-ordinated system, altered function will also occur at other sites. If this is amplified by repetitive loading through sport, soft tissue injury and, in some cases, cartilage damage may result.

Anatomic asymmetry, joint laxity and gait must therefore be carefully assessed in patients with chronic lower limb symptoms, and with backache in particular. Gait abnormalities may require a treadmill assessment, as abnormal patterns may not be apparent until the athlete runs or becomes fatigued.

Hyperpronation of the feet (Fig. 21.10) in the stance phase of running increases the risk of such disorders as shin splints, medial tibial stress fractures and Achilles tendon injury when repetitive loading occurs.

CLINICAL CONDITIONS

Tendon injury

The type of injury depends upon the levels of loading and the site of injury; where there is a tendon sheath, frictional tenosynovitis (a) or paratendinitis (b) can occur, particularly at the wrist (a) and ankle (b).

Mafulli and colleagues have referred to the importance of clinicians recognizing the degenerative nature of chronic tendinopathies[41]. The characteristic pathology of chronic overuse conditions of the patellar tendon, Achilles tendon and rotator cuff are of a non-inflammatory tendinosis with neovascularization (Table 21.7). The normally tight parallel bundles of collagen fibers are disturbed, with unequal and irregular crimping. There is an absence of inflammatory cells and the increased cell proliferation seen has been demonstrated by the presence of proliferating cell nuclear antigen (PCNA)[42].

In the early phase of tendinopathy it is possible that an inflammatory component is important and that chronic paratendinitis may affect vascularization and deeper tendon pathology. Acute paratendinitis (Table 21.8) may show marked inflammatory changes with paratendon effusion. The term 'tendinitis' is probably best restricted to primary inflammatory conditions such as B27-associated tendinitis, although usually the dominant problem is at the enthesis (enthesitis).

Overuse tenosynovitis

The sites commonly involved through sport are the flexor and extensor tendons in the hands, wrists and ankles and also in the shoulder. The features that are particularly important are tendinosis, deformity and triggering.

Tendinosis must still be excluded by ultrasound or magnetic resonance imaging (MRI) as it may be difficult to distinguish in the presence of tenosynovitis. It usually causes more pain and restriction of movement across a joint, such as the ankle. A history of a sudden snap must be taken very seriously if complete rupture is to be avoided.

Deformity, indicating rupture, must be noted. At the ankle, tibialis posterior rupture will cause flattening of the medial arch. In the fingers, extensor tendon rupture is particularly seen in catching sports such as baseball and cricket, and may occur at two common sites:

- the dorsum of the base of the middle phalanx, causing boutonnière deformity
- the dorsum of the base of the terminal phalanx, causing mallet deformity.

Triggering in the hand flexors of sportspeople may require surgery, as it implies either repeated synovitis, causing flexor tendon thickening,

usually at the metacarpophalangeal (MCP) joint, or a nodule caused by superficial rupture of the spiral tendon fibers.

Management

In early uncomplicated tenosynovitis, rest in a support is frequently sufficient. If not, a corticosteroid injection, avoiding direct intratendinous injection, is usually successful provided recurrence is not induced by too rapid a return to sport. However, in certain conditions, for example extensor tendon tenosynovitis due to repetitive rapid wrist movement in rowers and flexor tendon triggering, constriction of the tendon may be so marked that urgent decompression is essential, to avoid further damage to the tendon substance.

Ankle tenosynovitis will frequently reflect an abnormal running gait, for example tibialis posterior involvement and flattening of the medial longitudinal arch. Suitable orthotic advice is an important part of management.

Tibialis anterior tenosynovitis, on the other hand, is rare even in sportspeople. However, if present, it usually exemplifies the role of specific repetitive action in etiology, being seen particularly after long periods of downhill activity in hikers, long-distance runners and skiers.

Paratendinitis and tendinosis

At heavily loaded tendons without a tendon sheath, such as the patellar and Achilles tendons, there may be an associated inflammation in the paratendon (paratendinitis). 'Jumper's knee' is due to microtearing at the inferior patellar pole attachment and corresponds with Sinding–Larsen–Johansson syndrome in children (Table 21.5). Lesions can extend down the patellar tendon or can occasionally be localized to the mid-tendon region. They are best assessed by ultrasound scan (Fig. 21.11) or MRI (Fig. 21.12), although computerized tomography (CT) scanning (Fig 21.13) may still be utilized if MRI is not available.

Achilles tendinopathy

There are many types of Achilles tendon injury, and only the most common are described here.

Superficial injury: paratendinitis

The most treatable cause is due to chronic frictional irritation by the heel tab of the shoe, which can be avoided by wearing better shoes or cutting the heel tab. Paratendinitis or paratendon effusion can occur as a result of simple overuse.

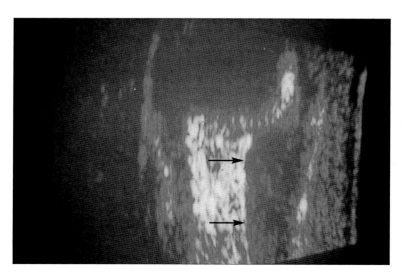

Fig. 21.11 Ultrasound of an abnormal patellar tendon with enlargement and reduced echogenicity of the tendon (arrows).

TABLE 21.7 PATHOLOGY OF TENDINOSIS

- Degenerative process within tendon
- Angioblastic reaction
- Lack of inflammatory cell infiltration

TABLE 21.8 PATHOLOGY OF PARATENDINITIS

- (Acute) edema and hyperemia
- Inflammatory cell infiltration
- ± Fibrinous exudate and associated crepitus

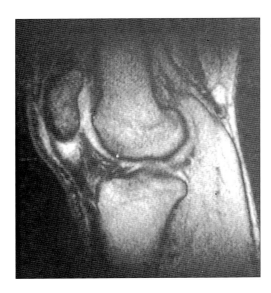

Fig. 21.12 Sagittal MRI in patellar pole tendinitis.

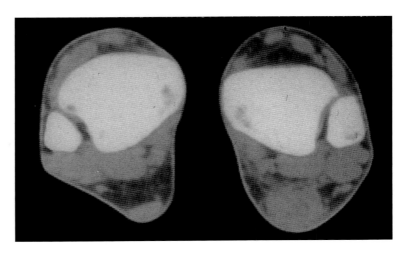

Fig. 21.14 Cross-sectional CT view of both lower legs showing a thickened left Achilles tendon with central necrosis.

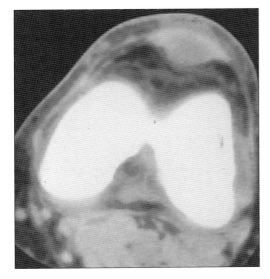

Fig. 21.13 CT scan showing large cystic lesion in mid patellar ligament.

Deep tendinosis

This is clinically likely with a history of recurrent achillodynia and, on examination, swelling with local tenderness at rest that decreases when the tendon is put under stretch by dorsiflexion. In this condition microtearing probably occurs as a result of accumulated impact loading, aggravated by the whipping action of the Achilles' tendon as the foot pronates, or of eccentric loading when the fatigued runner alters his/her gait.

Management includes a reduction of training level, especially on hills, use of a heel lift to decrease strain and supervised stretching. Nonsteroidal anti-inflammatory drugs (NSAIDs) may facilitate rehabilitation but corticosteroids should be avoided when central core changes have been confirmed by MRI, CT scanning (Fig. 21.14) or ultrasound imaging.

If there is an abnormal running pattern orthoses may be indicated, particularly for excessive pronation, and tibialis posterior should be strengthened. Surgical intervention and long-term prognosis has been well reviewed by Paavola and colleagues[43].

Bursitis

A pre-Achilles bursitis often presents with plantar flexion impingement pain and is associated with tenderness that is anterior to the tendon. Plantar flexion pain associated with os trigonum impingement was discussed earlier in this chapter.

Complete rupture

This is uncommon in young athletes, with a mean age of rupture of about 35 years. Although histology obtained from acute ruptures usually shows evidence of chronic changes, two-thirds of patients are asymptomatic until rupture. It is mainly seen in sports involving explosive forward movement. Kaalund and colleagues[44] showed that, of 96 ruptures seen in Denmark over a 2.5-year period, 40% were due to badminton and only 18% to soccer. Of those occurring in soccer players, 87% occurred in the middle or last period of the game, supporting the view that poor muscle coordination in tired players is an important risk factor. Following surgery, 46% resumed sport within 6 months and 82% by 1 year, but seven individuals did not return to sport.

Tendon injury in children

Traction apophysitis (see also injury factors in children)

Children are particularly prone to attachment injury (traction apophysitis) of which Osgood–Schlatter apophysitis of the tibial tubercle is the best known. The other common conditions and clinical features are set out in Table 21.5. Attachment injuries may be seen at any heavily loaded apophysis, for example ischial hamstring attachments in sprinters and dancers or medial elbow in javelin throwers.

Osgood–Schlatter apophysitis

This was previously typically seen in athletically active boys of 13–14 years of age. Now, with the increase in sporting activity, it is also being seen in girls aged 10–11 years (equivalent in skeletal maturity to boys of 13–14 years).

Pain is felt at the tibial tubercle, aggravated by heavy activity. The main signs are local tibial tubercle tenderness and swelling, with quadriceps tightness as part of the underlying cause. Bony enlargement persists when the painful period has settled.

Chronic symptoms of pain on activity may continue into adult life because of separated ossific bodies irritating the patellar tendon. Surgery is then often necessary and may need to include modification of any tubercle prominence, which may be much more obvious on CT scanning (Fig. 21.15).

Iliotibial band syndrome

The iliotibial band or tract is thickened fascia connecting the ilium with the lateral tibia (Fig. 21.16) and it receives part of the insertion of tensor fasciae latae and gluteus maximus. When the hip is flexed the tensor fasciae latae pulls the iliotibial band forwards but, when the hip is extended, the gluteus maximus pulls it backwards. Therefore, repetitive flexion and extension can lead to irritation of either the iliotibial band

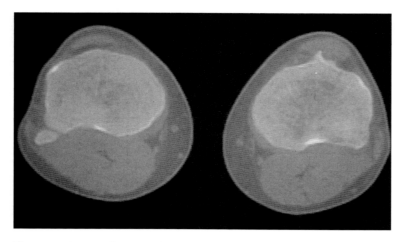

Fig. 21.15 CT scan showing tibial tubercle prominence due to previous Osgood–Schlatter disease that has caused patellar tendinopathy.

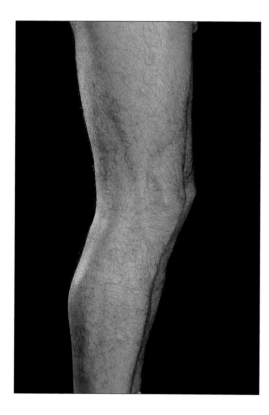

Fig. 21.16 Lateral view of the right leg showing the iliotibial band.

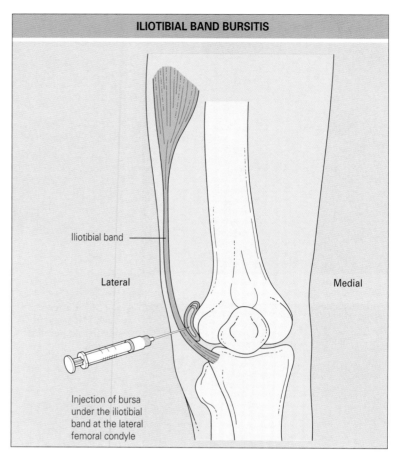

ILIOTIBIAL BAND BURSITIS

Iliotibial band

Lateral

Medial

Injection of bursa under the iliotibial band at the lateral femoral condyle

Fig. 21.17 Iliotibial band bursitis.

or its associated bursa over the lateral femoral condyle, usually as a result of high-intensity training, particularly if camber running (running on a sloping surface).

Pain usually takes some miles of running before it builds up and is localized to about 2 cm above the joint line. A stiff-legged gait may be adopted, as this relieves pain.

The signs include:

- local tenderness at the lateral femoral condyle
- pain on standing on the flexed (30–40%) knee
- tight iliotibial band detected by Ober's test: with the patient lying on the unaffected side with hip flexed, the affected knee is flexed and the hip abducted and extended to line up with the trunk. In now attempting to adduct the hip, it will be found that this is limited because the short iliotibial band will be caught on the greater trochanter.

Excess forefoot pronation or leg-length inequality may play a part in etiology and should be controlled with an orthotic before return to

sport. Reduction of mileage and avoidance of camber running may resolve the condition but local corticosteroid injection may be required, particularly if there is an associated bursitis (Fig. 21.17).

Bursitis

Superficial bursae are commonly affected by injury but deep frictional bursitis is frequently overlooked as a cause of symptoms.

Bursae have an indistinct synovial cell lining, with underlying fibrovascular tissue, and are situated between fascial planes or subcutaneously. They improve the gliding motion of two adjoining structures by reducing friction. Direct trauma causes a hemobursa and chronic irritation an inflammatory bursitis, often leading to chronic bursal thickening with calcium deposition.

A septic bursitis, usually due to staphylococci, should be suspected and excluded by aspiration/culture if the bursa is acutely inflamed, particularly if there is an overlying skin abrasion (e.g. olecranon or prepatellar). Gouty bursitis may also be exacerbated by trauma, so fluid must be sent for crystal examination by polarizing light microscopy.

Shoulder bursitis

In sportspeople, subacromial bursitis is usually due to repetitive overhead throwing, hitting or lifting, especially in tennis, swimming and weightlifting. Osteophytosis of the inferior aspect of the acromioclavicular joint may contribute to the impingement.

Elbow bursitis

Olecranon bursitis usually follows a fall on to a firm surface but may be due to repetitive bending, as in gymnastics.

Hip bursitis

Iliopsoas bursitis, with pain on hip extension, is an important condition in the differential diagnosis of groin pain.

Knee bursitis

Prepatellar bursitis (carpet-layer's or housemaid's knee)

This bursa is present in about 90% of the normal population. It is subcutaneous and anterior to the lower half of the patella and upper half of the patellar ligament. Following direct trauma or repetitive friction due to prolonged kneeling, a swelling may be noticed by the patient. It is not usually painful, except on pressure, and swelling is usually cool. In acute bursitis, other causes such as staphylococcal infection or gouty inflammation should be considered. Even in acute infective prepatellar bursitis, knee movement is usually well preserved, with pain at the end range of movement in flexion stretching the anterior soft tissues. It is essential when needle aspiration is performed that it is accurate and does not include aspiration of the knee joint, as this could convert a relatively benign infective bursitis into deep-seated joint infection. In joint sepsis severe restriction and irritability of the joint is usually found.

Deep infrapatellar bursitis

This small bursa lies between the upper part of the tibial tubercle and the ligamentum patellae. It is separated from the knee joint synovium by a fat pad (Fig 21.18). When it is inflamed, swelling can be noticed on either side of the patellar ligament insertion to the tibial tubercle. Infection is rare because this is a deeper bursa than the pre-patellar bursa, but inflammation may follow direct trauma or repetitive pressure (prayer bursitis) or irritation from debris following previous Osgood–Schlatter disease (Fig. 21.15).

Suprapatellar bursitis

The suprapatellar bursa of the knee communicates with the knee joint and will swell as part of joint effusion or synovitis.

Subcrural bursitis

The subcrural bursa, beneath the quadriceps tendon, usually communicates with the joint and therefore is affected by causes of joint swelling. Occasionally it may be affected independently when separated from the joint and presents as a horseshoe swelling around the patella distended with fluid.

Fat pad syndrome (Hoffa's disease)

The infrapatellar fat pad (Fig. 21.18) lies behind the patellar ligament. A portion of it is carried in between synovial folds and is frequently the site

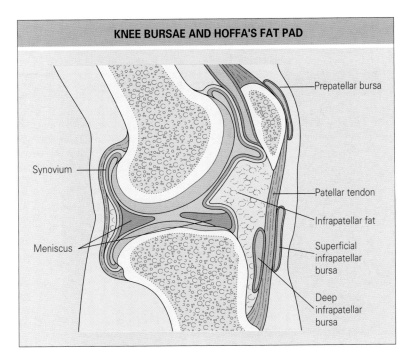

KNEE BURSAE AND HOFFA'S FAT PAD

Synovium
Meniscus
Prepatellar bursa
Patellar tendon
Infrapatellar fat
Superficial infrapatellar bursa
Deep infrapatellar bursa

Fig. 21.18 Knee bursae and Hoffa's fat pad.

of hypertrophy. The synovial membrane, which covers the deep surface of the infrapatellar fat pad, leads to a triangular fold passing upwards and backwards to be attached by its apex to the anterior tip of the intercondylar fossa. The fold is called the infrapatellar synovial fold (ligamentum mucosum) and its free margins are known as the alar folds (ligamenta alaria).

When the knee joint is extended, the patella is drawn up by quadriceps contraction and the infrapatellar fat pad follows, thus preventing its impingement between tibia and femur. However, when the fat pad is hypertrophied or the quadriceps has lost its tone the pad may be caught between the articular surfaces.

Treatment should include temporary restriction of full extension and injection if there is significant hypertrophy, particularly when associated with synovial thickening. In resistant cases partial surgical excision of the fat pad may be necessary.

Pes anserinus bursitis

The pes anserinus bursa, lying between the medial collateral ligament and the overlying pes anserinus (comprising the tendons of sartorius, gracilis and semitendinosus), is typically affected in swimmers ('breaststroker's knee') and runners.

Rupture of a popliteal cyst (Baker's cyst)

The patient presents with a classical history of sudden upper calf pain (the patient may often feel they have been kicked in the calf) with reduction of pre-existing knee swelling followed by generalized calf swelling, and there may be pitting edema from the dorsum of the foot to the calf. This has been termed the 'pseudothrombophlebitis syndrome'[45]. The most important differential diagnosis is from deep vein thrombosis although sometimes, because of secondary venous obstruction, a deep vein thrombosis can develop after cyst rupture. Patients with a popliteal cyst must be warned about this risk, particularly if flying, and prophylactic low-dose aspirin is generally indicated. When rupture has occurred, venous Doppler studies are the investigation of choice as venous occlusion cannot be excluded on clinical grounds alone.

Treatment of a ruptured cyst is treatment of the underlying cause. Aspiration and injection of the joint should be performed if there is a synovitis or management of an underlying mechanical cause within the knee causing recurrent effusion.

Semimembranosus bursitis

There are two posterior knee bursae, one between each of the heads of the gastrocnemii and the joint capsule. They often communicate with the joint.

The medial bursa (semimembranosus), lying between the medial head of gastrocnemius and the capsule, extends between the gastrocnemius and semimembranosus. Enlargement of this bursa forms as a swelling in the median aspect of the popliteal fossa and may follow repetitive knee flexion (gamekeeper's knee). It usually enlarges distally deep to the medial head of gastrocnemius and appears as an oval fluctuant swelling, limited laterally but less defined medially, in the popliteal space.

It tenses on extension and relaxes on flexion. If part of inflammatory joint disease it may respond to treatment of the underlying joint disease or injection. It must be distinguished from a Baker's cyst, which always communicates with the joint and if large and persistent will require surgical excision.

Popliteus bursitis

The popliteus bursa arises from the synovial membrane of the knee surrounding the popliteus tendon intra-articularly. When inflamed it can sometimes be seen as a rounded swelling behind the lateral condyle of the femur, deep to the biceps femoris and the iliotibial band.

Popliteus bursitis is usually seen as an overuse lesion and presents with pain on the posterolateral aspect of the knee. Examination of the knee is usually normal apart from resisted flexion reproducing the pain. Resisted external rotation may also be painful. Treatment is by deep friction, muscle rehabilitation and injection if persistent.

Plicae synoviales

The plicae synoviales are remnants of the embryological divisions within the knee. The development of knee arthroscopy and MRI has shown that these bands are present in over 20% of knees, with medial plicae more common than lateral. Symptoms can develop after repetitive activities or direct injury, but it is essential before considering intervention to be sure that the symptoms do relate to the plica. At arthroscopy many plicae are probably excised unnecessarily.

The medial patella plica, or medial shelf, appears to be the one most likely to cause clinical problems. This was first described by Lino in 1939[46] and well reviewed by Broom in 1986[47]. It runs obliquely from the medial border of the knee joint downwards, inserting into the synovium and covering the medial infrapatellar fat pad. During knee flexion, the plica glides over the medial condyle like a windscreen wiper. However, if the plica becomes thickened or inflamed due to trauma or synovitis it may cause sudden pain, as it is pinched between the patella and medial condyle of the femur. There may be pain and a feeling of a slight soft tissue block to full extension of the knee. A painful arc during flexion of the knee can occur if there is irregularity of the femoral condyle, for instance due to osteochondral damage and a thickened plica riding over this area.

The plica can often be felt if the examiner rolls the medial capsule of the knee under the thumb or index finger with the knee flexed to about 45° (Fig. 21.19). If this is painful and recognized by the patient as the pain previously felt, an injection should be given. If the symptoms persist, arthroscopic resection is occasionally indicated. Underlying synovitis of the knee joint may, however, be the associated cause and should be treated appropriately first. It should be stressed that the presence of a medial plica is a normal variant and, unless inflamed, with appropriate symptoms and clinical findings, arthroscopic resection should not be performed.

Ankle bursitis

Retrocalcaneal or pre-Achilles bursitis may be associated with a prominent os trigonum (Fig. 21.9) and is particularly seen in hill running.

Superficial Achilles bursitis ('pump bump') is frequently secondary to frictional irritation by inadequate footwear. Haglund's syndrome refers to pain in the posterior heel, characterized by a painful 'pump bump' and a typical radiographic configuration of the posterior border of the os calcis with convexity of the posterior soft tissues due to the bursitis. Failure to respond to modification of footwear and training may require surgical intervention.

Compartmental syndromes

These can be defined as an increase in tissue pressure, within a confined space or muscle compartment, that compromises local circulation and function.

Acute compartment syndrome

Acute compartment syndrome is a surgical emergency and may result from a direct blow to the muscle, from the trauma associated with a fracture or from prolonged pressure over a muscle compartment. It also occurs rarely following prolonged exertion. Acute compartment syndromes can lead to rapid and complete muscle necrosis. Early surgical decompression of the compartment may allow restoration of circulation to the muscle and preserve function. The clinical diagnosis of acute compartment syndrome is based on patients who have pain that is out of proportion to the injury or history of injury, swelling and firmness of the muscle compartment and pain on passive stretch. Later in the evolution of acute compartment syndrome, patients develop signs of decreased perfusion, including decreased pulses, decreased capillary refill and skin pallor. Neurologic symptoms may also appear.

Chronic compartment syndrome

This is the typical form seen in athletes and is characterized by a return to normal function between episodes of exercise-induced pain. It is most commonly seen in the lower leg.

The muscles of the leg are contained within four compartments separated by deep transverse fascia (Fig. 21.20). The athlete describes aching or cramping of the leg, roughly in the distribution of the involved compartment. The period from commencement of exercise to the onset of symptoms is variable and depends upon the type and intensity of exercise, but is usually within 10–30 minutes. Return to normal is also variable, taking minutes in most cases but in more severe cases occasionally taking hours for complete resolution. Neurologic symptoms may occur because of ischemia of nerves, particularly in the anterior tibial syndrome.

There are no diagnostic signs at rest, although fascial defects may be found in up to 40% of cases. After sufficient exercise, tenderness and

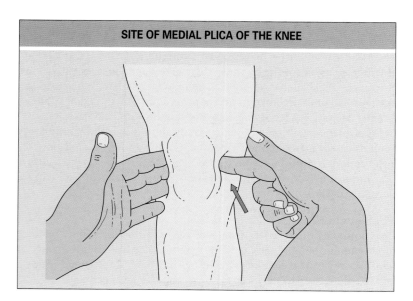

SITE OF MEDIAL PLICA OF THE KNEE

Fig. 21.19 Site of medial plica of the knee.

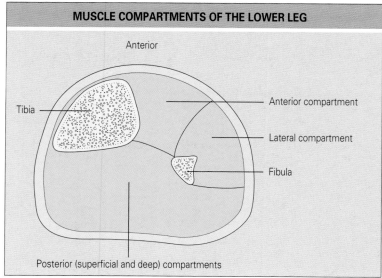

MUSCLE COMPARTMENTS OF THE LOWER LEG

Anterior

Tibia

Anterior compartment

Lateral compartment

Fibula

Posterior (superficial and deep) compartments

Fig. 21.20 Muscle compartments of the lower leg.

fullness will be found in the muscle compartment involved, most commonly the anterolateral.

Slit catheter measurement of intracompartmental pressure before and after exercise can be used to select patients suitable for surgical decompression, provided it is performed in a specialist center with reliable standardization. It is likely that MRI will prove of increasing importance in diagnosis, with the development of more sophisticated imaging techniques looking at biochemical shifts or pH changes.

Compartmental syndrome of the forearm is much less common but may be seen in weightlifters and rowers particularly. The deep fascia of the forearm encloses both the flexor and extensor muscles, which are separated by the radius, ulna and interosseus membrane. The deep flexor compartment of the forearm is the more common site.

Shin splints

The term 'shin splints' has been used to cover a variety of conditions causing lower medial tibial pain, but the American Medical Association's definition limits the use of the term to musculotendinous inflammation, causing pain or discomfort in the leg from repetitive running on hard surfaces or forcible excessive use of the foot dorsiflexors. It is therefore also referred to as 'medial tibial stress syndrome' and excludes stress fractures or ischemic disorders.

The history is initially of medial tibial pain at the beginning of a workout but later pain may become persistent and in severe cases may even develop in some everyday activities.

On examination, there is a 3–6cm area of tenderness on the posteromedial border of the distal third of the tibia that is much less localized than a stress fracture. The pain can only infrequently be aggravated by active plantar flexion and inversion of the foot against resistance. Radiographs are normal, but technetium bone scan may show increased longitudinal uptake involving the posteromedial tibial cortex (Fig. 21.21), unlike the more pisiform shape of the increased uptake of a typical stress fracture (Fig. 21.22).

Groin injury

Groin problems are particularly common in soccer and jumping sports. The term 'groin strain' is best avoided and specific localizing signs should be sought. The sites of pain and local tenderness, as well as pain on resisted stress or stretching, are important in defining injury to rectus femoris, iliopsoas and adductors. Limitation of hip movement because of hip disease, and referred pain due to spinal disorders must also be excluded.

Adductor tendon injury

This is characterized by pain when sprinting, pivoting or kicking. Symptoms may spread through compensation mechanisms to the opposite side. On examination there is tenderness in gracilis and adductor brevis, close to the insertion, with pain on resisted adduction and on abduction stretch. The risk of injury to the adductors appears to be increased by spinal problems, hip disorders and abdominal muscle insufficiency. Leg-length inequality or foot deformity may also be important factors in injury to the adductors and symphysis.

Symphysitis and symphysis instability must be excluded, particularly if there are bilateral groin and lower abdominal symptoms. However, plain radiographs frequently show symphysis irregularity in footballers without clinical or radiological signs of instability (Fig. 21.1).

True instability can be demonstrated by flamingo (stork) views, with movement of the pubic rami in relation to each other when the patient stands first on one leg, then on the other. Technetium isotope scan, with squat views following bladder emptying, may confirm symphysitis if there is focally increased uptake at the symphysis.

A long period of withdrawal from sport is often essential. In one series, time to recovery was 9.5 months in men and 7 months in women, with a 25% relapse rate in men[48]. Rarely, the symphysis is the site of

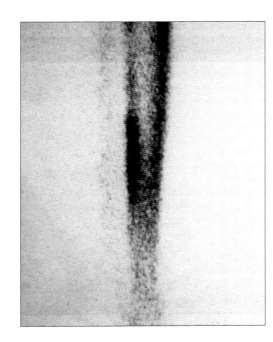

Fig. 21.21 Technetium scan showing diffuse medial tibial periosteal uptake.

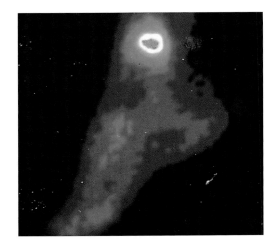

Fig. 21.22 Technetium scan showing focal uptake of a stress fracture of the lower tibia.

infection: urinary tract infection or associated staphylococcal skin sepsis should be sought.

Conjoint tendon injury of the inguinal ring

This should be considered, even in the absence of a defined hernia, when there is localized tenderness with cough-induced pain at the external ring, which on palpitation usually feels dilated. Concomitant adductor or symphysis symptoms may also be found and should be treated first before surgery is considered.

The term 'groin strain' is inadequate because, at surgical exploration, conjoint tendon injury is frequently found and appropriate repair usually allows return to full sporting activity. Herniogram is no longer generally recommended but direct scopic visualization and repair appears to offer the best chance of return to full sporting activity quickly. However, adequately controlled follow-up studies of this technique are needed to fully assess its value and the risk of recurrence.

Neuropathies

Neuropathies may occur following direct trauma or chronic repetitive loading, resulting in either a traction or compressive entrapment, including muscular hypertrophy affecting the nerve. Less common compression sites and the sports involved are summarized in Tables 21.9 and 21.10.

		TABLE 21.9 SPORT-INDUCED UPPER LIMB COMPRESSION NEUROPATHIES		
Site	**Nerve**	**Symptoms**	**Signs**	**Sport**
Shoulder Erb's point Scapular notch	Suprascapular	Traction injury Direct or repetitive injury	Infraspinatus Supraspinatus weakness Pain (sensory supply to posterior joint capsule)	Rugby
Spinoglenoid notch		Often pain-free (if compression distal to sensory branch to shoulder)	Infraspinatus only	Volleyball
Quadrilateral space	Axillary	Acute with shoulder dislocation Chronic	Deltoid weakness with sensory loss over deltoid	Throwing sports
	Long thoracic nerve of Bell	Acute more common than chronic	Serratus anterior weakness	
	Musculocutaneous	Weak elbow flexion	Biceps and/or brachialis weakness Sensation loss: lateral cutaneous nerve of forearm	
	Spinal accessory	Weak shoulder elevation	Trapezius and sternocleidomastoid weakness	
Elbow Pronator syndrome	Median	Forearm pain on activity Sensory symptoms but rarely at night Negative Tinel's sign	Weakness of flexor digitorum profundus and pronation Entrapment by muscular hypertrophy	Weightlifting
Radial tunnel syndrome	Radial	Pain, paresthesias and weakness	Weakness of wrist extension	
Posterior interosseus syndrome	Posterior interosseus	Motor symptoms only	Extensor carpi ulnaris weak: wrist dorsiflexes radially Weak extension at MCPs Normal extension at PIPs (intrinsics)	
Medial elbow	Ulnar	Pain Paresthesias of 4th and 5th digits	Local tenderness Positive Tinel's sign Elbow flexion test (3min of full flexion of elbow with wrist fully extended)	Throwing Racket sports Weightlifting Gymnastics
Wrist/hand Carpal tunnel	Median	Carpal tunnel syndrome Paresthesia at night or on use	Weakness of abductor pollicis brevis Sensory loss, especially in index and middle fingers	
Canal of Guyon Type I (proximal or first part of canal)	Ulnar	Weakness and paresthesias	Paresthesias; spares dorsal cutaneous branch to ulnar aspect of hand	Cycling Racket sports
Type II (distal canal and hook of hamate)	Ulnar	Pure motor symptoms	Reduced grip Froment's paper sign	Ball handling sports
Type III (distal canal, beyond hamate)	Ulnar	Pure sensory symptoms	Palmar loss of sensation in 4th and 5th digits	
Thumb Ulnar digital nerve to thumb, beyond hamate	Ulnar	Pure sensory symptoms Pain and paresthesias	Local tenderness Positive Tinel's sign	Bowling

The ulnar nerve illustrates best some of these injury risks. At the elbow, it is particularly vulnerable in racquet and throwing sports. These produce a valgus stress on the elbow in flexion such that a valgus laxity of the ulnar collateral ligament may develop, which alters the biomechanics of the elbow joint. In adolescents, before fusion of the secondary ossification center occurs, the growth plate of the medial epicondyle represents the weakest attachment of the flexor pronator muscle group, so repetitive stress may produce a traction apophysitis (Table 21.5). Valgus laxity, or osteophytes in older participants, may be a cause of ulnar traction and it has been reported that 16% of the population demonstrate recurrent dislocation of the ulnar nerve in flexion, which increases the traction risk to the nerve.

MANAGEMENT OF SPORT INJURY

General principles

It is crucial in dealing with individuals engaged in active sport who develop an injury to define:

- the exact anatomic site and type of injury
- the forces and training load involved in injury and modification of these following recovery to prevent recurrence
- abnormalities of running gait or sports technique that will require adjustment.

Management of acute injury

The team doctor, coach or physical therapist may be able to help in clarifying the likely injury by describing the 'event' and the observed forces of injury. If the injured athlete is seen immediately and has a joint injury, it is important to examine the joint before protective muscle spasm makes this impossible.

Immediate swelling of a joint at the time of injury implies hemarthrosis. In the knee this will usually be due to ACL tear or osteochondral damage. Urgent arthroscopy is important, followed by appropriate intensive rehabilitation where ACL rupture has occurred and cannot be repaired immediately. The anterior-cruciate-deficient knee requires a program of balanced hamstring and quadriceps muscle strengthening, with later secondary repair only if instability is a functional problem. An associated

TABLE 21.10 SPORT-INDUCED LOWER LIMB COMPRESSION NEUROPATHIES

Site	Nerve	Symptoms	Signs	Sport
Hindfoot Between deep fascia of abductor hallucis brevis and medial margin of quadratus plantae	First branch of lateral plantar	Chronic heel pain increased by walking, greatly increased by running	Tenderness deep to abductor hallucis brevis Foot may be hypermobile	Running Jogging
Tarsal tunnel (flexor retinaculum, medial calcaneum, talus and medial malleolus)	Posterior tibial	Burning paresthesias in sole of foot, spreading to toes Increased by standing/running and at night	Ankle injury prior to onset often recorded Positive Tinel's sign; eversion may increase, (exclude spinal)	Running
Medial arch and navicular tuberosity	Medial plantar	Medial arch pain	Foot eversion increased (excessive heel valgus on running – may be precipitated by use of arch support)	Jogging
At exit from deep fascia (local compartment)	Superficial peroneal	Pain in distal calf and lateral foot, increased by running	Tenderness at deep fascial exit Palpable fascial defect in 60% of cases History of chronic ankle sprains common	Running Hockey Tennis
Forefoot Microtrauma against distal edge of intermetatarsal ligament especially if pronation increased	Interdigital (neuromas) Plantar digital nerves especially in 3rd (or 2nd) web space	Plantar or forefoot pain on activity, often radiating to toes	Point tenderness between metatarsal heads Relief by removal of shoe, rest and massage	Running Ballet dancing

meniscal injury is frequently the cause of symptoms in an anterior-cruciate-deficient knee and should be treated first. Anterior cruciate tear is best assessed by the Lachman test and the pivot shift test (see Chapter 19).

Having excluded severe injuries such as fracture, dislocation and ligament rupture, in the less severe injuries without skin breakage the practitioner should advise the application of the principles of 'RICE'.

- **Rest**. Short-term immediate rest reduces bleeding and inflammation. It is essential to reintroduce activity after injury in a graduated way, and to avoid any training errors that may have contributed to the problem.
- **Ice.** Application of an ice pack (covered with a towel to prevent skin burning), decreases vascularity and inflammation and has an analgesic effect.
- **Compression** reduces bleeding and tissue swelling.
- **Elevation** reduces swelling.

Management after this early period is dependent on the type and severity of injury. Controlled stretching is important, particularly in hamstring and Achilles tendon injury. Early return to activity is advisable in mild ankle ligament injury but individuals should not return to sport until they are pain-free and full ankle control has been achieved. This involves a program of exercises to re-educate ankle proprioceptive muscle control, progressing through use of the wobble board.

General management of chronic injury
Local corticosteroid injections in chronic soft tissue injury
The use of local corticosteroid injections in chronic soft tissue injury in sportspeople has become a somewhat emotive issue. This seems generally to be based on inappropriate administration of corticosteroids by some clinicians and the variability of the results of published studies on the effects of corticosteroids on collagenous structures.

There is clear evidence from animal experiments that injection of some corticosteroid preparations into tendons or ligaments may cause alteration in their structure and behavior.[49,50] The injudicious use of corticosteroid injections, allowing too rapid a return to heavy loading, will almost inevitably lead to further microfailure in tendons weakened by injury. It is important to reduce activity in the period after injection and to use injections only as an adjunct to rehabilitation with restrengthening and stretching, essential before return to full active sport. Where corticosteroids have been allowed to enter the tendon substance, complete rupture may occur if the tendon is subjected to (very) heavy loading. Although very rare, this complication is usually only reported in athletes, particularly in the Achilles tendon, and the elderly.

Experimental effects of corticosteroids on tendons and ligaments
Carstram[51] and Wrenn and colleagues[52] showed that intramuscular cortisone inhibits the formation of adhesions in the healing process after tendon injury with some weakening of the tendon structure. Direct injection of corticosteroid into healthy tendons at doses comparable with those used therapeutically has produced variable experimental data, possibly partly reflecting differences in length of follow-up. Mackie and colleagues[53] and Phelps and colleagues[54] concluded that there were no significant changes in the mechanical properties of rabbit tendons injected in this way. Noyes and colleagues[49], however, showed clear evidence of decreases in the stiffness, failure load and energy absorption of ACL in monkeys following direct intracollagenous injection of methylprednisolone acetate, the changes persisting for up to 52 weeks. Kapetanos[50] confirmed that a long-acting corticosteroid (triamcinolone acetonide) injected into artificially injured rabbit Achilles tendons significantly decreased tendon weight, adhesion response, load to failure and energy to failure. Wesley McWhorter and colleagues[55], however, failed to show any difference, compared with controls, in the strength of rat Achilles tendon or consistent reduction of cell types recognized as components of the healing process after peritendinous hydrocortisone acetate injection.

Rational use of corticosteroid injections
When an inflammatory response in injured tendons is unresponsive to local treatment and is inhibiting rehabilitation, with inevitable loss of strength in the entire muscle–tendon complex, local peritendinous corticosteroid injection is justified, providing the following precautions are observed:

- short-acting preparations should be used
- great care must be taken to avoid injecting directly into tendon tissue – this can be ensured by careful siting of the needle and recognition that injection must never be forced in under pressure
- injection should be followed by a period of rest and then graduated restrengthening, on the basis that recovery of tendon strength takes considerably longer than generally recognized
- heavily loaded tendons should be adequately assessed by imaging because, in the apparently peritendinous injection, corticosteroid may travel into the tendon substance where there is a significant destructive lesion.

It is recommended that peritendinous injection of the Achilles tendon in athletes is not performed without a soft tissue scan to exclude deeper Achilles injury. Only in simple paratendinitis chronically resistant to treatment should peritendinous injection be considered.

Intra-articular corticosteroid injections should not be given to athletes unless a fully investigated primary rheumatologic condition, such as synovitis due to spondyloarthritis, has been proved.

Localized injection of deep frictional bursitis is less contentious but chronic superficial bursitis around the knee is usually poorly responsive to corticosteroid injection.

Non-steroidal anti-inflammatory drugs

These are of value in the active inflammatory phase, particularly where major pain and swelling inhibit muscle function and therefore adequate rehabilitation. Attention must always be paid to previous dyspeptic history, as NSAIDs may potentiate stress-induced gastric changes, particularly after endurance events. The cyclo-oxygenase (COX)-2-selective inhibitors appear to have a much lower risk of serious gastrointestinal toxicity, including ulcer bleeding and perforation. All NSAIDs may exacerbate asthma.

Experimental evidence from studies of wound healing points to the importance for adequate healing of the initial marked polymorphonuclear leukocyte infiltration. As experimental removal of the polymorphonuclear phase reduces fibroblastic proliferation and angiogenesis, medication inhibiting this process could be suspected of resulting in poorly healed soft tissue structures, with risk of further failure. For this reason, corticosteroids should not be given in the acute phase of injury response.

Local NSAID application by gel formulation or patch merits further analysis, particularly as combination with ultrasound may promote delivery to soft tissue sites. The occasional report of exacerbation of asthma by such preparations illustrates that their use should be initiated and supervised by a medical practitioner who has fully assessed the athlete.

Surgical treatment

General principles

Urgent surgical intervention is generally necessary for injuries in sports causing complete tendon or ligament rupture, and sometimes for muscle rupture with extensive bleeding. It has already been emphasized that a history of immediate joint swelling after trauma usually indicates hemarthrosis, an indication of major injury, for example rupture of the ACL of the knee, requiring immediate orthopedic referral. Intensive postoperative rehabilitation must be co-ordinated between the surgeon, therapist and patient.

Similarly, surgical intervention in chronic injury, after conservative treatment has failed, should only be undertaken as part of a defined program designed to restore as near normal co-ordinated musculoskeletal function as is possible. The aims and limitations of surgery must therefore be discussed with the athlete and a carefully planned rehabilitation program, commencing as soon after surgery as the procedure allows, must be defined by the therapist and patient. No guarantee of return to full athletic prowess should be given to the patient.

Surgical intervention in chronic injury should only be considered after failed rehabilitation and a clear diagnosis has been defined (often) confirmed by appropriate imaging:

- 'diagnostic arthroscopy' is no longer appropriate as MRI will generally define meniscal injury, osteochondral or bone bruising
- decompressive, for example, exploration and release of tendon, muscle or nerve constricted through injury
- reconstructive, involving secondary procedures designed to restore function, for example in ACL rupture

- corrective, where modification is attempted of normal variants or abnormalities of skeletal anatomy, which through the repetitive stresses of sport are causing pain and/or loss of function, for example in os trigonum impingement.

Arthroscopy

The development of arthroscopy, particularly as a day-case facility, has revolutionized the management of intra-articular knee and other joint pathology (Chapter 19). It provides not only an accurate diagnostic assessment, confirming or clarifying MRI findings, but also therapeutic intervention at the same time. This allows early treatment of symptomatic meniscal tears and other intra-articular pathology, without the frequently rapid loss of muscle function and risk of further, often more complex, injury.

A locked knee, where there is a block to full extension of the knee due to a meniscal tear, is a surgical emergency requiring urgent arthroscopy. ACL repair is now frequently performed using arthroscopic techniques and long-term follow-up results are awaited with interest.

Although the knee has been the focus for arthroscopic intervention over the past 10 years, the technique is playing an increasingly important role in the management of shoulder pathology, particularly in the treatment of resistant subacromial impingement and rotator cuff injury. Ankle arthroscopy has an important role in management of osteochondral injury of the talus.

Decompressive surgery

Decompressive surgery should be performed when injury has resulted in major constriction or compression of soft tissues, for example in tenosynovitis of the hands, wrists or ankles. Removal of necrotic tissue, inhibiting function in large tendons without tendon sheaths, allows the residual normal tendon tissue to return to more normal function and thus permits recovery of tendon strength through appropriate rehabilitation. Removal of bony projections caused by previous injury may be indicated where frictional irritation of overlying soft tissue structures is occurring.

Reconstructive surgery

Reconstructive surgery involves more major intervention and should only be considered when, for example, it is clear that a chronically deficient ligament is the cause of symptoms and cannot be compensated for by improvement in muscle function. Many sportspeople have been shown to be playing sport, often at top-class level, with unsuspected ACL injury. Frequently, knee symptoms in the ACL-deficient knee are due to meniscal tear, and the latter should be treated surgically before consideration of surgery for the ligament rupture. Indeed, many authors recommend up to 9 months' rehabilitation of balanced hamstring and quadriceps function before considering surgery in the chronically symptomatic ACL-deficient knee. Similarly, adequate recovery of proprioceptive function in the ankle by intensive rehabilitation usually precludes the need for surgery after ankle ligament injury, unless there is associated osteochondral injury.

Recurrent dislocation of the shoulder must be defined clearly as a real problem and non-responsive to compensatory restrengthening before further investigation, such as CT arthrography or MRI with a view to surgery, is discussed with the patient.

Corrective surgery

Corrective surgery is carried out to modify anatomic variants associated with symptoms through the repetitive stresses of sport. In the case of os trigonum impingement, the problem is relatively straightforward and the need for surgery is usually clearly defined. However, in other situations this can be a form of intervention fraught with potential problems. Only patients with severe and chronic symptoms unresponsive to conservative treatment, including physical therapy and, if appropriate, orthotic advice, should be considered for this type of surgery.

The problems of patellofemoral pain and patellar malalignment exemplify the risks of intervening in this type of condition. Long-term results should be analyzed as part of the overall problem of the management of anterior knee or patellofemoral knee pain.

Management of anterior knee pain in sportspeople

Patellofemoral pain is a common complaint of athletes, typically representing a quarter of all knee problems treated at a sports injury clinic. Chondromalacia patellae should not be used as a synonym for patellofemoral pain. Arthroscopy has shown that in patients with symptoms and signs thought to be clinically consistent with a diagnosis of chondromalacia patellae, up to 50% show no macroscopic abnormalities. Much attention has focused on the possibility that a great deal of patellofemoral pain, in athletes particularly, reflects extensor mechanism dysfunction (vastus medialis deficiency).

Conservative management must be given adequate time and should include:

- modification of activity, with avoidance of repetitive knee loading in flexion
- an NSAID if required, to permit adequate rehabilitation of vastus medialis obliquus
- patellar strapping
- orthotics, in patients in whom foot abnormalities are a factor.

However, many studies have shown that up to 20% of athletes fail to improve adequately with such regimens, and surgery should be considered in these cases.

Surgical intervention, for example lateral release of the patella[56], has produced variable results. The majority of studies show that over 80% of patients with chronic patellofemoral pain respond initially to this procedure but with increasing time there is diminishing long-term benefit. An analysis by Kolowich and colleagues[57] suggested that the ideal candidates for this procedure are patients with chronic anterior knee pain who on examination show tight lateral patellar soft tissues but a normal Q-angle (Fig. 21.7). Conversely, patients with excessive laxity of the patellar retinaculum and an abnormal Q-angle showed poor results. However, it is the patients who fall between these two extremes who present difficulty in prediction of response to surgery. This excellent study of the risk–benefit ratio of surgery in a broad group of patients is the type of critical analysis that should be applied to surgical intervention of this kind in the management of chronic sports injuries.

Sportspeople may opt for any intervention offered in a search for athletic success but it is essential that the clinician provides realistic goals.

REFERENCES

1. Morris JN, Everitt MG, Pollard R et al. Vigorous exercise in leisure-time: protection against coronary heart disease. Lancet 1980; 2: 1207–1210.
2. Department of Health. The health of the nation: a strategy for health in England. London: HMSO; 1992.
3. Jacobs JC, Berdon E, Johnson AD. LA-B27 associated spondyloarthritis and enthesopathy in childhood: clinical, pathological and radiographic observations in 58 patients. Pediatrics 1982; 100: 521–528.
4. Jacobs JC. Spondyloarthritis and enthesopathy. Arch Intern Med 1983; 143: 103–107.
5. International Federation of Sports Medicine. Physical exercise – an important factor for health. Br J Sports Med 1990; 24: 82.
6. Mack RP, ed. Biomechanics of running. In: American Academy of Orthopedics Symposium on the Foot and Leg in Running Sports. St Louis, MO: Mosby; 1982.
7. Lehman WL. Overuse syndromes in runners. Am Fam Physician 1984; 29: 157–164.
8. Stanitski CL. Common injuries in preadolescent and adolescent athletes: recommendations for prevention. Sports Med 1989; 7: 32–41.
9. Davidson RJL, Robertson JD, Galea G, Maughan RJ. Haematological changes associated with marathon running. Int J Sports Med 1987; 8: 19–25.
10. McCarthy DA, Dale MM. The leucocytosis of exercise – a review and model. Sports Med 1988; 6: 333–336.
11. Pedersen BK. Influence of physical activity on the cellular immune system: mechanisms of action. Int J Sports Med 1991; 12: 23–29.
12. Young A. Plasma creatinine kinase after the marathon – a diagnostic dilemma. Br J Sports Med 1984; 18: 269–267.
13. Strachan AF, Noakes TD, Kotzenberg G et al. C-reactive protein concentrations during long distance running. Br Med J 1984; 289: 1249–1251.
14. Farrell PA, Garthwaite TL, Gustafson AB. Plasma adrenocorticotropin and cortisol responses to submaximal and exhaustive exercise. J Appl Physiol 1983; 55: 1441–1444.
15. Bloom S, Johnson R, Park D et al. Differences in the metabolic and hormonal response to exercise between racing cyclists and untrained individuals. J Physiol 1976; 258: 1–18.
16. O'Connor PJ, Morgan WP, Raglin JS et al. Mood state and salivary cortisol levels following overtraining in female swimmers. Psychol Neurol Endocrinol 1989; 14: 303–310.
17. Roberts D, Smith DJ. Effects of high intensity exercise on serum ferritin and antitrypsin in trained and untrained men. Clin Sports Med 1989; 1: 63–71.
18. Carbon RJ, Macey MG, McCarthy DA et al. The effect of 30 min cycle ergometry on ankylosing spondylitis. Br J Rheumatol 1996; 35: 167–177.
19. Warme WJ, Feagin JA, Paul King PA et al. Injury statistics,1982–1993, Jackson Hole Ski Resort. Am J Sports Med 1995; 23: 597–600.
20. Stuart MJ, Aynsley Smith RN. Injuries in Junior A ice hockey: a three-year prospective study. Am J Sports Med 1995; 23: 458–461.
21. Sandelin J, Kiviluoto O, Santavirta S, Honkanen R. Outcome of sports injuries treated in a casualty department. Br J Sports Med 1985; 19: 103–106.
22. De Loës M. Medical treatment and costs of sports-related injuries in a total population. Int J Sports Med 1990; 11: 66–72.
23. Kvist M, Kujala UM, Heinonen OJ et al. Sports-related injuries in children. Int J Sports Med 1989; 10: 81–86.
24. Gibson T. Sports injuries. Baillière's Clin Rheumatol 1987; 13: 583–600.
25. Richardson AB, Jobe FW, Collins HR. The shoulder in competitive sports. Am J Sports Med 1980; 8: 159–163.
26. Dalton SE. Overuse injuries in adolescent athletes. Sports Med 1992; 13: 58–70.
27. Lane NE, Bloch DA, Jones HM et al. Long-distance running, bone density and osteoarthritis. JAMA 1986; 255: 1147–1151.
28. McBryde AM. Stress fractures in athletes. J Sports Med 1975; 3: 212–217.
29. Renstrom PAFH, Leadbetter WB. Tendinitis 1: basic concepts. Clin Sports Med 1992; 11: 493–671.
30. Archambault JM, Wiley JP, Bray RC. Exercise loading of tendons and the development of overuse injuries. Sports Med 1995; 20: 77–89.
31. Coombs RRH, Klenerman L, Narcisi P. Collagen typing in Achilles tendon rupture. J Bone J Surg 1980; 62B: 258.
32. De Stefano V. Pathogenesis and diagnosis of ruptured Achilles tendon. Orthop Rev 1975; 4: 17.
33. Noyes F, Trovik PJ, Hyde WB. Biomechanics of ligament failure (II): an analysis of immobilization, exercise and reconditioning effects in primates. J Bone J Surg 1974; 56A: 1406–1418.
34. Butler DL, Grood ES, Noyes FR, Zernkka RF. Biomechanics of ligaments and tendons. Exerc Sport Sci Rev 1978; 6: 125–181.
35. Kvist M, Järvinen M. Clinical, histochemical and biomechanical features in repair of muscle and tendon injuries. Int J Sports Med 1982; 3: 12–14.
36. Matheson GO, Clement DB, McKenzie DC et al. Stress fractures in athletes: a study of 320 cases. Am J Sports Med 1987; 15: 46–58.
37. Editorial. Athletic women, amenorrhea and skeletal integrity. Ann Intern Med 1985; 102: 258–9.
38. Grahame R, Bird KA, Child, A et al. The revised (Brighton 1998) criteria for the diagnosis of benign joint hypermobility syndrome. J Rheumatol 2000: 27: 1777–1779.
39. Larsson L-G, Baum J, Mudholkar GS. Hypermobility features in a Swedish population. Br J Rheumatology 1993; 32: 116–119.
40. Beighton P, Grahame R, Bird H. Hypermobility of joints. New York: Springer Verlag; 1983.
41. Mafulli N, Khan KM, Puddu G. Overuse tendon conditions: time to change a confusing terminology. Arthroscopy 1998, 14: 840–843.
42. Roolf CG, Fu BSC, Pau AI et al. Increased cell proliferation and associated expression of PDGFRB causing hypercellularity in patellar tendinosis. Rheumatology 2001; 40: 256–261.
43. Paavola M, Orava S, Lappilahti J et al. Chronic Achilles tendon overuse injury: complications after surgical treatment: an analysis of 432 consecutive patients. Am J Sports Med 2000; 28: 77–82.
44. Kaalund S, Lass P, Hogsaa B, Nøhr M. Achilles tendon rupture in badminton. Br J Sports Med 1989; 23: 102–104.
45. Katz RS, Zizic TM, Arnold WP, Stevens MB. The pseudothrombophlebitis syndrome. Medicine (Baltimore) 1977; 56: 151–164.
46. Iino S. Normal arthroscopic findings in the knee joint in adult cadavers, J Jpn Orthop Assoc 1936; 14: 467–523.
47. Broom MJ, Fulkerson JP. The plica syndrome: a new perspective, Orthop Clin North Am 1986; 17: 279–281.
48. Fricker PA, Taunton JE, Ammann W. Osteitis pubis in athletes. Infection, inflammation or injury? Sports Med 1991; 12: 266–279.
49. Noyes FA, Nussbaum NS, Tomk PJ, Cooper SM. Biomechanical and ultrastructural changes in ligaments and tendons after local corticosteroid injections. J Bone J Surg 1975; 57A: 876.
50. Kapetanos G. The effect of the local corticosteroids on the healing and biomechanical properties of the partially injured tendon. Clin Orthop Res 1982; 163: 170–179.

51. Carstram N. Prevention of experimental tendon adhesions by cortisone. Acta Orthop Scand 1952; 22: 15.
52. Wrenn RN, Goldner JL, Markee JL. An experimental study of the effect of cortisone on the healing process and tensile strength of tendons. J Bone J Surg 1954; 36A: 588–601.
53. Mackie JW, Goldin B, Foss M, Cockrill JL. Mechanical properties of rabbit tendons after repeated anti-inflammatory steroid injections. Med Sci Sports 1974; 6: 198–202.
54. Phelps D, Soustegard DA, Matthews LS. Corticosteroid injection effects on the biomechanical properties of rabbit patellar tendons. Clin Orthop 1974; 100: 345–348.
55. Wesley McWhorter J, Francis RS, Heckmann RA. Influence of local steroid injections of traumatized tendon properties: a biomechanical and histological study. Am J Sports Med 1991; 19: 435–439.
56. Ogilvie-Harris DJ, Jackson RW. The arthroscopic treatment of chondromalacia patellae. J Bone J Surg 1984; 66B: 660–665.
57. Kolowich PA, Paulos LE, Rosenberg TD, Farnsworth S. Lateral release of the patella: indications and contradictions. Am J Sports Med 1990; 18: 359–365.

RHEUMATOID ARTHRITIS AND OTHER SYNOVIAL DISORDERS

22 Clinical features of rheumatoid arthritis

Duncan A Gordon and David E Hastings

Classification

- The 1987 ARA criteria for the classification of rheumatoid arthritis (RA) highlight symmetric polyarthritis, nodules, radiographically evident erosions and rheumatoid factor
- Early on these may not be definitive criteria, as the subsequent course may indicate other diagnoses.

Inflammation

- Clinical evaluation is fundamental to the management of RA and includes examination for joint inflammation
- Unchecked RA inflammation may lead to clinical and radiologic evidence of damage and destruction
- In RA, inflammation primarily affects synovium, but bursae, tendon and other extra-articular features may evolve.

Course

- RA may be categorized as early, progressive or late
- Onset may be acute, gradual or insidious
- Subsequent course may be self-limited, episodic or progressive
- Health status self-report questions may be helpful for assessing the progress or prognosis of disease.

TABLE 22.1 THE 1987 AMERICAN RHEUMATISM ASSOCIATION REVISED CRITERIA FOR RHEUMATOID ARTHRITIS CLASSIFICATION [3]	
Criterion	Definition
1. Morning stiffness	Morning stiffness in and around the joints, lasting at least 1h before maximal improvement
2. Arthritis in three or more joint areas	At least three joint areas (out of 14 possible areas: right or left PIP, MCP, wrist, elbow, knee, ankle, MTP joints) simultaneously have had soft tissue swelling or fluid (not bony overgrowth alone) as observed by a physician
3. Arthritis of hand joints	At least one area swollen (as defined above) in a wrist, MCP or PIP joint
4. Symmetric arthritis	Simultaneous involvement of the same joint areas (as defined in 2) on both sides of the body (bilateral involvement of PIPs, MCPs or MTPs without absolute symmetry is acceptable)
5. Rheumatoid nodules	Subcutaneous nodules over bony prominences or extensor surfaces, or in juxta-articular regions as observed by a physician
6. Serum rheumatoid factor	Demonstration of abnormal amounts of serum rheumatoid factor by any method for which the result has been positive in fewer than 5% of normal controls
7. Radiographic changes	Radiographic changes typical of rheumatoid arthritis on posteroanterior hand and wrist radiographs, which must include erosions or unequivocal bony decalcification localized in, or most marked adjacent to, the involved joints (osteoarthritis changes alone do not qualify)

Note: For classification purposes, a patient has RA if at least four of these criteria are satisfied (criteria 1–4 must have been present for at least 6 weeks)
If at least four of these criteria are satisfied (1–4 for at least 6 weeks), the patient has RA. Patients should not be designated as having classic, definite or probable RA. MCP, metacarpophalangeal; MTP, metatarsophalangeal; PIP, proximal interphalangeal.

INTRODUCTION

Rheumatoid arthritis (RA) is a disease that affects at least twice as many women as men. Although it may begin at any age, its peak onset is in the fourth and fifth decades of life, increasing sharply with age thereafter. The onset of RA appears to be more frequent in the winter than in the summer months[1,2]. Its diagnosis is compatible with a variety of presentations and a clinical course that can last from a few weeks or months of discomfort to many years of profound disability. Although diagnostic criteria[3] may be helpful in diagnosis, in a given case they may not be definitive, because the diagnosis may become obvious only with the passage of time. This is because, initially, other causes of synovitis may be indistinguishable from RA. For example, the diagnosis of lupus, psoriatic arthritis or human leukocyte antigen HLA-B27 spondyloarthropathies may take months or years to become apparent[4].

Although we know much about the epidemiology, immunologic and genetic aspects of RA, it is a sporadic condition of unknown cause, and we have no idea what initiates or perpetuates it. Until the cause of RA becomes known, it cannot be precisely defined. A heterogeneous model for RA seems best, because it may be one disease with more than one cause, or more than one disease with a single cause[5]. At present, RA is best defined by the clinical description of the 1987 criteria of the American Rheumatism Association (ARA) (Table 22.1)[3].

These criteria were presented in two forms: a traditional one (Table 22.1) and a classification tree (Fig. 22.1). In the first, a patient fulfilling four of seven criteria is said to have RA. In the second scheme, criteria 1 and 5 were deleted, so that arthritis of three or more joints for 6 weeks or more with radiographic joint erosions or the presence of rheumatoid factor meets criteria for the diagnosis of RA. The entire criteria set strongly separates patients with RA from those with other conditions. Moreover, unlike the previous 1958 criteria, the classification tree format shows better accuracy in patients with disease duration of 1 year or less[3]. These new criteria include objective features seen in a majority of patients with RA but, unlike the former set, there are no exclusions[3].

The natural history of persons who meet criteria for classification of RA may also vary greatly from self-limited, to mild, to severe outcomes. For this reason, Pincus and Callahan[6] have suggested the need for subclassification according to different types of disease course.

When faced with a patient with polyarthritis, the physician must keep in mind the many other conditions resembling RA. It is important to distinguish such disorders from RA as soon as possible, because the correct diagnosis of RA is fundamental to the application of good management (see Chapters 23 and 24).

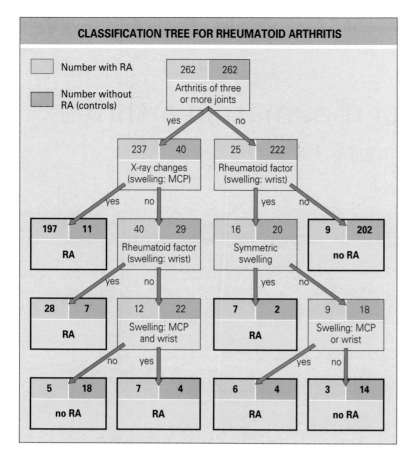

CLASSIFICATION TREE FOR RHEUMATOID ARTHRITIS

Fig. 22.1 A modified classification tree for rheumatoid arthritis[3]. The clinical criteria must have been observed by a physician and present for at least 6 weeks. Individuals can be classified as having or as not having RA (no RA). In parentheses are indicated surrogate variables that can be used when another variable (radiograph or rheumatoid factor test result) is not available.

CLINICAL EVALUATION

A careful clinical evaluation is the first step towards winning the patient's confidence and cooperation. It is also the most important step in the successful management of RA.

History

Making a diagnosis of RA depends on an accurate description of the patient's illness, obtained from a careful history (Table 22.2). Success in this endeavor requires effective communication with the patient and family, and this takes time. Diffuse symmetric joint pain and swelling affecting the small peripheral joints are the most common presenting symptoms. These symptoms are often associated with difficulty making a fist, and morning stiffness of variable duration.

A history of non-restorative sleep pattern may be informative in understanding the patient's morning stiffness and other diffuse aching. The symptoms should be interpreted in terms of the patient's functional ability to perform self-care and other daily home, work or sports activities (Table 22.3). It must be remembered that RA affects the patient's body as a whole, not just the articular system, and invariably has an impact on every aspect of the patient's physical and psychosocial life. In a large inception cohort of 332 patients, the onset of RA was associated with worse disability and joint damage in the elderly, especially postmenopausal women[7].

A history of RA in other members of the family should trigger suspicion of hereditary influences and heighten suspicion that the patient's symptoms could be an expression of early RA. It can be the case, however, that this knowledge has heightened the patient's anxiety about the symptoms, regardless of whether RA exists.

TABLE 22.2 CLINICAL EVALUATION OF RHEUMATOID ARTHRITIS – HISTORY OF PRESENT ILLNESS

Chronological account of illness from the onset

Onset: acute or gradual, with details

Location of pain (local or referred): precise anatomy, presence/absence of swelling

Pattern of joint involvement: axial, peripheral, symmetric

Type of pain: quality and character

Severity: pain threshold effects, interference with activities of daily living, range of joint movement

Radiation of pain: local or deep referred type

Clinical course: duration, frequency, periodicity, persistence

Modifying factors: aggravating, relieving, medication effects

Associated symptoms: fatigue, other systemic symptoms

Duration of morning stiffness: non-restorative sleep pattern

Present status: regional review of joints, extra-articular features, functional class, activities of daily living, psychologic state

TABLE 22.3 CLINICAL EVALUATION OF RHEUMATOID ARTHRITIS – FUNCTIONAL CAPACITY AND ACTIVITIES OF DAILY LIVING

Classification of functional capacity

Normal function without or despite symptoms

Some disability, but adequate for normal activity without special devices or assistance

Activities restricted, requires special devices or personal assistance

Totally dependent

Classification of activities of daily living

Mobility: walking, climbing, use of transport, bed–chair transfers

Personal care: eating, dressing, washing, grooming, use of toilet

Special hand functions: door handles, keys, coins, jar tops, carrying, pen, scissors

Work and play activities: work outside home, light and heavy work in house, hobbies, sports

It might be assumed that anxiety and depression would correlate with continuing disease activity, but it appears that socioeconomic factors may be greater determinants of depression than physical factors[8]. However, an episode of major depression before the onset of RA appears to predict greater pain in patients with continuing depression[9].

In other instances, patients who exhibit increased diffuse pain with decreased joint activity may show features of fibromyalgia syndrome, which explains this paradoxical reaction[10,11]. The role of physical trauma as a cause of RA is uncertain, but in someone with RA it may advance the course of disease or serve as an aggravating factor, delaying recovery[12]. A history of psychologic trauma or stress preceding the onset of RA should be sought. Although the relevance of psychological factors in RA is unproven, a retrospective study of a group of twins discordant for RA examined this aspect[13]. In each case the twin affected by arthritis had a background of psychologic entrapment not seen in the unaffected twin. Moreover, the role of environmental factors in the causation of RA is highlighted in twin studies, in which, in monozygotic twins discordant for RA, the genetic contribution to disease was only 15%[14]. Traditionally, pregnancy is considered to have a favorable effect on RA, but results of a prospective national UK study of 140 pregnant woman showed improvement in only 67% of cases, regardless of treatment[15].

A decreased risk of RA has been reported in women with previous pregnancies, and low androgen concentrations have implied a reduced incidence of RA in women taking oral contraceptives[16]. Interestingly, the proinflammatory effect of prolactin may explain why breast-feeding after the first pregnancy may increase the risk of RA[17].

The patient's educational background and occupation may affect management, and outcome and should be carefully documented. Notwithstanding genetic and sex factors, patients with more years of education seem to develop less severe disease[18]. Persons who are cigarette smokers – especially men – appear to be at increased risk for RA. Wolfe[19] has shown that this relationship exists between rheumatoid factor, nodules, radiographic progression, lung disease and overall severity of RA. Miners exposed to mineral dusts not only are at risk for RA but, once it has developed, are at increased risk of developing associated pneumoconiosis (Caplan's syndrome)[20].

The overall impact of RA on work status was well illustrated in a Swedish cohort of 106 patients with RA[21]. More than 50% of the patients were unable to continue working after 10 years of disease (Fig. 22.2). The major predictors for work disability were a high Health Assessment Questionnaire (HAQ) score at baseline, lower levels of education and older age.

Functional disability indices

A number of self-report questionnaires, such as the Stanford HAQ, Functional Disability Index, Arthritis Impact Measurement Scales and modifications thereof, have been developed for the evaluation of patients with RA (Table 22.4)[22–24]. These provide useful information not available by conventional means. They can be used to document the patient's functional status, with results similar to many traditional measures of RA activity. A reappraisal by Wolfe[25] of the major determinants of HAQ disability in RA were found to be associated with disease activity, pain and psychosocial factors, rather than with structural damage[25]. It is questionable, however, whether they can reliably assess problems of anxiety or depression in the patient with RA[24]. The value of these scales is attested by many rheumatologists who have incorporated them into their practice routines. Basic demographic variables are also part of this documentation.

Examination

As RA is a systemic condition, evaluation should include a complete physical examination that also documents the presence or absence of a

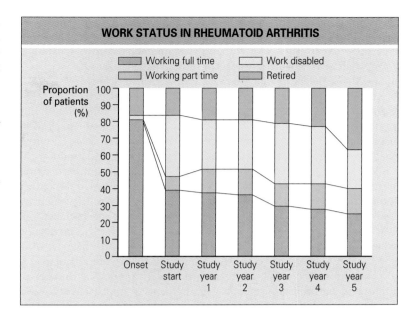

WORK STATUS IN RHEUMATOID ARTHRITIS

Fig. 22.2 **Work status in rheumatoid arthritis.** Changes in work status over time in 106 patients with RA participating in a prospective study. The chart shows conditions at disease onset, at study start on average 1 year later, and for another 5 years thereafter, for all the patients[21].

number of extra-articular features. These include subcutaneous nodules, digital vasculitis and the other systemic features described in Chapter 19. Any one of these may be mistaken for a non-rheumatoid condition, and their presence indicates a more ominous form of the disease. Various systemic features may also be the result of an adverse drug reaction. The joints shown in Figure 22.3 should be examined systematically, as described under the next five headings, to determine which ones are inflamed or damaged. The pattern of joint involvement, whether symmetric, axial or peripheral, should be recorded.

Joint inflammation

The key signs of early joint inflammation in RA are those of tenderness and swelling. These may be associated with local heat, but erythema is not a feature of rheumatoid inflammation. Heat and erythema may be seen with coincidental septic or gouty arthritis.

TABLE 22.4 SELF-REPORT QUESTIONNAIRE FOR RHEUMATOID ARTHRITIS				
Please check (✓) the ONE best answer for your abilities.				
At this moment, are you able to:	Without any difficulty	With some difficulty	With much difficulty	Unable to do
1. Dress yourself, including tying shoelaces and doing buttons?				
2. Get in and out of bed?				
3. Lift a full cup or glass to your mouth?				
4. Walk outdoors on flat ground?				
5. Wash and dry your entire body?				
6. Bend down to pick up clothing from the floor?				
7. Turn regular faucets (taps) on and off?				
8. Get in and out of a car?				
The questionnaire is used to make a quantitative assessment of the functional capacity of the patient to carry out the tasks of daily living[23]				

A joint is considered 'active' if it is tender on pressure or painful on passive movement, with stress or swelling other than bony proliferation. The presence or absence of pain and swelling are recorded separately. Joint swelling may be periarticular or intra-articular. The latter is associated with the detection of a joint effusion, described below.

A diagram depicting the joints (Fig. 22.3) may be used at each assessment, to record signs of disease activity or tender joint count. Joint effusions are recorded separately, because although the presence of an effusion usually indicates inflammation, this is not always the case. In any event, if fluid is detected, the matter can be settled by aspirating and examining it for leukocytosis or other signs of inflammation. At this juncture it is useful to mention the distinction between a tender 'joint count' and a tender 'point count'. Patients with RA or fibromyalgia may have widespread pain, and sometimes the two conditions coexist (see Chapter 20). In the case of RA, however, tenderness is related to one or more joints specifically, whereas fibromyalgia is defined as present in a patient if 11 or more of 18 specific soft tissue tender point sites are found that are not articular. It is also helpful to use a diagram to record tender points. The number of minutes of morning stiffness and measurements of grip strength using a blood pressure cuff manometer are other measures of disease activity.

Tenderness

Tenderness is elicited by direct palpation pressure over the joint. Firmer pressure on the tissues between or remote from the joints should not be tender, with the exception of the fibrositic tender points (see above). Testing for joint tenderness is particularly useful for detecting early and progressive disease activity in the wrist, finger and toe joints. Pain during the arc of movement in late-stage disease may, however, be caused by bare bone rubbing on bare bone from loss of articular cartilage, and is

not a reliable indication of the presence of inflammation. For this reason, the hips should be excluded from the routine simple joint count.

Stress pain

Stress pain is produced when a joint at the limit of its range of movement is nudged a little further. It is an especially useful symptom in the shoulder (limit of internal and external rotation), wrists, metacarpophalangeals and joints in the ankle region. To determine how hard to press in testing for stress pain, the general level of tenderness can be assessed by squeezing control sites in the midtrapezius and lower calf, and by pressing over the manubrium, metacarpals and proximal phalanges. Pressure on joints should be about 20% less than that required to reach the pain threshold over the control sites. When in doubt, it is best to record the joint as inactive.

Synovial effusion

The most reliable general sign of a synovial effusion in early and progressive disease is the demonstration of fluctuation: the hydraulic effect of an increase in fluid tension produced by pressure in one direction is transmitted equally in all three planes (Fig. 22.4). This is the four-finger

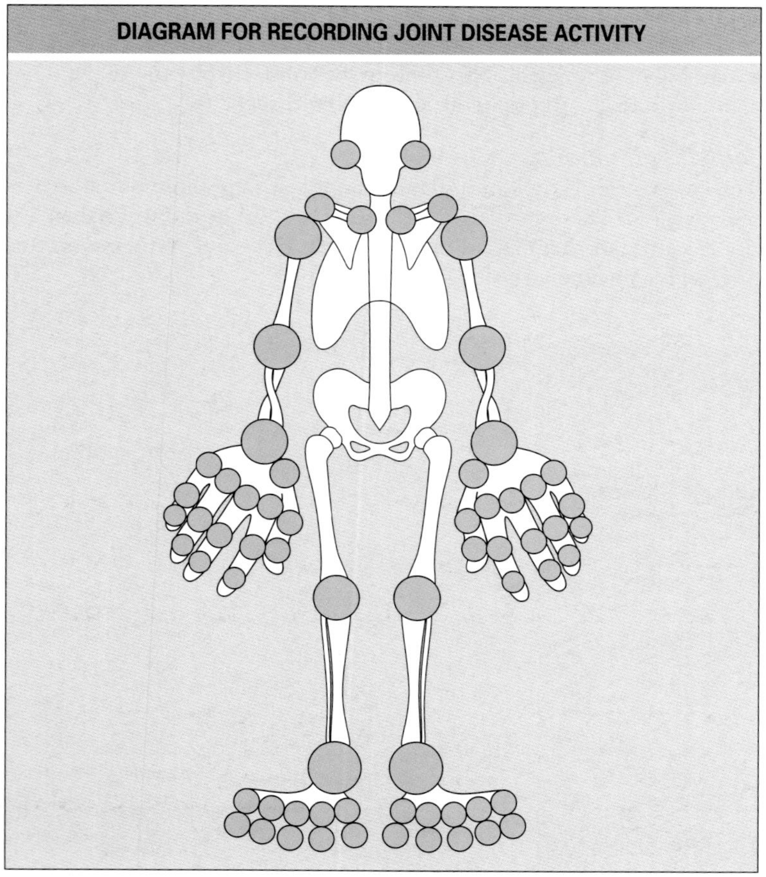

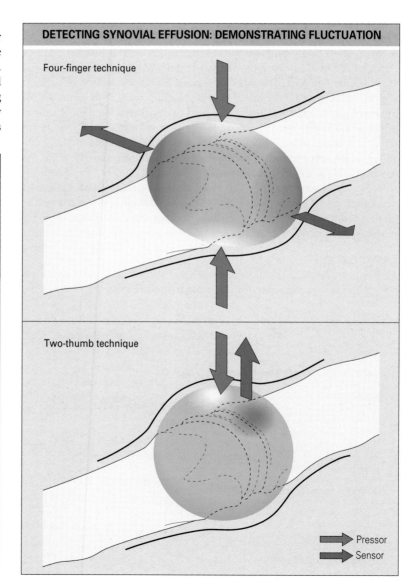

DETECTING SYNOVIAL EFFUSION: DEMONSTRATING FLUCTUATION

Four-finger technique

Two-thumb technique

Pressor
Sensor

Fig. 22.4 Detecting synovial effusion: demonstrating fluctuation. An increase in fluid tension induced by finger pressure in one area is transmitted so that the sensor finger(s) can detect it elsewhere. In the two-thumb (or two-finger) technique, the pressure should be in a direction slightly different from that of the sensor finger, to avoid false-positive results.

DIAGRAM FOR RECORDING JOINT DISEASE ACTIVITY

Fig. 22.3 Diagram for recording joint disease activity or destruction. The cartoon may be used on a printed form or rubber stamp to chart the joints that are active or deformed at the time of each assessment. The joints circled here should always be assessed.

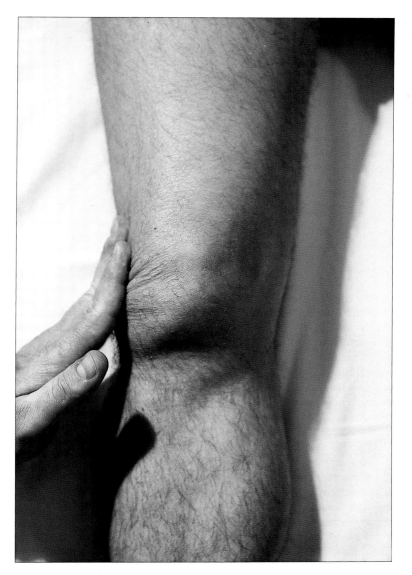

Fig. 22.5 Early RA of the knee, showing extension of a small effusion into the suprapatellar pouch.

TABLE 22.5 CLINICAL EVALUATION OF RHEUMATOID ARTHRITIS – EXAMINATION
Extra-articular features
Record presence of nodules, Raynaud's phenomenon, digital infarcts, episcleritis, peripheral neuropathy, palmar erythema, leg ulcers
Note tendon sheath involvement, or tendon nodules, subluxation or rupture
Check for anemia, splenomegaly, leukopenia, pleuritis or pericarditis, the sicca syndrome or renal involvement
Articular: measures of inflammatory activity
Check for tenderness, stress pain, synovial effusion, grip strength and duration of morning stiffness
Articular: measures of destruction and deformity
Check for lax collaterals, subluxation, malalignment, metatarsal prolapse, hammer toes and bone-on-bone crepitus

TABLE 22.6 FACTORS IN RHEUMATOID ARTHRITIS INDICATING AN UNFAVORABLE PROGNOSIS
Accumulated joint damage rate Uncontrolled polyarthritis Structural damage and deformity Functional disability
Presence of extra-articular features Local and/or systemic
Psychosocial problems
Rheumatoid factor seropositivity Presence of immune complexes
Immunogenetic testing for >1 HLA-DR4 cluster of RA susceptibility genes (DRB1* 0401, 0404, 0405)

technique – applicable only when the joint can be surrounded. For most joints, a two-finger or two-thumb technique must be used, one pressing downward, the other feeling an upward lift. These techniques can be practiced on a slightly softened grape. In the two-digit technique, the direction of pressure should differ slightly from the sensor finger to prevent false-positive scorings from lateral shifts of fat or tendons. Fat, being fluid at body temperature, may fluctuate. If it is subcutaneous, it can be pinched up in a way impossible with effusions; if deep, it is rarely exactly coextensive with the synovial space. Muscle will also fluctuate across the direction of the fibers, but not parallel with them. In the knee joint, small effusions are sometimes visible (Fig. 22.5), but may only be detectable by using the 'bulge sign'. This is a sensitive indication of a small effusion: the pouch of synovium medial to the patella is emptied of fluid by a gentle upward stroke, and refilled by a downward stroke on the lateral side. A sudden bulge can also be detected when a mildly affected elbow is gently moved to 90% of extension.

Joint damage and destruction

Joint destruction in progressive and late disease may be assessed clinically or radiologically (Table 22.5). Common clinical observations associated with joint disruption include a reduction in the range of movement, collateral instability, malalignment, subluxation or loss of articular cartilage causing bone-on-bone crepitus. No simple method of describing

these often complicated changes has yet achieved international acceptance. A separate, simple count of damaged joints is recommended.

The information obtained from clinical evaluation will reveal which joint structures are affected by inflammation, which are damaged and to what extent function is impaired. Nevertheless, even with training, standardization and refinement of these methods, a good deal of inter-observer variability exists when they are applied to clinical trials[26]. For this reason, it is a customary requirement for trials that sequential measurements in the same patient should be performed by the same examiner.

After the foregoing baseline evaluations have been accomplished, the diagnosis of RA can usually be confirmed and the patient can be categorized as having early, progressive or late disease.

Disease stages

Early disease

Patients who as yet exhibit no clinical evidence of joint damage or radiologic signs of cartilage loss or bone erosion may be described as having early disease. Our use of the term 'early disease' is synonymous with 'mild disease' activity. It is not intended to have any particular prognostic significance. Although it is unpredictable whether patients with early disease will eventually run a benign or malignant course, most exhibit an intermediate, smoldering activity[2]. Spontaneous remission may occur, especially if the onset of polyarthritis has been quite sudden[1]. Even though patients are categorized as having early disease, a number of prognostic factors should be sought (Table 22.6).

When a group in Manchester followed a primary-care cohort of 528 patients with early RA for 5 years, they found that the first anniversary HAQ score was the strongest predictor of disability at 5 years[27]. However, there was considerable individual variation among patients[28]. An earlier international study of 706 patients with RA of no more than 4 years duration showed that functional disability correlated best with joint count, female sex, erythrocyte sedimentation rate (ESR) and disease duration, but not rheumatoid factor, X-ray changes, age or education level[29]. Thus there are early disease factors that suggest a more unfavorable outlook requiring more aggressive treatment.

Often the diagnosis of RA is obvious, but frequently there are too few definite features and the diagnosis can only be tentative, in which case the patient may be placed in this early category. The ARA criteria for classification of RA may not always be helpful in diagnosis of patients at the earliest stage of disease. Over time, developments may show that a presumptive diagnosis of early RA was incorrect and features of another diffuse connective tissue disorder – such as systemic lupus erythematosus, scleroderma, or psoriatic arthritis – may evolve. Thus it may be a mistake to apply the RA 'label' to a patient too soon, because when new symptoms arise other diagnostic possibilities may not be considered.

Progressive disease

Some patients show a more progressive disease course from the outset; they have unrelenting, chronic disease activity despite treatment. In addition to persistent polyarthritis and systemic features, these individuals usually have an increased ESR, positive rheumatoid factor test and early radiographic evidence of joint erosions. Wolfe and Pincus[30] examined the relationship of inflammatory measures by ESR with duration of disease in 1897 patients with RA, based on 21 866 consecutive determinations. They found that, although ESR decreased by 4mm/h over the first 10 years, it remained stable or greater thereafter. They concluded that the level of inflammation in RA may be set early and remain stable thereafter.

Late disease

This category is used to describe patients whose disease has led to definite joint damage with all its attendant complications. In most cases, the disease is of many years' duration and its damaging effects are a reflection of its severity. Typically, these patients have been resistant to various disease-suppressive medications, although in some patients the disease may have 'burned itself out', leaving only residual joint damage. Work disability is a characteristic of patients in this category. Wolfe and Hawley[31] investigated this aspect in an 18 year longitudinal study of 823 patients with RA. They found that persistent ESR abnormalities, HAQ scores and pain from the outset of disease best predicted work disability.

INDIVIDUAL JOINTS – A REGIONAL APPROACH

Joint involvement in RA is symmetric, and whereas wrists, fingers, knees and feet are the most commonly affected joints in early disease, progressive disease is also associated with larger joints, such as the shoulders, elbows and knees. Articular indices weighted for size and amount of synovium, such as the historical Lansbury index[32], have been found to correlate better with the amount of inflammation than do simple joint counts[33]. The simultaneous presence of joint tenderness and swelling in early and progressive disease also show a greater correlation with joint inflammation than either variable alone[33]. Eventually, if unchecked, persistent inflammation leads to destruction of soft tissue, with ligamentous laxity and deformity.

The hands

Examination of the hands is important, because the features they exhibit are frequently a reflection of the patient's overall disease, whether early, late or progressive. Symmetric swelling of the metacarpophalangeal (MCP) and proximal interphalangeal (PIP) joints, with fusiform

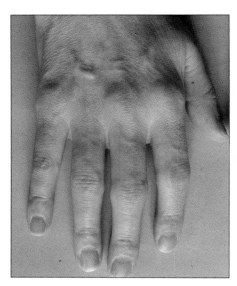

Fig. 22.6 The hand in early RA. View of the right hand, showing swelling of the MCP and PIP joints. Fusiform swelling of the PIP joints is typical of RA and associated with morning stiffness, difficulty making a fist, reduced grip strength and tenderness of the affected joints. The left hand showed similar changes. (Reproduced with permission from Dieppe et al. Slide atlas of clinical rheumatology. London: Gower Medical Publishing; 1983.)

swelling of the latter, are typical of RA (Fig. 22.6). Distal interphalangeal (DIP) involvement may be seen, but may indicate coincidental osteoarthritis. Tenderness on palpation will determine which of these joints are to be noted as 'active'. Effusion should be sought using the four-finger technique (Fig. 22.4). Hand assessment is incomplete without recording grip strength, but it is worth noting that poor grip strength may be as much a reflection of tendon involvement as of joint disease. Grip-strength testing is no longer included in the standard measures used in therapeutic trials in rheumatoid arthritis.

Although local swellings of the MCP and PIP joints are characteristic of RA, massive diffuse swelling of both hands, with a 'flipper' or 'boxing glove' appearance, may be associated with an acute onset. Pitting edema is characteristic of this swelling, and if a seronegative elderly person is affected, a more likely diagnosis is that of benign polyarthritis of the aged[34]. If diffuse swelling of one or both hands is associated with signs of sympathetic overactivity and shoulder stiffness, then reflex dystrophy may be a better explanation than RA. However, reflex dystrophy may coexist with RA or contribute to its disease expression. Interestingly, articular signs may be absent when RA develops in a patient with pre-existing hemiparesis[35]. The greater the paralysis, the less the degree of joint inflammation.

Inspection of the hands may reveal other extra-articular features. Raynaud's phenomenon may be seen in a minority of patients, and palmar erythema in more. Digital and nail-fold infarcts indicate more severe rheumatoid vasculitis.

A more detailed examination of joints and tendons is required to monitor progressive hand deformity in RA. Hasting's classification is helpful in identifying these problems (Table 22.7).

Metacarpophalangeal joints

Metacarpophalangeal involvement, with the development of volar subluxation and ulnar drift, is a characteristic deformity of progressive RA. A number of factors favor its occurrence and progression[37]. Synovitis within the MCP joints tends to weaken the dorsal and radial structures and relatively lengthen the collateral ligaments. Inherent mechanical factors then favor ulnar drift of the fingers. The power of hand grip pulls the tendons ulnarwards as the 5th metacarpal descends. The ulnar collateral ligaments are shorter and less oblique than the radial counterparts, and thus the elongation is greater on the radial than the ulnar side. The firm attachment of the volar plate also fixes the pull of the long flexors to the proximal phalanx and tends to displace the proximal phalanx in both an ulnar and a volar direction. The transverse linkage of the extensor tendons functions much like a clothesline, so that anything pulling the extensor tendon of the 5th finger in an ulnar

Individual joints – a regional approach

TABLE 22.7 HASTING'S CLASSIFICATION OF RHEUMATOID HAND DEFORMITIES		
Joint involvement	MCP joints	Synovitis Passively correctable ulnar drift Fixed volar subluxation, ulnar drift
	PIP joints	Synovitis Boutonnière deformity Swan-neck deformity Flail IP joint
	Thumb	Flail IP joint Boutonnière deformity Duckbill thumb (CMC) dislocation
	Wrist	Synovitis Carpal supination–subluxation Radiocarpal dislocation
Tendon involvement	Flexor tendon disease	Loss of active flexion Triggering Tendon rupture Median nerve involvement
	Extensor tendon disease	Synovitis – dorsal mass Extensor tendon rupture Extensor tendon dislocation

CMC, carpometacarpal. (Data from Hastings[36].)

direction will pull the other fingers the same way. An effect of radial deviation of the wrist must also be considered. In the presence of ulnar drift, a normal wrist will tend to deviate radially to compensate for that deformity. Moreover, any wrist involvement that produces radial deviation will tend to aggravate the tendency to ulnar drift of the fingers.

Proximal interphalangeal joints

Three deformities resulting from lack of collateral ligament support characterize PIP joint involvement – the boutonnière, the swan-neck (Fig. 22.7) and the unstable PIP joint. Synovitis in the PIP joint can produce any of these deformities. As noted, synovitis with joint effusion in early RA causes fusiform swelling. Synovitis may appear as a bulge on the dorsal aspect, often on each side of the extensor tendon.

A boutonnière deformity develops when there is relative laxity or attenuation of the central slip and the lateral bands move in a volar direction. This destroys the extensor balance of the fingers and extension is concentrated on the terminal phalanx, whereas the lateral bands actually become flexors of the PIP joints. The lack of passive flexion of the terminal interphalangeal (IP) joint with the PIP joint in extension is the earliest sign of this complication. It may be rapidly progressive. A swan-neck deformity represents the reverse of the boutonnière deformity and exists when the main extensor forces focus on the base of the proximal phalanx and the lateral bands sublux to a dorsal position. It may be a physiological deformity, the result of trauma, secondary to PIP joint disease or a result of MCP joint disease with secondary intrinsic contracture. In the early stages, the deformity seems relatively reversible, but

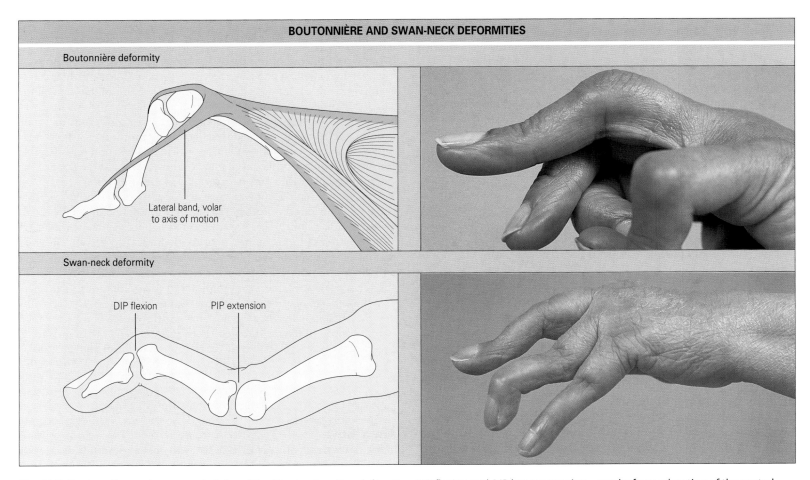

BOUTONNIÈRE AND SWAN-NECK DEFORMITIES

Boutonnière deformity

Lateral band, volar to axis of motion

Swan-neck deformity

DIP flexion   PIP extension

Fig. 22.7 Boutonnière and swan-neck deformities. The boutonnière deformity – PIP flexion and DIP hyperextension – results from relaxation of the central slip, with 'buttonholing' of the PIP joint between the lateral bands. The swan-neck deformity – MCP flexion, PIP hyperextension and DIP flexion – may be mobile, snapping or fixed. Its pathogenesis may be related primarily to PIP or MCP involvement. Combinations of MCP and PIP involvement are less frequent. (Adapted from Hastings DE and Welsh RP. Surgical reconstruction of the rheumatoid hand. Toronto: Orthopaedic Medical Management Corporation; 1979.)

as the lateral bands displace to the dorsal position, flexion becomes increasingly difficult. Often the movement is accomplished only by a snap, as the lateral bands move from the dorsal to the normal dorsal–lateral position. Once the lateral bands become fixed in a dorsal position, then flexion of the PIP joint is no longer possible.

Distal interphalangeal joints

Involvement of the DIP joint is not characteristic of RA, but probably occurs more frequently than appreciated[38]. It is never an initial or isolated manifestation of RA, and it is usually episodic and more likely to occur in seropositive RA. DIP disease must be distinguished from inflammatory osteoarthritis.

The rheumatoid thumb

Three deformities affect the thumb: the flail IP joint, the boutonnière thumb and the relatively rare duckbill thumb. The flail IP joint results from synovitis leading to the destruction of the collateral ligaments. Pinching pushes the terminal phalanx away and the patient begins to pinch against the proximal phalanx. The boutonnière thumb is the same deformity as that described earlier for the other fingers. MCP synovitis weakens the insertion of the extensor pollicis brevis to the base of the proximal phalanx and results in an MCP flexion deformity and a secondary IP hyperextension because of the unbalanced action of extensor pollicis longus. The duckbill thumb develops when the primary pathology is at the first carpometacarpal joint. This is a dislocation accompanied by an adduction deformity of the first metacarpal. The MCP joint is hyperextended and the IP joint flexed; the deformity is similar to a swan-neck deformity of the finger.

Flexor tendon involvement

Tendons, like joints, are sheathed with synovium; when they are inflamed the condition is known as tenosynovitis. Flexor tenosynovitis can take many different forms in early and progressive disease.

Loss of active flexion

If passive flexion of a finger exceeds active flexion, tenosynovitis is present. Crepitus can be felt in the palm as the fingers are extended and flexed. Adhesions between the superficial and deep tendons may limit the excursion of the profundus tendon and the patient will not be able to make a full fist. A trigger finger is a frequent feature of flexor tenosynovitis. The pathology is a thickening of the tendon (often by a rheumatoid nodule within the tendon), rather than stenosis of the tendon sheath.

Ruptures of flexor tendons occur, but are much less common than extensor rupture. The tendon most likely to rupture is the flexor pollicis longus. The cause is usually synovitis in the carpal tunnel and wrist disease, with encroachment of a spicule of carpal bone from the floor of the carpal tunnel.

Florid flexor tenosynovitis of the carpal tunnel leads to compression of the median nerve. Volar wrist pain may be confused with articular disease, but the weakness, finger tingling and thenar wasting point to nerve involvement that can be confirmed by electromyographic studies. Early RA can actually present with a carpal tunnel syndrome as the sole feature before polyarthritis becomes apparent[39]. Occasionally, triggering may develop in the carpal tunnel.

Extensor tendon involvement

Extensor tenosynovitis is frequently evident in early disease as swelling over the dorsum of the wrist, below the extensor retinaculum. Asking the patient to extend the fingers will accentuate the swelling – the 'tuck' sign (Fig. 22.8). This mass on the back of the wrist is usually only a painless cosmetic deformity. Painful finger extension, however, may indicate active tendon erosion. There may be a triggering effect, and with further erosion tendon rupture follows. This is usually the result of carpal supination–subluxation and attrition of the tendons over the distal ulna.

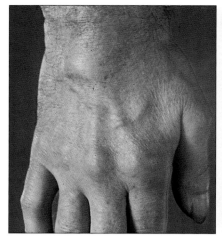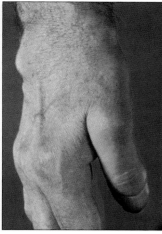

Fig. 22.8 Tenosynovial swelling from tenosynovitis – the 'tuck' sign. Tenosynovial swelling overlies the metacarpals of the right hand. Bulging becomes accentuated with full extension of all the fingers of the hand. Persistent tenosynovitis over the dorsal wrist may lead to extensor tendon erosion and rupture, particularly of the tendons of the 4th and 5th fingers.

It is important to differentiate an extensor tendon rupture from an extensor tendon dislocation at the MCP joints. At first, the latter is passively correctable, but it soon becomes fixed. Examination will reveal the intact extensor tendon over the dorsum of the hand. Another rare complication is the loss of finger extension caused by an entrapment neuropathy of the posterior interosseous branch of the radial nerve, as a result of rheumatoid synovitis about the elbow[40].

The wrist

Symmetrical disease of the wrists is almost invariably present in RA[36]. Ulnar styloid swelling and loss of wrist extension indicate early involvement. Synovitis commonly affects the weakest support of the wrist on the ulnar side. Attenuation of the weak triangular ligament allows displacement of the wrist in a volar direction. The wrist also tends to rotate around the stronger radial dorsal ligament, promoting a deformity known as carpal supination–subluxation. This subluxation is responsible for the prominence of the distal ulna, causing erosion of the floor of the extensor compartments and extensor tendon rupture. As the wrist rotates into supination, subluxation of the extensor carpi ulnaris occurs, so that this tendon no longer functions as a dorsiflexor. Contracture of the extensor carpi radialis longus and brevis leads to unopposed radial dorsiflexion with ulnar translocation of the carpus. With disease progression, the volar and ulnar aspect of the radius erodes, with the carpus moving in a volar and ulnar direction. This strains the extensor carpi radialis brevis and if this tendon ruptures, the wrist progresses to volar dislocation. The intercarpal ligaments may also be affected, with wrist collapse. This accentuates the instability. Rarely, synovitis appears to promote fibrous and then bony ankylosis of the carpal bones. Then stiffness, rather than instability, becomes the problem. Rarely, severe resorption of finger and wrist joints may progress to a condition known as arthritis mutilans. A prospective 20-year review of 103 patients with seropositive erosive RA seen at the Rheumatism Foundation Hospital, Heinola, Finland found a 4.4% prevalence of arthritis mutilans affecting MCP, PIP and wrist joints[41].

The elbow

This joint is frequently involved in RA, with loss of extension as an early sign. Even with extensive involvement, elbow function is usually well maintained. When loss of flexion occurs, however, it interferes with the patient's self-care activities. Elbow effusions are visible and palpable in the dimple between the tip of the olecranon and the head of the radius. When small effusions are not visible, gentle extension to 90% may show

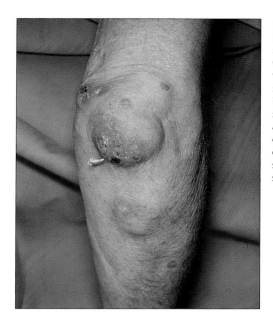

Fig. 22.9 Olecranon bursitis and subcutaneous nodule. Olecranon swelling with erythema from septic bursitis after incision and drainage. A subcutaneous nodule appears distal to the olecranon bursa. Either of these lesions may serve as a portal for systemic infection.

a sudden bulge. Periarticular cysts may be associated with elbow effusion and, as in the knee, may rupture (into the forearm), with inflammatory swelling. With persistent synovitis, erosive changes first develop in the humeroulnar joint. Because the radius is linked to the ulna by an interosseous membrane, the two move as a unit. When the cartilage between the humerus and the ulna is lost, the head of the radius moves proximal to the capitellum, blocking flexion and extension. Loss of elbow extension precedes loss of flexion. Constant abutment of the radial head produces typical lateral pain, limited supination and crepitus with pronation and supination. Medial swelling of the elbow joint with damage and destruction may be associated with an ulnar entrapment neuropathy. In addition, synovitis of the lateral elbow joint may cause entrapment of the posterior interosseous branch of the radial nerve[40].

Subcutaneous nodules

Subcutaneous nodules overlying the extensor aspect of the proximal ulna are present in about 30% of patients with RA. Not only is the nodule a cardinal diagnostic feature of RA, but it may break down, forming a cyst and serving as a site for local infection (Fig. 22.9) or as a portal for complicating systemic infection causing septic arthritis. Vasculitis of the skin overlying the nodule may also contribute to these complications. Subcutaneous nodules or rheumatoid nodulosis may form over other pressure locations, such as the occiput, palms of the hands, sacrum or tendo Achillis, and may become infected. They should be sought in any patient with RA who appears to have sepsis.

The olecranon bursa

Bursae should not be overlooked in the evaluation of any joint region, as they may be a site of rheumatoid activity[42]. There are about 80 bursae on each side of the body, and they are lined by a synovial membrane that secretes synovial fluid and may develop rheumatoid synovitis. Only occasionally do they communicate with an adjacent joint space. Involvement of the olecranon bursa by RA is an obvious example of bursitis. Pain and swelling may be manifestations of synovitis or infection (Fig. 22.9). Whereas septic arthritis is almost invariably the result of hematogenous spread of bacteria, septic olecranon bursitis is always a consequence of a skin break, with direct entry from outside. Skin vasculitis overlying bursal swelling can contribute to this septic complication. Occasionally the bursa ruptures and causes diffuse forearm edema.

Other bursae that may be similarly affected include the subacromial, trochanteric, iliopsoas, gastrocnemius, semimembranosus, subachilles and posterior calcaneal. Sometimes, multiple bursae may be affected by rheumatoid granulomas[43].

The shoulder

Involvement of the shoulder joint in RA is variable, but is usually only a feature in patients who have progressive or late disease. Often, shoulder symptoms do not arise until joint destruction has become advanced. This is because adaptive mechanisms – the hands, wrists and elbows – are sufficiently good that daily self-care activities can be maintained for a long time.

Synovitis leads to erosion and damage of both the humeral head and the glenoid fossa. When shoulder effusions develop, they appear anteriorally below the acromion. Subacromial bursal swelling may also appear as a pouch that is independent of the glenohumeral joint. The bursa may also rupture. The long head of the biceps may also rupture in patients with RA. This can be detected as a biceps bulge when the patient flexes the elbow against resistance.

The rotator cuff is also lined with synovium, and may show inflammation and destruction, with monoarticular pain and limitation sufficiently acute to mimic septic arthritis. Frequently, there is weakening and loss of attachment of the rotator cuff, with secondary upward migration of the humeral head.

Acromioclavicular joint disease is frequently found in RA and may be the prime source of shoulder pain. It also correlates with the degree of glenohumeral disease.

The temporomandibular joint

This joint is commonly involved, with tenderness and painful limitation of mouth opening. It may eventually become associated with a receding or 'gump jaw' deformity.

The cricoarytenoid joint

Involvement of this joint in progressive disease is commonly associated with hoarseness. Superimposed upper respiratory infections may lead to upper airway obstruction with respiratory stridor, requiring a life-saving tracheostomy[44]. Limitation of cricoarytenoid movement may also be associated with lung aspiration and its complications.

Ossicles of the ear

Ankylosis of these joints may be associated with hearing loss independent of a medication-induced effect.

Sternoclavicular and manubriosternal joints

These joints possess synovial and cartilage portions and are more commonly affected than is appreciated. Subluxation and actual dislocation of the manubriosternal joint may occur[45].

The cervical spine

The neck is an important target in RA, particularly at the C1–C2 level. The space between the odontoid process and the arch of the atlas normally measures 3mm or less. If this space exceeds 3mm, the condition is defined as atlantoaxial subluxation. It can often exceed 10mm. Cervical subluxation at any level is common in severe erosive RA and may be found in 30% of patients in this category[46]. Although neck stiffness is common in RA, the majority of patients with atlantoaxial subluxation are not much affected by severe neck pain. When neck pain does occur, it is usually high in the cervical spine, with radiation into the occiput or occasionally into temporal and retro-orbital regions. Sometimes, atlantoaxial subluxation is associated with a frightening 'clunking' sensation on neck extension.

When considering the cervical spine at the C1–C2 level, it is helpful to divide the space through the arch of the atlas into thirds: one-third for the odontoid process, one-third for the spinal cord and one-third free. If a C1–C2 slip exceeds 10mm, the free third is lost and cervical cord

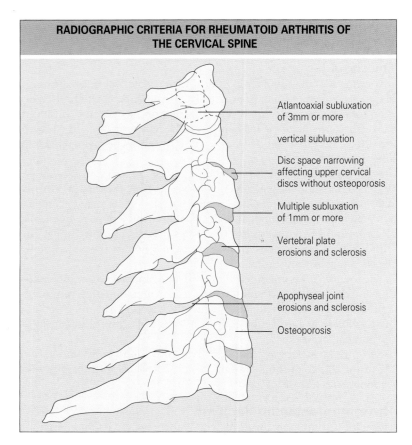

RADIOGRAPHIC CRITERIA FOR RHEUMATOID ARTHRITIS OF THE CERVICAL SPINE

- Atlantoaxial subluxation of 3mm or more
- vertical subluxation
- Disc space narrowing affecting upper cervical discs without osteoporosis
- Multiple subluxation of 1mm or more
- Vertebral plate erosions and sclerosis
- Apophyseal joint erosions and sclerosis
- Osteoporosis

Fig. 22.10 Radiographic criteria for rheumatoid arthritis of the cervical spine. (Modified after Winfield et al.[46])

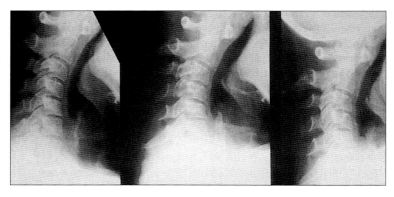

Fig. 22.11 Serial radiographs of the cervical spine, showing progression after the appearance of subluxation within 2 years of disease onset[46].

damage becomes a risk (Figs 22.10 & 22.11). There is a synovial articulation between the transverse ligament of the atlas and the posterior aspect of the odontoid. This transverse ligament prevents a forward slip of C1 on C2, and continuing synovitis in this articulation compromises the ligament and may produce erosions of the dens. Synovial involvement may also affect the apophyseal joints in the occipitoatlantal area. If this causes loss of bone and change in shape, the odontoid may move up through the foramen magnum, producing basilar invagination and threatening the upper cervical cord and medulla. In these patients, sudden death may occur after unexpected vomiting or physical trauma. Basilar–vertebral vascular insufficiency may also occur in these patients, with syncope after downward gaze. The usual indication for neurosurgical intervention in these individuals is either intractable neck pain or pyramidal tract weakness of the arms and legs. RA of the apophyseal joints and disk spaces may cause subluxation at other levels, which

may slowly lead to quadriparesis[47]. Fortunately, these complications are rare.

In patients with cervical symptoms despite negative radiographic findings, contrast enhanced magnetic resonance imaging may be of value in characterization of the craniocervical region[48].

When a patient with RA requires surgery, the presence of cervical subluxation presents a general anesthetic risk. Preoperative assessment by lateral flexion cervical radiographs is essential to exclude this possibility. If cervical involvement is detected, then special precautions are required perioperatively to prevent cervical cord damage.

The thoracic and lumbar spine

Involvement of the thoracic and lumbar spine is very uncommon in RA. Apophyseal synovitis may rarely present as an epidural mass, and lumbar spinal stenosis has been reported. Compression fractures secondary to the osteoporosis of RA aggravated by corticosteroids are common in the thoracic region. Compression fractures in the lumbar region are not characteristic of RA and suggest that other underlying causes, such as osteomyelitis or cancer, should be considered.

The sacroiliac joints

Radiographic changes of the sacroiliac joints may be seen in advanced RA; usually they consist of erosions and osteopenia. However, ankylosing spondylitis and RA may occasionally coexist, usually in men, just as RA may be seen in patients with psoriasis, gout or osteoarthritis[49].

The hip

Early symptoms of hip involvement may be an abnormal gait or groin discomfort. Even with progressive RA, however, the hips are often spared. Moreover, the onset of hip disease in patients with RA is subtle, because patients maintain a pain-free range of hip movement until synovitis causes a progressive loss of cartilage space. Once this symmetric erosive process becomes established, bilateral protrusion of the acetabulae is inevitable[50]. Alternatively, with collapse of the femoral head from osteonecrosis, the deformity is lateral migration, rather than protrusion into the pelvis. The stiffness and pain of these complications interfere with the patient's ability to walk. A previous history of glucocorticosteroid use is often noted in these individuals.

Iliopsoas bursa

Synovitis and effusion of the iliopsoas bursa (Fig. 22.12) may present with a unilateral or bilateral inguinal mass, or with lower extremity swelling without obvious relationship to the hip[51]. The bursa lies

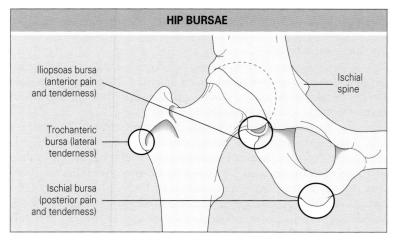

HIP BURSAE

- Iliopsoas bursa (anterior pain and tenderness)
- Ischial spine
- Trochanteric bursa (lateral tenderness)
- Ischial bursa (posterior pain and tenderness)

Fig. 22.12 Hip bursae that may be affected by rheumatoid granuloma. Involvement of the iliopsoas bursa is associated with an inguinal mass that may be mistaken for a hernia, lymphadenopathy or aneurysm[51].

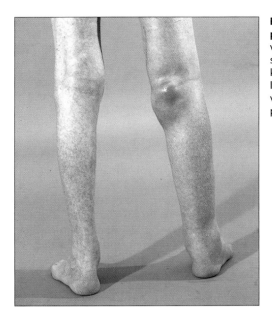

Fig. 22.13 Baker's popliteal cyst. Posterior view showing rheumatoid swelling behind the right knee. Swelling of the lower limb was related to venous compression by popliteal synovitis.

between the capsule of the hip and the iliopsoas muscle lateral to the femoral vessels. It rarely communicates with the hip joint and it is the largest bursa around the hip. Symptoms that may be mistaken for a hernia, lymphadenopathy or aneurysm arise from the inguinal mass. Femoral vein compression may lead to lower limb edema and a picture resembling deep-vein thrombosis.

Trochanteric and ischial bursae

Bursitis of the trochanteric bursa is more common than that of the ischial bursa. Either may be mistaken for true hip joint involvement (Fig. 22.12).

The knee

Obvious involvement of the knee is common in early and progressive RA. Sometimes, however, meniscal surgery has been performed in patients before the diagnosis of RA became apparent. Small effusions of the knee joint are detectable in early disease by means of the 'bulge' sign (Fig. 22.5). This sign is useful for detecting small amounts of fluid, but it does not necessarily confirm an inflammatory process without analysis of the synovial fluid. The normal skin temperature of the knee is significantly lower than that of the thigh or tibia. This is the basis of the 'cool patella' sign[52]. In the case of knee inflammation, palpation over the thigh, patella and calf with the back of the hand shows the temperature

over the patella to be equal to the heat over the thigh and tibia (i.e. a loss of the cool patella sign).

With an increase in the amount of the knee effusion, the fluid bulge sign disappears and positive ballottement or the patellar tap sign develops. The patient tends to assume a more comfortable position with the knee flexed and, if this becomes a habit, a loss of full knee extension eventually results. In full extension, the recumbent patient will be unable to push the popliteal surface of the knee into the examiner's hand.

Popliteal (Baker's) cysts

Knee extension lag may be associated with popliteal fullness caused by a Baker's cyst. The cyst can extend from its location in the gastrocnemius bursa down into the medial aspect of the calf. This is seen best by observing the standing patient from behind (Fig. 22.13). Sometimes these cysts extend into the medial ankle region. The Baker's popliteal cyst arises as an extension from the joint cavity; synovial tissue acts as a ball-valve, allowing fluid accumulation without means for decompression[53]. Exertion sufficient to increase the intra-articular knee joint pressure can lead to rupture of the synovial cyst, with extravasation of inflammatory synovial fluid into the calf, presenting a picture that mimics acute thrombophlebitis[53]. A hemorrhagic 'crescent' sign in the skin about the ankle below the malleoli is characteristic of synovial rupture and is not a feature of thrombophlebitis[54].

Rarely, after inflammation from a rupture into the calf has subsided, another rupture may cause posterior thigh extravasation and hemorrhage (Fig. 22.14). Anterolateral joint cysts may also extend below the knee, but this is a very rare occurrence[55].

Later disease

Eventually, destruction of the knee by RA leads to limitation in walking, similar to the disability seen with the rheumatoid hip. With loss of cartilage comes laxity of the collateral and cruciate ligaments. This is detected by stressing the knee joint for lateral and medial collateral stability with the knee cradled in the arms of the examiner at 15% of flexion. Cruciate anterior–posterior instability is detectable by means of the 'drawer' sign. A special problem arises in women with physiologic valgus. This produces increasing loading on the lateral compartment of the knee joint, with erosion of the tibial plateau and progressive valgus deformity. As the valgus increases so does the loading, so that a vicious cycle is produced. Less common is the same set of circumstances in a varus position. With varus there is often collapse or fracture of the medial plateau and more severe deformity.

Occasionally, inflammation results in binding of the collateral ligaments to the side of the femoral condyle. This destroys the normal

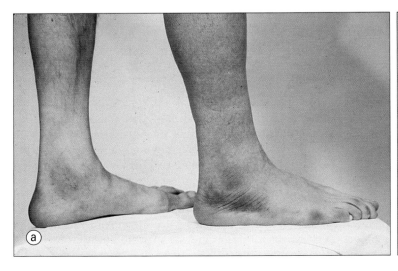

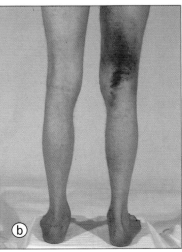

Fig. 22.14 Acute synovial rupture. A 51-year-old man with RA of 3 years' duration developed a right knee effusion after an evening of square-dancing. Two days later, he noted progressive pain and swelling of the right calf. (a) Six days later, there was bluish discoloration of both sides of the ankle. (b) A few weeks later, after more dancing, he noted posterior thigh pain and swelling that soon became associated with purple discoloration of his right posterior thigh[54].

anteroposterior gliding motion of the tibia on the femur and leads to a relative posterior subluxation of the tibia. This is usually associated with fixed flexion of the knee, and as the tibia tries to extend, it digs into the femoral condyle, producing a bony block anteriorly.

The ankle

The ankle joint (tibial–talar articulation) is not as frequently involved as the subtalar and midtarsal joints of the hindfoot. Persistent synovitis of the ankle joint leads to loss of cartilage and bone-on-bone contact. However, ankle involvement is not usually a cause of great disability, because the joint remains quite stable. Sometimes a stress fracture of the distal fibula may masquerade as a flare of ankle arthritis[56].

The foot

Hindfoot involvement

The subtalar and talonavicular joints are commonly affected in RA, but this is not always appreciated. Synovitis of these joints causes pain and stiffness, and sometimes subtalar dislocation. Secondary peroneal muscle spasm develops and tends to immobilize the subtalar joint. The spasm promotes a valgus deformity and causes a peroneal spastic flat foot. As cartilage loss and bone erosion develop, valgus deformity increases, with progressive flattening of the longitudinal arch. Eventually the os calcis abuts against the lateral malleolus with collapse through the midfoot, producing pressure points over the head of the talus. At this stage the joint may spontaneously fuse without further progression.

Although heel pain is a characteristic of the spondyloarthropathies, it can be a particular problem in RA. It can arise from a subachilles or retrocalcaneal bursitis associated with a nodule in the tendo Achillis. Rupture of this tendon may also complicate the picture[57]. Persistent heel pain caused by a calcaneal stress fracture is sometimes misinterpreted as subtalar or ankle synovitis.

The forefoot

Disease of the metatarsal heads is common in RA, causing much pain and disability. Forefoot deformity usually starts with synovitis of the MTP joints and involvement of the flexor tendons within their sheath. Because of volar pain, the patient tends to walk on the heels with maximum dorsiflexion. This leads to reactivity of the extensor digitorum longus, with clawing of the toes and the eventual dorsal dislocation of the MTP joint (Fig. 22.15). With this comes a secondary depression and erosion of the metatarsal heads and widening of the entire forefoot.

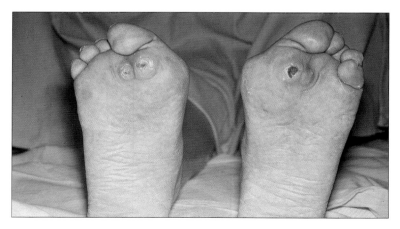

Fig. 22.15 Rheumatoid forefoot. Plantar view of the feet in a patient with RA. Hallux valgus, MTP subluxation and bursal swelling under weight-bearing areas are seen. Subluxation of the metatarsal head is associated with clawing of the toes, cock-up digital deformities and over-riding of the toes. The ulcerated bursae under the left metatarsal head may become associated with a chronic synovial fistula and secondary infection[58].

Metatarsus primus varus is commonly seen in women with RA, and this leads to a severe hallux valgus deformity.

Forefoot fistulae

Chronic synovitis of the metatarsal heads may be associated with severe progressive erosive changes and the formation of bony cysts known as geodes. Spread of the synovial granuloma and bony breakdown causes calluses or bunions to form over these areas. Further breakdown of tissue leads to a chronic cutaneous fistula as synovial fluid tracks from the MTP joint to the dorsal or plantar surface of the foot[58]. Secondary infection along this fistulous track is a hazard that may require surgery extending back into the MTP joint. Although chronic fistulous rheumatism is seen most often with metatarsal synovitis, chronic cutaneous fistulae may develop in relation to any rheumatoid joint. Diffuse pitting edema of the feet may be the result of local venous insufficiency, obstruction of lymphatics or veins from a swollen ankle, knee or hip, or it may even relate to cardiac disease, such as RA pericarditis. Numbness of the medial aspect of the forefoot may result from a tarsal tunnel entrapment neuropathy of the medial peroneal nerve.

NATURAL HISTORY

Disease onset

The clinical course of RA follows an onset of disease that may be abrupt and acute, or gradual and insidious, or subacute between these extremes[1,2]. For this reason, the measurement of disease activity in RA is not easily defined[59]. A gradual onset is most common (at least 50% of cases), whereas a sudden onset is much less common (10–25%)[1,2]. RA begins predominantly as an articular disease and one or many joints may be affected. It may also start with an extra-articular or non-articular presentation, such as a local bursitis, tenosynovitis, carpal tunnel syndrome, or as a systemic presentation with diffuse polyarthralgia or polymyalgia. Although the onset is predominantly articular, it is frequently associated with a variety of extra-articular features, including generalized weakness, anorexia, weight loss or fever. In some cases, fatigue alone or diffuse nonspecific aching with other extra-articular features, such as pulmonary disease, may herald – by weeks or months – the onset of polyarthritis[2,20].

Pattern of presentation

Gradual onset

The most common early presentation is a gradual or insidious one affecting small peripheral joints such as the wrists, MCPs, PIPs, ankles or MTPs. It is defined as one that the patient can date only to the nearest month. It is usually symmetric, with considerable morning stiffness and the patient complaining of difficulty making a fist and poor grip strength. The morning stiffness may last minutes to hours.

Slow, monoarticular presentation

Less common is a slow monoarticular presentation affecting larger joints such as shoulders or knees. The symptoms may remain confined to one or two joints, but frequently spread over the ensuing days and weeks additively, to affect wrists, fingers, ankles or feet in a widespread fashion.

Abrupt, acute polyarthritis

Less frequently, RA presents as an abrupt acute polyarthritis of the shoulders, elbows, wrists, fingers, hips, knees, ankles and feet, with intense joint pain, diffuse swelling and limitation leading to incapacitation. A sudden onset is defined as one for which the patient can give a specific date. This type of onset may affect patients at any age, but has particular significance in the elderly. Older men, especially, may develop a syndrome of 'remitting, seronegative, symmetric, synovitis with pitting edema (RS3PE syndrome)'[34] that may be confused with RA. A similar subgroup of elderly British males showed an acute 'stormy' onset, with resolution usually within a year – 'benign RA of the aged'[60].

Acute monoarthritis

An acute monoarthritis of a knee, shoulder or hip can present a picture suggesting a septic, pseudogout or gouty process, although this presentation is rare. Joint pain more severe than that found in RA is characteristic of the last two conditions, which may resemble or even complicate RA. The results of synovial fluid analysis should settle any diagnostic confusion in these cases. An acute monoarticular presentation may proceed to more widespread involvement with any of the preceding patterns.

Tenosynovitis or bursitis may also be associated with mono- or polyarthritis and subcutaneous nodules over extensor surfaces, such as the elbow, sacrum or tendo Achillis.

Palindromic rheumatism

Another variation of the abrupt onset of polyarthritis is known as 'palindromic rheumatism'[61]. Here, variable episodes of polyarthritis suddenly affect one or more large or peripheral joints, last a few hours or a few days, and then spontaneously subside, with complete clearing of all rheumatic signs between attacks. These short-lived episodes may recur over weeks or months, with increasing frequency and severity, and may herald the onset of persistent polyarthritis. At least 33% of these palindromic cases evolve into typical RA, and in one review of 653 patients only 15% became symptom-free after 5 years[62].

Local extra-articular features

As noted, bursitis and tenosynovitis may be associated with RA. Sometimes, however, the earliest manifestation and presentation of RA may be a median nerve compression (carpal tunnel syndrome) from volar wrist tenosynovitis[38]. Similarly, other local extra-articular features may be the presenting feature.

Systemic extra-articular features

Elderly patients, in particular, may present with polyarthralgias and polymyalgias affecting the neck and shoulders or hips and knees and profound fatigue. Although these features, especially in association with fever and high ESR lasting several weeks, suggest a diagnosis of polymyalgia rheumatica, this picture may be a forerunner of full-blown RA. The notion has been advanced that seronegative RA in the elderly has more in common with polymyalgia rheumatica than typical seropositive erosive RA[63].

Pattern of progression

No matter what the onset or presentation, the patient's subsequent progress may follow several different patterns. It may be a course that is brief and self-limited, or episodic (palindromic), or prolonged and progressive, or something intermediate. The severity may vary from mild to intense. Attacks may be prolonged and smoldering or prolonged and progressive. With continuing disease activity, the patient's daily activities and functional capacity are affected to a greater or lesser extent. Although disability is usually proportional to the amount of painful joint involvement, in men who do physically hard work there is sometimes progressive joint dysfunction and disability without much pain. The physical abilities of patients who have this 'neuropathic' picture may dwindle insidiously before the work impairment or daily activities decline and the seriousness of the situation becomes apparent. This highlights the importance of careful evaluation and re-evaluation of the patient's condition. For this reason, good records are essential, to document the patient's progress and response to treatment, and these records should incorporate the features contained in the American College Rheumatology (ACR) criteria for clinical remission in RA (Table 22.8)[64]. The criteria include features believed to predict a favorable outcome, and are mostly inflammatory articular characteristics of RA. Unlike the self-report questionnaires, these criteria do not take into account the patient's present functional state, which is frequently a better predictor of the patient's future condition[25]. Moreover, when a patient is not responding to treatment as expected, it is important

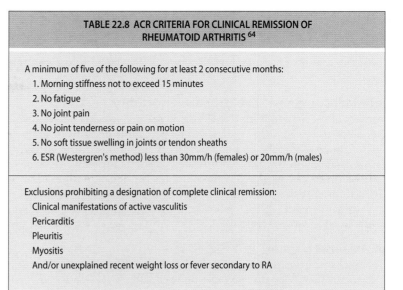

TABLE 22.8 ACR CRITERIA FOR CLINICAL REMISSION OF RHEUMATOID ARTHRITIS [64]

A minimum of five of the following for at least 2 consecutive months:
1. Morning stiffness not to exceed 15 minutes
2. No fatigue
3. No joint pain
4. No joint tenderness or pain on motion
5. No soft tissue swelling in joints or tendon sheaths
6. ESR (Westergren's method) less than 30mm/h (females) or 20mm/h (males)

Exclusions prohibiting a designation of complete clinical remission:
Clinical manifestations of active vasculitis
Pericarditis
Pleuritis
Myositis
And/or unexplained recent weight loss or fever secondary to RA

to be aware of all the factors that may adversely affect outcome. The patient's systemic reaction, extra-articular features and serologic status may in fact be more important than the articular features and their complications. Alternatively, the patient may be showing an adverse reaction to one or more medications.

Few studies have examined the natural history of a group of patients with well-defined RA over a long period of time. One such representative study is that by Masi et al.[65], who followed 50 patients with early RA for almost 6 years and described three articular patterns (Fig. 22.16):

- Monocyclic pattern: a single cycle with remission for at least 1 year, seen in 20% of patients
- Polycyclic pattern: seen in 70% of patients with either intermittent or continuing subtypes. The latter group showed smoldering activity with incomplete remission or progression
- Progressive pattern: with increasing joint involvement seen in about 10% of patients.

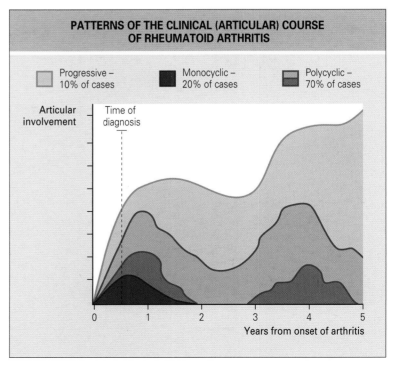

PATTERNS OF THE CLINICAL (ARTICULAR) COURSE OF RHEUMATOID ARTHRITIS

Progressive – 10% of cases   Monocyclic – 20% of cases   Polycyclic – 70% of cases

Articular involvement

Time of diagnosis

Years from onset of arthritis

Fig. 22.16 Patterns of the clinical (articular) course of rheumatoid arthritis. Articular patterns in 50 patients with RA. (Data from Masi et al.[65])

Patients with malignant RA would come into this last category. Most authorities would agree with these general observations, but many current ideas on the natural history of RA must remain speculative until the results of more longitudinal population-based studies become available.

Clinical course – morbidity and mortality

Studies of the natural history of RA could provide insights into outcome variables and prognosis. Understanding prognosis helps us to evaluate better the psychosocial and compensation implications for estimating work disability in RA. It is worthwhile considering whether the type of disease onset and patterns of presentation previously outlined can be used to predict the subsequent course of RA. A generally held view is that an acute onset forecasts a favorable prognosis, whereas an insidious onset heralds a worse outlook.

Acute onset pattern

In a series of 102 early cases of adult RA, Fleming et al.[1] reported that 11 patients with sudden disease onset showed, after 5 years, a better functional outcome than did 69 patients with a slow onset of disease. However, in a later series of 100 patients, Jacoby et al.[2] observed that, after an 11-year follow up, there was no difference in functional class whether disease onset was acute, subacute or gradual. In the past, cases with acute onset as a result of a reactive or viral polyarthritis may have been mistaken for RA. Another explanation for a better outcome in acute patients is that they are more likely to seek prompt medical attention. The favorable course of mild, transient or self-limited RA, however, has not attracted much attention, because rheumatologists are mostly concerned with progressive RA.

Gradual onset pattern

In Fleming's report[1], a worse prognosis was found in patients with disease that was gradual in onset and associated with large-joint involvement (shoulders, elbows, wrists, knees) in addition to involvement of the first and second MTPs. In the Jacoby series[2], the type of onset was not predictive of functional status after 11 years; moreover, in a later Finnish study of 235 patients with RA[66], radiographically evident damage

after 7 years was the same whether the onset had been acute (69), subacute (55) or gradual (111).

General variables

A number of variables are believed to have prognostic implications (Table 22.6). In a large Finnish population survey of 7217 adults, the detection of rheumatoid factor in 15 of 21 patients with seropositive RA antedated the onset of RA usually by 5 years[67]. Thus, in spite of the factors cited in Table 22.6, better markers are needed for detecting early disease and identifying at an early stage those patients who are likely to pursue a progressive course. Ideally, some of the newer immunogenetic, synovial or imaging methods may fulfill these needs. It should also be noted that patients with RA are at risk for other chronic diseases. In a Dutch study, 27% of a cohort of 186 patients were reported to show coexisting non-rheumatic conditions[68]. These were mostly cardio-respiratory, and most were pre-existing.

Health status questionnaire assessments

For the assessment of prognosis, a number of variable health status self-report questionnaires have been developed[22-25]. Data obtained by rheumatologists using these self-report assessments suggest that the overall long-term prognosis in patients with RA may be worse than previously estimated[21]. Wolfe and Cathey[69] assessed functional disability using the Stanford HAQ and Functional Disability Index in 1274 patients with RA followed longitudinally for up to 12 years. Half the patients showed loss of function that was moderate within 1–2 years, severe in 2–6 years and very severe in 10 years. The progression of disability was most rapid in the early years and then tapered off. The disease worsened more quickly in women and was associated with a longer duration of disease, decreased grip strength, and worse pain, global severity and psychologic scores. Older patients also showed more systemic features associated with greater functional loss[69].

In another longitudinal study, from Santa Clara County, California, patients with disease for more than 20 years deteriorated more rapidly than those with disease of a shorter duration[70]. The Stanford HAQ disability index also revealed more rapid deterioration in women, in

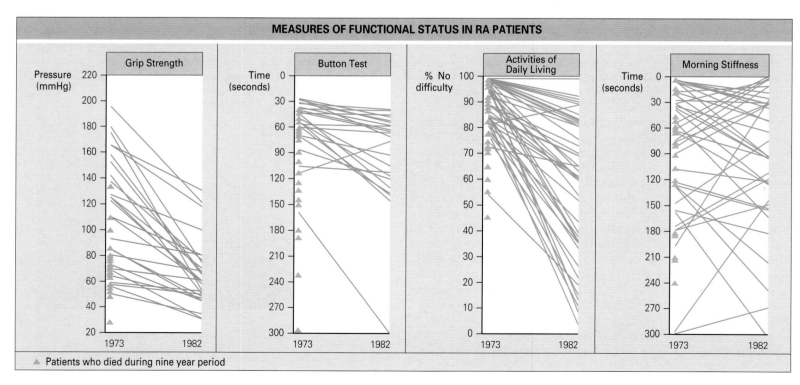

Fig. 22.17 Measures of functional status in RA patients. (Data from Pincus et al.[76] and Pincus and Callahan[77].)

patients with fewer years of education and those with increased age. The same investigators showed that the Stanford HAQ disability index is a useful prognosticator of duration of survival[71]. Patients with more severe disease are more likely to receive prednisone, and its long-term use was a risk factor associated with greater disability and premature death[71]. Severity measured by these prognostic factors may predict, not only morbidity, but also a twofold increase in mortality rate that is comparable to that of malignant conditions such as Hodgkin's disease or chronic heart disease[72]. Moreover, when Gabriel et al.[73] examined mortality among persons living in Rochester, Minnesota, over four decades, they found a greater mortality among patients with RA than was expected[73]. A much larger population-based cohort of 46 917 patients with RA in Sweden followed from 1964 to 1995 also showed increased mortality rates in RA patients compared with the general population[74]. However, in contrast to the Mayo study, the Karolinska analysis revealed a decreasing mortality rate among RA patients from 1975.

Estimates of functional status using these questionnaires appear to provide a better-estimate long-term prognosis than can be obtained with radiographic or serologic measures[75]. Moreover, these prognostic analyses confirm that RA is a marker for the development of many comorbid chronic conditions, such as bacterial infections and cardiovascular and renal diseases.

Although self-report questionnaires have proved valuable, patients with limited education find them difficult to use, and rheumatologists are reluctant to rely on questionnaire data alone. Pincus et al.[76] studied three simple measures of functional status – grip strength, walking time and a button test. Their results were comparable to laboratory measures, showed reliable reproducibility and were similar to self-report questionnaires in their capacity to predict outcome[77] (Fig. 22.17). Although patients with poor long-term outlook have attracted the attention of hospital-based rheumatologists, these severely affected patients may not be representative of RA as a whole. This is because of the view that RA in the community may be a milder disease than was believed in the past[78]. This idea is supported by the results of an inception cohort of 622 Dutch patients with RA followed over 10 years from onset of their disease[79]. The investigators found no excess mortality over expected, and functional capacity of patients remained constant during the first 6 years, after an initial improvement. Risk factors for death were seen only in men and patients with an older age at onset. Perhaps methotrexate is having a favorable effect on prognosis never seen before its widespread use.

REFERENCES

1. Fleming A, Crown JM, Corbett M. Early rheumatoid disease. I. Onset. II. Patterns of joint involvement. Ann Rheum Dis 1976; 35: 357–363.
2. Jacoby RK, Jayson MIV, Cosh JA. Onset, early stages and prognosis of rheumatoid arthritis: a clinical study of 100 patients with 11 year follow-up. BMJ 1973; 2: 96–100.
3. Arnett FC, Edworthy SM, Bloch DA et al. The American Rheumatism Association 1987 revised criteria for the classification of rheumatoid arthritis. Arthritis Rheum 1988; 31: 315–324.
4. Anderson RJ. Rheumatoid arthritis B. Clinical and laboratory features. In: Klippel JH, ed. Primer on the rheumatic diseases, 12E. Atlants: Arthritis Foundation; 2001: 218–225.
5. Weyand CM, Goronzy JJ. Inherited and noninherited risk factors in rheumatoid arthritis [review]. Curr Opin Rheumatol 1995; 53: 206–213.
6. Pincus T, Callahan LF. How many types of patients meet classification criteria for rheumatoid arthritis [editorial]? J Rheumatol 1994; 21: 1385–1389.
7. Kuiper S, van Gestel AM, Swinkels HL et al. Influence of sex, age, and menopausal state on the course of early rheumatoid arthritis. J Rheumatol 2001; 28: 1809–1816.
8. Hawley DJ, Wolfe F. Anxiety and depression in patients with rheumatoid arthritis: a prospective study of 400 patients. J Rheumatol 1988; 15: 932–941.
9. Fifield J, Tennen H, Reisine S, McQuillan J. Depression and the long-term risk of pain, fatigue, and disability in patients with rheumatoid arthritis. Arthritis Rheum 1998; 41: 1851–1857.
10. Moldofsky H, Chester WJ. Pain and mood patterns in patients with rheumatoid arthritis. Psychosom Med 1970; 32: 309–318.
11. Wolfe F, Cathey MA, Kleinkeksel SM et al. Psychological status in primary fibrositis and fibrositis associated with rheumatoid arthritis. J Rheumatol 1984; 11: 500–506.
12. Wallace DJ. Does stress or trauma cause or aggravate rheumatic disease? Baillière's Clin Rheumatol 1994; 8: 149–159.
13. Meyerowitz S, Jacox RF, Hess DW. Monozygotic twins discordant for rheumatoid arthritis. Arthritis Rheum 1968; 11: 1–21.
14. Silman AJ, MacGregor AJ, Thomson W et al. Twin concordance rates for rheumatoid arthritis: results from a nationwide study. Br J Rheumatol 1993; 32: 903–907.
15. Barrett JH, Brennan P, Fiddler M et al. Does rheumatoid arthritis remit during pregnancy and relapse post-partum? Results from a nationwide study in the United Kingdom performed prospectively from late pregnancy. Arthritis Rheum 1999; 42: 1219–1227.
16. Hazes JMW, Dijkmans AC, Vandenbroucke JP et al. Pregnancy and the risk of developing rheumatoid arthritis. Arthritis Rheum 1990; 33: 1770–1775.
17. Brennan P, Silman AJ. Breast-feeding and the onset of rheumatoid arthritis. Arthritis Rheum 1994; 37: 808–813.
18. Leigh JP, Fries JF. Education level and rheumatoid arthritis: evidence from five data centers. J Rheumatol 1991; 18: 24–34.
19. Wolfe F. The effect of smoking on clinical, laboratory, and radiographic status in rheumatoid arthritis. J Rheumatol 2000; 27: 630–637.
20. Gordon DA, Hyland RH, Broder I. Rheumatoid arthritis. In: Cannon GW, Zimmerman GA, eds. The lung in rheumatic diseases. New York: Marcel Dekker; 1990: 229–259.
21. Fex E, Larsson B-M, Nived K et al. Effect of rheumatoid arthritis on work status and social and leisure time activities in patients followed 8 years from onset. J Rheumatol 1998; 25: 44–50.
22. Anderson JJ, Felson DT, Meenan RF, Williams HJ. Which traditional measures should be used in rheumatoid arthritis clinical trials? Arthritis Rheum 1989; 32: 1093–1099.
23. Pincus T, Callahan LF, Brooks RH et al. Self-report questionnaire scores in rheumatoid arthritis compared with traditional physical, radiographic, and laboratory measures. Ann Intern Med 1989; 110: 259–266.
24. Hagglund KJ, Roth DL, Haley WE, Alarcon GS. Discriminant and convergent validity of self-report measures of affective distress in patients with rheumatoid arthritis. J Rheumatol 1989; 16: 1428–1432.
25. Wolfe F. A reappraisal of HAQ disability in rheumatoid arthritis. Arthritis Rheum 2000; 43: 2751–2761.
26. Klinkhoff AV, Bellamy N, Bombardier C et al. An experiment in reducing interobserver variability of the examination for joint tenderness. J Rheumatol 1988; 15: 492–494.
27. Wiles NJ, Dunn G, Barrett EM et al. One year followup variables predict disability 5 years after presentation with inflammatory polyarthritis with greater accuracy than at baseline. J Rheumatol 2000; 27: 2360–2366.
28. Wiles N, Barrett J, Barrett E et al. Disability in patients with early inflammatory polyarthritis cannot be 'tracked' from year to year: an examination of the hypothesis underlying percentile reference charts. J Rheumatol 1999; 26: 800–804.
29. Smedstad LM, Moum T, Guillemin F et al. Correlates of functional disability in early rheumatoid arthritis: a cross-sectional study of 706 patients in four European countries. Br J Rheumatol 1996; 35: 746–751.
30. Wolfe F, Pincus T. The level of inflammation in RA is determined early and remains stable over the long-term course of the illness. J Rheumatol 2001; 28: 1817–1824.
31. Wolfe F, Hawley DJ. The longterm outcomes of rheumatoid arthritis: work disability: a prospective 18 year study of 823 patients. J Rheumatol 1998; 25: 2108–2117.
32. Lansbury J, Haut DD. Quantitation of the manifestations of rheumatoid arthritis. Area of joint surfaces as an index to total joint inflammation and deformity. Am J Med Sci 1956; 232: 150–155.
33. Thompson PW, Silman AJ, Kirwan JR, Currey HLF. Articular indices of joint inflammation in rheumatoid arthritis. Correlation with the acute phase response. Arthritis Rheum 1987; 30: 618–623.
34. McCarty DJ, O'Duffy JD, Pearson L, Hunter JB. Remitting seronegative symmetrical synovitis with pitting edema (RS3PE syndrome). JAMA 1985; 2545: 2763–2767.
35. Thompson M, Bywaters EGL. Unilateral rheumatoid arthritis following hemiplegia. Ann Rheum Dis 1961; 21: 370–377.
36. Hastings DE. In Gordon DA, ed. Rheumatoid arthritis – contemporary management series, 2E. New York: Medical Examination Publishing; 1985: 147–149.
37. Hastings DE, Evans JA. Rheumatoid wrist deformities and their relation to ulnar drift. J Bone Joint Surg 1975; 57A: 930–934.
38. Jacob J, Sartorius D, Kursunoglu S et al. Distal interphalangeal joint involvement in rheumatoid arthritis. Arthritis Rheum 1986; 29: 10–15.
39. Chamberlain A, Corbett M. Carpal tunnel syndrome in early rheumatoid arthritis. Ann Rheum Dis 1970; 29: 149–152.
40. Chang LW, Gowans JDC, Granger CV et al. Entrapment neuropathy of the posterior interosseous nerve. Arthritis Rheum 1972; 15: 350–352.
41. Yoshida M, Belt EA, Kaarela K et al. Prevalence of mutilans-like hand deformities in patients with seropositive rheumatoid arthritis: a prospective 20-year study. Scand J Rheumatol 1999; 28: 38–40.
42. Bywaters EGL. The bursae of the body. Ann Rheum Dis 1965; 24: 215–218.
43. Yasuda M, Ono M, Naono T, Nobunaga M. Multiple rheumatoid bursal cysts. J Rheumatol 1989; 16: 1986–1988.

44. Polisar I, Burbank B, Levitt LM *et al*. Bilateral midline fixation of cricoarytenoid joints as a serious medical emergency. JAMA 1960; 172: 901–906.
45. Khong TK, Rooney PJ. Manubriosternal joint subluxation in rheumatoid arthritis. J Rheumatol 1982; 9: 712–715.
46. Winfield J, Young A, Williams P *et al*. A prospective study of the radiological hanges in the cervical spine in early rheumatoid disease. Ann Rheum Dis 1981; 40: 109–114.
47. Nakano KK, Schoene WC, Baker RA, Dawson DM. The cervical myelopathy associated with rheumatoid arthritis: an analysis of 32 patients, with 2 postmortem cases. Ann Neurol 1978; 3: 144–151.
48. Stiskal MA, Neuhold A, Szolar DH *et al*. Rheumatoid arthritis of the craniocervical region by MR imaging: detection and characterization. Am J Roentgenol 1995; 165: 582–592.
49. Fallet GH, Barnes CG, Berry H *et al*. Coexisting rheumatoid arthritis and ankylosing spondylitis. J Rheumatol 1987; 14: 1135–1138.
50. Hastings DE, Parker SM. Protrusio acetabuli in rheumatoid arthritis. Clin Orthop 1975; 108: 76–83.
51. Underwood PL, McLeod RA, Ginsburg WW. The varied clinical manifestations of iliopsoas bursitis. J Rheumatol 1988; 15: 1683–1685.
52. Menard HA, Paquette D. Skin temperature of the knee: an unrecognized physical sign of inflammatory disease of the knee. Can Med Assoc J 1980; 122: 439–440.
53. Gerber NJ, Dixon AStJ. Synovial cysts and juxta-articular bone cysts. Semin Arthritis Rheum 1974; 3: 323–348.
54. Kraag G, Thevathasan EM, Gordon DA, Walker IH. The hemorrhage crescent sign of acute synovial rupture. Ann Intern Med 1976; 85: 477–478.
55. Thevenon A, Hardouin P, Duquesnoy B. Popliteal cyst presenting as an anterior tibial mass. Arthritis Rheum 1985; 28: 477–478.
56. Wei N. Stress fractures of the distal fibula presenting as monoarticular flares in patients with rheumatoid arthritis. Arthrits Rheum 1994; 37: 1555–1556.
57. Rask MR. Achilles tendon rupture owing to rheumatoid disease. JAMA 1978; 239: 435–436.
58. Shapiro RF, Resnick D, Castles JJ *et al*. Fistulization of rheumatoid joints. Spectrum of identifiable syndromes. Ann Rheum Dis 1975; 34: 489–498.
59. Boers M, van Riel PL, Felson DT, Tugwell P. Assessing the activity of rheumatoid arthritis [review]. Baillières Clin Rheumatol 1995; 9: 305–317.
60. Corrigan AB, Robinson RG, Terenty TR *et al*. Benign rheumatoid arthritis of the aged. BMJ 1974; 1: 444–446.
61. Schumacher HR. Palindromic onset of rheumatoid arthritis. Clinical, synovial fluid and biopsy studies. Arthritis Rheum 1982; 25: 361–369.
62. Guerne P-A, Weisman WH. Palindromic rheumatism: part of or apart from the spectrum of rheumatoid arthritis? Am J Med 1992; 93: 451–460.
63. Healey LA, Sheets PK. Polymyalgia rheumatica and seronegative rheumatoid arthritis may be the same entity. J Rheumatol 1992; 19: 270–272.
64. Pinals RS, Masi AF, Larsen RA *et al*. Preliminary criteria for clinical remission in rheumatoid arthritis. Bull Rheum Dis 1982; 32: 7–10.
65. Masi AT, Feigenbaum SL, Kaplan SB. Articular patterns in the early course of rheumatoid arthritis. Am J Med 1983; 75(suppl 6A): 16–26.
66. Luukkainen R, Isomaki H, Kajander A. Prognostic value of the type of onset of rheumatoid arthritis. Ann Rheum Dis 1983; 42: 274–275.
67. Aho K, Heliovaara M, Maatela J *et al*. Rheumatoid factors antedating clinical rheumatoid arthritis. J Rheumatol 1991; 18: 1282–1284.
68. Kroot E-JJA, van Gestel AM, Swinkels HL *et al*. Chronic comorbidity in patients with early rheumatoid arthritis: a descriptive study. J Rheumatol 2001; 28: 1511–1157.
69. Wolfe F, Cathey MA. The assessment and prediction of functional disability in rheumatoid arthritis. J Rheumatol 1991; 18: 1298–1306.
70. Leigh JP, Fries JF, Parikh N. Severity of disability and duration of disease in rheumatoid arthritis. J Rheumatol 1992; 19: 1906–1911.
71. Leigh JP, Fries J. Mortality predictors among 263 patients with rheumatoid arthritis. J Rheumatol 1991; 18: 1307–1312.
72. Wolfe F, Mitchell DM, Sibley JT *et al*. The mortality of rheumatoid arthritis. Arthritis Rheum 1994; 37: 481–494.
73. Gabriel SE, Crowson CS, O'Fallon WM. Mortality in RA: have we made an impact in 4 decades? J Rheumatol 1999; 26: 2529–2533.
74. Bjornadel L, Baecklund E, Yin L *et al*. Decreasing mortality in patients with rheumatoid arthritis: results from a large population-based control in Sweden 1964–1995. J Rheumatol 2002; 29: 906–912.
75. Pincus T, Brooks RH, Callahan LF. Prediction of long-term mortality in patients with rheumatoid arthritis according to simple questionnaire and joint count measures. Ann Intern Med 1994; 120: 26–34.
76. Pincus T, Brooks RH, Callahan LF. Reliability of grip strength, walking time and button test performed according to a standard protocol. J Rheumatol. 1991; 18: 997–1000.
77. Pincus T, Callahan LF. Predictive value of quantitative physical and questionnaire measures of functional status for 9-year morbidity in rheumatoid arthritis. J Rheumatol 1992; 19: 1051–1057.
78. Hakala P, Nieminen O, Koivisto O. More evidence from a community based series of better outcome in rheumatoid arthritis. Data on the effect of multidisciplinary care on the retention of functional ability. J Rheumatol 1994; 21: 1432–1437.
79. Kroot EJA, Van Leeuwen MA, van Rijswijk MH *et al*. No increased mortality in patients with RA: up to 10 years of follow up from disease onset. Ann Rheum Disease 2000; 59: 954–958.

23 Evaluation and management of early inflammatory polyarthritis

Mark A Quinn, Michael J Green and Paul Emery

- Early features of rheumatoid arthritis are often non-specific
- A problem-orientated approach to management may be optimal – i.e. is it inflammatory/will it be persistent, etc.)
- American College of Rheumatology classification criteria are misleading early in the disease course particularly in the first 12 weeks
- Investigations, including blood tests and X-rays, may be normal at outset
- Optimal management should aim to eliminate inflammation
- Early identification of non-responders/inadequate responders should allow targeted use of more aggressive treatment regimens

TABLE 23.1 IMPORTANT QUESTIONS IN EARLY INFLAMMATORY POLYARTHRITIS
• Is it inflammatory?
• Is it persistent (<3 months symptom duration)?
• Is it severe?

INTRODUCTION

Rheumatoid arthritis (RA) is a common condition, affecting around 1% of the population. Once initiated, the persistent synovitis, characteristic of RA, causes progressive joint destruction and deformity with resultant deterioration in quality of life and high cost to society (estimated at £1.3 billion annually in the UK)[1]. The conventional approach to treatment of RA has been a protocol starting with the least toxic but least effective therapies, and followed by more effective but more toxic drugs, i.e. the classic treatment pyramid. It was therefore common practice that the more effective disease modifying anti-rheumatic drugs (DMARDs) were only initiated when patients had demonstrable radiological damage and in effect 'had earned their treatment'. This treatment approach was based on the notion that RA is 'mild', with joint damage and disability occurring only slowly. Radiological outcome studies however have demonstrated that damage occurs very early in disease and 90% of patients have radiological evidence of damage by the end of 2 years[2]. More recent studies using imaging techniques such as magnetic resonance imaging (MRI) and ultrasonography have confirmed evidence of damage within weeks of onset of symptoms[3,4]. Over and above these considerations there is increasing scientific evidence that mortality rates are significantly increased when RA is poorly controlled[5]. In view of these findings the old fashioned pyramid approach would seem no longer justifiable, especially since it tended to delay the use of effective therapies to a time when the disease is possibly more resistant to drug interventions. There is now a wide range of published studies demonstrating that DMARDs improve clinical outcome measures when used in patients with early RA and that delaying treatment is detrimental[6]. It is now generally agreed that therapy with a DMARD should be instituted at the time of diagnosis of RA (Table 23.1).

There are however inherent difficulties in making an accurate diagnosis of RA in the very early stages. The most characteristic feature of this disorder is chronicity and this by definition takes time to occur. The lack of a disease-specific feature or test means that the diagnosis of RA remains a composite of clinical and investigational features which when used in the early stages of disease assessment may be confusing and even potentially misleading[7,8]. Furthermore, labeling a patient as having RA in the early stages of an inflammatory arthritis may not be the most important step. It may be more relevant to establish the presence or absence of synovitis and to assess an individual patient's likely prognosis (and possibly response to therapy).

A logical implication of the above is that if treatment can be commenced before RA is fully developed (i.e. before persistence is established), even greater benefits may be possible. This requires patients with potentially persistent, more severe disease to be identified and treated effectively in the very earliest stages of the disease. Rapid patient access to assessment and therapy therefore is the first and perhaps most important issue when managing patients with early arthritis. There are now numerous local and nationwide initiatives, both in Europe and the USA, designed to reduce this delay. The CARE (collaboration to assess and refer early) initiative was established to meet the need for simplified referral criteria to allow early assessment of suspected RA for specialist assessment and further treatment[9]. The guidelines are designed to encourage early referral and will be widely distributed through specialist organizations and is endorsed by the European League Against Rheumatism (EULAR).

WHICH PATIENTS SHOULD BE SEEN EARLY BY A SPECIALIST?

At presentation to primary care physicians the exact diagnosis may be unclear with a number of potential diagnoses (Table 23.2). Further investigations at this stage are often not diagnostic. For example in patients who eventually develop RA up to 60% of patients may have a normal acute phase response, 70% have normal joint X-rays and 60% do not have a positive rheumatoid factor even at the time of presentation to secondary care (Table 23.3)[10]. The diagnosis and the decision to refer patients with an inflammatory arthritis therefore cannot be based on investigations alone, as negative results may delay the referral of appropriate patients. Referral for specialist opinion should be based on the appropriate history and presence of clinical features suggestive of inflammatory disease (Table 23.4). For the optimal management of patients with early inflammatory polyarthritis, a system of early referral is crucial and agreed protocols for referral need to be developed between primary and secondary care physicians.

TABLE 23.2 DIFFERENTIAL DIAGNOSIS OF A PATIENT WITH POLYARTHRITIS

Inflammatory arthritis

- Rheumatoid arthritis
- Postviral arthritis
- Psoriatic arthritis
- Reactive arthritis
- Ankylosing spondylitis
- Enteropathic arthritis
- Polyarticular gout/pseudogout (calcium pyrophosphate disease)

Connective tissue diseases

- Systemic lupus erythematosus
- Scleroderma
- Behçet's disease
- Polyarteritis nodosa
- Undifferentiated connective tissue disease

Non-inflammatory joint conditions

- Generalized osteoarthritis
- Soft tissue rheumatism/fibromyalgia

Important differential diagnoses

- Septic arthritis
- Polymyalgia rheumatica
- Paraneoplastic syndrome
- Subacute bacterial endocarditis

TABLE 23.3 DIFFICULTIES ENCOUNTERED IN ASSESSING EARLY INFLAMMATORY POLYARTHRITIS

- In the earliest stages NSAID response may be marked and it can erroneously appear that the disease is cured
- RA clinical features are non-specific – self limiting arthritis can fulfill ACR RA classification criteria; i.e. RA is distinguished only by chronicity
- Blood tests and X-rays may be negative at onset
- RA can co-exist with other diseases and X-rays may therefore be confusing, e.g. patients with osteoarthritis who develop RA may initially only have X-ray evidence of osteoarthritis

TABLE 23.4 IMPORTANT FEATURES OF EARLY INFLAMMATORY POLYARTHRITIS

- Joint swelling
- Metacarpophalangeal and metatarsophalangeal involvement
- A good anti-inflammatory response
- A symmetrical distribution of symptoms
- Family history
- Significant early morning stiffness

WHICH PATIENTS REQUIRE DISEASE-MODIFYING THERAPY?

There is now substantial evidence (discussed below), including randomized controlled trials, indicating that the early institution of DMARD therapy is beneficial whether it be in patients with early RA or in those with unselected polyarthritis. The currently used 'diagnostic criteria' for diseases including RA are unsuitable, particularly early in disease, and the fulfillment of these criteria does not guarantee a homogeneous outcome[7,8]. It would therefore appear reasonable to consider DMARD therapy for all patients with an early inflammatory polyarthritis where it has been established that persistent disease activity is likely. Recent studies have consistently demonstrated that the single most important determinant of persistence is disease duration and a period of 12 weeks of joint symptoms would appear to be pivotal[7,11,12]. For those patients presenting with a polyarthritis prior to this stage, the outlook is good, with as many as 50% of patients having a longstanding remission following a single dose of corticosteroids. However, in patients who present more than 12 weeks after the onset of symptoms, the likelihood of persistent disease is increased fivefold[7] (Fig. 23.1).

CAN SEVERITY OF DISEASE BE PREDICTED AT ONSET?

After establishing persistence, the next steps are to obtain an accurate assessment of the patients' likely prognosis and an idea of how they will respond to various potential therapies. As discussed above the clinical and laboratory features available at the time of disease onset cannot consistently predict the outcome of patients. Frustratingly the best predictor of poor disease is the progression of disease from one time point to the next. Some of the better predictors of prognosis have therefore been combined in the form of algorithms in an attempt to help guide management decisions (Table 23.5). These can improve the specificity for selecting patients with severe disease, however, when tested in clinical practice they still only correctly predict outcome in 70–80% of patients[13].

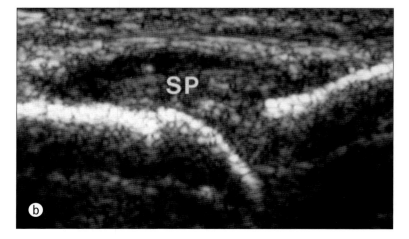

Fig. 23.1 Symmetrical small joint arthritis. (a) Clinical appearance – RA or benign self-limiting disease? (b) Longitudinal ultrasound section of the second metacarpophalangeal joint demonstrating synovial hypertrophy and joint effusion.

TABLE 23.5 RECOGNIZED PROGNOSTIC FACTORS IN EARLY RA

- Autoantibodies – rheumatoid factor/anti-CCP antibodies
- Genetic factors – shared epitope
- Acute phase markers – CRP/ESR/PV
- Sex – female
- Imaging
  - evidence of damage (ultrasound/MRI/X-ray)
  - severity and localization of inflammatory disease (ultrasound/MRI)
- Functional impairment – health assessment questionnaire (HAQ)

The use of better imaging techniques may further improve these algorithms (Fig. 23.2), by ensuring a homogenous study population. Distribution of inflammatory disease found using MRI of the hands has already demonstrated prognostic utility in early inflammatory polyarthritis. The inflammatory process in self-limiting disease has a predominantly extracapsular distribution, whereas persistent disease and true RA have predominantly synovial-based pathology[14] (Fig. 23.3).

The currently available prognostic markers alone are not able to determine how aggressive the disease is (i.e. whether to introduce biologics at presentation), particularly in the very early stages.

While accepting the weaknesses of algorithms a pragmatic approach using a system called PISA (persistent inflammatory symmetrical arthritis) has been adopted as an aid to making clinical decisions, and to standardize the characteristics of cohorts of patients for clinical studies. This is a system of severity assessment based on the most consistent predictors of prognosis and has been specifically developed for the staging of patients with an early inflammatory polyarthritis[10]. It requires patients to have persistent symmetrical small joint arthritis of at least 12 weeks duration. The extension of the time limit to 12 weeks from the 6 weeks included in the ACR criteria reduces the possibility that a self-limiting arthritis is erroneously included in the persistent group[7]. The PISA approach aims to exclude those patients who manage to fulfill clinical criteria for RA but who are likely to have self-limiting disease or a better prognosis if treated early with adequate therapy. This approach utilizes a numerical scoring system where the presence of a number of clinical and laboratory factors are used to predict poor prognosis disease (Table 23.6). These markers have consistently been associated with a poor outcome, measured in terms of radiographic damage and function. Patients with a composite score of greater than 3 at the initial assessment have been shown to have a particularly poor outcome and therefore more aggressive therapy may be required at an early stage[15]. Thus, while this system may be helpful in the majority of patients, an early review of all patients with a diagnosis of RA is advocated to assess the response to therapy and/or whether a change in disease phenotype has taken place. A central issue is whether what is observed is a change in disease or a simply a lack of response to therapy.

LEEDS EARLY ARTHRITIS PROJECT (LEAP) TREATMENT PROTOCOL FOR EARLY INFLAMMATORY POLYARTHRITIS

Figure 23.4 outlines a pragmatic approach to management decisions in the early stages of an inflammatory arthritis. Where possible this is based on the best available evidence. Where an evidence base is lacking it has been developed based on our own experience of the management of patients with an early inflammatory arthritis. Management decisions are made at three levels, i.e.

- which patients should be screened (discussed above)
- how to treat those patients not requiring DMARD therapy initially
- those patients who require the commencement of DMARD therapy.

WHAT IF DISEASE MODIFYING ANTI-RHEUMATIC DRUG THERAPY IS NOT INITIALLY INDICATED?

Patients first presenting to rheumatologists often fail to satisfy disease classification criteria and present with atypical symptoms and signs. This group includes patients either

- in the very early stages of disease
- who appear to have a mild disease (assessed by prognostic criteria)
- asymmetrical disease or
- those with an oligoarthritis (fewer than five joints involved).

A proportion of these patients represent disease in evolution while others will be self-limiting.

At present there are no agreed guidelines for the initial management of patients with mild early inflammatory arthritis. One approach, described in two recent publications, involves the use of a single dose of corticosteroids given at presentation[7,17].

For such patients there is sufficient uncertainty about their prognosis that a short delay in initiating definitive DMARD therapy is felt to be acceptable. The approach suggested is a single dose of corticosteroids given either intramuscularly (120mg methylprednisolone or 80mg if under 60kg) or intra-articularly followed by an early review (2–4 weeks) to assess response. The abolition of symptoms and signs at this early stage indicates a good long-term prognosis. Furthermore, persistent synovitis following this initial intervention indicates a high risk of a long-term arthritis, with the implication that DMARD therapy should be started without further delay.

A large proportion of these mild inflammatory polyarthritis patients have self-limiting disease and universal DMARD therapy would unnecessarily expose a considerable number to the risk of drug toxicity. Traditionally, management has involved a watch and wait policy, perhaps leading to a delay in intervention. The new approach, using a single dose of corticosteroid, facilitates a more informed decision regarding the use of DMARD therapy

THE THERAPEUTIC APPROACH TO EARLY INFLAMMATORY ARTHRITIS

Once the diagnosis of persistent synovitis or RA has been made, what is the best therapeutic approach? Non-steroidal anti-inflammatory drugs (NSAIDs) comprise the most commonly prescribed group of drugs for arthritis; both in primary and secondary care settings. Disease modifying anti-rheumatic drugs have historically been reserved for patients with persistent inflammatory disease after NSAID treatment or patients with evidence of damage at outset. This reluctance to prescribe DMARDs early was fueled by concerns regarding the risk of toxicity and the requirements for monitoring. However, current evidence would suggest this reluctance to be unfounded. In practice, 90% of patients diagnosed with RA will receive DMARDs within 3 years of diagnosis and thus delay does not reduce patient exposure to these drugs[15].

It is possible to calculate a toxicity index derived from symptoms, abnormal laboratory values and hospitalizations related to treatment for these drugs. When compared to NSAIDs, intramuscular gold and hydroxychloroquine have toxicity indices considerably lower than some commonly used NSAIDs, and methotrexate and azathioprine have equivalent indices. In context, DMARD toxicity is no worse than that of long-term use of the traditionally used NSAIDs[18,19]. At present the improved safety profile of the newer cyclo-oxygenase (COX)-2-selective NSAIDs has yet to be tested versus DMARDs.

Further support for the early introduction of DMARDs comes both from studies comparing early versus delayed DMARD use in early RA[20,21] and also placebo-controlled trials[22–26]. In an analysis of 1435 patients from 11 different studies, disease duration was of foremost importance in

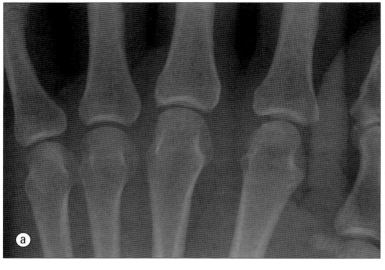

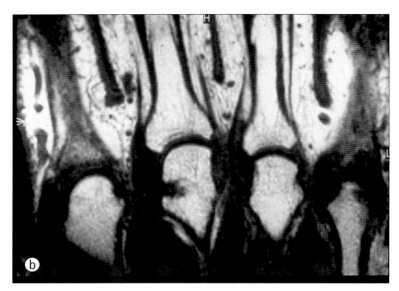

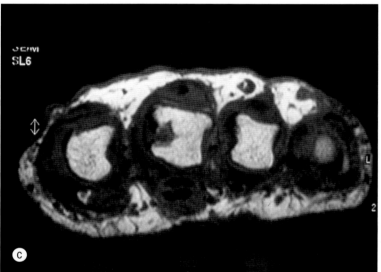

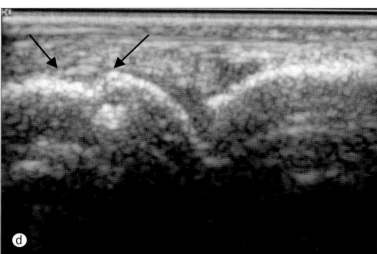

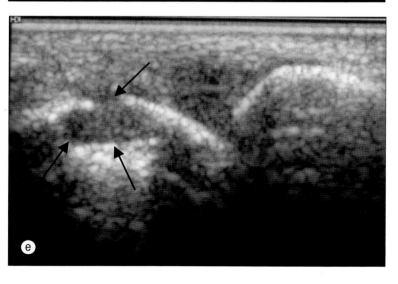

Fig. 23.2 Plain radiographs, enhanced MRI and ultrasound of a patient with early RA. (a) Normal plain radiograph of the metacarpophalangeal joints – 70% are normal at time of first presentation with RA. (b, c) Magnetic resonance images of metacarpophalangeal joints of the same patient in axial and coronal plains demonstrating an early erosion of the third metacarpophalangeal joint. (d, e) Ultrasound images of a metacarpophalangeal joint demonstrating the evolution of a joint erosion in a patient with a normal radiograph.

predicting response to DMARD therapy with 53% of patients with disease duration less than 1 year responding to therapy, whereas patients with longer duration showed diminished response[27].

With toxicity data and the ever-growing clinical data demonstrating that early intervention reduces structural damage[28], long-term disability[29] and mortality[5], the prompt introduction of DMARDs is now advocated for patients with persistent synovitis.

NON-STEROIDAL ANTI-INFLAMMATORY DRUGS

These are usually the first drugs prescribed following symptom onset and in most part prior to assessment by a rheumatology specialist. As mentioned previously, NSAIDs can have a dramatic effect in early inflammatory arthritis to the extent of masking symptoms and signs of inflammatory polyarthritis, which may offer false reassurance or result

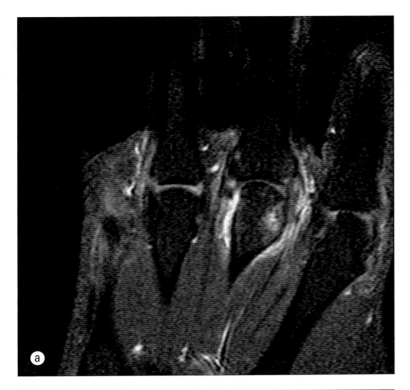

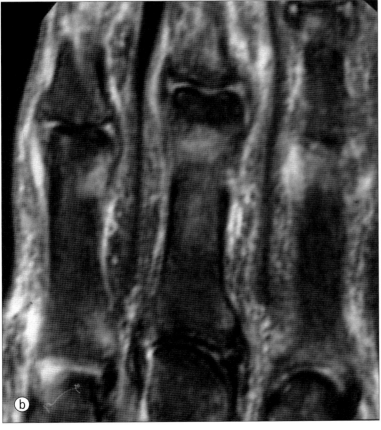

Fig. 23.3 MR images demonstrating the different appearances of self-limiting and persistent disease. (a) RA; predominant intra-articular inflammatory disease. (b) Self-limiting disease with predominant extracapsular pathology.

TABLE 23.6 PERSISTENT INFLAMMATORY SYMMETRICAL ARTHRITIS (PISA) SCORING SYSTEM		
Prognostic factor	**Score**	**Patient score**
Rheumatoid factor positive	1	
HLA DR1/DR4/DR10	1	
C-reactive protein >20mg/l	1	
Female sex	1	
Health assessment questionnaire raw score >4 =11	1	
Health assessment questionnaire raw score >11	2	
Total score	7	

A score of ≥3 indicates poor prognosis.

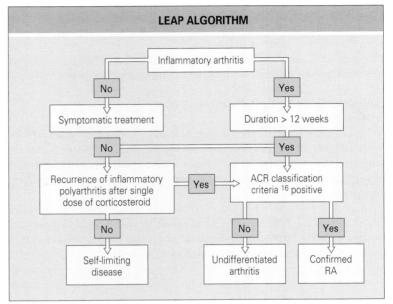

Fig. 23.4 LEAP algorithm. Leeds Early Arthritis Project algorithm for the management of early inflammatory polyarthritis.

in a delay in diagnosis[30]. If there is clinical uncertainty as to the inflammatory nature of a patient's condition, the patient should be reviewed off NSAID therapy. True inflammatory disease will almost certainly deteriorate with NSAID withdrawal and clinical signs may become more apparent. A similar approach may be adopted in patients with remission or near remission on DMARDs, where successful withdrawal of NSAIDs without worsening of symptoms reflects satisfactory disease suppression.

Numerous NSAIDs are available and new compounds are continuously being developed offering improved safety and efficacy profiles. Individual response can be very varied. In general a long acting preparation is to be preferred for efficacy, primarily in order to alleviate prolonged early morning stiffness, with the added benefit of ease of administration, while short acting agents may have advantages for safety. Agents combined with gastroprotectants should be considered where patients are thought to be at risk or the COX-2-selective drugs where efficacy is comparable with reduced gastric toxicity compared to conventional NSAIDs[31,32].

DISEASE MODIFYING ANTI-RHEUMATIC DRUGS

The practice of early introduction of DMARD therapy is now widely accepted, based on favorable results from long-term functional and radiographic outcome studies. Ideally, the treatment of choice should be effective, well tolerated, easy to administer and inexpensive. In addition to selecting which agent should be used first, there is the question of whether these agents should be used alone or in combination.

Multiple strategies have been employed for the treatment of RA, including the conventional pyramid approach, the inverse pyramid, step-up, step-down, saw tooth and a number of hybrid approaches. Data have made clear that no strategy is suitable for all patients and therapy must be tailored to suit the individual.

Combination therapy in early disease has been increasingly used in the hope of complete suppression of synovitis, reduction in radiographic damage, and decrease in functional disability and joint deformity. However, studies have failed to show a consistent benefit of combination therapy over mono-therapy[33–36]. Data in favor of combination therapy is only reliably seen when corticosteroids form part of the combination of DMARDs used. For the most part, however, benefit lasts only for the duration of corticosteroid use and toxicity data is scant. As a result combination therapy cannot be recommended for all patients at disease outset. Disease outcome remains highly variable and therapeutic response and ultimate prognosis cannot be predicted. For the purpose of clinical trials where poor prognosis patients may be selected, such variability in response to therapy diminishes the power to show a difference. The failure to respond to therapy remains the best predictor of poor prognosis. The emphasis should be on early review and rapid identification of poor or non-responders in order for patients to be targeted with appropriately aggressive treatment strategies. Such an approach allows therapy to be tailored to the individual patient's need.

Selection of the first disease modifying anti-rheumatic drug

Whereas there have been a number of studies comparing one DMARD with another in an attempt to demonstrate greater effectiveness, the interpretation of results can be confusing. The majority of studies demonstrate equivalence of therapies for clinical and radiographic outcomes[6].

In a 48-week double-blind placebo-controlled trial, sulfasalazine proved significantly more effective at retarding radiographic progression compared with hydroxychloroquine[37], however no significant differences in clinical and laboratory variables were shown[38].

From efficacy, tolerability and safety data, methotrexate and sulfasalazine emerge as the best first-line agents with hydroxychloroquine being useful for the patients with very mild disease or osteoarthritis with an inflammatory component. With the availability of biological agents an argument could be made in favor of methotrexate as it can be used as the universal 'anchor' therapy to which old and new therapies may be added and also has marginally better long term tolerance over sulfasalazine.

Leflunomide has demonstrated similar efficacy and tolerability to sulfasalazine with a more rapid rate of onset and significantly greater reduction in functional disability over 24 weeks[39]. When compared with methotrexate over 2 years in 999 patients, methotrexate showed improved clinical efficacy in the first year with similar rates of radiographic progression. In the second year there was significantly greater reduction in radiographic progression with methotrexate[40]. Such data suggest that leflunomide may offer an alternative to sulfasalazine and methotrexate as a first-line agent in RA, but at present it is not licensed for combination therapy which limits its flexibility when compared to methotrexate.

THE ROLE OF CORTICOSTEROIDS

The role of corticosteroid in the management of RA remains controversial. It is highly effective in suppressing both COX-2, proinflammatory cytokines and proteases and thus has a number of uses in the management of RA, including an induction regimen (prior to onset of effective DMARD action), rescue therapy when patients have an acute flare of disease and at low dosage as part of maintenance therapy. The aim is to use the minimum dose necessary for effective disease suppression without unnecessarily exposing patients to the well-documented long-

term side effects. There is some evidence that the use of low dose prednisolone (7.5mg) in addition to conventional DMARDs slows radiographic progression[41]. However when therapy was blindly stopped and the cohort reanalyzed after 1 year, the rate of radiographic progression rate in the steroid group was similar to that of the placebo arm[42]. Furthermore this study failed to demonstrate functional benefit from corticosteroid addition.

Intra-articular corticosteroids can effectively suppress synovitis and are commonly used in the clinic as adjunct therapy. The ultimate aim of therapy remains remission. In an attempt to achieve this, early RA patients selected for poor prognosis, were randomized to aggressive therapy (methotrexate + cyclosporin A with intra-articular injections to all active joints) versus a more conventional regimen (sulfasalazine with aspiration + injection of significant joint effusions only). The results did not show a significant additional benefit for the aggressive approach[35].

The COBRA study group reported a step-down therapeutic approach of sulfasalazine + methotrexate + high-dose prednisolone versus sulfasalazine alone[43]. Although significant radiographic benefits were seen at 80 weeks, disease activity was comparable in the two groups after the steroid therapy was stopped. There was also a trend towards greater bone density loss in a sub-group of the steroid-treated group. A cost-effectiveness analysis, however, tended to favor the combination group[44].

Corticosteroids are undoubtedly effective, but are limited long-term by toxicity, the severity of which is difficult to quantify. The two studies that used the most aggressive corticosteroid approaches[35,43] suggested a rate of bone loss (measured by bone densitometry) proportional to steroid dose used. More worrying is the fact that early exposure correlates with bone loss at 2 years[35], long after steroid dosing has ceased, suggesting bone density loss is sustained. Other side effects tend to be later and harder to quantify such as accelerated cardiovascular disease, glucose intolerance and alteration of the adrenal axis. Moreover, in RA, where osteoporosis and skin thinning are already a problem of the disease, additional toxicity from corticosteroids can be particularly harmful.

More aggressive treatment regimens that include corticosteroids[34,35,41,43] therefore appear to reduce damage for the duration of suppression of inflammation, but there is no evidence for a qualitative change in the disease mechanisms. Using the oncological analysis, it is clear that initial aggressive regimens result in initial debulking of disease with improvement in damage and altering the early outcome, yet the disease process continues. A quantitative improvement can therefore be attained, but as yet the qualitative change in outcome, which had been hoped for, has not been demonstrated. Activity returns when treatment is reduced. Effective suppression of disease using DMARD therapy is therefore the principal aim with steroids used for bridging purposes prior to the onset of DMARD action, for rescue in cases of disease flare and using intra-articular injections for local resistant disease. There may also be a role in early disease to differentiate IP from non-inflammatory disease and also to determine whether the inflammation is consistent.

The optimum mode of administration of corticosteroids is open for debate, but the intramuscular route has several advantages over oral. It is often a single dose, lasts up to 8 weeks, and negates problems with compliance, dependence and variable bioavailability of oral corticosteroids.

BIOLOGICAL AGENTS

Biological therapies which block the action of tumor necrosis factor (TNF)-α are now licensed and therapies blocking the effect of other proinflammatory cytokines are in various stages of development.

The majority of studies to date have assessed the safety and efficacy of these drugs in established RA, but studies in early disease are now emerging. In a study of 632 patients with active early RA (<3 years), the etanercept group demonstrated significant clinical differences in the first

6 months when compared to methotrexate, highlighting the rapid action of etanercept[45], as well as demonstrating the ability to significantly reduce erosions in the first year of treatment.

In a sub-analysis of early patients (<3 years) from the ATTRACT study[46], where patients resistant to methotrexate received either methotrexate + placebo or methotrexate + infliximab 3mg or 10mg/kg every 4 or 8 weeks, significant radiographic improvement was seen in all infliximab treated patients[47]. Radiographic progression was effectively halted in the infliximab treated patient groups.

At this stage there is insufficient evidence fully to assess the impact of these new agents in the management of early RA and the optimal way in which to use them has yet to be found. It is not feasible or logical to currently recommend these agents for all patients, and specific contraindications such as previous malignancy, chronic suppurative disease and previous tuberculosis prevent them from being a panacea. However, it is clear that these treatments have already had a major impact on the way in which RA is managed and their role will need to be regularly reassessed.

REFERENCES

1. Pincus T, Callahan LF. What is the natural history of rheumatoid arthritis? Rheum Dis Clin North Am 1993; 19: 123–151.
2. Emery P. The optimal management of early rheumatoid disease: the key to preventing disability. Br J Rheum 1994; 33: 765–768.
3. McGonagle D, Conaghan PG, O'Connor P et al. The relationship between synovitis and bone changes in early untreated rheumatoid arthritis. Arthritis Rheum 1999; 42: 1706–1711.
4. Wakefield RJ, Gibbon WW, Conaghan PG et al. The value of sonography in the detection of bone erosion in patients with rheumatoid arthritis: A comparative study with conventional radiography. Arthritis Rheum 2000; 43: 2762–2770.
5. Symmons D, Jones MA, Scott DL, Prior P. Long term mortality outcome in patients with rheumatoid arthritis: early presenters continue to do well. J Rheumatol 1998; 25: 1072–1077.
6. Quinn MA, Conaghan PG, Emery P. The therapeutic approach of early intervention for rheumatoid arthritis: what is the evidence? Rheumatology 2001; 40: 1211–1220.
7. Green MJ, Marzo-Ortega H, McGonagle D et al. Persistence of mild early inflammatory arthritis: The importance of disease duration, rheumatoid factor and the shared epitope. Arthritis Rheum 1999; 42: 2184–2188.
8. Harrison BJ, Symmons DPM, Barrett EM, Silman AJ. The performance of the 1987 ARA classification criteria for rheumatoid arthritis in a population based cohort of patients with early inflammatory arthritis. J Rheumatol 1998; 25: 2324–2330.
9. Emery P, Breedveld F, Dougados M et al. Early referral recommendation for newly diagnosed rheumatoid arthritis: evidence-based development of a clinical guide. Ann Rheum Dis 2002; 61: 290–297.
10. Emery P. Prognosis in inflammatory arthritis: the value of HLA genotyping and oncological analogy. The Dunlop Dotteridge Lecture. J Rheumatol 1997; 24: 1436–1442.
11. Harrison B, Thomson W, Symmons D et al. The influence of HLA-DRB1 alleles and rheumatoid factor on disease outcome in an inception cohort of patients with early inflammatory arthritis. Arthritis Rheum 1999; 42: 2174–2183.
12. Tunn EJ, Bacon PA. Differentiating persistent from self-limiting symmetrical synovitis in an early arthritis clinic. Br J Rheum 1993; 32: 97–103.
13. Van Zeben D, Hazes JM, Zwinderman AH et al. Factors predicting outcome of rheumatoid arthritis, results of a follow up study. J Rheumatol 1993; 20: 1288–1296.
14. McGonagle D, Gibbon WW, O'Connor P et al. An anatomical explanation for good prognosis rheumatoid arthritis. Lancet 1999; 353: 123–124.
15. Emery P, Salmon M. Early rheumatoid arthritis: time to aim for remission? Ann Rheum Dis 1995; 4: 944–947.
16. Arnett FC, Edworthy SM, Bloch DA et al. The American Rheumatism Association 1987 revised criteria for the classification of rheumatoid arthritis. Arthritis Rheum 1988; 31: 315–324.
17. Green M, Marzo-Ortega H, Wakefield RJ et al. Predictors of outcome in patients with oligoarthritis: results of a protocol of intraarticular corticosteroids to all clinically active joints. Arthritis Rheum 2001; 44: 1177–1183.
18. Fries JF, Williams CA, Bloch DA. The relative toxicity of non-steroidal antiinflammatory drugs. Arthritis Rheum 1991; 34: 1353–1360.
19. Fries JF, Williams CA, Ramey D, Bloch DA. The relative toxicity of disease-modifying antirheumatic drugs. Arthritis Rheum 1993; 36: 297–306.
20. Egsmose C, Lund B, Borg G et al. Patients with early arthritis benefit from early 2nd line therapy: 5 year follow-up of a prospective double blind placebo controlled study. J Rheumatol 1995; 22: 2208–2213.
21. Van der Heide A, Jacobs JWG, Bijlsma JWJ et al. The effectiveness of early treatment with 'second-line' anti-rheumatic drugs. A randomised controlled trial. Ann Intern Med 1996; 124: 699–707.
22. Hannonen P, Mottenen T, Hakola M, Oka M. Sulfasalazine in early rheumatoid arthritis. A 48 week double-blind, prospective, placebo-controlled study. Arthritis Rheum 1993; 36: 1501–1509.
23. The Australian Multicentre Clinical Trial Group. Sulfasalazine in early RA. J Rheumatol 1992; 19: 1672–1677.
24. Davis MJ, Dawes PT, Fowler PD et al. Should disease modifying drugs be used in mild rheumatoid arthritis? Br J Rheum 1991; 30: 451–454.
25. Borg G, Allander E, Lund B et al. Auranofin improves outcome in early rheumatoid arthritis. Results from a 2 year double-blind, placebo controlled study. J Rheumatol 1988; 15: 1747–1754.
26. The HERA study group. A randomized trial of hydroxychloroquine in early rheumatoid arthritis: the HERA study. Am J Med 1995; 98: 156–168.
27. Anderson JJ, Wells G, Verhoeven AC et al. Factors predicting response to treatment in rheumatoid arthritis. The importance of disease duration. Arthritis Rheum 2000; 43: 22–29.
28. Abu-Shakra M, Toker R, Flusser D et al. Clinical and radiographic outcomes of rheumatoid arthritis patients not treated with disease modifying drugs. Arthritis Rheum 1998; 41: 1190–1195.
29. Fries J, Williams CA, Morfield D et al. Reduction in long-term disability in patients with rheumatoid arthritis by disease-modifying antirheumatic drug-based treatment strategies. Arthritis Rheum 1996; 39: 616–622.
30. Marzo-Ortega H, Green MJ, Karim Z et al. Non-steroidal anti-inflammatory drugs alter the presentation of early inflammatory arthritis. Rheumatology 2000; 39 (suppl 1): 42.
31. Simon LS, Weaver AL, Graham DY et al. Anti-inflammatory and upper gastrointestinal effects of celecoxib in rheumatoid arthritis: a randomized controlled trial. J Am Med Assoc 1999; 282: 1921–1928.
32. Bombardier C, Laine L, Reicin A et al. Comparison of upper gastrointestinal toxicity of rofecoxib and naproxen in patients with rheumatoid arthritis. N Engl J Med 2000; 343: 1520–1528.
33. Dougados M, Combe B, Cantagrel A et al. Combination therapy in early rheumatoid arthritis: a randomised, controlled, double blind 52 week clinical trial of sulphasalazine and methotrexate compared with the single components. Ann Rheum Dis 1999; 58: 220–225.
34. Haagsma CJ, Van Riel PLCM, De Jong AJL, Van de Putte LBA. Combination of sulphasalazine and methotrexate versus the single components in early rheumatoid arthritis: A randomised, controlled, double-blind, 52 week clinical trial. Br J Rheumatol 1997; 36: 1082–1088.
35. Mottenen T, Hannonen P, Leirisalo-Repo M et al. Comparison of combination therapy with single drug-therapy in early rheumatoid arthritis: a randomised trial. Lancet 1999; 353: 1568–1573.
36. Proudman S, Conaghan P, Richardson C et al. Treatment of poor prognosis early rheumatoid arthritis a randomised study of methotrexate, cyclosporin A and intraarticular corticosteroids compared with sulfasalazine alone. Arthritis Rheum 2000; 43: 1809–1819.
37. Van der Heijde DM, Van Riel PL, Nuver-Zwart IH et al. Effects of hydroxychloroquine and sulphasalazine on progression of joint damage in rheumatoid arthritis. Lancet 1989; 1: 1036–1038.
38. Nuver-Zwart IH, Van Riel PLCM, Van de Putte LBA, Gribnau FWJ. A double blind comparative study of sulfasalazine and hydroxychloroquine in rheumatoid arthritis: evidence of an earlier effect of sulphasalazine. Ann Rheum Dis 1989; 48: 389–395.
39. Smolen JS, Kalden JK, Scott DL et al. Efficacy and safety of leflunomide compared with placebo and sulphasalazine in active rheumatoid arthritis: a double-blind, randomised, multicentre trial. Lancet 1999; 353: 259–266.
40. Emery P, Breedveld FC, Lemmel EM et al. A comparison of the efficacy and safety of leflunomide and methotrexate for the treatment of rheumatoid arthritis. Rheumatology 2000; 39: 655–665.
41. Kirwan JR and the ARC low dose glucocorticoid study group. The effect of glucocorticoids on joint destruction in rheumatoid arthritis. N Engl J Med 1995; 333: 142–146.
42. Hickling P, Jacoby RK, Kirwan JR and the Arthritis and Rheumatism Council low dose glucocorticosteroid group. Joint destruction after glucocorticoids are withdrawn in early rheumatoid arthritis. Br J Rheum 1998; 37: 930–936.
43. Boers M, Verhoeven AC, Markusse HM et al. Randomised comparison of combined step-down prednisolone, methotrexate and sulphasalazine with sulphasalazine alone in early rheumatoid arthritis. Lancet 1997; 350: 309–318.
44. Verhoeven AC, Bibo JC, Boers M et al. for the COBRA trial group. Cost-effectiveness and cost-utility of combination therapy in early rheumatoid arthritis: randomized comparison of combined step-down prednisolone, methotrexate and sulphasalazine with sulphasalazine alone. Br J Rheumatol 1998; 37: 1102–1109.
45. Bathon JM, Martin RW, Fleischmann RM et al. A comparison of etanercept and methotrexate in patients with early rheumatoid arthritis. N Eng J Med 2000; 343: 1586–1593.
46. Lipsky PE, van der Heijde DMFM, St Clair EW et al. Infliximab and methotrexate in the treatment of rheumatoid arthritis. N Engl J Med 2000; 43: 1594–1602.
47. Emery P, Maini RN, Lipsky PE et al. Infliximab plus methotrexate prevents structural damage, reduces signs and symptoms and improves disability in patients with active early rheumatoid arthritis. Ann Rheum Dis 2000; 59(suppl 1): 48.

24 Management of rheumatoid arthritis: synovitis

Barry Bresnihan

- Inflammation and structural damage in rheumatoid arthritis are associated with complex pathophysiological pathways
- The potential for joint damage is present during the earliest phases of disease
- Early introduction of effective treatment to maximally inhibit the inflammatory and destructive mechanisms is recommended
- Methotrexate is generally the preferred treatment for most patients – ensure optimal dosage and mode of administration
- Combination with other disease-modifying antirheumatic drugs, or with low-dose prednisolone, should be considered if response to methotrexate is suboptimal
- Targeted biologic therapies are recommended for aggressive disease categories

THE MANIFESTATIONS OF SYNOVITIS IN RHEUMATOID ARTHRITIS

Clinical appearances

In rheumatoid arthritis (RA), the symptoms of articular synovitis usually develop gradually over weeks to months[1]. In about 15% of patients, the symptoms may develop more acutely over days. The most prominent initial symptoms are stiffness, pain and swelling, usually affecting several joints at the same time. The joints most frequently involved early in the course of the disease are the small joints of the feet and hands, commonly in a symmetric distribution, with gradual progression to the larger joints of the upper and lower limbs and often the cervical spine and temporomandibular joints. Tendon sheath synovitis, involving in particular the flexor tendon sheaths of the hand, is another common feature. A significant degree of functional impairment may accompany persistent synovitis. The clinical course may be severe and progressive in some patients, mild and self-limiting in a small minority, or intermediate with gradual deterioration in most. Ultimately, the long-term functional outcome will mainly depend on the degree of matrix degradation that occurs in cartilage and bone.

Macroscopic appearances

The gross changes that are characteristic of RA result from chronic synovial inflammation[2]. Typically, the surface of the synovium becomes hypertrophic and edematous, with an intricate system of prominent villous fronds that extend into the joint cavity. Contemporary imaging modalities, such as magnetic resonance imaging and ultrasonography, possess the capability to further characterize and quantify macroscopic synovial inflammation, joint effusion, cartilage integrity and bone erosion[3,4]. In addition, the macroscopic appearances of synovitis may be quantified at arthroscopy[5].

Microscopic appearances

The characteristic microscopic appearances of RA include marked synovial lining layer hyperplasia and the accumulation of macrophages, T cells, B cells, plasma cells, natural killer (NK) cells, dendritic cells, mast cells and neutrophils in the sublining layer[6]. Large numbers of neutrophils traffic through the intimal layer into the synovial fluid[7]. Many proinflammatory mediators and tissue-degrading products such as reactive oxygen species and reactive nitrogen species, prostaglandins, cytokines, autoantibodies and proteases are secreted into the synovial compartment by the infiltrating cell populations. A knowledge of the histopathologic appearances of RA, the pathophysiologic mechanisms they represent and the alterations that occur with therapeutic interventions should enable greater rationalization in the selection of therapy and facilitate the future identification of novel therapeutic targets.

The dominant cells in the synovial lining layer are the fibroblast-like synoviocyte and the macrophage[6]. They release an array of proinflammatory cytokines and their inhibitors, which may promote further intra-articular perturbations. There is abundant production of matrix metalloproteinases (MMPs), cysteine proteases and other tissue-degrading mediators that accumulate in the synovial fluid and augment joint damage by directly interacting with exposed cartilage matrix. These features are present very early in the disease course. Increased lining layer macrophage accumulation and perivascular mononuclear infiltration are prominent days after the onset of symptoms[8] and are also present in clinically uninvolved joints[9]. CD68+ macrophage accumulation in the synovium is more prominent in symptomatic joints[10,11]. Abundant protease gene expression is also observed in synovial tissue obtained only weeks after the onset of symptoms, emphasizing the very early potential for joint destruction in RA[12].

T cells and plasma cells are prominent in the synovial sublining layer. Lymphocyte aggregates are observed in 50–60% of patients. These aggregates can be surrounded by plasma cells. In addition, macrophages and lymphocytes infiltrate the areas between the lymphocyte aggregates. In some patients, areas with granulomatous necrobiosis are apparent[13]. These areas may include fibrinoid necrosis that may be lined by a collar of epithelioid histiocytes and granulation tissue. Macrophages often constitute the majority of inflammatory cells in the synovial sublining layer. Local disease activity is particularly associated with their number and with the expression of cytokines, such as tumor necrosis factor (TNF)-α and interleukin (IL)-6[11,14]. The synovial sublining macrophages produce a variety of mediators of joint destruction[6].

There are two basic patterns of T-cell infiltration[15]. First, perivascular lymphocyte aggregates can be found, which consist predominantly of CD4+ cells in association with B cells, a few CD8+ cells and dendritic cells. The second pattern of T-cell infiltration is the diffuse infiltrate of T cells scattered throughout the synovium. A subset of the CD4+ T cells is activated.

A possible biologic effect of the activated T-cell population is transformation of migrating macrophages through direct cell contact. This mechanism is known to stimulate macrophage production of cytokines and MMPs *in vitro*[16,17]. A factor in human serum, identified as apolipoprotein (apo)A1, was shown to inhibit contact-mediated stimulation of monocytes by activated T lymphocytes *in vitro*[18]. It was speculated that apo A1 might play an important role in modulating T-lymphocyte-mediated effects in both acute and chronic inflammation. Many T cells in synovial tissue are, on the other hand, in a state of hyporesponsiveness[15,19]. Interdigitating dendritic cells, which are potent antigen presenting cells, are located in proximity to CD4+ T cells in the lymphocyte aggregates and near the intimal lining layer[20].

B cells constitute a small proportion of the total number of lymphocytes in the synovial sublining layer. However, numerous plasma cells may be present throughout the synovium, sometimes exceeding the number of infiltrating T cells. A considerable number of the plasma cells synthesize and secrete rheumatoid factors and other autoantibodies[21]. Follicular dendritic cells are observed in the same areas in proximity to proliferating B cells. They are thought to play a crucial role in isotype switching and final differentiation of B cells towards plasma cells or memory B cells[22,23].

Cells producing TNF-α are prominent in the lining layer of most, but not all, RA tissue samples[24]. TNF-α-producing cells are also present to a lesser degree in the sublining interaggregate areas and in the lymphoid aggregates. The impressive therapeutic effects of TNF-α blockade in RA may result from inhibition of the pathogenetic effects of TNF-α produced by synovial tissue macrophages. Cells that are immunoreactive for IL-1 and IL-1 receptor antagonist (IL-1Ra) are also present in the lining and sublining layers[24,25]. The distribution of IL-1Ra gene expression and protein production in RA differs from osteoarthritis, with notably less in the lining layer of RA synovium[26]. This observation is consistent with a relative deficiency of IL-1Ra production by RA synovial macrophages[27]. Studies of synovium from patients with late-stage RA suggest that TNF-α, IL-1α, IL-1β, their inhibitors and receptors are produced by most, but possibly not all, tissue samples. However, it is possible that the detection of cytokine production might depend on the site of biopsy. This was examined in multiple samples using reverse transcriptase polymerase chain reaction. TNF-α was expressed in all samples from all biopsy sites but at very low levels in the tissues of some. IL-1β was expressed in all samples from most sites[28].

There has been extensive analysis of proteolytic enzyme production by synovial tissue samples and primary synoviocyte cultures selected from non-carpophalangeal joint sites in established RA[6]. These studies have demonstrated MMP-1, MMP-3 and tissue inhibitor of metalloproteinase (TIMP) mRNA in the lining layer cells, including both macrophage and fibroblast-like synoviocyte populations, and in some sublining layer cell populations. Other MMPs, including MMP-9 (gelatinase B), have also been demonstrated in RA synovial tissue[29]. The tissue distribution of MMP-9 was localized to sites of synovial inflammation, particularly the lining layer, endothelium and tissue macrophages. MMP-13 has been cloned from RA synovial tissue[30]. MMP-13 mRNA and protein was demonstrated in lining layer fibroblast-like synoviocyte and not macrophages in most late-stage RA tissue samples. It seems likely that the degree of cartilage and bone degradation will depend on excessive MMP activity over the inhibitors in the synovium, especially within the pannus. In addition to MMPs, cathepsin B and cathepsin L production by synovial lining layer cells has also been demonstrated[31,32].

TREATMENT OF SYNOVITIS IN RHEUMATOID ARTHRITIS

Early treatment to prevent joint damage

The potential importance of recognizing and treating RA in its earliest stages has been argued forcefully[33]. It is assumed intuitively by many that effective early suppression of synovial inflammation will directly prevent the progression of cartilage and bone degradation and associated functional impairment. However, this assumption has been challenged and awaits confirmation[34]. For example, the possible dissociation between mechanisms of inflammation and progressive structural damage was highlighted by the study of infliximab treatment, which suggested, in a subset of patients, that the protective effects on joint damage were independent of effects on disease activity as measured by American College of Rheumatology (ACR) 20% response criteria[35]. Irrespective of whether there is or is not a direct association between the mechanisms of synovial inflammation and cartilage and bone matrix degradation, early prevention of joint damage should be a primary motivation when selecting the optimal treatment strategy for each patient with RA.

Most clinicians choose a therapeutic approach that is most likely to rapidly alleviate the symptoms of joint inflammation. Non-steroidal anti-inflammatory drugs (NSAIDs) and low-dose corticosteroids can often provide satisfactory rapid relief of pain and stiffness. The disease-modifying antirheumatic drugs (DMARDs) usually provide more sustained relief of symptoms. However, in choosing which therapeutic agent to prescribe first to patients with early RA, an understanding of its capacity to slow the rate of progressive structural damage is also important. Unfortunately, the classification of DMARDs that effectively decrease the rate of progressive structural damage remains controversial, as many of the earlier randomized clinical trials of drugs such as gold salts, D-penicillamine and azathioprine were either not designed to evaluate this aspect adequately or used radiologic outcome measures that were not validated. Therefore, the attempted classification of drugs into categories such as symptom-modifying antirheumatic drugs (SMARDs), DMARDs and disease-controlling antirheumatic treatments (D-CARTs) was based on limited evidence to support the inclusion of some conventional non-targeted drugs.

When evaluating the efficacy of novel treatments, it is appropriate to evaluate morphologic changes in synovial tissue samples obtained from the primary site of inflammation rather than changes in cell populations from other compartments, such as peripheral blood and synovial fluid. This point was highlighted in a study of Campath-1H treatment in which synovial tissue demonstrated persistent T-lymphocyte infiltration at a time when circulating lymphocytes were markedly depleted[36]. Therefore, this discussion will include some reference to studies that have evaluated treatment-related changes in synovial morphology.

Methotrexate

While there may be some differences between countries in the initial choice of DMARD for treating persistently active RA, low-dose methotrexate is ordinarily the first choice of most rheumatologists. The initial dose is usually 7.5mg or 10mg administered orally either in a single dose or in divided doses on 1 day each week. The dose may be escalated in increments of 2.5 or 5mg/week each month until the usual maintenance dose of 15–25mg/week is reached. A weekly methotrexate dose of 25–30mg is considered the maximum by most rheumatologists. The therapeutic effect may be delayed for up to 4 months.

The clinical benefits of methotrexate extend to significant retardation of structural damage[37]. Patients should be advised to limit their alcohol intake strictly while receiving methotrexate, and supplemental folic acid is recommended for as long as treatment is continued. Laboratory monitoring of white cell and platelet counts, and liver function tests is mandatory. Monitoring practices tend to vary considerably, but a reasonable approach is to check the laboratory parameters at monthly intervals for the first 6 months and at 1–2-monthly intervals thereafter, depending on the dose and assuming an absence of early toxicity. Methotrexate dosage should be reduced or discontinued if the white cell or the platelet counts fall significantly, or if there is significant or persistent transaminases elevations. Criteria for monitoring of liver enzymes and indications for surveillance liver biopsies have been published by the ACR[37,38]. Liver biopsies are not thought to be necessary by most clinicians unless there is repetitive elevation of liver transaminases or low serum albumin over time.

Severe nausea, usually maximal on the day after taking weekly methotrexate, is experienced by a minority of patients. Prescribing prophylactic antinausea medication, administering folic or folinic acid or converting from oral to subcutaneous or intramuscular administration facilitates the continuation of treatment for many patients.

Some consideration needs to be given to prescribing methotrexate to younger patients in the context of possible pregnancy. Methotrexate in doses of up to 30mg/week does not appear to affect female fertility adversely, but may cause reversible male sterility[39]. It is embryotoxic, so that women of childbearing age should use adequate contraception if methotrexate is recommended. Women who wish to conceive should discontinue methotrexate before attempting conception. Certainly, women should discontinue methotrexate for at least one menstrual cycle but some recommend discontinuation for at least 3–6 months. Women who discontinue methotrexate in order to conceive should be advised to continue folic acid supplementation because of the association between folate deficiency, which is induced by methotrexate, and neural tube defects in the fetus. Similarly, it is recommended by some rheumatologists that males should discontinue methotrexate at least 3 months before conception is attempted. Methotrexate is contraindicated during pregnancy and lactation.

After treatment with methotrexate, a decrease in synovial tissue inflammation was observed histologically[40]. Moreover, a selective decrease in collagenase but not stromelysin or *TIMP1* gene expression was demonstrated. It was concluded that these effects were indirect and due to alterations in the synovial tissue cytokine milieu. This was confirmed in a study that demonstrated a decrease in cell infiltration and expression of IL-1β and TNF-α in biopsy specimens from patients who responded to methotrexate treatment[41].

Other conventional disease-modifying antirheumatic drugs

Having once been the mainstay of DMARD therapy in RA, gold salts, D-penicillamine and azathioprine are now rarely considered drugs of first choice. Sulfasalazine, especially in some European countries, may be the DMARD of first choice for some rheumatologists in early RA. There is some evidence that it can reduce the rate of structural damage[42]. Sulfasalazine is best commenced in a dose of 0.5g/day, and increased in increments of 0.5g/day every 4–7 days to a maintenance dose of 2g/day, or sometimes 3g/day. The clinical effect is usually apparent in about 8 weeks. Laboratory monitoring is mandatory, especially during the first 3 months of therapy, when monthly blood counts and liver function tests should be examined. Some recommend that laboratory monitoring should occur monthly for 6 months and 3-monthly thereafter for as long as treatment is continued. Sulfasalazine is likely to be favored in milder cases, or in younger patients, when issues of fertility, pregnancy or lactation have to be considered.

Sulfasalazine does not adversely affect female fertility[39]. In males, it induces reversible infertility due to oligospermia, impaired sperm motility and increased spermatozoal abnormalities. Sulfasalazine and its metabolite, sulfapyridine, readily cross the placenta to the fetal circulation. Fetal blood concentrations are approximately similar to maternal concentrations. However, during pregnancy, sulfasalazine does not appear to adversely affect either fetal or maternal well-being so that treatment may be continued. The drug should be administered with caution to breastfeeding mothers as adverse events have been reported in some infants.

Hydroxychloroquine, like sulfasalazine, is sometimes the DMARD of first choice in selected patients with relatively mild disease. The initial dose is often 400mg/day, with a reduction to a maintenance dose of 200mg/day often possible after 3–6 months if a good clinical effect is seen. There is no convincing evidence that hydroxychloroquine slows the rate of structural damage in RA. Laboratory monitoring during treatment is not required. Unlike some other antimalarial compounds, irreversible retinopathy is extremely rare, particularly when the daily dosage does not exceed 6.5mg/kg. Hydroxychloroquine may be safe to use during pregnancy.

The effects of conventional DMARDs on synovitis have been described by several groups. Gold salts and D-penicillamine resulted in reduced T-cell and B-cell infiltration and human leukocyte antigen (HLA)-DP and DQ expression, particularly in those patients demonstrating a clinical response to treatment[43,44]. In addition, a significant decrease in the number of intimal layer monocytes and subintimal CD68[+] macrophages after treatment with gold salts was observed[45]. These histologic changes were associated with a significant decrease in the expression of proinflammatory cytokines, including IL-1α, IL-1β, IL-6 and TNF-α.

Cyclosporin

Cyclosporin treatment is usually recommended for patients who require second-line drugs and have failed other therapies. There is some evidence that cyclosporin slows the rate of joint damage[46] but not all studies agreed with this observation[47]. It must be prescribed with caution to patients over the age of 65 years or those who have a history of hypertension or renal disease or have premalignant conditions or infection. Cyclosporin should not be prescribed for pregnant women, nursing mothers or women who might become pregnant.

Before commencing cyclosporin, patients should have a screening blood count and liver profile, at least two separate blood pressure readings, and two baseline serum creatinine measurements. If the serum creatinine levels are elevated, a creatinine clearance test should be performed. The recommended initial dose of cyclosporin is 2.5–3.5mg/kg/day in a twice-daily regimen. After 4–8 weeks the dose may be increased in increments of 0.5–1.0mg/kg/day at 1–2-monthly intervals to a maximum of 5mg/kg/day. A clinical response is usually apparent at approximately 3 months. If a response has not occurred within 6 months the drug should be discontinued as ineffective. If possible, NSAIDs should be discontinued during cyclosporin treatment.

Monitoring during cyclosporin therapy is mandatory. The serum creatinine and blood pressure should be measured every 2 weeks for at least 3 months, and then every month if the recordings remain stable. If the creatinine increases to 30% above the baseline level, the dose should be decreased by 0.5–1.0mg/kg/day. If hypertension develops, the dose should be decreased or the hypertension treated, preferably with a calcium channel blocker.

Low-dose corticosteroids

The effects of low-dose corticosteroid therapy (prednisolone 7.5mg/day or less; see Chapter 11) on the symptoms and signs of RA can be immediate and dramatic. In current clinical practice, low-dose corticosteroids are frequently prescribed in early RA to provide adequate relief of symptoms while awaiting full expression of the beneficial effects of methotrexate or other DMARDs. The prednisolone dosage may then be reduced, or even discontinued, depending on the clinical course. In addition to the effects on the symptoms and signs of RA, low-dose prednisolone may have important beneficial effects in the prevention of joint damage[48]. High-dose prednisolone is commonly prescribed for vasculitis, mononeuritis multiplex, and acute pericarditis and pleurisy.

The following is a reasonable approach to prescribing low-dose prednisolone for some patients with RA[49]. In patients with active disease for

TABLE 24.1 SUGGESTED PATIENTS SUITABLE FOR TREATMENT WITH LOW-DOSE PREDNISOLONE

	Time since diagnosis (years)		
	0–2	3–5	>5
Erosions present	Treat	Probably treat	Probably do not treat
Erosions absent	Treat	Do not treat	Do not treat

(With permission from Lim and Kirwan[49].)

less than 2 years, low-dose prednisolone may reduce the rate of articular damage, whether or not erosions are already established (Table 24.1). In patients with active RA for 3–5 years, it may be prudent to add low-dose prednisolone to reduce the risk of developing further erosions, but prednisolone should not be added if erosions are not present, as the likelihood of new erosions developing in these patients is extremely small. There are few indications for prescribing low-dose prednisolone to patients with RA for more than 5 years. Low-dose prednisolone may be prescribed to pregnant women who have had to discontinue an effective DMARD, those with persistent active disease, or those who suffer a disease flare during or immediately after pregnancy.

Patients with worse RA are likely to receive higher cumulative doses of corticosteroids. The combination of more severe disease and greater corticosteroid exposure increases the risk of progressive loss of bone density. Therefore, monitoring of bone density and effective prevention of osteoporosis is essential.

The clinical response to intra-articular corticosteroid therapy was associated with histologic improvement and decreased gene expression of collagenase and TIMP-1[50]. The effects of pulse methylprednisolone included a rapid decrease in tissue levels of IL-8 and TNF-α but no effect on IL-1β or IL-1 receptor antagonist (IL-1Ra)[51]. Alterations in TNF-α expression correlated with the clinical response and with subsequent relapse.

Leflunomide

Leflunomide is a new DMARD with clinical efficacy that is broadly similar to sulfasalazine and methotrexate[52–55]. Leflunomide is indicated for the treatment of adults with active RA to improve the signs and symptoms and to retard structural damage[56]. A dose of 10–20mg/day is generally used. Leflunomide may be taken in combination with NSAIDs or corticosteroids. Special precautions are required in patients with renal impairment and the drug is not recommended in patients with significantly impaired renal function.

Leflunomide is contraindicated during pregnancy and lactation[39]. Women of childbearing age must use adequate contraception. A negative pregnancy test before commencing therapy is advisable. Women who receive leflunomide and wish to become pregnant must be informed that a 2-year interval between discontinuing treatment and attempting conception is recommended. Alternatively, if this is impractical, patients may undergo a washout procedure, which involves the administration of either cholestyramine 8g three times daily for 11 days or 50g of activated charcoal administered four times daily for 11 days. In addition, following either washout procedure, verification by two separate tests at an interval of at least 14 days and a waiting period of 6 weeks between the first occurrence of a plasma concentration less than 0.02mg/l and conception is required. Women receiving leflunomide who suspect they may be pregnant should inform their physician immediately. Men receiving leflunomide should also use adequate contraception.

Leflunomide treatment resulted in reduced numbers of synovial tissue macrophages and reduced intercellular adhesion molecule (ICAM)-1 and vascular cell adhesion molecule (VCAM)-1 expression[57]. In addition, a decreased MMP-1:TIMP-1 ratio in the synovial membrane was reported. In the patients who demonstrated the most clinical benefit, the reduced expression of ICAM-1, VCAM-1, IL-1β and MMP-1 was greatest.

Combination therapy

Methotrexate is considered by most rheumatologists to be the drug of choice in RA because of its safety profile and its potential to reduce symptoms and signs and prevent progressive structural damage[58]. However, a significant number of patients treated with methotrexate in monotherapeutic regimes fail to achieve optimal disease control. This failure has resulted in the development of several DMARD combination regimes, both in Europe and the USA, which usually include methotrexate. As previously highlighted, combining two or more DMARDs with different modes of action has the potential to produce a range of outcomes in relation to both efficacy and toxicity[59]. The ideal outcome of combination DMARD therapeutic strategies is one that is synergistic for efficacy and lacking any additive effects on toxicity.

Much consideration has been given to the indications for use of combination DMARD regimes in RA. Some studies have evaluated the role of combination therapy as the initial approach to treatment in early RA. Others have examined the effects of introducing combination regimes to patients who have failed to respond adequately to maximal doses of methotrexate. One protocol that successfully demonstrated significant long-term symptomatic and radiographic benefits from the early introduction of combination therapy included high-dose prednisolone, which was rapidly reduced and discontinued after 28 weeks, low-dose methotrexate and sulfasalazine in patients with RA for less than 2 years[60]. Studies that compared the combination of methotrexate and sulfasalazine to monotherapy regimes of the same compounds failed to demonstrate significant differences[61,62]. A study that evaluated the early introduction of triple combination DMARD therapy in RA compared methotrexate, sulfasalazine, hydroxychloroquine and low-dose prednisolone to sulfasalazine with or without prednisolone. The triple combination regime was associated with a superior rate of remission after 2 years[63].

Patients who fail to achieve an adequate response to methotrexate treatment, usually given orally in escalating doses that reach a maximum of 15–30mg/week, or who relapse after an initial satisfactory response, may benefit from weekly subcutaneous administration of methotrexate, because gastrointestinal absorption can be highly variable. Unfortunately, a considerable number of patients who receive adequate doses of methotrexate fail to demonstrate acceptable relief of symptoms or retardation of structural damage. Several studies have evaluated the effects of combining other DMARDs to maintenance methotrexate treatment in patients exhibiting a partial response to methotrexate alone. The first of these studies used a cyclosporin/methotrexate combination protocol[64]. The combination of cyclosporin and methotrexate was significantly superior to maintenance methotrexate monotherapy after 6 months, but cyclosporin dosage adjustments due to elevations in serum creatinine levels were necessary in some. Moreover, continued use of cyclosporin was associated with a high rate of withdrawal, most commonly due to elevated creatinine levels, hypertension and lack of sustained efficacy. Methotrexate has also been studied in combination regimes with sulfasalazine and hydroxychloroquine in patients with established RA. In one study, three therapeutic strategies were compared: the triple combination, sulfasalazine and hydroxychloroquine, and methotrexate monotherapy[65]. The triple combination demonstrated significantly greater efficacy, as well as fewer withdrawals.

The combination of methotrexate and leflunomide has also been studied in patients demonstrating an inadequate clinical response to methotrexate monotherapy (mean dose 17mg/week)[66]. A total of 77% of the patients completed 1 year of combination therapy and 53% met the ACR 20% response criteria. In general, treatment was well tolerated, with the exception of raised liver enzyme levels, but 10% of the patients withdrew because of persistently elevated serum transaminases.

Finally, the use of methotrexate in combination with targeted cytokine inhibition has been associated with impressive clinical and radiographic benefits, which are discussed below. An exciting possibility for future therapeutic advancement is the combination of targeted treatments that modulate the biologic effects of more than one cytokine, or other critical mediators, in the complex pathophysiologic pathways associated with RA.

Biologic agents

Tumor necrosis factor-α inhibition

Therapies targeting TNF-α that are currently approved for clinical use include infliximab, a chimeric monoclonal anti-TNF-α antibody[35,67], and etanercept, a recombinant human TNF receptor (p75)-Fc fusion protein[68,69]. Infliximab is approved, in combination with methotrexate, for the reduction of signs and symptoms in patients with moderately or severely active RA who have had an inadequate response to methotrexate monotherapy. Infliximab is also approved for the inhibition of progressive structural damage. The recommended maintenance dose is 3mg/kg given by intravenous infusion every 8 weeks, after three initial infusions in the same dosage administered at successive intervals of 2 and 4 weeks. The recommended dosage has proved to be inadequate for some patients, and higher doses of 5 or 6mg/kg, or more frequent administration at 6-weekly intervals, is sometimes employed in order to achieve an optimal response. Infusion reactions, consisting of nausea and headache, occur in approximately 15–20% of patients. The infusion reactions are transient and controlled by slowing the rate of infusion or treatment with acetaminophen (paracetamol) or antihistamines. Following a report of tuberculosis in 70 patients who received infliximab therapy for a median of 12 weeks, it is important to screen for latent tuberculosis or disease before commencing treatment[70]. Antinuclear antibodies and antibodies to double-stranded DNA are associated with infliximab treatment[35].

The effects of infliximab treatment on synovial tissue demonstrated a significant reduction in the intensity of T-cell infiltration and in the expression of VCAM-1 and E-selectin[71]. It was suggested that the decrease in cellular infiltration and the associated clinical response resulted from reduced migration of inflammatory cells into the joint secondary to inhibition of TNF-α-induced VCAM expression. In a further study, treatment with anti-TNF-α monoclonal antibody resulted in rapidly reduced synovial tissue synthesis of TNF-α[72].

Etanercept is approved for the reduction of signs and symptoms and the inhibition of progressive structural damage in patients with moderately or severely active RA[68,69]. Etanercept may be used alone or in combination with methotrexate in patients who do not respond adequately to methotrexate alone. Etanercept is also approved for the reduction of signs and symptoms of moderately or severely active polyarticular juvenile idiopathic arthritis in patients who have had an inadequate response to one or more DMARD. The recommended dose of etanercept for adults is 25mg administered by subcutaneous injection twice weekly. Injection-site reactions occur in about 40% of patients treated with etanercept. Reactions are confined to the skin and consist of raised urticarial lesions that are limited to the site of the injection. They rarely require discontinuation of treatment. The reactions usually begin to occur soon after the initiation of treatment. They are generally mild and self-limiting, and decrease and resolve with repeated dosing. Specific

treatment of the reactions is rarely required, but antihistamines or corticosteroids may be given topically if necessary.

Caution is advised in the use of infliximab and etanercept in patients with chronic infection or a history of recurrent infection. Neither should be administered to patients with a clinically important, active infection. Patients who develop a new infection while receiving TNF-α inhibitors should be monitored closely. Treatment should be discontinued if a serious infection or sepsis occurs. TNF-targeted treatments should not be administered to patients with multiple sclerosis.

Interleukin-1 inhibition

Anakinra is a recombinant human IL-1 receptor antagonist. It is a specific competitive inhibitor of IL-1β and prevents activation of target cells by binding to IL-1 receptors[73]. It is approved, either by itself or in combination with other DMARDs including methotrexate, for the reduction of signs and symptoms in patients with moderately or severely active RA[74,75]. In addition to proven efficacy in reducing signs and symptoms, there is convincing evidence from a randomized, placebo-controlled trial that anakinra reduces the rate of progressive joint damage[74,76]. The recommended dose for clinical use is 100mg/day, given by subcutaneous injection. Injection-site reactions are similar to the reactions that occur with etanercept and rarely require treatment. In the reported clinical trials, anakinra was not associated with an increased risk of serious infection[75,76], but continued caution is required when prescribing to patients with a history of recurring infection.

Synovial tissue samples have been evaluated before and after anakinra treatment[77]. There was a reduction in intimal layer macrophages and subintimal macrophages and lymphocytes following treatment. In contrast, increased cellular infiltration was observed in patients who received placebo. Downregulation of E-selectin, VCAM-1 and ICAM-1 expression was also associated with anakinra treatment. It was concluded that these observations represented inhibition of several biologically relevant IL-1β-mediated pathogenetic effects.

How does the efficacy of anakinra, which inhibits IL-1-mediated pathways, compare with the available TNF-α-targeted therapies? It is difficult to reliably compare published clinical trials that employed different study designs, patient selection criteria and outcome measures[78]. Three clinical trials that evaluated different cytokine-targeted therapies in combination with effective therapeutic doses of methotrexate have now been published[35,68,75]. Both the anakinra and etanercept studies were conducted over 24 weeks. The infliximab study continued for 54 weeks, although the clinical responses observed at the end of the study appeared to be similar to those at 24 weeks. The numbers of patients recruited into the anakinra and infliximab studies were similar, and were considerably greater than the number in the etanercept study. There were some demographic and clinical differences between the three study populations. The mean methotrexate doses were similar. The numbers of patients in the placebo groups that achieved an ACR 20 response ranged between 17% in the infliximab study and 27% in the etanercept study. The numbers of patients that achieved ACR 20 responses on completion ranged between 42% in both the anakinra (1mg/kg/day) and infliximab (3mg/kg/8-weekly) studies and 71% in the etanercept study, increases approximately 2–2.5-fold more than the respective placebo groups. ACR 50 responses were achieved by 24% of patients in the anakinra study, 21% in the infliximab study, and 39% in the etanercept study. ACR 70 responses were observed in 10–15% in the three studies. The magnitude of the ACR responses to each of the three different cytokine-targeted therapies, when administered in combination with effective therapeutic doses of methotrexate, were similar to the responses reported in other studies, which evaluated etanercept and anakinra in monotherapeutic regimes[69,74] and infliximab in combination with low-dose methotrexate[67].

Among the challenges that face rheumatologists in the new era of targeted therapies is how to choose the optimal regime for each patient. At present, there are no reliable predictors of response to one or other cytokine-targeted approach. There are no data to suggest that patients who are unresponsive to TNF-α-targeted therapy might respond to IL-1 inhibition, or that patients who respond inadequately to anakinra might be candidates for TNF-α-blockade. This issue represents a potentially very rewarding area for future clinical research.

CURRENT RECOMMENDATIONS

Current recommendations for the treatment of RA may be considered in the context of both initial treatment of early disease and treatment of established disease when methotrexate fails to provide an adequate response[59]. In most circumstances, the optimal treatment of early disease is methotrexate, commencing with a dose of 7.5–10mg/week and escalating in doses of 2.5–5mg/week at monthly intervals until a maintenance dose of 15–20mg/week is achieved (Table 24.2). Prednisolone 5–10mg/day is sometimes added in order to achieve rapid symptom relief while awaiting final expression of the methotrexate effect. Prednisolone should be reduced to a minimal maintenance dose, or discontinued if possible, after 4–6 months. An incomplete therapeutic effect should be followed by aggressive step-up to a combination DMARD regime, which could

include hydroxychloroquine, sulfasalazine or leflunomide. In the more severe disease categories, or when combination DMARD treatment is unsatisfactory, the introduction of targeted treatments that inhibit TNF-α or IL-1 should be considered in appropriate patients. Similarly, in patients with established RA who fail to respond to oral and/or subcutaneous methotrexate, an aggressive step-up to combination DMARD therapy, or a switch to targeted therapy in combination with methotrexate is advised.

TABLE 24.2 CURRENT RECOMMENDATIONS FOR THE TREATMENT OF RA SYNOVITIS

Early disease	Suboptimal methotrexate responses
Rapid escalation of methotrexate dose + low-dose corticosteroid	Aggressive step-up combination
Aggressive step-up combination (add hydroxychloroquine and/or sulfasalazine)	Switch to targeted cytokine inhibition + methotrexate
Switch to targeted cytokine inhibition + methotrexate	

(With permission from O'Dell[59].)

REFERENCES

1. Harris ED. Clinical features of rheumatoid arthritis. In: Kelley WN, Harris ED, Ruddy S, Sledge CB, eds. Textbook of rheumatology. Philadelphia, PA: WB Saunders; 1997: 898–931.
2. Hough AJ, Sokoloff L. Pathology. In: Utsinger PD, Zvaifler NJ, Ehrlich GE, eds. Rheumatoid arthritis: etiology, diagnosis, management. Philadelphia, PA: JB Lippincott; 1985: 49–69.
3. Peterfy CG. Magnetic resonance imaging in rheumatoid arthritis: current status and future directions. J Rheumatol 2001; 28: 1134–1142.
4. Backhaus M, Burmester G-R, Gerber T et al. Guidelines for musculoskeletal ultrasound in rheumatology. Ann Rheum Dis 2001; 60: 641–649.
5. Veale DJ, Reece RJ, Parsons W et al. Intra-articular primatised anti-CD4: efficacy in resistant rheumatoid knees. A study of combined arthroscopy, magnetic resonance imaging, and histology. Ann Rheum Dis 1999; 58: 342–349.
6. Tak PP, Bresnihan B. The pathogenesis and prevention of joint damage in rheumatoid arthritis. Advances from synovial biopsy and tissue analysis. Arthritis Rheum 2000; 43: 2619–2633.
7. Youssef PP, Cormack J, Evill CA et al. Neutrophil trafficking into inflamed joints in patients with rheumatoid arthritis and the effect of methylprednisolone. Arthritis Rheum 1996; 39: 216–225.
8. Schumacher HR, Kitridou RC. Synovitis of recent onset. A clinicopathologic study during the first month of disease. Arthritis Rheum 1972; 15: 465–485.
9. Soden M, Rooney M, Cullen A et al. Immunohistological features in the synovium obtained from clinically uninvolved knee joints of patients with rheumatoid arthritis. Br J Rheumatol 1989; 28: 287–292.
10. Pando JA, Duray P, Yarboro C et al. Synovitis occurs in some clinically normal and asymptomatic joints in patients with early arthritis. J Rheumatol 2000; 27: 1848–1854.
11. Kraan MC, Versendaal H, Jonker M et al. Asymptomatic synovitis precedes clinically manifest arthritis. Arthritis Rheum 1998; 41: 1481–1488.
12. Cunnane G, FitzGerald O, Hummel KM et al. Collagenase, cathepsin B and cathepsin L gene expression in the synovial membrane of patients with early inflammatory arthritis. Rheumatol 1999; 38: 34–42.
13. Klimiuk PA, Goronzy JJ, Bjornsson J et al. Tissue cytokine patterns distinguish variants of rheumatoid synovitis. Am J Pathol 1997; 151: 1311–1319.
14. Tak PP, Smeets TJM, Daha MR et al. Analysis of the synovial cellular infiltrate in early rheumatoid synovial tissue in relation to local disease activity. Arthritis Rheum 1997; 40: 217–225.
15. Firestein GS, Zvaifler NJ. How important are T cells in chronic rheumatoid synovitis? Arthritis Rheum 1990; 33: 768–773.
16. Vey E, Zhang JH, Dayer J-M. IFN-gamma and 1,25(OH)$_2$D$_3$ induce on THP-1 cells distinct patterns of cell surface antigen expression, cytokine production, and responsiveness to contact with activated T cells. J Immunol 1992; 149: 2040–2046.
17. Lacraz S, Isler P, Vey E et al. Direct contact between T lymphocytes and monocytes is a major pathway for induction of metalloproteinase expression. J Biol Chem 1994; 269: 22027–22033.
18. Hyka N, Dayer J-M, Modoux C et al. Apolipoprotein A-1 inhibits the production of interleukin-1β and tumor necrosis factor by blocking contact-mediated activation of monocytes by T lymphocytes. Blood 2001; 97: 2381–2389.
19. Maurice MM, Nakamura H, Van der Voort EAM et al. Evidence for the role of an altered redox state in hyporesponsiveness of synovial T cells in rheumatoid arthritis. J Immunol 1997; 158: 1458–1465.
20. Pettit AR, MacDonald KPA, O'Sullivan B, Thomas R. Differentiated dendritic cells expressing nuclear Re1B are predominantly located in rheumatoid synovial tissue perivascular mononuclear cell aggregates. Arthritis Rheum 2000; 43: 791–800.
21. Otten HG, Dolhain RJ, de Rooij HH, Breedveld FC. Rheumatoid factor production by mononuclear cells derived from different sites of patients with rheumatoid arthritis. Clin Exp Immunol 1993; 94: 236–240.
22. Krenn V, Schalhorn N, Greiner A et al. Immunohistochemical analysis of proliferating and antigen-presenting cells in rheumatoid synovial tissue. Rheumatol Int 1996; 15: 239–247.
23. Schroder AE, Greiner A, Seyfert C, Berek C. Differentiation of B cells in the nonlymphoid tissue of the synovial membrane of patients with rheumatoid arthritis. Proc Natl Acad Sci USA 1996; 93: 221–225.
24. Ulfgren A-K, Lindblad S, Klareskog L et al. Detection of cytokine producing cells in the synovial membrane from patients with rheumatoid arthritis. Ann Rheum Dis 1995; 54: 654–661.
25. Deleuran BW, Chu CQ, Field M et al. Localization of tumor necrosis receptors in the synovial tissue and cartilage–pannus junction in patients with rheumatoid arthritis. Arthritis Rheum 1992; 35: 1170–1178.
26. Firestein GS, Berger AE, Tracey DE et al. IL-1 receptor antagonist protein production and gene expression in rheumatoid arthritis and osteoarthritis synovium. J Immunol 1992; 149: 1054–1062.
27. Firestein GS, Boyle DL, Yu C et al. Synovial interleukin-1 receptor antagonist and interleukin-1 balance in rheumatoid arthritis. Arthritis Rheum 1994; 37: 644–652.
28. Kirkham B, Portek I, Lee CS et al. Intraarticular variability of synovial membrane histology, immunohistology, and cytokine mRNA expression in patients with rheumatoid arthritis. J Rheumatol 1999; 26: 777–784.
29. Ahrens D, Koch AE, Pope RM et al. Expression of matrix metalloproteinase 9 (96kd gelatinase B) in human rheumatoid arthritis. Arthritis Rheum 1996; 39: 1576–1587.
30. Wernicke D, Seyfert C, Hinzmann B, Gromnica-Ihle E. Cloning of collagenase 3 from synovial membrane and its expression in rheumatoid arthritis and osteoarthritis. J Rheumatol 1996; 23: 590–595.
31. Keyszer GM, Heer AH, Kriegsmann J et al. Comparative analysis of cathepsin L, cathepsin D, and collagenase gene expression in synovial tissues of patients with rheumatoid arthritis and osteoarthritis by in situ hybridization. Arthritis Rheum 1995; 38: 976–984.
32. Keyszer G, Redlich A, Haupl T et al. Differential expression of cathepsins B and L compared with matrix metalloproteinases and their respective inhibitors in rheumatoid arthritis and osteoarthritis: a parallel investigation by semiquantitative reverse transcriptase-polymerase chain reaction and immunohistochemistry. Arthritis Rheum 1998; 41: 1378–1387.
33. Kim JM, Weisman MH. When does rheumatoid arthritis begin and why do we need to know? Arthritis Rheum 2000; 43: 473–484.
34. Mulherin D, FitzGerald O, Bresnihan B. Clinical improvement and radiological deterioration in rheumatoid arthritis: evidence that the pathogenesis of synovial inflammation and articular erosion may differ. Br J Rheumatol 1996; 35: 1263–1268.
35. Lipsky P, van der Heijde DMFM, St. Clair EW et al. Infliximab and methotrexate in the treatment of rheumatoid arthritis. N Engl J Med 2000; 343: 1594–1602.
36. Ruderman EM, Weinblatt ME, Thurmond LM et al. Synovial tissue response to treatment with Compath-1H. Arthritis Rheum 1995; 35: 254–258.

37. Kremer JM, Alarcon GS, Lightfoot RW et al. Methotrexate for rheumatoid arthritis: suggested guidelines for monitoring liver toxicity. Arthritis Rheum 1994; 37: 316–328.

38. American College of Rheumatology Subcommittee on Rheumatoid Arthritis Guidelines. Guidelines for the management of rheumatoid arthritis 2002 Update. Arthritis Rheum 2002; 46: 328–346.

39. Bresnihan B. Treatment of early rheumatoid arthritis in the younger patient. J Rheumatol 2001; 28(suppl 62): 4–9.

40. Firestein G S, Paine MM, Boyle DL. Mechanism of methotrexate action in rheumatoid arthritis. Selective decrease in synovial collagenase gene expression. Arthritis Rheum 1994; 37: 193–200.

41. Dolhain RJEM, Tak PP, Dijkmans BAC et al. Methotrexate treatment reduced inflammatory cell numbers, expression of monokines and of adhesion molecules in synovial tissue of patients with rheumatoid arthritis. Br J Rheumatol 1998; 37: 502–508.

42. Van der Heijde DM, van Riel PL, Nurrer-Zwart IH et al. Effects of hydroxychloroquine and sulfasalazine on progression of joint damage in rheumatoid arthritis. Lancet 1989; 1: 1036–1038.

43. Rooney M, Whelan A, Feighery C, Bresnihan B. Changes in lymphocyte infiltration of the synovial membrane and the clinical course of rheumatoid arthritis. Arthritis Rheum 1989; 32: 361–369.

44. Walters MT, Smith JL, Moore K et al. An investigation of the action of disease modifying anti-rheumatid drugs on the rheumatic synovial membrane: reduction in T lymphocyte subpopulations and HLA-DP and DQ antigen expression after gold or penicillamine therapy. Ann Rheum Dis 1987; 30: 1–10.

45. Yanni G, Nabil M, Farahat MR et al. Intramuscular gold decreases cytokine expression and macrophage numbers in the rheumatoid synovial membrane. Ann Rheum Dis 1994; 53: 315–322.

46. Forre O and the Norwegian Arthritis Study Group. Radiologic evidence of disease modification in rheumatoid arthritis patients treated with cyclosporine: results of a 48-week multicenter study comparing low-dose cyclosporine with placebo. Arthritis Rheum 1994; 37: 1506–1512.

47. Landewe RBM, Goie The HS, van Rijthoven AAM et al. A randomized, double-blind, 24-week controlled study of low-dose cyclosporine versus chloroquine in early rheumatoid arthritis. Arthritis Rheum 1994; 37: 637–643.

48. Kirwan J and the Arthritis and Rheumatism Council Low-Dose Glucocorticoid Study Group. The effect of glucocorticoid on joint destruction in rheumatoid arthritis. N Engl J Med 1995; 333: 142–146.

49. Lim K, Kirwan JR. Do corticosteroids have a disease-modifying role in rheumatoid arthritis? In: van de Putte LBA, Furst DE, Williams HJ, van Riel PLCM, eds. Therapy of systemic rheumatic disorders. New York: Marcel Dekker; 1998: 277–288.

50. Firestein GS, Paine MM, Littman BH. Gene expression (collagenase, tissue inhibitor of metalloproteinases, complement, and HLA-DR) in rheumatoid arthritis and osteoarthritis synovium. Quantitative analysis and effect of intraarticular corticosteroids. Arthritis Rheum 1991; 34: 1094–1105.

51. Youssef PP, Haynes DR, Triantafillou S et al. Effects of pulse methylprednisolone on inflammatory mediators in peripheral blood, synovial fluid, and synovial membrane in rheumatoid arthritis. Arthritis Rheum 1997; 40: 1400–1408.

52. Mladenovic V, Domljan Z, Rozman B et al. Safety and effectiveness of leflunomide in the treatment of patients with active rheumatoid arthritis: results of a randomized, placebo-controlled, phase II study. Arthritis Rheum 1995; 38: 1595–1603.

53. Strand V, Cohen S, Schiff M et al. Treatment of active rheumatoid arthritis with leflunomide compared to placebo and methotrexate. Arch Intern Med 1999; 159: 2542–2550.

54. Smolen JS, Kalden JR, Scott DL et al. Efficacy and safety of leflunomide compared with placebo and sulfasalazine in active rheumatoid arthritis: a double-blind, randomised, multicentre trial. Lancet 1999; 353: 259–266.

55. Emery P, Breedveld FC, Lemmel EM et al. A comparison of the efficacy and safety of leflunomide and methotrexate for the treatment of rheumatoid arthritis. Rheumatology 2000; 39: 655–665.

56. Sharp JT, Strand V, Leung H et al. Treatment with leflunomide slows radiographic progression of rheumatoid arthritis: results from three randomized controlled trials of leflunomide in patients with active rheumatoid arthritis. Arthritis Rheum 2000; 43: 495–505.

57. Kraan MC, Reece RJ, Barg EC et al. Modulation of inflammation and metalloproteinase expression in synovial tissue by leflunomide and methotrexate in patients with active rheumatoid arthritis. Findings in a prospective, randomized, double-blind, parallel-design clinical trial in thirty-nine patients at two centres. Arthritis Rheum 2000; 43: 1820–1830.

58. Weinblatt ME, Polisson R, Blotner SD. The effects of drug therapy on radiographic progression of rheumatoid arthritis. Results of a 36-week randomized trial comparing methotrexate and auranofin. Arthritis Rheum 1993; 36: 613–616.

59. O'Dell JR. Combination disease-modifying anti-rheumatic drug (DMARD) therapy. In: Tsokos GC, ed. Modern therapeutics in rheumatic diseases. Totoya, NJ: Humana Press; 2001: 147–158.

60. Boers M, Verhoeven AC, Markusse HM et al. Randomized comparison of combined step-down prednisolone, methotrexate and sulphasalazine with sulphasalazine alone in early rheumatoid arthritis. Lancet 1997; 350: 309–318.

61. Haagsma CJ, van Riel PLCM, de Jong AJL, van de Putte LBA. Combination of sulphasalazine and methotrexate versus the single components in early rheumatoid arthritis: a randomized, controlled, double-blind, 52 week clinical trial. Br J Rheumatol 1997; 36: 1082–1088.

62. Dougados M, Combe B, Cantagrel A et al. Combination therapy in early rheumatoid arthritis: a randomised, controlled, double-blind 52-week clinical trial of sulphasalazine and methotrexate compared with the single components. Ann Rheum Dis 1999; 58: 220–225.

63. Mottonen T, Hannonsen P, Leirisalo-Repo M et al. Comparison of combination therapy with single-drug therapy in early rheumatoid arthritis: a randomised trial. Lancet 1999; 353: 1568–1573.

64. Tugwell P, Pincus T, Yocum D et al. Combination therapy with cyclosporine and methotrexate in severe rheumatoid arthritis. N Engl J Med 1995; 333: 137–141.

65. O'Dell JR, Haire CE, Erikson N et al. Treatment of rheumatoid arthritis with methotrexate alone, sulfasalazine, hydroxychloroquine, or a combination of all three medications. N Engl J Med 1996; 334: 1287–1291.

66. Weinblatt ME, Kremer JM, Coblyn JS et al. Pharmacokinetics, safety, and efficacy of combination treatment with methotrexate and leflunomide in patients with active rheumatoid arthritis. Arthritis Rheum 1999; 42: 1322–1329.

67. Maini RN, Breedveld FC, Kalden JR et al. Therapeutic efficacy of multiple intravenous infusions of anti-tumor necrosis factor a monoclonal antibody combined with low-dose weekly methotrexate in rheumatoid arthritis. Arthritis Rheum 1998; 41: 1552–1563.

68. Weinblatt ME, Kremer JM, Bankhurst AD et al. A trial of etanercept, a recombinant tumor necrosis factor receptor: Fc fusion protein, in patients with rheumatoid arthritis receiving methotrexate. N Engl J Med 1999; 340: 253–259.

69. Bathon JM, Martin RW, Fleischmann RM et al. A comparison of etanercept and methotrexate in patients with early rheumatoid arthritis. N Engl J Med 2000; 343: 1586–1593.

70. Keane J, Gershon S, Wise RP et al. Tuberculosis associated with infliximab, a tumor necrosis factor α-neutralizing agent. N Engl J Med 2001; 345: 1098–1104.

71. Tak PP, Taylor PC, Breedveld FC et al. Decrease in cellularity and expression of adhesion molecules by anti-tumor necrosis factor α monoclonal antibody treatment in patients with rheumatoid arthritis. Arthritis Rheum 1996; 39: 1077–1081.

72. Ulfgren A-K, Andersson U, Engstrom M et al. Systemic anti-tumor necrosis factor a therapy in rheumatoid arthritis down-regulates synovial tumor necrosis factor a synthesis. Arthritis Rheum 2000; 43: 2391–2396.

73. Dayer J-M, Feige U, Edwards CK III, Burger D. Anti-interleukin-1 therapy in rheumatic diseases. Curr Opin Rheumatol 2001; 13: 170–176.

74. Bresnihan B, Alvaro-Garcia JM, Cobby M et al. Treatment of rheumatoid arthritis with recombinant human interleukin-1 receptor antagonist. Arthritis Rheum 1999; 41: 2196–2204.

75. Cohen S, Hurd E, Cush J et al. Treatment of rheumatoid arthritis with anakinra, a recombinant human interleukin-1 receptor antagonist (IL-1ra), in combination with methotrexate. Arthritis Rheum 2002; 46: 614–624.

76. Jiang Y, Genant HK, Watt I et al. A multicenter, double-blind, dose-ranging, randomized and placebo controlled study of recombinant human interleukin-1 receptor antagonist in patients with rheumatoid arthritis: radiologic progression and correlation of Genant and Larsen scoring methods. Arthritis Rheum 2000; 43: 1001–1009.

77. Cunnane G, Madigan A, Murphy E et al. The effects of treatment with interleukin-1 receptor antagonist on the inflamed synovial membrane in rheumatoid arthritis. Rheumatology 2001; 40: 62–69.

78. Dayer J-M, Bresnihan B. Targeting interleukin-1 in the treatment of rheumatoid arthritis. Arthritis Rheum 2002; 46: 574–578.

PEDIATRIC RHEUMATOLOGY

25 Evaluation of musculoskeletal complaints in children

Helen Emery

Evaluating the child with musculoskeletal complaints requires a careful history and physical examination, after which the diagnosis is usually clear. Judicious use of investigations will contribute to confirming the cause of the symptoms. If the diagnosis is not obvious after this, a broader search to establish the cause of symptoms must be initiated.

IMPORTANT POINTS IN TAKING THE HISTORY

A co-operative child makes it much easier to obtain the history and perform the physical examination necessary in reaching a diagnosis. Children often feel threatened by a visit to the doctor, so a child-friendly environment in the waiting area and examination room with age-appropriate games or activities will help them feel more comfortable. Parents can rehearse the visit with the child, and a toy doctor kit will help the child become familiar with equipment and procedures, and facilitate co-operation. Even young children appreciate being talked with directly – after all, the problem is theirs, not their parents'. Start the visit with an explanation of what will happen to the child during the visit. You will be asking lots of questions, examining the child and then following up with a discussion of what may be going on, why it is happening and what you plan to do about it. It is important that everyone is honest with the child about what will happen – do not promise that there will be no blood tests if in fact they may be necessary, or that something won't hurt when it might. Even very young children should participate in providing the history, although their sense of time may not be accurate and they may have difficulty localizing pain. The parents should be able to provide the remainder of the history. However, if the child is sometimes in the care of a babysitter or relative, or is in school, it is important to seek input from whoever first sees the child in the morning, during sports and activities, and after school.

Pain

Details about the onset of the pain, pattern, site and radiation, duration, precipitating factors such as sports or other activities, relieving factors and severity must be obtained. Children may not complain directly about pain but may avoid activities that precipitate or exacerbate it. Using a smiling/frowning face visual aid may allow a child to express his discomfort, and pointing to the site of pain on themselves or on a body diagram may help localize it[1,2] (Fig. 25.1). Older children can use the more standard 1–10 visual analog scale, and any apparent discrepancy, for example the child smiling while saying the pain is a 10, should be noted. Remember that children may not localize pain well, and consider the possible alternate sites of origin of the pain. For example, hip joint pain may be felt in the groin but often the complaint is of anterior thigh or knee discomfort; likewise hip pain may originate from pathology in the spine or pelvis. Severe pain, crescendo pain, pain unrelieved by common analgesics such as acetaminophen (paracetamol) or ibuprofen, or requiring narcotics raises concern about an infectious or malignant process. A history of swelling, warmth and redness or discoloration of the joint or other structures should be noted.

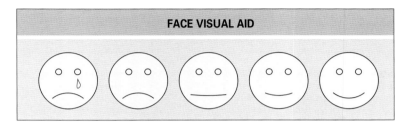

FACE VISUAL AID

Fig. 25.1 Face visual aid. A child can point to the face that best describes the severity of his pain.

Presence of morning stiffness most commonly points to an inflammatory process, and its duration and relief with heat and movement correlates well with the degree of activity of the inflammation, although it may be reported by an observer rather than the child. However, morning stiffness is also characteristic of fibromyalgia.

Crescendo pain, i.e. pain that becomes progressively worse, suggests an infectious or malignant process. Pain that wakes a child at night is also cause of concern about a malignant process, especially if it is associated with diminished activity during the day. However, 'growing pains' and benign tumors such as osteoid osteomas are also characterized by night pain.

Trauma

Trauma is often invoked as the cause of musculoskeletal complaints, although injuries are common in children and minor incidents such as falls from play equipment are often blamed when they are only coincidental. Children usually recover rapidly from injuries, and persistent swelling or pain should encourage pursuit of other causes. On the other hand, child abuse can present with musculoskeletal pain and injuries inconsistent with the history provided, or a child may have diffuse pain as a result of psychological, physical or sexual abuse[3].

Other important questions include the history of preceding illnesses, such as viral syndromes, sore throats or diarrheal illnesses. Immunization history should always be obtained, both in order to know if the child is protected against infections such as *Streptococcus pneumoniae*, *Haemophilus influenzae* and hepatitis, and to discover if there is any possibility of vaccine-induced arthritis, for example after administration of rubella vaccine.

Fever

Fever and its pattern can be very helpful in distinguishing the cause of musculoskeletal pain. The characteristic fever pattern of systemic onset juvenile arthritis is a single evening spike to at least 38.5° with return to normal or below between the spikes. Chills and malaise often precede the fever spikes, and the typical migratory erythematous rash may also appear during the fevers (Fig. 25.2). Profuse sweating often accompanies the break of the fever. Although there are variations on this theme – some children have a morning rather than evening spike or, rarely, two

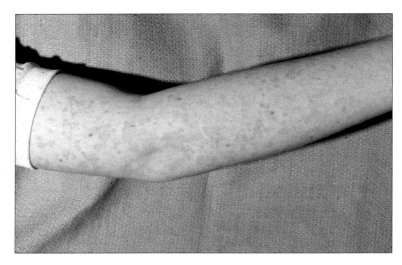

Fig. 25.2 The classic erythematous macular rash of systemic juvenile arthritis. This rash is usually non-pruritic and rapidly migratory, most prominent when the child is febrile.

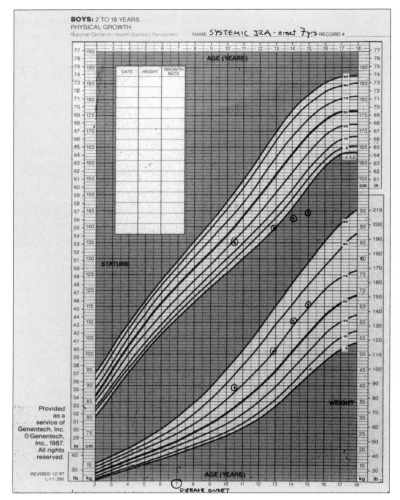

Fig. 25.3 Growth curve showing the failure of linear growth in a boy with systemic onset juvenile arthritis. Similar changes may be seen in other inflammatory diseases, even in the absence of treatment with corticosteroids.

spikes a day – a predictable fever pattern with return to baseline is part of the criteria for systemic onset juvenile arthritis. This fever pattern may be altered by the use of antipyretics, and observing the child for 24–48 hours without medication may be necessary to establish the true pattern. Persistent fevers are more likely to be associated with infection, inflammatory conditions such as inflammatory bowel disease, malignancies, or a rheumatic disease such as systemic lupus erythematosus (SLE) or vasculitis.

Fevers lasting a few days associated with musculoskeletal complaints are most commonly caused by intermittent viral infections. True periodic fevers associated with arthritis or arthralgias should raise suspicions of rare conditions such as familial Mediterranean fever; periodic fever with aphthous stomatitis, pharyngitis and adenitis (PFAPA syndrome), Behçet's disease, hyper-IgD syndrome or Hibernian fever[3,4].

Travel

Travel to areas known to be endemic for certain illnesses, such as Lyme disease or Ross River arthritis, should be considered. Consumption of foods possibly contaminated by organisms such as *Salmonella*, *Shigella*, *Listeria* or *Brucella* spp. should be considered.

Family history

A family history of rheumatic diseases, psoriasis or familial conditions such as arthrogryposis should be sought. Exploring in more depth for a history of family members with back pain, inflammatory bowel disease, reactive arthritis (formally called Reiter's syndrome) or eye problems such as acute iritis may lead to a history of HLA-B27 disease. Ethnicity and consanguinity of the parents may suggest the likelihood of certain conditions such as familial Mediterranean fever or autosomal recessive conditions[5,6].

Growth and development

Growth and development should be assessed to ascertain if it has progressed normally. If motor milestones are not reached at the appropriate age, or are lost – for instance if a child had started walking but then resumed crawling – a musculoskeletal or neurologic disorder is most likely to be responsible. Failure to gain height and weight may also reflect inflammation, and the onset of the inflammatory process may coincide with the change in growth curve (Fig. 25.3).

Social history

Social history should include family constellation, who is with the child (caretakers other than the parents may offer information unknown to

them, as well as opportunities for unexplained injury). School attendance may give clues as to how children have been affected by their symptoms, although a history of learning difficulties, drop in school performance or peer problems at school should lead to a discussion of whether a child is exhibiting physical symptoms as part of a school avoidance pattern.

Sleep history can lead to a history of non-restorative sleep consistent with fibromyalgia, although the child who wakes at night with pain may have 'growing pains' or a malignancy of some kind, such as an osteoid osteoma or leukemia.

Functional impairments

Functional impairments such as being unable to keep up with peers, easy fatigability or having to take extra naps may be clues to an underlying illness. Alteration in activities of daily living (ADLs) must also be assessed, and an understanding of appropriate expectations for children of different ages is also essential. For example, a 3-year-old should be able to ride a tricycle and dress independently except for buttons and shoelaces; a 6-year-old should be able to tie shoelaces and ride a two-wheeled bike; a no-hands situp is generally a 5-year-old skill. Difficulty with handwritten school assignments is common in children with hand and wrist involvement.

Previous treatments

Previous treatments and response to them is also important information. Many parents will give analgesics such as acetaminophen or ibuprofen for fever or pain. How frequently these have been administered may give a sense of the severity of symptoms. Anti-inflammatory agents given in lower doses may provide an analgesic effect but if given routinely in full therapeutic doses (i.e. 40–50 mg/kg per day of ibuprofen or 20mg/kg per day of naproxen) is likely to modify the fever of systemic onset juvenile arthritis or inflammatory joint disease. Treatment with corticosteroids may alter the picture of infectious, malignant or inflammatory processes, and starting a patient on steroids without a diagnosis carries a significant risk of modifying the picture, or masking or exacerbating the process.

Systems review

A full review of systems, including general questions as well as those more specific to rheumatic diseases, should be undertaken. Symptoms of Raynaud's syndrome in a prepubertal child strongly suggests an underlying rheumatic disease (generally not juvenile arthritis), although adolescent females may develop primary Raynaud's as well as Raynaud's secondary to an underlying disease (Fig. 25.4). Sjögren's symptoms are also strongly associated with rheumatic diseases in children.

Taking a history from teenagers (or sometimes even younger children) may involve obtaining confidential information. Provide an opportunity to ask sensitive questions by taking the initial history from the patient and parent together, then ask the parent to leave the room for the examination, during which confidential issues such as sexual behaviors, drug or alcohol use or social stressors may be raised. It is wise to precede this part of the interview with teenagers with a reassurance that the material discussed will be confidential, with the exception of information dangerous to the patient or others.

IMPORTANT POINTS ON PHYSICAL EXAMINATION

Every child should have complete vital signs checked, including blood pressure with an appropriately sized cuff, and these should be compared with normal values for age[7]. The height and weight should be plotted on a racially appropriate growth grid and compared with the child's previous growth record, as a decrease in percentile for either height or weight may reflect inflammation, the effect of steroids or poor nutritional intake.

The child should be undressed for the examination, although some children will allow only partial undressing at a time. Many children resist putting on hospital gowns; compromising on shorts and a tank top usually allows adequate access.

Examining a child can be a challenge. Much can be learned from observing children as they walk (or are carried) into the examination room, the way they change into a gown and climb on to the examination table. Incorporate moves into the examination like getting up from the floor and playing with the examination equipment, for example, to determine whether the child has the fine motor skills and hand strength to open a drawer, take out the tongue blade and remove it from the paper wrapping.

If the child has an obviously painful area, it is wise to examine that part last. Giving the child choices about which part to examine first – 'shall we start at the top or the toes?' and playing games the child is likely to know – 'this little pig went to market' with the toes, or 'where is thumbkin' for fingers, is the most effective way to get the child's cooperation. Almost all the pediatric examination can be performed in the parent's lap if this is less intimidating to the child, and towards the end of the examination the child may feel relaxed enough to sit on the examination table or floor to complete it.

Skin

Skin abnormalities can provide invaluable evidence about the cause of musculoskeletal pain, and all skin and mucus membranes should be examined closely for any rashes or other eruptions. The classic migratory lesions of erythema marginatum are seldom seen but very helpful in confirming rheumatic fever. Erythema nodosum leads to consideration of infectious causes, inflammatory bowel disease, drug-induced illness, sarcoidosis or vasculitic diseases (Fig. 25.5). Extensor surfaces should be checked for psoriasis, although occult lesions may be found in the scalp or navel; nailplate changes such as pitting or dystrophic changes may be the only clues to that disease. Examination of the nailbed may reveal the erythema and telangiectasias common in juvenile dermatomyositis and other forms of vasculitis (Fig. 25.6), while capillary dropout suggests scleroderma.

Vasculitic rashes such as palpable purpura or ecchymotic lesions can be seen with immune-complex-mediated conditions such as neisserial infections or in subacute bacterial endocarditis as well as in the primary vasculitic syndromes such as Henoch–Schönlein purpura (Fig. 25.7). The distribution, pattern of appearance and resolution (such as the recurrent crops with fading over a week usually seen in Henoch–Schönlein purpura) can be helpful.

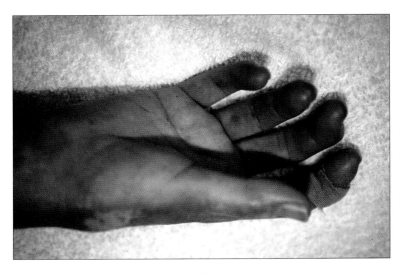

Fig. 25.4 Raynaud's phenomenon in children is nearly always associated with an underlying rheumatic disease.

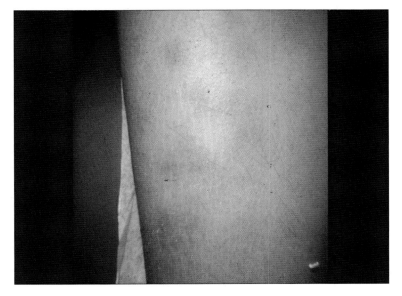

Fig. 25.5 Erythema nodosum. This rash usually occurs in the periorbital region. When found with arthritis, the differential diagnosis includes infections, drug reactions, sarcoidosis and vasculitic diseases.

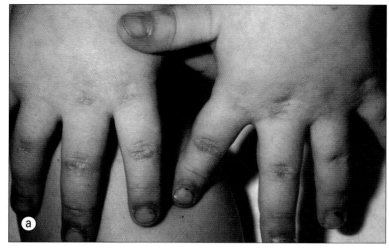

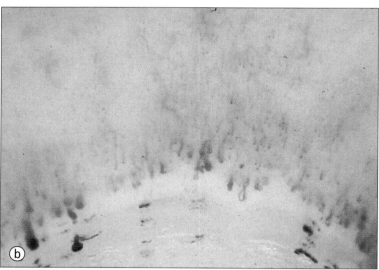

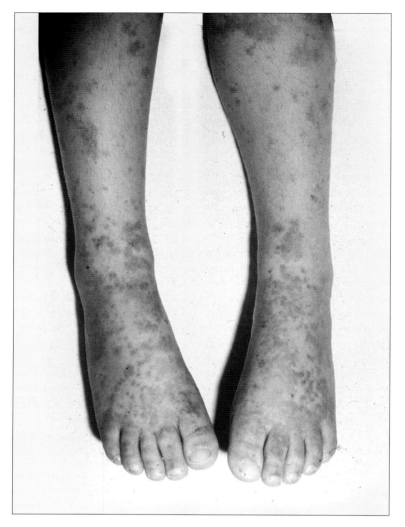

Fig. 25.6 Juvenile dermatomyositis. (a) Juvenile dermatomyositis causes typical erythematous lesions on the extensor surfaces of the hands. (b) The nailbed capillary dilatation and tortuosity correlate with the risk of vasculitis in the gastrointestinal tract.

Fig. 25.7 Lower extremity vasculitic rash usually found in Henoch–Schönlein purpura. However, it may be seen in other vasculitic disorders such as microscopic polyarteritis or Wegener's granulomatosis.

Subcutaneous nodules associated with juvenile rheumatoid arthritis are generally found over the elbows or other pressure areas in patients who are rheumatoid-factor-positive (only 10% of children with juvenile arthritis) or sometimes with SLE or mixed connective tissue disease. A variant histologically indistinguishable from rheumatoid nodules is benign rheumatoid nodules, part of the spectrum of granuloma annulare, which are usually found on the anterior tibia, foot or scalp rather than the classic extensor locations.

Some rashes are very helpful in making the diagnosis of a rheumatic disease – the migratory macular non-pruritic rash accompanying the fevers of systemic juvenile arthritis; the purple eyelid and scaly rashes on the extensor surfaces of the elbows, knuckles, knees and ankles seen in dermatomyositis; the classic malar rash or hard palate erythema or ulcerating nasal lesions of systemic lupus; the 'pepper and salt' papules of sarcoidosis.

Musculoskeletal examination

When considering the causes of musculoskeletal pain, the joint examination is critical. Especially in the pudgy child, warmth and swelling may be difficult to detect. Simple tests like whether the shin is warmer than the patella (the reverse suggests inflammation) or asymmetry of the extremities, including limb length discrepancy, suggest acute or chronic inflammation. Learning what is normal for a child (young

children especially are expected to be more flexible), as well as understanding what ranges are likely to be lost first (e.g. internal rotation at the hip and shoulder, supination at the elbow, extension at the knee and wrist, lateral flexion and extension at the cervical spine) gives helpful pointers to possible inflammatory changes. Children are very skilled at compensating for lost range, so stabilizing the surrounding structures, especially the joint above and below the site being examined, is essential. This is particularly true at the hip and shoulder, where excessive scapular rotation or pelvic tilt will mask loss of range at the joint. Palpation of the joints for swelling (both synovitis and effusions) and the bones and muscles for tenderness, is the best guide to the underlying process.

Playing tug of war can be helpful in assessing grip and arm strength, and pushing the examiner away with the feet is a good test of lower extremity strength. Squeezing a squeaky toy can encourage a child to actively obtain full range as well as testing strength (e.g. hand, elbow and knee flexion); getting up from the floor or a low stool tests hip girdle strength. Children under 5 usually cannot do situps but older children should be able to do several and hold sustained resistance against the examiner in muscle strength assessment. Formal manual muscle testing can be taught to most children over the age of 4 or 5 years.

Gait should be observed both walking and running if possible. An antalgic pattern of short stance phase and limp are common but also look for lack of rotation or extension at the hip, the big toe pulled into extension as a sign of ankle or metatarsophalangeal pain, or the flat-footed gait seen with hip or knee flexion contractures. Leg length should be measured from the anterior superior iliac spine to the medial malleolus of the ankle to determine if there is overgrowth (more common on the affected side of a child with oligoarticular juvenile arthritis).

Eyes

Examination of the eyes can give helpful information suggesting a rheumatic disease. A history of redness, pain or photophobia is consistent with acute iritis consistent with HLA-B27-associated diseases. Vasculitides such as Kawasaki disease and Wegener's granulomatosis may also present with non-purulent conjunctivitis or episcleritis. Cotton wool spots may also be seen in vasculitis, either a primary syndrome or associated with SLE or dermatomyositis. The chronic anterior uveitis associated particularly with early-onset oligoarticular juvenile arthritis is usually asymptomatic. Formation of synechiae may result in an irregular pupil or a fixed pupil and, rarely, band keratopathy can be seen (a band of calcium deposit over the cornea following the palpebral fissure). However, early signs of inflammation can usually only be found by a slit lamp examination. Prepare the child for this with a rehearsal at home or in the examination room by having the child get used to following a light in the dark and resting the chin on a table or the back of the chair. A pediatric ophthalmologist experienced with these examinations in children is most likely to get a complete and cooperative study.

Neurological examination

Pain or weakness may have a neurological origin, so a careful evaluation including reflexes, sensory and developmental testing should be performed, especially if an obvious musculoskeletal cause cannot be identified. Sometimes spinal cord processes such as Guillain–Barré syndrome or malignancies may present with lower extremity pain and loss of function.

General examination

Non-specific signs such as enlargement of the liver, spleen or lymph nodes suggest a more systemic origin of the musculoskeletal pain. Careful cardiovascular examination can indicate valvular changes such as those found in rheumatic fever or SLE, or pulse changes or bruits consistent with a large-vessel vasculitis such as Takayasu's arteritis. Thyroid enlargement (some is normal in adolescents) may suggest hyper- or hypothyroidism as the etiology of musculoskeletal pain. Abdominal tenderness or perirectal changes suggest that further evaluation for inflammatory bowel disease is indicated.

DEVELOPING A DIFFERENTIAL DIAGNOSIS

The major groups of conditions that may cause musculoskeletal pain should be considered:

- Does this child have an infection-related process?
- Does this child have a malignancy?
- Does the child have an injury?
- Does this child have a mechanical or non-inflammatory condition?
- Does this child have a metabolic problem?
- Does this child have a pain amplification syndrome?
- Does this child have a rheumatic disease?

The first two are not necessarily the most common but, because they are potentially the most serious and require early appropriate and aggressive intervention, they should be considered first. It is important to remember that rheumatic diseases are diagnosed partly on the basis of positive history and physical findings but also on the basis of exclusion of conditions that could mimic a rheumatic disease.

Acute bacterial infections

A child may develop an acute bacterial infection in a bone, joint, vertebral disc or soft tissue structures (cellulitis or rarely pyomyositis). Typically, children with a septic process are febrile, toxic and in significant pain. These infections usually originate from hematogenous seeding of the structures because children experience bacteremia more frequently than adults and have vasculature that permits bacteria to lodge in sites not generally affected in adults, such as the metaphysis of long bones or the intervertebral disc.

An infectious process shows steadily increasing crescendo pain, compared with the pattern of morning stiffness, improvement with activity, then evening pain and fatigue seen in juvenile arthritis. A septic joint usually shows marked warmth, diffuse tenderness, muscle guarding around the joint and extremely limited range of movement. Osteomyelitis[8] will have a similar pain pattern but the point of maximum tenderness is over the bone (the process usually originates in the metaphysis) rather than the joint and the range of movement is better preserved, although a sympathetic effusion may be detectable in the adjacent joint. Rarely, osteomyelitis may perforate into the joint space causing a simultaneous septic joint, especially where the capsular attachment is on the metaphyseal side of the epiphysis, such as in the shoulder and hip. Diskitis[9] may present with back pain and a rigid spine, although abdominal, hip or buttock pain are also common. Occasionally, multiple sites of infection may occur.

The bacteria likely to be responsible will depend on a number of factors, including the age of the child and host immune factors. Fortunately the availability of immunizations against previously important pathogens, e.g. *Streptococcus pneumoniae* and *Haemophilus influenzae* has reduced the incidence and altered the spectrum of bacterial infections where large-scale vaccination programs have been undertaken.

Important factors

Age of the child

- **Newborns and infants up to 6 months of age** are intrinsically poorly protected against bacterial infections and may develop overwhelming sepsis, although signs may include temperature instability rather than fever, and non-specific findings such as irritability, poor feeding and jaundice, especially in the first month of life. The likely bacteria are staphylococci, enteric organisms, group B streptococci and, if maternally exposed, *Neisseria gonorrhoeae*. Localizing findings may include pain on movement, for instance during a diaper change, or pseudo-paralysis. Because of the open blood flow through the metaphysis and epiphysis in children this age, the growth plate is often significantly damaged by infection and permanent growth abnormalities frequently result.
- **Children 6–48 months old** are more likely to develop pneumococcal or *Haemophilus influenzae* septic arthritis than older children.
- In **children over 4 years old**, over 90% of bone and joint infections are caused by *Staphylococcus aureus*.
- **Older children and teenagers** are most commonly infected by *S. aureus*, but may also be at risk for sexually transmitted diseases that may cause joint problems, such as *N. gonorrhoeae* and *Chlamydia* infections.

Host immune factors

Complement deficiencies may be inherited. C3 deficiency predisposes to susceptibility to pneumococcal organisms; late complement component deficiencies predispose to inability to form the terminal attack complex and kill *Neisseria* organisms. Acquired complement deficiency (as in active SLE) may also predispose a child to infections from encapsulated organisms, such as the pneumococcus and meningococcus.

Hemoglobinopathies including sickle-cell disease (HbSS)[10] and HbSC have been long recognized as predisposing patients to increased risk of osteomyelitis caused by both *S. aureus* and *Salmonella* species.

Immunodeficiencies[11-13], including agammaglobulinemia, may present with multiple joint arthritis, often with failure to thrive and a history of recurrent, deep or difficult-to-clear infections. Patients with common variable immunodeficiency may develop arthritis and vasculitis as a late manifestation.

The child who is immunosuppressed by a chemotherapy regime may develop septic foci from enteric or fungal organisms. The associated neutropenia may reduce the local inflammatory response, making localization of the site more difficult.

Previous antibiotic treatment

As most cases of septic arthritis and osteomyelitis are hematogenously spread, the initial site, for example impetigo or otitis media, could be cleared rapidly by administration of oral antibiotics. However, if the child was bacteremic, infection at the deeper site would not be eradicated by the usual doses of oral antibiotics, while the acuity and severity of the deeper infection may be masked. Therefore, it is essential to inquire about previous antibiotic treatment when evaluating musculoskeletal pain.

Penetrating bone or joint injury

Children may fall on to objects such as sticks or metal, or tread on sharp objects that penetrate their shoes. Whatever organisms are carried on the object, the skin, the shoes and the socks will be injected into the subcutaneous tissues, bones or joints of the child. These infections are commonly caused by multiple organisms, including unusual Gram-negative organisms such as *Pseudomonas* or *Serratia* species. The infection may be insidious, and becomes apparent sometimes weeks to months after the punctum has healed and sometimes the original injury has been forgotten.

Specific organisms

Tuberculosis is no longer common in many parts of the world but a history of exposure (often to disease in a close relative) or residence in an endemic area should raise concern. The bone, joint or tendon sheath infection is usually described as a 'cold' infection – slow and insidious, and usually very destructive to the bone or joint before the diagnosis is suspected.

Lyme disease[14,15] was originally identified because of an outbreak of oligoarticular juvenile arthritis in children. Typically, a tick bites the child; shortly thereafter malaise, fever, constitutional symptoms and the classic target lesion (erythema chronicum migrans) begins around the site of the bite. The arthritis is usually a late phenomenon, usually months or sometimes years after the original tick bite. Large joints, predominantly in the lower extremities, are affected in a slowly migratory pattern. At least a third of children do not recall a tick bite or rash, resulting in the misdiagnosis of juvenile arthritis.

Neisseria species, both *N. meningitidis* and *N. gonorrhoeae*, can cause an immune-complex-mediated arthritis. *N. gonorrhoeae* should be suspected in sexually active teenagers or in possible child abuse, and appropriate genital and throat cultures should be taken[16]. Disseminated *Neisseria* infection warrants investigation for an underlying complement component deficiency.

Postinfectious arthritis and myositis

A classic postinfectious arthritis is rheumatic fever, the sequel of pharyngitis caused by certain strains of group A streptococcus. The arthritis usually begins about 10 days after the throat infection, affects primarily large joints (knees, ankles, wrists, elbows) and is rapidly migratory, seldom lasting more than a few days in any joint. Even without treatment it is likely to resolve altogether within a month. While present it is very painful, with hot, intensely swollen and tender joints, but resolves rapidly with aspirin and other anti-inflammatory agents. Other supporting features are the presence of other Jones criteria.

Some patients with streptococcal infections also develop a more persistent reactive arthritis affecting small joints without other features of rheumatic fever[17].

Some enteric organisms such as *Salmonella*, *Shigella*, *Campylobacter* or *Yersinia* species precipitate a reactive arthritis a couple of weeks after the initial infection. In predisposed individuals (HLA-B27 is linked to this phenomenon), this arthritis may not be self-limiting but progress to a more classic spondyloarthropathy.

A number of common childhood viral illnesses, including parvovirus B 19, rubella, some strains of Coxsackie virus and, rarely, immunization strains, can cause a transient arthritis with primarily large joint involvement. Initially, this may appear indistinguishable from juvenile arthritis but will usually resolve within weeks, one of the reasons that the definition of juvenile arthritis is a minimum of 6 weeks duration of joint signs, which generally excludes postinfectious/reactive arthritis patterns.

Ross River arthritis is a mosquito-borne virus that causes large joint arthritis.

Viral myositis syndromes, caused most commonly by influenza, rubella and Coxsackie virus, are characterized by muscle pain, tenderness and tightness and elevated creatinine phosphokinase levels. These generally resolve within a week or two.

Approach to a child with suspected musculoskeletal infection

Early identification of the site and the organism responsible is essential to proper treatment. Typically, bacterial processes cause non-specific elevation of the white blood cell count with neutrophilia and elevated ESR and acute phase reactants such as C reactive protein. Blood cultures in children have a higher positive rate than in adults and two or three should be drawn in a febrile child. Imaging studies[18] may be helpful – plain radiographs are of limited use early in a septic process as they may take up to 2 weeks to show abnormalities and are used mainly to exclude other processes. Technetium bone scan will help to identify areas of increased uptake in the metaphyseal region of long bones, the usual site of osteomyelitis. Magnetic resonance imaging (MRI) may help to localize an infectious process but is less readily available and more expensive.

If septic arthritis is suspected, the best test is immediate joint fluid aspiration for culture, Gram stain and white blood cell count. Besides providing essential diagnostic information, the aspiration reduces intraarticular pressure that may damage cartilage and lead to avascular necrosis. Open drainage may be necessary to minimize the risk of long-term joint damage, especially in the hip (Fig. 25.8). If *N. gonorrhoeae* or

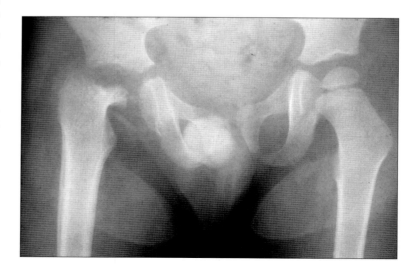

Fig. 25.8 This child was evaluated for fever and knee pain. Unfortunately the source of the referred pain (a septic hip) was not recognized for more than 24 hours, resulting in severe damage to the cartilage and femoral head.

Chlamydia trachomatis is suspected, cultures of genitalia and urine polymerase chain reaction (PCR) may be helpful.

Lyme disease is diagnosed by elevated titers to the causative organism, *Borrelia burgdorferi*, on both the enzyme-linked immunosorbent assay (ELISA) and the Western blot on the blood. PCR can also be performed on the joint fluid.

Most viral and postviral arthritis is diagnosed by excluding other causes, and passage of time, although specific titers may be positive.

Malignancies

Both primary and secondary malignancies may present with musculoskeletal pain.

Clinical clues include pain out of proportion to physical findings, pain at rest, and night pain, with absence of typical arthritis morning stiffness.

Primary tumors

A common benign tumor is osteoid osteoma, which commonly occurs around the pelvis and, while difficult to see on plain radiographs, displays markedly increased uptake on bone scan. These tumors are often more painful at night and often respond well to a trial of non-steroidal anti-inflammatory agents. Most other benign tumors are painless and are identified by incidental radiologic abnormalities, unless they are large enough to cause pathologic fractures.

Malignant primary bone tumors include osteogenic sarcoma; chondrosarcoma and Ewing's sarcoma. These are usually easily visualized on plain films as poorly demarcated lesions with mixed lytic and sclerotic pattern elevation of the periosteum and new bone formation (Codman's triangle), and also sometimes present with pathogenic fractures. Immediate referral to a pediatric oncology center is indicated for biopsy, staging and management.

Synovial cell tumors are rare – sarcomas and pigmented villonodular synovitis may present with joint swelling or bloody joint fluid. MRI is the best method of delineating the lesion and guiding the site for biopsy of affected tissue.

Systemic malignancies

Childhood leukemias and, less commonly, lymphomas may present with a clinical picture mimicking juvenile-onset arthritis[19,20]. Frequently, pain either in the bone or in the joint is the most pronounced complaint, although prominent synovial or periarticular swelling may sometimes be present. Useful clues are pain out of proportion to physical findings, pain at rest, or pain waking the child at night. However, sometimes the joint signs and symptoms may be migratory like those of rheumatic fever, or there may be pain and tenderness at the metaphysis rather than over the joint.

If the blood smear shows primitive cells, the diagnosis is easy; however the rheumatologist is more likely to see the child who does not have the typical peripheral blood changes. Suspicion should be raised if there is leukopenia (most children with juvenile arthritis have normal to high white blood cell counts) or thrombocytopenia (elevated platelet counts are typical of active inflammation). Anemia can be prominent in systemic-onset juvenile arthritis but should also trigger concern about an infiltrative or hemolytic process. Laboratory abnormalities may include elevated markers of cell turnover, such as increased uric acid and lactose dehydrogenate levels. Plain radiographs may show the classic leukemic lines at the end of long bones (zones of rarefaction adjacent to the epiphysis, representing uncalcified osteoid tissue), suggesting severe metabolic disturbance (Fig. 25.9). If there is any suspicion of leukemia or lymphoma, a bone marrow aspirate and biopsy must be performed and imaging of the major lymph node regions (with biopsy of atypical areas) undertaken.

Corticosteroids may temporarily reduce the signs and symptoms of a malignancy but are likely to delay making the correct diagnosis and significantly decrease the likelihood of the tumor responding to chemotherapy when the correct diagnosis is made. Therefore it is essen-

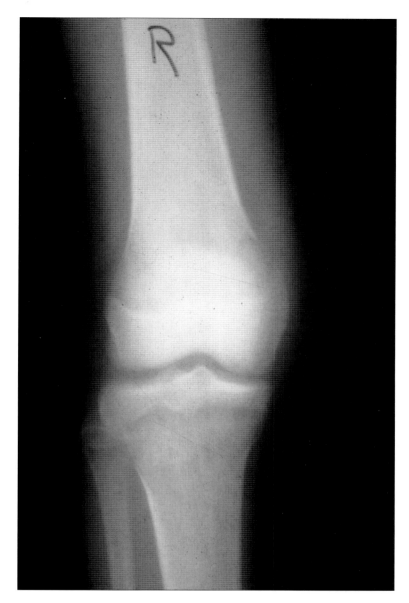

Fig. 25.9 Leukemic lines.

tial that steroids are never started until the possibility of a malignant condition has been excluded.

Secondary malignancies

Neuroblastoma is another childhood malignancy that can cause bone and joint complaints. Typically affected children are under the age of 7 and may have an abdominal mass. Swelling around the eyes is common as the tumor has a predilection for secondary lesions around the orbit. Plain films and technetium bone scan are helpful in identifying the bony lesions; catecholamine excretion in the urine is usually elevated.

Other childhood tumors such as germinal cell tumors may metastasize to bone. Back pain is atypical in most forms of childhood arthritis and spinal or perispinal involvement resulting from a malignancy should always be considered in a child with back pain.

Systemic conditions that may present with musculoskeletal pain

Inflammatory bowel disease is uncommon under the age of 4 years but may present with joint signs and symptoms months to years before complaints of abdominal pain, diarrhea or blood in the stool are identified. In children, growth failure can be an excellent marker for active systemic inflammation, and weight loss, or dropping across the percentile lines on the growth grid, strongly indicates consideration of underlying bowel pathology. Low serum albumin levels, anemia, positive tests for blood in the stool and elevated erythrocyte sedimentation rate (ESR) are often found. Endoscopy and barium studies of the bowel confirm the diagnosis[21].

Hypertrophic pulmonary osteoarthropathy, most commonly associated with chronic hypoxic conditions or liver disease, can cause clubbing of the fingers and toes and painful tender changes adjacent to the metaphyses of long bones. Plain films show elevation of the periosteum and new bone formation.

Cystic fibrosis is also associated with hypertrophic pulmonary osteoarthropathy but may involve a true arthritis, although immune-complex-mediated secondary to the frequent infections experienced by these patients[22].

Juvenile diabetes may be associated with chronic loss of extension at the metacarpophalangeal and interphalangeal joints (diabetic cheiroarthropathy). This pattern correlates with poorly controlled diabetes and elevated levels of hemoglobin A1c[23].

Thyroid disease in children, as in adults, may be associated with joint pain, myalgias and weakness[24].

Orthopedic non-inflammatory conditions

The lack of morning stiffness and absence of signs of an inflammatory process characterize these congenital or acquired conditions. Note that many of these processes occur around the hip and that any process that involves a single hip alone is unlikely to be caused by juvenile arthritis.

Conditions that may affect any part of the skeleton

Trauma is common in active children, so musculoskeletal complaints are often attributed to injuries. However, if the injury was not observed or if the injury appeared to be improving and then symptoms worsened, or if complaints seem disproportionate to the traumatic event, other causes for the symptoms should be considered. Plain radiographs are able to reveal fractures, although epiphyseal fractures may be difficult to identify.

In situations of child abuse the explanation of the injury may not seem compatible with the findings. A whole body skeletal survey using plain radiographs or bone scan may reveal evidence of previous injuries. Particularly suspicious are spiral fractures of long bones, fractures of varying ages and multiple sites of callus formation or periosteal changes. Most hospitals have a child abuse team, which will interview the child and parents and arrange for protection for the child if warranted. In the USA and many other countries, physicians are mandated to report suspected child abuse to the appropriate authorities.

Overuse syndromes are common in child athletes, and the child and family should be questioned carefully about activities and relationship to the symptoms. Throwing sports are stressful to the immature elbow and shoulder; track events may stress the knees and ankles, and gymnasts and dancers often try to achieve positions of extreme range of movement, leading to pain[25]. Musicians and players of computer games may also experience overuse syndromes.

Hypermobility[26] can be found in about 8% of children under the age of 5, and many older children experience persistent symptoms related to joint laxity. Typically these children have pain related to activity and may have small joint effusions in the absence of morning stiffness or other signs of inflammation[27]. Symptoms typically respond to rest and analgesics, although strengthening the muscle groups around the affected joints, teaching joint protection techniques and occasionally using bracing or taping during activities is helpful. The most common form of this syndrome is benign familial hypermobility, an autosomal

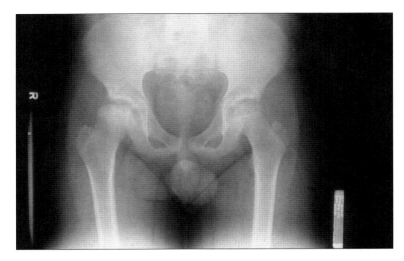

Fig. 25.10 Avascular necrosis. This is best recognized early on MRI. Late changes visible on plain radiographs include collapse of the femoral head and remodeling of the acetabulum.

dominant condition also known as Ehlers–Danlos syndrome type 3, although extreme hypermobility should lead to consideration of other true connective tissue disorders.

Avascular necrosis may occur at several sites. The most common site is the hip (Legg–Calvé–Perthes disease), more frequent in boys, peak age 6 years, and usually presenting with limp and knee pain[28]. About one-third of affected children have a history of transient synovitis in the same hip preceding the onset of the avascular necrosis, reflecting susceptibility to this process because of the non-distensible nature of the hip capsule and the tenuous blood supply to the femoral head through the ligamentum teres. Prolonged corticosteroid use is also a risk factor for this condition, as is the presence of antiphospholipid antibodies. Other sites affected include the talonavicular joint, the second metatarsal head and the wrist. Bone scans identify early changes of reduced blood flow to the affected area; MRI also will demonstrate the area of hypoperfusion and surrounding edema. Plain films may not show changes until extensive sclerosis and collapse have occurred (Fig. 25.10).

Osteochondritis desiccans is a condition, more common in boys, that causes the cartilage to flake off the joint surface, especially in the elbow and knee. The resulting loose body causes pain, catching or locking in the affected joint. This condition can be seen on plain films, especially views that highlight the joint surface (e.g. the tunnel or sunrise view of the knee, taken in flexion with both the femoral and patellar surfaces emphasized) or on MRI. Sometimes these cartilage fragments can become 'joint mice', free bodies in the joint.

Common conditions affecting a specific region

Back pain

Mechanical back pain is unusual in a child and consideration of processes such as spinal cord problems or malignancy is warranted. However, musculoskeletal problems such as spondylolisthesis (defect in the pars articularis at the lower lumbar region, sometimes with displacement) are more common in girls who hyperextend the spine. Oblique films of the spine will demonstrate the characteristic slip. Scheuermann's disease (juvenile kyphosis) is also recognized radiologically by anterior wedging of the vertebrae.

Hip

Slipped capital femoral epiphysis is most common in obese adolescent boys and presents with limp and knee pain[29]. Plain radiographs demon-

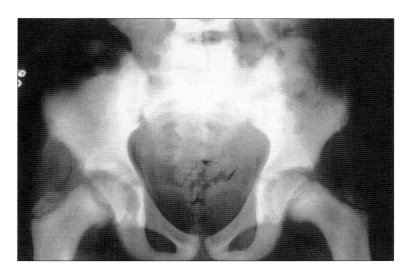

Fig. 25.11 Bilateral slipped femoral epiphyses, seen on plain radiograph.

strate the separation of the femoral epiphysis (Fig. 25.11). This condition requires the child be made immediately non-weight-bearing in an effort to prevent further slip, and surgical pinning to restore the femoral head to the correct position. Subsequent complications include avascular necrosis and chondrolysis[30]. A history of slipped femoral epiphysis on one side markedly increases the risk of a slip on the other side.

Knee pain

Patellofemoral syndrome occurs most commonly in athletes and in teenage girls and is caused by an irregular immature cartilage on the posterior aspect of the patella. Accompanying this is an easily subluxable patella and weakness of the medial quadriceps muscle. Complaints are of knee pain, most commonly after exercise that stresses the quadriceps mechanism or after sitting with the knees bent. Small effusions may be found. The physical findings are of lax patella and a positive apprehension test (pain and crepitus when the patella is held down on the femoral articular surface while the quadriceps is contracted).

Plica, a thickening of structures (possibly a congenital residual fold of tissue in the medial knee joint capsule) can also cause medial joint line pain and tenderness.

Meniscal injuries are rare before adolescence, although a congenital discoid meniscus can cause knee pain and swelling. These anatomic findings are best identified on MRI.

Osgood–Schlatter disease is a form of osteochondritis affecting the tibial tuberosity, with pain and tenderness over the site of the patellar tendon insertion. This can mimic the enthesitis seen at this site in the spondyloarthropathies.

Shin splints are usually found in athletes. The history is of pain and tenderness over the muscle insertions in to the anterior tibia, possibly with microscopic stress fractures.

Ankle and foot pain

Idiopathic Achilles tendinitis and plantar fasciitis may be found in active children but an enthesitis associated with a spondyloarthropathy should also be considered. Sever's disease is pain with radiographic density in the calcaneus that usually resolves spontaneously over time.

Metabolic and genetic conditions

Chromosome abnormalities

Children with trisomy 21 (Down's syndrome) may have a number of skeletal problems including hypermobility, cervical spinal stenosis and subluxation, and a multiple joint inflammatory arthritis[31]. They are also predisposed to autoimmune mediated thyroid disease and celiac disease, as well as leukemia, all of which may be associated with joint symptoms.

Immunodeficiency syndromes

A number of other chromosomally linked immune abnormalities are also associated with tendency to autoimmune phenomena, such as Di George's syndrome (22q deletion) and ataxia telangiectasia. Before the advent of intravenous administration of gammaglobulin, children with X-linked agammaglobulinemia may have multiple joint arthritis. Children with acquired immunodeficiency syndrome (AIDS) may also have arthritis, usually in association with adenopathy, hepatosplenomegaly and a history of multiple infections. Isolated IgA deficiency is identified in about 2% of children with arthritis, and arthralgias may also be associated with IgA deficiency.

Blood disorders

Any cause of recurrent bleeding into the joint may lead to a proliferative synovitis and joint destruction, most commonly in hemophilia A[32]. Children with sickle-cell disease or other hemoglobinopathies may also have joint pain and be susceptible to osteonecrosis and infections (*Staphylococcus* and *Salmonella* spp.). Thalassemia causes bony expansion from marrow hypertrophy and subsequent bone pain.

Storage diseases

Storage diseases[33] should be considered in children who have organomegaly, skin changes and abnormal joint findings with or without developmental delay. These include the sphingolipidoses (Gaucher's disease, Fabry's disease and Farber's disease), the metabolic bases of which are now understood; specific enzyme replacement therapy is available.

Other conditions

Gout is rare in children and is almost invariably associated with an inborn error in the purine pathway (for example Lesch–Nyhan syndrome), renal disease or severe polycythemia. Although uric acid nephropathy is a risk of the tumor lysis syndrome associated with childhood malignancies, gout almost never occurs.

Inborn errors of collagen, such as Stickler's syndrome, may also present with arthritis and/or multiple joint complaints. Clues to this group of disorders include other skeletal abnormalities such as a high-arched palate, eye findings, dysmorphic features or radiologic changes.

Pain syndromes

Benign limb pain ('growing pains')

A common complaint heard from parents of young children (usually aged 3–8 years) is known as growing pains, although the relationship with growth is tenuous. Typically, after an active day, the child wakes at night with deep thigh or calf pain that responds to analgesics, massage and heat. There may be a family history of similar problems in one of the parents[34]. Helpful in distinguishing this from a more serious cause of night pain is the normal physical examination, normal screening laboratory tests (complete blood count ESR) and the history that the child resumes full normal activities immediately after the episode.

Benign chest or costochondral pain

Some children, especially teenagers, have brief episodes of sharp chest pain, which leaves them feeling that they cannot take a deep breath but in fact is improved by deep breathing. This pain is localized to the chest wall, although many children have gone to the Emergency Department and had extensive cardiac evaluation because of fears of heart pain. The pain can be reproduced by pressure on the costochondral joints.

Reflex sympathetic dystrophy

This syndrome is uncommon in children. The presentation is usually exquisite pain, hypersensitivity even to very light touch, coolness, cyanosis and refusal to use the affected extremity. About half of these episodes have a preceding identifiable trigger such as trauma; the remainder appear to have a psychogenic origin. Laboratory studies are normal, although bone scans may show diminished flow to the affected area[35].

Fibromyalgia

Symptoms of joint pain and morning stiffness are similar to those of juvenile arthritis but the physical examination and laboratory studies do not show signs of inflammation. Sleep disturbance is common – either waking during the night or waking in the morning feeling unrefreshed, and many of these patients are stressed, high-achieving individuals[36,37]. The pressure points found in adult patients with this syndrome are also found in children.

Conversion reactions

Gait patterns that do not make anatomic sense, refusal to walk with no obvious abnormalities to explain non-ambulation, shifting or non-reproducible patterns of complaints, or disabling pain that has not been diagnosed in spite of extensive evaluation should always raise the issue of psychogenic origin. Many children who have these patterns have been abused, physically, psychologically or sexually. It is very important not to dismiss the child as a malingerer but to take the symptoms seriously and investigate for the underlying stressors causing them.

Rare diseases of unknown etiology

Sarcoid is uncommon in childhood and may present as a familial form (Blau's syndrome), or an infantile form (onset under the age of 5 years) with panuveitis, erythema nodosum and arthritis[38]. Adolescents are more likely to have the typical adult presentation, including lung involvement. The synovitis is usually more proliferative than that seen in juvenile arthritis, prompting biopsy to identify the granulomata.

Neonatal-onset multisystem inflammatory disease begins with an illness at birth that mimics systemic-onset juvenile arthritis, with high fevers, migratory rash, hepatosplenomegaly, progressive joint tightness and failure to thrive[39].

Chronic recurrent osteomyelitis is characterized by multiple sites of apparent infection at the end of long bones from which no organisms can be cultured.

Drug-induced joint pain

The use of minocycline for acne has been associated in many teenagers with joint symptoms and arthritis[40] that resolves with withdrawal of the drug.

Rheumatic diseases

All the rheumatic diseases of childhood are associated with musculo-skeletal pain and typically have morning stiffness, decreased activity and sometimes loss of developmental motor milestones. These include juvenile rheumatoid arthritis, juvenile-onset spondyloarthropathies, psoriasis-related arthritis, SLE, juvenile dermatomyositis, childhood-onset vasculitic syndromes and sclerodermas. While all of these have positive features that help characterize the condition, all require careful exclusion of conditions that may mimic rheumatic disease.

REFERENCES

1. Merkel S, Malviya S. Pediatric pain, tools, and assessment. J Perianesth Nurs 2000; 15: 408–414.
2. Varni JW. Evaluation and management of pain in children with juvenile rheumatoid arthritis. Rheumatology Suppl 1992; 33: 32–35.
3. McBeth J, Macfarlane GJ, Benjamin S et al. The association between tender points, psychological distress, and adverse childhood experiences: a community-based study. Arthritis Rheum 1999; 42: 1397–1404.
4. Drenth JP, van der Meer JW. Hereditary periodic fever. N Engl J Med 2001; 345: 1748–1757.
5. Hull KM, Kastner DL, Balow JE. Hereditary periodic fever. N Engl J Med 2001; 346: 1415–1416.
6. Thomas KT, Feder HM Jr, Lawton AR, Edwards KM. Periodic fever syndrome in children. J Pediatr 1999; 135: 15–21.
7. Harriet Lane Service. Normal values: blood pressure. In: Harriet Lane Handbook, 15th ed. St Louis, MO: Mosby; 1999: 171–178.
8. Wall EJ. Childhood osteomyelitis and septic arthritis. Curr Opin Pediatr 1998; 10: 73–76.
9. Tay BK, Deckey J, Hu SS. Spinal infections. J Am Acad Orthop Surg 2002; 10: 188–197.
10. Chambers JB, Forsythe DA, Bertrand SL et al. Retrospective review of osteoarticular infections in a pediatric sickle cell age group. J Pediatr Orthop 2000; 20: 682–685.
11. Uluhan A, Sager D, Jasin HE. Juvenile rheumatoid arthritis and common variable hypogammaglobulinemia. J Rheumatol 1998: 25; 1205–1210.
12. Thakar YS, Chande C, Dhanvijay AG et al. Analysis of immunoglobulin deficiency cases: a five year study. Indian J Pathol Microbiol 1997; 40: 309–313.
13. Sullivan KE, McDonald-McGinn DM, Driscoll DA et al. Juvenile rheumatoid arthritis-like polyarthritis in chromosome 22q11.2 deletion syndrome (DiGeorge anomalad/velocardiofacial syndrome/conotruncal anomaly face syndrome). Arthritis Rheum 1997; 40: 430–436.
14. Steere AC, Malawista SE, Snydman DR et al. Lyme arthritis: an epidemic of oligoarticular arthritis in children and adults in three Connecticut communities. Arthritis Rheum 1977; 20: 7–17.
15. Huppertz HI. Lyme disease in children. Curr Opin Rheumatol 2001; 13: 434–440.
16. Ingram DL. Neisseria gonorrhoeae in children. Pediatr Ann 1994; 23: 341–345.
17. Li EK. Rheumatic disorders associated with streptococcal infections. Baillière's Best Pract Res Clin Rheumatol 2000; 14: 559–578.
18. Kothari NA, Pelchovitz DJ, Meyer JS. Imaging of musculoskeletal infections. Radiol Clin North Am 2001; 39: 653–671.
19. Trapani S, Grisolia F, Simonini G et al. Incidence of occult cancer in children presenting with musculoskeletal symptoms: a 10-year survey in a pediatric rheumatology unit. Semin Arthritis Rheum 2000; 29: 348–359.
20. Cabral DA, Tucker LB. Malignancies in children who initially present with rheumatic complaints. J Pediatr 1999; 134: 53–57.
21. Lindsley CB, Schaller JG. Arthritis associated with inflammatory bowel disease in children. J Pediatr 1974; 84: 16–20.
22. Massie RJ, Towns SJ, Bernard E et al. The musculoskeletal complications of cystic fibrosis. J Paediatr Child Health 1998; 34: 467–470.
23. Infante JR, Rosenbloom AL, Silverstein JH et al. Changes in frequency and severity of limited joint mobility in children with type 1 diabetes mellitus between 1976–78 and 1998. J Pediatr 2001; 138: 33–37.
24. Keenan GF, Ostrov BE, Goldsmith DP, Athreya BH. Rheumatic symptoms associated with hypothyroidism in children. J Pediatr 1993; 123: 586–588.
25. Small E. Chronic musculoskeletal pain in young athletes. Pediatr Clin North Am 2002; 49: 655–662.
26. Grahame R, Bird HA, Child A. The revised (Brighton 1998) criteria for the diagnosis of benign joint hypermobility syndrome (BJHS). J Rheumatol 2000; 27: 1777–1779.
27. Murray KJ, Woo P. Benign joint hypermobility in childhood. Rheumatology (Oxford) 2001: 40: 485–487.
28. Skaggs DL, Tolo VT. Legg–Calvé–Perthes disease. J Am Acad Orthop Surg 1996; 4: 9–16.
29. Loder RT, Greenfield ML. Clinical characteristics of children with atypical and idiopathic slipped capital femoral epiphysis: description of the age-weight test

and implications for further diagnostic investigation. J Pediatr Orthop 2001; 21: 481–487.

30. Rattey T, Piehl F, Wright JG. Acute slipped capital femoral epiphysis. Review of outcomes and rates of avascular necrosis. J Bone Joint Surg 1996; 78A: 398–402.

31. Olson JC, Bender JC, Levinson JE et al. Arthropathy of Down syndrome. Pediatrics 1990; 86: 931–936.

32. Hilgartner MW. Current treatment of hemophilic arthropathy. Curr Opin Pediatr 2002; 14: 46–49.

33. Chalom EC, Ross J, Athreya BH. Syndromes and arthritis. Rheum Dis Clin North Am 1997; 23: 709–727.

34. Oberklaid F, Amos D, Liu C et al. 'Growing pains': clinical and behavioral correlates in a community sample. J Dev Behav Pediatr 1997; 18: 102–106.

35. Sherry DD. Pain syndromes in children. Curr Rheumatol Rep 2000; 2: 337–342.

36. Siegel DM, Janeway D, Baum J. Fibromyalgia syndrome in children and adolescents: clinical features at presentation and status at follow-up. Pediatrics 1998; 101: 377–382.

37. Schanberg LE, Keefe FJ, Lefebvre JC et al. Social context of pain in children with Juvenile Primary Fibromyalgia syndrome: parental pain history and family environment. Clin J Pain 1998; 14: 107–115.

38. Lindsley CB, Petty RE. Overview and report on international registry of sarcoid arthritis in childhood. Curr Rheumatol Rep 2000; 2: 343–348.

39. Prieur AM. A recently recognised chronic inflammatory disease of early onset characterised by the triad of rash, central nervous system involvement and arthropathy. Clin Exp Rheumatol 2001; 19: 103–106.

40. Elkayam O, Yaron M, Caspi D. Minocycline-induced autoimmune syndromes: an overview. Semin Arthritis Rheum 1999; 28: 392–397.

INFECTION-RELATED RHEUMATIC DISORDERS

26 Septic arthritis and osteomyelitis

Lars Lidgren

- The skeleton is affected by a wide variety of different infections with distinct etiology, pathogenesis, clinical features and management
- Staphylococci are the most common cause of musculoskeletal sepsis
- Streptococcal and mycobacterial infections are increasing in prevalence
- Antibiotic resistance, especially in prosthetic infections of low virulence caused by coagulase-negative staphylococci, is an increasing problem
- The adherence of bacteria to biomaterials used in joint replacement remains a major unresolved problem

HISTORY

'Laudable pus' was identified by Galen as being part of the healing process in open fractures, and allowing spontaneous healing was the treatment of choice in most centers in Europe until the 19th century[1].

Hippocrates understood the importance of the reduction of fractures and the appliance of wound dressings but it was not until Lister had, as a surgeon, accepted Pasteur's findings that both antisepsis and asepsis slowly became standard practice. Bone infection in osteomyelitis is described in Greek, Roman and Arab texts from AD 500–1200, and limited sequestrectomy was an accepted treatment. Chemotherapy in osteomyelitis was first used in 1936[2] and rapidly gained popularity as penicillin was introduced.

EPIDEMIOLOGY

The annual incidence of bacterial arthritis and acute osteomyelitis in Sweden is 10/100 000[3,4]. The incidence is higher in warm and humid geographic areas and is probably also related to socioeconomic conditions. In Western Australia, among European children, there are twice as many cases of acute osteomyelitis as in, for example, Scotland or Sweden.

In New Zealand the Maori have four times, and in Australia the Aborigines 12 times, as many hospital admissions for acute osteomyelitis as Europeans in both Australia and Europe[5]. The number of acute bone infections that develop into chronic infection has been drastically reduced, by early antibiotic treatment and surgical decompression, from 10–20% to less than 2%[6].

The number of new cases of chronic osteomyelitis of post-traumatic, postoperative and hematogenous origin in various European countries during the past decade has been estimated to be 15–30/100 000 population[3,5,7]. However, the number of cases of hematogenous origin is expected to reduce substantially. In a recent study (1990–97) acute hematogenous osteomyelitis in children was found to be becoming rare, with only 2.9/100 000/year in Scotland. The annual incidence of vertebral osteomyelitis is estimated to be 0.5–1.0/100 000 population[8,9].

Postoperative diskitis occurs in about 1%[10,11] and only rarely is hematogenous diskitis seen, especially in the cervical spine in children.

Currently, at least 1.8 million joint prosthetic implants and 2 million devices for hip fractures per year are implanted all over the world. In the 1970s, before any preventive measures were taken, about 10% of all major surgical hip procedures involving an implant resulted in infection.

Improvements in surgical techniques, pre- and perioperative routines and antibiotic prophylaxis, as well as treatment against hematogenous spread from infectious foci in, for instance, the skin, have led to a reduction of the infection rate to less than 0.5% in hip surgery and 1% in knee prosthetic surgery[12].

CLINICAL FEATURES AND PATHOGENESIS

Septic arthritis

Clinical features

The presentation of septic arthritis varies with age. In infancy, the symptoms are usually systemic rather than local[13,14]. Small children develop high, septic-pattern fever (Table 26.1) and are usually ill. The clinical features are more those of sepsis than of local arthritis. Older children are also febrile and unwell but the local signs are more prominent. Distention of the joint capsule and increased intra-articular pressure contribute to pain. If the hip joint is involved it is usually held in flexion, as this position gives maximum compliance. Adults and elderly patients with osteoarthritis or rheumatoid arthritis (RA) are at greater risk of an acute septic arthritis. The lower extremities are more often

	Fever	Local pain	Inflammatory signs	Purulent drainage	Reduced function
TABLE 26.1 CLINICAL FEATURES OF SEPTIC BONE AND JOINT LESIONS					
Septic arthritis	+	+	+	− to (+)	(+) to +
Prosthetic joint infection	(+) to +	(+) to +	(−) to (+)	−	(−) to +
Septic bursitis	(+) to +	(+)	(+) to +	−	(−) to (+)
Acute osteomyelitis	+	+	(+) to +	−	− to (+)
Pelvic osteomyelitis	+	+	(−) to (+)	− to +	(+) to +
Chronic osteomyelitis	− to (+)	− to (+)	(−) to (+)	− to (+)	− to (+)
Osteitis	− to (+)	(+)	(−) to (+)	−	− to (+)
Spondylitis	(−) to +	(−) to (+)	(−)		− to +
− = absent (−) = low-grade (+) = moderate + = high-grade					

affected, particularly the hip and knee joints. Patients generally have severe pain and are reluctant to move and put weight on the joint[15].

The joint capsule is distended, warm and often reddened and edematous (Fig. 26.1). If the infection is detected and treated during the first 2–3 days the outcome is favorable and there is no mortality. A delay in diagnosis, particularly in septic arthritis of the hip in children, often results in joint destruction[16] (Fig. 26.2).

Pathogenesis

A prerequisite for the development of septic arthritis is that bacteria can reach the synovial membrane. This can take place in different ways (Fig. 26.3).

Firstly, bacteria may reach the joint from a remote infectious focus via the hematogenous route. Such foci are usually abscesses or infected wounds in the skin, infections in the teeth, upper or lower respiratory tract infections, urinary or intestinal tract infections or endocarditis. In some cases no obvious primary focus is noted – a common experience in septicemia. The bacteria reach the deep vascular plexus terminating in the looped capillary anastomosis (circulus articularis vasculosus)[16,17].

A second route, particularly common in small children, is a dissemination of bacteria from an acute osteomyelitic focus in the metaphysis or epiphysis. The vessels through the physis and epiphysis are not occluded as is usually the case above 1 year of age[18]. Above this age, spread of bacteria can occur from the metaphysis of the humerus and femur or in the elbow, where the joint capsule covers parts of the metaphysis, allowing bacteria to penetrate through the cortical bone and the periosteum to the joint cavity. In adults with closed growth plates there is a re-established connection between the meta-

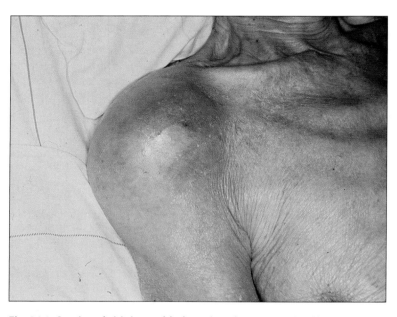

Fig. 26.1 Septic arthritis in an elderly patient, here recognized by distention, increased skin temperature and tenderness. The septic arthritis does not always differ from other kinds of arthritis.

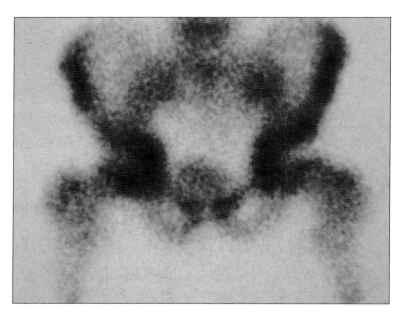

Fig. 26.2 Segmental femoral head necrosis in septic arthritis of the left hip.

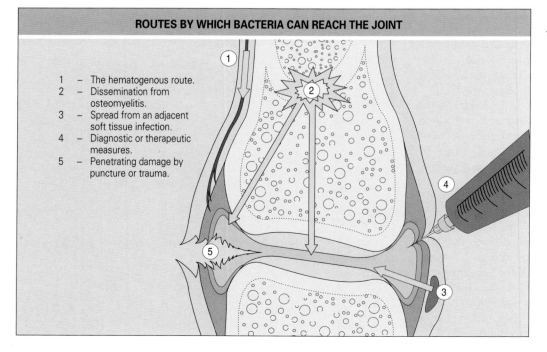

ROUTES BY WHICH BACTERIA CAN REACH THE JOINT

1 – The hematogenous route.
2 – Dissemination from osteomyelitis.
3 – Spread from an adjacent soft tissue infection.
4 – Diagnostic or therapeutic measures.
5 – Penetrating damage by puncture or trauma.

Fig. 26.3 Routes by which bacteria can reach the joint.

physis and the epiphysis and spread of infection to the synovial plexus is possible.

Third, an infection in the vicinity of the joint can progress to the joint or spread via the lymphogenic route. This is most often seen in non-penetrating traumatic and postoperative wound infections and in skin and soft tissue infections around the joint, particularly the knee joint.

A fourth possibility is iatrogenic infection caused by joint puncture for a diagnostic or therapeutic purpose. Although extremely rare, this has not yet been completely eradicated.

Lastly, penetrating trauma, usually caused by dirty objects or by animal or human bites, often gives rise to a severe infection because of the high inoculate of bacteria and the lacerated tissue. After joint surgery, perioperatively implanted bacteria can cause a postoperative infection.

In hematogenous infection, once the bacteria have reached the synovial membrane an inflammatory reaction starts. Leukocytes migrate to the focus and inflammatory proteins exude to the infectious focus. The synovial membrane proliferates and becomes tender, and the blood flow increases. There is exudation of bacteria, cells and proteins into the joint cavity. The bacteria in the joint fluid can be killed by phagocytes. The joint becomes swollen and the joint pressure rises and can cause cartilage damage. The enzymes elastase and collagenase are liberated from polymorphonuclear leukocytes and synovial cells degrade the cartilage. The infection and inflammation can spread in the subchondral bone[19]. Joint cartilage loses its resilience, tolerating only about a third of the normal pressure. The tissue changes become irreversible, often in a few days (Fig. 26.4)[20]. A proliferating pannus tissue will often result from persistent infection.

Prosthetic joint infection

Clinical features

The symptoms can differ in the early and late postoperative period. If an infection presents soon after surgery, staphylococci and streptococci are more common and the symptoms are more intensive, with high fever, general malaise and a wound discharging pus[21]. Later on, when the wound has healed or a sinus has developed, the patient may still have pain with soft tissue swelling (Fig. 26.5). In postoperative infections presenting late the general symptoms are usually not impressive and the local signs can be rather discrete, with slight tenderness and pain. In

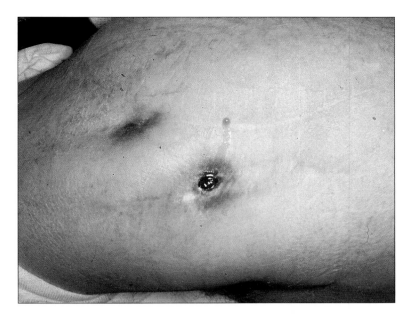

Fig. 26.5 In spite of a severe deep infection around a prosthesis, the only external signs may be a fistula and edema.

some cases of hip joint infection with joint effusion, the pressure can be so high that dislocation occurs[12]. In hematogenous infections the onset is usually acute, with high, septic fever and increasing pain even at rest. A hematogenous prosthetic joint infection is serious, with high morbidity and mortality, especially in fragile patients (RA) and with *Staphylococcus aureus* infection[22].

Pathogenesis

Low-virulence bacteria such as coagulase-negative staphylococci are the dominating pathogens in infections around prosthetic materials[23]. Patients with an implanted large foreign body are often elderly, which increases the risk of infection. Bacteria, particularly the staphylococci, are apt to adhere to a foreign biomaterial surface. This colonization, 'a race for the surface'[24], is the first step in a process that results in chronic infection in a prosthetic joint. Bacteria compete with host-tissue cells for the ability to produce proteins and polysaccharides and furthermore to be integrated with the surface of biomaterial. A biofilm is established. The bacteria are embedded in slime, a glycocalyx that protects them from antimicrobial agents and the cellular and humoral host defenses. Physical forces and hydrophobic interactions, non-specific chemical bindings and specific bacterial receptor–host component bindings mediated by ligands facilitate a strong attachment of bacteria to the foreign material[25,26,27].

Septic bursitis

The superficial subcutaneous olecranon, prepatellar and infrapatellar bursae are the most common sites affected by bacterial infections[28]. Antecedent trauma, mostly occupation-related, to the infected bursa is found in the majority of patients. Some underlying conditions, e.g. diabetes mellitus, rheumatoid arthritis, chronic alcohol abuse, may be contributing factors. Associated septicemia in cases of septic bursitis is uncommon

Acute bacterial bursitis is most common at the elbow and knee. Adults are mostly affected. The onset is rapid, often after repeated trauma. High fever, sometimes with chills, and swelling of the bursa with increased warmth, redness and pain are characteristic (Fig. 26.6). Joint function is generally not affected. In cases with olecranon bursitis without trauma, diabetes mellitus is a frequent underlying disease. The prognosis is good, with few sequelae[29].

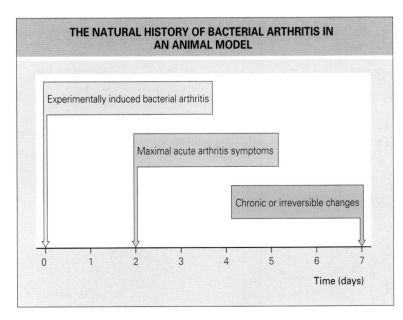

Fig. 26.4 **The natural history of bacterial arthritis in an animal model.** This is similar to development in the clinical case. (Data from Goldenberg and Reed[20].)

THE NATURAL HISTORY OF BACTERIAL ARTHRITIS IN AN ANIMAL MODEL

Experimentally induced bacterial arthritis

Maximal acute arthritis symptoms

Chronic or irreversible changes

Time (days)

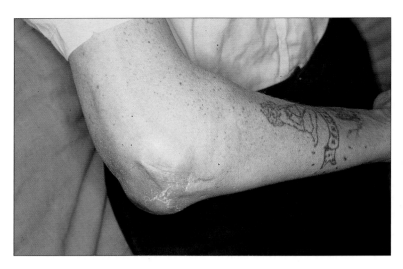

Fig. 26.6 Bursitis symptoms are similar to arthritis but a diagnostic puncture of the bursa containing purulent material in septic bursitis is easy to do.

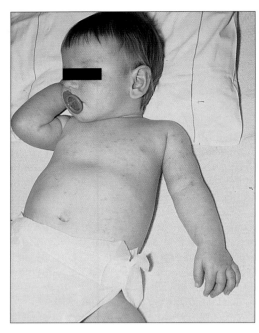

Fig. 26.7 An acute osteomyelitis in the proximal metaphysis of the left humerus. The child is not willing to move the affected limb. The roseola is consistent with a *Salmonella* infection, which was confirmed by fecal cultures.

Acute osteomyelitis

Clinical features

This type of infection principally affects children and young adults[15]. In children below 1 year of age acute osteomyelitis presents with arthritis in about 75% of cases and septicemia in almost all[14]. The epiphysis is sometimes involved[30]. Older children will not move or weight-bear on the affected limb (Fig. 26.7). The metaphysis, mostly in the lower extremities around the knee joint, in the trochanter region or in the humerus, is tender to the touch and can be swollen and warm. In the proximal humerus and femur the joint may be involved because of the insertion of the joint capsule below the metaphysis. If the infection is diagnosed and treated during the first 2–3 days after onset the prognosis is good and chronic complications are rare.

Pathogenesis

The metaphysis has a rich blood supply and a slow circulation time. By contrast, the perfusion is slow through the venous sinusoids. The endothelial cells of the sinusoids have a reduced phagocytic activity[31,32]. These factors are favorable for bacterial adherence and multiplication in the metaphysis (Fig. 26.8). The ensuing inflammatory reaction increases the intraosseous pressure, and microthrombi of the small vessels obstruct the blood flow. The result is an intraosseous inflammatory focus with abscess formation under high pressure, and a reduced blood supply resulting in the destruction of osseous trabeculae by osteoclasts followed by osteoblastic activity forming new bone tissue[33]. In chickens it has been shown that bacteria deposit in the growth plate and bacterial proliferation occludes the blood vessels within 24 hours[34]. Abscess formation usually occurs within 2–3 days. When the purulent infection has penetrated laterally through haversian channels to the subperiosteal area and/or down to the medullary cavity, the lesion becomes chronic.

Pelvic osteomyelitis

Clinical features

In younger athletic individuals this disease presents as an acute hematogenous infection around the symphysis or the sacroiliac joints and is caused by *S. aureus*[35]. In women with obstetric or gynecologic pelvic infections a different clinical picture is seen, with subacute onset and contiguous dissemination from the pelvis.

The symptoms can be diffuse and difficult to attribute to a skeletal infection; pain and fever are the most prominent symptoms. The condition may be difficult to detect and the diagnosis is often delayed. However, the prognosis is good and sequelae are rare.

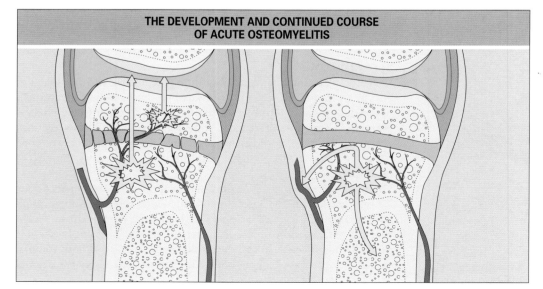

THE DEVELOPMENT AND CONTINUED COURSE OF ACUTE OSTEOMYELITIS

Fig. 26.8 The development and continued course of acute osteomyelitis. This differs with age. In infants below 1 year of age the epiphysis is nourished by penetrating arteries through the physis, allowing development of the condition within the epiphysis. In children up to 15 years of age the infection is restricted to below the epiphysis because of interruption of the vessels.

Pathogenesis

In young people, mostly men, *S. aureus* can usually reach the pelvic bones via the blood. The sacroiliac joints, the symphysis and the acetabulum are commonly affected. Osteomyelitis has been noted in athletes, and it is possible that skin lesions with colonizing *S. aureus* are the source of bacteria[35].

In women during the childbearing period, bacteria, usually Gram-negative intestinal organisms and/or anaerobes[12], may spread contiguously from an infectious focus in the pelvic region as a complication of pregnancy or gynecologic disease.

Chronic and subacute osteomyelitis

Clinical features

Chronic osteomyelitis can be intermittent or continuous. The hematogenous form caused by *S. aureus* is now mainly found in elderly people who became infected before the antibiotic era[36], and chronic osteomyelitis in adults is usually post-traumatic or postoperative. The long tubular bones in the lower extremities are most often affected in both forms. The intermittent type presents symptoms either in the form of pain, swelling and increased skin temperature around the affected area, and possibly a moderate rise in body temperature, or as a sinus continuously discharging pus without swelling and often with only slight pain. Subacute Brodie's abscess is another type of osteomyelitis that presents with pain, often without inflammatory signs (Fig. 26.9).

There is almost no mortality in chronic osteomyelitis but the relapse frequency is high (10–20%) and definitive healing is rare even after adequate treatment.

Pathogenesis

Chronic osteomyelitis can develop from an untreated acute osteomyelitis or, more commonly, as a complication of an infected fracture or postoperative infection. Often the vessels are lacerated. The massive bacterial invasion of a vast area promotes propagation of the infection, often in the whole diaphysis. Destruction of the bone tissue is prominent and sequestra and circumscribed abscesses arise. Lysis is followed by new bone deposition. This can grow centrifugally or encroach on the medullary cavity[12].

Sinus formation originating from intraosseous cavities is common, with discharge of pus, infected material and small bone pieces to the skin surface. Defective healing and skeletal malformation are common.

Osteitis

Clinical features

Infections of short and flat bones, particularly common in the feet but also occurring in the hands, and usually discrete, give rise to symptoms and are initiated by infections in the skin and/or soft tissue. The patients often have underlying diseases such as diabetes mellitus or arteriosclerosis. Because of the limited bone infection, fever is not common and pain and other symptoms commonly seen in osteomyelitis are not severe. Sometimes a thin fistula or an abrasion down to the bone surface can be the result of a penetrating infectious process. The chances of retaining the affected region intact are low as the condition usually requires varying degrees of resection or amputation[12].

Pathogenesis

If bacteria disseminate from a contiguous focus in the skin or soft tissues, the cortical bone can be affected. Most often such infections occur in the feet. The short, cancellous bones are the site of low-virulence infection. Destruction is seen but new bone formation is not as pronounced as in osteomyelitis of the long tubular bones.

Septic spondylitis

Clinical features

The symptoms of septic spondylitis are often not distinct and may be misinterpreted. However, there is often tenderness over the affected vertebrae. With the exception of postoperative diskitis[37], which rarely proceeds to spondylitis, the route of infection is hematogenous. Spondylitis is most common in the elderly (50–70 years) and located in the lumbar spine. The onset can be insidious, with increasing fever and uncharacteristic back pain or pain radiating to the thorax or abdomen. In such cases the condition is often misinterpreted as myocardial infarction, pleuropneumonia, cholecystitis or appendicitis[38]. Sometimes the onset is acute, with high body temperature, chills and severe back pain.

The process often starts at the endplate, the vertebrae often becoming affected later (Fig. 26.10) with abscess formation; the nerve roots can be involved, resulting in paresis. The purulent infection can also spread to the surrounding soft tissue, and an associated epidural abscess is also possible (Fig. 26.11). Neurologic or disabling sequelae occur in a small

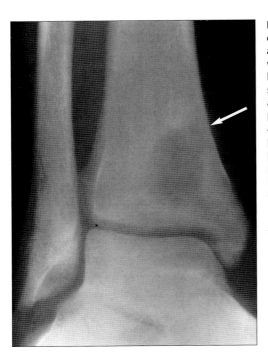

Fig. 26.9 Subacute osteomyelitis (Brodie's abscess). The well-defined oval lucency in the distal tibia shows fading sclerosis along its margins in a pattern typical of a bone abscess. Note the small projection of the upper pole of the lesion pointing to the medial metaphysis, where a subtle periosteal reaction is beginning to form (arrow). This identifies the site where this lesion may ultimately drain.

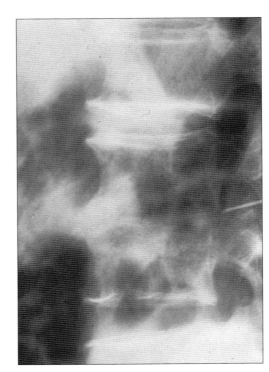

Fig. 26.10 Septic spondylitis of L3 and L4 with destruction of the disc and the adjacent end plates. The aspiration needle for culture and histology is seen. The position of the needle should always be documented with a radiograph.

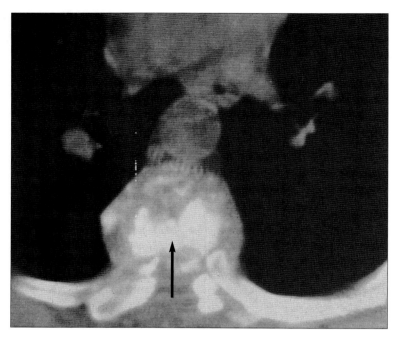

Fig. 26.11 Computed tomography scan showing osteomyelitic destruction of the fourth thoracic vertebral body with soft tissue swelling.

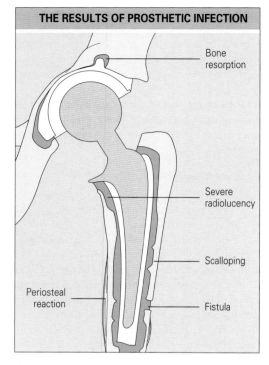

THE RESULTS OF PROSTHETIC INFECTION

Bone resorption

Severe radiolucency

Scalloping

Periosteal reaction

Fistula

Fig. 26.12 The results of prosthetic infection. Periosteal reaction, scalloping, severe radiolucency at the interface, fistula through the bone and severe bone resorption are illustrated. All these changes can also be seen in severe prosthetic mechanical loosening but do not progress as rapidly as in infection.

percentage of cases, but the prospects for complete healing of the infection are good. Serious sequelae are more likely to follow tuberculous infection.

Pathogenesis

Bacteria reach the vertebrae almost exclusively after hematogenous dissemination from a known infectious or cryptogenic focus, as in the case of acute osteomyelitis. The intervertebral space is commonly infected first, with subsequent spread to the adjacent vertebrae. Destruction of the endplate follows and the disk and the vertebrae become compressed. Later, this is often followed by spontaneous interbody vertebral fusion. Local spread of infection is common, with the formation of abscess masses localized in the epidural space or in the soft tissues.

DIAGNOSTIC PROCEDURES AND INVESTIGATIONS

The definite diagnosis of deep, late, especially hematogenous infection may sometimes be difficult. Erythrocyte sedimentation rate (ESR) together with C-reactive protein (CRP) are usually quite sensitive in non-rheumatoid patients, especially in infections associated with joint prostheses. The presence of radiographic changes indicates that an infection has been present for 2–3 weeks or more. Plain radiographs, although not specific, often show a rapidly developing irregular resorption zone around implants, sometimes with an extensive periosteal reaction (Fig. 26.12).

Scintigraphy employing sequential technetium-99m phosphate (three-phase bone scan) is diagnostic aid before radiographic changes appear. In acute hematogenous osteomyelitis with cold lesions caused by a deficient blood supply in a tubular bone, the scan can be repeated after 2–3 days. Computed tomography (CT) and magnetic resonance imaging (MRI) are helpful for the diagnosis but ideal diagnostic tests are still lacking. Indium-111-labeled leukocytes have been used in a few studies and have shown high specificity and sensitivity. In a recent study indium-111 was compared with technetium-99m nanocolloid in 35 patients with suspected infection; nanocolloid showed a sensitivity of 90% and a specificity of 80%, compared to indium[12]. In clinical prac-tice, however, technetium-99m nanocolloid scanning has the advantage of being completed in a day, whereas indium requires the use of autologous granulocytes and a 2-day procedure (Fig. 26.13).

In acute septic arthritis the microbes are generally localized to the synovia, particularly in the initial stage. Bacteria can be killed by phagocytes and thus there is a risk of obtaining negative cultures from the aspirated joint fluid. It is advisable to dilute the aspirated material in a blood-culture bottle in a proportion of about 1:10 to inhibit the bactericidal components of the joint fluid[12]. Repeated aspiration increases both sensitivity and specificity, especially in prosthetic infection.

In addition to cultures it is advisable to make smears for direct microscopy. If it is possible to perform an arthroscopy, or when a synovectomy is indicated, tissue samples should be used for culture[39]. The same procedures are recommended in prosthetic joint infections. Quantification of cultures, with positive tissue biopsies, is important for a clinical diagnosis of infection[12]. Ultrasonication of the implant or tissue has given a higher rate of positive culture. Recently polymerase chain reaction (PCR) techniques with genetic probes for identifying bacteria have been developed but further clinical evaluation is needed before they become general practice.[40–42].

In suspected acute osteomyelitis, pelvic osteomyelitis, sacroiliitis and spondylitis, samples for culture and direct microscopy can often be obtained by needle aspiration or open biopsy[43]. In all these acute infections cultures from blood and suspected infectious foci can facilitate the etiologic diagnosis.

In chronic osteomyelitis and osteitis with fistulae it is not adequate to take cultures from the superficial orifice. This area is usually colonized by irrelevant bacteria[12]. During the surgical exploration of the infectious focus, tissue biopsies are suitable for culture. Blood cultures and cultures from other foci in the body are not indicated, since chronic infection is restricted to the bone.

In spondylitis, puncture and aspiration of the intervertebral space (Fig. 26.10) or of a vertebra under fluoroscopy, for a smear and culture, is a rapid diagnostic method for determining the causative agent[12]. If the patient has septic fever or a focus of origin, blood cultures and a sample from the lesional area should be taken.

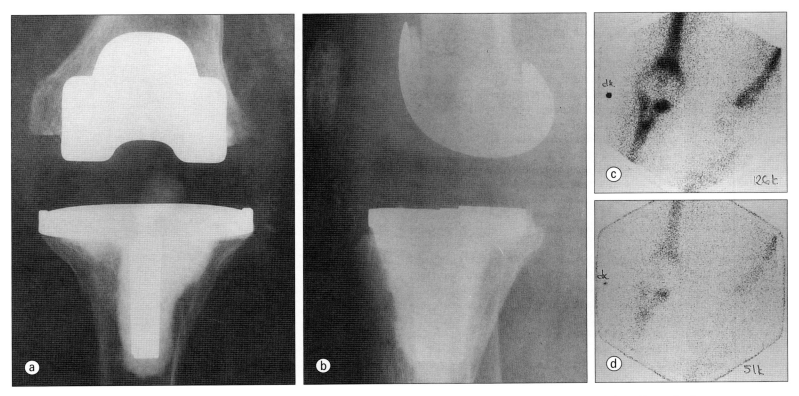

Fig. 26.13 A knee prosthesis 1 year after surgery in a patient with RA and severe pain at rest and on weight-bearing. (a, b) The radiographs show no abnormalities and no radiolucency. (c) Technetium-99m nanocolloid scintigraphy shows obviously increased uptake corresponding to the distal femur and proximal medial tibia. (d) The uptake with indium-111 leukocyte scintigraphy was increased in a similar distribution.

Recommended bacteriologic investigations for acute febrile conditions and chronic conditions are, respectively:

- blood culture, culture from primary foci, smear and culture from the local infectious focus
- representative samples from the deep infectious focus: aspirate or biopsy.

ETIOLOGY

The bacterial etiology in bone and joint infections depends on the type and route of infection. Significant factors are the course of the infection (acute or chronic), pathogenesis (hematogenous or contiguous), the localization of the infection (Table 26.2), the age of the patient and underlying disease. Of great importance also for verifying the etiology are the conditions for sampling and culturing: type and amount of material, media used, accessibility to the laboratory and the quality of the laboratory[12].

With regard to the different bacteria it is difficult to compare various patient materials and to state the relative frequency of microorganisms. *Staphylococcus aureus* is always common in all entities. It is the most common bacteria found in osteomyelitis in all ages and is almost the sole cause of chronic hematogenous osteomyelitis[36]. Coagulase-negative staphylococci and skin anaerobes are opportunistic bacteria but are common in the presence of foreign material. Beta-hemolytic Streptococcus group B is more often seen in neonatal osteomyelitis[44].

TABLE 26.2 BACTERIOLOGIC FINDINGS IN BONE AND JOINT INFECTIONS								
	Acute septic arthritis	Prosthetic joint infection	Bursitis	Acute hematogenous osteomyelitis	Chronic osteomyelitis	Pelvic osteomyelitis	Spondylitis	Diabetic osteitis
Staphylococcus aureus	+++	+++	+++	+++	+++	+++	+++	++
Coagulase-negative staphylococci		+++			+			
Hemolytic streptococcus	++	++	++	++			++	++
Other streptococci	+	+		+			+	+
Skin anaerobes	+	+++		+	+			++
Gram-negative cocci	+			+				
Haemophilus influenzae	+	+		+				
Gram-negative aerobes	+	++	+	+	+	++	++	++
Pseudomonas aeruginosa	+	+		+	+		+	
Salmonella	+	+		+	+		+	
Intestinal anaerobes		+			+	++		++
Mycobacteria	+	+			+		+	
+++ = very common (30% or more)		++ = common (5–30%)			+ = occurs in some circumstances (age, underlying disease, foreign material)			

Haemophilus influenzae is common in hematogenous arthritis in children of 1 month to 5 years of age[45]. This agent, however, is now becoming less common through vaccination of children against infections caused by capsulated *H. influenzae*. *Escherichia coli* was common some years ago in neonatal arthritis and osteomyelitis but as a result of better hygiene it is now less common and is mostly seen in neonatal arthritis[40]. Gram-negative intestinal bacteria are more frequent in the elderly in conditions such as diabetic osteitis, spondylitis and prosthetic joint infections. *Pseudomonas aeruginosa* is found in drug addicts with arthritis and spondylitis, and after trauma. In post-traumatic osteomyelitis, Gram-negative aerobes are becoming increasingly common compared to Gram-positive bacteria. *Salmonella* spp. are more common in developing countries in osteomyelitis, particularly in association with sickle cell anemia, and in arthritis in children[45]. Anaerobes are found almost exclusively in diabetic osteitis and prosthetic joint infections.

Many types of microorganism are found in orthopedic infections but most of them occur only sporadically. *Mycoplasma* spp. and *Ureaplasma* spp. are rare and can cause infections in immunocompromised patients[46]. Mycobacteria, including atypical varieties, can cause arthritis, spondylitis and osteomyelitis. Overall, the global incidence of tuberculosis is rising, which will be reflected in joint and bone infections[47]. In prosthetic joint infections some unusual bacteria spread by the hematogenous route are sometimes found[48]. Moreover, in joint replacement infections, the occurrence of problematic bacteria due to high antibiotic resistance is feared. Bacteria that pose problems include methicillin-resistant *Staphylococcus aureus*, coagulase-negative staphylococci and *Enterococcus faecium*, some species of which are vancomycin-resistant.

Clavicular osteomyelitis can be caused by *S. aureus*, but *Propionibacterium acnes* is also reported as a putative agent[49].

MANAGEMENT OF BACTERIAL INFECTIONS IN BONE AND JOINTS

It has been shown that a dedicated team approach with participation of an infectious disease specialist and an orthopaedic surgeon enhances outcomes of osteomyelitis treatment[12,50]. Prerequisites for successful antibiotic therapy in acute hematogenous osteomyelitis are susceptible causative bacteria, sufficient penetration of drugs to the bone tissue and the affected area and the availability of appropriate forms of administration, i.e. parenteral and well-absorbed oral formulations[12].

In acute hematogenous osteomyelitis, the penetration of antibiotic therapy is impaired as the intraosseous pressure rises and the blood vessels become occluded by edema and microthrombi. At the time when an abscess has developed, the access of antibiotics to the infectious focus is very limited. Therefore, the antibiotics should be instituted within 2–3 days of onset of the clinical symptoms[51].

Factors contributing to decreased efficacy of antibiotics in chronic osteomyelitis are diminished blood flow secondary to deranged bone structure, trauma and sclerosis, the presence of abscesses, sequestra and foreign material, and the development of glycocalyx[26] (Fig. 26.14). *Staphylococcus aureus* can bind to blood and tissue components such as fibrinogen, immunoglobulin G, complement, fibronectin, collagen, vitronectin, laminin and sialoprotein II[52].

Certain strains of *S. aureus*, such as phage-group I strains, are difficult to eradicate and there is an increase in penicillinase-producing or methicillin-resistant staphylococci[35]. The antimicrobial therapy recommendations made below are relevant for countries in which both the frequency of methicillin-resistant staphylococci and the bacterial resistance against antibiotics are lower than 1% (e.g. the Nordic countries). In countries where methicillin-resistance is common, drugs such as vancomycin, teicoplanin, aminoglycosides,

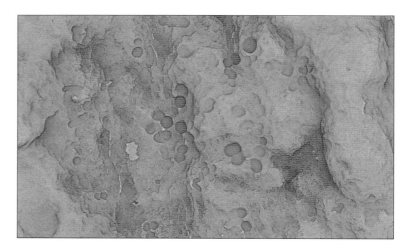

Fig. 26.14 **Bone sequestra found in chronic osteomyelitis have no blood supply and function as foreign bodies with a rough, irregular surface.** In this scanning electron microscopy picture adherent cocci (*S. aureus*) and a few rods (*E. coli*) are displayed.

rifampin (rifampicin), fusidic acid and quinolones must be used, either in single therapy or, preferably, in combination guided by susceptibility.

Septic arthritis, bursitis and prosthetic joint infections

Early and aggressive therapy is imperative to prevent destruction, especially in childhood[53], and mortality, particularly in elderly patients with RA or diabetes. The history, age and underlying diseases are valuable guides in the choice of antibiotic treatment. In all these entities *S. aureus* and other Gram-positive cocci are common and in some countries *H. influenzae* is still predominant in children under 3 years of age with acute arthritis. The occurrence of Gram-negative organisms in the elderly with predisposing diseases, as well as *S. aureus* in RA, must be taken into account[36].

Isoxazolyl penicillins in suspected Gram-positive infection and a cephalosporin in suspected Gram-negative infection are effective in the ordinary acute case. Parenteral cloxacillin 2g t.i.d. or 100mg/kg/day in Gram-positive infections, and cefuroxime 1.5g t.i.d. or 75–80mg/kg/day in Gram-negative infections is recommended. The duration of parenteral therapy should be 7–10 days and thereafter oral drugs, flucloxacillin 1.5g t.i.d. or 75–80mg/kg/day or a cephalosporin, are given for a total of up to 6 weeks[12,54,55].

In prosthetic joint infections a combination of oral clindamycin and ciprofloxacin are alternatives, depending on the bacteriologic findings. This combination may be used for the treatment of coagulase-negative staphylococci often methicillin resistant, which is the most common finding. Other useful combinations are rifampin and ciprofloxacin or rifampin and fusidic acid[56]. In such cases, which are often treated operatively, local treatment with antibiotic-containing bone cement or other vehicles could be used between the first and second operation in a two-stage procedure[12]. Because of methicillin resistance, vancomycin 1g twice daily may also be used, although its use should be restricted because of the high risk of inducing resistance among enterococci.

Bursitis can be treated with drainage and a short course of parenteral cloxacillin or benzyl penicillin, depending on the microbiological findings. In two-thirds of cases *S. aureus* or streptococci will be the dominant microorganism and subsequent oral treatment should be given for only 1–2 weeks[28].

In septic arthritis of the hip, surgical drainage of the joint is effective and necessary. In case of infection in other joints, repeated aspiration should be performed if no pus is found initially. However, if aspiration

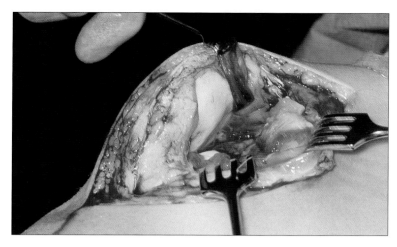

Fig. 26.15 Particularly in postoperative and post-traumatic arthritis with no response to antibiotic treatment, a pannus formation, as seen here on the femoral condyle, may develop.

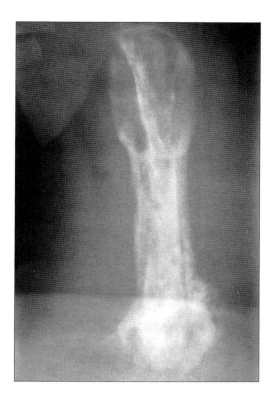

Fig. 26.16 Chronic osteomyelitis with sequestrum and involucrum in an 18-month-old boy.

is unsuccessful or if the symptoms increase within the first 24–48 hours, an arthrotomy is necessary. Arthroscopy has been used as an alternative and is also effective for irrigation of the joint. The early use of devices for passive motion has reduced the need for surgical mobilization after bacterial arthritis. The joint is protected from weight-bearing for an average of 6 weeks. However, the patient is mobilized as soon as the pain has subsided normally within the first week. Late synovectomy has been performed in the knee joint to prevent cartilage destruction and subsequent osteoarthritis[39] (Fig. 26.15).

The treatment of infected joint implants is complicated. Factors influencing the choice of treatment include the condition of the patient and the adjacent joint soft tissue, the quality of the bone stock, the type of primary revision implants, the type and sensitivity of the infected organism, the patient's daily activity requirements and finally the rarity of the problem. The treatment of these patients should be centralized, especially decisions on definitive treatment from among long-term antibiotics, revision arthroplasty, arthrodesis and, rarely, amputation.

The surgical procedure in itself, involving meticulous removal of all foreign material in a staged procedure before the insertion of a new prosthesis, also calls for centralized treatment. The fusion rate in arthrodesis and the healing rate of an infected knee prosthesis is improved if the patient is treated at an experienced center[57]. The septic complication in a joint implant carries an overall mortality from 5% in knee prostheses up to 15% for hip prostheses[57].

Acute hematogenous osteomyelitis

Streptococci and S. aureus dominate in juveniles and adults[58]. In addition to these, H. influenzae and E. coli can also occur in neonatal osteomyelitis, and E. coli and other intestinal bacteria in the elderly.

Beta-lactam antibiotics, clindamycin, fusidic acid, certain quinolones, such as ciprofloxacin, and rifampin are known to penetrate bone tissue in sufficient amounts. Erythromycin and aminoglycosides have inadequate penetration properties[12].

Administration of parenteral antibiotics is indicated initially in acute hematogenous osteomyelitis, followed by an oral regime. Penicillins with a spectrum against Gram-positive bacteria or cephalosporins against Gram-positive and Gram-negative bacteria are the drugs of choice for acute hematogenous osteomyelitis. Clindamycin, fusidic acid and ciprofloxacin are alternatives in specified situations, based on bacteriologic findings and/or penicillin hypersensitivity. Combinations containing erythromycin, aminoglycosides and rifampin have been used but are second choices.

Staphylococcus aureus must be covered in all age groups. A combination of benzyl penicillin and isoxazolyl penicillin, or a corresponding drug, is recommended. The former is more effective against penicillin-sensitive S. aureus and streptococci and the latter against penicillinase-producing staphylococci. High doses should be used, preferably 150mg/kg/day and 100mg/kg/day respectively, in three divided doses[12].

In acute hematogenous osteomyelitis, abscesses should be drained, since decompression prevents further obstruction of blood vessels and resulting bone necrosis. Drainage also results in a dramatic improvement in the patient's general condition. If antibiotic treatment has not been started early and decompression has not been carried out, the trabecular bone may be sequestered and eventually embedded in new bone (Fig. 26.16). Weight-bearing on the extremity should be avoided until radiographic signs of bone restoration are present because there is a high risk of pathologic fracture[12].

When culture results become available, one of the two antibiotics can be withdrawn. The duration of therapy has been discussed in several articles and is proposed to be 3 weeks[34]. However, there are great difficulties involved in keeping children in hospital to receive intravenous antibiotics for such a long time. Parenteral treatment can be limited to 1 week, followed by oral treatment for up to a total of about 2 months[12].

In age groups in which H. influenzae or Gram-negative intestinal bacteria are suspected as being the cause of acute hematogenous osteomyelitis, cloxacillin should be combined with ampicillin or, preferably, a cephalosporin effective against this flora, e.g. cefuroxime, should be chosen. This drug also has sustained effect against Gram-positive bacteria. In cases of unknown etiology and in which either Gram-positive or Gram-negative bacteria are possible, cefuroxime is again the more suitable choice[12].

In elderly patients, in whom Gram-negative bacteria are common as a consequence of urinary, biliary, intestinal and lower respiratory infections or invasive diagnostic procedures at these sites, treatment with broad-spectrum antibiotics, e.g. broad-spectrum penicillins, cefuroxime, cefotaxime or trimethoprim–sulphamethoxazole, is indicated.

Parenteral treatment should be given until fever and the local signs of infection have disappeared, which usually takes 7–10 days. Laboratory variables such as ESR or CRP should be monitored, and normalization of these variables may be interpreted as evidence of the effectiveness of the antibiotic treatment. If chronic osteomyelitis with radiographic changes develops, treatment should be continued for up to 6 months, particularly in cases of staphylococcal etiology[36]. By instituting early systemic antibiotic treatment, it is possible to prevent the development of radiographic changes. The prognosis is directly related to the time at which antibiotic therapy was instituted[51]. Only when an abscess is demonstrable is operative drainage superior to antibiotic treatment[59].

Spondylitis and pelvic osteomyelitis

The evolution of spondylitis is often slow and the prognosis mostly good. There is therefore no need for haste in instituting antibiotic therapy. It is better to first attain a confirmed diagnosis and establish the etiology as far as possible. Usually, acute spondylitis with intensive symptoms such as fever, pain and disability is treated in the same way as acute hematogenous osteomyelitis, depending on disease history and bacterial findings. In the case of progressing neurology, surgical decompression is necessary. MRI is helpful in showing epidural abscess, which sometimes calls for immediate surgery. In hematogenous pelvic osteomyelitis *S. aureus* is the most common agent, particularly in patients under 50 years of age, and the onset is often more acute.

In cases of Gram-positive and *E. coli* infection, antibiotic therapy for 2–3 months is often sufficient if the radiographic findings are discrete. *Salmonella*-induced and tuberculous spondylitis are more difficult to heal, and a longer period of treatment – 6–12 months – is often needed[12].

Chronic osteomyelitis

The treatment of chronic osteomyelitis is more difficult and less well standardized than that of acute infection. Recurrences of infection are common in chronic osteomyelitis, and extensive surgery and debridement is an important part of successful therapy.

Bacteriologic and pharmacologic data make isoxazolyl penicillins the drugs of choice in chronic hematogenous osteomyelitis. They are tolerated well even in high doses, with a low rate of toxic side effects; rash and diarrhea are seen only in a few cases. There is a low risk of developing chromosomal resistance but this has not been a problem despite general long-term treatment. Generally oral drugs, such as flucloxacillin 1.5g t.i.d, could be used[12]. Probenecid, 1g b.d., enhances the serum concentration and lowers the protein binding of isoxazolyl penicillins. Clindamycin, fusidic acid and cephalosporins with effect against Gram-positive bacteria are alternatives for the treatment of patients with penicillin allergy. If the treatment fails, rifampin 0.6–0.9g daily, which penetrates into the granulocytes and kills intracellularly localized staphylococci, may be added in combination with isoxazolyl penicillin. Parenteral antibiotics should be used only for 1–2 days perioperatively in connection with the surgery, giving oral drugs for the rest of the long-term treatment period. Prolonged parenteral antibiotic therapy is not necessary but the total period of treatment should be extended. The doubling time and the metabolism of the bacteria are very slow in osteomyelitis, which necessitates prolonged treatment[60].

The long-term results are very good, and high-dose oral antibiotics for at least 6 months are tolerable and sufficient in combination with surgery. In cases where surgery is contraindicated or not accepted by the patient, antibiotics alone are usually sufficient.

Radiographic changes are already present, so careful planning is required in order to decide whether or not a sequestrum is present and whether surgical intervention is necessary. This could include procedures ranging from a simple sequestrectomy and removal of granulation tissue up to removal of an entire section of tubular bone followed by subsequent bone transplantation. Intramedullary reaming has been used for chronic hematogenous osteomyelitis with severe pain at rest, in order to re-establish a new medullary cavity and improve endosteal circulation[61].

REFERENCES

1. Bick EM. Source book of orthopedics. Hafner: New York; 1968.
2. Le Cocq JF, le Cocq E. Use of neoarsphenamine in treatment of acute *S. aureus* septicaemia and osteomyelitis. J Bone Joint Surg 1941; 23: 596–597.
3. Lidgren L, Lindberg L. Orthopedic infections during a 5-year period. Acta Orthop Scand 1972; 43: 325–334.
4. Danielsson L, Uden A. Diagnostik och behandling av akut hematogen osteit hos barn. Lakartidningen 1981; 4: 241–244.
5. Gillespie WJ, Nade S. Musculoskeletal infections. Oxford: Blackwell Scientific Publications; 1987.
6. Smith I. *Staphylococcus aureus*. In: Mandell GL, Douglas R, Bennett JE, eds. Principles and practice of infectious diseases. New York: John Wiley & Sons; 1979: 1530–1532.
7. Boda A. The problem of osteomyelitis in Hungary. In: Meeting of the European study group on bone and joint infections, Vienna, 27 August 1983.
8. Digby JM, Kersley JB. Pyogenic non-tuberculous spinal infection: an analysis of thirty cases. J Bone Joint Surg 1979; 61B: 47–55.
9. Silverthorn KM, Gillespie WJ. Pyogenic vertebrae osteomyelitis. NZ Med J 1986; 99: 62–65.
10. El-Gindi S, Aref S, Salama M, Andrew J. Infection of intervertebral discs after operation. J Bone Joint Surg 1976; 57A: 1104–1106.
11. Lindholm T S, Pylkkanen P. Discitis following removal of intervertebral disc: a report on 120 patients. Spine 1982; 7: 618–622.
12. Hedström SÅ, Lidgren L. Orthopedic infections. Lund: Studentlitteratur; 1988.
13. Fox L, Sprunt K. Neonatal osteomyelitis. Pediatrics 1978; 62: 535–542.
14. Welkon CJ, Long SS, Fischer MC, Alburger PD. Pyogenic arthritis in infants and children: a review of 95 cases. Infect Dis 1986; 5: 669–676.
15. Mitchell M, Howard B, Haller J *et al*. Septic arthritis. Radiol Clin North Am 1988; 26: 1295–1313.
16. Griffin PP. Acute septic arthritis of the hip in childhood: its pathogenesis and treatment. Hip 1979; 4: 89–104.
17. Freeland AE, Senter BS. Septic arthritis and osteomyelitis. Hand Clin 1989; 5: 533–552.
18. Alderson M, Speers D, Emslie KR, Nade S. Acute hematogenous osteomyelitis and septic arthritis – a single disease. A hypothesis based upon the presence of transphyseal blood vessels. J Bone Joint Surg 1986; 68B: 268–274.
19. Lane Smith R, Schurman DJ, Kajiyama G *et al*. The effect of antibiotics on the destruction of cartilage in experimental infectious arthritis. J Bone Joint Surg 1987; 69A: 1063–1068.
20. Goldenberg DL, Reed JI. Bacterial arthritis. N Engl J Med 1985; 312: 764–771.
21. Powers KA, Terpenning MS, Voice RA, Kauffman CA. Prosthetic joint infections in the elderly. Am J Med 1990; 88: 9N–13N.
22. Dubost JJ, Soubrier M, De Champs C *et al*. No changes in the distribution of organisms responsible for septic arthritis over a 20 year period. Ann Rheum Dis 2002; 61: 267–269.
23. Lidgren L. Joint prosthetic infections: A success story. Acta Orthop Scand 2001; 72(6): 553–556.
24. Gristina AG. Biomaterial-centered infection: microbial adhesion versus tissue integration. Science 1987; 237: 1588–1595.
25. Garvin KL, Hanssen AD. Infection after total hip arthroplasty. Past, present, and future. J Bone Joint Surg 1995; 77A: 1576–1588.
26. Gristina AG, Shibata Y, Giridhar G *et al*. The glycocalyx, biofilm, microbes, and resistant infections. Semin Arthroplasty 1994; 5: 160–170.
27. Trampuz A, Osmon DR, Hanssen AD, et al Molecular and antibiofilm approaches to prosthetic joint infection. Clin Orthop Rel Res 2003;414:69-88.
28. Zimmerman III B, Mikolich DJ, Ho G. Septic bursitis. Semin Arthritis Rheum 1995; 24: 391–410.
29. Söderqvist B, Hedström SÅ. Predisposing factors, bacteriology and antibiotic therapy in 35 cases of septic bursitis. Scand J Infect Dis 1986; 18: 305–311.
30. Sandberg-Sørensen T, Hedeboe J, Rostgaard-Christensen E. Primary epiphyseal osteomyelitis in children. J Bone Joint Surg 1988; 70B: 818–820.
31. Fitzgerald RH. Pathogenesis of musculoskeletal sepsis. In: Hughes SPF, Fitzgerald RH, eds. Musculoskeletal infections. Chicago, IL: Year Book Medical Publishers; 1986: 14–33.
32. Wald ER. Risk factors for osteomyelitis. Am J Med 1985; 78: 206–212.
33. Peterson HA. Hematogenous osteomyelitis in children. Instr Course Lect 1983; 32: 33–37.
34. Emslie KR, Nade S. Acute hematogenous staphylococcal osteomyelitis. A description of the natural history in an avian model. Am J Pathol 1983; 110: 3333–45.
35. Hedström SÅ, Lidgren L. Acute hematogenous pelvic osteomyelitis in athletes. Am J Sports Med 1982; 1: 44–46.

36. Hedström SÅ. Staphylococcal problems in orthopedic infections. In: Hedström SÅ, ed. Advances of staphylococcal infections. Södertälje: Astra Alab AB; 1987: 87–99.

37. Dall BE, Rowe DE, Odette WG, Batts DH. Postoperative discitis. Diagnosis and management. Clin Orthop 1987; 224: 138–146.

38. Musher DM, Thorsteinsson SB, Minuth JN, Luchi RJ. Vertebral osteomyelitis: still a diagnostic pitfall. Arch Intern Med 1976; 136: 105–110.

39. Törholm C, Hedström SÅ, Sundèn G, Lidgren L. Synovectomy in bacterial arthritis. Acta Orthop Scand 1983; 54: 748–753.

40. Lidgren L, Knutson K, Stéfansdóttir A. Infection of prosthetic joints. Best Pract Res Clin Rheumatol 2003;17:209-218.

41. Tunney MM, Patrick S, Gorman SP, et al. Improved detection of infection in hip replacements: a currently underestimated problem. J Bone Joint Surg 1998;80-B: 568-572.

42. Mariani BD, Martin DS, Levine MJ, et al. Polymerase chain reaction detection of bacterial infection in total knee arthroplasty. Clin Orthop Rel Res 1996;331:11-22.

43. Kasser JR. Hematogenous osteomyelitis. Untangling the diagnostic confusion. Postgrad Med 1984; 76: 79–86.

44. Jackson MA, Nelson JD. Etiology and management of acute suppurative bone and joint infections in pediatric patients. J Pediatr Orthop 1982; 2: 315–319.

45. Cavell B, Hedström SÅ. Septic *Salmonella* bone and joint infections in 2 infants. Opuscula Medica 1989; 34: 53–54.

46. Jorup-Rönström C, Ahl T, Hammarström L *et al.* Septic osteomyelitis and polyarthritis with *Ureaplasma* in hypogammaglobulinemia. Infection 1989; 17: 301–303.

47. Jellis JE. Bacterial infections: bone and joint tuberculosis. Baillière's Clin Rheumatol 1995; 9: 151–159.

48. Hedström SÅ, Lidgren L. Les infections hèmatogènes sur prothèses articulaires et leur prèvention. In: L'infection en chirurgie ortopèdique GEEIOA, ed. Expansion Scientifique Francaise (SOFCOT) no. 37: Paris; 1990: 102–105.

49. Alessi DM, Sercarz JA, Calcaterra TC. Osteomyelitis of the clavicle. Arch Otolaryngol Head Neck Surg 1988; 114: 1000–1002.

50. Ziran BH, Rao N, Hall RA. A dedicated team approach enhances outcomes of osteomyelitis treatment. Clin Orthop Rel Res 2003;414:31-36.

51. Vaughan PA, Newman NM, Rosman MA. Acute hematogenous osteomyelitis in children. J Pediatr Orthop 1987; 7: 652–655.

52. Rydén C. Studies on interactions between staphylococcal cells and some connective tissue components. Thesis, University of Uppsala, 1987.

53. Shaw BA, Kasser JR. Acute septic arthritis in infancy and childhood. Clin Orthop 1990; 257: 212–225.

54. Mader JT, Wang J, Calhoun JH. Antibiotic therapy for musculoskeletal infections. An Instructional Course Lecture, American Academy of Orthopaedic Surgeons. J Bone Joint Surg 2001;83-A(12):1878-1890.

55. Osmon DR. Antimicrobial resistance: guidelines for the practicing orthopaedic surgeon. An Instructional Course Lecture, American Academy of Orthopaedic Surgeons. J Bone Joint Surg 2001;83-A(12): 1891-1901.

56. Stengel D, Bauwens K, Sehouli J, Ekkernkamp A, Porzsolt F. Systematic review and meta-analysis of antibiotic therapy for bone and joint infections. Lancet Infectious Diseases 2001; 1: 175–188.

57. Knutson K, Lindstrand A, Lidgren L. Arthrodesis for failed knee arthroplasty. A report of 20 cases. J Bone Joint Surg 1985; 67B: 47–52.

58. Armstrong EP, Rush DR. Treatment of osteomyelitis. Clin Pharm, 1983; 2: 213–224.

59. LaMont RL, Anderson PA, Dajani AS, Thirumoorthi MC. Acute hematogenous osteomyelitis in children. J Pediatr Orthop 1987; 7: 579–583.

60. Zak O, Reilly TO. Animal models as predictors of the safety and efficacy of antibiotics. Eur J Clin Microbiol Inf Dis 1990; 9: 472–478.

61. Lidgren L, Törholm C. Intramedullary reaming in chronic diaphyseal osteomyelitis. Clin Orthop 1980; 151: 215–221.

27 Lyme disease

Allen C Steere

Definition

- A tick-borne infection caused by the spirochete *Borrelia burgdorferi*, *B. afzelii* or *B. garinii* leading to multisystem illness primarily in the skin, joints, nervous system and/or heart

Clinical features

- Peak onset in the summer months in endemic areas in North America, Europe or Asia
- First clinical sign usually a slowly expanding skin lesion, erythema migrans, which occurs at the site of the tick bite
- Disseminated infection often associated with characteristic manifestations in the skin, joints, nervous system and/or heart
- Diagnosis usually based on characteristic clinical findings and a positive IgG serologic test for *B. burgdorferi*
- Treatment with oral antibiotics except for objective neurologic abnormalities, which seem to require intravenous antibiotic therapy

LYME DISEASE

History

Lyme disease was described as a separate entity in 1976 because of geographic clustering of children in Lyme, Connecticut who were believed to have juvenile rheumatoid arthritis[1]. The rural setting of the case clusters and the identification of erythema migrans as a feature of the illness suggested that the disorder was transmitted by an arthropod. It soon became apparent that Lyme disease was a multisystem illness that affected primarily the skin, nervous system, heart or joints[2]. Epidemiologic studies of patients with erythema migrans implicated certain *Ixodes* ticks as vectors of the disease[3].

In addition to providing clues about the cause of the illness, erythema migrans linked Lyme disease with certain syndromes in Europe. Early in this century, Afzelius in Sweden and Lipschutz in Austria[4] described a characteristic expanding skin lesion, called erythema migrans or erythema chronicum migrans, which they attributed to *Ixodes ricinus* tick bites. Many years later, it was recognized that erythema migrans could be followed by a chronic skin disease, acrodermatitis chronica atrophicans, which had already been described as a separate entity[5]. In the 1940s, Bannwarth in Germany defined a syndrome, also called tick-borne meningo-polyneuritis, that consisted of radicular pain followed by chronic lymphocytic meningitis and sometimes cranial or peripheral neuritis[6]. These various syndromes were brought together conclusively in 1982 and 1983 with the recovery of a previously unrecognized spirochete from the tick vector[7] and from infected patients[8].

Lyme disease or Lyme borreliosis is now recognized as an important infectious disease in North America, Europe and Asia[9]. In the USA, the infection is caused by *Borrelia burgdorferi*, whereas in Europe it is caused primarily by *Borrelia afzelii* and *Borrelia garinii*, and only these two species are responsible for the illness in Asia[10].

Epidemiology

Since surveillance for Lyme disease was begun by the Centers for Disease Control and Prevention in 1982, the number of reported cases has increased dramatically. Currently, about 15 000 cases are reported each year, making Lyme disease the most common vector-borne disease in the USA[11]. The disorder occurs primarily in three distinct foci: in the northeast from Maine to Maryland, in the midwest in Wisconsin and Minnesota, and in the west in northern California and Oregon (Fig. 27. 1). In Europe, Lyme borreliosis is widely established in forested areas[12]. The highest reported frequencies of the disease are in middle Europe and Scandinavia, particularly in Germany, Austria, Slovenia and Sweden. The infection also occurs in Russia, China and Japan.

Lyme borreliosis is transmitted by ticks of the *Ixodes ricinus* complex, including *I. scapularis* in the northeastern and north central USA, *I. pacificus* in the western states, *I. ricinus* in Europe and *I. persulcatus* in Asia[13]. These ticks, which are nearly identical in appearance, have larval, nymphal and adult stages; they require a blood meal at each stage (Fig. 27.2). The risk of infection in a given area depends largely on the density of these ticks, and on their feeding habits and animal hosts, which have evolved differently in different geographic locations.

In the north eastern and north central USA, *I. scapularis* (also called *I. dammini*) ticks are abundant, and a highly efficient cycle of

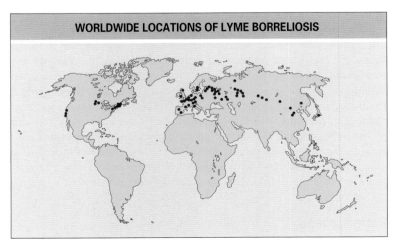

WORLDWIDE LOCATIONS OF LYME BORRELIOSIS

Fig. 27.1 Worldwide locations of Lyme borreliosis. The red markers show affected locations in North America, Europe and Asia.

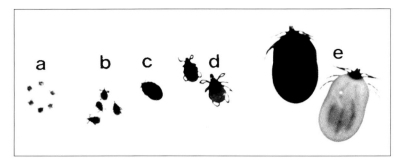

Fig. 27.2 The life-cycle stages of *Ixodes scapularis*, the tick that transmits Lyme disease in the northeastern and north central USA. (a) Tiny larval ticks, which are <1mm in diameter. (b) Unengorged nymphal ticks, which are only 1–2mm in diameter. This stage of the tick is primarily responsible for transmission of the spirochete to humans during the late spring and early summer. (c) An engorged nymphal tick. (d) Unengorged adult male (black) and female (orange) ticks. (e) Engorged adult male and female ticks. (From Steere AC. Lyme desease. N Engl J Med 1989; 321:586–596. © 1989. With permission of Massachusetts Medical Society. All rights reserved.)

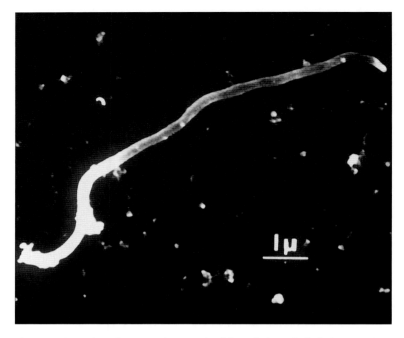

Fig. 27.3 Scanning electron micrograph of *Borrelia burgdorferi*. The *Borrelia* spp. are longer and more loosely coiled than the other spirochetes. Of the *Borrelia* spp., *B. burgdorferi* is the longest (20–30μm) and narrowest (0.2–0.3μm).

B. burgdorferi transmission occurs between immature larval and nymphal *I. scapularis* and white-footed mice[14], resulting in high infection rates in nymphal ticks and a high frequency of human Lyme disease during the late spring and summer months[11]. The vector ecology of *B. burgdorferi* is quite different on the West coast in northern California and Oregon[15]. There, the frequency of Lyme disease is low because nymphal *I. pacifius* ticks often feed on lizards rather than rodents, and lizards are not susceptible to *B. burgdorferi* infection. Similarly, in the southeastern USA, nymphal *I. scapularis* feed primarily on lizards, and *B. burgdorferi* infection occurs rarely, if at all, in that part of the country. There, a skin rash resembling erythema migrans, which is not caused by *B. burgdorferi*, has been associated with the bite of the Lone-Star tick[16].

Etiologic agent

As with all spirochetes, the *Borrelia* species have a protoplasmic cylinder surrounded by periplasm containing the flagella, which is surrounded, in turn, by an outer membrane (Fig. 27.3).[17] The unique feature of *Borrelia* species is that a number of their outer membrane proteins are encoded by plasmid genes. Recently, the complete genome of *B. burgdorferi* sensu stricto (strain B31) was sequenced[18]. The genome is quite small (approximately 1.5 megabases) and consists of a highly unusual linear chromosome of 950kb, in addition to nine linear and 12 circular plasmids.

The remarkable aspect of the *B. burgdorferi* genome is the large number of sequences for predicted or known lipoproteins[18], including the plasmid-encoded outer-surface proteins (Osp) A–F. These and other differentially expressed outer-surface proteins presumably help the spirochete to adapt to and survive in markedly different arthropod and mammalian environments[19]. In addition, during early, disseminated infection, a surface-exposed lipoprotein, called VlsE, has been reported to undergo extensive antigenic variation[20]. The organism has a minimal number of proteins with biosynthetic activity and apparently depends on the host for much of its nutritional requirements[18]. The genome contains no homologs for systems specialized in the secretion of toxins or other virulence factors. The only known virulence factors of *B. burgdorferi* are surface proteins that allow spirochetal attachment to mammalian cells.

Pathogenesis

To maintain its complex life enzootic cycle, *B. burgdorferi* must adapt to two markedly different environments, the tick and the mammalian host[21]. In the midgut of the tick, the spirochete expresses OspA and OspB, two closely related proteins[22]. When the blood meal is taken, OspC is upregulated as the organism traverses to the tick salivary gland and to the mammalian host[23]. After injection by the tick, the spirochete usually spreads locally in the skin, and within days to weeks it may disseminate. *B. burgdorferi* has a number of mechanisms that may aid dissemination. For example, OspC sequences vary considerably among strains, and only a few of the OspC sequence groups are associated with disseminated disease[24]. Spread through skin and other tissue matrices may be facilitated by the spirochete's binding of human plasminogen and its activators to its surface[25]. The organism migrates through the endothelium primarily at intracellular junctions, but may also penetrate through the cytoplasm of the cell[26]. During dissemination and homing to specific sites, the organism attaches to certain host integrins[27], matrix glycosaminoglycans[28] and extracellular matrix proteins[29]. For example, *Borrelia* decorin binding proteins A and B bind decorin, a glycosaminoglycan on collagen fibrils, which may explain why the organism is commonly aligned with collagen fibrils in the extracellular matrix in the heart, nervous system or joints[30]. Decorin-deficient mice have lesser bacterial colonization of joints and milder arthritis than normal mice of the same strain that express decorin[31].

As shown definitively in murine models, proinflammatory innate immune responses are critical in the control of early, disseminated infection[32,33]. Spirochetal lipoproteins, which bind the CD14 molecule and Toll-like receptor-2 on macrophages, are potent activators of the innate immune response, leading to the production of macrophage-derived proinflammatory cytokines[34]. In addition, T helper 1 cells (Th1), which are a part of the adaptive immune response, are prominent early in the murine infection[35]. In humans, infiltrates of macrophages and T cells in erythema migrans lesions express mRNA for both proinflammatory (Th1) and anti-inflammatory (Th2) cytokines[36]. Particularly in disseminated infection, adaptive T and B cell responses in lymph nodes lead to antibody production to many components of the organism[37,38].

Spread of *B. burgdorferi* within the nervous system has been demonstrated in non-human primates[39], which are the only known animal model of neuroborreliosis. In immunosuppressed monkeys, which had a larger spirochetal burden than immunocompetent animals, *B. burgdorferi* localized to the leptomeninges, motor and sensory nerve roots and dorsal root ganglia, but not to the brain parenchyma[40]. In the peripheral nervous system, spirochetes were seen in the perineurium, the connective tissue sheath surrounding each bundle of peripheral nerve fibers.

During attacks of arthritis in human patients, innate immune responses are found to *B. burgdorferi* lipoproteins, and $\gamma\delta$ T cells in joint fluid may aid in this response[41]. In addition, marked adaptive immune responses are seen to many spirochetal proteins[38,42]. A borrelia-specific, proinflammatory Th1 response is concentrated in joint fluid[43,44], but anti-inflammatory (Th2) cytokines are also present[44]. Furthermore, patients with Lyme arthritis usually have higher borrelia-specific antibody titers than patients with any other manifestation of the illness, including late neuroborreliosis[38,45]. In the murine infection, antibody responses are critical in the resolution of arthritis[46,47], whereas cellular responses are the dominant factor in resolution of the cardiac lesion[48,49].

Compared with patients with treatment responsive arthritis, those with a treatment-resistant course have an increased frequency of HLA-DRBI*0401 or related alleles, and they more often have cellular and humoral immune responses to OspA[42,50]. It has been proposed that autoimmunity may develop within the proinflammatory milieu of affected joints in patients with treatment-resistant arthritis because of molecular mimicry between an immunodominant T cell epitope of OspA (OspA$_{165-173}$) of *B. burgdorferi* and a similar sequence in a human protein, perhaps human lymphocyte function associated antigen-1 (hLFA-1$\alpha_{332-340}$)[51], an adhesion molecule that is highly expressed on T

cells in synovium[52]. OspA$_{165-173}$-reactive T cells are concentrated in the joints of these patients[53]. When hLFA-1$\alpha_{332-340}$ is processed and presented by the DRB1*0401 molecule, this self peptide may behave as a partial agonist for such cells[54]. However, hLFA-1 may not be the only, or even the most important, autoantigen in treatment-resistant Lyme arthritis.

Clinical features

As with syphilis, Lyme disease generally occurs in stages, with different clinical manifestations at each stage. Early infection consists of stage 1 (localized erythema migrans), followed within days to weeks by stage 2 (disseminated infection particularly affecting the nervous system, heart or joints), followed within weeks to months by late infection (stage 3, persistent infection)[55]. The basic outlines of the disease are similar worldwide, but there are regional variations, primarily between America and Eurasia (Table 27.1).

Skin manifestations

Erythema migrans and early disseminated infection, and acrodermatitis

In 80% or more of American patients, Lyme disease begins with a slowly expanding skin lesion, erythema migrans, which occurs at the site of the tick bite (Fig. 27.4)[56]. As the area around the center expands, most lesions develop bright red outer borders with partial central clearing. The centers of early lesions sometimes become intensely erythematous and indurated, vesicular or necrotic. In Europe, erythema migrans is often an indolent, localized infection, whereas this lesion in the USA is associated with more intense inflammation and signs that often

TABLE 27.1 COMPARISON OF LYME DISEASE IN NORTH AMERICA AND EURASIA		
Systems affected	North America (*B. burgdorferi*)	Europe and Asia (*B. afzelii* or *B. garinii*)
Skin		
Acute phase	Erythema migrans faster spreading, more intensely inflamed, and of briefer duration; frequent, possibly widespread hematogenous dissemination	Erythema migrans slower spreading, less intensely inflamed and of longer duration; less frequent hematogeneous dissemination, but possible regional or contiguous spread to other sites
Chronic phase	Acrodermatitis rarely reported	Acrodermatitis chronica atrophicans, caused primarily by *B. afzelii*
Nervous system		
Acute phase	Meningitis, severe headache, mild neck stiffness, less prominent radiculoneuritis	Severe radicular pain and pleocytosis, less prominent headache and neck stiffness, caused particularly by *B. garinii*
Chronic phase	Subtle sensory polyneuropathy without acrodermatitis Subtle encephalopathy, cognitive disturbance, slight intrathecal antibody production	Subtle sensory polyneuropathy within areas affected by acrodermatitis Severe sensory polyneuropathy within areas affected by acrodermatitis Severe encephalomyelitis, spasticity, cognitive abnormalities, and marked intrathecal antibody production, caused primarily by *B. garinii*
Cardiac		
Acute phase	Atrioventricular block and subtle myocarditis	Atrioventricular block and subtle myocarditis
Chronic phase	None reported	Dilated cardiomyopathy
Arthritis		
Acute phase	More frequent oligoarticular arthritis, more intense joint inflammation	Less frequent oligoarticular arthritis, less intense joint inflammation
Chronic phase	Treatment-resistant arthritis in about 10 percent of patients, probably due to autoimmune mechanism	Persistent arthritis rare, probably not due to an autoimmune mechanism
Asymptomatic infection		
	In about 10 percent of patients	In more than 10 percent of patients
Antibody response		
	Expansion of response to many spirochetal proteins	Expansion of response to fewer spirochetal proteins

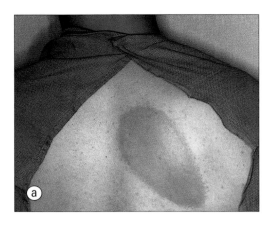

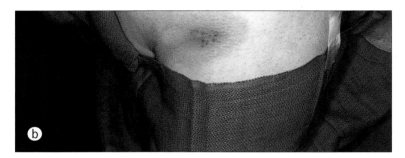

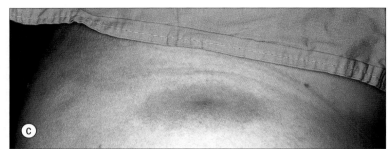

Fig. 27.4 Erythema migrans of Lyme disease. Lyme disease usually begins with a slowly expanding skin lesion, erythema migrans, that occurs at the site of a tick bite. (a) Classic erythema migrans skin lesion (10cm in diameter) on the back. The lesion has a redder outer border, with slight central clearing. (b) Pale lesion (7cm in diameter) with several vesicles in the center, near the groin. (c) Pale lesion (5cm in diameter) with a target center over the iliac crest. In each instance, *B. burgdorferi* was isolated from a skin biopsy sample of the lesion. (Courtesy of Dr Vijay Sikand, East Lyme, CT, USA.)

suggest dissemination of the spirochete[57]. In one study, spirochetes were cultured from plasma samples in 50% of American patients with erythema migrans[58].

Although the list of the possible manifestations of the disease is long (Table 27.2), disseminated infection is often associated with characteristic symptoms in the skin, nervous system or musculoskeletal sites[55,56]. Excruciating headache, particularly in the back of the head, and mild neck stiffness are common – a picture that raises the possibility of meningitis. Among 12 patients who had such symptoms associated with erythema migrans, eight had a positive test for *B. burgdorferi* DNA in cerebrospinal fluid, but none had a spinal fluid pleocytosis at that time[59]. The musculoskeletal pain is often migratory in joints, bursae, tendons, muscle or bone, lasting only hours in a given location. Fever, if present, is typically low grade, except in young children. At this stage, patients often have debilitating malaise and fatigue.

In European patients, especially elderly women with *B. afzelii* infection, a chronic, slowly progressive skin condition called acrodermatitis chronica atrophicans may develop on sun-exposed acral surfaces[60]. These lesions, which may be the presenting manifestation of the disease, may last for many years, and *B. burgdorferi* has been cultured from such lesions as late as 10 years after disease onset[61].

Neurologic manifestations

Within weeks, during or shortly after the period of early disseminated infection, about 15% of untreated patients in the USA develop objective signs and symptoms of acute neuroborreliosis[55,62]. Possible manifestations include lymphocytic meningitis with episodic headache and mild neck stiffness, subtle encephalitis with difficulty with mental functioning, cranial neuropathy (particularly unilateral or bilateral facial palsy), motor or sensory radiculoneuritis, mononeuritis multiplex, cerebellar ataxia or myelitis[62–64]. In Europe, the first neurologic sign is often radicular pain, which is followed by the development of a pleocytosis in cerebrospinal fluid, but meningeal or encephalitic signs are more often absent[65]. In children, the optic nerve may also be affected because of inflammation or increased intracranial pressure, which may lead to blindness[66]. However, even in untreated patients, acute neurologic involvement typically improves or resolves within weeks to months.

In 5% or fewer of untreated patients, *B. burgdorferi* may cause chronic neuroborreliosis, sometimes after long periods of latent infection[67]. In both America and Europe, a chronic axonal polyneuropathy may develop, manifested primarily as spinal radicular pain or distal paresthesias[65,67,68]. Electromyograms typically show diffuse involvement of both proximal and distal nerve segments. In Europe, *B. garinii* may cause chronic encephalomyelitis, characterized by spastic paraparesis, cranial neuropathy, or cognitive impairment with marked intrathecal antibody production to the spirochete[65]. In the USA, a mild, late neurologic syndrome has been reported, called Lyme encephalopathy, manifested primarily by subtle cognitive disturbances[67,69,70]. Although inflammatory changes are lacking in cerebrospinal fluid, intrathecal production of antibodies to the spirochete can often be demonstrated. One unusual case of *B. burgdorferi*-induced meningoencephalitis and cerebral vasculitis has been reported that was unresponsive to antibiotics[71]. In this case, a T cell clone recovered from cerebrospinal fluid responded both to spirochetal epitopes and autoantigens.

Carditis

Within several weeks after disease onset, about 5% of untreated patients have acute cardiac involvement, most commonly fluctuating degrees of atrioventricular block, or occasionally acute myopericarditis, mild left ventricular dysfunction or, rarely, cardiomegaly or fatal pancarditis[55,72]. The duration of cardiac abnormalities is usually brief (between 3 days and 6 weeks); complete heart block usually does not persist for longer than 1 week, and insertion of a permanent pacemaker is not necessary[73]. One elderly patient, who was co-infected with *B. burgdorferi* and *Babesia microtii*, died from cardiac involvement of the infection[74]. In Europe, *B. burgdorferi* has been isolated from endomyocardial biopsies of several patients with chronic dilated cardiomyopathy[75,76]. However, this complication has not been observed in the USA[77].

Joint involvement

Months after the onset of illness, about 60% of untreated patients in the USA have intermittent attacks of joint swelling and pain, primarily in large joints, especially the knee, over a period of several years (Fig. 27.5)[55,78]. However, other large and small joints, the temporomandibular joint or

	Early infection		Late infection
System	Localized Stage 1	Disseminated Stage 2	Persistent Stage 3
Skin	Erythema migrans	Secondary annular lesions Malar rash Diffuse erythema or urticaria Evanescent lesions Lymphocytoma	Acrodermatitis chronica atrophicans Localized scleroderma-like lesions

Musculoskeletal		Migratory pain in joints, tendons
		   bursae, muscle, bone
		Brief arthritis attacks
		Myositis
		Osteomyelitis
		Panniculitis
			Prolonged arthritis attacks
			Chronic arthritis
			Peripheral enthesopathy
			Periostitis or joint subluxations below lesions of
			   acrodermatitis

Neurologic		Meningitis Cranial neuritis, Bell's palsy Motor or sensory radiculoneuritis Subtle encephalitis Mononeuritis multiplex Myelitis Chorea Cerebellar ataxia	Chronic encephalomyelitis Subtle encephalopathy Chronic axonal polyradiculopathy
Lymphatic	Regional lympadenopathy	Regional or generalized Lymphadenopathy Splenomegaly	
Heart		Atrioventricular nodal block Myopericarditis Pancarditis	
Eyes		Conjunctivitis Iritis Choroiditis Retinal hemorrhage or detachment Panophthalmitis	Keratitis
Liver		Mild hepatitis	
Respiratory		Non-exudative sore throat	
Kidney		Microscopic hematuria or proteinuria	
Genitourinary		Orchitis	
Constitutional symptoms	Minor	Severe malaise and fatigue	Fatigue

The systems are listed from the most to the least commonly affected. The staging system provides a guideline for the expected timing of the different manifestations of the illness, but this may vary in an individual case. (From Steere AC. Lyme disease. N Engl J Med 1989; 321:586–596. © 1989. With permission of Massachusetts Medical Society. All rights reserved.)

periarticular sites are sometimes affected (Table 27.3). Affected knees may be very swollen and warm, but not particularly painful. Baker's cysts may form and rupture early. Attacks of arthritis, which usually affect only one or a few joints at a time, last from a few weeks to months, separated by longer periods of complete remission. The total number of patients who continue to have recurrent attacks of arthritis decreases by about 10–20% each year. A clinical course with arthritis as the only feature of the illness may be more common in children than in adults, and joint involvement may be milder in young children than in older children[79-81].

Usually, after several brief attacks of arthritis, about 10% of untreated patients develop chronic Lyme arthritis, defined as 1 year or more of continuous joint inflammation[78]. Similarly, in about 10% of patients, particularly those with human leukocyte antigen-DRB1*0401 or related alleles[82,83], the arthritis persists in knees for months or even several years after intravenous or oral antibiotic treatment for 30 or 60 days, respectively[84]. Polymerase chain reaction (PCR) tests for *B. burgdorferi* DNA in synovium or joint fluid are usually negative after this treat-

ment[85,86], suggesting that live spirochetes have been eradicated by it. An autoimmune pathogenesis has been proposed to explain this treatment-resistant course[42,51]. However, even chronic Lyme arthritis eventually remits spontaneously[78].

In Europe, the pattern of arthritis is similar with that in the USA, but the frequency of arthritis and the intensity of joint inflammation are less, and chronic arthritis is rare[87,88].

Investigations

B. burgdorferi can be cultured in a complex liquid medium called Barbour–Stoenner–Kelly medium[8], which permits definitive diagnosis. However, except in a few cases, positive cultures have been obtained only early in the illness, primarily from biopsies of erythema migrans lesions[89], less often from plasma samples[58] and only occasionally from cerebrospinal fluid samples in patients with meningitis[64]. The principal role for PCR testing in Lyme disease is in the detection of *B. burgdorferi* DNA from joint fluid[85], which is greatly superior to culture for this purpose. Although *B. burgdorferi* DNA has been detected in cere-

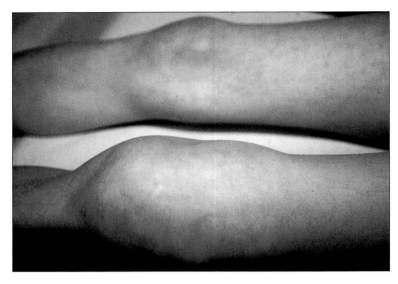

Fig. 27.5 The swollen knee of a 9-year-old child with Lyme arthritis. In the USA, affected knees may be very swollen and warm, but not particularly painful. In Europe and Asia, the amount of joint swelling is often less.

TABLE 27.3 JOINT AND PERIARTICULAR INVOLVEMENT IN LYME DISEASE. JOINTS AND PERIARTICULAR SITES AFFECTED IN 28 UNTREATED PATIENTS WITH LYME DISEASE

Joint	No. of patients (n=28)	Periarticular site	No. of patients (n=28)
Knee	27	Tendons	
Shoulder	14	Back	9
Ankle	12	Neck	6
Elbow	11	Bicipital	4
Temporomandibular	11	Lateral epicondyle	2
Wrist	10	Lateral collateral	1
Hip	9	De Quervain's	1
Metacarpophalangeal	4	Bursae	
Proximal interphalangeal	4	Prepatellar	4
Distal interphalangeal	4	Subacromial	2
Metatarsophalangeal	4	Infraspinatus	2
Sternoclavicular	1	Olecranon	2
		Sausage digits	2
		Heel pain	2

(With permission from Steere[78].)

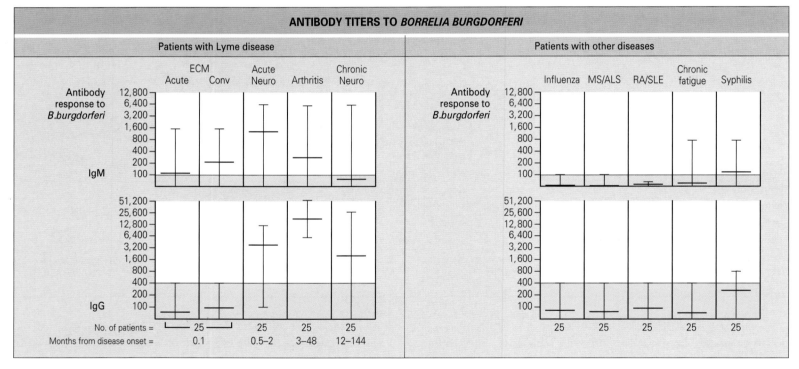

Fig. 27.6 Antibody titers to *Borrelia burgdorferi*. Titers acquired by ELISA in patients from the USA with various manifestations of Lyme disease and in control individuals. Horizontal bars, mean; vertical bars, range; hatched bars, normal range derived from sera from 50 normal control individuals. Acute neuro, meningitis; ALS, amyotrophic lateral sclerosis; Chronic neuro, encephalopathy or polyneuropathy; Conv, convalescent phase; EM, erythema migrans; MS, multiple sclerosis; RA, rheumatoid arthritis; SLE, systemic lupus erythematosus. (With permission from Dressler *et al.*[45])

brospinal fluid by PCR among patients with acute or chronic neuroborreliosis[90,91], it is a low-yield procedure. The Lyme urine antigen test, which has given grossly unreliable results[92], should not be used to support the diagnosis of Lyme disease.

In patients in the USA, the diagnosis is usually based on the recognition of a characteristic clinical picture, together with exposure in an endemic area and, except in those with erythema migrans, a positive antibody response to *B. burgdorferi* by enzyme-linked immunosorbent assay (ELISA) and western blot, interpreted according to the Centers for Disease Control/Association of State and Territorial Public Health

Laboratory Directors' criteria (Figs 27.6 & 27.7, Table 27.4)[45,93,94]. In Europe, where there is less expansion of the antibody response, no single set of criteria for immunoblot interpretation give high levels of sensitivity and specificity in all countries[95].

Serodiagnosis is insensitive during the first several weeks of infection. In the USA, approximately 20–30% of patients have positive responses, usually of the IgM isotype, during this period[45,96], but by convalescence 2–4 weeks later, about 70–80% have seroreactivity, even after antibiotic treatment. After 1 month, the great majority of patients with active infection have positive IgG antibody responses[45]. In persons with illness

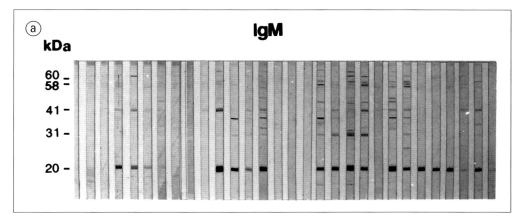

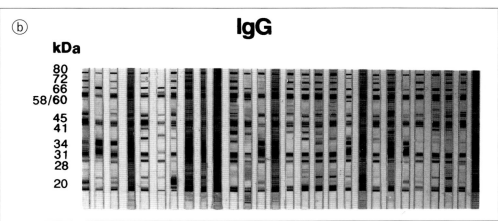

Fig. 27.7 Western blots showing positive responses for antibody to *B. burgdorferi*. (a) IgM western blot in 25 patients with erythema migrans. (b) IgG western blot in 25 patients with Lyme arthritis. In patients with erythema migrans, the IgM response is directed particularly against the 23kDa OspC protein and the 41kDa flagellar protein of the spirochete. Months to years after disease onset, in patients with Lyme arthritis, the IgG response is directed against many spirochetal proteins. Molecular mass markers (kDa) are shown at the left. (With permission from Dressler *et al*.[45])

TABLE 27.4 LYME DISEASE NATIONAL SURVEILLANCE CASE DEFINITION*

A case of Lyme disease is defined as follows:
1. A person with erythema migrans, observed by a physician.
   This skin lesion expands slowly over days to weeks to form a large round lesion, often with central clearing. To be counted for surveillance purposes, a solitary lesion must reach a size of at least 5cm
2. A person with at least one later manifestation and laboratory evidence of infection.
   Nervous system: Lymphocytic meningitis, cranial neuritis, radiculoneuropathy or, rarely, encephalomyelitis, alone or in combination. For encephalomyelitis to be counted for surveillance purposes, there must be evidence of intrathecal antibody production against *B. burgdorferi* in cerebrospinal fluid
   Cardiovascular system: Acute-onset, high-grade (2nd or 3rd degree) atrioventricular conduction defects that resolve in days to weeks and are sometimes associated with myocarditis
   Musculoskeletal system: Recurrent, brief attacks (weeks to months) of objective joint swelling in one or a few joints, sometimes followed by chronic arthritis in one or a few joints
3. Laboratory evidence.
   Isolation of *B. burgdorferi* from tissue or body fluid or detection of diagnostic levels of antibody to the spirochete by the two-test approach of ELISA and western blot, interpreted according to the Centers for Disease Control/Association of State and Territorial Public Health Laboratory Directors' criteria.*

* In a person with acute disease of less than 1 month duration, IgM and IgG antibody responses should be measured in acute and convalescent serum samples. An IgM western blot is considered positive if at least two of the following three bands are present: 23, 39 or 41kDa. An IgG blot is considered positive if at least five of the following 10 bands are present: 18, 23, 28, 30, 39, 41, 45, 58, 66 or 93kDa. Only the IgG response should be used to support the diagnosis after the first 1 month of infection. After that time, an IgM response alone is likely to be a false-positive result

(Adapted from recommendations made by the Centers for Disease Control and Prevention[92,93]; From Steere AC. Lyme disease. N Engl J Med 2001; 345:115–125. © 2001. With permission of Massachusetts Medical Society. All rights reserved.)

---

for longer than 1 month, a positive IgM test alone is likely to be a false-positive result, and therefore this response should not be used to support the diagnosis of Lyme disease after the first 1 month of infection. Several second-generation tests that use recombinant spirochetal proteins or synthetic peptides have shown promising results[97,98].

In patients with neuroborreliosis, especially in those with meningitis, intrathecal production of IgM, IgG or IgA antibody to *B. burgdorferi* may often be demonstrated by antibody capture enzyme immunoassay[99]. In patients with peripheral nervous system involvement, electromyograms typically show an axonal polyneuropathy or radiculoneuropathy, with diffuse involvement of both proximal and distal nerve segments[68]. Neither single photon emission computed tomography scanning of the brain[100] nor neuropsychological tests of memory[101] have sufficient specificity to be helpful in diagnosis.

Patients with Lyme carditis usually have fluctuating degrees of atrioventricular nodal block or, sometimes, more generalized repolarization abnormalities, including ST segment or T-wave changes[72,73]. Occasionally, they may have radionuclide evidence of mild left ventricular dysfunction and, rarely, chest radiographs may reveal cardiomegaly.

Among patients with Lyme arthritis, joint fluid white cells counts range from 500 to 110 000 cells/mm³, most of which, in patients with high white cell counts, are polymorphonuclear leukocytes[78]. Although tests for rheumatoid factor and antinuclear antibodies are usually negative, small amounts of rheumatoid factor[102] or antinuclear antibodies in low titer[81] may be detected. The most common radiographic finding is knee joint effusion[103]. Later in the illness, the joints of some patients with chronic arthritis show the typical changes of an inflammatory arthritis, including juxta-articular osteoporosis, cartilage loss and cortical or marginal bone erosions. Before antibiotic treatment, PCR tests for *B. burgdorferi* DNA in joint fluid are usually positive[85]. *B. burgdorferi* DNA may be detected more readily in synovial tissue than in synovial fluid[104,105]. The spirochete has been cultured only rarely from affected joints[106].

After antibiotic treatment, antibody titers decrease slowly, but IgG and even IgM responses may persist for many years after treatment[107]. Thus even a positive IgM response cannot by interpreted as showing recent infection or reinfection unless the appropriate clinical picture is present. *B. burgdorferi* may also cause asymptomatic infection in approximately 10% of patients in the USA[108], and in a greater percentage in Europe[109]. In tests that use whole sonicated spirochetes as the antigen preparation, vaccination for Lyme disease may cause positive IgG results by ELISA, but vaccine-induced or infection-induced antibody responses may usually be differentiated by western blotting[108]. If patients with past or asymptomatic infection or vaccine-induced immunity have symptoms caused by another illness, the danger is that they may be attributed incorrectly to Lyme disease.

Differential diagnosis

Coinfection

I. scapularis ticks transmit not only *B. burgdorferi*, but also other infectious agents, including a red blood cell parasite, *Babesia microtii,* and the agent of human granulocytic ehrlichiosis, *Anaplasma phagocytophila.* Ehrlichiosis may cause a flu-like illness associated with high fever, particularly in elderly individuals[110]. *Babesia microti* usually causes only mild or asymptomatic infection, but in elderly or asplenic individuals, it may result in a severe, malaria-like illness[111]. Of 240 patients diagnosed with Lyme disease in Connecticut, 26 (11%) were coinfected with *Babesia*[112]. Of 52 persons with IgG titers positive for *B. burgdorferi,* two (4%) had IgG antibodies to the human granulocytic ehrlichia agent[113]. When patients are coinfected with *B. burgdorferi* and one or both of these other tick-borne pathogens, they may have more severe illness[112].

Evidence for these infections includes the identification of ehrlichia or babesia DNA by PCR in blood tests or IgG seroconversion between acute and convalescent serum samples, determined by indirect immunofluorescence. Serologic diagnosis is confounded by the fact that ehrlichia infection may produce a false-positive IgM western blot for Lyme disease[114]. Neither *Babesia* nor *Ehrlichia* is known to cause chronic disease such as occurs with untreated *B. burgdor*feri infection.

Positive Lyme serology and non-specific symptoms

Patients may develop pain, fatigue or neurocognitive syndromes soon after contracting Lyme disease, and in some cases these symptoms may persist for years[115,116]. These patients have an array of subjective symptoms, including debilitating fatigue, diffuse musculoskeletal pain, cognitive difficulty and sleep disturbance, usually accompanied by normal neurologic and neurocognitive test results. This clinical picture, which is sometimes called post-Lyme disease or chronic Lyme disease syndrome, is similar to chronic fatigue syndrome or fibromyalgia. This post-infectious syndrome occurs more frequently in patients whose symptoms are suggestive of early dissemination of the spirochete to the nervous system, particularly if treatment is delayed[117,118]. However, in one large study, the frequency of symptoms of pain and fatigue was no greater in patients who had had Lyme disease than in age-matched individuals who had not had this infection[119]. In contrast with the experience with chronic neuroborreliosis, these syndromes are not cured by further antibiotic treatment[120].

Lyme arthritis or other rheumatic disease?

Lyme arthritis typically causes marked joint swelling and pain in one or a few joints at a time, with minimal systemic symptoms[78]. This clinical picture is most like reactive arthritis (Reiter's syndrome) in adults, or pauciarticular juvenile rheumatoid arthritis in children. Lyme arthritis does not cause chronic, symmetrical polyarthritis and therefore distinguishing Lyme arthritis from rheumatoid arthritis is not difficult. Fibromyalgia and chronic fatigue syndrome are commonly

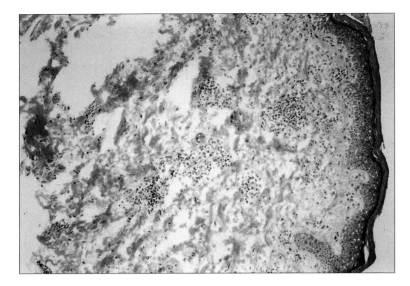

Fig. 27.8 Histopathology of lesional skin in patient with erythema migrans. The lesion shows a moderate infiltration of mononuclear cells, primarily lymphocytes, macrophages and, sometimes, a few plasma cells in the papillary rather than the reticular dermis. Section stained with hematoxylin and eosin. Original magnification × 100.

misdiagnosed as Lyme disease[115,121,122]. In contrast with Lyme arthritis, patients with fibromyalgia often have marked fatigue, severe headache, diffuse musculoskeletal pain, stiffness and pain in many joints, diffuse dysesthesias, difficulty with concentration and sleep disturbance. On physical examination, such patients have several symmetric tender points in characteristic locations, but they lack evidence of joint inflammation.

Histology

B. burgdorferi has been seen in small numbers in most affected tissues. Histologically, these tissues usually show an infiltration of lymphocytes and macrophages with some plasma cells (Fig. 27.8)[36,123,124]. Synovial tissue from patients with chronic Lyme arthritis shows synovial hypertrophy, vascular proliferation, stromal deposition of fibrin and infiltration of mononuclear cells, sometimes with pseudolymphoid follicles (Fig. 27.9)[125,126]. This picture is similar to that found in the various forms of chronic inflammatory arthritis, including rheumatoid arthritis. However, compared with other synovial diseases, some degree of vascular damage, including obliterative microvascular lesions, seem to be found only in Lyme synovia.

Management

Evidence-based treatment recommendations for Lyme disease were recently presented by the Infectious Diseases Society of America[127] (Table 27.5). In general, Lyme disease can be treated effectively with appropriate oral antibiotic agents, except for neurologic abnormalities, which seem to require treatment with intravenous antibiotics. The American College of Physicians has also developed an algorithm to guide testing and treatment, depending on the pretest probability of Lyme disease[128]. According to this algorithm, empirical antibiotic therapy without serologic testing is recommended for patients with a high pre-test probability of Lyme disease (such as those with erythema migrans), two-step testing (by ELISA and, if positive, by western blot) is recommended for patients with an intermediate pre-test probability (such as those with recurrent oligoarticular arthritis), and neither testing nor treatment is recommended for those with a low pre-test probability (such as those with non-specific symptoms of myalgia, arthralgias and fatigue).

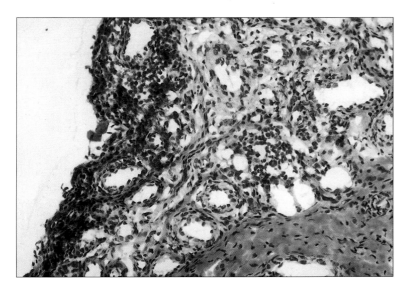

Fig. 27.9 Cellular architecture and infiltrating cells in synovial tissue from a patient with treatment-resistant Lyme arthritis. The tissue shows villous hypertrophy, synovial cell hyperplasia, vascular proliferation and an infiltration of mononuclear cells. Section stained with hematoxylin and eosin. Original magnification ×200.

Early localized or disseminated infection

For early localized or disseminated infection, doxycycline for 14 to 21 days is recommended in persons older than 8 years of age, except for pregnant women (Table 27.5). An advantage of doxycycline is its efficacy against the agent of human granulocytic ehrlichiosis, a possible coinfecting agent. Amoxicillin, the second-choice alternative, should be used in children or pregnant women. In case of allergy, cefuroxime axetil is a third-choice alternative. Erythromycin or its cogeners, which are fourth-choice alternatives, are recommended only for patients who are unable to take doxycycline, amoxicillin or cefuroxime axetil. Because maternal–fetal transmission of *B. burgdorferi* seems to occur rarely, if at all[129], standard treatment for the manifestation of the illness is recommended.

In multicenter studies of patients with erythema migrans, similar results were obtained with doxycycline, amoxicillin and cefuroxime axetil, and more than 90% of patients had satisfactory outcomes[130,131]. Although some patients had subjective symptoms after treatment, objective evidence of persistent infection or relapse was rare, and retreatment was usually not needed. Intravenous ceftriaxone, although effective, was not superior to oral agents as long as the patient did not have objective neurological involvement[132]. In contrast with second- and third-generation cephalosporin antibiotics, first-generation cephalosporins, such as cephalexin, were ineffective[133].

Neurologic abnormalities

For patients with objective neurologic abnormalities, 2- to 4-week courses of intravenous ceftriaxone are most commonly given[67,70,134] Parenteral treatment with cefotaxime or penicillin G may be a satisfactory alternative[135]. The signs and symptoms of acute neuroborreliosis usually resolve within weeks, but those of chronic neuroborreliosis improve slowly over a period of months. Objective evidence of relapse is rare after a 4-week course of treatment. In Europe, oral doxycycline may be adequate treatment for acute neuroborreliosis[136]. Although this medication may be used successfully in patients with facial palsy alone in the USA, it is important to assess whether such patients have more diffuse involvement of the nervous system, which is best treated with intravenous therapy. Lyme encephalopathy may be treated successfully with a 1-month course of intravenous ceftriaxone[70], but immune-mediated or postinfectious phenomena may also play a part in the pathogenesis of these syndromes.

TABLE 27.5 TREATMENT REGIMENS FOR LYME DISEASE

Early infection (local or disseminated)

Adults
Doxycycline, 100mg orally twice daily for 14–21 days
Amoxicillin, 500mg orally three times daily for 14–21 days
or (alternatives in case of doxycycline or amoxicillin allergy):
Cefuroxime axetil, 500 mg orally twice daily for 14–21 days
Erythromycin, 250 mg orally 4 times a day for 14–21 days
Children (age 8 years or less)
Amoxicillin, 250mg orally three times a day or 50mg/kg per day in three divided doses for 14–21 days
or (alternatives in case of penicillin allergy):
Cefuroxime axetil, 125mg orally twice daily or 30mg/kg per day in two divided doses for 14–21 days
Erythromycin, 250mg orally three times a day or 30mg/kg per day in three divided doses for 14–21 days

Neurologic abnormalities (early or late)

Adults
Ceftriaxone 2g i.v. once a day for 14–28 days
Cefotaxime, 2g i.v. every eight hours for 14–28 days
Na penicillin G, 3.3 × 10⁶U i.v. every 4h for 14–28 days
or (alternative in case of ceftriaxone or penicillin allergy):
Doxycycline, 100mg orally three times a day for 30 days, but this regimen may be ineffective for late neuroborreliosis
Facial palsy alone: oral regimens may be adequate
Children (age 8 years or less)
Ceftriaxone, 75–100mg/kg per day (maximum 2g) i.v. once a day for 14–28 days
Cefotaxime, 150mg/kg per day in three or four divided doses (maximum 6g) for 14–28 days
Na penicillin G, 200 000–400 000U/kg per day in six divided doses for 14–28 days

Arthritis (intermittent or chronic)

Oral regimens listed above for 30–60 days
or
i.v. regimens listed above for 14–28 days

Cardiac abnormalities

First-degree atrioventricular block: oral regimens, as for early infection
High-degree atrioventricular block (P–R interval >0.3s): i.v. regimens and cardiac monitoring
Once the patient has stabilized, the course may be completed with oral therapy

Pregnant women

Standard treatment for manifestation of the illness. Avoid doxycycline

i.v., intravenous

Antibiotic recommendations are based on the guidelines from the Infectious Diseases Society of America[127]. (From Steere AC. Lyme disease. N Engl J Med 2001; 345:115–125. © 2001. With permission of Massachusetts Medical Society. All rights reserved.)

Carditis

In patients with high-degree atrioventricular nodal block (P–R interval >0.3s), intravenous treatment for at least part of the course and cardiac monitoring are recommended, but insertion of a permanent pacemaker is not necessary. Once the patient's condition has stabilized, the course may be completed with oral treatment.

Arthritis

Either oral or intravenous regimens are usually effective for the treatment of Lyme arthritis[84,134]. Oral treatment is easier to administer, it is associated with fewer side effects and it is considerably less expensive[137].

Its disadvantage is that some patients treated with oral agents have subsequently manifested overt neuroborreliosis, which may require intravenous therapy for successful treatment[84]. Despite treatment with either oral or intravenous antibiotics, about 10% of patients in the USA have persistent joint inflammation for months or even several years after at least 2 months of oral antibiotics or at least 1 month of intravenous antibiotics[84]. If patients have persistent arthritis despite this treatment, and if the results of PCR testing of joint fluid are negative, such patients may be treated with anti-inflammatory agents or arthroscopic synovectomy.

Post-Lyme disease syndrome

Patients with post-Lyme disease syndrome are best treated symptomatically, rather than with prolonged courses of antibiotics. In a study of patients with this syndrome who received either intravenous ceftriaxone for 30 days followed by oral doxycycline for 60 days or intravenous and oral placebo preparations for the same duration, there were no significant differences between the groups in the percentage of patients who felt that their symptoms had improved, worsened or stayed the same[119]. Prolonged ceftriaxone therapy for unsubstantiated Lyme disease has resulted in biliary complications[138] and, in one reported case, prolonged cefotaxime administration resulted in death[139].

Prevention

Protection against tick bites

The risk of tick bites in high-risk areas may be reduced by simple measures. These include avoidance of tick infested areas, protective clothing, use of repellants and acaracides, tick checks and landscape modifications of periresidential environments[140].

Studies have shown the frequency of Lyme disease after a recognized tick bite to be only about 1%[141], perhaps because at least 24 hours of tick attachment seems to be necessary for transmission to occur[142]. Thus, if an attached tick is removed quickly, no other treatment is usually necessary. However, a single 200mg dose of doxycycline effectively prevents Lyme disease when given within 72 hours after the tick bite occurs[143].

Vaccination

A vaccine for Lyme disease, consisting of recombinant OspA in adjuvant, was commercially available in the USA, but it was recently withdrawn by the manufacturer. In a phase III efficacy and safety trial, vaccine efficacy in the prevention of definite Lyme disease was 49% after two injections, and 76% after three injections[108]. The most important factor in protection was the strength of the antibody response to the protective antibody epitope of OspA. Injection of the vaccine was associated with mild-to-moderate local or systemic reactions lasting a median duration of 3 days. Although T cell responses to OspA have been associated with treatment-resistant Lyme arthritis[42,51], vaccine or placebo recipients did not differ significantly in the development of arthritis or any other late syndrome after vaccination. Thus, the conditions necessary for the induction of autoimmunity in joints in the natural infection seemed not to be duplicated with vaccination. Although the vaccine is no longer available, the experience gained with it has proven the feasibility of vaccination for the prevention of this complex, tick-borne infection.

REFERENCES

1. Steere AC, Malawista SE, Snydman DR et al. Lyme arthritis: an epidemic of oligoarticular arthritis in children and adults in three Connecticut communities. Arthritis Rheum 1977; 20: 7–17.
2. Steere AC, Malawista SE, Hardin JA et al. Erythema chronicum migrans and Lyme arthritis: the enlarging clinical spectrum. Ann Intern Med 1977; 86: 685–698.
3. Steere AC, Broderick TF, Malawista SE. Erythema chronicum migrans and Lyme arthritis: epidemiologic evidence for a tick vector. Am J Epidemiol 1978; 108: 312–321.
4. Lipschutz B. Uber eine seltene Erythemform (Erythema chronicum migrans). Arch Dermatol Syph 1913; 118: 349–356.
5. Buchwald A. Ein fall von diffuser idiopathischer Hautatrophie. Arch Dermatol Syph 1883; 10: 553.
6. Bannwarth A. Zur Klinik und Pathogenese der 'chronischen lymphocytaren Meningitis'. Arch Psychiatr Nervenkrankh 1944; 117: 161–185.
7. Burgdorfer W, Barbour AG, Hayes SF et al. Lyme disease – a tick-borne spirochetosis? Science 1982; 216: 1317–1319.
8. Steere AC, Grodzicki RL, Kornblatt AN et al. The spirochetal etiology of Lyme disease. N Engl J Med 1983; 308: 733–740.
9. Steere AC. Lyme disease. N Engl J Med 2001; 345: 115–125.
10. Baranton G, Postic D, Saint Girons I et al. Delineation of Borrelia burgdorferi sensu stricto, Borrelia garinii sp. nov., and group VS461 asssociated with Lyme borreliosis. Int J Syst Bacteriol 1992; 42: 378–383.
11. Orloski KA, Hayes EB, Campbell GL, Dennis DT. Surveillance for Lyme disease – United States, 1992–1998. MMWR Morb Mortal Wkly Rep 2000; 49: 1–11.
12. Stanek G, Satz N, Strle F, Wilske B. Epidemiology of Lyme borreliosis. In: Weber K, Burgdorfer W, eds. Aspects of Lyme borreliosis. Berlin, Heidelberg: Springer-Verlag; 1993: 358–370.
13. Lane RS, Piesman J, Burgdorfer W. Lyme borreliosis: relation of its causative agent to its vectors and hosts in North America and Europe. Annu Rev Entomol 1991; 36: 587–609.
14. Spielman A. The emergence of Lyme disease and human babesiosis in a changing environment. Ann NY Acad Sci 1994; 740: 146–156.
15. Brown RN, Lane RS. Lyme disease in California: a novel enzootic transmission cycle of Borrelia burgdorferi. Science 1992; 256: 1439–1442.
16. Campbell GL, Paul WS, Schriefer ME et al. Epidemiologic and diagnostic studies of patients with suspected early Lyme disease, Missouri, 1990–1993. J Infect Dis 1995; 172: 470–480.
17. Barbour AG, Hayes SF. Biology of Borrelia species. Microbiol Rev 1986; 50: 381–400.
18. Fraser CM, Casjens S, Huang WM et al. Genomic sequence of a Lyme disease spirochete, Borrelia burgdorferi. Nature 1997; 390: 580–586.
19. de Silva AM, Fikrig E. Arthropod- and host-specific gene expression by Borrelia burgdorferi. J Clin Invest 1997; 100: S3–S5.
20. Zhang J-R, Norris SJ. Genetic variation of the Borrelia burgdorferi gene VlsE involves cassette-specific, segmental gene conversation. Infect Immun 1998; 66: 3698–3704.
21. Akins DR, Bourell KW, Caimaro MJ et al. A new animal model for studying Lyme disease spirochetes in a mammalian host-adapted state. J Clin Invest 1998; 101: 2240–2250.
22. Montgomery RR, Malawista SE, Feen KJM, Bockenstedt LK. Direct demonstration of antigenic substitution of Borrelia burgdorferi ex vivo: exploration of the paradox of the early immune response to outer surface proteins A and C in Lyme disease. J Exp Med 1996; 183: 261–269.
23. Schwan TG, Piesman J, Golde WT et al. Induction of an outer surface protein on Borrelia burgdorferi during tick feeding. Proc Natl Acad Sci USA 1995; 92: 2909–2913.
24. Seinost G, Dykhuizen DE, Dattwyler RJ et al. Four clones of Borrelia burgdorferi sensu stricto cause invasive infection in humans. Infect Immun 1999; 67: 3518–3524.
25. Coleman JL, Gebbia JA, Pieman J et al. Plasminogen is required for efficient dissemination of B. burgdorferi in ticks and for enhancement of spirochetemia in mice. Cell 1997; 89: 1111–1119.
26. Thomas DD, Comstock LE. Interaction of Lyme disease spirochetes with cultured eucaryotic cells. Infect Immun 1989; 57: 1324–1326.
27. Coburn J, Chege W, Magoun L et al. Characterization of a candidate Borrelia burgdorferi β3-chain integrin ligand identified using a phage display library. Mol Microbiol 1999; 34: 926–940.
28. Parveen N, Leong JM. Identification of a candidate glycosaminoglycan-binding adhesin of the Lyme disease spirochete Borrelia burgdorferi. Mol Microbiol 2000; 35: 1220–1234.
29. Probert WS, Johnson BJB. Identification of a 47 kDa fibronectin-binding protein expressed by Borrelia burgdorferi isolate B31. Mol Microbiol 1998; 30: 1003–1015.
30. Guo BP, Brown EL, Dorward DW et al. Decorin-binding adhesins from Borrelia burgdorferi. Mol Microbiol 1998; 30: 711–723.
31. Brown EL, Wooten M, Johnson BJB et al. Resistance to Lyme disease in decorin-deficit mice. J Clin Invest 2001; 107: 845–852.
32. Weis JJ, McCracken BA, Ma Y et al. Identification of quantitative trait loci governing arthritis severity and humoral responses in the murine model of Lyme disease. J Immunol 1999; 162: 948–956.
33. Barthold SW, de Souza M. Exacerbation of Lyme arthritis in beige mice. J Infect Dis 1995; 172: 178–184.
34. Hirschfeld M, Kirschning CJ, Schwandner R et al. Cutting edge: inflammatory signaling by Borrelia burgdorferi lipoproteins is mediated by Toll-like receptor 2. J Immunol 1999; 163: 2382–2386.
35. Kang I, Barthold SW, Persing DH, Bockenstedt LK. T-helper-cell cytokines in the early evolution of murine Lyme arthritis. Infect Immun 1997; 65: 3107–3111.
36. Muellegger RR, McHugh G, Ruthazer R et al. Differential expression of cytokine mRNA in skin specimens from patients with erythema migrans or acrodermatitis chronica atrophicans. J Invest Derm 2000; 115: 1115–1123.

37. Krause A, Brade V, Schoerner C et al. T cell proliferation induced by Borrelia burgdorferi in patients with Lyme borreliosis. Arthritis Rheum 1991; 34: 393–402.

38. Akin E, McHugh GL, Flavell RA et al. The immunoglobin (IgG) antibody response to OspA and OspB correlates with severe and prolonged Lyme arthritis and the IgG response to P35 correlates with mild and brief arthritis. Infect Immun 1999; 67: 173–181.

39. Roberts ED, Bohm RPJ, Lowrie RCJ et al. Pathogenesis of Lyme neuroborreliosis in the rhesus monkey: the early disseminated and chronic phases of disease in the peripheral nervous system. J Infect Dis 1998; 178: 722–732.

40. Cadavid D, O'Neill T, Schaefer H, Pachner AR. Localization of Borrelia burgdorferi in the nervous system and other organs in a nonhuman primate model of Lyme disease. Lab Invest 2000; 80: 1043–1054.

41. Vincent MS, Roessner K, Sellati T et al. Lyme arthritis synovial $\gamma\delta$ T cells respond to Borrelia burgdorferi lipoproteins and lipidated hexapeptides. J Immun 1998; 161: 5762–5771.

42. Chen J, Field JA, Glickstein L et al. Association of antibiotic treatment-resistant Lyme arthritis with T cell responses to dominant epitopes of outer-surface protein A (OspA) of Borrelia burgdorferi. Arthritis Rheum 1999; 42: 1813–1822.

43. Gross DM, Steere AC, Huber BT. Dominent T helper 1 response is antigen specific and localized to synovial fluid in patients with Lyme arthritis. J Immun 1998; 160: 1022–1028.

44. Yin Z, Braun J, Neure L et al. T cell cytokine pattern in the joints of patients with Lyme arthritis and its regulation by cytokines and anticytokines. Arthritis Rheum 1997; 40: 69–79.

45. Dressler F, Whalen JA, Reinhardt BN, Steere AC. Western blotting in the serodiagnosis of Lyme disease. J Infect Dis 1993; 167: 392–400.

46. Barthold SW, Feng S, Bockenstedt LK et al. Protective and arthritis-resolving activity in sera of mice infected with Borrelia burgdorferi. Clin Infect Dis 1997; 25: S9–S17.

47. Feng S, Hodzic E, Barthold SW. Lyme arthritis resolution with antiserum to a 37-kilodalton Borrelia burgdorferi protein. Infect Immun 2000; 68: 4169–4173.

48. Kelleher Doyle M, Telford SR, Criscione L et al. Cytokines in murine Lyme carditis: Th 1 cytokine expression follows expression of proinflammatory cytokines in susceptible mouse strain. J Infect Dis 1998; 177: 242–246.

49. Barthold SW, Beck DS, Hansen GM et al. Lyme borreliosis in selected strains and ages of laboratory mice. J Infect Dis 1990; 162: 133–138.

50. Kalish RA, Leong JM, Steere AC. Association of treatment resistant chronic Lyme arthritis with HLA-DR4 and antibody reactivity to OspA and OspB of Borrelia burgdorferi. Infect Immun 1993; 61: 2774–2779.

51. Gross DM, Forsthuber T, Tary-Lehman M et al. Identification of LFA-1 as a candidate autoantigen in treatment-resistant Lyme arthritis. Science 1998; 281: 703–706.

52. Akin E, Aversa J, Steere AC. Expression of adhesion molecules in synovia of patients with treatment- resistant Lyme arthritis. Infect Immun 2001; 69: 1774–1780.

53. Meyer AL, Trollmo C, Crawford F et al. Direct enumeration of Borrelia-reactive CD4$^+$ T cells ex vivo by using MHC class II tetramers. Proc Natl Acad Sci USA 2000; 97: 11433–11438.

54. Trollmo C, Meyer AI, Steere AC et al. Molecular mimicry in Lyme arthritis demonstrated at the single cell level: LFA-1α L is a partial agonist for OspA-reactive T cells. J Immunol 2001; 166: 5286–5291.

55. Steere AC. Lyme disease. N Engl J Med 1989; 321: 586–596.

56. Steere AC, Bartenhagen NH, Craft JE et al. The early clinical manifestations of Lyme disease. Ann Intern Med 1983; 99: 76–82.

57. Strle F, Nadelman RB, Cimperman J et al. Comparison of culture-confirmed erythema migrans caused by Borrelia burgdorferi sensu stricto in New York state and by Borrelia afzelii in Slovenia. Ann Intern Med 1999; 130: 32–36.

58. Wormser GP, Bittker S, Cooper D et al. Comparison of the yields of blood cultures using serum or plasma from patients with early Lyme disease. J Clin Microbiol 2000; 38: 1648–1650.

59. Luft BJ, Steinman CR, Neimark HC et al. Invasion of the central nervous system by Borrelia burgdorferi in acute disseminated infection. JAMA 1992; 267: 1364–1367.

60. Asbrink E, Hovmark A. Early and late cutaneous manifestations of Ixodes-borne borreliosis (erythema migrans borreliosis, Lyme borreliosis). Ann NY Acad Sci 1988; 539: 4–15.

61. Asbrink E, Hovmark A. Successful cultivation of spirochetes from skin lesions of patients with erythema chronica migrans afzelius and acrodermatitis chronica atrophicans. Acta Pathol Microbiol Immunol Scand 1985; 93: 161–163.

62. Pachner AR, Steere AC. The triad of neurologic manifestations of Lyme disease: meningitis, cranial neuritis, and radiculoneuritis. Neurology 1985; 35: 47–53.

63. Reik L, Steere AC, Bartenhagen NH et al. Neurologic abnormalities of Lyme disease. Medicine (Baltimore) 1979; 58: 281–294.

64. Coyle PK, Goodman JL, Krupp LB et al. Lyme disease: continuum: lifelong learning in neurology, vo. 5, No.4, part A. Philadelphia: Lippincott Williams & Wilkins; 1999.

65. Oschmann P, Dorndorf W, Hornig C et al. Stages and syndromes of neuroborreliosis. J Neurology 1998; 245: 262–272.

66. Rothermel H, Hedges TR III, Steere AC. Optic neuropathy in children with Lyme disease. Pediatrics 2001; 108: 477–481.

67. Logigian EL, Kaplan RF, Steere AC. Chronic neurologic manifestations of Lyme disease. N Engl J Med 1990; 323: 1438–1444.

68. Logigian EL, Steere AC. Clinical and electrophysiologic findings in chronic neuropathy of Lyme disease. Neurology 1992; 42: 303–311.

69. Halperin JJ, Luft BJ, Anand AK et al. Lyme neuroborreliosis: central nervous system manifestations. Neurology 1989; 39: 753–759.

70. Logigian EL, Kaplan RF, Steere AC. Successful treatment of Lyme encephalopathy with intravenous ceftriaxone. J Infect Dis 1999; 180: 377–383.

71. Hemmer B, Gran B, Zhao Y et al. Identification of candidate T-cell epitopes and molecular mimics in chronic Lyme disease. Nat Med 1999; 5: 1375–1382.

72. Steere AC, Batsford WP, Weinberg M et al. Lyme carditis: cardiac abnormalities of Lyme disease. Ann Intern Med 1980; 93: 8–16.

73. McAlister HF, Klementowicz PT, Andrews C et al. Lyme carditis: an important cause of reversible heart block. Ann Intern Med 1989; 110: 339–345.

74. Marcus LC, Steere AC, Duray PH et al. Fatal pancarditis in a patient with coexistent Lyme disease and babesiosis: demonstration of spirochetes in the myocardium. Ann Intern Med 1985; 103: 374–36.

75. Stanek G, Klein J, Bittner R, Glogar D. Isolation of Borrelia burgdorferi from the myocardium of a patient with longstanding cardiomyopathy. N Engl J Med 1990; 322: 249–252.

76. Lardieri G, Salvi A, Camerini F et al. Isolation of Borrelia burgdorferi from myocardium [letter]. Lancet 1993; 342: 8869.

77. Sonnesyn SW, Diehl SC, Johnson RC et al. A prospective study of the seroprevalance of Borrelia burgdorferi infection in patients with severe heart failure. Am J Cardiol 1995; 76: 97–100.

78. Steere AC, Schoen RT, Taylor E. The clinical evolution of Lyme arthritis. Ann Intern Med 1987; 107: 725–731.

79. Szer IS, Taylor E, Steere AC. The long-term course of children with Lyme arthritis. N Engl J Med 1991; 325: 159–163.

80. Huppertz H-I, Karch H, Suschke H-J et al. Lyme arthritis in European children and adolescents. Arthritis Rheum 1995; 38: 361–368.

81. Eichenfield AH, Goldsmith DP, Benach JL et al. Childhood Lyme arthritis: experience in an endemic area. J Pediatr 1986; 109: 753–758.

82. Steere AC, Dwyer E, Winchester R. Association of chronic Lyme arthritis with HLA-DR4 and HLA-DR2 alleles. N Engl J Med 1990; 323: 219–223.

83. Steere AC, Baxter-Lowe LA. Association of chronic, treatment-resistant Lyme arthritis with rheumatoid arthritis (RA) alleles [abstract]. Arthritis Rheum 1998; 41: S81.

84. Steere AC, Levin RE, Molloy PJ et al. Treatment of Lyme arthritis. Arthritis Rheum 1994; 37: 878–888.

85. Nocton JJ, Dressler F, Rutledge BJ et al. Detection of Borrelia burgdorferi DNA by polymerase chain reaction in synovial fluid in Lyme arthritis. N Engl J Med 1994; 330: 229–234.

86. Carlson D, Hernandez J, Bloom BJ et al. Lack of Borrelia burgdorferi DNA in synovial samples in patients with antibiotic treatment-resistant Lyme arthritis. Arthritis Rheum 1999; 42: 2705–2709.

87. Herzer P, Wilske B, Preac-Mursic V et al. Lyme arthritis: clinical features, serological, and radiographic findings of cases in Germany. Klin Wochenschr 1986; 64: 206–215.

88. Hovmark A, Asbrink E, Olsson I. Joint and bone involvement in Swedish patients with Ixodes ricinus-borne Borrelia infection. Zentralbl Bakt Hyg 1986; A263: 275–284.

89. Berger BW, Johnson RC, Kodner C, Coleman L. Cultivation of Borrelia burgdorferi from erythema migrans lesions and perilesional skin. J Clin Microbiol 1992; 30: 359–361.

90. Nocton JJ, Bloom BJ, Rutledge BJ et al. Detection of Borrelia burgdorferi DNA by polymerase chain reaction in cerebrospinal fluid in patients with Lyme neuroborreliosis. J Infect Dis 1996; 174: 623–627.

91. Lebech AM, Hansen K, Rutledge BJ et al. Diagnostic detection and direct genotyping of Borrelia burgdorferi by polymerase chain reaction in cerebrospinal fluid in Lyme neuroborreliosis. Mol Diagn 1998; 3: 131–141.

92. Klempner MS, Schmid C, Hu L et al. Intralaboratory reliability of serologic and urine testing in Lyme disease. Am J Med 2001; 110: 217–219.

93. Case definitions for public health surveillance. MMWR Morb Mortal Wkly Rep 1990; 39: 19–21.

94. Second International Conference on serologic diagnosis of Lyme disease. Recommendations for test performance and interpretation. MMWR Morb Mortal Wkly Rep 1995; 44: 590–591.

95. Robertson J, Guy E, Andrews N et al. A European multicenter study of immunoblotting in serodiagnosis of Lyme borreliosis. J Clin Microbiol 2000; 38: 2097–2102.

96. Engstrom SM, Shoop E, Johnson RC. Immunoblot interpretation criteria for serodiagnosis of early Lyme disease. J Clin Microbiol 1995; 33: 419–427.

97. Gomes-Solecki MJ, Dunn JJ, Luft BJ et al. Recombinant chimeric Borrelia proteins for diagnosis of Lyme disease. J Clin Microbiol 2000; 38: 2530–2535.

98. Liang FT, Steere AC, Marques AR et al. Sensitive and specific serodiagnosis of Lyme disease by enzyme-linked immunosorbent assay with a peptide based on an immunodominant conserved region of Borrelia burgdorferi VlsE. J Clin Microbiol 1999; 37: 3990–3996.

99. Steere AC, Berardi VP, Weeks KE et al. Evaluation of the intrathecal antibody response to Borrelia burgdorferi as a diagnostic test for Lyme neuroborreliosis. J Infect Dis1990; 161: 1203–1209.

100. Logigian EL, Johnson KA, Kijewski MF et al. Reversible cerebral hypoperfusion in Lyme encephalopathy. Neurology 1997; 49: 1661–1670.

101. Kaplan RF, Jones-Woodward L. Lyme encephalopathy: a neuropsychological perspective. Semin Neurol 1997; 17: 31–37.

102. Axford JS, Rees DH, Mageed RA et al. Increased IgA rheumatoid factor and V(H)1 associated cross reactive idiotype expression in patients with Lyme arthritis and neuroborreliosis. Ann Rheum Dis 1999; 58: 757–761.

103. Lawson JP, Steere AC. Lyme arthritis: radiologic findings. Radiology 1985; 154: 37–43.

104. Jaulhac B, Chary-Valckenaere I et al. Detection of Borrelia burgdorferi by DNA amplification in synovial tissue samples from patients with Lyme arthritis. Arthritis Rheum 1996; 39: 736–745.

105. Priem S, Burmester GR, Kamradt T et al. Detection of Borrelia burgdoferi by polymerase chain reaction in synovial membrane, but not in synovial fluid from patients with persisting Lyme arthritis after antibiotic therapy. Ann Rheum Dis 1998; 57: 118–121.

106. Snydman DR, Schenkein DP, Berardi VP et al. Borrelia burgdorferi in joint fluid in chronic Lyme arthritis. Ann Intern Med 1986; 104: 798–800.

107. Kalish RA, McHugh G, Granquist J et al. Persistence of IgM or IgG antibody responses to Borrelia burgdorferi 10 to 20 years after active Lyme disease. Clin Infect Dis 2001; 33: 780–785.

108. Steere AC, Sikand VK, Meurice F *et al*. Vaccination against Lyme disease with recombinant *Borrelia burgdorferi* outer-surface lipoprotein a with adjuvant. N Engl J Med 1998; 339: 209–215.

109. Gustafson R, Svenungsson B, Gardulf A *et al*. Prevalence of tick-borne encephalitis and Lyme borreliosis in a defined Swedish population. Scand J Infect Dis 1990; 22: 297–306.

110. Goodman JL, Nelson C, Vitale B *et al*. Direct cultivation of the causative agent of human granulocytic ehrlichiosis. N Engl J Med 1996; 334: 209–215.

111. Ruebush TK 2nd, Juranek DD, Chisholm ES *et al*. Human babesiosis on Nantucket Island. Evidence for self-limited and subclinical infections. N Engl J Med 1977; 297: 825–827.

112. Krause PJ, Telford SR, Spielman A *et al*. Concurrent Lyme disease and babesiosis: evidence for increased severity and duration of illness. JAMA 1996; 275: 1657–1660.

113. DeMartino SJ, Carlyon JA, Fikrig E. Coinfection with *Borrelia burgdorferi* and the agent of human granulocytic ehrlichiosis. N Engl J Med 2001; 345: 150–151.

114. Wormser GP, Horowitz HW, Nowakowski J *et al*. Positive Lyme disease serology in patients with clinical and laboratory evidence of human granulocytic ehrlichiosis. Am J Clin Pathol 1997; 107: 142–147.

115. Sigal LH. Summary of the first 100 patients seen at a Lyme disease referral center. Am J Med 1990; 88: 577–581.

116. Dinerman H, Steere AC. Lyme disease associated with fibromyalgia. Ann Intern Med 1992; 117: 281–285.

117. Shadick NA, Phillips CB, Sangha O *et al*. Musculoskeletal and neurologic outcomes in patients with previously treated Lyme disease. Ann Intern Med 1999; 131: 919–926.

118. Kalish RA, Kaplan RF, Taylor E *et al*. Evaluation of study patients with Lyme disease, 10–20 year follow-up. J Infect Dis 2001; 183: 453–460.

119. Seltzer EG, Gerber MA, Cartter ML *et al*. Long-term outcomes of persons with Lyme disease. JAMA 2000; 283: 609–616.

120. Klempner MS, Hu LT, Evans J *et al*. Two controlled trials of antibiotic treatments in patients with persistent symptoms and a history of Lyme disease. N Engl J Med 2001; 345: 85–92.

121. Steere AC, Taylor E, McHugh GL, Logigian EL. The overdiagnosis of Lyme disease. JAMA 1993; 269: 1812–1816.

122. Burdge DR, O'Hanlon DP. Experience at a referral center for patients with suspected Lyme disease in an area of nonendemicity: first 65 patients. Clin Infect Dis 1993; 16: 558–560.

123. Duray PH. The surgical pathology of human Lyme disease: an enlarging picture. Am J Surg Path 1987; 11: 47–60.

124. Vallat JM, Hugon J, Lubeau M *et al*. Tick-bite meningoradiculoneuritis: clinical, electrophysiologic, and histologic findings in 10 cases. Neurology 1987; 37: 749–753.

125. Johnston YE, Duray PH, Steere AC *et al*. Lyme arthritis: spirochetes found in synovial microangiopathic lesions. Am J Path 1985; 118: 26–34.

126. Steere AC, Duray PH, Butcher EC. Spirochetal antigens and lymphoid cell surface markers in Lyme synovitis: comparison with rheumatoid synovium and tonsillar lymphoid tissue. Arthritis Rheum 1988; 31: 487–495.

127. Wormser GP, Nadelman RB, Dattwyler RJ *et al*. Practice guidelines for the treatment of Lyme disease. Clin Infect Dis 2000; 31: S1–S14.

128. Nichol G, Dennis DT, Steere AC *et al*. Test-treatment strategies for patients suspected of having Lyme disease: a cost-effectiveness analysis. Ann Intern Med 1998; 128: 37–48.

129. Williams CL, Stobino B, Weinstein A *et al*. Maternal Lyme disease and congenital malformations: a cord blood serosurvey in endemic and control areas. Paediatr Perinat Epidemiol 1995; 9: 320–330.

130. Dattwyler RJ, Volkman DJ, Conaty SM *et al*. Amoxycillin plus probenecid versus doxycycline for treatment of erythema migrans borreliosis. Lancet 1990; 336: 1404–1406.

131. Nadelman RB, Luger SW, Frank E *et al*. Comparison of cefuroxime axetil and doxycycline in the treatment of early Lyme disease. Ann Intern Med 1992; 117: 273–280.

132. Dattwyler RJ, Luft BJ, Kunkel MJ *et al*. Ceftriaxone compared with doxycycline for the treatment of acute disseminated Lyme disease. N Engl J Med 1997; 337: 289–294.

133. Nowakowski J, McKenna D, Nadelman RB *et al*. Failure of treatment with cephalexin for Lyme disease. Arch Fam Med 2000; 9: 563–567.

134. Dattwyler RJ, Halperin JJ, Volkman DJ, Luft BJ. Treatment of late Lyme borreliosis – randomized comparison of ceftriaxone and penicillin. Lancet 1988; 1: 1191–1194.

135. Pfister HW, Preac-Mursic V, Wilske B, Einhaupl KM. Cefotaxime vs penicillin G for acute neurologic manifestations of Lyme borreliosis: a prospective randomized study. Arch Neurol 1989; 46: 1190–1194.

136. Karlsson M, Hammers-Berggren S, Lindquist L *et al*. Comparison of intravenous penicillin G and oral doxycycline for treatment of Lyme neuroborreliosis. Neurology 1994; 44: 1203–1207.

137. Eckman MH, Steere AC, Kalish RA, Pauker SG. Cost effectiveness of oral as compared with intravenous antibiotic therapy for patients with early Lyme disease or Lyme arthritis. N Engl J Med 1997; 337: 357–363.

138. Ettestad PJ, Campbell GL, Weibel SF *et al*. Biliary complications in the treatment of unsubstantiated Lyme disease. J Infect Dis 1995; 171: 356–361.

139. Patel R, Grogg KL, Edwards WD *et al*. Death from inappropriate therapy for Lyme disease. Clin Infect Dis 2000; 31: 1107–1109.

140. Centers for Disease Control and Prevention. Recommendations for the use of Lyme disease vaccine. MMWR Morb Mortal Wkly Rep 1999; 48: 1–21.

141. Shapiro ED, Gerber MA, Holabird NB *et al*. A controlled trial of antimicrobial prophylaxis for Lyme disease after deer-tick bites. N Engl J Med 1992; 327: 1769–1773.

142. Piesman J. Dynamics of *Borrelia burgdorferi* transmission by nymphal *Ixodes dammini* ticks. J Infect Dis 1993; 167: 1082–1085.

143. Nadelman RB, Nowakowski J, Fish D *et al*. Single dose doxycycline prophylaxis for prevention of Lyme disease after an *Ixodes scapularis* tick bite. N Engl J Med 2001; 345: 79–84.

SPONDYLOARTHROPATHIES

28 Clinical features of ankylosing spondylitis

Muhammad Asim Khan

Definition

- A chronic systemic inflammatory rheumatic disorder with predilection for axial skeletal involvement, and inflammation at sites of bony insertions for tendons and ligaments (enthesitis)
- Sacroiliitis is its hallmark
- Strong genetic predisposition associated with HLA-B27

Clinical features

- Chronic inflammatory low back pain and stiffness
- Limitation of spinal mobility and chest expansion
- Acute anterior uveitis or other less common extra-articular manifestations in some patients
- Association with psoriasis, chronic inflammatory bowel disease and reactive arthritis in some patients
- Characteristic radiographic findings
- Generally good symptomatic response to anti-inflammatory doses of non-steroidal anti-inflammatory drugs

INTRODUCTION

Ankylosing spondylitis (AS) is a chronic systemic inflammatory rheumatic disorder of uncertain etiology that primarily affects the axial skeleton (sacroiliac joints and spine); sacroiliac joint involvement (sacroiliitis) is its hallmark[1–3] (Fig. 28.1). The name is derived from the Greek roots *angkylos* = 'bent' (although the word ankylosis now means joint stiffening or fusion) and *spondylos* = spinal vertebra. However, spinal ankylosis appears only in late stages of the disease and may not occur at all in some patients with mild disease.[1–12] Hip and shoulder joints and less commonly the peripheral (limb) joints may also be involved. There can also be involvement of some extra-articular structures. The disease is approximately two to three times more common in males than females in developed countries[2,12].

Historical aspects

This disease has affected mankind since antiquity,[4] but the earliest anatomical descriptions of skeletons with abnormalities typical of AS are attributed to Realdo Colombo in 1559, and Bernard Connor in 1693[6]. Bernard Connor described an ankylosed skeleton consisting of fused pelvis, spine and ribs that was unearthed by French farmers in a cemetery. He wrote that the bones were 'so straitly and intimately joined, their ligaments perfectly bony, and their articulations so effaced, that they really made but one uniform continuous bone'.

The first clinical descriptions of the disease were reported in the mid to late 19th century and medical interest in AS was stimulated by a series of publications between the years 1893 and 1899 by Vladimir von Bechterew (1857–1927) in St Petersburg, Russia[6]. Other clinical reports on AS were published by Adolf Strümpell (1853–1926) and Pierre Marie

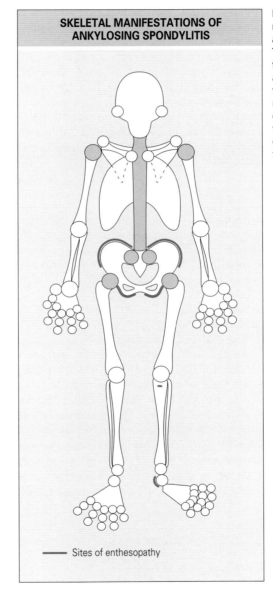

SKELETAL MANIFESTATIONS OF ANKYLOSING SPONDYLITIS

—— Sites of enthesopathy

Fig. 28.1 Skeletal manifestations of ankylosing spondylitis. The axial skeletal sites frequently involved in AS are colored pink, while the blue coloration marks some of the sites of enthesopathy, such as the heels, iliac crest and gluteal and tibial tuberosities.

(1853–1940). Therefore, AS has been known by many different names, including 'morbus Bechterew' (Bechterew's disease), 'Marie–Strümpell disease' and 'morbus Strümpell–Marie–Bechterew'. The earliest X-ray examination of a patient with AS was described in 1899, and Walter Geilinger[7] in 1917 provided one of the first clear radiographic descriptions of the typical syndesmophytes that lead to spinal fusion in AS. Krebs, Scott, Forestier and others, many years later in the 1930s, clearly delineated other radiographic manifestations of AS, including sacroiliitis[6].

During the first half of the 20th century the disease was inappropriately also known as 'rheumatoid spondylitis', particularly in the USA, because of the false belief that it was a variant of rheumatoid arthritis (RA). It was only in 1963 that the American Rheumatism Association officially adopted the term ankylosing spondylitis in preference to rheumatoid spondylitis. In Europe, on the other hand, the term ankylosing spondylitis, or its variants 'spondylitis ankylosans' and 'spondylarthritis ankylopoietica', have been in wide use for more than 100 years[6–9].

Spondyloarthropathies

Ankylosing spondylitis mostly occurs alone without any associated disease but it may sometimes be associated with inflammatory bowel disease (IBD; ulcerative colitis and Crohn's disease), psoriasis or reactive arthritis – so-called 'secondary' AS. The arthritis observed in AS or in association with these related diseases is frequently referred to collectively as 'spondyloarthropathy' because sacroiliitis, spondylitis and inflammatory peripheral arthritis are their frequent manifestations[5,10–15]. By definition, the term 'primary', 'uncomplicated' or 'pure' AS implies exclusion of the other spondyloarthropathies; it is typically a disease predominantly involving the axial skeleton and is generally considered to be the commonest and most typical form of spondyloarthropathy in developed countries[10–12]. Some authors add a prefix 'seronegative' to the term 'spondyloarthropathy' to denote the lack of association of this group of diseases with IgM rheumatoid factor in the serum of patients.

CLINICAL FEATURES

Ankylosing spondylitis usually begins with back pain and stiffness in late adolescence and early adulthood. The average age of onset in developed countries varies between 24 and 26 years, and disease onset after age 45 is very rare[1,2,5,6,9,13]. A variety of clinical presentations due to enthesitis, peripheral arthritis or acute anterior uveitis may antedate back symptoms in some patients[11–26] (Table 28.1).

About 15% of patients have onset of their disease in childhood (before age 16) but this percentage may be as high as 40% in some developing countries[14,15,23–26]. Many of these children, often boys, have 5–10 years of persistent or recurrent bouts of enthesitis and/or lower extremity oligoarthritis (seronegative enthesopathy and arthritis, SEA syndrome) before definite symptoms and signs of axial disease develop. The SEA syndrome and juvenile-onset forms of AS and related spondyloarthropathies account for about 20% of all cases of juvenile arthritis seen by pediatric rheumatologists[24,25]. They are relatively more commonly observed among North American native populations and Mexican mestizos, and in many developing countries[14,15,23,26].

The clinical features of AS can be divided into musculoskeletal and extraskeletal manifestations (Table 28.1). The earliest, most typical

TABLE 28.1 CLINICAL FEATURES OF AS

Skeletal	Axial arthritis, e.g. sacroiliitis and spondylitis
	Arthritis of 'girdle joints' (hips and shoulders)
	Peripheral arthritis uncommon
	Others: enthesitis, osteoporosis, vertebral fractures, spondylodiscitis, pseudoarthrosis
Extraskeletal	Acute anterior uveitis
	Cardiovascular involvement
	Pulmonary involvement
	Cauda equina syndrome
	Enteric mucosal lesions
	Amyloidosis, miscellaneous

and consistent findings of AS result from sacroiliitis and enthesitis (Fig. 28.2)[27–32]. There is often associated inflammation of discovertebral, apophyseal, costovertebral and costotransverse joints of the spine, and of the paravertebral ligamentous structures. This can result in fibrous and bony ankylosis after many years, perhaps as a secondary consequence of the primary inflammatory process[29,30,32] (Fig. 28.3).

Musculoskeletal manifestations

Chronic low back pain and stiffness

The most common and characteristic initial symptoms are chronic low back pain and stiffness, usually of insidious onset and dull in character. Many patients complain of pain in the buttock region as their earliest symptom but are unable to localize it precisely[5,6,12,16]. The pain probably represents sacroiliac joint involvement and is felt deep in the gluteal region, but some patients may note radiation of pain down the upper part of posterior thigh region, which can be misdiagnosed as 'lumbago' or 'sciatica', although neurologic examination is within normal limits. The pain may be unilateral or intermittent at first, or may alternate, first in one buttock and then the other, but it generally becomes persistent and bilateral within a few months, and the lower lumbar area becomes stiff and painful. This may be accompanied by sacroiliac and/or spinal tenderness.

The back pain and stiffness can be quite severe at this early stage and the pain tends to be accentuated on coughing, sneezing or maneuvers that cause a sudden twist of the back. Sometimes, pain and stiffness in the midthoracic or cervical region, or chest pain, may be the initial symptom, rather than the more typical low backache[10–12,17]. Back symptoms tend to worsen after prolonged periods of inactivity ('gel phenomenon'), and are therefore worse in the morning. The pain and stiffness tend to be eased by moving about ('limbering up') and with mild physical activity or exercise, and a hot shower. Some patients may wake-up at night to exercise or move about for a few minutes before returning to bed. The patient often experiences difficulty in getting out of bed because of pain and stiffness and may roll sideways off the bed, trying not to flex or rotate the spine.

Because of the high prevalence of back pain in the population at large, it is helpful to elicit from the patient's clinical history certain features that help in differentiating the non-inflammatory causes from the inflammatory back pain of AS and related spondyloarthropathies[6,16]. Characteristically, the onset of inflammatory back symptoms is insidious rather than abrupt, and the patient often cannot precisely date the onset of symptoms because they may be trivial or fleeting aches and pains in the beginning. The onset is usually in young individuals in their late teens and early twenties. It is very uncommon for the disease to begin after 45 years of age[6,13]. As the symptoms become chronic (defined as persistence for at least 3 months), the patient notices prominent back pain and stiffness in the morning that usually lasts for half an hour or more. The symptoms improve with physical activity or exercise but not with rest, and they get worse on prolonged rest.

Occasionally, back pain may be absent or too mild to impel the patient to seek medical care. Some may complain only of back stiffness, fleeting muscle aches or musculotendinous tender spots. These symptoms may become worse on exposure to cold or dampness[2,16,33], and some of these patients may be misdiagnosed as having fibromyalgia. Mild constitutional symptoms, such as anorexia, malaise, weight loss and low-grade fever, may occur in some patients in the early stages of their disease, and are relatively more common among patients with juvenile-onset AS, especially in developing countries[2,16,23,25,26].

Sleep disturbance and daytime fatigue

In many patients the back pain and stiffness may interrupt sleep, especially in the early morning hours, rather than at earlier times in the

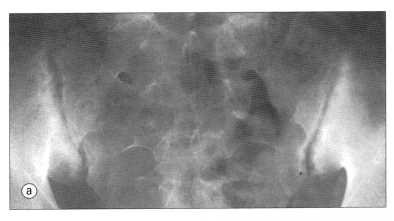

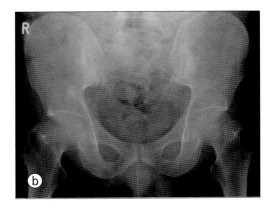

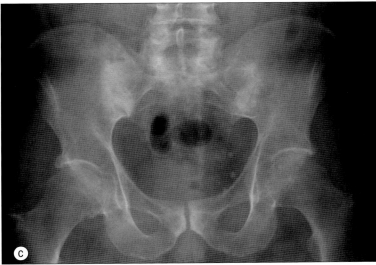

Fig. 28.2 Radiographic changes of sacroiliitis. (a) Early radiographic changes of sacroiliitis in AS consist of bony erosions ('postage stamp serrations') and adjacent bony sclerosis. These changes are typically seen first, and tend to be more prominent, on the iliac side of the sacroiliac joints. (b) Pelvic radiograph showing bilateral sacroiliitis (grade 2–3), with erosions, bony sclerosis and joint width irregularities. (c) Pelvic radiograph showing bilateral sacroiliitis (grade 3), with definite erosions, severe juxta-articular bony sclerosis and blurring of the joint. Radiographic changes of osteitis pubis are also present. (b & c Courtesy of M Rudwaleit and J Sieper.)

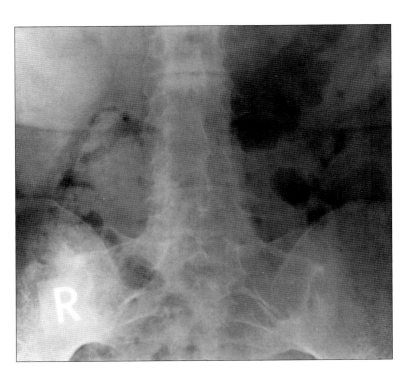

Fig. 28.3 Radiographic changes of advanced AS with fused sacroiliac joints. The ankylosis has also involved the lower lumbar spine ('bamboo spine'). Discogenic disease with end-plate bone changes is present at the L2, L3 level.

night. Therefore inadequate sleep and daytime somnolence and fatigue can be major complaints, and they are closely related to pain and stiffness at bedtime and during the night. A recent study found that 80% of the female and 50% of the male AS patients complained of too little sleep, primarily because of pain, compared to less than 30% of the general population[34].

Enthesitis

Enthesitis can result in extra-articular or juxta-articular bony tenderness, a major or presenting complaint in some patients, especially among those with juvenile-onset AS[20–30]. Enthesitis may appear alone or with arthritis, and can cause tenderness of costosternal junctions, spinous processes, iliac crests, greater trochanters, ischial tuberosities, tibial tubercles or sites of attachments of ligaments and tendons to calcaneus and tarsal bones of the feet. Plantar fasciitis or less often Achilles tendinitis can result in heel pain and tenderness over the inferior and posterior surfaces of the calcaneus respectively[20–24].

Hip and shoulder involvement

Sometimes the first symptoms may result from involvement of 'root' or 'girdle' joints (the hips and the shoulders). An accurate assessment of the range of motion of these joints should be recorded, because their involvement can result in severe functional limitation and disability. These joints may be involved at some stage of disease in one-third of the patients but this is relatively more common among those with juvenile-onset of AS[24–26,29]. If hip involvement has not occurred in the first 10 years of disease, it is very unlikely to occur later. However, some degree of fixed flexion contracture may be noted at later stages of the disease, and that can give rise to a characteristic rigid gait with some flexion at the knees to maintain an erect posture.

Hip joint involvement is usually bilateral, insidious in onset and potentially more crippling than involvement of any other joint of the extremities. It typically results in symmetric concentric joint space narrowing[29] (Fig. 28.4). The pain is typically felt in the groin but in some it may be felt in the ipsilateral knee or the thigh. Some patients with juvenile onset of AS may present with recurrent episodes of unilateral or bilateral painful but reversible contractures of their hip flexor muscles.

Involvement of the shoulder girdle (glenohumeral, acromioclavicular or sternoclavicular joints) may only lead to relatively minor limitations, mostly resulting from some loss of shoulder joint and thoracoscapular movement[35]. Erosive enthesitis of the supraspinatus tendon insertion is the characteristic shoulder lesion in AS patients[29] (Fig. 28.5). Primary involvement of the glenohumeral joint is rare but it can result in complete ankylosis of the joint[29].

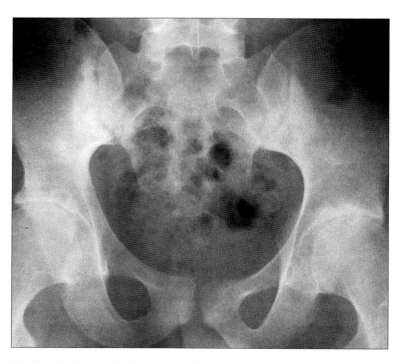

Fig. 28.4 Radiographic changes resulting from bilateral hip joint involvement in moderately advanced stages of AS.

Peripheral joint involvement

Involvement of peripheral joints other than hips and shoulders is infrequent in primary AS in developed countries, although sites affected may include the knees, wrists, elbows and feet. When present, involvement is usually asymmetric, monoarticular or oligoarticular; it is normally mild, rarely persistent or erosive and tends to resolve without any residual joint deformity in most patients[1,2,6,11,12]. However, peripheral joint involvement is relatively more frequent in developing countries, and also among patients who have associated psoriasis or inflammatory bowel disease, or those with juvenile onset of AS[13–15, 21–26]. Peripheral joint involvement can occasionally occur after the axial disease has become inactive. Rare occurrence of inflammatory edema of distal extremities together with peripheral arthritis and enthesitis has been reported[13].

Intermittent knee hydroarthrosis is occasionally the presenting manifestation of juvenile-onset AS[23,25]. Tarsal joint involvement in the feet, primarily reported in Mexican mestizo children, can be an unusual presenting manifestation of juvenile AS. It can ultimately lead to bony ankylosis of joints of the feet and is therefore called 'tarsal ankylosing enthesitis' or 'ankylosing tarsitis'[23].

Chest and spinal involvement

Involvement of the thoracic spine (including the costovertebral and costotransverse joints), enthesitis at costosternal areas and inflammation of manubriosternal junction or sternoclavicular joints may cause chest pain[17,21,29]. The pain may be accentuated on coughing or sneezing and at times may even mimic symptoms of atypical angina or pericarditis. Many patients give a history of having complained of chest pain to a physician before AS has been diagnosed. Some patients notice an inability to expand the chest fully on inspiration. Stiffness and pain in the cervical spine generally tend to develop after some years but occasionally occur in the early stages of the disease. Some patients may get recurrent episodes of stiff neck (torticollis).

Physical examination

As in other diseases where the etiology is not clearly defined, the diagnosis of AS is based on clinical and radiographic features[16,29–31,36–39]. A thorough physical examination, particularly of the musculoskeletal system, is needed. Clinical signs are sometimes minimal in the early stages of the disease. Examination of the sacroiliac joints and the spine (including the neck), measurement of chest expansion and range of motion of the hip and shoulder joints, and a search for signs of enthesitis are critical in making an early diagnosis of AS[16,31,39]. Important physical findings due to enthesitis that can be present in many patients but are often overlooked include tenderness over vertebral spinal processes, iliac crest, anterior

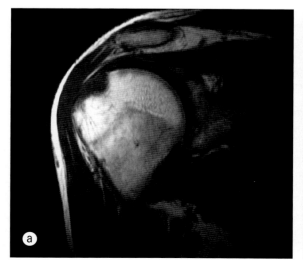

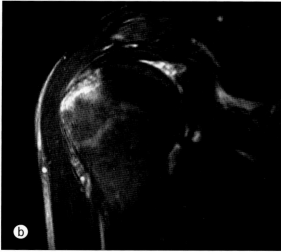

Fig. 28.5 Magnetic resonance images showing enthesitis at the rotator cuff insertion into the superolateral aspect of the humeral head. (a) T1-weighted image, coronal section, demonstrating loss of the marrow fat signal in the greater tuberosity of the humeral head.
(b) T2-weighted image, coronal section, demonstrating diffuse edema in the greater tuberosity of the humerus adjacent to the supraspinatus enthesis. (Courtesy of W Maksymowych.)

chest wall, calcaneus (plantar fasciitis and/or Achilles tendinitis), ischial tuberosities, greater trochanters and sometimes tibial tubercles[5,22–25].

Direct pressure over the sacroiliac joint frequently, but not always, elicits pain if there is active sacroiliitis (Fig. 28.6). Sometimes sacroiliac pain may be elicited by pressure over the anterior superior iliac spines and on compressing the two iliac bones towards each other or forcing them away from each other. The pain can also be elicited by pressure over the lower half of the sacrum, with the patient lying prone, or by compressing the pelvis with the patient lying on one side. Hyperextension of the lumbar spine or hyperextension of one hip joint while applying counterpressure on the iliac crest by the other hand, with the patient lying supine, can also be painful. Other maneuvers include maximal flexion of one hip joint and hyperextension of the other, or maximal flexion, abduction and external rotation of the hip joints (Figs 28.7 & 28.8). All these maneuvers are then repeated on the opposite side. However, these tests will also elicit pain in the presence of hip joint involvement by itself.

If two or more of these maneuvers elicit pain in the region of the sacroiliac joints, the likelihood of the presence of active sacroiliitis (in the presence of appropriate clinical symptoms) is quite strong, and this must be confirmed by radiographic imaging[29–31] (Fig. 28.2). These clinical signs, however, may be absent in some patients despite sacroiliitis because the sacroiliac joints have strong ligaments that limit their

motion, and also these tests are not specific for sacroiliitis. In addition, these physical signs become negative in late stages of the disease, as fibrosis and bony ankylosis replace inflammation. Clinical detection of flexion contracture of the hip joint is illustrated in Figure 28.9 and limitation of shoulder range of motion in Figure 28.10.

Tenderness and stiffness of the paraspinal muscles often accompany the inflammation of the axial skeleton, and the initial loss of spinal mobility is usually due to pain and muscle spasm rather than bony ankylosis. Therefore, marked improvement in spinal mobility can occur

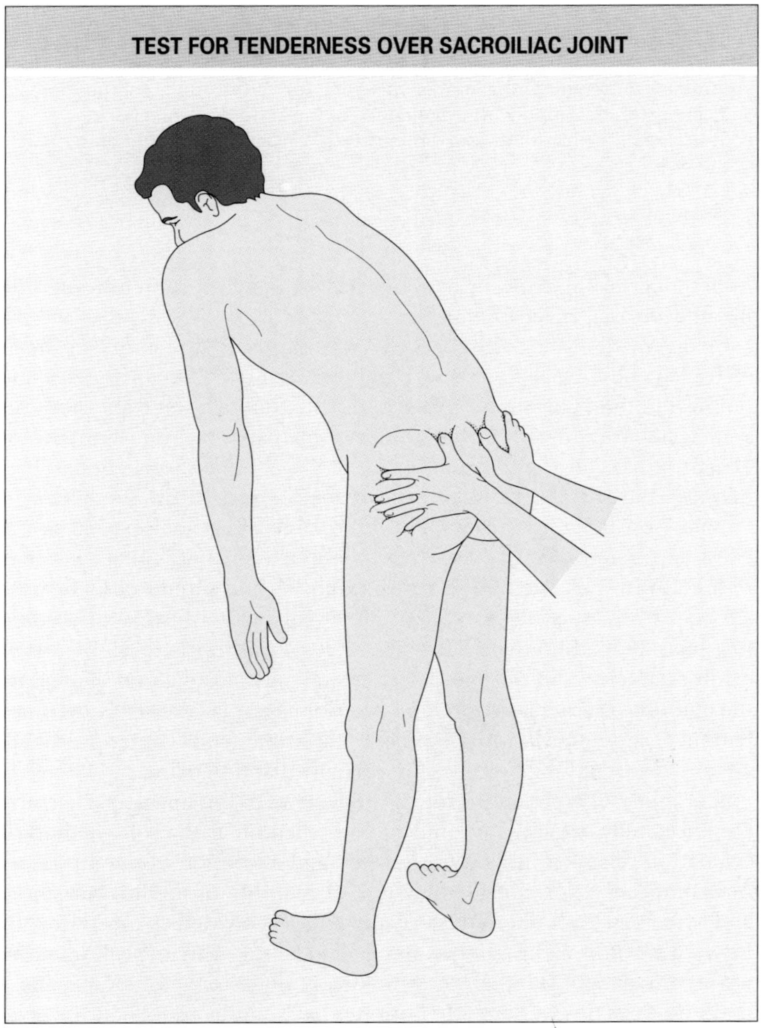

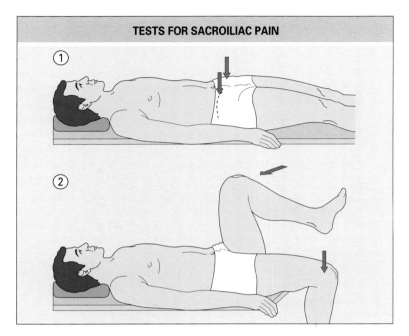

Fig. 28.7 Tests for sacroiliac pain. Two procedures that may cause pain in the sacroiliac area in patients with sacroiliitis. Application of direct pressure on the anterior superior iliac spines, along with attempts to force the iliac spines laterally apart (1); and forced flexion of one hip maximally towards the opposite shoulder, with hyperextension of the contralateral hip joint (2).

TEST FOR TENDERNESS OVER SACROILIAC JOINT

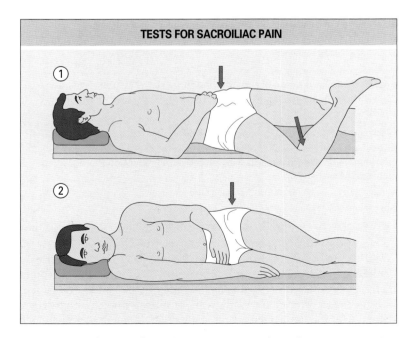

Fig. 28.6 Test for tenderness over sacroiliac joint. Application of firm pressure by thumb (or fist) directly over the sacroiliac joints can elicit tenderness in many patients. The figure also illustrates the patient's inability to touch the floor. The decrease in spinal mobility is often more readily recognized on hyperextension (dorsiflexion) or lateral flexion of the spine.

Fig. 28.8 Tests for sacroiliac pain. Two more procedures that may cause pain in the sacroiliac area in patients with sacroiliitis. Application of downward pressure on the flexed knee, with hip flexed, abducted and externally rotated (1); and compression of the pelvis with the patient lying on one side (2).

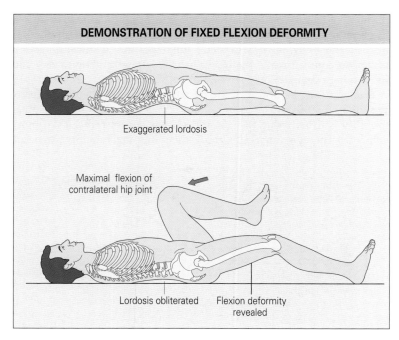

DEMONSTRATION OF FIXED FLEXION DEFORMITY

Exaggerated lordosis

Maximal flexion of contralateral hip joint

Lordosis obliterated   Flexion deformity revealed

Fig. 28.9 Demonstration of fixed flexion deformity. Fixed flexion deformity of the hip joint can be revealed as the contralateral hip joint is maximally flexed to obliterate the exaggerated compensatory lumbar lordosis.

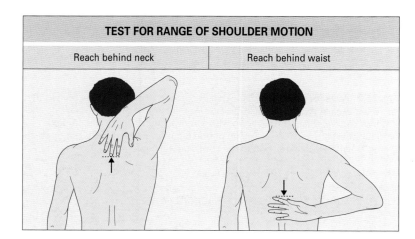

TEST FOR RANGE OF SHOULDER MOTION

| Reach behind neck | Reach behind waist |

Fig. 28.10 Test for range of shoulder motion. Relatively subtle limitation of motion of the shoulder joint can easily be detected. The patient is asked to bring the arm behind the waist (to test internal rotation) and reach up along the spine as high as possible, then to bring the arm behind the neck and reach down along the spine as far as possible (to test external rotation). In individuals with the normal range of motion of the shoulder joints, these reaches overlap, but in patients with limited range of motion there is a gap between these reaches.

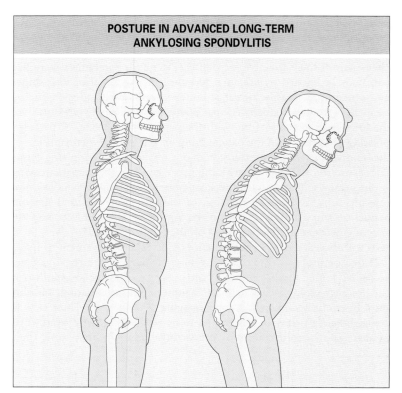

POSTURE IN ADVANCED LONG-TERM ANKYLOSING SPONDYLITIS

Fig. 28.11 Posture in advanced long-term ankylosing spondylitis. Progressive flattening of the lumbar spine and forward stooping of the thoracic and cervical spine, along with prominence of the abdomen, mild flexion contracture of the hip joints and diminution of vertical height after many years of the disease process.

after treatment with non-steroidal anti-inflammatory drugs (NSAIDs) and intensive physical therapy at an early stage of the disease.

With longer disease duration and disease progression, there is a gradual loss of mobility of the lumbar spine. The entire spine becomes increasingly stiff, with loss of spinal mobility in all planes. The patient loses normal posture after many years of disease progression; there is flattening of the lumbar spine and gradual development of accentuated dorsal (thoracic) spinal kyphosis (Fig. 28.11). The inflammatory process can extend to involve the cervical spine, and assessment of its range of motion, particularly the lateral flexion, axial rotation and hyperextension, should not be neglected[39]. Temporomandibular joint pain and

local tenderness may occur in about 10% of patients, sometimes resulting in decreased range of motion of this joint.

Involvement of the costovertebral and costotransverse joints results in restricted chest expansion. Severe limitation of chest expansion is a late physical finding but mild to moderate reduction of chest expansion can be detectable at an early stage of AS in some patients. The normal chest expansion is 5cm or greater, although it is age- and sex-dependent. It is measured at the fourth intercostal space (or just below the breast in females) on maximal inspiration after forced maximal expiration. A chest expansion of less than 2.5cm is abnormal (unless there is other reason for it, such as emphysema or scoliosis), and should raise the possibility of AS, especially in young individuals with a history of chronic low back pain. Because of the presence of enthesitis, patients often exhibit tenderness of the anterior chest wall over costochondral areas or the manubriosternal junction. The anterior chest wall gradually becomes flattened, shoulders become 'stooped', the abdomen becomes protuberant and the breathing becomes increasingly diaphragmatic.

The ability of a patient to touch the floor with the fingertips, keeping the knees fully extended, should not be relied on as the sole method of evaluation of spinal mobility. A good range of motion of the hip joints can compensate for considerable loss of mobility of the lumbar spine, and *vice versa*. Schober's test is quite useful to detect limitation of forward flexion of the lumbar spine (Fig. 28.12). This is performed by having the patient stand erect (with knees fully extended) and placing a mark on the skin overlying the fifth lumbar spinous process at the level of the posterior superior iliac spines (the 'dimples of Venus'). A second mark is placed 10cm above in the midline. The patient is then asked to maximally bend the spine forward without bending the knees. The 10cm distance between the two marks on the skin expands by 5cm or more in normal healthy individuals through stretching of the skin overlying the

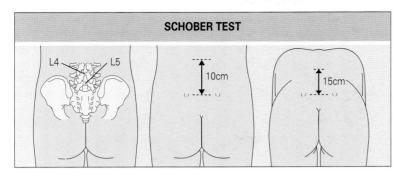

Fig. 28.12 Schober test. This measures the ability to flex the lumbar spine (see text).

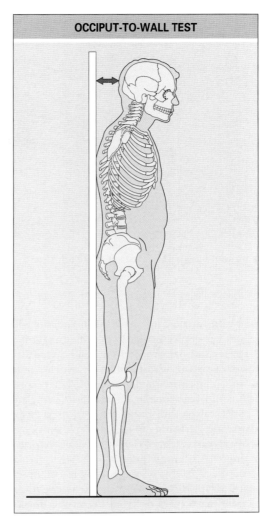

Fig. 28.13 Occiput-to-wall test.

mobile lumbar spine. An increase of less than 3cm indicates diminished lumbar spinal mobility. Limitations of lateral flexion as well as hyperextension of the spine also accompany and often precede this diminished spinal mobility on forward flexion.

Although spinal ankylosis develops at a variable rate and pattern, the typical spinal deformities of AS usually evolve after 10 or more years. However, the disease may occasionally remain confined to one part of the spine. Involvement of the cervical spine, usually one of the last musculoskeletal manifestations, results in progressive limitation of neck motion with a decreased ability to turn or extend the neck fully and a gradual development of forward stooping of the neck after many years (Fig. 28.11). The stooping of the neck can be measured by the occiput-to-wall test (Fig. 28.13). The patient, while standing erect with the buttocks against a wall and the back of the heels touching the wall, attempts to touch the wall with the back of the head while keeping a horizontal gaze. Any gap between the occiput and the wall is measured.

At this advanced stage the presence of disease is readily apparent because of the characteristic gait and posture and the way the patient sits or rises from the examining table. At this stage the pain from spinal involvement diminishes and there is less morning stiffness, but some degree of inflammatory pain is usually present. In extreme cases, the entire spine may be fused in a flexed position and the field of vision becomes limited, making it difficult for some patients to look ahead as they walk. Similarly, the hip joints may become ankylosed and the patient may need to stand with knees flexed to maintain posture. Such patients may injure themselves more readily because the rigid spine impairs their ability to balance themselves after sudden changes of position.

The deep tendon reflexes in the lower extremities are normal and the straight-leg-raising test is negative. Convincing evidence for involvement of skeletal muscles in AS is lacking. The muscle weakness and sometimes marked muscle wasting seen in some patients with advanced disease probably results from disuse, although some ultrastructural changes in muscle and a persistent modestly raised level of serum creatine kinase have occasionally been observed[2,16]. However, in addition to any myopathy, one should not overlook the presence of any myelopathy in such patients.

Extraskeletal manifestations

Ocular manifestations

Acute anterior uveitis is the most common extra-articular feature of AS, occurring in 25–40% of patients at some time in the course of their disease[40–45]. It is an acute inflammation of the iris and ciliary body and is therefore also called 'acute iritis' or 'iridocyclitis'. It is relatively more common in those AS patients who possess HLA-B27, or have peripheral joint involvement[41,45]. In North America and western Europe, close to 95% of patients with AS and acute anterior uveitis possess HLA-B27,

and approximately 50% of all patients with isolated acute anterior uveitis are HLA-B27-positive. It is the most common definable type, representing about 15% of all kinds of uveitis. Occasionally, the uveitis may be the presenting symptom that draws attention to the diagnosis of AS or related spondyloarthropathy[40,42].

It is typically unilateral, but has a tendency to recur, not infrequently in the contralateral eye. The symptoms usually begin acutely with eye pain, increased lacrimation, photophobia and some blurring of vision. The eye is inflamed, there is circumcorneal congestion (Fig. 28.14), the pupil is small, the iris is edematous and it may appear slightly discolored compared to the contralateral side. There is copious exudate in the anterior chamber of the eye, which can be seen on slit-lamp examination. The inflammatory cells adhere to the endothelial lining cells of the cornea, forming small aggregates called keratitic precipitates. Ophthalmologists characterize these findings as 'non-granulomatous' to distinguish them from what is usually seen in uveitis of sarcoidosis and some of the other granulomatous diseases.

The individual attack of acute uveitis usually subsides within a few weeks without any sequelae, but residual visual impairment may occur if treatment is inadequate or delayed. The pupil may become irregular if the inflamed iris gets stuck to the cornea (anterior synechiae) or to the lens (posterior synechiae). This can result in secondary glaucoma and cataract in the long run. In rare cases, the posterior chamber may also be involved, resulting in cystoid macular edema; and one should look for the presence of associated IBD or psoriais if the uveitis begins insidiously, lasts longer than 6 months, is bilateral or involves the posterior uveal tract[43,44].

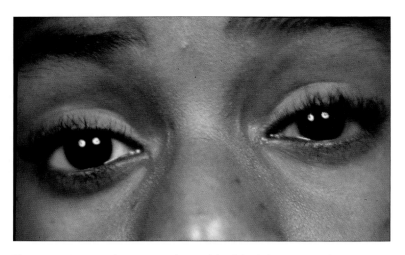

Fig. 28.14 Untreated acute anterior uveitis of the left eye. Note the circumcorneal congestion.

Cardiac manifestations
Recent studies suggest that cardiovascular involvement in patients with AS is more common than was previously realized[46–48]. Inflammation at the aortic root (aortitis) causes intimal proliferation and adventitial scarring of the vasa vasorum. This can lead to fibrosis, which results in hemodynamically unimportant consequences. However, in some patients, it results in aortic incompetence due to a dilated aortic ring and thickened and shortened aortic valves with nodularities of their cusps. The fibrotic process can also cause thickening of the adjacent ventricular septum and the basal part of anterior leaflet of the mitral valve to form a characteristic 'subaortic bump'. This 'bump' and/or thickened valvular cusps can be detected in more than 30% of AS patients by transthoracic and transesophageal echocardiography. However, most such patients are without any clinically apparent heart disease. Extension of the fibrotic process into the atrioventricular conduction bundle can, however, cause partial or complete heart block[47].

The risk of occurrence of aortic insufficiency and cardiac conduction disturbances increases with the age of the patient, the duration of AS, the presence of HLA-B27 and peripheral joint involvement[47]. For example, cardiac conduction disturbances occur in up to 3% of those with disease of 15 years' duration but up to 9% after 30 years. Complete heart block causing Stokes–Adam's attacks may supervene in some patients, necessitating implantation of cardiac pacemakers. The aortic regurgitation follows a chronic but relentless course to heart failure, usually over several years, necessitating valvular replacement. Sometimes acute aortic (and rarely even mitral) insufficiency with rapid deterioration of cardiac function can occur in relatively young patients with minimal spondylitis[46].

Studies in Sweden have described the occurrence of the cardiac syndrome of 'lone aortic incompetence plus pacemaker-requiring bradycardia' in men without spondyloarthropathy as an HLA-B27-associated inflammatory condition[47]. Among 91 patients with the combination of heart block and aortic insufficiency, 88% had HLA-B27 but only about 20% of them had AS or related spondyloarthropathy. There is no association between HLA-B27 and lone aortic incompetence in the absence of complete heart block or spondyloarthropathy. However, HLA-B27 was found to be more prevalent (17%) among 83 patients with isolated complete heart block (without any clinical or radiographic evidence of associated spondyloarthropathy) than the 6% prevalence in normal controls.

Pulmonary manifestations
Rigidity of the chest wall in patients with AS results in inability to expand the chest fully on inspiration and can result in mild restrictive lung func-

tion impairment. However, this does not usually result in ventilatory insufficiency because of increased diaphragmatic contribution. Pleuropulmonary involvement can occur as a rare and late extraskeletal manifestation, in the form of a slowly progressive and usually bilateral apical pulmonary fibrobullous disease in 1–2% of patients. It appears as linear or patchy opacities on chest radiographs and they can eventually become cystic[49]. These cavitations may mimic tuberculosis lesions and may become colonized by *Aspergillus* species, with the formation of mycetoma. The patient may complain of cough, increasing dyspnea and occasionally hemoptysis.

Newer imaging modalities, such as thin-section high-resolution computed tomography (CT), indicate that there is general under-recognition of the pulmonary parenchymal involvement in AS[50,51]. An uncontrolled study of 26 AS patients revealed a high incidence of lung abnormalities on high-resolution CT of the lungs, including four patients with interstitial lung disease that has hitherto not been associated with AS[51]. The abnormalities observed are usually subtle and subclinical, mostly comprising thickening of the interlobular septa, mild bronchial wall or pleural thickening, pleuropulmonary irregularities and linear septal thickening. Moreover, they do not correlate with functional and clinical impairment.

Gastrointestinal manifestations
Apart from the well known association of chronic IBD with AS, there is also a high prevalence of other forms of spondyloarthropathies, unrelated to the extent of the bowel disease[52–55]. However, sacroiliitis, both symptomatic and asymptomatic, is related to the disease duration. In a recent study of a population-based cohort of 521 patients with IBD seen 6 years after diagnosis, 6% of patients with Crohn's disease and 2.6% of those with ulcerative colitis were found to have AS[54]. The overall prevalence of spondyloarthropathy was 22%, and 2% had radiological sacroiliitis without clinical features of spondyloarthropathy.

Clinically 'silent' (asymptomatic) enteric mucosal inflammatory lesions, both macroscopic and microscopic, have been detected in the terminal ileum and proximal colon on ileocolonoscopic studies in more than 50% of AS patients with no gastrointestinal symptoms[52]. Follow-up studies of such patients indicate that 6% of them will develop IBD and, among those with histologically 'chronic' inflammatory gut lesions, between 15% and 25% will develop clinically obvious Crohn's disease[52]. This suggests that the latter group of patients initially had a subclinical form of Crohn's disease when they presented with arthritis, and supports the existence of a pathogenic link between gut inflammation and AS that is independent of HLA-B27.

Osteoporosis
Spinal osteoporosis is frequently observed, especially in patients with severe AS of long duration, partly as a result of lack of spinal mobility due to ankylosis, but it may also be related to mineralization defect[56,57] (Fig. 28.15). A marked reduction in bone mineral density of the lumbar spine and femoral neck has been reported by dual energy X-ray absorptiometry (DEXA) measurement in a group of young patients with early AS. It may result from proinflammatory cytokines and contributes to spinal fractures and progressive spinal deformity in some patients. Bone biopsies and assessment of biochemical markers of bone metabolism have shown that both diminished bone formation and enhanced bone resorption are involved[56,57].

Spondylodiscitis and spinal fractures
An aseptic spondylodiscitis, mostly in the midthoracic spine and usually asymptomatic, can occur without any physical trauma and is relatively more common in the patients whose spondylitis also involves the cervical spine[58]. There is also an increased prevalence of anterior compression of the vertebral body, discovertebral destructive lesions (so-called Andersson lesions) and spinal fractures[59–65].

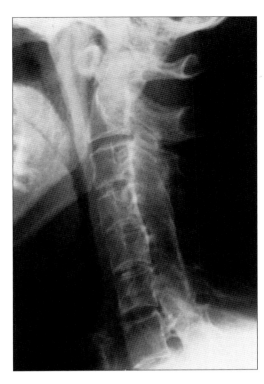

Fig. 28.15 Radiograph of cervical spine, lateral view, showing marked osteopenia and bony fusions at multiple levels. Osteitis of the corners of the vertebral bodies is best demonstrated at C6–C7 level anteriorly, causing 'shiny corners' (Romanus lesions) due to reactive bone sclerosis. There is associated bony resorption that results in 'squared' vertebral bodies and formation of a vertical bony 'bridging' (syndesmophyte formation) between the two vertebral bodies. There is extensive fusion of the apophyseal joints posteriorly from C3 to C7 level. There is no subluxation at the atlantoaxial junction.

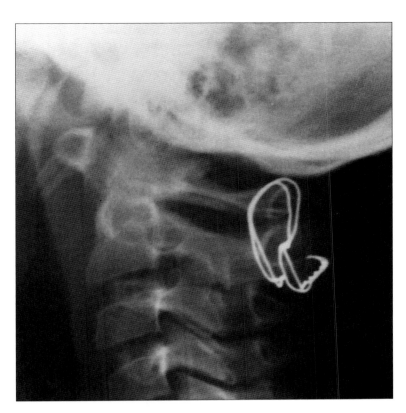

Fig. 28.16 Radiograph of the cervical spine, lateral view, of a young boy with juvenile ankylosing spondylitis. He had undergone surgery for spontaneous severe atlantoaxial subluxation, and the radiograph shows incomplete reduction of the subluxation following surgery.

The ankylosed spine breaks like a long bone and the fracture line is usually transverse; it is more often transdiscal (i.e. across syndysmophytes) than transvertebral. The rigid osteoporotic spine is unduly susceptible to fracture even after a relatively minor trauma, including events that may not be remembered or recalled by the patient[59,60]. One should exclude the possibility of spinal fracture in any patient with advanced AS who complains of new onset of neck or back pain, even in the absence of a definite trauma.

The fracture of cervical spine, usually at the C5–6 or C6–7 level, can result in quadriplegia, especially if associated with dislocation, and is a very serious complication with a high morbidity and mortality[59,65]. Sometimes the undiagnosed or improperly treated fracture results in spondylodiscitis and pseudoarthrosis, and can lead to severe kyphotic deformities[59–64]. The diagnosis of these fractures may be difficult in a 'bamboo spine', and focal spinal abnormalities on bone scans can be a clue to the presence of fracture or pseudarthrosis[60,63]. Magnetic resonance imaging (MRI) is important in detecting and evaluating complications of fractures or pseudoarthrosis, as well as changes in the dura mater, soft tissue and longitudinal ligaments[64].

Atlantoaxial subluxation

Erosions of the odontoid process and the transverse ligament can result in spontaneous atlantoaxial subluxation, usually anteriorly (Fig. 28.16). It can present as occipital pain, with or without signs of spinal cord compression, and is relatively more commonly observed in those with peripheral joint involvement, and also possibly among Mexican patients[66]. It generally occurs in the later stages of the disease, although it can be an early manifestation[67]. Rarely vertical (upward migration of the odontoid process into the brainstem (platybasia)), rotatory, posterior atlantoaxial, or subaxial subluxations, and fracture of the odontoid process have been reported[29,68].

Neurological manifestations

Neurological involvement may occur in patients with AS and is related most often to fracture dislocation of the spine, cauda equina syndrome or atlantoaxial subluxation. A slowly progressive cauda equina syndrome is a rare but significant complication of long-standing AS and results from fibrous entrapment and scarring of the sacral and lower lumbar nerve roots resulting from chronic adhesive arachnoiditis[69,70]. It is associated with dural calcification, erosions of the spinal canal associated with enlarged dural sacs (dural ectasia), and dorsal dural diverticula, which are characteristic of this condition and can be demonstrated by CT and MRI. It can result in sensory loss in the sacral and lower lumbar dermatomes ('saddle anesthesia') and decreased rectal and/or urinary sphincter tone, and may also cause some pain and weakness in the legs. Occurrence of a multiple-sclerosis-like syndrome has also been reported in AS patients but proper epidemiological studies are needed to verify if there is any association[71–73].

Renal manifestations

Renal disease, with or without any impairment of renal function, can occur in patients with AS for various reasons and usually presents with proteinuria and microscopic hematuria, sometimes detected on routine urinalysis[74–79]. Secondary amyloidosis (AA type) is now rarely observed among patients with AS or related spondyloarthropathies in the USA and is also decreasing in some other countries. This is possibly because of more widespread use of NSAIDs and other drugs now available to better control chronic inflammation[78,79]. However, amyloidosis often remains undiagnosed until late in its course because of its slow evolution and relative rarity. This complication should, however, be considered in the differential diagnosis of proteinuria with or without progressive azotemia. Biopsies of abdominal fat pad or rectal mucosa in one European study detected presence of amyloidosis in 10 of 137 unselected patients with AS (approximately 7%), but only two had clinical amyloidosis with proteinuria[77]. However, three more patients developed clinical amyloidosis after a mean of 5.4 years of follow-up.

An increased incidence of IgA nephropathy has also been reported in patients with AS and related spondyloarthropathies[76,80]. Interestingly, an elevated level of serum IgA is frequently observed in patients with AS[81].

Renal disease can also result from chronic NSAID use, and there are a few old reports of a somewhat higher incidence of chronic non-specific prostatitis among patients with AS.

Other clinical manifestations

Preliminary reports indicate that patients with AS and related spondyloarthropathies have an increased incidence of Sjögren's syndrome[82,83]. A possible association with vitiligo has also been suggested[84]. There are a few case reports of co-occurrence of relapsing polychondritis, sarcoidosis, familial Mediterranean fever, Behçet's disease, or retroperitoneal fibrosis in patients with AS and related spondyloarthropathies[85–88], and there is one study suggesting a higher incidence of varicoceles in AS patients[89]. Some spondylitis patients with associated IBD may get pyoderma gangrenosum, erythema nodosum, or sclerosing cholangitis, which are well-recognized extraintestinal manifestations of IBD[90].

INVESTIGATIONS

The most useful investigations are from musculoskeletal imaging (see below), although a number of other laboratory tests are informative. An elevated erythrocyte sedimentation rate (ESR) or serum C-reactive protein (CRP) is present in up to 70% of patients with active AS[6]. However, there is a lack of clear correlation with clinical disease activity, and levels of these acute phase reactants seem to have only limited clinical usefulness[6,91]. A normal ESR and/or CRP does not exclude the presence of clinically active AS. Both may relate more to peripheral arthropathy than the axial disease in AS. Generally speaking, the finding of an elevated ESR or serum CRP in a person with inflammatory back pain increases the likelihood of AS.

A mild normocytic normochromic anemia is present in 15% of patients, depending on the severity of the inflammatory process. Mild to moderate elevations of serum concentration of IgA are observed in 50–60% of patients with AS, and the serum IgA level correlates with acute phase reactants, disease activity and the presence of peripheral arthritis in particular[2,16,81]. Serum complement levels are normal or elevated. Some investigators have detected circulating immune complexes in the serum of patients with AS, while others have not confirmed these findings.

Positive tests for rheumatoid factor and antinuclear antibodies do not occur more frequently in patients with AS than in healthy controls[2,8]. Modest elevations of serum alkaline phosphatase (primarily derived from bone) are seen in some patients but are unrelated to the activity or the duration of the disease and their clinical significance is unclear[16]. The synovial fluid in AS patients does not show markedly distinctive features compared to other inflammatory arthropathies. Mild elevation of cerebrospinal fluid protein has been noted in some patients, perhaps as a result of mild arachnoiditis.

Pulmonary function tests show no ventilatory insufficiency even in advanced cases of AS; an increased diaphragmatic contribution helps to compensate for the rigidity of the chest wall. Vital capacity and total lung capacity are moderately reduced, reflecting the restricted chest wall movement; residual lung volume and functional residual capacity are usually, but not always, increased; and airflow measurements are normal.

Musculoskeletal imaging

Characteristically, the radiographic changes of AS are seen in the axial skeleton, especially in the sacroiliac, discovertebral, apophyseal, costovertebral and costotransverse joints, and they evolve slowly over many years[21,29,30]. The earliest, most consistent and most characteristic radiographic findings are seen in the sacroiliac joints. Various methods have been used to examine the sacroiliac joints radiographically; none is ideal

because of the complex configuration and individual variations of these joints. The radiographic interpretation of early sacroiliitis can be difficult, partly due to the presence of degenerative changes. A plain anteroposterior radiograph of the pelvis or one aimed 30° cephalad (Ferguson's view) is usually adequate to visualize these joints, and an oblique view is not recommended.[92]

The radiographic findings of sacroiliitis are usually bilateral and symmetric. They are first seen in the lower third (synovial part) of the joint, mostly on the iliac side and consist of blurring of the subchondral bone plate[29]. In more advanced disease, erosions ('postage stamp serrations') and sclerosis of the adjacent bones are seen at both joint margins (Fig. 28.2). Progressive subchondral bone erosions at both joint margins can result in 'pseudo-widening' of the sacroiliac joint space. Later erosions become less obvious but the subchondral sclerosis persists and may become more prominent.

There is gradual fibrosis, calcification, interosseous bridging and ossification of the sacroiliac joints. Ultimately (usually after several years) there may be complete bony fusion across the joint and resolution of the adjacent bony sclerosis (Fig. 28.3). Other pelvic abnormalities that may occur include sclerosis and bony erosions at the pubic symphysis (osteitis pubis), and cortical irregularities and osteitis ('whiskering') at sites of osseous attachment of tendons and ligaments (enthesitis), particularly at the ischial tuberosities, iliac crest and femoral trochanters[29].

The evaluation of the sacroiliac joints has been studied by infrared thermography, radionuclide scintigraphy (bone scan), conventional tomography and single photon emission CT (SPECT) in patients with early disease in whom standard radiography of the sacroiliac joints may show normal or equivocal changes. CT of the sacroiliac joint is a more sensitive technique than conventional radiography but both only detect chronic changes (Fig. 28.17). Infrared thermography is not useful and conventional tomography and scintigraphy also need not be performed for diagnosis in such patients because conventional tomography is inferior to CT, and scintigraphy is too non-specific to be of much clinical value in this situation[29,30,93].

Sacroiliac plane radiographs are less reliable in detecting sacroiliitis in children and adolescents, and these patients may require dynamic (gadolinium-enhanced) MRI, which produces, without any ionizing radiation, excellent but more costly computer-generated imaging[6,9,30,94–96]. Dynamic MRI and the use of 'STIR' and other fat suppression techniques can demonstrate the inflammatory response associated with enthesitis[9,20,30,96] (Figs 28.18–28.20). The inflammatory reaction involves not only the adjacent soft tissues but also the underlying bone

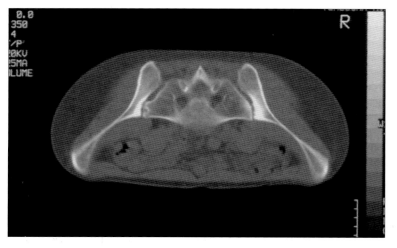

Fig. 28.17 CT of the sacroiliac joints demonstrating definite bilateral sacroiliitis (erosions and sclerosis). (Courtesy of M Rudwaleit and J Sieper.)

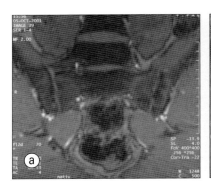
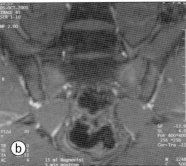
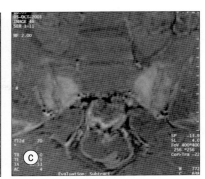

Fig. 28.18 Imaging of inflammatory changes. (a) MRI of the sacroiliac joints. (b) Bilateral inflammatory changes visualized by gadolinium enhancement (5 minutes after gadolinium injection). (c) MRI subtraction evaluation; enhancement of synovial part of sacroiliac joints and juxta-articular bone (reflecting inflammatory changes in the bone, the so called 'bone edema') are clearly visible. (Courtesy of M Rudwaleit and J Sieper.)

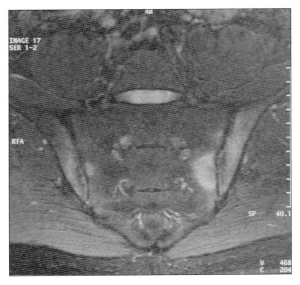

Fig. 28.19 MRI of the sacroiliac joints. This image uses a fat suppression technique (STIR) to visualize inflammatory changes in the bone ('bone edema'), which are more marked on one side. (Courtesy of M Rudwaleit and J Sieper.)

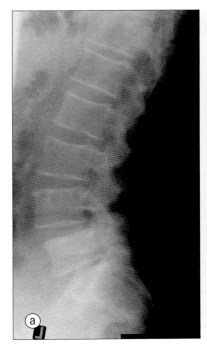
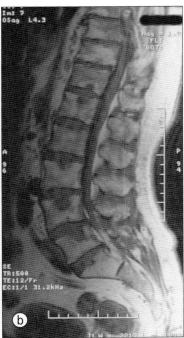

Fig. 28.20 Imaging of AS. (a) Radiograph (lateral view) of the lumbar spine showing a typical Andersson lesion (spondylodiscitis) of the 4th lumbar vertebra. (b) Sagittal T1-weighted MRI of the same patient reveals multisegmental involvement that was not visible on plain radiographs. Moreover, it also shows fat deposition in several vertebral bodies, reflecting degenerative or postinflammatory changes. (Courtesy of M Rudwaleit and J Sieper.)

marrow, and it can sometimes extend to a considerable distance away from the involved enthesis insertion. This utilization of MRI in detecting the inflammatory response at an early stage is not sufficiently well characterized to recommend its widespread use at present[36].

Studies of families with AS have demonstrated that HLA-B27-positive individuals who have typical inflammatory back symptoms or chest pain can lack any radiographic evidence of sacroiliitis or spondylitis[97]. It may take an average of 9 years before sacroiliitis can be detected by plain radiography in such patients, according to one study[98]. In a study of long-term follow-up of undifferentiated spondyloarthropathy, a majority (68%) of such patients developed AS[99]. Dynamic MRI is more sensitive than CT in detecting early sacroiliitis in such patients[9,30,96], and it is also very helpful in detecting spinal fractures and dural diverticuli associated with cauda equina syndrome in AS[63,70].

A study compared CT and MRI in 24 patients with clinical evidence of AS but uncertain radiologic findings, and 12 controls[100]. CT was found to be more specific but less sensitive than MRI; contrast-enhanced MRI especially is more likely to detect early lesions. CT detected sacroiliitis in 38% of the 24 patients and none of the controls. MRI detected sacroiliitis in 54% of the patients, but 17% of controls. Additional studies are required before dynamic MRI can be accepted as a substitute for conventional radiography for detecting sacroiliitis or for monitoring disease activity or progression[95,101]. Ultrasonography is useful in detecting enthesitis and associated bursitis, tendinitis and tenosynovitis (Fig. 28.21), but its accuracy varies, depending on the operator's experience[13,102].

The inflammatory lesions in the vertebral column affect the apophyseal (posterior intervertebral) joints, the superficial layers of the annulus fibrosus at their attachment to the corners of vertebral bodies, and the intervertebral ligaments. Marginal erosive lesions of the corner of the vertebral body with adjacent reactive bone sclerosis can be seen radiographically as 'highlighted corners' (Romanus lesion) (Figs 28.15 & 28.22), but they are better demonstrated by contrast-enhanced (dynamic) MRI[9,20,29,30,94]. Subsequent bone resorption (erosions) can result in 'squaring' of the vertebral body, and this can be followed by a gradual ossification of the superficial layers of the annulus fibrosus and eventually 'bony bridging' between the adjacent vertebrae[29,32]. These vertical bony bridges are called syndesmophytes (Figs 28.23 & 28.24). They begin at the angles of the involved vertebral bodies and are called 'marginal' syndesmophytes. They usually start forming initially in the lower thoracic and the adjacent lumbar spine and then start appearing in the upper thoracic and ultimately the cervical spine.

Radiographic changes identical to those seen in 'primary' AS are generally also seen in those with 'secondary' AS in association with

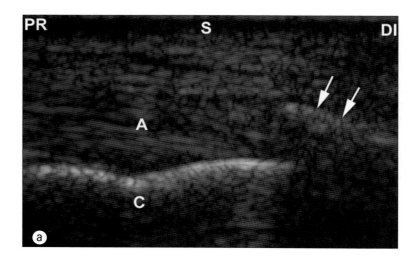

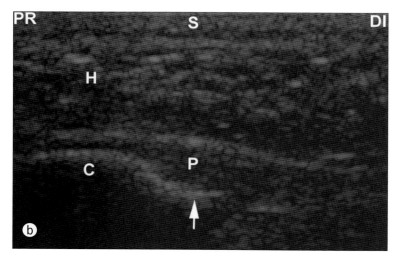

Fig. 28.21 Imaging of the foot. (a) Longitudinal ultrasound scan showing Achilles tendinitis (enthesitis); the tendon is marked as A, and the arrows indicate the presence of an enthesophyte. PR, proximal part of the tendon; DI, distal part; C, calcaneus; S, skin. (b) Longitudinal ultrasound scan showing plantar fasciitis; the enthesophyte is marked by an arrow. C, calcaneus; H, heel fat pad; S, skin. (Courtesy of P Balint and D Kane.)

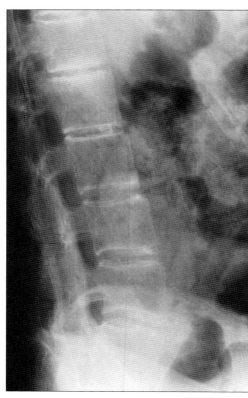

Fig. 28.22 Radiograph of lumbar spine. Lateral view, showing 'shiny corners' (Romanus lesions) and 'squared' vertebral bodies. Mild discogenic disease (discitis) is present between the T12 and L1 vertebrae.

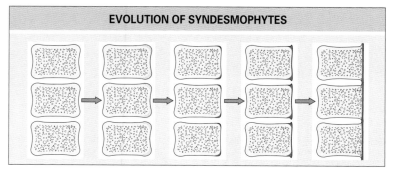

Fig. 28.23 Evolution of syndesmophytes. Lateral view of lumbar spinal vertebral bodies. Osteitis of the corners of the vertebral bodies anteriorly, causing reactive sclerosis ('shiny corners'), shown in red, leads to local bone resorption and resultant 'squared' vertebral bodies. This is followed by vertical bony 'bridging' (syndesmophyte formation), resulting from ossification of the superficial layers of the annulus fibrosus. (Modified from Khan[103].)

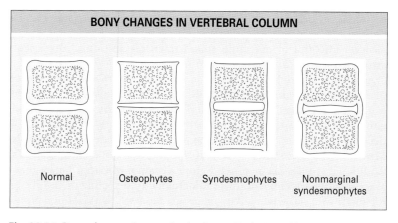

Fig. 28.24 Bony changes in vertebral column. Evolution of bony changes observed in degenerative disc disease (osteophytes), ankylosing spondylitis (syndesmophytes) and psoriatic spondylitis (non-marginal syndesmophytes), affecting the lumbar spine (anteroposterior view).

ulcerative colitis and Crohn's disease[1,2,29]. In contrast, patients with spondylitis in association with reactive arthritis and psoriasis tend to develop random, asymmetric and bulky syndesmophytes (Figs 28.24 & 28.25). These are often called 'non-marginal' syndesmophytes because they do not just extend from one vertebral angle to the other but may start from the middle of one vertebral body and extend to the same area of the adjacent vertebral body. Differentiation of the various forms of spondylo-arthropathy in the end, of course, is based on accompanying clinical features rather than any radiographic differences[5,16,31,103,104] (Table 28.2).

There are often concomitant inflammatory changes and resultant ankylosis in the apophyseal joints, and ossification of some of the spinal ligaments. There is involvement of the costovertebral and costotransverse joints, which can gradually result in limitation of chest expansion. Patients with long-standing severe AS ultimately develop a virtually complete fusion of the vertebral column ('bamboo spine'), which often includes the cervical spine (Fig. 28.26). Some patients may develop spondylodiscitis at one or multiple levels in the spine; it causes discovertebral destructive changes (Andersson lesion), a circumscribed aseptic destructive process and sclerosis affecting intervertebral discs and the adjacent bone plates of the vertebral bodies[29,58,105] (Fig. 28.3).

Spinal osteopenia is frequently observed, which increases the risk of vertebral compression and/or transverse spinal fracture and pseudo-

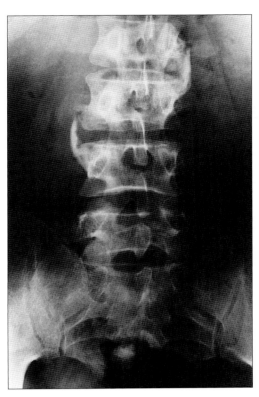

Fig. 28.25 Radiograph of lumbar spine, antero-posterior view, showing bulky, asymmetric non-marginal syndesmophytes in a patient with reactive arthritis. These non-marginal syndesmophytes are identical to those seen in some patients with psoriatic spondylitis, and they can occur in the absence of radiologically ascertainable sacroiliitis. The sacroiliac joints do not show any erosive disease in this patient.

Hip joint involvement has been correlated with early age at onset for AS and is a bad prognostic sign[106] (Fig. 28.4). It leads to symmetric concentric joint space narrowing, irregularity of the subchondral bone plate with subchondral sclerosis, osteophyte formation at the outer margins of the articular surfaces (both the acetabulum and the femoral head) and ultimately bony ankylosis[29]. Shoulder girdle involvement can result in erosions on the superolateral aspect of the humeral head due to erosive enthesitis of the supraspinatus tendon (Fig. 28.5). Involvement of the glenohumeral joint is less common, and it causes concentric joint space narrowing and can lead to bony fusion. There is a relative absence of periarticular osteopenia in the involved hip or shoulder girdles in early stages, as compared to RA. There can be erosive abnormalities or osseous ankylosis of the acromioclavicular joint. Periosteal osseous proliferation leads to a shaggy contour of the marginal bone, and also at sites of bony attachment of ligaments and tendons ('enthesophytes'), such as at the acromial attachment of the acromioclavicular ligament ('bearded acromion')[29].

DIAGNOSIS

The clinical diagnosis of AS depends primarily on the history and physical examination and is confirmed by radiographic examination[5,16,30]. The patient's symptoms, the family history and the articular and extra-articular physical findings offer the best clues to diagnosis. On initial evaluation of a patient, certain features of the patient's history and physical examination raise the index of suspicion, and finding radiographic evidence of bilateral sacroiliitis markedly heightens the probability of AS[16].

It needs to be emphasized, however, that sacroiliitis is not unique to AS and does occur in other spondyloarthropathies. Therefore, although radiography of the pelvis is a useful test for differentiating AS from other causes of back pain, the occurrence of sacroiliitis alone does not necessarily represent definite AS, which requires the added presence of one or more clinical feature(s).

The first internationally accepted classification criteria for AS were proposed in Rome in 1961 and were revised 5 years later in New York, when the presence of radiographic evidence of sacroiliitis was proposed to be necessary for the diagnosis[12,36,107]. These criteria have subsequently been modified[108] (Table 28.3) but there may be a need to further revise them in light of recent progress in our understanding of the broader spectrum of disease. All these criteria greatly depend on the radiographic evidence of sacroiliitis, which is the best non-clinical indicator of the presence of AS. A patient can be classified as having AS if sacroiliitis is associated with at least one clinical criterion, other causes of sacroiliitis having been excluded. These criteria are designed to be highly specific and they may therefore lack sensitivity if used for clinical diagnosis because not all patients with mild or early disease may meet the criteria[9–12,109–113].

The diagnosis of AS is unfortunately often delayed, usually by 5 or more years[109–113]. Some patients may not have any chronic inflammatory low back pain or sacroiliitis at an early stage, when they may present with symptoms resulting from enthesitis or acute iritis[5,24,42]. Others may get intermittent episodes of stiff neck, shoulder pain or chest tenderness[5,16,17]. This is more likely to occur in children/adolescents and women because of an atypical or incomplete clinical picture due to arthritis and/or enthesitis[5,12,25,110–113]. For example, the presenting symptom in some children may be intermittent knee effusions, pain in the groin (hip joint), or painful ankle or foot and resultant limp[23–25]. Some patients may suffer from psoriasis or IBD, or have a family history of these diseases, or of AS and related diseases, including acute iritis. Multiple referrals of such patients for the same complaint often do not result in a correct diagnosis, and during this prolonged diagnostic delay many unnecessary and invasive investigations are performed[5].

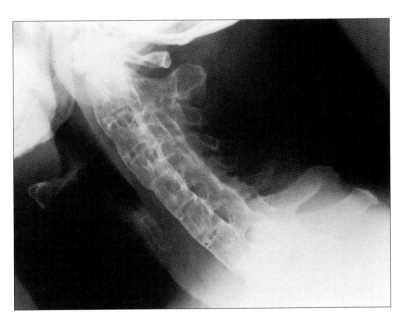

Fig. 28.26 Spinal fusion. Radiograph (lateral view) of the cervical spine showing complete fusion in a patient who had suffered from ankylosing spondylitis for more than 40 years. He later sustained a neck fracture (C6–7 level) after a relatively trivial fall.

arthrosis[56–65]. DXA, quantitative CT and quantitative ultrasound measurements can detect the presence of decreased bone mineral density of the lumbar spine and the femoral neck[57]. However, the presence of marked syndesmophytes in advanced disease may yield normal or increased value for the bone mineral density of the lumbar spine.

Magnetic resonance imaging is important in detecting and evaluating complications of fractures or pseudoarthrosis, as well as changes in the duramater, soft tissue and spinal ligaments[64]. The fractures or pseudoarthrosis give a pattern of either low signal on T1-weighted and high signal on T2-weighted images, or low signal on both T1- and T2-weighted images.

TABLE 28.2 COMPARISON OF ANKYLOSING SPONDYLITIS AND RELATED DISORDERS

Characteristic	Disorder				
	Ankylosing spondylitis	Reactive arthritis	Juvenile spondyloarthropathy	Psoriatic arthropathy*	Enteropathic arthropathy†
Usual age at onset	Young adult age <40	Young to middle-aged adult	Childhood onset, ages 8–16 years	Young to middle-aged adult	Young to middle-aged adult
Sex ratio	Three times more common in males	Predominantly males	Predominantly males	Equally distributed	Equally distributed
Usual type of onset	Gradual	Acute	Variable	Variable	Gradual
Sacroiliitis or spondylitis	Virtually 100%	<50%	<50%	~20%	<20%
Symmetry of sacroiliitis	Symmetric	Asymmetric	Variable	Asymmetric	Symmetric
Peripheral joint involvement	~25%	~90%	~90%	~95%	15–20%
HLA-B27 (in Whites)	~90%	~75%	~85%	<50%‡	~50%‡
Eye involvement§	25–30%	~50%	~20%	~20%	≤15%
Cardiac involvement	1–4%	5–10%	Rare	Rare	Rare
Skin or nail involvement	None	<40%	Uncommon	Virtually 100%	Uncommon
Role of infectious agents as triggers	Unknown	Yes	Unknown	Unknown	Unknown

* About 5–7% of patients with psoriasis develop arthritis, and psoriatic spondylitis accounts for about 10% of all patients with psoriatic arthritis. † Associated with chronic inflammatory bowel disease. ‡ B27 prevalence is higher in those with spondylitis or sacroiliitis. § Predominantly conjunctivitis in reactive and psoriatic arthritis, and acute anterior uveitis in the other three disorders listed. (Adapted from Arnett et al.[104])

TABLE 28.3 THE MODIFIED NEW YORK CRITERIA FOR AS
1. Low back pain of at least 3 months duration improved by exercise and not relieved by rest
2. Limitation of lumbar spinal motion in sagittal (sideways) and frontal (forward and backward) planes
3. Chest expansion decreased relative to normal values for the same sex and age
4. Bilateral sacroiliitis grade 2–4 *or* unilateral sacroiliitis grade 3 or 4
Definite ankylosing spondylitis is present if criterion 4 *and* any one of the other criteria is fulfilled.

Use of HLA-B27 typing as an aid to diagnosis

The radiographic evidence of sacroiliitis is the best non-clinical indicator of the disease presence. However, the status of the sacroiliac joints on routine pelvic radiographs may not always be easy to interpret in the early phase of the disease, especially in adolescents. There is a place for a less expensive and non-invasive laboratory test in such clinical situations to help minimize the degree of uncertainty of the diagnosis. HLA-B27 typing can be of value in such a situation, or where an unusual or atypical clinical presentation of AS is suspected, or in the diagnosis of early undifferentiated spondyloarthropathy[112,113] (Fig. 28.27).

However, the clinical usefulness of this test may differ appreciably among ethnic and racial groups[2,16,112]. HLA-B27 is present in approximately 8% of the normal white population (of western European extraction) and in more than 90% of patients with 'primary' AS, indicating that HLA-B27 typing as a test for AS is highly specific (100 − 8 = 92%) and also highly sensitive (more than 90%)[5,45,112]. In other words, the test is 8% 'false-positive' (i.e. presence of HLA-B27 is unrelated to the clinical problem) and less than 10% 'false-negative' (i.e. fewer than 10% of patients with 'primary' AS lack HLA-B27). Therefore, as with other clinical tests that are neither 100% sensitive nor 100% specific, the clinical usefulness (predictive value) of HLA-B27 test depends on the clinical situation in which it is ordered[112]. The test is most useful when the physician faces a clinical 'toss-up' situation, i.e. the pretest probability of AS is approximately 0.5, in the presence of equivocal findings on sacroiliac radiography[16,112,113] (Table 28.4).

The clinical usefulness (predictive value) of a positive test result will be highest in those population groups that have a low general prevalence of HLA-B27, and yet HLA-B27 has a strong association with AS in such a population. This is the case among the Japanese; they show a strong association (>85%) of HLA-B27 with AS but this gene is present in less than 1% of the population[112–114]. On the other hand, a positive test result will be relatively less useful among Inuits – in spite of a strong association of HLA-B27 (>90%) with AS – because there is a high prevalence of HLA-B27 (25–40%) in the Inuit population[112–114]. If the HLA-B27 test is ordered in an Inuit patient in whom the pretest probability of AS or a related spondyloarthropathy is very low, and the test result is positive, the probability that the patient has the disease still remains relatively low.

Among African-Americans, on the other hand, HLA-B27 is present in 2–4% of the general population but in only about 50% of AS patients[16,112–114]. Therefore, if the HLA-B27 test were ordered because of a reasonable suspicion of AS ('toss-up' situation), the likelihood of the disease being present would be markedly strengthened by a positive test result. However, a negative test result would not be of value in excluding the disease because 50% of African-American patients with AS lack this gene.

The HLA-B27 test cannot be thought of as a 'routine', 'diagnostic', 'confirmatory' or 'screening' test for AS in patients presenting with back pain or arthritis. As a rule, in those patients in whom history and physical examination suggest AS but whose radiographic findings do not

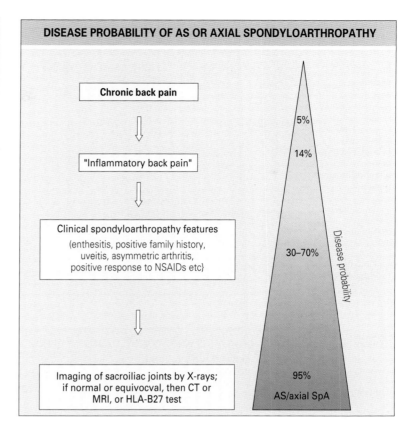

DISEASE PROBABILITY OF AS OR AXIAL SPONDYLOARTHROPATHY

Chronic back pain → 5%

"Inflammatory back pain" → 14%

Clinical spondyloarthropathy features (enthesitis, positive family history, uveitis, asymmetric arthritis, positive response to NSAIDs etc) → 30–70%

Imaging of sacroiliac joints by X-rays; if normal or equivocval, then CT or MRI, or HLA-B27 test → 95% AS/axial SpA

Disease probability

Fig. 28.27 Disease probability of AS or axial spondyloarthropathy. A single clinical feature is not sufficient to make the diagnosis: the more features typical of the disease are present the higher the diagnostic probability. In the typical chronic low back pain population presenting to their primary care physician, presence of at least two of the following four features increases the probability of AS or axial spondyloarthropathy by a factor of three, rising from less than 5% at baseline to more than 14%. These clinical features are: (a) back pain and stiffness every morning that lasts at least 30 minutes; (b) symptoms improve with exercise but not with rest; (c) presence of alternating or bilateral buttock pain; and (d) the symptoms interrupt sleep in the early morning hours more so than at other times in the night. Then on top of that, if the patient manifests additional clinical feature(s) (some of them are listed in this figure), the probability of disease presence easily reaches or can even exceed a 'toss-up' clinical situation, i.e. 30–70% range. The diagnosis can be established when radiographic evidence of sacroiliitis is present. However, back pain due to AS often precedes unequivocal radiographic signs of sacroiliitis by several years. Therefore, the status of the sacroiliac joints on a pelvic radiograph may not always be easy to interpret in the early phase of the disease, particularly in adolescent patients. Newer imaging modalities (see text) can help to detect early sacroiliitis in this clinical situation. Alternatively, an early diagnosis of AS or axial spondyloarthropathy can be made with much less uncertainty when test for HLA-B27 is positive in this 'toss-up' situation (Table 28.4), although the diagnosis will be a little presumptive because the criteria for AS (Table 28.3) greatly depend on the radiographic evidence of sacroiliitis, which is the best non-clinical indicator of the disease presence[112,113]. (Courtesy of M Rudwaleit and J Sieper [Adapted with permission]).

permit this diagnosis to be made, the HLA-B27 test may allow the presumptive diagnosis of AS to be accepted or rejected with less uncertainty[112–114]. In patients with back pain or arthritis in whom AS is suggested neither by the history nor by physical examination, HLA-B27 testing is inappropriate because a positive result would still not permit the diagnosis of AS to be made.

An overwhelming majority of patients with AS can be readily diagnosed clinically on the basis of the history, physical examination and radiographic findings, and they do not need to be tested for HLA-B27. Moreover, it does not help to distinguish between AS, reactive arthritis and other spondyloarthropathies, because all these diseases are associated with HLA-B27, although the strength of the association varies

TABLE 28.4 POST-TEST PROBABILITIES OF ANKYLOSING SPONDYLITIS IN WHITES

Pre-test probability	Probability given positive test result	Probability given negative test result
0.01	0.100	0.001
0.05	0.380	0.005
0.10	0.560	0.010
0.20	0.740	0.020
0.30	0.830	0.030
0.40	0.880	0.050
0.50	0.920	0.080
0.60	0.950	0.120
0.70	0.960	0.170
0.80	0.980	0.260
0.90	0.990	0.440
0.95	0.995	0.620
0.99	0.999	0.900

(Adapted from Khan and Khan[112].)

TABLE 28.5 ASSOCIATION OF HLA-B27 AND SPONDYLOARTHROPATHIES (IN WHITES)

Disease	Approximate HLA-B27 prevalence (%)
Ankylosing spondylitis	~90
Reactive arthritis	40–80
Juvenile spondyloarthropathy	~70
Enteropathic spondyloarthritis	35–75
Psoriatic spondyloarthritis	40–50
Undifferentiated spondyloarthropathy	~70
Acute anterior uveitis (acute iritis)	~50
Aortic incompetence with heart block	~80
General healthy population	~8

among them (Table 28.5). Differentiation between these diseases is based primarily on clinical features (Table 28.2).

Although HLA-B27 typing can define the population at higher risk of AS and related spondyloarthropathies, it is of very limited practical value for that purpose because no effective means of prevention are currently available. Moreover, most HLA-B27-positive people in the general population never develop AS or a related disease. HLA-B27 typing may help ophthalmologists to better define a patient presenting with acute uveitis and refer HLA-B27-positive patients for rheumatology consultation, especially those with associated musculoskeletal symptoms, because up to 75% of them have or will develop AS or a related spondyloarthropathy[40,42,43,113].

Familial aggregation of AS and related spondyloarthropathies, acute anterior uveitis, aortic incompetence plus heart block, and hip joint involvement are more common in patients with HLA-B27 and they tend to have a younger age of onset[2,41]. Moreover, the presence of HLA-B27 is associated with the development of more severe and prolonged joint symptoms in reactive arthritis and an increased risk of sacroiliitis and spondylitis. However, knowledge of HLA-B27 status at disease onset is of uncertain value in predicting the patient's long-term prognosis.

HLA-B27 itself is not an allele but a family of at least 26 different alleles – HLA-B*2701 to HLA-B*2725 (there is no B*2722 allele, and B*2705 itself comprises three variants: B*27052, B*27053, B*27054), based on sequence-based typing methods[31,114,115]. These alleles, also called subtypes, differ from each other by one or more amino-acid substitutions, mostly resulting from changes in exons 2 and 3, which encode the $\alpha 1$

and $\alpha 2$ domains, respectively, that from the peptide-binding cleft. Their assignment to the HLA-B27 family is based on nucleotide sequence homology, and nearly all members of the family can by typed by the traditional serologic methods. However, certain subtypes, such as B*2712, B*2715 and B*2723 may show no serological reactions with B27-specific antisera; but they can be detected by polymerase chain reaction sequence-specific primer (PCR-SSP) method updated to enable the detection of all the subtypes, or by sequence-based typing.

The most widely distributed subtype around the world is HLA-B*2705, and it is clearly associated with AS and related spondyloarthropathies except in the west African population of Senegal and Gambia. HLA-B*2704, another strongly disease-associated subtype, is predominant among the Chinese and Japanese[114,115]. Occurrence of AS has been observed in individuals possessing any one of the first 10 relatively more common HLA-B27 subtypes except HLA-B*2706 and HLA-B*2709[116,117]. Disease occurrence has not been studied in most of the remaining subtypes that are all quite rare, but occurrence of AS has been documented in individuals possessing B*2713, B*2714, B*2715 or B*2719. Data from south-east Asia indicate that HLA-B*2706 may not be associated with AS and related spondyloarthropathies, but occurrence of AS has been documented in HLA-B*2706 individuals who also have one of the disease associated subtypes, B*2705 or B*2704[117]. HLA-B*2709, a subtype primarily observed among residents of the island of Sardinia, seems to lack any association with AS among Sardinians, although a few patients with undifferentiated spondyloarthropathy have been reported from the Italian mainland[118,119].

Differential diagnosis

Low back pain with stiffness is the most common presenting symptom in patients with AS, although a variety of other presentations may antedate back symptoms in many patients. However, backache is one of the most common health problems and results from multiple causes, and AS is not its most common cause in the general population[18,19,120]. These various causes may be divided into two main subtypes:

- spondylogenic: traumatic, structural (degenerative and discogenic), inflammatory, metabolic, infective and neoplastic or other bone lesions
- non-spondylogenic: neurologic, vascular, viscerogenic, psychogenic.

Fibromyalgia, which affects 2–4% of women between 20 and 60 years of age, can also cause diagnostic confusion because the primary complaint in some AS patients, especially women, may be fleeting muscle aches and pains or musculotendinous tender areas in the back, fatigue and disturbed sleep. Moreover, just as in many patients with fibromyalgia, these symptoms may become worse on exposure to cold or dampness[33].

The back pain from many of the non-inflammatory spondylogenic causes that can be confused radiologically with AS, particularly in patients with widespread degenerative disc disease (at multiple discovertebral junctions and apophyseal joints) and ankylosing hyperostosis. However, the non-inflammatory type of back pain is generally aggravated by physical activity and relieved by rest. Moreover, there is generally no limitation of chest expansion (corrected for age), the lateral spinal flexion is usually within normal limits and the ESR is frequently normal. The sacroiliac joint radiographs are usually normal or show only mild degenerative changes; the typical bony erosions and marked subchondral sclerosis of sacroiliitis are absent.

The typical osteophytes of severe degenerative disc disease are easily distinguishable from syndesmophytes[21,29] (Fig. 28.24). However, diagnostic confusion can occur in some AS patients who have concomitant degenerative disc disease at the time the syndesmophytes are forming. In some elderly patients with severe degenerative changes of the sacroiliac joint, such as joint space narrowing, subchondral bone sclerosis and

TABLE 28.6 FEATURES DIFFERENTIATING BETWEEN ANKYLOSING HYPEROSTOSIS AND AS		
Feature	Ankylosing hyperostosis	Ankylosing spondylitis
Usual age of onset (years)	>50	<40
Thoracolumbar kyphosis	±	++
Limitation of spinal mobility	±	++
Pain	±	++
Limitation of chest expansion	±	++
Radiographic features:		
Hyperostosis	++	+
Sacroiliac joint erosion	– –	++
Sacroiliac joint (synovial) obliteration	±	++
Sacroiliac joint (ligamentous) obliteration	±	++
Apophyseal joint obliteration	– –	++
Anterior longitudinal ligament ossification	++	±
Posterior longitudinal ligament ossification	+	?
Syndesmophytes	– –	++
Enthesopathies (whiskerings) with erosions	– –	++
Enthesopathies (whiskerings) without erosions	++	+

(Adapted from Yagan and Khan[121].)

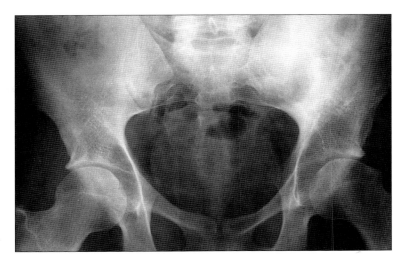

Fig. 28.28 Radiograph of the pelvis (anteroposterior view) of a patient with SAPHO syndrome. Osteitis involving the left sacroiliac joint.

bridging osteophytes in the lower part of the joints may erroneously suggest sacroiliitis on pelvic radiography, but not on CT.

The posture of patients with spinal stenosis may be confused with AS; this condition is usually seen in elderly patients with degenerative disc disease[120]. These patients have varying degrees of pain, worsened by standing erect, walking downhill or lying on the back, and eased by forward stooping or lying on the side with the hip flexed. There is pseudoclaudication, often involving the L4 nerve root, and neurologic findings are variable.

Ankylosing hyperostosis, also called Forestier's disease or diffuse idiopathic skeletal hyperostosis (DISH), usually occurs in elderly individuals and is characterized by hyperostosis affecting the anterior longitudinal ligament and bony attachments of tendons and ligaments; there is no association with HLA-B27[121]. The differentiating features between AS and DISH are listed in Table 28.6. Ossification of the posterior longitudinal ligament has on rare occasion been observed in DISH as well as in AS[122]. Occasionally, severe hyperostotic and degenerative changes of the sacroiliac joints can occur, such as capsular ossifications, joint space narrowing and subchondral bone sclerosis. These changes can give an appearance superficially resembling sacroiliitis or fused sacroiliac joints on the anteroposterior pelvic radiogram. Chronic treatment with retinoids (synthetic derivatives of vitamin A) for skin diseases such as acne and psoriasis can sometimes cause bone abnormalities mimicking spondyloarthropathies or DISH[123]. The sacroiliac joints, however, are typically unaffected.

Osteitis condensans ilii, a self-limiting and often asymptomatic condition that is seen primarily in young multiparous women and shows no association with HLA-B27, should not be confused with sacroiliitis[19,29]. It is characterized by radiographic evidence of a triangular area of dense sclerotic bone adjacent to the lower half of the sacroiliac joints, primarily on the iliac side. The sacroiliac joint itself, however, is normal.

Infections of the spine such as septic (pyogenic) sacroiliitis or disc space infection, tuberculous spondylitis and spondylitis due to brucellosis should not be confused with AS[120,124,125]. Sacroiliac joint changes

suggesting sacroiliitis, and even complete fusion of these joints, can sometimes be observed in paraplegics and quadriplegics[126]. The osteoarticular manifestations of sternocostoclavicular hyperostosis and chronic aseptic osteomyelitis, often multifocal and recurrent, sometimes in association with acne conglobata, acne fulminans, hidradenitis suppurativa or palmoplantar pustulosis, can involve several spondyloarthropathic features, especially on long-term follow-up[127,128]. These include anterior chest wall involvement, seronegative asymmetric oligoarthritis and enthesopathies, but sacroiliac joint involvement is primarily unilateral and there is no association with HLA-B27 and no familial aggregation (Fig. 28.28). An eponym, SAPHO syndrome (synovitis–acne–pustulosis–hyperostosis–osteitis), is now being widely used for this clinical condition[127].

Miscellaneous other conditions that might be confused radiographically with AS because of sacroiliac joint abnormalities or syndesmophyte-like appearance of the spine include primary and secondary hyperparathyroidism, dialysis-associated spondyloarthropathy, Scheuermann's disease, congenital kyphoscoliosis, fluorosis, chondrocalcinosis, ochronosis and Paget's disease affecting pelvis or spine[29,120,129,130]. Other causes of back pain include spinal osteoporosis with or without compression fractures and sacral insufficiency fractures, axial osteomalacia, multiple myeloma, metastatic prostate cancer and other malignancies, chronic pelvic inflammatory disease, referred pain from abdominal viscera and retroperitoneal fibrosis[29,120,131,132].

A late-onset undifferentiated spondyloarthropathy syndrome that occurs in men that are over 50 years of age has recently been described[13]. This arthropathy may sometimes resemble the syndrome of remitting seronegative symmetric synovitis with pitting edema (RS3PE). At onset, the patients may show little or no clinical involvement of the axial skeleton, but many of them later develop bilateral sacroiliitis or even go on to develop AS.

The distinction of AS from RA is usually not difficult. Patients with RA usually have polyarthritis that is symmetric in distribution and affects small and large joints of the extremities; involvement of the sacroiliac, apophyseal and costovertebral joints is very rare. In AS, on the other hand, any involvement of peripheral joints (other than hip and shoulder joints) is usually oligoarticular and asymmetric, affecting more often the larger joints of lower extremities; serologic tests for rheumatoid factor are negative; and subcutaneous nodules are absent. There are rare instances of concurrent AS and RA, primarily seen in individuals who have co-inherited the genetic predisposing factors for both diseases, i.e. HLA-B27 for AS and HLA-DR4 for RA.

NATURAL HISTORY

The course of AS is highly variable, with no predictable pattern of progression[6,12,134,135]. It can be characterized by spontaneous remissions and exacerbation, particularly in early disease[2,134]. Daily pain and stiffness generally persist for many decades for most patients, rarely going into long-term remission. However, the outcome can be generally favorable in many patients because the disease may remain relatively mild or limited to the sacroiliac joints and the lumbar spine. Those who have mild disease with only limited spinal involvement maintain good functional ability. Patients with persistent severe disease can get progressive functional impairment associated with spinal fusion, including the cervical spine, and associated kyphosis.

Although the axial disease is more severe in males, the overall pattern seems to be similar in both sexes[6,12,135]. Pregnancy does not improve the symptoms of AS; either no change or only temporary aggravation of activity is observed during pregnancy[135]. Hormonal status, fertility and course of pregnancy and childbirth have been reported to be normal in women with AS.

The clinical assessment of disease activity in patients with AS is difficult, especially in uncomplicated disease confined to the sacroiliac joints and spine. However, the newly developed composite assessment criteria, now known as the WHO/ILAR/OMERACT core set for clinical and functional assessment of AS, have been found to be very useful[36,133] (Table 28.7). They can be used for evaluating therapy with symptom-modifying and disease-controlling antirheumatic drugs and physical therapy, and for clinical record keeping in daily practice. A preliminary definition of short-term improvement in AS has also been published[36]. Moreover, a recently proposed instrument (18 item questionnaire that takes about 4 minutes to complete) for assessing quality of life (ASQoL) provides a valuable tool for assessing the impact of therapeutic interventions for AS.

Disability

Most with AS patients remain gainfully employed, despite having severely restricted spinal mobility[6,137–142]. A recent large study of age- and sex-matched German patients with AS and RA seen at tertiary rheumatological centers shows that they have similar levels of pain and impaired wellbeing, but AS less often leads to early termination of gainful employment[137]. Only 3% of AS patients in one European study were unable to work after 2 decades of disease[138]. The disease in women was somewhat milder, but the patients' self-ratings did not show a more favorable overall outcome because their self-ratings of pain and impaired activities of daily living were worse than those in men[137].

Although it is difficult to predict the ultimate outcome for an individual patient, some factors, particularly occurring during the first 10 years of the disease, are particularly important with respect to subsequent outcome[6,106,135]. Patients with hip joint involvement, who more often have a younger age of onset, or those with a completely ankylosed cervical spine with kyphosis, are more likely to become disabled. The results of total hip arthroplasty in recent years have been very gratifying in preventing partial or total disability in many such patients. Poor response or intolerance to NSAIDs, and the presence of severe extra-articular complications worsen the prognosis. The stage of AS at the time of its diagnosis and initiation of the appropriate therapy, severity of early stages of the disease, the quality of medical management, and the degree of patient compliance with the suggested treatment, also influence the overall prognosis.

A recent American study indicates that functional disability in AS progresses more rapidly in older patients and smokers, and less rapidly in those who have better social support and are able to perform back exercises regularly[141]. In a Norwegian study, cessation of work was associated with low level of education, complete ossification of the spine, acute anterior uveitis, female sex and the co-existence of non-rheumatic diseases[134]. Patients with physically demanding jobs are more likely to change their type of work, decrease their work hours or experience temporary or permanent work disability than those with jobs that are physically less demanding[139]. Functional disability is the most important predictor of total healthcare (direct and indirect).

Disease heterogeneity

There is ample evidence to suggest disease heterogeneity of AS, best exemplified by the difference between the HLA-B27-positive and HLA-B27-negative patients[41,45,114,143]. Even although there are many similarities, generally speaking, HLA-B27-negative AS is somewhat later in its onset, significantly less often complicated by acute anterior uveitis and more frequently accompanied by psoriasis, ulcerative colitis and Crohn's disease, and less often shows familial aggregation[41,45,114,144]. In fact, it is unusual among people of northern European extraction to observe families with two or more first-degree relatives affected with HLA-B27-negative AS in the absence of psoriasis or chronic IBD in the family.

Detailed studies are under way to understand the genetic aspects of susceptibility, severity, and clinical expression in ankylosing spondylitis[114,144]. HLA-B27-positive twins show more than 50% pairwise concordance rate for AS if they are monozygotic versus only 20% if they are dizygotic[2,144]. The ongoing genome-wide studies indicate that, besides HLA-B27 and some additional genes in the MHC region on the short arm of chromosome 6, a few more genes on other chromosomes seem to be involved as well[114,143–146]. Thus it is very likely that several genes may influence susceptibility to AS, and others may influence disease severity and phenotypic expression[144].

Life span

An excess mortality was observed in the past, primarily ascribed to amyloidosis and complications of spinal irradiation (excess malignancies, especially a fivefold increase in leukemias)[147,148]. In subsequent studies an excess mortality was observed among non-irradiated patients seen at tertiary care centers, primarily due to cardiopulmonary causes, but only

---

TABLE 28.7 ASSESSMENT OF DISEASE ACTIVITY IN PATIENTS WITH AS

Domain	Instrument
Physical function	BASFI *or* Dougados Functional Index
Pain	Visual analog scale (VAS) – last week/spine/at night/due to AS *and* VAS – last week/spine/due to AS
Spinal mobility	Chest expansion test *and* modified Schober's test *and* occiput to wall distance test
Patient global	VAS – last week
Stiffness	Duration of morning stiffness – spine/last week
Peripheral joints	Number of swollen joints (44 joint count)
Entheses	No preferred instrument is yet available
Acute phase reactants	ESR
X-ray spine	Anteroposterior + lateral lumbar spine *and* Lateral cervical spine *and* X-ray pelvis (sacroiliac and hip joints)
X-ray pelvis	(see under X-ray spine above)
Fatigue	No preferred instrument is yet available

The SM-ARD/PT core set comprises the following five components: Physical function, Pain, Spinal mobility, Patient global, Stiffness. These components are also included in the other two core sets, i.e. for DC-ART and clinical record keeping. The additional components for clinical record keeping are: Peripheral joints, Entheses, Acute phase reactants. The core set for DC-ART, in addition to the above mentioned eight components, requires: X-ray spine, X-ray pelvis and Fatigue.
Specific instruments for each domain in core sets for symptom-modifying (SM-ARD) and disease controlling antirheumatic drugs (DC-ART), and for physical therapy (PT) and clinical record-keeping.

more than 20 years after their disease diagnosis[149–151]. These studies consisted of patients with disease severe enough to both impel the patients to seek specialized care and to be correctly diagnosed at a time when AS was felt to be a rare disease[150]. It is quite likely that the survival of those patients with mild disease, who form the majority of patients with AS, is comparable to that of the general population. However, spinal fracture, cardiopulmonary involvement, associated medical conditions, including ulcerative colitis and Crohn's disease, as well as complications of medical and surgical treatment, may contribute to premature mortality in some patients.

REFERENCES

1. Moll JMH, ed, Ankylosing spondylitis. Edinburgh: Churchill Livingstone; 1980.
2. Calin A, Taurog J, eds. The spondylarthritides. Oxford: Oxford University Press; 1998.
3. Braun J, Khan MA, Sieper J. Entheses and enthesopathy: what is the target of the immune response. Ann Rheum Dis 2000; 59: 985–994.
4. Feldtkeller E, Lemmel E-M, Russell AS. Ankylosing spondylitis in the pharaohs of ancient Egypt. Rheumatol Int 2003; 23: 1–5.
5. Khan MA. Update on spondyloarthropathies. Ann Intern Med 2002; 135: 896–907.
6. Sieper J, Braun J, Rudwaleit M, Boonen A, Zink A. Ankylosing spondylitis: an overview. Ann Rheum Dis 2002; 61 (Suppl 3): iii 8–iii 18.
7. Geilinger W. Ankylosierenden Spondylitis. Druck Der Union Deutsche Verlagsgesellschaft, Stuttgart, [German Edition] 1917.
8. Khan MA. Five classical clinical papers on ankylosing spondylitis. In Dieppe P, Wollheim FA, Schumacher HR (Eds.). Classical Papers in Rheumatology. Martin Dunitz Ltd., London, 2002, pp. 118–133.7.
9. Braun J, Sieper J (Eds). Spondylitis ankylosans. Unimed Verlag AG, Bremen [German Edition] 2002.
10. Khan MA, van der Linden SM. A wider spectrum of spondyloarthropathies. Semin Arthritis Rheum 1990; 20: 107–113.
11. Khan MA (Ed.): Spondyloarthropathies. Rheum Dis Clin North Am. 1992; 18: 1–276.
12. van der Linden SJ, van der Heijde D. Spondylarthropathies. Ankylosing spondylitis. In: Ruddy S, Harris ED, Sledge CB, (Eds). Kelly's textbook of rheumatology, 6th ed. Philadelphia, PA: WB Saunders; 2000: 1039–1053.
13. Olivieri I, Ciancio G, Pedula A et al. Ankylosing spondylitis and undifferentiated spondyloarthropathies: a clinical review and description of a disease subset with older age at onset. Curr Opin Rheumatol 2001; 13: 280–284.
14. Boyer GS, Templin DW, Bowler A et al. Spondyloarthropathy in the community: clinical syndromes and disease manifestations in Alaskan Eskimo populations. J Rheumatol 1999; 26: 1537–1544.
15. Boyer GS, Templin DW, Bowler A et al. A comparison of patients with spondyloarthropathy seen in specialty clinics with those identified in a community wide epidemiologic study: has the classic case misled us? Arch Intern Med 1997; 157: 2111–2117.
16. Khan MA, Kushner I. Diagnosis of ankylosing spondylitis. In: Cohen AS, ed. Progress in clinical rheumatology 1. Orlando, FL: Grune & Stratton; 1984: 145–178.
17. Van der Linden SM, Khan MA, Rentsch HU et al. Chest pain without radiographic sacroiliitis in relatives of patients with ankylosing spondylitis. J Rheumatol 1988; 15: 836–839.
18. Blackburn WD Jr, Alarcón GS, Ball GV. Evaluation of patients with back pain of suspected inflammatory nature. Am J Med 1988; 85: 766–770.
19. Khan MA. Back and neck pain. In: Fitzgerald F, ed. Current practice of medicine, 2nd ed. Philadelphia, PA: Current Medicine; 1999: 187–203.
20. McGonagle D, Khan MA, Marzo-Ortega H et al. Entheitis in ankylosing spondylitis and related spondyloarthropathies. Curr Opin Rheumatol 1999; 11: 244–250.
21. Khan MA, ed. Ankylosing spondylitis and related spondyloarthropathies. Spine: state of the art reviews. Philadelphia, PA: Hanley & Belfus; 1990.
22. Yu D, ed. Spondyloarthropathies. Rheum Dis Clin North Am 1998; 24: 663–915.
23. Burgos-Vargos R, Vasquez-Mellado J. The early clinical recognition of juvenile-onset ankylosing spondylitis and its differentiation from juvenile rheumatoid arthritis. Arthritis Rheum 1995; 38: 835–844.
24. Rosenberg AM, Petty RE. A syndrome of seronegative enthesopathy and arthropathy in children. Arthritis Rheum 1982; 25: 1041–1047.
25. Cassidy JT, Petty RE, eds. Textbook of pediatric rheumatology, 4th ed, Philadelphia, PA: WB Saunders; 2001.
26. Baek HJ, Shin KC, Lee YJ et al. Juvenile onset ankylosing spondylitis (JAS) has less severe spinal disease course than adult onset ankylosing spondylitis (AAS): clinical comparison between JAS and AAS in Korea. J Rheumatol 2002; 29: 1780–5.
27. Maksymowych W. Ankylosing spondylitis: at the interface of bone and cartilage. J Rheumatol 1999; 27: 2295–2301.
28. François RJ, Braun J, Khan MA. Entheses and enthesitis: a histopathological review and relevance to spondyloarthropathies. Curr Opin Rheumatol 2001; 13: 255–264.
29. Resnick D, Niwayama G. Ankylosing spondylitis. In: Resnick D, ed. Diagnosis of bone and joint disorders. 3rd Edition. Philadelphia: WB Saunders; 1995:1008–74.
30. Braun J, Bollow M, Sieper J. Radiologic diagnosis and pathology of the spondyloarthropathies. Rheum Dis Clin North Am 1998; 24: 697–735.
31. Khan MA: Spondyloarthropathies. In: Hunder G, ed. Atlas of Rheumatology. 3rd Edition. Philadelphia, PA: Current Medicine 2002, pp. 141–167.
32. Aufdermaur M. The morbid anatomy of ankylosing spondylitis. Doc Rheumatol Geigy 1957: 1–70.
33. Challier B, Urlacher F, Vancon G et al. Is quality of life affected by season and weather conditions in ankylosing spondylitis? Clin Exp Rheumatol 2001; 19: 277–281.
34. Hultgren S, Broman JE, Gudbjornsson B et al. Sleep disturbances in outpatients with ankylosing spondylitis: a questionnaire study with gender implications. Scand J Rheumatol 2000; 29: 365–369.
35. Will R, Kennedy G, Elswood J et al. Ankylosing spondylitis and the shoulder: commonly involved but infrequently disabling. J Rheumatol 2000; 27: 177–182.
36. Braun J, van der Heijde D, Dougados M et al. Staging of patients with ankylosing spondylitis: a preliminary proposal. Ann Rheum Dis 2002; 61 (Suppl 3): iii19–iii23.
37. Deyo RA, Jarvik JG. Diagnostic evaluation of low back pain with emphasis on imaging. Ann Intern Med. 2002; 137: 586–597.
38. Blower PW, Griffin AJ. Clinical sacroiliac tests in ankylosing spondylitis and other causes of back pain – 2 studies. Ann Rheum Dis 1984; 43: 192–195.
39. Viitanen JV, Kokko ML, Heikkila S, Kautiainen H. Neck mobility assessment in ankylosing spondylitis: a clinical study of nine measurements including new type methods for cervical rotation and lateral flexion. Br J Rheumatol 1998; 37: 377–381.
40. Banares A. Hernandez-Garcia C, Fernandez-Gutierrez B, Jover JA. Eye involvement in the spondyloarthropathies. Rheum Dis Clin North Am 1998; 24: 771–784.
41. Khan MA, Braun WE, Kushner I. Comparison of clinical features of HLA-B27 positive and negative patients with ankylosing spondylitis. Arthritis Rheum 1977; 20: 909–912.
42. Pato E, Banares A, Jover JA et al. Undiagnosed spondyloarthropathy in patients presenting with anterior uveitis. J Rheumatol 2000; 27: 2198–2202.
43. Smith JR. HLA-B27–associated uveitis. Ophthalmol Clin North Am 2002; 15: 297–307.
44. Uy HS, Christen WG, Foster CS. HLA-B27 associated uveitis and cystoid macular edema. Ocul Immunol Inflamm 2001; 9: 177–183.
45. Feldtkeller E, Khan MA, van der Heijde D, van der Linden S, Braun J. Age at disease onset and diagnosis delay in HLA-B27 negative vs. positive patients with ankylosing spondylitis. Rheumatol Int 2003 in press.
46. Lautermann D, Braun J. Ankylosing spondylitis – cardiac manifestations. Clin Exp Rheumatol 2002; 20 (Suppl. 28) S11–S15.
47. Bergfeldt L. HLA-B27 associated cardiac disease. Ann Intern Med 1997; 127: 621–629.
48. Sun JP, Khan MA, Farhat AZ, Bahler RC: Alterations in cardiac diastolic function in patients with ankylosing spondylitis. Intl J Cardiol 37; 65–72, 1992.
49. Boushea DK, Sundstrom WR. The pleuropulmonary manifestations of ankylosing spondylitis. Semin Arthritis Rheum 1989; 18: 277–281.
50. Turetschek K, Ebner W, Fleischmann D et al. Early pulmonary involvement in ankylosing spondylitis: assessment with thin-section CT. Clin Radiol 2000; 55: 632–636.
51. Casserly IP, Fenlon HM, Breatnac HE, Sant SM. Lung findings on high-resolution computed tomography in idiopathic ankylosing spondylitis. Correlation with clinical findings, pulmonary function testing and plain radiography. Br J Rheumatol 1997; 36: 677–682.
52. De Keyser F, Baeten D, Van Den Bosch F et al. Gut inflammation and spondyloarthropathies. Curr Rheumatol Rep. 2002; 4: 525–532.
53. Baeten D, De Keyser F, Mielants H, Veys EM. Immune linkage between inflammatory bowel and spondyloarthropathies. Curr Opin Rheumatol 2002; 14: 342–347.
54. Palm Oyvind, Moum B, Ongre A, Gran JT. Prevalence of ankylosing spondylitis and other spondyloarthropathies among patients with inflammatory bowel disease: a population study (The IBSEN Study). J Rheumatol 2002; 29: 511–515.
55. Salvarani C, Vlachonikolis IG, van der Heijde DM et al. Musculoskeletal manifestations in a population based cohort of inflammatory bowel disease patients. Scand J Gastroenterol 2001; 36: 1307–1313.
56. Gratacos J, Collado A, Pons F et al. Significant loss of bone mass in patients with early, active ankylosing spondylitis: a followup study. Arthritis Rheum 1999; 42: 2319–2324.
57. Toussirot E, Michel F, Wendling D. Bone density, ultrasound measurement and body composition in early ankylosing spondylitis. Rheumatol 2001; 40: 882–888.
58. Kabaskal Y, Garrett SL, Calin A. The epidemiology of spondylodiscitis in ankylosing spondylitis, a controlled study. Br J Rheumatol 1996; 35: 660–663.
59. Hitchon PW, From AM, Brenton MD, Glaser JA, Torner JC. Fractures of the thoracolumbar spine complicating ankylosing spondylitis. J Neurosurg 2002; 97(2 Suppl): 218–222.
60. Finkelstein JA, Chapman JR, Mirza S. Occult vertebral fractures in ankylosing spondylitis. Spinal Cord 1999; 37: 444–447.
61. Mitra D, Elvins DM, Speden DJ, Collins AJ. The prevalence of vertebral fractures in mild ankylosing spondylitis and their relationship to bone mineral density. Rheumatology (Oxford) 2000; 39: 85–89.
62. Cooper C, Carbone L, Michet CJ et al. Fracture risk in patients with ankylosing spondylitis: a population based study. J Rheumatol 1994; 21: 1877–1882.
63. Resnick D, Williamson S, Alazraki N. Focal spinal abnormalities on bone scans in ankylosing spondylitis: a clue to the presence of fracture or pseudarthrosis. Clin Nucl Med 1995; 6: 213–217.
64. Shih TT, Chen PQ, Li YW, Hsu CY. Spinal fractures and pseudoarthrosis complicating ankylosing spondylitis: MRI manifestation and clinical significance. J Comput Assist Tomogr 2001; 25: 164–170.

65. Tico N, Ramon S, Garcia-Ortun F *et al*. Traumatic spinal cord injury complicating ankylosing spondylitis. Spinal Cord 1998; 36: 349–352.
66. Ramos-Remus C, Gomez-Vargas A, Guzman-Guzman JL *et al*. Frequency of atlantoaxial subluxation and neurologic involvement in patients with ankylosing spondylitis. J Rheumatol 1995; 22: 2120.
67. Thompson GH, Khan MA, Bilenker RM. Spontaneous atlantoaxial subluxation as a presenting manifestation of juvenile ankylosing spondylitis. Spine 1982; 7: 78–79.
68. Little H, Swinson DR, Cruickshank B. Upward subluxation of the axis in ankylosing spondylitis. Am J Med 1976; 60: 279–285.
69. Tullous MW, Skerhut HEI, Story JL *et al*. Cauda equina syndrome of long-standing ankylosing spondylitis. Case report and review of the literature. J Neurosurg 1990; 73: 441–447.
70. Bilgen IG, Yunten N, Ustun EE *et al*. Adhesive arachnoiditis causing cauda equina syndrome in ankylosing spondylitis: CT and MRI demonstration of dural calcification and a dorsal dural diverticulum. Neuroradiology 1999; 41: 508–511.
71. Khan MA, Kushner I. Ankylosing spondylitis and multiple sclerosis: a possible association. Arthritis Rheum 1979; 22: 784–786.
72. Hanrahan PS, Russell AS, McLean DR. Ankylosing spondylitis and multiple sclerosis: an apparent association. J Rheumatol 1988; 15: 1512–1514.
73. Cellerini M, Gabbrielli S, Bongi SM. Cerebral magnetic resonance imaging in a patient with ankylosing spondylitis and multiple sclerosis-like syndrome. Neuroradiology 2001; 43: 1067–1069.
74. Strobel ES. Fritschka E. Renal diseases in ankylosing spondylitis: review of the literature illustrated by case reports. Clin Rheumatol 1998; 17: 524–530.
75. Vilar MJP, Cury SE, Ferraz MB *et al*. Renal abnormalities in ankylosing spondylitis. Scand J Rheumatol 1997; 26: 19–23.
76. Lai KN, Li PKT, Hawkins B, Lai FM-M. IgA nephropathy associated with ankylosing spondylitis: occurrence in women as well as in men. Ann Rheum Dis 1989; 48: 435–437.
77. Gratacos J, Orellana C, Sanmarti R *et al*. Secondary amyloidosis in ankylosing spondylitis: a systematic survey of 137 patients using abdominal fat aspiration. J Rheumatol 1997; 24: 912–925.
78. Ahmed Q, Chung-Park M, Mustafa K, Khan MA. Psoriatic spondyloarthropathy with secondary amyloidosis. J Rheumatol 1996; 23: 1107–1110.
79. Laiho K, Tiitinen S, Kaarela K *et al*. Secondary amyloidosis has decreased in patients with inflammatory joint disease in Finland. Clin Rheumatol 1999; 18: 122–123.
80. Satko SG, Iskandar SS, Appel RG. IgA nephropathy and Reiter's syndrome. Report of two cases and review of the literature. Nephron 2000; 84: 177–182.
81. Mackiewicz A, Khan MA, Reynolds TL *et al*. Serum IgA and acute phase proteins in ankylosing spondylitis. Ann Rheum Dis 1989; 48: 99–103.
82. Scotto di Fazano C, Grilo RM, Vergne P, *et al*. Is the relationship between spondyloarthropathy and Sjogren's syndrome in women coincidental? A study of 13 cases. Joint Bone Spine 2002; 69: 383–387.
83. Brandt J, Rudwaleit M, Eggens U *et al*. Increased frequency of Sjogren's syndrome in patients with spondyloarthropathy. J Rheumatol 1998; 25: 718–724.
84. Padula A, Ciancio G, La Civita L *et al*. Association between vitiligo and spondyloarthritis. J Rheumatol 2001; 28: 313–314.
85. Pazirandeh M, Ziran BH, Khandelwal BK *et al*. Relapsing polychondritis and spondyloarthropathies. J Rheumatol 1988; 15: 630–632.
86. Abouzahir A, El Maghraoui A, Tabache F *et al*. Sarcoidosis and ankylosing spondylitis. A case report and review of the literature. Ann Med Interne (Paris) 2002; 153: 407–10. [Article in French]
87. LeBlanc CM, Inman RD, Dent P *et al*. Retroperitoneal fibrosis: An extra-articular manifestation of ankylosing spondylitis. Arthritis Rheum 2002; 47: 210–214.
88. Bezza A, Maghraoui AE, Ghadouane M *et al*. Idiopathic retroperitoneal fibrosis and ankylosing spondylitis. A new case report. Joint Bone Spine. 2002; 69: 502–505.
89. Ozgocmen S, Kocakoc E, Kiris A, Ardicoglu A, Ardicoglu O. Incidence of varicoceles in patients with ankylosing spondylitis evaluated by physical examination and color duplex sonography. Urology. 2002; 59: 919–922.
90. Bernstein CN, Blanchard JF, Rawsthorne P, Yu N The prevalence of extraintestinal diseases in inflammatory bowel disease: a population based study. Am J Gastroenterol 2001; 96: 1116–1122.
91. Spoorenberg A, van der Heijde D, de Klerk E *et al*. Relative value of erythrocyte sedimentation rate and C-reactive protein in assessment of disease activity in ankylosing spondylitis. J Rheumatol 1999; 26: 980–984.
92. Battistone MJ, Manaster BJ, Reda DJ, Clegg DO. Radiographic diagnosis of sacroiliitis – Are sacroiliac views really better? J Rheumatol 1998; 25: 2395–401.
93. Miron SD, Khan MA, Wiesen E *et al*. The value of quantitative sacroiliac scintigraphy in detection of sacroiliitis. Clin Rheumatol 1983; 2: 407–414.
94. Jevtic V, Kos-Golja M, Rozman B, McCall I. Marginal erosive discovertebral 'Romanus' lesions in ankylosing spondylitis demonstrated by contrast enhanced Gd-DTPA magnetic resonance imaging. Skeletal Radiol 2000; 29: 27–33.
95. Yu W, Feng F, Dion E *et al*. Comparison of radiography, computed tomography and magnetic resonance imaging in the detection of sacroiliitis accompanying ankylosing spondylitis. Skeletal Radiol 1998; 27: 311–320.
96. Bollow M, Braun J, Biedermann T *et al*. Use of contrast-enhanced MR imaging to detect sacroiliitis in children. Skeletal Radiol 1998; 27: 606–616.
97. Khan MA, van der Linden S, Kushner I *et al*. Spondylitic disease without radiographic evidence of sacroiliitis in relatives of HLA-B27 positive ankylosing spondylitis patients. Arthritis Rheum 1985; 28: 40–43.
98. Mau W, Zeidler H, Mau R *et al*. Clinical features and prognosis of patients with possible ankylosing spondylitis: results of a 10 year follow-up. J Rheumatol 1988; 15: 1109–1114.
99. Kumar A, Bansal M, Srivastva DN *et al*. Long-term outcome of undifferentiated spondyloarthropathy. Rheumatol Int 2001; 20: 221–224.
100. Hanly, JG, Mitchell, MJ, Barnes DC *et al*. Early recognition of sacroiliitis by magnetic resonance imaging and computed tomography. J Rheumatol 1994; 21: 2088.
101. Oostveen J, Prevo R, den Boer J, van de Laar M. Early detection of sacroiliitis on magnetic resonance imaging and subsequent development of sacroiliitis on plain radiography. A prospective, longitudinal study. J Rheumatol 1999; 26: 1953–1958.
102. Balint PV, Kane D, Wilson H, McInnes IB, Sturrock RD. Ultrasonography of entheseal insertions in the lower limb in spondyloarthropathy. Ann Rheum Dis. 2002; 61: 905–910.
103. Khan MA. Ankylosing spondylitis: the facts. Oxford University Press, Oxford, UK, 2002; pp. 1–193.
104. Arnett FC, Khan MA, Wilkens RF. Are you missing ankylosing spondylitis? Patient Care 1986; 20: 51–78.
105. Dihlmann W, Delling G. Disco-vertebral destructive lesions (so-called Andersson lesions) associated with ankylosing spondylitis. Skeletal Radiol 1983; 3: 10–16.
106. Amor B, Santos RS, Nahal R *et al*. Predictive factors for the longterm outcome of spondyloarthropathies. J Rheumatol 1994; 21: 1883–1887.
107. Kellgren JH, ed. The epidemiology of chronic rheumatism, vol. II. Oxford: Blackwell Scientific; 1963.
108. van der Linden S, Valkenburg HA, Cats A. Evaluation of diagnostic criteria for ankylosing spondylitis. A proposal for modification of the New York criteria. Arthritis Rheum 1984; 27: 361–367.
109. Kidd BL, Cawley MI. Delay in diagnosis of spondarthritis. Br J Rheumatol 1988; 27: 230–232.
110. Mader R. Atypical clinical presentation of ankylosing spondylitis. Semin Arthritis Rheum 1999; 29: 191–196.
111. Gran JT, Ostensen M. Spondyloarthritides in females. Baillière's Clin Rheumatol 1998; 12: 695–715.
112. Khan MA, Khan MK. Diagnostic value of HLA-B27 testing in ankylosing spondylitis and Reiter's syndrome. Ann Intern Med 1982; 96: 70–76.
113. Khan MA. Thoughts concerning the early diagnosis of ankylosing spondylitis and related diseases. Clin Exp Rheumatol 2002; 20 (Suppl. 28): S6–S10.
114. Khan MA, Ball EJ. Ankylosing spondylitis and genetic aspects. Baillière's Best Pract Res Clin Rheumatol 2002 (in press).
115. Ball E, Khan MA. HLA-B27 polymorphism. Joint Bone Spine 20001; 68: 378–382.
116. Ramos M, De Castro JA. HLA-B27 and the pathogenesis of spondyloarthritis. Tissue Antigens 2002; 60: 191–205.
117. Feltkamp TEW, Mardjuadi A, Huang F, Chou C-T. Spondyloarthropathies in eastern Asia. Curr Opin Rheumatol 2001; 13: 285–290.
118. D'Amato M, Fiorillo MT, Galeazzi M *et al*. Frequency of the new HLA-B*2709 allele in ankylosing spondylitis patients and healthy individuals. Dis Markers 1995; 12: 215–217.
119. Olivieri I, Ciancio G, Padula A *et al*. The HLA-B*2709 subtype confers susceptibility to spondylarthropathy. Arthritis Rheum 2002; 46: 553–554.
120. Deyo RA, Weinstein JN. Low back pain. N Engl J Med 2001; 344: 363–370.
121. Yagan R, Khan MA. Confusion of roentgenographic differential diagnosis of ankylosing hyperostosis (Forestier's disease) and ankylosing spondylitis. Spine: State of the Art Reviews 1990; 4: 561–575.
122. Yagan R, Khan MA, Bellon EM. Spondylitis and posterior longitudinal ligament ossification in the cervical spine. Arthritis Rheum 1983; 26: 226–230.
123. Kaplan G, Haettich B. Rheumatological symptoms due to retinoids. Baillière's Clin Rheumatol 1991; 5: 77–97.
124. Hetem SF, Schils JP. Imaging of infections and inflammatory conditions of the spine. Semin Musculoskeletal Radiol 2000; 4: 329–347.
125. Stabler A, Reiser MF. Imaging of spinal infection. Radiol Clin North Am 2001; 39: 115–135.
126. Khan MA, Kushner I, Freehafer AA. Sacroiliac joint abnormalities in paraplegics. Ann Rheum Dis 1979; 38: 317–319.
127. Kahn M-F, Khan MA. SAPHO syndrome. Baillière's Clin Rheumatol 1994; 8: 333–326.
128. Hayem G, Bouchaud-Chabot A, Benali K *et al*. SAPHO syndrome: a long-term follow-up study of 120 cases. Semin Arthritis Rheum 1999; 29: 159–171.
129. Theodorou DJ, Theodorou SJ, Resnick D. Imaging in dialysis spondyloarthropathy. Semin Dial 2002; 15: 290–6.
130. Wenger DR, Frick SL. Scheuermann kyphosis. Spine 1999; 24: 2630–2639.
131. Nelson AM, Riggs BL, Jowsey JO. Atypical axial osteomalcia: report of four cases with two having features of ankylosing spondylitis. Arthritis Rheum 1978; 21: 715–722.
132. Akkus S, Tamer MN, Yorgancigil H. A case of osteomalacia mimicking ankylosing spondylitis. Rheumatol Int 2001; 20: 239–242.
133. Dougados M, van der Heijde D. Ankylosing spondylitis: how should the disease be assessed? Best Pract Res Clin Rheumatol 2002; 16: 605–18.
134. Gran JT, Skomsvoll JF. The outcome of ankylosing spondylitis: a study of 100 patients. Br J Rheumatol 1997; 36: 766–771.
135. Ostensen M, Ostensen H. Ankylosing spondylitis – the female aspect. J Rheumatol 1998; 25: 120–124.
136. Doward LC, Spoorenberg A, Cook SA *et al*. Development of the ASQoL: a quality of life instrument specific to ankylosing spondylitis. Ann Rheum Dis 2003; 62: 20–26.
137. Zink A, Braun J, Listing J, Wollenhaupt J. Disability and handicap in rheumatoid arthritis and ankylosing spondylitis–results from the German Rheumatological database. J Rheumatol 2000; 27: 613–622.
138. Boonen A, de Vet H, van der Heijde D, van der Linden S. Work status and its determinants among patients with ankylosing spondylitis. A systematic literature review. J Rheumatol 2001; 28: 1056–1062.
139. Ward MM, Kuzis S. Risk factors for work disability in patients with ankylosing spondylitis. J Rheumatol 2001; 28: 315–321.
140. Chorus AM, Boonen A, Miedema H, van der Linden S. Employment perspective in patients with ankylosing spondylitis. Ann Rheum Dis 2002; 61: 693–699.
141. Ward MM. Predictors of the progression of functional disability in patients with ankylosing spondylitis. J Rheumatol 2002; 29: 1420–1425.

142. Boonen A, Severens JL. Ankylosing spondylitis: what is the cost to society, and can it be reduced? Best Pract Res Clin Rheumatol 2002; 16: 691–705.

143. Lopez-Larrea C, Mijiyawa M, Gonzalez S et al. Association of ankylosing spondylitis with HLA-B*3403 in a West African population. Arthritis Rheum 2002; 46: 2968–2971.

144. Brown MA, Crane AM, Wordsworth BP. Genetic aspects of susceptibility, severity, and clinical expression in ankylosing spondylitis. Curr Opin Rheumatol 2002; 14: 355–360.

145. Brown MA, Wordsworth BP, Reveille JD. Genetics of ankylosing spondylitis. Clin Exp Rheumatol 2002; 20(Suppl. 28): S43–S49.

146. Laval SH, Timms A, Edwards S et al. Whole-genome screening in ankylosing spondylitis: evidence of non-MHC genetic-susceptibility loci. Am J Hum Genet 2001; 68: 916–926.

147. Kaprove RE, Little AH, Graham DC, Rosen PS. Ankylosing spondylitis. Survival in men with and without radiotherapy. Arthritis Rheum 1980; 23: 57–61.

148. Smith PG, Doll R. Mortality among patients with ankylosing spondylitis after a single treatment course with x-rays. Br Med J 1982; 284: 449–460.

149. Lehtinen K. Cause of death in 79 patients with ankylosing spondylitis. J Rheumatol 1980; 9: 145–147.

150. Khan MA, Khan MK, Kushner I. Survival among patients with ankylosing spondylitis: a life-table analysis. J Rheumatol 1981; 8: 86–90.

151. Braun J, Pincus T. Mortality, course of disease and prognosis of patients with ankylosing spondylitis. Clin Exp Rheumatol 2002; 20(Suppl. 28): S16–S22.

29 Ankylosing spondylitis: management

Ian Haslock

- Early diagnosis, patient education and physical therapy are essential for the successful management of ankylosing spondylitis
- The goals of physical therapy are to restore and maintain posture and movement to as near normal as possible
- Self-management with exercises must be continued on a lifelong basis
- Non-steroidal anti-inflammatory drugs relieve pain and stiffness and facilitate physical therapy
- Sulfasalazine and methotrexate have some effect, particularly in peripheral joint disease
- Anti-tumor necrosis factor-α therapy appears to offer both symptom relief and the possibility of true disease modification

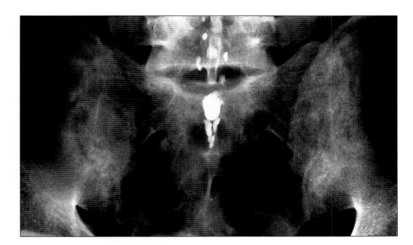

Fig. 29.1 Sacroiliac joint radiograph of a man with AS. Sacroiliitis is shown, along with residual contrast material from a previous myelogram.

INTRODUCTION

The cornerstones of treatment of all rheumatic diseases are early, accurate diagnosis and effective patient education. These are probably more important in ankylosing spondylitis (AS) than in any other condition. Early diagnosis enables treatment before permanent rigidity and deformity have taken place. It also enables patients to develop an appropriate lifestyle as early as possible. The patient's long-term cooperation is the single most crucial factor leading to successful management of AS. It is unlikely that the degree of long-term cooperation and commitment needed to develop a therapeutic lifestyle will be achieved unless the patient has a thorough understanding of the disease and the rationale behind its management.

As soon as the diagnosis of AS is made, the patient must be given a clear description of the nature of spondylitis. In particular, AS must be differentiated from mechanical back pain, and the differences in therapeutic approach to these conditions must be clearly stated. The advice can be reinforced with written material, such as that produced by the Arthritis Research Campaign (ARC) and National Ankylosing Spondylitis Society (NASS) in the UK and the Arthritis Foundation and the Spondylitis Society of America in the USA. Evaluation of the ARC leaflets confirmed their effectiveness in conveying information[1], but it is also important that this is reinforced by other members of the multidisciplinary team, especially the clinic nurses and physical therapists. Many patients now look for information on the internet. All the organizations mentioned above have informative, accurate web sites, but not all information given on the web is unbiased and accurate[2] and healthcare professionals managing patients with spondylitis must be prepared both to give advice regarding appropriate web sites and to refute misinformation given by others.

Unfortunately, many patients suffer from delay in diagnosis[3] and may have been given alternative diagnoses before the accurate one is made. The patient whose radiograph is shown in Figure 29.1 is typical of many patients with AS. His sacroiliac pain had been diagnosed as 'sciatica' and he had investigations including myelography and exploratory surgery in

order to find the cause of his symptoms. His sacroiliitis was clearly visible, but unreported, on many previous films. Such patients are justifiably suspicious of a totally new diagnosis, especially one which requires a radically different approach to treatment compared with previous advice. There is evidence that delays in diagnosis are decreasing. A survey of the 14 000 members of the German ankylosing spondylitis society, the Deutsche Vereinigung Morbus Bechterew (DVMB), showed that the average time to diagnosis had decreased from 15 years in those with a disease onset in the 1950s to 7.5 years for those with disease onset in 1975–79. It did not appear that further improvements were occurring at later dates[4].

OBJECTIVES OF TREATMENT

Initially, the objective is to reduce the patients' pain and stiffness, if possible by self-management. Where movement has been lost, there is an urgent need to restore as much as possible. The long-term objectives are to maintain symptom relief, maintain posture and movement, including chest wall and peripheral joint movement, and enable a full work capacity unimpeded by sickness absenteeism. In enabling these objectives, medication should be minimal and self-care maximal.

MANAGEMENT TECHNIQUES

Physical therapy

Physiotherapy is widely recognized as the single most important aspect of management of AS. There is some evidence that exercise alone can produce adequate symptom relief in many patients with AS; 178 of 236 patients from the armed forces followed long-term achieved symptom control by this means alone[5]. Controlled studies of physical therapy are

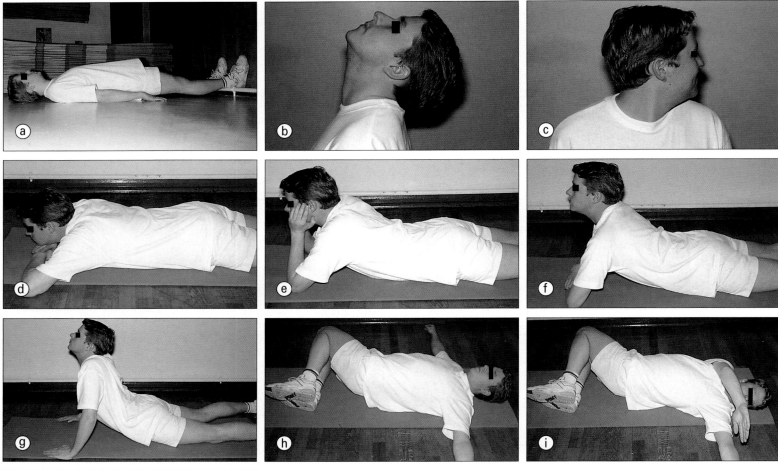

Fig. 29.2 An exercise sequence in AS. (a) Initially, posture is checked and corrected. Cervical spine exercises include full flexion (b), extension (c) and rotation (d–g). A full sequence of back extension is followed by rotation in (h, i) lying and (j) upright kneeling positions. Finally, breathing using thoracic muscles is checked and practiced.

rare, although significant benefit from exercise and education can be demonstrated over relatively short periods[6] and manipulative therapy has also been shown to increase range of movement in the short term[7]. Physical therapy takes two forms; that provided within the physical therapy department, and the patients' own home exercise regimes.

At the time of diagnosis of AS, the patient should have an immediate referral to a physical therapist, whose aims will be to restore posture and movement to as near normal as possible. Hydrotherapy is particularly valuable in producing the appropriate environment in which movement can be maximized[8]. A variety of pain relief methods such as pulsed short-wave therapy, local heat or cold, interferential therapy, local ultrasound or transcutaneous nerve stimulation[9] may be useful in facilitating movement. Non-steroidal anti-inflammatory drugs (NSAIDs) in high doses also may be needed during this phase of treatment, again with the objective of diminishing pain to a degree sufficient to allow full mobilization. Regaining lost movement at this time may cause discomfort, which results in apprehension in many patients, especially those who have been previously misdiagnosed and instructed to rest if pain increases. The attending physician must be sensitive to the patient's anxieties and willing to produce the greatest possible degree of analgesia to facilitate increased range of movement. Chest expansion and breathing exercises are also important. Local enthesopathy may need systemic drug treatment, local corticosteroid injection or local treatment by the physical therapist, using modalities such as ultrasound.

The initial period of treatment must be combined with an intensive education program. The patient must be told repeatedly that long-term success in disease management is dependent on the regularity of their home exercise regime; extra discomfort must be seen as a need for extra exercise, not extra rest. In teaching patients their home exercise regime, it is essential that therapists recognize that doing regular exercises is time-consuming and boring. It is therefore essential to try to incorporate as much appropriate exercise as possible into the patient's lifestyle by encouraging recreational exercises such as swimming and lighter sports such as badminton. Postural correction often involves undoing ingrained habits, particularly sitting in slouched positions. Good chest movement and breathing technique have to be taught, not assumed, and all these patients should be strongly advised not to smoke.

The initial period of physical therapy is a time of intense activity for the therapist and the patient. If treatment has been started before a significant amount of fixed deformity has occurred, and if the patient has proved cooperative with the treatment program, both therapist and patient will be rewarded by improved movement and decreased symptoms. The fact that this period of disease management is short and that the gains made are often quite dramatic, makes it a popular time for all concerned. However, unless the instant gratification of this exciting period can be translated into commitment to a long-term management program, the progess made is likely to be transient.

The patient's own efforts are the key to long-term success. Persuading all patients with AS that a daily exercise program must become as automatic a part of their day as cleaning their teeth or combing their hair calls for a major educational effort and constant reinforcement. The program the therapist teaches must be realistic physically, taking into account the degree of deformity that has already become fixed, and must have a time commitment that can be accommodated within the patient's everyday life (Fig. 29.2). Unrealistic expectations produce negative reactions that sabotage the entire program. The exercise and lifestyle program should also aim at cardiovascular fitness, as this has been shown to be important in maintaining work capacity, even if chest wall rigidity has occurred[10].

Lifelong regular exercise

Supervision of exercise regimes long-term by physical therapists has been shown to improve persistence with exercises and result in better outcomes than simple encouragement to persist with a home exercise regime[11]. Internal self-motivation involves frequent reinforcement of the need to exercise, coupled with clear explanation of its value in disease management. External motivation from spouses and family members is important. Joining a self-help group such as NASS often provides the spur needed to undertake regular exercise, although objective evidence of benefit from membership in a self-help group is lacking[12]. The provision of devices giving feedback regarding the effectiveness of home exercises can also be helpful in maintaining the impetus to continue them effectively[13].

Reinforcement of the exercise program is the responsibility of all health professionals coming into contact with the patient. The understanding, help and support of family members is also important, and securing their cooperation is a vital part of the educational process. Every consultation, for whatever purpose, should include the questions, 'Are you still doing all the exercises the physical therapist showed you?' and 'How often are you doing them?'. Any deterioration in posture should also be noted and commented on, with an attempt made to find the cause and remedy the problem.

Many patients with AS do not require regular prescriptions, and some mechanism must exist to ensure that they are seen and assessed regularly by their physical therapist, or family or hospital doctor. A chart showing progressive change in objective measurements, which the patient keeps, is a good method of documenting progression for both the patient and the clinical team. Even patients with late disease benefit from techniques such as appropriately applied passive stretching[14], and once demonstrated to be effective, techniques such as this can be taught to the patient for use with the assistance of a helper. Supervised training periods, including sessions in a hydrotherapy pool undertaken at weekly intervals, have also been shown to maintain mobility and function over prolonged periods, although no untreated control group was available for comparison[15]. However, the measured retention of movement and posture over a 5-year period using this regime provides a useful benchmark for alternative strategies.

A particularly intensive approach to physical treatment has been used in the AS unit at Bath, England[16]. Patients there were admitted to hospital each year for an intensive 3-week period of physiotherapy and hydrotherapy, accompanied by an educational program and reinforcement of their home exercise regime. Short-term benefit was found by comparing measurements made at the beginning with those at the end of each in-patient period. It was concluded that, even in advanced disease, small but worthwhile benefits could be achieved. A similar regime provided similar results over a slightly longer follow-up period[17], but whether such a highly expensive use of resources is justified, especially in comparison with intensive outpatient regimes, remains open to question.

For more everyday practice, one reliable way of reinforcing exercises and lifestyle is through a patient-run group. Most branches have arrangements for regular assessment and exercise sessions, usually staffed by volunteer physical therapists. Each session incorporates a warm-up and stretching period followed by exercise sessions, including hydrotherapy where available, and often culminating in light-heartedly competitive games. The meetings give the opportunity for discussion of problems with the therapist, and more formal educational sessions to improve the patient's knowledge of their disease and its management. Also, patient groups such as NASS provide a rich source of knowledge[4] and opinion, in addition to a focus of pressure for better diagnostic and treatment facilities.

The end-product of these efforts should be knowledgeable, active patients with a postural and exercise program built in to their daily lives, enabling them to be fit and active with minimal symptoms.

OCCUPATIONAL THERAPY

In the case of patients with early disease, occupational therapists will probably limit their interventions to the educational part of patient management. This will particularly involve advice about posture, especially appropriate seating, and recreation. The psychologic training of occupational therapists often makes them the most appropriate team member to lead the development of pain control strategies with patients[18].

For those in whom disease is more advanced, assessment of activities of daily living and ergonomic assessment of the home and the work place become more important, and may lead to the provision of aids if deformity produces significant practical problems. Patients with spondylitis often find that their decreased bending ability causes problems with dressing, and items such as elastic laces and stocking aids become essential for independence. Raised chair seats and toilet seats, showers in place of baths and other more complex home modifications may be needed as disease advances. Mobility is vital to all patients with arthritis; and car adaptations including wide-view mirrors, and modified controls may be required by those with more advanced spondylitis. For patients with very severe fixed spinal deformity, prismatic spectacles may be the only method of achieving an adequate amount of forward vision.

Other members of the multidisciplinary team, such as podiatrists and social workers, will also become involved with any patient whose disease progresses. Work is an area of particular importance to patients with AS, as many are on the thresholds of their careers when the diagnosis is made, and a realistic discussion about the possibility of disease progression may be an important part of their career choice. Those in employment may need skilled career advice to facilitate changing to more suitable occupations, but for most this can be achieved without a significant diminution in their job satisfaction or income[19]. Studies undertaken in the armed forces demonstrate the ability of fit, active, well-motivated people to follow a physically demanding career despite AS. Unfortunately, the persuasive talents of the Marine drill sergeant regarding regular exercise have no equal in civilian life. In general, the greatest problems for AS patients lie in jobs involving prolonged work in a single position, especially desk or computer work. Work posture is vital, as is the need to change position regularly and, preferably, to undertake some form of exercise such as a brisk walk, during the lunchbreak.

DRUG TREATMENT

Simple analgesics are usually considered to have a limited role in treating inflammatory rheumatic diseases. They are, however, quite widely used, about 33% of patients taking them, often as over-the-counter rather than prescribed medication. This reflects patients' desire for pain relief as their most important objective of drug treatment[20]. Health professionals are not good at appreciating the severity of patients' pain. Aggregated data from clinical trials suggested that both doctors and nurses assessed the patients' pain as about 20% less than the patients did. This is probably because of a combination of the poverty of the tools used to assess pain routinely, coupled with a societal prejudice to applaud stoicism, and difficulty by the professional in accepting the inadequacies of their prescribed treatments. Patients also desire their medication to be as risk-free as possible[21], and the extensive publicity regarding NSAID-induced gastrointestinal bleeding seems to have had a considerable effect on patients' perceptions of these drugs, which enhances the desire to stick with simple analgesics, or no drugs at all, whenever possible. It also contributes to the popularity of 'alternative' therapy, which promises safety in addition to a degree of efficacy unobtainable by allopathic means.

Non-steroidal anti-inflammatory drugs

The NSAIDs are used extensively to provide symptom relief to patients with AS. Overall, the objective of NSAIDs is to relieve pain sufficiently to allow free movement, especially for the exercise program essential to the spondylitic patient. During early stages of the disease they are often used in full dosage to cover the entire day. This schedule is particularly important when initial physical therapy is being used to maximize movement. Subsequently, morning stiffness is often the only symptom, or the predominant one, and a single sustained-release or long-acting night-time dose such as modified-release indomethacin 75mg, modified-release diclofenac 100mg or naproxen 500mg is often the preparation of choice, allowing freedom of movement in the morning. Many patients find that even this level of medication is needed only on an occasional basis, provided they maintain their regular exercises. Others will require either prolonged night-time medication or the continued use of divided doses to give more sustained symptom relief.

Choice of NSAID

The traditional 'best' NSAID is phenylbutazone, which has been claimed for many years to have particular benefit in patients with AS. For this reason, although phenylbutazone has been banned for general use in many countries, some may still permit its prescription by hospital consultants only, specifically in the treatment of AS. Despite the continuing availability of this medication for AS, it is now little used in the UK and USA and there is no convincing evidence that its 'special' efficacy has been missed. This view is not shared in much of continental Europe, where it remains the treatment of choice in AS for many physicians.

Indomethacin is probably the most widely used NSAID in AS, and has adopted the role of phenylbutazone as being especially valuable for patients with seronegative spondyloarthritis. A large study of more than 1300 British patients with AS showed that indomethacin was both the NSAID most commonly and continuously used, and the one that was most likely to be taken over a prolonged period[22]. It has the advantage of several dosage forms and sizes, making it flexible in use. Single modified-release 75mg doses at night are an effective way of diminishing morning stiffness. Suppositories have been used for this purpose in the mistaken belief that they deliver a sustained action by virtue of slower absorption; this is untrue, the morning activity being related to the greater dose in the suppositories (100mg) rather than to differences in absorption rate. Indomethacin has a reputation as a drug with a high incidence of side effects. Central nervous system toxicities, especially headache, do limit its use. These appear to be associated with peak plasma concentrations, and are reduced by modified-release preparations. The belief that indomethacin is particularly toxic as far as the upper gastrointestinal tract is concerned is not borne out by endoscopic studies[23] and, in any case, spondylitic patients are usually in a younger age group, with less risk of serious side effects in the gut, at their time of maximal NSAID need.

Naproxen is the second most popular NSAID[22]. It has a long half-life, giving relief of morning stiffness from a 500mg night-time dose, or whole-day symptom relief from a twice-daily dosage. The dose may be increased to 1.5g daily to relieve symptoms from acute exacerbations.

Almost all other NSAIDs are also used in treating AS. Selection is always a balance of effectiveness and tolerance. Patients' responses, both positive and adverse, are highly individual and far exceed the overall statistical differences between drugs. It has been suggested that summation of these apparently idiosyncratic differences can result in an overall 'pecking order' of NSAIDs being constructed that might give guidance for selection, taking into account factors such as age and sex in addition to individual diagnoses[24].

The effects of NSAIDs have been attributed to their ability to inhibit prostaglandins involved in the inflammatory process, with the side effects relating to the simultaneous inhibition of protective prostaglandins. It has been demonstrated that the target enzyme cyclo-oxygenase (COX) exists in two isoforms: a constitutive form, COX1, being responsible for the protective action in areas such as maintenance of gastric defences, and an inducible form, COX2, involved in the inflammatory process. This observation has enabled an understanding of differences in toxicity in the conventional NSAIDs, with higher ratios of COX1:COX2 inhibition being associated with greater toxicity. It has also led to the development of so-called 'specific' COX2 inhibitors or 'coxibs', which, in normal therapeutic doses, have little or no COX1-inhibiting activity. Two such compounds are now available – rofecoxib and celecoxib – and they appear to have borne out the theoretical prediction that their efficacy would be similar to that of conventional NSAIDs while the amount of serious upper gastrointestinal toxicity would be diminished. Experience of their use in AS is limited, but there is evidence of short-term efficacy in this disease[25]. Long-term studies in AS and comparisons with a range of NSAIDs, including newer ones with higher COX2:COX1 ratios than current drugs, and comparisons between individual coxibs, are still required before their definitive role can be assessed.

Two aspects of NSAID use in AS deserve particular attention. First, their proven action is restricted to relief of symptoms such as pain and stiffness. Any increase in spinal movement is related to an increased ability to exercise because of this symptom relief, rather than to any intrinsic action of the drug. Secondly, clinical trials of NSAIDs in AS must be studied with considerable attention to the details of the trial procedures. Many trials allow physical therapy to continue during drug treatment if the patient was being treated with it on entry to the study. Physical therapy is such an important part of AS management that the results of any study that allows inconsistent physical therapeutic input should be rejected. Many trial procedures are also of insufficient duration to give optimal information regarding efficacy and tolerability[26].

There are also two ways in which NSAIDs might have a more specific role in AS. A retrospective analysis of a small number of patients taking phenylbutazone suggested that this drug inhibited the calcification of syndesmophytes[27]. Similar suggestions have been made regarding indomethacin[28]. These observations have not been explored using prospective placebo-controlled studies, but it has been suggested that AS has become less severe since the introduction of NSAIDs[29]. It is thus unknown whether NSAIDs should be used in the symptomatic fashion outlined above, or whether they should be taken on a long-term basis irrespective of symptoms. The effects of NSAIDs on the upper gastrointestinal tract are well recognized, but more recently their effects in the small bowel have been recognized as being both common and important. When these observations are coupled with the observation of silent lesions in the same area observed by ileocolonoscopy and scintigraphy[30] in patients with seronegative spondyloarthropathies, the potential for NSAIDs to have an adverse effect on the disease must be considered.

Disease-modifying treatment

In contrast to the claims made in rheumatoid arthritis (RA), no claim has yet been made that any drug has a true disease-modifying effect on AS. Almost all the second line drugs used in the management of RA have been tried at some time in AS. The majority have been disappointing, with gold, penicillamine and antimalarials proving ineffective.

Sulfasalazine

Sulfasalazine has particular properties that command attention, with interest based on its widespread use in the treatment of inflammatory bowel disease. Although it was generally accepted that AS is an hereditary accompaniment to inflammatory bowel disease[31], rather than being caused by it, as is the case with enteropathic arthritis, this view received challenge from the work of Mielants and colleagues. They undertook colonoscopy and visual examination of the terminal ileum, initially in patients with reactive arthritis after enteric infection. They observed inflammatory lesions in the small bowel, and later extended their observations to idiopathic AS, in which similar lesions were again demonstrated[32]. Although clinically silent, these lesions bear a striking histologic similarity to Crohn's disease, and some of the patients who have them go on to develop florid clinical Crohn's disease. Their relationship to etiology is thus a continuing source of speculation. Under these circumstances, use of sulfasalazine combines the serendipitous logic of extrapolation from RA to AS with a scientific logic suggested by these observations.

Several studies of sulfasalazine have now been undertaken both in patients with peripheral joint synovitis and in those with spinal disease alone. An initial meta-analysis confirmed both the efficacy and safety of sulfasalazine in AS in the short term[33]. A more recent re-evaluation of published trials suggested that the spinal and peripheral joints are affected differently, and that sulfasalazine should be considered as a safe and well-tolerated therapy for persistent, active peripheral synovitis[34]. There is some evidence that the effect is greater in those with early disease than those in whom disease is more advanced, this being defined by the presence of fixed or bony deformity[35]. There is also some evidence that clinical improvement is accompanied by decreases in C-reactive protein (CRP) concentration and erythrocyte sedimentation rate (ESR), a combination of events that in RA is considered indicative of disease-modifying action. As sulfasalazine is a drug with which there is considerable clinical experience, including its safe use over many years, it would seem reasonable to introduce it early in the treatment of patients whose disease shows signs of poor control by physical treatment coupled with NSAIDs. Incremental doses starting at 0.5g twice daily and increasing to 1.5g twice daily have been used, although slightly higher doses are sometimes used to treat inflammatory bowel disease and are logical if partial response occurs.

Sulfasalazine may reduce the sperm count, and a warning about this is part of the information given to all men taking it. In practice, there seems to be little effect except in those in whom infertility is proving a problem. In contrast, sulfasalazine is probably the safest drug treatment for a woman contemplating pregnancy.

Methotrexate

Methotrexate has been given to patients with AS in low dosages (7.5–25mg oral or intramuscular weekly pulsed doses) similar to those used in RA, and appears to have a beneficial effect on both peripheral joints and spinal disease[36], although few placebo-controlled studies have yet been published. Many of the patients to whom methotrexate might be of particular value are young people with severe, active disease that is unremittingly progressive despite cooperation with an exercise regime. Some of these patients wish to start a family, and the potentially teratogenic effect in both men and women taking this drug has proved a significant practical problem.

All patients taking methotrexate must be warned explicitly about its teratogenic risks. Men must be reminded of the need to ensure adequare contraceptive precautions during intercourse while they are taking methotrexate and for 3 months thereafter. Women taking methotrexate must ensure they take reliable contraceptive precautions during treatment and for 3 months after stopping treatment, and must also be warned that termination of pregnancy may be needed should they accidentally conceive. In practice, these constraints have proved an inhibition to many patients contemplating the use of methotrexate.

Other immunosuppressive agents

Cyclophosphamide, given intravenously in 200mg doses on alternate days for 3 weeks, followed by a 100mg oral dose weekly for 3 months, has been used successfully on an open basis, producing a reduction in peripheral joint synovitis and spinal pain, although no improvement in spinal movement[37]. This was accompanied by a significant decrease in ESR, but no controlled studies have been undertaken. There is also anecdotal evidence that azathioprine is helpful in intractable enthesopathy, but again controlled observations do not exist.

Pamidronate

The major use of bisphosphonates has been in the treatment of osteoporosis and other bone disorders such as Paget's disease. Recent work suggests that they may suppress the formation of proinflammatory cytokines such as interleukin (IL)-1, IL-6 and tumor necrosis factor (TNF)-α. An open study in patients with AS used two regimes of intravenous pamidronate, 30mg monthly for 3 months then 60mg monthly for a further 3 months, compared with 60mg monthly for 3 months. Both groups showed clinical improvement and the 6-month regime also produced a reduction in ESR[38]. The only significant side effect of treatment was a post-injection flare, especially after the first infusion. This occurred in 50% of patients, which will produce difficulty with double-blind evaluation against placebo. This form of treatment could also have an effect on the osteoporosis found in AS, mediated both by its anti-inflammatory and antiresorptive actions.

Thalidomide

Thalidomide also affects proinflammatory cytokines, particularly IL-12 and TNF-α. Open studies in AS at doses of up to 300mg daily produced both significant clinical improvement and a decrease in CRP[39].

Tumor necrosis factor-α blockade

The TNF-α blocking drugs, infliximab and etanercept, have proved dramatically effective in the treatment of rheumatoid arthritis and also Crohn's disease. There is less experience in AS, but the findings of a number of studies are now available[40,41] that suggest a high level of effectiveness in AS. The short-term efficacy demonstrated in early studies[42] appears to be maintained after follow-up for 1 year[43]. These drugs appear to act on both spinal and peripheral joints, and offer hope of genuine disease retardation, with prevention or delay of spinal ankylosis. This possibility is supported by the improvement in magnetic resonance imaging (MRI) appearances of both sacroiliitis and enthesitis during etanercept treatment[44]. A clinical and MRI study using infliximab also showed improvement in MRI appearance in both early and advanced disease[45]. Experience of early treatment, which would be predicted to be of maximum benefit, is small at present, but the 11 patients in one study[46] had a mean disease duration of 5 years (range 0.5–13 years), and showed very considerable improvement. Of the 10 patients who completed the regimen of three infliximab infusions, nine showed improvement of 50% or more in activity, function and pain scores. There were significant decreases in both CRP and IL-6. SF36 scores showed improvement, and two of three patients with MRI evidence of inflammation showed improvement.

The potential for effective, truly disease-modifying, but expensive and potentially toxic, therapy in AS produces some important questions[47]. Who should be treated? The majority of patients with AS do well with regular exercises and non-steroidal drugs. It would seem inappropriate to introduce anti-TNF treatment at an early stage in these patients. However, prognostic factors in early AS are not well defined, so picking an appropriate cohort for early aggressive treatment rationally is at present difficult. A 10-year longitudinal study of 151 patients with AS was carried out in an attempt to determine poor prognostic factors[48]. It found that hip arthritis, increased ESR (more than 30mm in the first 1 hour), poor response to NSAIDs, limitation of spinal movement and oligoarthritis, occurring in the first 2 years of disease, plus onset at age 16 years or less, were poor prognostic factors. At present, the criterion used for any extension of therapy is the failure of simple treatment, which might be inappropriately vague if optimal gain is to be achieved from these drugs. How early is early? Delays in diagnosis of AS are still measured in years, with little sign of recent improvement. If timely early treatment is the most effective, there will be difficulty recruiting patients for convincing clinical trials and, if successful, difficulty improving early diagnosis at primary care level. In summary, the exact place of this treatment remains to be defined, but this definition is needed urgently, as it offers what is, at present, the best potential treatment for a disease that can have catastrophic long-term consequences.

Corticosteroids

Long-term treatment with systemic corticosteroids has little part to play in the management of AS, although rare patients exist in whom no other form of treatment proves effective. Despite its appearance of overossification, the spine in AS contains vertebrae that are significantly osteoporotic, possibly as a result of diversion of mechanical stress from the vertebral bodies to the surrounding syndesmophyte bridges, in addition to the effect of proinflammatory cytokines. The effect of long-term corticosteroids on this osteoporosis is unproved, but on theoretic grounds might be expected to increase it. Figure 29.3 shows the bone mineral density (BMD) of an active man with AS who had a good exercise record and had been treated with low-dose corticosteroids for 21 years. The osteoporosis seen puts him at significant risk of spinal fracture.

Parenteral low-dose corticotropin proved ineffective when added to an inpatient rehabilitation regime[49]. Intravenous pulsed methylprednisolone is undoubtedly effective in reducing severe symptoms[50]. The indications for its use are poorly defined, but experience suggests it is an extremely effective way of controlling symptoms on a short-term basis. The period of reduced symptoms produced by this treatment should always be utilized for intensive physical therapy, in order to maximize movement and correct posture as much as possible. Local corticosteroid injections are useful both for peripheral joint disease and for local treatment of enthesopathy.

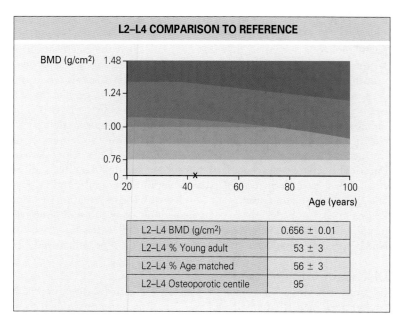

Fig. 29.3 Bone mineral density with corticosteroid treatment. Result from dual-energy X-ray absorptiometer scan of a 42-year-old man with AS. He had been treated with prednisolone for 21 years. His *Z* score for vertebral height was –2.44.

L2–L4 BMD (g/cm²)	0.656 ± 0.01
L2–L4 % Young adult	53 ± 3
L2–L4 % Age matched	56 ± 3
L2–L4 Osteoporotic centile	95

Radiation therapy

Radioactive synovectomy, using yttrium-90 especially, is a useful treatment for chronic synovitis, particularly in the knee. This treatment should be reserved for those who have completed their family, because of the small risk of chromosome change through irradiation of the groin lymphatics.

External radiotherapy aimed at the spine and sacroiliac joints was widely used until the publication of work by Court-Brown and Doll[51], which demonstrated an increased incidence of leukemia in patients treated in this way. Since then, radiotherapy has been largely discarded, although it is possible that carefully targeted treatment using modern equipment would give benefit with a degree of safety comparable to that of some disease-modifying antirheumatic drugs – certainly the doses and frequency of treatment used in the 1940s were well in excess of those that would be used now. Patients who had been treated with radiotherapy also illustrate the need for persisting with exercises, irrespective of the quality of symptom control. Many of these patients were told they had been cured, and hence their regular exercise regimes were no longer needed. Although many remained pain-free, the progression of spinal fusion and the disability caused by it continued unabated.

Local radiotherapy is still accepted as having a small place in the management of AS. Any isolated joints or entheses unresponsive to systemic and local treatment might be considered for this form of treatment, but in practice it is almost exclusively reserved for the treatment of painful heels. Although an apparently 'minor' problem, painful heels can be the source of considerable disability. Enthesitis at the insertion of the tendo Achillis or the plantar fascia into the calcaneum may also be accompanied by calcaneal periostitis (Fig. 29.4). Although this usually occurs in established AS, it may be either the presenting symptom or, rarely, the sole manifestation of the disease. Treatment with sorbo insoles and local physiotherapy may be effective. Local steroid injections can be dramatically effective, although injection of Achilles tendinitis and paratendinitis may lead to tendon rupture[52]. Resistant cases usually respond rapidly to local radiotherapy[53], preferably with superficial orthovoltage radiation or, if this is unavailable, electrons of appropriate energy (6–9McV) from a suitable linear accelerator. The localized area treated and the relatively

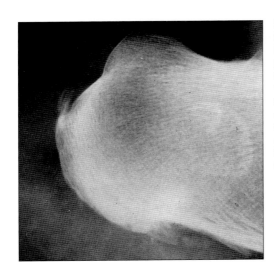

Fig. 29.4 Radiographic features in the heel of a patient with spondyloarthropathy. 'Whiskering' is present at the insertion of the tendo Achilles, and plantar aponeurosis periostitis can be seen along the inferior and posterior aspects of the calcaneus.

small dose needed (6–12Gy) mean that complications are extremely unlikely, and this form of treatment can, therefore, be recommended under these circumstances.

OSTEOPOROSIS IN ANKYLOSING SPONDYLITIS

The development of thick bony bridges between vertebrae and the apparent tendency of patients with AS to be prone to heterotopic new bone formation after surgery have given the impression that AS is a disease characterized by thick and excessive bone. In addition, treatment with prolonged weight-bearing exercise should provide the stimulus for maximal bone formation. Despite this, many patients with AS show evidence of significant spinal osteoporosis[54]. This is presumably related to deviation of mechanical stresses away from the vertebral bodies by the syndesmophytic bridges, although the local relationship between bridging and porosis has not yet been ascertained. Local inflammatory disease may also contribute to local bone loss from a mechanism similar to the juxta-articular bone loss in RA[55]. There is certainly an association with active inflammation[56], but there is still some doubt as to the exact mechanisms involved, as most patients show normal markers of bone formation and resorption[57]. Osteoporosis may contribute to the vulnerability of the AS spine when subjected to trauma.

It would seem reasonable for all patients with AS to undergo bone densitometry, usually by dual-energy X-ray absorptiometry scanning, to ascertain their degree of osteoporosis, with follow-up scans at regular intervals of not less than 2 years. Hip measurement is especially important in those in whom the presence of syndesmophytes artificially increases the spinal density. Where significant osteoporosis is found, the usual investigations of this condition, remembering that many of the patients are male, should be undertaken. Treatment recommendations are at present speculative, but if a patient has osteoporosis, and no non-spondylitic cause for this has been found, the treatment of choice is probably a bisphosphonate such as alendronate or risedronate in post-menopausal women and in men. There is at present no information on the effect that inflammatory lesions in the gut of the spondylitic patient have on either calcium absorption or the development of osteoporosis, although idiopathic inflammatory bowel disease is associated with excess bone loss[58].

NON-LOCOMOTOR DISEASE

Eye disease is the most common extralocomotor complication of AS with at least 20% of patients suffering isolated or repeated attacks of iritis (anterior uveitis). As there is no close temporal relationship between the severity of iritis and spondylitis, the eye disease is usually treated as a separate entity, although there is some evidence that sulphasalazine may produce a reduction in both the severity and frequency of anterior uveitis[59]. The most important aspect of treatment is to ensure that the patients seek immediate medical advice on developing a painful red eye. The consequences of delayed or inadequate treatment are the formation of synechiae, which are adhesions from the back of the iris. Secondary glaucoma may then supervene.

Anterior uveitis associated with AS is usually unilateral. In most cases, topical treatment with corticosteroid eye drops and mydriatics is all that is required. The eye may need to be protected from the light to ensure comfort during the period of pupillary dilatation. Administration of corticosteroids orally or by intraocular injection is required when local treatment fails to relieve the inflammation. In children with treatment-resistant uveitis, etanercept has been shown to be beneficial[60], but a retrospective study in adults with a variety of rheumatic diseases, including AS and psoriatic spondylitis, showed that, in contrast to 100% showing a decrease in articular inflammation, only 38% showed improvement of their uveitis. Neither of the patients with spondylitis showed improvement in their eyes, the patient with psoriatic spondylitis actually developing eye disease during etanercept treatment[61]. Three patients with chronic unilateral anterior uveitis were included in one study of infliximab[45]. Two were described as showing 'noticeable improvement', whereas the third suffered a flare after initial improvement. More work is obviously needed to define the role of anti-TNF drugs in the management of this potentially serious condition.

Iritis is, on occasions, the presenting symptom of AS, especially in those in whom back pain is mild or stiffness has occurred insidiously. Those treating apparently idiopathic anterior uveitis, especially when unilateral, should always consider the possibility of this diagnosis. One study of 514 consecutive patients with anterior uveitis attending a specialist uveitis clinic[62] showed that 117 (22.7%) had a seronegative spondyloarthritis, with ankylosing spondylitis being the most common (75 patients). In 62 of the spondylarthritis patients, including 35 with AS, uveitis was the presenting symptom.

The two major internal organs involved in AS are the heart and the lungs. Diseases such as aortic valve disease are treated identically to similar diseases in non-spondylitic patients. Extra precautions may be needed at the time of any surgery, as neck rigidity can produce difficulties for anesthesia. Long-term anticoagulation after valve surgery complicates the treatment of the joint disease because of interactions with NSAIDs, which displace warfarin from protein binding and thus alter anticoagulant need. Also, patients who are in need of cardiac surgery, and hence anticoagulation, are usually older, and so come into the age group in which the risk of major bleeding produced by NSAIDs is increased. It is prudent in these patients to avoid non-selective NSAIDs if at all possible, and if symptom relief cannot be obtained in any other way, to use COX2-selective inhibitors. These may be useful in this situation, as they do not inhibit platelet function and have been shown to be associated with a lower risk of gastrointestinal bleeding. An alternative approach is cotherapy with proton-pump inhibitors.

Upper zone lung fibrosis is, at least in part, caused by inadequate aeration of this area, especially in those with rigid chest walls who rely on diaphragmatic breathing. Inclusion of breathing exercises in the routine for patients with AS is an important part of prevention of this complication. When it occurs, diagnostic confusion with tuberculosis may occur, especially where cavitation occurs (Fig. 29.5). Such cavities may become colonized with *Aspergilla*.

No specific treatment is available for the lung disease of AS. Stopping smoking and regular breathing exercises are obviously essential. Incidental infections and fungal colonization require appropriate specific treatment, which should be given promptly in order to minimize further lung damage.

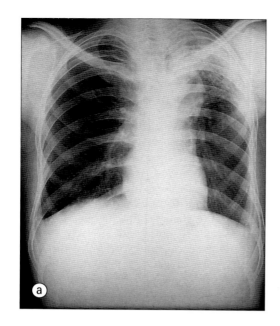
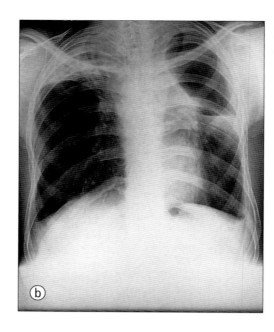

Fig. 29.5 (a) Upper lobe lung fibrosis leading to (b) cavitation in AS. This cavity became colonized with *Aspergilla*.

MANAGEMENT OF WOMEN WITH ANKYLOSING SPONDYLITIS

Until relatively recently, conventional teaching was that ankylosing spondylitis is rare in women. This led to situations typified by the patient shown in Figure 29.6. When she presented with symptoms typical of AS, that diagnosis was not considered as it was 'well known' that this disease did not occur in women. As a result, she was treated with a corset, which certainly made her spinal rigidity worse. Despite her clinically obvious AS, this diagnosis had still not been considered because she was able to touch her toes – as she illustrates, this is easily

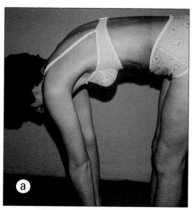

Fig. 29.6 AS in women.
(a) This woman with AS was misdiagnosed because of her ability to touch her toes. Thorough examination revealed (b) her full range of extension (c) and her side flexion to be virtually nil. More accurate observation and the performance of a Schober test (Fig. 29.12) revealed that her forward flexion took place almost entirely from her hips.

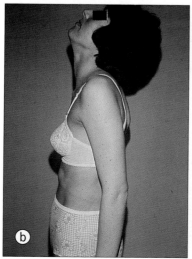
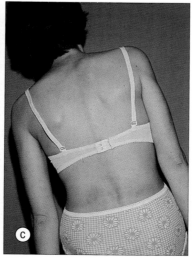

possible for someone with a rigid back who has mobile hips and well-stretched hamstrings, and is a perfect example of the reason why finger–floor distance is an inappropriate measure.

Pregnancy in women with AS requires particular consideration for five reasons:

- Genetic counselling. AS is known to be a disease with a strong genetic component. Many patients require discussion of the implications of this before embarking on pregnancy
- Effects of treatment on conception. AS itself does not appear to affect fertility adversely, but some drugs used to treat AS, such as methotrexate, are potentially teratogenic, and appropriate advice about this must be given to all women of childbearing age
- Effects of pregnancy on disease activity. About 75% of women with RA have amelioration of their disease during pregnancy. This is not the case in AS, when at most 25% improve during pregnancy, the majority being the same or worse at this time[63]. Carefully planned physical therapy based on that used for all AS patients is important for these patients, in addition to the usual regime of antenatal exercises. All medication should be kept to a minimum, but many will need at least intermittent NSAIDs in order to maintain function
- Delivery. Given that the sacroiliac joints, and sometimes the hips, are targets for inflammation in AS, some problems with delivery might be anticipated. Although the majority of women with AS are able to have normal vaginal deliveries, the cesarean section rate does appear to be greater than in women who do not have AS, with the AS cited as the reason for section in more than 50%[64].
- Postpartum disease flares. Over 50% of the patients surveyed by Ostensen and Ostensen[64] reported a flare of their disease during the 6 months postpartum. This was sufficient to interfere with baby care in many of them. There was a strong correlation between flares of disease postpartum and active disease at the time of conception. This raises the question as to whether women with AS should be advised not to become pregnant during periods of disease activity.

The underlying principles of management of men and women with AS are identical although, compared with men, women report more pain and more need for medication, especially sulphasalazine and corticosteroids, despite having less severe spinal X-ray changes overall and a lesser incidence of iritis[4]. It is apparent, however, that women with AS require more awareness amongst heathcare professionals that they do suffer from AS, and that their disease presents some specific problems in management that require specific interventions over and above those of their male counterparts.

ANKYLOSING SPONDYLITIS ASSOCIATED WITH OTHER DISEASES

As the central member of the seronegative spondyloarthropathies, AS may be associated with other diseases in the group, particularly psoriasis and inflammatory bowel disease. The treatment of the skin and joint components of AS associated with psoriasis are separate, except that methotrexate might have a beneficial effect on both aspects of the disease (see Chapter 32). When AS is associated with inflammatory bowel disease, it must be remembered that NSAIDs may cause exacerbation of the bowel disease[65] and must be used with care. The propensity for fenamates to cause diarrhea makes them particularly unsuitable. There is speculation that modified-release formulations, which are designed to release small quantities of drug throughout the length of the gut, might be particularly problematic, although at present this is unproved. The effect of sulfasalazine on both gut and joints makes it a particularly good choice under these circumstances, although the salicylate-only medications such as mesalamine (mesalazine) that are now being used to treat inflammatory bowel disease have no direct effect on joint disease.

SURGERY

The rigid, flexed cervical spine and immobile chest wall of the patient with AS may produce significant technical difficulties for the anesthesiologist and a need for immaculate perioperative management by the physical therapist. Prolonged recumbancy is a time of great danger to the AS patient. Despite this, surgery can be an extremely valuable part of their management. Spinal surgery involves two areas particularly: the cervical spine, where atlantoaxial subluxation may require attention or where osteotomy can improve posture and forwards vision; and the dorsolumbar spine, where the paradoxical operation of spinal fusion may be needed for a 'last joint' problem, or where osteotomy may be used to improve spinal posture.

Atlantoaxial subluxation is less common in AS than in RA. Patients with RA can have significant degrees of atlantoaxial slip with no symptoms, because of the general ligamentous laxity and erosion of bones

that accompany this pathology. In contrast, the bone and ligaments in AS are rigid and unyielding, with neurologic sequelae being consequently more common. In such patients, cervical fusion may be necessary in order to retain neurologic integrity and control symptoms such as referred occipital pain (Fig. 29.7).

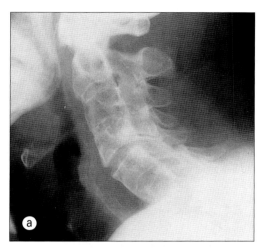

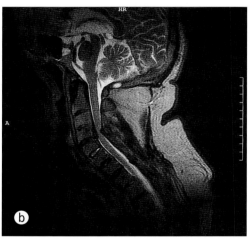

Fig. 29.8 Last-joint syndrome in AS. Although this usually occurs in the dorsolumbar spine, the example shown here is in the cervical spine. (a) On X-ray. (b) On MRI.

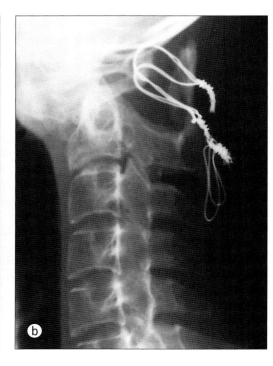

Fig. 29.7 Before and after cervical fusion. (a) The atlantoaxial subluxation seen preoperatively was accompanied by severe pain and numbness over the occiput. (b) The symptoms were completely relieved by cervical fusion.

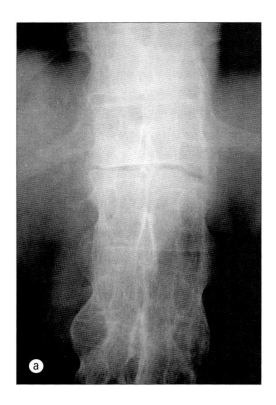

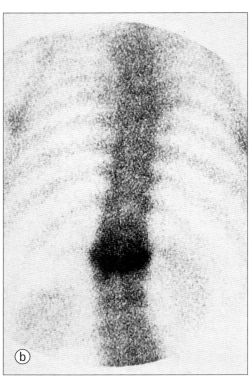

Fig. 29.9 Last-joint syndrome in AS.
(a) X-ray appearance showing the 'last joint' with discitis. (b) Discitis demonstrated by isotope scanning.

The 'last-joint' syndrome, in which bridging ossification of syndesmophytes has taken place at every level except one (Fig. 29.8), presents a cruel dilemma: on the one hand, exercise continues to be important in maintaining posture, even when extensive fusion has taken place; on the other, the sole mobile segment is exposed to considerable stresses during activity, with pain, which may be severe, and sometimes the development of discitis (Fig. 29.9). Treatment is initially by rest, sometimes by the use of a corset or brace[66]. Surgical fusion is required where the pain is unrelieved by conservative means, or where discitis is so severe that healing under external immobilization fails to occur.

Spinal surgery may also be indicated when the posture of a fixed spondylitic spine is so extreme that forward vision can only be achieved with prismatic spectacles. A wedge osteotomy produces a less stooped posture, with a consequent ability to see ahead. This surgery may be sited at the cervical or dorsolumbar area, and is accompanied by a risk of neurologic damage, which must be balanced against the potential improvement in lifestyle produced by postural correction and enhanced forward vision. This type of surgery should only be undertaken by a skilled spinal surgeon, anesthesiologist, nursing and physical therapy team in theaters equipped for intraoperative spinal monitoring. In this and all surgery on AS patients, the period of postoperative immobilization should be kept to a minimum and the physical therapist should ensure that the patient maintains the fullest possible range of movements compatible with any necessary postoperative fixation. Attention to breathing is particularly important if postoperative chest infection is to be avoided. New techniques for the insertion of cement into osteoporotic wedged vertebrae to restore their anatomy are now available, but there is as yet insufficient experience with them to know if they have any place in spondylitis.

The root joints (those at the 'roots' of the limbs – i.e. the shoulders and hips), particularly the hips, are frequently involved in AS, and total hip replacement is indicated in those in whom severe pain or severe limitation of movement occurs. Loss of range at the hips may reveal a greater than expected degree of disability caused by spinal fusion, forward flexion, in particular, being entirely dependent on hip movement in some patients.

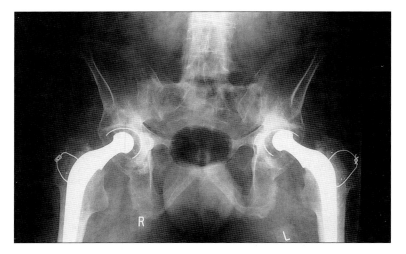

Fig. 29.10 Total hip replacement in AS. These prostheses had been inserted 13 years before this X-ray was taken.

Two anxieties have been expressed regarding hip replacement in patients with AS. As many are young and active, it has been suggested that mechanical failure produced by high use might be a major problem. There is also anxiety that patients with AS may be particularly prone to extra-articular ossification, causing loss of movement in the replaced joint. Long-term follow-up suggests that these are not common problems, with a high degree of short-term and long-term value accruing from the operation[67]. It should be noted, too, that patients followed long-term in these studies had replacement with conventional cemented hips (Fig. 29.10), rather than the cementless ones that are now sometimes selected for younger, more active patients, or the more limited resurfacing prostheses such as the McMinn.

DETERMINATION OF IMPROVEMENT OR DETERIORATION

There are many approaches to assessing treatment response in AS. As with many inflammatory diseases, determination of ESR, plasma

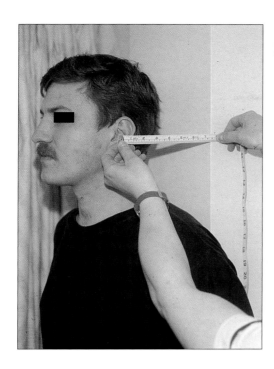

Fig. 29.11 Measurement of wall–tragus distance.

tant in AS, as measurements will be needed over long periods of time and are unlikely to be undertaken by the same observer throughout.

Measurement of movement should ideally cover all areas of the spine, in addition to peripheral joints, and incorporate all planes of movement. Because the different planes are affected to the same extent, measurement of one usually suffices as a surrogate for the others in everyday practice. The simplest technique is Macrae's modification of Schober's technique[69], which measures forward flexion of the lumbar spine. The lumbosacral junction is identified between the dimples of Venus, and marks are made 5cm below it and 10cm above. Because the lower point is adjacent to the tethered skin over the coccyx and the upper point is free to move, flexion causes distraction of the two marks (Fig. 29.12). The result is usually expressed as the amount of skin distraction, this in turn being related to true spinal motion in a linear fashion. Methods of measuring side flexion and rotation have been devised but are rarely used, most assessments being by eye or by simple clinical means such as the distance reached by the fingertips down the lateral thigh. Provided precautions are taken to ensure that no flexion takes place simultaneously, measurement of this distance using a tape measure is reliable and correlates well with instrumental measurement using an inclinometer. One frequently used measure that deserves unequivocal condemnation is measuring the fingertip–floor distance on forward flexion. This measures an inconsistent combination of spinal and hip movement, although it is frequently suggested as being a useful measure of spinal flexion. In some patients, the fingertips or even the full palm can be placed on the floor in the absence of any true spinal flexion, and this measurement should be discarded because of its practical imprecision and the imprecision in thought that often accompanies its use.

Chest expansion is reduced when the costovertebral joints are involved in the inflammatory process. Simple measurement with a tape measure at the level of the 4th rib anteriorly provides useful and simple quantification. Although an arbitrary 2.5cm expansion is used in some epidemiologic definitions of AS, there is considerable overlap between AS patients and controls (Fig. 29.13), and a significant decrease in

viscosity or CRP may be valuable in the initial diagnosis and in following subsequent progress. However, the relationships between these measurements and disease progression are imprecise and insufficient to produce an adequate description of disease state[68]. Symptoms are mainly pain and stiffness, which can be measured by a variety of techniques such as visual analog scales. No technique exists for measuring spinal stiffness objectively.

Clinical measures

Posture is easier to visualize than to quantify. Serial photographs may produce a telling record of disease progression. Simpler methods include wall–occiput or wall–tragus measurements (Fig. 29.11), which are easy to undertake with a tape measure and have a reasonable level of intra- and interpersonal reliability. Interobserver error is particularly impor-

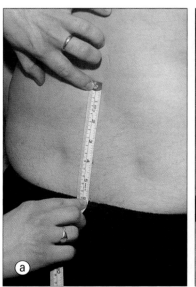
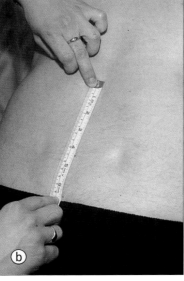

Fig. 29.12 Macrae's modification of Schober's test. (a) The lumbosacral junction is identified between the dimples of Venus, and measurement made 5cm below and 10cm above. (b) The distraction of these marks is proportional to true lumbar flexion. In the example shown, the patient has AS and skin distraction is limited.

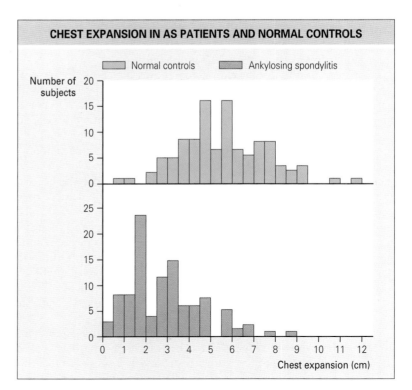

Fig. 29.13 Chest expansion in AS patients and normal controls. Although patients with AS have significantly less chest expansion than normal controls, the overlap is considerable. (Data from Moll and Wright[70].)

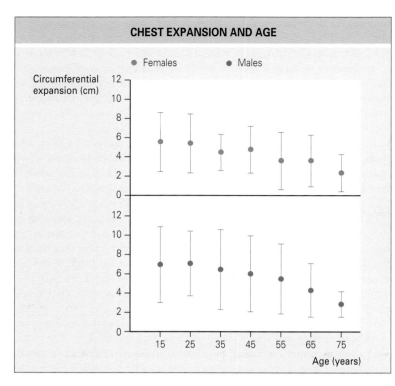

Fig. 29.14 Chest expansion and age. Chest expansion decreases with age, and this must be taken into account when considering the normality of an individual clinical measurement. (Data from Moll and Wright[71].)

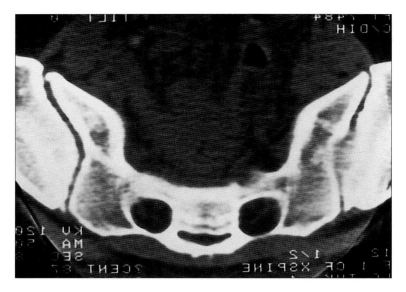

Fig. 29.15 Sacroiliac MRI. Sacroiliitis in a woman with a normal X-ray. This shows both small erosions and early fusion.

normal chest expansion with age (Fig. 29.14). These factors make chest expansion a more useful measure of progression than an absolute point measurement.

Some relatively simple instruments have been designed that facilitate measurement of spinal movement. The spondylometer, introduced in 1949[72], is a protractor with a long articulated arm. Flexion produces a composite measure of lumbar and dorsal movement, the design of the instrument automatically giving more weight to flexion in the clinically more important lumbar area. Inclinometers have also been used, the most sophisticated being the arthrospinometer, which incorporates a magnetic compass as a standard reference, thus increasing its versatility[73]. Although used episodically in drug trials, none of these has become part of routine use. However, there is now an increasing need to document the long-term results of the treatment of rheumatic disease, and the low intraobserver errors of instruments such as the spondylometer may produce a resurgence of interest in them as everyday clinical tools.

Flexion of the dorsal spine is incorporated into spondylometer and inclinometer measurements, and the arthrospinometer may also be used to measure dorsal rotation, although the technique is too cumbersome and time consuming to be used other than for research. Cervical spine movement has proved difficult to measure except by eye, and although a number of gadgets to enhance measurement have been devised, none has yet found a place in routine clinical practice. As neck rotation appears to be an important parameter contributing to overall disability, a simple measure of it may be an important facet of overall assessment of the patient with AS. Use of a protractor has proved a reliable method[74], and should probably be more widely used.

Enthesopathy is a characteristic of all the seronegative spondyloarthropathies. An enthesitis index has been devised[75] that has proved useful in assessing the results of drug treatments. It is suggested that this index reflects changes in disease activity better than traditional anthropometric measures, although the Assessment of Ankylosing Spondylitis working group were unable to recommend any currently available instrument for measuring enthesitis[76].

Imaging

Sacroiliac inflammation is an important feature of AS, but its measurement has proved difficult. There are many clinical tests for the presence of sacroiliitis, but these prove unreliable in practice[77] and at best facilitate only a 'present or absent' judgment, rather than allowing gradation of response. Scintigraphy has advocates as a diagnostic method, although it has not achieved universal acceptance. Personal experience suggests that it is a useful aid to diagnosis in carefully selected patients, but there is no evidence of its utility in measuring progression. Thermography has been shown to be capable of detecting sacroiliac inflammation and of detecting change in response to drugs. It is, however, an expensive, cumbersome and time-consuming technique, and is unsuited to routine practice. MRI is a sensitive way of detecting sacroiliitis before radiological change is apparent (Fig. 29.15)[78]. Its cost has hitherto made it more useful for early diagnosis rather than evaluation of disease progression, but the need for rigorous evaluation of expensive treatments such as anti-TNF-α has changed this balance, and it has been used successfully to demonstrate improvement using such treatment[44,45].

Radiological changes are characteristic features of AS. A number of radiological assessment instruments have been developed, including the Stoke Ankylosing Spondylitis Spine Score (SASSS)[79] and the Bath Ankylosing Spondylitis Radiology Index (BASRI)[80]. Overall radiological assessments are of more value over long rather than short time periods[81] and it is probably now inappropriate to rely on measures involving repeated exposure to ionizing radiation, despite their convenience and relatively low cost, when alternatives exist.

Patient-centered outcomes

A number of newer indices have patient questionnaires at their heart. This approach combines economy, as an external metrologist is not required, with an increasing appreciation of the importance of the patient's perception of their own disease. The Health Assessment Questionaire, which is widely used in evaluating RA, has been modified (HAQ-S) with the aim of extending its role into the management of patients with spondyloarthritis[82]. The Dougados Functional Index (DFI) combines both a questionnaire and an articular index specifically designed for spondyloarthritis. This provides an evaluation of both the disease and its response to treatment[83].

The Bath group have developed an extensive repertoire of indices that explore different aspects of the patient's disease[84]. Three self-administered questionnaires evaluate disease status (Bath Ankylosing

Spondylitis Disease Activity Index, BASDAI), disability (Bath Ankylosing Spondylitis Functional Index, BASFI) and the patient's perception of the effects of disease on their well-being (Bath Ankylosis Spondylitis Patient Global Score, BAS-G). A set of physical measures are added (Bath Ankylosis Spondylitis Metrology Index, BASMI), and the package gives a broad view of the patient's disease, and also gives insight into the complexity of comprehensiveness in assessment. The full set of Bath indices seems likely to have more of a place in research than in routine practice.

The BASFI has been compared with the DFI and the HAQ-S, and was shown to be more responsive than the other two indices in situations both of improvement and of deterioration in functional performance[85]. This must be interpreted with some caution, as all three indices showed means towards the lower end of the scale. A comparison of the DFI and the HAQ-S suggested that the HAQ-S showed greater construct validity and sensitivity to change than the DFI, although it showed little advantage over the unmodified HAQ[86]. One important finding of this study was that the six measures of physical function (cervical rotation, occiput to wall distance, chest expansion, Schober test, Smythe's test and intermalleolar straddle) that were used to assess construct validity explained a maximum of 24% (HAQ-S) of the instruments they were evaluating. This illustrates well the importance of looking beyond pure physical measurements in evaluating AS. The literature regarding the DFI and the BASFI was reviewed on behalf of the Assessments in Ankylosing Spondylitis working group[87]. The conclusion was that each had value, but that there were insufficient head-to-head comparisons under different circumstances to choose an overall 'best' instrument. A modification of the DFI, replacing its 3-point Likert scale with a 5-point one, was evaluated for the same working party, and no significant differences were found between it and the BASFI[88]. Both are, therefore, included as recommended tools by the Assessments in Ankylosing Spondylitis working group[76].

QUALITY OF LIFE

Despite its reputation as a mild disease, AS can have considerable effects on the quality of life of those who have it. Even in those with mild disease, the intrusive effects of regular exercises, however 'good for you' they may be, coupled with the need to take medication with its consequent side effects, and the knowledge that there is a strong genetic component to the disease, all take their toll. Severe disease with constant pain, restriction of movement, social dysfunction, work loss, deformity and fatigue has an all too obvious effect. There have been few attempts to measure this aspect of AS, although a review for the Outcome Measures in Rheumatology group (OMERACT) showed that they have been used more frequently recently[89] and the need to justify the increased cost of expensive new therapies has meant that evaluations such as the SF36 before and after treatment are now being used increasingly[46]. Despite this, the totality of the disease burden to the individual, their family and society is still relatively unexplored.

CONCLUSION

Epidemiologic studies of AS have suggested that the disease is becoming milder and its age of onset later. This conflicts with anecdotal experience by the author from a general rheumatology department, which suggests that an increasing number of people have severe, aggressive disease that is failing to respond to the simple NSAID plus exercise programs that have appeared to be so successful in the past. The team approach to treatment, often utilizing the physical therapist as the focal point for the patient, remains a valid way of delivering care. However, there is a need to develop better prognostic markers early in the course of the disease, so that intensive drug treatment can be started early in those patients for whom it is appropriate. Development of strategies based on this need, while maintaining the primacy of physical treatment and patient education, remains a priority for the development of AS therapy. Research is still needed regarding all aspects of treatment, from the optimum use of NSAIDs and the most effective physical therapy and exercise regimes to the place of modern, expensive treatments in this disease. The burden of disease needs more formal evaluation, and, above all, professional education must be a priority if genuine early diagnosis of AS is to become a reality.

REFERENCES

1. Lubrano E, Helliwell P, Moreno P et al. The assessment of knowledge in AS patients by a self-administered questionnaire. Br J Rheumatol 1998; 37: 437–41.
2. Suarez-Almazor M, Kendall CJ, Dorgan M. Surfing the net – information on the world wide web for persons with arthritis: patient empowerment or patient deceit? J Rheumatol 2001; 28: 185–191.
3. Kidd BL, Cawley MID. Delay in diagnosis of spondarthritis, Br J Rheumatol 1988; 27: 230–232.
4. Feldtkeller E, Bruckel J, Khan MA. Scientific contributions of ankylosing spondylitis patient advocacy groups. Curr Opin Rheumatol 2000; 12: 239–247.
5. Wynn Parry CB. Physical measures of rehabilitation. In: Moll JMH, ed. Ankylosing spondylitis. Edinburgh: Churchill Livingstone; 1980: 214–226.
6. Kraag G, Stokes B, Groh J et al. The effects of comprehensive home physiotherapy and supervision on patients with ankylosing spondylitis – a randomised controlled trial. J Rheumatol 1990; 17: 228–233.
7. Ormos G, Domjan L, Balint G. A controlled trial for assessing the effect of manual therapy on cervical spine mobility. Hung Rheumatol 1987; (suppl): 177–180.
8. Tishier M, Brotovski Y, Yaron M. Effect of spa therapy on patients with ankylosing spondylitis. Clin Rheumatol 1995; 14: 21–25.
9. Gemignani G, Olivieri I, Rujo G, Pasero G. Transcutaneous elecrical nerve stimulation in ankylosing spondylitis: a double-blind study. Arthritis Rheum 1991; 34: 788–789.
10. Fisher LR, Cawley MID, Holgate ST. Relation between chest expansion, pulmonary function, and exercise tolerance in patients with ankylosing spondylitis. Ann Rheum Dis 1990; 49: 921–925.
11. Hidding A, van der Linden S, Gielen X et al. Continuation of group physical therapy is necessary in ankylosing spondylitis. Arthritis Care Res 1994; 7: 90–96.
12. Russell P, Unsworth A, Haslock I. The effect of exercise on ankylosing spondylitis: a preliminary study. Br J Rheumatol 1993; 32: 498–506.
13. Kraag G, Stokes B, Groh J et al. The effects of comprehensive home physiotherapy and supervision on patients with ankylosing spondylitis – an 8-month follow up. J Rheumatol 1994; 21: 261–263.
14. Bulstrode SJ, Barefoot J, Harrison RA, Clarke AK. The role of passive stretching in the treatment of ankylosing spondylitis. Br J Rheumatol 1987; 26: 40–42.
15. Rassmussen JO, Hansen TM. Physical training for patients with ankylosing spondylitis. Arthritis Care Res 1989; 2: 25–27.
16. Roberts WN, Larson MG, Liang MH et al. Sensitivity of anthropometric techniques for clinical trials in ankylosing spondylitis. Br J Rheumatol 1989; 28: 40–45.
17. Vitanen JV, Lehtinen K, Suni J, Kantiainen H. Fifteen months follow-up of intensive in-patient physiotherapy and exercise in ankylosing spondylitis. Clin Rheumatol 1995; 14: 413–419.
18. Buckelew SP, Parker JC. Coping with arthritis pain. Arthritis Care Res 1989; 2: 136–145.
19. Wordsworth BP, Mowat AG. A review of 100 patients with ankylosing spondylitis with particular reference to socio-economic effects. Br J Rheumatol 1986; 25: 175–180.
20. Pal B. Use of simple analgesics in the treatment of ankylosing spondylitis. Br J Rheumatol 1987; 26: 207–209.
21. O'Brien BJ, Elswood J, Calin A. Perception of prescription drug risks: a survey of patients with ankylosing spondylitis. J Rheumatol 1990; 17: 503–507.
22. Calin A, Elswood J. A prospective nationwide cross-sectional study of NSAID usage in 1331 patients with ankylosing spondylitis. J Rheumatol 1990; 17: 801–803.
23. Henry D, Lim LL-Y, Rodriguez LAG et al. Variability in risk of gastrointestinal complications with individual non-steroidal anti-inflammatory drugs: results of a collaborative meta-analysis. BMJ 1996; 312: 1563–1566.
24. Cox NL, Doherty SM. Non-steroidal anti-inflammatories: out-patient audit of patient preferences and side-effects in different diseases. In: Rainsford KD, Velo GP, eds. Side effects of anti-inflammatory drugs. Part 1: Clinical and epidemiological aspects. Lancaster: MTP Press; 1987: 137–150.
25. Dougados M, Behier JM, Jolchine et al. Efficacy of Celecoxib, a COX-2 specific inhibitor, in ankylosing spondylitis: a placebo and conventional NSAID controlled study. Arthritis Rheum 2001; 44: 180–185.
26. Dougados M, Gueguen A, Nakache J-P et al. Ankylosing spondylitis: what is the optimum duration of a clinical study? A one year versus a 6 weeks non-steroidal anti-inflammatory drug trial. Rheumatology 1999; 38: 235–244.

27. Boersma JW. Retardation of ossification of the lumbar vertebral column in ankylosing spondylitis by means of phenylbutazone. Scand J Rheumatol 1976; 5: 60–64.

28. Lehtinen R. Clinical and radiological features of ankylosing spondylitis in the 1950s and 1976 in the same hospital. Scand J Rheumatol 1979; 8: 57–61.

29. Saraux A, Guedes C, Allain J et al. Prevalence of rheumatoid arthritis and spondyloarthropathy in Brittany, France. J Rheumatol 1999; 26: 22–27.

30. Alonso J C, Soriano A, Rubio C et al. Technetium-99m-HMPAO-labeled leukocyte imaging in patients with seronegative spondylarthropathies. J Nucl Med Technol 1999; 27: 204–206.

31. Moll JMH, Haslock I, Macrae IF, Wright V. Associations between ankylosing spondylitis, psoriatic arthritis, Reiter's disease, the intestinal arthropathies and Behçet's syndrome. Medicine (Baltimore) 1974; 53: 343–364.

32. Mielants H, Veys EM, de Vos M, Cuvelier C. Gut inflammation in the pathogenesis of idiopathic forms of reactive arthritis and in the peripheral joint involvement of ankylosing spondylitis. In: Spondyloarthropathies: involvement of the gut. Mielants H, Veys EM, eds Amsterdam: Excerpta Medica; 1989: 11–12.

33. Ferraz MB, Tugwell P, Goldsmith CH, Atra E. Meta-analysis of sulfasalazine and ankylosing spondylitis. J Rheumatol 1990; 17: 1482–1486.

34. Clegg DO, Reda D J, Abdellatif M. Comparison of sulfasalazine and placebo for the treament of axial and peripheral articular manifestations of the seronegative spondylarthropathies: a Department of Veterans Affairs cooperative study. Arthritis Rheum 1999; 42: 2325–2329.

35. McConkey B. Sulphasalazine and ankylosing spondylitis. Br J Rheumatol 1990; 29: 2–5.

36. Creemers MCW, Franssen MJAM, van der Putte LBA et al. Methotrexate in severe ankylosing spondylitis: an open study. J Rheumatol 1995; 22: 1104–1107.

37. Sadowska-Wroblewska M, Garwolinska H, Maczynska-Rusiniak B. A trial of cyclophosphamide in ankylosing spondylitis with involvement of peripheral joints and high disease activity. Scand J Rheumatol 1986; 15: 259–264.

38. Maksymowych WP, Jhangri GS, Leclercq S et al. An open study of pamidronate in the treatment of refractory ankylosing spondylitis. J Rheumatol 1998; 25: 714–717.

39. Breban M, Gombert B, Amor B, Dougados M. Efficacy of thalidomide in the treatment of refractory ankylosing spondylitis. Arthritis Rheum 1999; 42: 580–581.

40. Gorman J D, Sack K E, Davis J C. Etanercept in the treatment of ankylosing spondylitis: a randomised double-blind placebo-controlled study. Arthritis Rheum 2000; 43(suppl): Abstract 2020.

41. Brandt J, Haibel H, Thriene W et al. Quality of life improvement in patients with severe ankylosing spondylitis upon treatment with anti-TNF-α. Arthritis Rheum 2000; 43(suppl): Abstract 2001.

42. Van den Bosch P, Kruithof E, Baeten D et al. Effects of a loading dose regimen of three infusions of chimeric monoclonal antibody to tumour necrosis factor α (infliximab) in spondyloarthropathy: an open pilot study. Ann Rheum Dis 2000; 59: 428–433.

43. Kruithof E, Van den Bosch F, Baeten D et al. TNF-α blockade with infliximab in patients with active spondyloarthropathy: follow up of one year maintenance regimen. J Rheumatol 2001; 28(suppl 63): Abstract T88.

44. Marzo-Ortega H, McGonagle D, O'Connor P et al. A clinical and MRI assessment of the efficacy of the recombinant TNF alpha receptions: Fc fusion protein etancercept in the treatment of resistant spondyloarthropathy. Arthritis Rheum 2000; 43(suppl): Abstract 209.

45. Stone M, Salonen D, Lax M et al. Clinical and imaging correlates of response to treatment with infliximab in patients with ankylosing spondylitis. J Rheumatol 2001; 28: 1605–1614.

46. Brandt J, Haibel H, Cornely D et al. Successful treatment of active ankylosing spondylitis with the anti-tumour necrosis factor α monoclonal antibody infliximab. Arthritis Rheum 2000; 43: 1346–1352.

47. Braun J, Sieper J. Anti-TNF-α: a new dimension in the pharmacotherapy of the spondyloarthropathies? Ann Rheum Dis 2000; 59: 404–406.

48. Amor B, Silva-Santos R, Nahal R et al. Predictive factors of the long term outcome of spondylarthopathies. J Rheumatol 1994; 21: 1883–1887.

49. Wordsworth BP, Pearcy MJ, Mowat AG. In-patient regime for the treatment of ankylosing spondylitis: an appraisal of improvement in spinal mobility and the effects of corticotrophin. Br J Rheumatol 1984; 23: 39–43.

50. Peters N D, Ejstrup L. Intravenous methylprednisolone pulse therapy in ankylosing spondylitis. Scand J Rheumatol 1992; 21: 134–138.

51. Court-Brown WM, Doll R. Mortality from cancer and other causes after radiotherapy for ankylosing spondylitis. BMJ 1965; ii: 1327–1332.

52. Gibson T. Is there a place for corticosteroid injection in the management of Achilles tendon lesions? Br J Rheumatol 1991; 30: 436.

53. Grill V, Smith M, Ahern M, Littlejohn G. Local radiotherapy for pedal manifestations of 2 HLA B27 related arthopathies. Br J Rheumatol 1988; 27: 390–392.

54. Will R, Palmer R, Bhalla A et al.et al. Osteoporosis in early ankylosing spondylitis: a primary pathological event? Lancet 1989; ii: 1483–1485.

55. Marhoffer W, Stracke H, Masoud I et al. Evidence of impaired cartilage/bone turnover in patients with active ankylosing spondylitis. Ann Rheum Dis 1995; 54: 556–559.

56. Gratacos J, Collado A, Pons F et al. Significant loss of bone mass in patients with early, active ankylosing spondylitis. Arthritis Rheum 1999; 42: 2319–2324.

57. Bronson WD, Walker SD, Hillman LS et al. Bone mineral density and biochemical markers of bone metabolism in ankylosing spondylitis. J Rheumatol 1998; 25: 929–935.

58. Roux C, Abitbol V, Chaussade S et al. Bone loss in patients with inflammatory bowel disease: a prospective study. Osteoporos Int 1995; 5: 156–160.

59. Dougados M, Berenbaum F, Maetzel A, Amor B. The use of sulfasalazine for the prevention of attacks of acute anterior uveitis associated with spondylarthropathy. Rev Rheum (Engl Ed) 1993; 60: 80–82.

60. Reiff A, Takei S, Sadeglic S et al. Etanercept therapy in children with treatment-resistant uveitis. Arthritis Rheum 2001; 44: 1411–1415.

61. Smith JR, Levinson RD, Holland GN et al. Differential efficacy of tumor necrosis factor inhibition in the management of inflammatory eye disease and associated rheumatic disease. Arthritis Care Res 2001; 45: 252–257.

62. Pato E, Banares A, Jover JA et al. Underdiagnosis of spondyloarthropathy in patients presenting with anterior uveitis. J Rheumatol 2000; 27: 2198–2202.

63. Ostensen M, Husby G. Ankylosing spondylitis and pregnancy. Rheum Dis Clin N Am 1989; 15: 241–254.

64. Ostensen M, Ostensen H. Ankylosing spondylitis; the female aspect. J Rheumatol 1998; 25: 120–124.

65. Somerville RW, Hawkey CJ. Non-steroidal anti-inflammatory drugs and the gastrointestinal tract. Postgrad Med J 1986; 62: 23–28.

66. Dunn N, Preston B, Lloyd Jones K. Unexplained acute backache in longstanding ankylosing spondylitis. BMJ 1985; 291: 1632–1634.

67. Calin A, Elswood J. The outcome of 138 total hip replacements and 12 revisions in ankylosing spondylitis: high success rate after a mean follow-up of 7.5 years. J Rheumatol 1989; 16: 955–958.

68. Ruof J, Stucki G. Validity aspects of erythrocyte sedimentation rate and C-reactive protein in ankylosing spondylitis: a literature review. J Rheumatol 1999; 26: 966–970.

69. Macrea IF, Wright V. Measurement of back movement. Ann Rheum Dis 1969; 28: 584–593.

70. Moll JMH, Wright V. The pattern of chest and spinal mobility in ankylosing spondylitis. Rheumatol Rehab 1973; 12: 115–134.

71. Moll JMH, Wright V. An objective study of chest expansion. Ann Rheum Dis 1972; 31: 1–8.

72. Dunham WF. Ankylosing spondylitis: measurement of hip and spinal movements. Br J Phys Med 1949; 12: 126–129.

73. Domjan L, Balint G. A new goniometer for measuring spinal and peripheral joint mobility. Hung Rheumatol 1987; 71–76.

74. Pile RD, Laurent MR, Salmond CE et al. Clinical assessment of ankylosing spondylitis: a study of observer variation in spinal measurements. Br J Rheumatol 1991; 17: 29–34.

75. Mander N, Simpson JN, McLellan A et al. Studies with an enthesis index as a method of clinical assessment in ankylosing spondylitis. Ann Rheum Dis 1987; 46: 197–202.

76. van der Heijde D, van der Linden S, Dougados M, Bellamy N, Russel AS, Edmonds J. Ankylosing spondylitis: plenary discussion and results of voting on selection of domains and some specific instruments. J Rheumatol 1999; 26: 997–1002.

77. Rudge SR, Swannel AJ, Rose DH, Todd JH. The clinical assessment of sacro-iliac joint involvement in ankylosing spondylitis. Rheumatol Rehab 1982; 21: 15–20.

78. Oostveen J, Prevo R, den Boer J, van de Laar M. Early detection of sacroiliitis on magnetic resonance imaging and subsequent development of sacroiliitis on plain radiography. A prospective, longitudinal study. J Rheumatol 1999; 26: 1953–1958.

79. Dawes P. Stoke Ankylosing Spondylitis Spine Score. J Rheumatol 1999; 26: 993–996.

80. Calin A, Mackay K, Santos H, Brophy S. A new dimension to outcome: application of the Bath Ankylosing Spondylitis Radiology Index. J Rheumatol 1999; 26: 988–992.

81. Spoorenberg A, de Vlam K, van der Heijde D et al. Radiological scoring methods in ankylosing spondylitis: reliability and sensitivity to change over one year. J Rheumatol 1999; 26: 997–1002.

82. Daltroy LH, Larson MG, Roberts WN, Liang MH. A modification of the Health Assessment Questionnaire for the spondyloarthropathies. J Rheumatol 1990; 17: 946–950.

83. Dougados M, Gueguen A, Nakache J-P et al. Evaluation of a functional index and an articular index in ankylosing spondylitis. J Rheumatol 1988; 15: 302–307.

84. Calin A. The individual with ankylosing spondylitis: defining disease status and the impact of the illness. Br J Rheumatol 1995; 34: 663–672.

85. Ruof J, Sangha O, Stucki G. Comparative responsiveness of 3 functional indices in ankylosing spondylitis. J Rheumatol 1999; 26: 1959–1633.

86. Ward MM, Kuzis S. Validity and sensitivity to change of spondylitis-specific measures of functional disability. J Rheumatol 1999; 26: 121–127.

87. Ruof J, Stucki G. Comparision of the Dougados Functional Index and the Bath Ankylosing Spondylitis Functional Index. A literature review. J Rheumatol 1999; 26: 955–960.

88. Spoorenberg A, van der Heijde D, de Klerk E et al. A comparative study of the usefulness of the Bath Ankylosing Spondylitis Functional Index and the Dougados Functional Index in the assessment of ankylosing sponylitis. J Rheumatol 1999; 26: 961–965.

89. Ortiz Z, Shea B, Dieguez M G et al. The responsiveness of generic quality of life instruments in rheumatic diseases. A systematic review of randomized controlled trials. J Rheumatol 1999; 26: 210–216.

30 Reactive arthritis: clinical features and treatment

Auli Toivanen

Definition

- A sterile joint inflammation that develops after a distant infection
- The disease is systemic and not limited to the joints
- Triggering infections most commonly originate in the throat, urogenital organs or gastrointestinal tract
- The disease also occurs without obvious preceding infection, e.g. in association with inflammatory bowel disease

Clinical features

- Arthritis, enthesopathy, tendinitis, tenosynovitis, osteitis and muscle pains
- Skin and mucous membrane lesions are frequent
- Eye inflammations, e.g. uveitis and conjunctivitis
- Visceral involvement, such as nephritis or carditis, is relatively rare
- Severity ranges from mild arthralgia to disabling disease
- Spontaneous recovery is common and the prognosis is, in general, good
- Later, many patients suffer arthralgias and recurrences, and some develop ankylosing spondylitis
- Susceptibility to the disease is strongly linked to possession of the HLA-B27 antigen

HISTORICAL BACKGROUND

Reiter's syndrome, frequently considered as the most typical example of reactive arthritis was named after Hans Reiter (1881–1969) who, in 1916, described an officer suffering from a dysenteric illness with arthritis, urethritis and conjunctivitis[1]. Reiter did not actually recognize that the arthritis and conjunctivitis were related to the dysentery, but called the disease 'spirochaetosis arthritica'. However, as early as the 16th century, Pierre van Forest, and in the 17th century, Martinière, had recognized arthritis as a complication of urethritis. The first description of 'reactive arthritis' is attributed to Sir Benjamin Brodie (1783–1862)[2].

At the end of the Second World War, in Finland, Ilmari Paronen observed 344 cases of arthritis in connection with an outbreak of *Shigella* that occurred on the Karelian isthmus[3]. In 1969, Sairanen and coworkers published a follow-up study of 100 of these patients, detailing the prognosis of the disorder[4]. The term 'reactive arthritis' was introduced in 1976 by Aho *et al.*[5], and has gained wide use, even though it does not indicate the systemic character of the disease. The term 'Reiter's syndrome' is still in general use and refers to the triad of arthritis, urethritis and conjunctivitis, with 'incomplete Reiter's syndrome' used to describe conditions in which only two of these features are present. Both complete and incomplete Reiter's syndrome should be considered to be identical with reactive arthritis.

Observations of family clustering were soon confirmed by the finding that reactive arthritis is strongly associated with human leukocyte antigen (HLA)-B27. Great research interest has been focused on reactive arthritis, partly because the information gained may elucidate pathogenetic processes involved in the development of other rheumatic diseases, such as rheumatoid arthritis and ankylosing spondylitis.

EPIDEMIOLOGY

Because the clinical severity of reactive arthritis varies greatly and milder cases apparently go unnoticed, the true incidence of reactive arthritis is hard to assess. Certainly, growing awareness of reactive arthritis as a diagnostic possibility has increased the number of cases recognized. According to a Finnish estimation[6,7], the annual incidence of arthritis after bowel or urogenital infection is 30 per 100 000 adults, to which must be added a proportion of cases of seronegative oligoarthritis, some of which are probably reactive arthritis, the incidence of which is 40/100 000 (Table 30.1). Reactive arthritis apparently affects all populations. Typically, it is a disorder of young adults, rare in small children and in older people; most patients are aged between 20 and 40 years[2,8]. Rheumatic fever, which also can be considered a type of reactive arthritis, occurs often in developing countries, but has practically disappeared elsewhere.

Reactive arthritis affects males and females with the same frequency. Genetic factors play a part in susceptibility to the disease, most patients reporting a family history of a similar disease. Between 65% and 96% of those affected are positive for HLA-B27. Indeed, HLA-B27 is a strong risk factor for developing reactive arthritis[9–12], with the increase in risk as high as 50-fold[5]. However, the association is not absolute: HLA-B27-positive individuals do not always develop reactive arthritis, even after a suitable infection, and the arthritis can occur also in HLA-B27-negative individuals. This is illustrated by observations by van Bohemen *et al.*[13] in connection with an outbreak of bacillary dysentery in The Netherlands: in three families, some but not all HLA-B27-positive members developed reactive arthritis after verified infection. The disease is more severe and the tendency to chronic development is greater in HLA-B27-positive individuals[12,14,15], although HLA-B27-negative individuals can have a chronic or prolonged course of the disease[16].

TABLE 30.1
EPIDEMIOLOGY OF REACTIVE ARTHRITIS

- Most commonly affects young adults
- Equally frequent in males and females
- Annual incidence 30–40/100 000
- Probably worldwide
- Genetic associations
  Family clustering
  Strongly associated with HLA-B27
- Frequency in connection with infection, (e.g. enteric) varies

Recently, it has been suggested that two forms of the disease – HLA-B27 associated and non-associated – should be distinguished[17]. These two forms also are triggered by different infectious agents, as discussed below.

The frequency of reactive arthritis after enteric infections caused by *Salmonella*, *Shigella* and *Campylobacter* has been reported to be 1–4% in unselected populations[18–20]. In some *Yersinia* outbreaks, the frequency of this complication has been quite high and in others negligible[21,22]. The fact that bacteria of the same genus, or species even, vary in their capacity to trigger reactive arthritis is of considerable interest.

CLINICAL FEATURES

Reactive arthritis has generally been defined as sterile synovitis developing after a distant infection. The detection of microbial components, including microbial DNA and RNA in the joints of patients with this disease has led to worldwide reconsideration of the definition. However, at present there are no generally accepted diagnostic criteria available for use by clinicians[23,24].

History

Typically, the first symptoms are of joint discomfort. A careful history may indicate symptoms of enteric or urogenital infection a few days to a couple of weeks previously, and often the patient reports such symptoms in other family members. Sometimes, abdominal pains in the few days before the appearance of joint symptoms may be suspected to be due to acute appendicitis or salpingo-oophoritis; this is especially the case in young adults. They may even have undergone laparotomy, in which case usually only mesenteric lymphadenitis has been found. Yet it is remarkable that patients requiring hospital care for severe enteritis caused by, for example, *Yersinia*, have rarely developed reactive arthritis. A common clinical experience is that the symptoms of the triggering infection have often been mild and, in about 10% of cases, the infection has passed unnoticed[25,26].

Infections most commonly preceding reactive arthritis are those caused by *Salmonella*, *Shigella*, *Yersinia*, *Campylobacter*, *Chlamydia trachomatis* or *C. pneumoniae*, *Borreliae*, *Neisseria* and streptococci. Several viruses have been implicated; those most often mentioned in connection with joint inflammation are rubella, hepatitis and parvovirus. It is apparent that the disease triggered by enteric or urogenital infection is usually HLA-B27-associated, but this is not the case for reactive arthritis caused by several other infectious agents such as *Borrelia*, meningococci, streptococci or viruses[17,27,28]. It is important to note that *Salmonella*, *Borrelia* and *Neisseria* can cause true septic arthritis in addition to reactive arthritis. It is not unusual, however, that a triggering infection cannot be identified, and in these cases the diagnosis remains uncertain. Non-infectious inflammatory bowel diseases may be associated with reactive arthritis[29,30] – for example, after intestinal bypass operation for morbid obesity. It is obvious, however, that in these conditions the intestinal microbial flora or the mucosal defense mechanisms are altered[26]. The same may apply to reactive arthritis occurring after a pseudomembranous colitis associated with overgrowth of *Clostridium difficile*[31].

General symptoms

Reactive arthritis is a systemic disease (Fig. 30.1), although the severity varies greatly. Frequently, general symptoms such as malaise, fatigue and fever are seen.

Joint and musculoskeletal symptoms

The most prominent symptoms are usually those in the joints. They vary from mild arthralgias to severely disabling polyarthritis[2,12,15,25]. Typically, there is asymmetric monoarthritis or oligoarthritis. The weight-bearing joints are most often affected: knees (Fig. 30.2), ankles

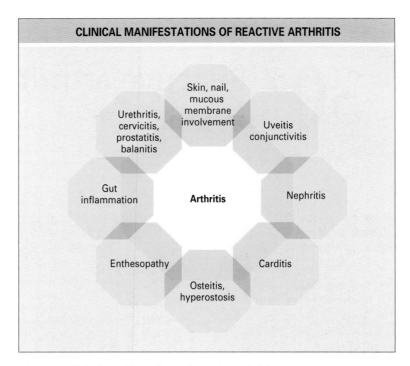

CLINICAL MANIFESTATIONS OF REACTIVE ARTHRITIS

Skin, nail, mucous membrane involvement

Urethritis, cervicitis, prostatitis, balanitis

Uveitis conjunctivitis

Gut inflammation

Arthritis

Nephritis

Enthesopathy

Carditis

Osteitis, hyperostosis

Fig. 30.1 Clinical manifestations of reactive arthritis.

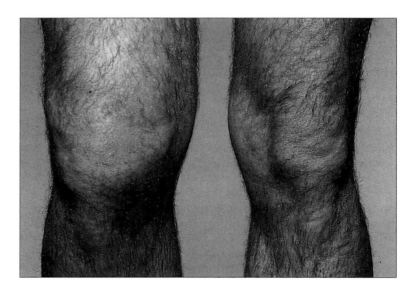

Fig. 30.2 Reactive arthritis of the knee.

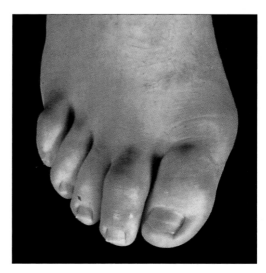

Fig. 30.3 Dactylitis in reactive arthritis.

and hips – but quite commonly other large joints, such as the shoulders, elbows and wrists, and small joints of the hands and feet may also be involved. The inflammation may vary from day to day and shift from one joint to another. The joints involved may be red and warm, and occasionally there is also *erythema nodosum*. Dactylitis is not uncommon (Fig. 30.3), and sometimes the condition may mimic rheumatoid arthritis, with stiffness on inactivity. Especially in the later stages, patients often complain of pains in the sacroiliac region.

A diagnosis cannot be made on the basis of physical examination alone, because the findings vary greatly and may mimic any other disease involving joint inflammation, including gout, rheumatoid arthritis or true purulent arthritis[32].

Reactive arthritis is not limited to the joints: enthesopathies, tenosynovitis, or both, are present in a high proportion of cases. Thus plantar fasciitis, Achilles tendinitis or bursitis of the ankle region often results in difficulties in walking. Pain on palpation is frequent at the sites where tendons attach to bones, and this enthesopathy may also limit movement. In severe cases, muscle wasting may be quite prominent. Unusually severe cases may become bedridden. Rarely, the disease renders the patient quite helpless and disabled. The outcome, however, is not related to the initial severity of the disease.

Skin and mucous membrane symptoms

The skin lesion most commonly attributed to reactive arthritis is *keratoderma blenorrhagicum* (Fig. 30.4), often referred to as '*pustulosis palmoplantaris*'. The lesions are indistinguishable from psoriasis, both clinically and histologically. The same holds for the nail lesions seen in both reactive arthritis and psoriasis. This similarity has not gained wide attention, but may be of interest when the pathogenesis of reactive arthritis and psoriatic arthropathy are considered. *Erythema nodosum*, often seen after *Yersinia* infection, is not common in the course of reactive arthritis and is not associated with HLA-B27.

When reactive arthritis is triggered by urogenital infection such as gonorrhea or chlamydial urethritis, it is called uroarthritis. Sterile urogenital inflammation can also be part of the reactive disease. Thus 'sterile urethritis' has been tacitly included in the triad classically recognized as Reiter's syndrome. Circinate balanitis (Fig. 30.5), which is also psoriatic in nature, and cystitis and prostatitis may be present, and can sometimes lead to complications such as shrinking of the bladder. Further, it seems that pelvic inflammatory disease, including salpingitis, may arise in women with reactive arthritis[33]. Inflammation of the urogenital tract has a tendency to relapse.

Various lesions are seen in the mouth. Wright and Moll[2] describe these as painless shiny patches, occurring on the palate, tongue and

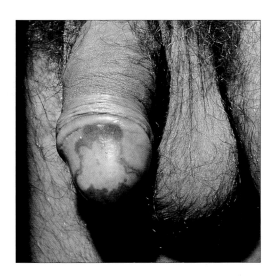

Fig. 30.5 Circinate balanitis in a man with reactive arthritis. (Courtesy of Professor VK Havu, Department of Dermatology, University of Turku.)

mucosa of the cheeks and lips. Erythema of the soft palate, uvula and tonsillar region has been described occasionally.

Gastrointestinal symptoms

Enteric infections or inflammatory diseases can, like urogenital infections, be the etiologic triggering event. It has become apparent that, as in the urogenital system, the epithelium of the intestine may form part of the reactive disease itself. Patients may complain of occasional abdominal pains and diarrhea, but at this stage no pathogens can be isolated from stool cultures. When ileocolonoscopy has been carried out in patients with established reactive arthritis, either macroscopically or microscopically detectable lesions resembling ulcerative colitis or Crohn's disease have been seen[29,30].

Ocular lesions

Inflammatory eye lesions form a classic part of the clinical picture. They may be either unilateral or bilateral. Conjunctivitis with sterile discharge is frequently seen. It usually subsides, but may progress to produce episcleritis, keratitis or even corneal ulcerations[2]. Acute uveitis, especially anterior uveitis (iritis), is also common. The ocular lesions may be the only or the first manifestation of reactive arthritis. They have a strong tendency to recur. Patients with reactive iritis most commonly complain of redness, photophobia and pain, and some have diminution of vision and increased lacrimation[34]. In patients with ocular complaints, it is advisable to undertake careful ophthalmologic examination, because if ocular lesions are left undiagnosed and untreated, permanent damage to the vision may follow.

Other systemic manifestations

Carditis is classically associated with rheumatic fever, and in developing countries valvular disease as a late sequel is a major problem. In reactive arthritides seen after enteric or urogenital infections, cardiac involvement is not as prominent. With increasing awareness it has become apparent, however, that conduction disturbances, even requiring pacemaker treatment, may occur[2,12].

Mild renal and urinary pathology, such as proteinuria, microhematuria and aseptic pyuria, are seen in about 50% of patients with reactive arthritis. Severe glomerulonephritis and IgA nephropathy are rare and hardly ever lead to permanently impaired renal function.

INVESTIGATIONS

In most cases of reactive arthritis, the patient seeks medical help for joint symptoms or for eye inflammation. The history and findings at the physical examination may immediately suggest the diagnosis, but confirmation requires laboratory and radiologic investigations (Table 30.2).

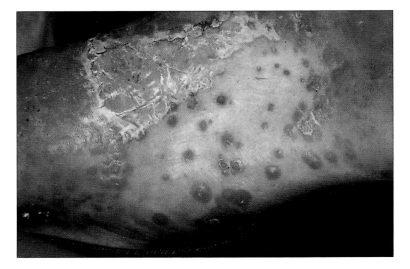

Fig. 30.4 Skin lesions (keratoderma blenorrhagicum) in reactive arthritis.

TABLE 30.2 INVESTIGATION OF REACTIVE ARTHRITIS
• ESR
• C-Reactive protein
• Blood cell count
• Liver function tests, e.g. ALT, AST, GGT
• Kidney function tests, e.g. serum creatinine or blood urea nitrogen
• Rheumatoid factor tests
• Urine analysis
• Electrocardiogram
• Joint fluid sample with analysis of:
Cell count
Exclusion of crystals
Gram stain
Bacterial culture
• Bacterial culture of:
Feces
Urine or urethral swab
Cervical sample
Throat
• Blood culture (not always necessary)
• Antibody determination at admission
• HLA-B27 antigen (or HLA typing) after 2–4 weeks
• Radiograph of affected joints
• Ophthalmologic examination if eye symptoms present

ALT, serum alanine-aminotransferase; ESR, erythrocyte sedimentation rate; GGT, serum gamma glutamyltransferase.

Laboratory investigations

The erythrocyte sedimentation rate is markedly increased in most cases of acute reactive arthritis, and values exceeding 60mm/h are commonly seen. The C-reactive protein is similarly increased at the onset of the disease. At a later stage, patients with chronic symptoms nevertheless have normal erythrocyte sedimentation rate and C-reactive protein values. The blood cell count may reveal moderate leukocytosis and mild anemia.

Urine analysis should be carried out at diagnosis and should be repeated during the follow-up, in order to detect possible aseptic pyuria resulting from urethritis. It is advisable to check renal function, for example by serum creatinine or blood urea nitrogen tests, and liver function by serum alanine aminotransferase or serum gamma glutamyltransferase. Tests for rheumatoid factor are usually negative.

Electrocardiography should be performed and repeated in patients who have a prolonged disease course, to exclude possible conduction disturbances. When endocarditis is suspected, especially in cases of rheumatic fever, it is essential also to assess cardiac function by echocardiography.

Joint fluid should always be aspirated when possible. Gram stain and bacterial culture should be performed to exclude septic arthritis[32]. In reactive arthritis, bacteria are not demonstrable either by staining or even extensive culturing. Microbial components have been detected, however, in the synovial membrane or in synovial fluid, by the use of special techniques not suitable for routine clinical work; these include immunofluorescence, immunoelectronmicroscopy, immunoblotting and polymerase chain reaction (PCR) techniques. In the early stages of reactive arthritis, the cell count in the synovial fluid can be quite high, and polymorphonuclear leukocytes can dominate the picture[32,35]. Later, lymphocytosis can develop. Demonstrations of specific antibodies in the synovial fluid, and of synovial mononuclear cells specifically responding to an infectious agent may be of diagnostic significance. However, these methods require elaborate techniques not available in most hospitals. Microscopy under polarized light should be performed, to exclude gout or pseudogout. Blood culture is not routinely necessary, but should be undertaken if joint infection is suspected.

Microbiologic and serologic studies form a cornerstone of diagnosis. Every effort should be made to isolate the causative microorganism from the throat, feces or urogenital tract. For detection of *Chlamydia*, application of PCR to first voided urine samples is a practical method. Isolation of *Yersinia* requires special methods, and it is easily missed in routine fecal culture. In most cases, however, results are negative, which emphasizes the role of serology. The serologic tests to be considered include antibody assays against *Salmonella*, *Yersinia*, *Campylobacter*, *Chlamydia*, *Neisseria gonorrhoeae*, *Borrelia burgdorferi* and β-hemolytic streptococci. Increase in and persistence of IgA class antibodies are especially characteristic, and these antibodies are not reliably detected by bacterial agglutination[36].

Depending on the infection history of the patient, antibodies against various viruses may yield a specific diagnosis.

It should be stressed that the list of microorganisms triggering reactive arthritis is steadily growing, and it is assumed that more remain to be identified. Thus negative serology does not rule out a diagnosis of reactive arthritis; furthermore, in some patients the antibodies increase slowly and yield a positive result only a few weeks after the onset of disease.

Detection of the HLA-B27 antigen is helpful in the diagnosis and in considering the treatment and follow-up of the patient. As noted before, however, the disease may also occur, and even have a chronic course, in HLA-B27-negative individuals.

Radiography and other imaging

Radiographic studies of symptomatic joints should be undertaken not so much to confirm the diagnosis of reactive arthritis as to rule out erosive disease, for example rheumatoid arthritis. The findings in reactive arthritis are usually rather scant, such as juxta-articular osteoporosis and soft tissue swelling. In patients with recurrent and chronic disease, erosions may be observed. More often, periosteal reaction and proliferation, especially at the insertion sites of tendons, are seen. Thus plantar spurs are a common sign in chronic cases. Magnetic resonance imaging has proved useful for the detection of joint effusion, enthesitis and tendinitis, but the benefit for routine clinical practice is small.

Chronic or recurring reactive arthritis also often leads to sacroiliitis and spondylitis that may be radiographically indistinguishable from ankylosing spondylitis, which is more easily detected by magnetic resonance imaging.

Radionuclide scintigraphy is a sensitive technique for demonstrating inflammation and is superior to radiography, especially in cases of enthesopathy, periostitis or early sacroiliitis[2,37].

Other investigations

Synovial biopsy is not of diagnostic value, as the inflammation is nonspecific. On occasion, exclusion of alternative diagnoses such as pigmented villonodular synovitis or tuberculous arthritis may be valuable.

In patients with reactive arthritis, inflammatory bowel disease (ulcerative colitis or Crohn's disease) may be a background factor. Ileocolonoscopy has revealed that, in many patients, either macroscopic or microscopic lesions of these conditions are present, in the absence of subjective symptoms[29,30]. Scintigraphy using radiolabeled leukocytes is used to search for inflammatory sites in the bowel area, especially in the terminal ileum. Neither this procedure nor endoscopy or radiographic investigation of the colon are routinely recommended.

In those with eye symptoms, it is advisable to refer the patient to an ophthalmologist, because uveitis requires rapid diagnosis for prompt and correct treatment. Without a slit-lamp examination, the uveitis may remain undiagnosed and result in permanent damage to the vision.

DIFFERENTIAL DIAGNOSIS

The most important question at presentation is whether the patient has reactive arthritis or true septic infection of the joint[32]. This may be extremely difficult to resolve, but it is especially crucial to do so in children, in whom a purulent arthritis may rapidly lead to destruction of the joint. Therefore it is advisable to proceed with blind antimicrobial treatment on the basis of a presumptive diagnosis of septic arthritis in uncertain cases. Joint inflammation may be sufficiently intense to produce redness reminiscent of erysipelas.

Gout or pseudogout may present with symptoms and findings similar to those of reactive arthritis, but careful history taking, analysis of crystals in the joint fluid and serum urate determination clarify the situation in most instances.

Rheumatoid arthritis, psoraitic arthritis and ankylosing spondylitis can often only be differentiated from reactive arthritis on prolonged follow-up.

ETIOLOGY

There is no disagreement that infection is central to the etiology of reactive arthritis. A previously healthy but genetically predisposed individual contracts a suitable triggering infection and, after some time, reactive arthritis develops. This pathogenetic process spans the incubation time of the triggering infection and its clinically overt phase, and thereafter a few days to a couple of weeks until the full-blown reactive arthritis[17]. With increasing awareness of this condition, the list of the causative agents is still growing. Although efforts have been made to characterize the microorganisms linked to reactive arthritis, no common or definite feature has so far emerged. Many of the bacteria implicated are Gram-negative, have cell membranes that contain lipopolysaccharide and peptidoglycan, and are intracellularly invasive – that is, able to enter cells and to survive (and even multiply) intracellularly[38]. Many are quite common in the environment, and infection does not necessarily lead to reactive arthritis. In most instances, the triggering infection affects the throat, the intestine or the urogenital tract. Therefore it appears that mucosal immune defense mechanisms must be of importance – but how and why are not known[39]. The frequency of reactive arthritis with outbreaks of *Yersinia*, *Salmonella* and *Shigella* varies quite considerably. The fact that several different microbes lead to a similar clinical entity demonstrates that the classical Koch postulates do not apply in this instance.

The available evidence implies that some features of a microbe are important for its arthritogenicity[13,38,39].

PATHOGENESIS

The pathogenesis of reactive arthritis is interesting not only in itself but also, given the time course, as a putative model of other inflammatory diseases of the joints and connective tissue. By contrast, rheumatoid arthritis and ankylosing spondylitis develop slowly, and when the diagnosis can be established with the accuracy necessary for research work, several months and even years have lapsed. At such a late stage, it is difficult to gain information on the early triggering or pathogenetic events. Reactive arthritis has a sudden onset, within days or a few weeks of the triggering infection, which often can be identified, and thus studies on its pathogenesis are possible. The joint inflammation develops some time after the actual triggering infection and it is apparent that immunologic defense mechanisms have a central role. Much new information has been gained, and several groups are working on the pathogenesis.

Role of HLA-B27

An important factor associated with the susceptibility to reactive arthritis is the HLA-B27 antigen. Although not all HLA-B27-positive individuals develop reactive arthritis after a suitable triggering infection, and some B27-negative individuals may do so, this tissue antigen indisputably has an important role. For more than two decades, extensive efforts have been devoted by several groups to clarify the mechanisms behind this association. The different HLA-B27 loci have been character-

ized in minute detail and the peptides bound by this structure have been analysed. Yet it remains unknown how HLA-B27 works in the pathogenetic process.

A theory that has gained wide attention is that of molecular mimicry – that is, 'trigger' microorganisms share a structure with the HLA-B27 molecule[40]. Sequencing of genes for HLA-B27 and microbial antigens has further made it possible to carry out comparisons at the nucleotide and amino acid levels. Indeed, molecular mimicry in the form of amino acid homology has been observed between HLA-B27 and microbial antigens[41]; however, this apparently is not restricted to disease-associated microorganisms. Work using synthetic peptides and their capacity to generate a response by either B or T cells has raised suspicions about the biological importance of this homology. Therefore the role of molecular mimicry in the pathogenesis of reactive arthritis or ankylosing spondylitis needs critical re-evaluation[38,42].

Recently, mouse and rat strains carrying a transgene for HLA-B27 have been developed. These may help to elucidate the role of HLA-B27 in the pathogenesis of reactive arthritis and ankylosing spondylitis.

Immune response

In studies of the immune reaction against the triggering microorganisms, several interesting findings have been obtained. As an example, the results for *Yersinia*-triggered reactive arthritis are presented in Table 30.3.

In follow-up studies, the immune responses of patients developing reactive arthritis have been compared with those recovering without postinfectious complications[12,36]. The most characteristic feature of patients with reactive arthritis is a strong and persisting IgA antibody response. With time, the antibodies increase in avidity, indicating a maturation of the response. Considering the short half-life of IgA, this indicates prolonged antigenic stimulation. The observation that the antibodies recognize a multitude of antigenic epitopes of *Yersinia* suggests that the driving force might be either whole microbes or large components of them.

The T cell responses against *Yersinia* antigens are weak in peripheral blood samples of patients with reactive arthritis, compared with those of persons who do not develop postinfectious complications[36]. However, at the synovial level, a strong but relatively non-specific response of T cells is seen[43]. It seems that T cells with slightly different specificities can be cloned from the synovial fluid, indicating that local stimulation may play a part[44–46].

Yersinia infection always causes formation of immune complexes. Such complexes composed of *Yersinia* antigen and specific antibody have been demonstrated in the blood and synovial fluid of patients with reactive arthritis[47].

All these observations suggest that, in patients with reactive arthritis, the microorganism may persist somewhere in the body, for example in

---

TABLE 30.3
IMMUNE RESPONSE IN YERSINIA-TRIGGERED REACTIVE ARTHRITIS

- Initially, weak IgM-class antibody production
- Later, strong and persisting IgG and especially IgA antibody production
- IgA antibodies increase in avidity with time
- Antibodies are directed against several antigenic epitopes of Yersinia
- Non-specific immune complexes are always found in serum
- Specific immune complexes containing Yersinia and anti-Yersinia antibody may be found in serum and in synovial fluid
- Peripheral blood T cells show weak response to Yersinia
- T cells in the synovial fluid show vigorous but somewhat non-specific response to Yersinia (or other arthritis-triggering microorganism)

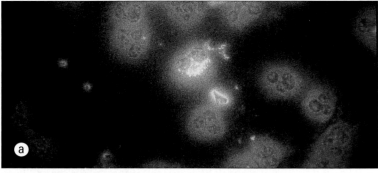
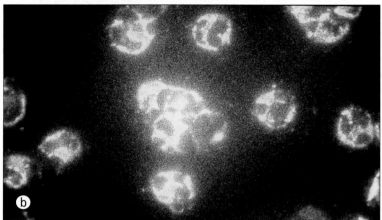

Fig. 30.6 Microbial material in synovial fluid cells. (a) In a patient with *Yersinia*-triggered reactive arthritis. (b) In a patient with chronic *Yersinia*-triggered reactive arthritis. There is positive immunofluorescence staining by an antiserum obtained by immunizing a rabbit with live *Yersinia*. Most of the cells are polymorphonuclear granulocytes and, in the chronic case, nearly all are strongly positive. (Granfors K *et al. Yersinia* antigens in synovial-fluid cells from patients with reactive arthritis. N Engl J Med 1989; 320:216–221. © 1989. With permission of Massachusetts Medical Society. All rights reserved.)

the intestinal mucosa or in the mesenteric lymph nodes. Furthermore, microbial components might actually enter the site of inflammation itself – that is, the synovium or the synovial fluid. Using immuno-fluorescence (Fig. 30.6) and immunoblotting techniques, in addition to immunoelectronmicroscopy, positive reactions have been obtained in reactive arthritis triggered by *Chlamydia*, *Salmonella*, *Yersinia* and *Shigella*[48–54]. Moreover, PCR methodology has resulted in positive demonstration of chlamydia DNA and RNA in the synovial fluid of patients with reactive arthritis[55–57]. It must be stressed, however, that viable organisms have not been isolated, in spite of extensive efforts.

Currently it seems, therefore, that reactive arthritis involves persistence of the triggering microorganism in the host, and the spread of its components either as parts of immune complexes or within phago-cytosing cells into the joints, where they activate the inflammatory cascade[58–61].

MANAGEMENT

Acute reactive arthritis

There are some general considerations in the management of reactive arthritis. First, the disease most commonly affects previously healthy, young adults. Secondly, the severity of the disease varies from mild arthralgias to a severe arthritis, and hence treatment has to be adjusted accordingly[62,63]. The patient may be afraid of having a chronic, progressively destructive disease. Correct information is the cornerstone of the treatment, to relieve unnecessary anxiety and to achieve the patient's compliance with suggested treatments.

TABLE 30.4
TREATMENT OF ACUTE REACTIVE ARTHRITIS
• Antibiotics if infection is still present • Rest • Non-steroidal anti-inflammatory drugs • Intra-articular corticosteroids • Systemic corticosteroids • Rarely, disease modifying antirheumatic drugs

Obviously, suitable rest is advisable. Even within a few weeks after recovery, the patient should not use the joints too vigorously, as non-specific factors and minor traumas may lead to recurrences. When several joints are affected, muscle wasting may occur unless physiotherapy is given.

Non-steroidal anti-inflammatory drugs (NSAIDs) form the basis of treatment (Table 30.4). They should be used regularly over some time in order to achieve maximum anti-inflammatory effect, and patients should be informed of this, otherwise they consider the drug as an analgesic. During recovery, insufficient analgesia may lead to limited use of the joints and actually prolong the rehabilitation. There is no definite drug of choice, because patients' responses differ (see Chapter 10). In the case of enthesopathies, locally applied NSAID ointments may be useful.

Corticosteroids are a valuable asset in the treatment of reactive arthritis. In many cases, intra-articular administration gives prompt relief. However, septic arthritis must be excluded before the injection. Systemic treatment with corticosteroids has also proved effective. They should be used in patients in whom NSAIDs have not had a sufficient effect and in whom many joints are affected. The treatment can be started with a relatively high dose, 30–50mg daily of prednisolone or its equivalent, tapering down according to the improvement. Oral corticosteroids should be withdrawn slowly, but with NSAIDs continuing. Corticosteroids should not be used for more than 2–4 months (see Chapter 11).

Antibiotic treatment

As persistence of the triggering microbe and presence of microbial components at the sites of inflammation have been demonstrated, the role of antibiotic treatment has become a central question. Many physicians do indeed give the patients with reactive arthritis at least a short course of antibiotics. However, there is no clinical evidence supporting this practice.

Antibiotic treatment should be given if a microbe is isolated. This is more to diminish spread of the infection than to influence the continuing course of the disease. In two instances antibiotics have been proven to be useful. In rheumatic fever they are used for primary or secondary prevention. However, they do not have a role in the treatment of the rheumatic fever itself. The treatment of borreliosis to minimize the impact of Lyme disease is discussed in Chapter 27. Clinical and experimental data exist to indicate that, if antibacterial treatment of reactive arthritis can be started very early during the pathogenetic process, the disease can be prevented or the prognosis improved. However, it is obvious that, at the time of the first joint symptoms – which is when the patient usually comes to the physician – the pathogenic process is probably not reversible. All available clinical evidence indicates that, in fully developed reactive arthritis, short term antibacterial treatment has no beneficial effect, and overall the results with long-term administration of antibacterial agents are also poor[63–66]. Studies using an experimental model of reactive arthritis in rats have yielded similar results[66,67]. In some instances, sulphasalazine has proven beneficial, probably because of its antirheumatic effect rather than its antibacterial effect. In addition, tetracyclines have sometimes been found to have an effect on reactive arthritis, but, again, this is probably due to their anti-inflammatory action rather than any antibacterial effect[63,66,68].

Cases with chronic symptoms

Recurrences of reactive arthritis are treated in the same way as the acute disease. Chronic arthralgias are a difficult therapeutic problem. With time, the patients often derive less and less benefit from the various NSAIDs, and side effects become more common with prolonged use. Nevertheless, these drugs are the best of the alternatives. Physical therapy may give some patients relief, but does not have a long-term effect. In chronic cases, corticosteroids are not advisable, because their therapeutic effect in this situation is not very good, and the prognosis is in any case good in almost all patients.

As in acute reactive arthritis, in chronic reactive arthritis antibiotics have also not proven useful, even when administered for a 3-month period[66,69]. Sulfasalazine is of interest because of the observation that patients with reactive arthritis often have more or less asymptomatic inflammation of the bowel. However, results regarding the effect of sulphasalazine are somewhat contradictory[70-73]. In some instances, it may give good results. The drug should be started at low dose, increasing to 2g/day, or even 3g/day if tolerated by the patient. Unfortunately, some patients cannot continue with the drug because of gastrointestinal intolerance.

When the symptoms of chronic reactive arthritis resemble rheumatoid arthritis, classic antirheumatic treatment, for example gold salts (injected or by mouth), may prove quite useful and lead to rapid improvement. In these patients the treatment can be stopped after some months without the disease relapsing. There have been some reports regarding the use of methotrexate or azathioprine, but the results of controlled trials with a large number of patients are not yet available[63].

Extra-articular disease

Ocular inflammation must be diagnosed and treated promptly, otherwise irreversible damage to eyesight may occur. If possible, the patient should be referred to an ophthalmologist, because the diagnosis of uveitis requires the use of a slit-lamp. Treatment consists of corticosteroids in the form of eye drops or even systemically, and of mydriatics. The patient should be informed about the strong possibility of recurrence.

Excluding the endocarditis of rheumatic fever, the most common cardiac complications are conduction disturbances. In these instances, a cardiac pacemaker may be indicated.

The nephritis that can be associated with reactive arthritis is usually mild, subsides spontaneously and does not require any treatment. Skin lesions, which are considered identical to psoriasis by many dermatologists, are treated accordingly. In mild cases, keratinolytic agents such as salicylic acid ointment or topical corticosteroid may be used. In more severe cases, methotrexate or retinoids are often beneficial.

PROGNOSIS

The prognosis of reactive arthritis is generally good. The duration of an episode varies from a few days to several weeks. Even patients who are severely incapacitated and bedridden can look forwards to full recovery. However, recurrences are frequent, and they can be triggered not only by new infections but also by non-specific stress factors. Urogenital and eye inflammations, particularly, have a tendency to recur. Many patients complain of abdominal discomfort and occasional diarrhea for months and even years after the initial attack of the disease. Back pain and arthralgia are common, and also frank synovitis may be seen. Tendinitis and enthesopathy may lead to erosion or proliferation of bone at the tendon insertions. These joint symptoms may be precipitated by rather non-specific factors, such as changes in the weather, and many patients report discomfort during the fall and winter seasons. Conversely, a new infection by bacteria known to trigger the disease may pass without any sequelae. The non-symptomatic period between recurrences may last for several years. It remains an open question whether degenerative changes, such as osteoarthritis, develop more readily in a joint that has been affected by reactive arthritis.

Follow-up studies of reactive arthritis suggest that 20–70% of patients later suffer some joint discomfort or other symptoms[74,75]. For the individual patient, it is important to know that, in spite of unpleasant symptoms, severe destructive disease as a sequel of reactive arthritis is extremely rare. Similarly, follow-up has not revealed reactive arthritis to be a precurser of rheumatoid arthritis. Thus, of 100 patients who were studied 20 years after a *Shigella*-triggered reactive arthritis, none had rheumatoid arthritis[4], and in another follow-up study of 60 patients, only one definite case of rheumatoid arthritis was found[74]. Although both clinical and radiographic sacroiliitis typical of ankylosing spondylitis can occur on follow-up, even in these cases the disease usually remains mild. With this knowledge, the patient may tolerate the discomfort and learn to live with the disease rather well.

REFERENCES

1. Reiter H. Uber eine bisher unerkannte Spirochäteninfektion (*Spirochaetosis arthritica*). Dtsch Med Wochenschr 1916; 42: 1535–1536.
2. Wright V, Moll JMH, eds. Seronegative polyarthritis. Amsterdam: North Holland Publishing Company; 1976.
3. Paronen I. Reiter's disease. A study of 344 cases observed in Finland. Acta Med Scand 1948; (suppl 212): 1–112.
4. Sairanen E, Paronen I, Mähönen H. Reiter's syndrome: a follow-up study. Acta Med Scand 1969; 185: 57–63.
5. Aho K, Ahvonen P, Lassus A *et al*. *Yersinia* arthritis and related diseases: clinical and immunogenetic implications. In: Dumonde DC, ed. Infection and immunology in the rheumatic diseases. Oxford: Blackwell Scientific Publications; 1976: 341–344.
6. Isomäki H, Raunio J, von Essen R *et al*. Incidence of inflammatory rheumatic diseases in Finland. Scand J Rheumatol 1978; 7: 188–192.
7. Aho K. Bowel infection predisposing to reactive arthritis. In: Rooney PJ, ed. Baillière's clinical rheumatology, vol 3. London: Baillière Tindall; 1989: 303–319.
8. Leino R, Kalliomäki JL. Yersiniosis as an internal disease. Ann Intern Med 1974; 81: 458–461.
9. Aho K, Ahvonen P, Lassus A *et al*. HLA-B27 in reactive arthritis: a study of *Yersinia* arthritis and Reiter's disease. Arthritis Rheum 1974; 17: 521–526.
10. Laitinen O, Leirisalo M, Skylv G. Relation between HLA-B27 and clinical features with *Yersinia* arthritis. Arthritis Rheum 1977; 20: 1121–1124.
11. Keat A. HLA-linked disease susceptibility and reactive arthritis. J Infect 1982; 5: 227–239.
12. Lahesmaa-Rantala R, Toivanen A. Clinical spectrum of reactive arthritis. In: Toivanen A, Toivanen P, eds. Reactive arthritis. Boca Raton: CRC Press; 1988: 1–13.
13. van Bohemen CG, Lionarons RJ, van Bodegom P *et al*. Susceptibility and HLA-B27 in post-dysenteric arthropathies. Immunology 1985; 56: 377–379.
14. Calin A, Fries JF. An 'experimental' epidemic of Reiter's syndrome revisited. Follow-up evidence on genetic and environmental factors. Ann Intern Med 1976; 84: 564–566.
15. Leirisalo M, Skylv G, Kousa M *et al*. Follow-up study on patients with Reiter's disease and reactive arthritis with special reference to HLA-B27. Arthritis Rheum 1982; 25: 249–259.
16. Laivoranta S, Ilonen J, Tuokko J *et al*. HLA frequencies in HLA-B27 negative patients with reactive arthritis. Clin Exp Rheumatol 1995; 13: 637–640.
17. Toivanen P, Toivanen A. Two forms of reactive arthritis? Ann Rheum Dis 1999; 58: 737–741.
18. Håkansson U, Löw B, Eitrem R *et al*. HLA-B27 and reactive arthritis in an outbreak of salmonellosis. Tissue Antigens 1975; 6: 366–367.
19. Simon DG, Kaslow RA, Rosenbaum J *et al*. Reiter's syndrome following epidemic shigellosis. J Rheumatol 1981; 8: 969–973.
20. Eastmond CJ, Rennie JAN, Reid TMS. An outbreak of *Campylobacter* enteritis – a rheumatological follow-up survey. J Rheumatol 1983; 10: 107–108.
21. Tertti R, Granfors K, Lehtonen O-P *et al*. An outbreak of *Yersinia pseudotuberculosis* infection. J Infect Dis 1984; 149: 245–250.
22. Tertti R, Vuento R, Mikkola PGK *et al*. Clinical manifestations of *Yersinia pseudotuberculosis* infection in children. Eur J Clin Microbiol Infect Dis 1989; 8: 587–591.
23. Gran JT. Classification and diagnosis of seronegative spondylarthropathies. Scand J Rheumatol 1999; 28: 332–335.
24. Toivanen A, Toivanen P. Reactive arthritis. Curr Opin Rheumatol 2000; 12: 300–305.
25. Ahvonen P. Human yersiniosis in Finland. II. Clinical features. Ann Clin Res 1972; 4: 39–48.

26. Leino R, Toivanen A. Arthritis associated with gastrointestinal disorders. In: Toivanen A, Toivanen P, eds. Reactive arthritis. Boca Raton: CRC Press; 1988: 77–86.
27. Toivanen P, Toivanen A. Role of micro-organisms in the pathogenesis of arthritis: lessons from reactive and Lyme arthritis. Scand J Rheumatol 1995; 24(suppl 101): 191–197.
28. Toivanen A, Toivanen P. Aetiopathogenesis of reactive arthritis. Rheumatol Eur 1995; 24: 5–8.
29. De Vos M, Cuvelier C, Mielants H et al. Ileocolonoscopy in seronegative spondylarthropathy. Gastroenterology 1989; 96: 339–344.
30. Mielants H, Veys EM. The gut and reactive arthritis. Rheumatol Eur 1995; 24: 9–11.
31. Nikkari S, Yli-Kerttula U, Toivanen P. Reactive arthritis in a patient with simultaneous parvovirus B19 infection and Clostridium difficile diarrhoea. Br J Rheumatol 1997; 36: 143–144.
32. Toivanen P, Toivanen A. Bacterial or reactive arthritis? Rheumatol Eur 1995; 24(suppl 2): 253–255.
33. Yli-Kerttula UI, Vilppula AH. Reactive salpingitis. In: Toivanen A, Toivanen P, eds. Reactive arthritis. Boca Raton: CRC Press; 1988: 125–131.
34. Saari KM. The eye and reactive arthritis. In: Toivanen A, Toivanen P, eds. Reactive arthritis. Boca Raton: CRC Press; 1988: 113–124.
35. Shmerling RH, Delbanco TL, Tosteson ANA et al. Synovial fluid tests. What should be ordered? JAMA 1990; 264: 1009–1014.
36. Toivanen A, Granfors K, Lahesmaa-Rantala R et al. Pathogenesis of Yersinia-triggered reactive arthritis: immunological, microbiological and clinical aspects. Immunol Rev 1985; 86: 47–70.
37. Isomäki H, Anttila P. Radiology of reactive arthritis. In: Toivanen A, Toivanen P, eds. Reactive arthritis. Boca Raton: CRC Press; 1988: 133–138.
38. Sieper J, Braun J. Pathogenesis of spondylarthropathies. Persistent bacterial antigen, autoimmunity, or both? Arthritis Rheum 1995; 38: 1547–1554.
39. Toivanen A, Toivanen P. Epidemiologic aspects, clinical features, and management of ankylosing spondylitis and reactive arthritis. Curr Opin Rheumatol 1994; 6: 354–359.
40. Oldstone MBA. Molecular mimicry and autoimmune disease. Cell 1987; 50: 819–820.
41. Schwimmbeck PL, Oldstone MBA. Klebsiella pneumoniae and HLA B27-associated diseases of Reiter's syndrome and ankylosing spondylitis. Curr Topics Microbiol Immunol 1989; 145: 45–56.
42. Lahesmaa R, Skurnik M, Toivanen P. Molecular mimicry: any role in the pathogenesis of spondyloarthropathies? Immunol Res 1993; 12: 193–208.
43. Gaston JSH, Life PF, Granfors K et al. Synovial T lymphocyte recognition of organisms that trigger reactive arthritis. Clin Exp Immunol 1989; 76: 348–353.
44. Hermann E, Mayet W-J, Poralla T et al. Salmonella-reactive synovial fluid T-cell clones in a patient with post-infectious salmonella arthritis. Scand J Rheum 1990; 19: 350–355.
45. Hermann E, Yu DT, Meyer zum Büschenfelde K-H et al. HLA-B27-restricted CD8 T cells derived from synovial fluids of patients with reactive arthritis and ankylosing spondylitis. Lancet 1993; 342: 646–650.
46. Herrmann E. T cells in reactive arthritis. APMIS 1993; 101: 177–186.
47. Lahesmaa-Rantala R, Granfors K, Isomäki H et al. Yersinia specific immune complexes in the synovial fluid of patients with Yersinia-triggered reactive arthritis. Ann Rheum Dis 1987; 46: 10–14.
48. Granfors K, Jalkanen S, von Essen R et al. Yersinia antigens in synovial-fluid cells from patients with reactive arthritis. N Engl J Med 1989; 320: 216–221.
49. Toivanen A, Lahesmaa-Rantala R, Ståhlberg T et al. Do bacterial antigens persist in reactive arthritis? Clin Exp Rheum 1987; 5(suppl 1): 25–27.
50. Keat A, Thomas B, Dixey J et al. Chlamydia trachomatis and reactive arthritis – the missing link. Lancet 1987; i: 72–74.
51. Schumacher HR Jr, Magge S, Cherian PV et al. Light and electron microscopic studies on the synovial membrane in Reiter's syndrome. Immunocytochemical identification of chlamydial antigen in patients with early disease. Arthritis Rheum 1988; 31: 937–946.
52. Granfors K, Jalkanen S, Lindberg AA et al. Salmonella lipopolysaccharide in synovial cells from patients with reactive arthritis. Lancet 1990; 335: 685–688.
53. Hammer M, Zeidler H, Klimsa S et al. Yersinia enterocolitica in the synovial membrane of patients with Yersinia-induced arthritis. Arthritis Rheum 1990; 33: 1795–1800.
54. Merilahti-Palo R, Söderström K-O, Lahesmaa-Rantala R et al. Bacterial antigens in synovial biopsy specimens in Yersinia-triggered reactive arthritis. Ann Rheum Dis 1991; 50: 87–90.
55. Taylor-Robinson D, Gilroy CB, Thomas BJ et al. Detection of Chlamydia trachomatis DNA in joints of reactive arthritis patients by polymerase chain reaction. Lancet 1992; 340: 81–82.
56. Gérard HC, Branigan PJ, Schumacher HR Jr et al. Synovial Chlamydia trachomatis in patients with reactive arthritis/Reiter's syndrome are viable but show aberrant gene expression. J Rheumatol 1998; 25: 734–742.
57. Hughes RA, Keat AC. Reiter's syndrome and reactive arthritis: a current view. Semin Arthritis Rheum 1994; 24: 190–210.
58. Lipsky PE, Davis LS, Cush JJ et al. The role of cytokines in the pathogenesis of rheumatoid arthritis. Springer Semin Immunopathol 1989; 11: 123–162.
59. Ziff M. Role of endothelium in chronic inflammation. Springer Semin Immunopathol 1989; 11: 199–214.
60. Toivanen A, Toivanen P. Pathogenesis of reactive arthritis. In: Toivanen A, Toivanen P, eds. Reactive arthritis. Boca Raton: CRC Press; 1988: 167–178.
61. Simon AK, Seipelt E, Sieper J. Divergent T-cell cytokine patterns in inflammatory arthritis. Proc Natl Acad Sci USA 1994; 91: 8562–8566.
62. Toivanen A, Toivanen P. Epidemiologic, clinical, and therapeutic aspects of reactive arthritis and ankylosing spondylitis. Curr Opin Rheumatol 1995; 7: 279–283.
63. Toivanen A. Managing reactive arthritis. Rheumatology 2000; 39: 117–121.
64. Sieper J, Fendler C, Laitko S et al. No benefit of long-term ciprofloxacin treatment in patients with reactive arthritis and undifferentiated oligoarthritis. Arthritis Rheum 1999; 42: 1386–1396.
65. Yli-Kerttula T, Luukkainen R, Yli-Kerttula U et al. Effect of a three-month course of ciprofloxacin on the outcome of reactive arthritis. Ann Rheum Dis 2000; 59: 565–570.
66. Toivanen A. Bacteria-triggered reactive arthritis. Implications for antibacterial treatment. Drugs 2001; 61: 343–351.
67. Zhang Y, Toivanen A, Toivanen P. Experimental Yersinia-triggered reactive arthritis; effect of a 3-week course with ciprofloxacin. Br J Rheumatol 1997; 36: 541–546.
68. Lauhio A, Leirisalo-Repo M, Lähdevirta J et al. Double-blind, placebo controlled study of three-month treatment with lymecycline in reactive arthritis, with special reference to Chlamydia arthritis. Arthritis Rheum 1991; 34: 6–14.
69. Toivanen A, Yli-Kerttula T, Luukkainen R et al. Effect of antimicrobial treatment on chronic reactive arthritis. Clin Exp Rheumatol 1993; 11: 301–307.
70. Mielants H, Veys EM. HLA-B27 related arthritis and bowel inflammation. Part 1. Sulphasalazine (Salazopyrin) in HLA-B27 related reactive arthritis. J Rheumatol 1985; 12: 287–293.
71. Trnavský K, Peliskóvá Z, Vácha J. Sulphasalazine in the treatment of reactive arthritis. Scand J Rheumatol 1988; (Suppl 67): 76–79.
72. Egsmose C, Hansen TM, Andersen LS et al. Limited effect of sulphasalazine treatment in reactive arthritis. A randomised double blind placebo controlled trial. Ann Rheum Dis 1997; 56: 32–36.
73. Clegg DO, Reda DJ, Abdellatif M. Comparison of sulphasalazine and placebo for the treatment of axial and peripheral articular manifestations of the seronegative spondylarthropathies. Arthritis Rheum 1999; 42: 2325–2329.
74. Kalliomäki JL, Leino R. Follow-up studies of joint complications in yersiniosis. Acta Med Scand 1979; 205: 521–525.
75. Yli-Kerttula T, Tertti R, Toivanen A. Ten-year follow up study of patients from a Yersinia pseudotuberculosis III outbreak. Clin Exp Rheumatol 1995; 13: 333–337.

31 Psoriatic arthritis: clinical features

Ian N Bruce

- Definition: An inflammatory arthritis associated with psoriasis, which is usually negative for rheumatoid factor
- Prevalence: 0.04–0.1%
- Sex distribution: equal
- 15% develop psoriasis AFTER onset of arthritis
- Nail changes have the strongest association with arthropathy, particularly affecting the distal interphalangeal joints
- Typical clinical features:
  - Distal interphalangeal joint involvement
  - Asymmetric sacroiliitis/spondylitis
  - Dactylitis
  - Enthesitis
- Number of joints involved can increase with disease duration
- Polyarticular involvement tends to have poorer long-term outcomes

HISTORY

Psoriatic arthritis can be defined as 'an inflammatory arthritis associated with psoriasis, which is usually negative for rheumatoid factor' (RF)[1]. Alibert first described the association between psoriasis and arthritis in 1818, although the term 'psoriasis arthritique' was first used by Bazin in 1860. Bourdillon developed a more detailed description of the condition in 1888[1]. It has only been since the 1950s that psoriatic arthritis has been systematically studied. Wright[2] noted that patients with psoriasis and erosive arthritis had a low frequency of RF positivity. In addition, he also pointed out the predilection for involvement of the distal interphalangeal (DIP) and sacroiliac joints, the frequent asymmetric nature of the arthritis and the tendency to severe joint destruction – 'arthritis mutilans'.

In 1964, the American Rheumatism Association recognized psoriatic arthritis as a distinct entity[3]. In the past 40 years, our understanding of the clinical spectrum of psoriatic arthritis has expanded as a result of detailed analysis of large clinic series and improvements in imaging techniques. Considerable controversy continues, however, as to the distinctiveness of psoriatic arthritis as a discrete entity.

EPIDEMIOLOGY

The association of psoriasis and arthritis (Tables 31.1 and 31.2)

Several studies have demonstrated that psoriasis is more common in patients with inflammatory arthritis and also that inflammatory arthritis occurs more commonly in cases with psoriasis than in the background population. In a retrospective clinic series, Dawson and Tyson[4] noted psoriasis in 2.6% of patients with inflammatory polyarthritis, compared with 0.3% of those with osteoarthritis. In a population study, Hellgren[5] found psoriasis in 4.5% of patients with 'rheumatoid arthritis (RA)', compared with 2.7% of controls. When RF status is taken into account, the association between psoriasis and inflammatory arthritis is greatest

TABLE 31.1 INCREASED PREVALENCE OF INFLAMMATORY POLYARTHRITIS IN PSORIASIS

Author	Year	IPA in psoriasis (%)	IPA in controls (%)	Comments
Leczinsky[8]	1948	6.8	0.7	Controls had other skin conditions
Hellgren[5]	1969	9	2.3	IPA defined as possible – classic RA
Van Romunde et al.[9]	1984	5	2.2	Only 41 psoriasis patients studied

IPA, inflammatory polyarthritis.

TABLE 31.2 INCREASED PREVALENCE OF PSORIASIS IN INFLAMMATORY POLYARTHRITIS, ESPECIALLY SERONEGATIVE ARTHROPATHIES

Author	Year	Controls (%)	All IPA (%)	Seropositive IPA (%)	Seronegative IPA (%)
Dawson and Tyson[4]	1938	0.3	2.6		
Baker[6]	1966	1.5		1.2	20.2
Mongan and Atwater[7]	1968			2.8	12.5
Hellgren[5]	1969	2.7	4.5		
Harrison et al.[10]	1997		5	1.7	5.6

IPA, inflammatory polyarthritis.

TABLE 31.3 PREVALENCE AND INCIDENCE OF PSORIATIC ARTHRITIS				
Author	Year	Country	Prevalence (%)	Incidence/year
Lomholt[13]	1963	Faroe Islands	0.04	
Van Romunde[9]	1984	Netherlands	0.05	
Shbeeb et al.[14]	2000	USA	0.1	
Kaipiainen-Seppanen[15]	1996	Finland		6/100 000
Harrison et al.[10]	1997	UK		3.6/100 000 (males)
				3.4/100 000 (females)
Shbeeb et al.[14]	2000	USA		6/100 000

amongst seronegative patients[6,7]. In one study psoriasis occurred in 1.3% of controls and 1.2% of those with seropositive arthritis, whereas 20.2% of patients with seronegative inflammatory arthritis had psoriasis[6] (Table 31.2). With regard to the presence of inflammatory arthritis in patients with psoriasis, a similar association has been noted. In Hellgren's study[5], 9% of patients with psoriasis had 'RA', compared with 2.3% of controls. Similarly, Leczinsky[8] found that 6.8% of patients with psoriasis had inflammatory arthritis, compared with 0.7% of controls with other skin complaints (Table 31.1). Other uncontrolled clinic surveys of patients with psoriasis have suggested a 30–35% prevalence of inflammatory arthritis[11,12]. These higher estimates may reflect the more detailed evaluation of axial and peripheral joints undertaken, although awareness and selection biases cannot be excluded. Overall, there is an increased association between inflammatory arthritis and psoriasis. Several explanations for this association can be suggested. First, psoriasis may be a risk factor for inflammatory arthritis. Secondly, psoriasis and inflammatory arthritis may share a common etiologic trigger. Finally, a distinct entity of psoriatic arthritis may exist. The last of these is generally accepted to be true, but until more is known about psoriatic arthritis, the first two explanations cannot be completely discounted.

Incidence and prevalence of psoriatic arthritis

There have only been a few studies estimating the prevalence of psoriatic arthritis in the general population, giving rates of between 0.04 and 0.1%[9,13,14] (Table 31.3). These likely underestimate the true prevalence of psoriatic arthritis, because the dermatological or rheumatological criteria applied will often lead to exclusion of some cases. In addition, it is difficult to account for patients who have minimal or no psoriasis at the time of study. The incidence of psoriatic arthritis has recently been estimated in Europe and the USA[10,14,15]. In the Norfolk Arthritis Registry of recent onset inflammatory arthritis (a community-based cohort), the incidence of psoriatic arthritis was estimated to be 3.6 per 100 000 per annum in men and 3.4 per 100 000 per annum in women. This study did not include patients presenting with monoarthritis or spondyloarthropathy only. The incidence in Olmsted County, Minnesota, USA was reported as 6.6 per 100 000 per annum, for both sexes combined[14]. Again, only patients with a dermatologist-confirmed diagnosis of psoriasis were included.

Additional observations

In contrast to RA, which has a female preponderance, the overall sex distribution of psoriatic arthritis is 1:1[10,14,16]. The mean age at onset of psoriatic arthritis is in the range of 30–55 years[10,16,17]. With regard to the timing of skin and joint disease, approximately 67% of patients develop psoriasis before the onset of arthritis[11,16,17]. In about 16%, the two conditions occur within 12 months of each other[11,16], and in the remainder, arthritis precedes the onset of psoriasis by more than 1 year[11,16]. The timing of onset may not be randomly distributed across all patients with psoriasis. Rahman et al.[18] found that, in patients with type 1 psoriasis (age of onset <40 years old), the skin disorder preceded the onset of arthritis by a

mean of 9 years. In contrast, in older patients with type 2 psoriasis (age of onset >40 years old), arthropathy developed at a mean period of 1 year after the onset of skin disease, suggesting that a greater proportion of older patients have a near synchronous onset of the two conditions.

Relationship to HIV infection

An association of HIV infection with susceptibility to psoriatic arthritis has long been suggested. Indeed, the prevalence of psoriatic arthritis in HIV infection is greater than expected in the general population[19]. This has particular implications for the incidence and prevalence of psoriatic arthritis in Africa. Historically, seronegative arthropathies are uncommon in sub-Saharan Africa because of the low prevalence of human leukocyte antigen (HLA)-B27[20]. A recent study from Zambia found that spondyloarthropathies are now the most common group of inflammatory arthritis observed in this population[21]. The prevalence of spondyloarthropathies was 180/100 000 among HIV-positive populations, compared with 15/100 000 in HIV-negative populations[21]. A subsequent study from the same region found that 27 of 28 patients (96%) with psoriatic arthritis were HIV-positive, compared with 30% of the background population[22]. Several studies in North American HIV cohorts have found a prevalence of psoriatic arthritis of 0.4–2%[19,23,24]. In the context of HIV infection, severe skin and polyarticular joint disease, which often occur simultaneously, have been reported[22,25,26]. The spectrum of severity is wide, and in some cases improvement of arthritis with the onset of AIDS has been observed[22].

CLINICAL FEATURES

Psoriatic arthropathy is classified within the group of seronegative spondyloarthropathies, on the basis of work by Moll and Wright[1] and others that has demonstrated many clinical and familial associations between psoriatic arthritis and other conditions in this group, such as reactive arthritis and ankylosing spondylitis. The inclusion of psoriatic arthritis within the spondyloarthropathies is also reflected in the European Spondylarthropathies Study Group (ESSG) criteria[27].

Articular involvement

Joint involvement in psoriatic arthritis can vary considerably, from an isolated monoarthritis to extensive destructive arthritis. It can involve peripheral joints and the axial spine with varying frequencies. The most

TABLE 31.4 THE MOLL AND WRIGHT CLASSIFICATION OF PSORIATIC ARTHRITIS[1]
• Arthritis with distal interphalangeal joint involvement predominant
• Arthritis mutilans
• Symmetric polyarthritis – indistinguishable from RA
• Asymmetric oligoarticular arthritis
• Predominant spondylitis

TABLE 31.5 RELATIVE FREQUENCY OF VARIOUS SUBTYPES OF PSORIATIC ARTHRITIS						
Author	Disease duration (years)	Frequency (%)				
		DIP predominant	Oligoarticular	Polyarticular	Spondyloarthropathy	Arthritis mutilans
Jones et al.[17]	Onset	2*	63†	25	10	0
Veale et al.[28]	4 (median)	16	43	33	4	2
Gladman et al.[16‡]	9 (mean)	12	14	40	2	16
Jones et al.[17]	12 (mean)	1*	26	63	6	4

* Defined as DIP only, in this series. † Includes mono- and oligoarticular onset. ‡ The balance in this series had overlapping patterns.

Findings of selected clinic series are displayed according to disease duration of the cohort studied. (Note: Jones et al.[17] described patterns at onset and follow-up.)

widely used classification is that proposed by Moll and Wright[1], which identifies five major subtypes of psoriatic arthritis (Table 31.4). There have been many further attempts to revise and modify this system, but these have not been widely adopted. Applying this system has, however, provided some valuable insights into the nature of psoriatic arthritis and provides a framework in which to consider many of the key features of psoriatic arthritis. There is a high degree of overlap between categories within this classification, and hence it has limitations in practice. For example, spondyloarthropathy may be the dominant feature in only a minority of patients, whereas clinical and radiological involvement of the spine can be detected in approximately one-third of cases[16]. Similarly, exclusive involvement of the DIP joint is less common than involvement of this joint as part of a general peripheral arthritis[17,28]. It is thus not surprising that series have shown quite marked differences in their relative proportions of these subtypes. This is partly related to the entry criteria to these cohorts, as well as to some differences in the definitions for each subgroup used. In addition, the disease duration at the time of study has a significant influence (Table 31.5, Fig. 31.1). Thus Jones et al.[17] found that, whereas the majority of patients described mono- or oligoarticular disease at onset, after a mean follow-up of 12.1 years, 63% of patients had polyarthritis. Marsal et al.[29] also found that the median number of joints affected at onset of disease was 2 (range 0–8), compared with a median of 10 (range 2–19) after a follow-up period of 8 years. Arthritis mutilans is also a feature of prolonged disease[17]. In addition, there is a tendency for the frequency of spinal involvement to increase with time[30]. A more pragmatic classification based simply on peripheral or axial involvement has therefore been suggested, and may be justified[29].

Symmetry of involvement in psoriatic arthritis

Wright[2] identified asymmetry as a common feature of psoriatic arthritis. In particular, asymmetric involvement was typical of the oligoarticular pattern[1]. Other investigators have also found that the majority of patients with oligoarticular arthritis have an asymmetric pattern[16,17]. In contrast, the majority of patients with polyarticular disease have symmetric involvement[17,31]. Symmetry may, however, be largely a function of the total number of joints involved in the inflammatory process. In a comparison of patients with early and late RA and psoriatic arthritis, after correction for the total number of involved joints there was no difference in the degree of joint symmetry observed between these conditions[32].

Distal interphalangeal joint involvement

Involvement of the DIP joints in psoriatic arthritis is considered a distinctive feature of this condition (Fig. 31.2). These joints are thus involved more frequently in those with psoriatic arthritis than in patients with inflammatory arthritis without psoriasis[33]. In a community-based survey of early inflammatory arthritis, a DIP-predominant pattern at onset was found in 3.9% of patients with psoriasis, compared with 0.3% of patients without psoriasis[10]. Several large hospital series have noted *involvement* of the DIP joints, as part of a polyarthritis, in up to 54% of patients with psoriatic arthritis[16,17,28]. In contrast, the 'DIP-predominant' subgroup of those with psoriatic arthritis represents a much smaller proportion of cases (1–16%). As the DIP joints may be the first to be involved, the DIP predominant pattern can occur early in the disease course[1,28]. DIP joint involvement is also commonly associated with two other significant features of psoriatic arthritis, namely dactylitis[16,28] and nail dystrophy[2].

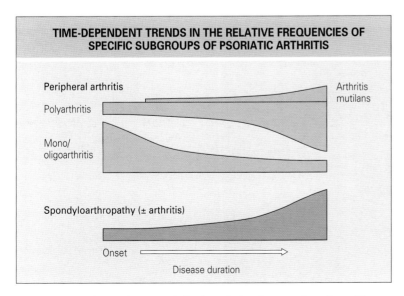

Fig 31.1 Time-dependent trends in the relative frequencies of specific subgroups of psoriatic arthritis. ±, with or without.

TIME-DEPENDENT TRENDS IN THE RELATIVE FREQUENCIES OF SPECIFIC SUBGROUPS OF PSORIATIC ARTHRITIS

Peripheral arthritis

Arthritis mutilans

Polyarthritis

Mono/ oligoarthritis

Spondyloarthropathy (± arthritis)

Onset

Disease duration

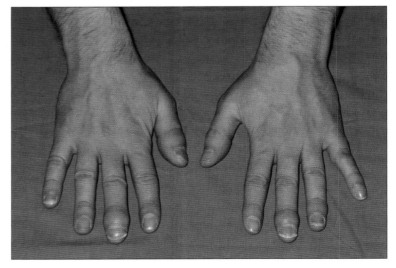

Fig. 31.2 Psoriatic arthritis with predominant involvement of the DIP joints. (Copyright University of Manchester.)

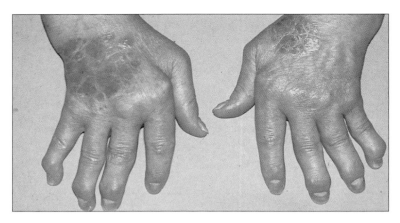

Fig. 31.3 **Symmetric polyarthritis resembling RA.**

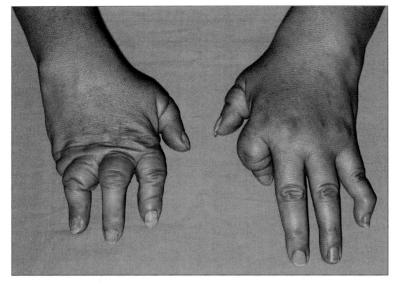

Fig. 31.4 **Arthritis mutilans.** Note shortening of the thumbs and left index finger (the right 5th finger has been amputated). (Copyright University of Manchester.)

Mono- and oligoarticular arthritis

The frequency of these forms of psoriatic arthritis is highly variable across different series, ranging in prevalence from 11% to 70%[1,16]. Indeed, in a community-based study of psoriatic arthritis in Olmsted County, Minnesota USA, 90% of patients with psoriatic arthritis had an oligoarticular pattern at onset[14]. As pointed out earlier, mono- and oligoarthritis are the most common presenting patterns[14,17,29]. A high proportion will, however, progress towards additional joint involvement[17]. In addition to involvement of the lower limb joints, this pattern of arthritis can frequently affect the small joints of the hands, including the proximal interphalangeal and DIP joints. This pattern also has a male predominance[28].

Symmetric polyarthritis

Symmetric polyarthritis involves the small joints of the hands and feet, in addition to larger joints (Fig. 31.3). It has a female preponderance[16,28,34] and can be clinically indistinguishable from RA[2,31]. The exact frequency of this pattern is again controversial. Shbeeb *et al.*[14] described a 3% prevalence of polyarthritis at onset. The frequency in hospital clinics can range from 15% to 61%, and may in part reflect the referral base that these clinics serve[1,16,34]. Polyarthritis also tends to develop over time, and patients with polyarticular disease have a longer disease duration than the other more discrete patterns[17,28]. Regardless of the precise frequency of the polyarthritis, it is patients with this condition who have more evidence of erosive joint damage[28,29].

Arthritis mutilans

There is no clear definition of this commonly used term. In general, it describes the end stage of a destructive erosive arthritis, with disorganization of joints leading to subluxation, 'flail' joints and digital telescoping – the so-called 'doigt en lorgnette' (opera glass finger)[2] (Figs 31.4 & 31.5). In most series, the prevalence is less than 5%[1,17,28]. Arthritis mutilans is associated with long-standing disease and a female preponderance[17,29]. An association with sacroiliac joint involvement has also been described[1,29].

Spondyloarthropathy

The spondyloarthropathy of psoriatic arthritis is uncommon as a predominant feature, and only accounts for approximately 5% of cases[1,16]. Careful clinical and radiological assessment, however, reveals involvement of the axial spine in 20–40% of cases[16,28,34], increasing to as many as 51% at long-term follow-up[30]. Involvement of the sacroiliac joints can be symmetric or asymmetric. In patients with bilateral sacroiliitis, there is a stronger association with HLA B27[34]. During follow-up, although the radiographic changes in the spine tend to progress, spinal mobility is preserved or improves, and this form of spinal disease carries a better prognosis than pure ankylosing spondylitis[35]. This may partly reflect the

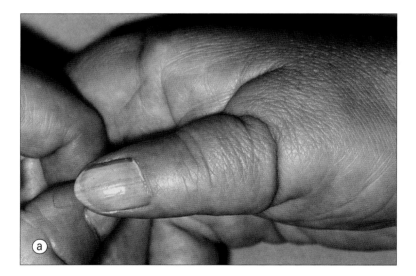
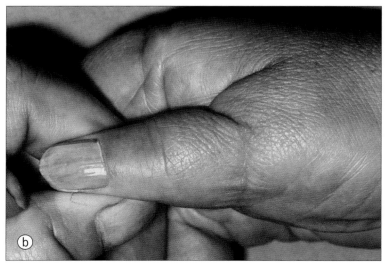

Fig. 31.5 **Digital telescoping in arthritis mutilans.** (Copyright University of Manchester.)

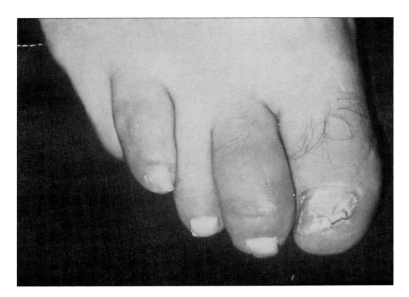

Fig. 31.6 Dactylitis of the second toe.

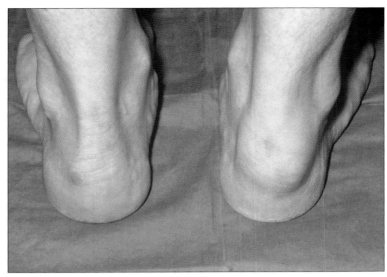

Fig. 31.7 Enthesitis involving the insertion of the right tendo Achilles.

random nature of spinal involvement that is observed, in addition to a lower frequency of zygoapophyseal joint fusion seen in psoriatic arthritis[36,37]. The cervical spine is also a common site of involvement in psoriatic arthritis. This can occur as part of a more widespread axial disease or as the sole site of axial involvement. Cervical spine disease becomes more frequent with time[38]. Two main types of cervical spine changes are described[38,39]: an ankylosing type, similar to that seen in ankylosing spondylitis, and an erosive/inflammatory type that can result in atlantoaxial or subaxial instability. Since cervical spine involvement can be clinically silent, patients with psoriatic arthritis, particularly those with long-standing disease, should have cervical spine radiographs before a general anesthetic[38].

Other musculoskeletal features

Dactylitis

Dactylitis or 'sausage digit' is a feature of the seronegative spondyloarthropathies in general. It represents a complete swelling of a single digit in the hand or foot. Dactylitis is a common feature of psoriatic arthritis, occurring in 30–40% of patients during the course of their disease[16,28]. It most commonly involves one or two digits at a time, and the feet are affected more commonly than the hands[40] (Fig. 31.6). There is an association with DIP joint involvement[16,28]. Radiologically, patients with a history of dactylitis more frequently develop erosive damage[29,40]. Magnetic resonance imaging (MRI) has revealed dactylitis to be strongly associated with flexor tenosynovitis, whereas active synovitis during an episode is not a universal finding[41,42].

Enthesitis

Inflammatory lesions at the insertion of tendon into bone are a hallmark clinical feature of spondyloarthropathies and, indeed, it has been postulated that it is this inflammatory lesion that is the key central pathogenic process in all seronegative spondyloarthropathies[43]. Symptomatic enthesitis occurs in 20–40% of patients with psoriatic arthritis[44,45]. It has been reported to be a presenting feature in 4%[44]. Common sites of enthesitis include the tendo Achilles (Fig. 31.7), the plantar fascia insertion into the calcaneum, and ligamentous insertions into pelvic bones.

Peripheral edema

Peripheral edema of one or more distal extremities is an increasingly recognized feature of several inflammatory conditions, including psoriatic arthritis. In contrast to the remitting seronegative symmetric synovitis with peripheral edema syndrome, distal extremity swelling in

psoriatic arthritis is frequently asymmetric and preferentially affects the lower limbs. It can occur at any time and may be a presenting feature of the disease[45]. Clinically and radiologically, it is associated with extensor tenosynovitis and local enthesitis, and the edema is often along the course of the involved tendon[45]. Peripheral edema is usually responsive to oral steroids. Several cases of lymphedema associated with psoriatic arthritis have also been reported[46,47]. Although generally less painful, lymphedema can become more extensive, and has been associated with progression of erosive damage[46]. The response to steroids and disease-modifying antirheumatic drugs is varied, and it can be an additional source of disability in these patients[46,47].

Synovitis, acne, pustulosis, hyperostosis and osteitis syndrome

The syndrome of synovitis, acne, pustulosis, hyperostosis and osteitis (SAPHO) is an uncommon but recognized subgroup of psoriatic arthritis. Clinically, fewer than 3% of patients with psoriatic arthritis present in this fashion. Nevertheless, at least 67% of all patients with SAPHO have psoriasis vulgaris or palmoplantar pustulosis[48]. Scintigraphy suggests that involvement of the anterior chest wall may occur with a much greater frequency in patients with psoriatic arthritis than is clinically recognized[31].

Psoriatic onycho-pachydermo-periostitis

Several case reports of the rare manifestation of psoriatic arthritis known as psoriatic onycho-pachydermo-periostitis have been described. The key features include severe involvement of one or more terminal phalanges, with associated severe nail dystrophy, soft tissue swelling and marked periosteal reaction of the distal phalanx radiologically. The involvement of the DIP joint appears variable, but is difficult to assess because of the marked local inflammation[49,50]. Involvement of the great toe had been particularly described in this condition, and marked periostitis may eventually result in the radiological phenomenon of the 'ivory phalanx'[51].

Associated nail and skin changes

Skin changes

There is a suggestion that patients with psoriatic arthritis may have more extensive psoriasis than patients with uncomplicated psoriasis only[52], but, in general, most patients with psoriatic arthritis have only mild to moderate skin disease[53]. There is also no correlation between the extent of skin disease and total joint scores in patients with psoriatic arthritis[17,53]. Nevertheless, 30–40% of patients with psoriatic arthritis report

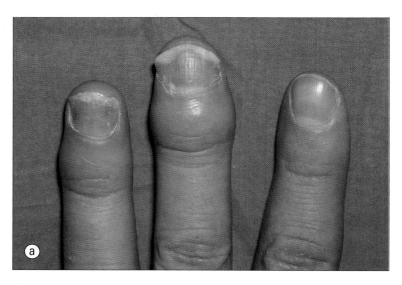 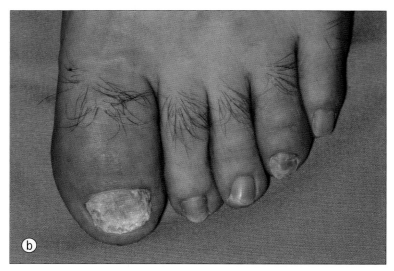

Fig. 31.8 Involvement of the joint and adjacent nail. (a) In the right hand. (b) In the foot. Note the lack of involvement of the right 4th finger and nail. (Copyright University of Manchester.)

synchronicity of flares of their joint and skin disease, although the validity of this observation has not been formally tested[2,16,52]. No subtype of psoriasis is over-represented in patients with psoriatic arthritis, although an association between palmoplantar pustulosis and the SAPHO syndrome is described.

Nail involvement

In contrast to skin disease, there is a close association between nail and joint involvement in psoriatic arthritis. Anatomically, the nail is closely related to the distal phalanx by Sharpey's fibers that insert into bone in a manner similar to an enthesis. This close association may help explain the clinical observations. Nail involvement is seen in 20–40% of patients with uncomplicated psoriasis, whereas 60–80% of patients with psoriatic arthritis have nail involvement[16,17,28]. All the typical nail changes of psoriasis can be observed in psoriatic arthritis, including pitting, ridging, hyperkeratosis and onycholysis[1]. A closer temporal association between the onset of nail and joint disease has been described compared with the onset of skin and joint disease. Although skin disease may precede arthropathy by an average of 7–10 years, the onset of nail changes often occurs only 1–2 years before the onset of arthropathy[2]. The association between nails and joints is particularly marked in the presence of DIP joint arthritis, and 80–100% of such patients have nail involvement that frequently occurs at the adjacent nail[2,17,28] (Fig. 31.8). Patients with DIP joint involvement also have more severe nail changes[17,33], and patients with nail disease have more DIP joint involvement[53]. There is also a closer synchronicity between flares of DIP joint disease and worsening of nail involvement than is reported for flares of skin and joint disease[2].

Other extra-articular features

There is an overlap between the extra-articular features observed in psoriatic arthritis and those of the other seronegative spondyloarthropathies. Ocular inflammation can occur, most frequently presenting as conjunctivitis. However, iritis has also been described in 7% of those affected by psoriatic arthritis[16]. Additional uncommon complications such as oral ulceration, urethritis and aortic valve disease have also been reported[54].

JUVENILE PSORIATIC ARTHRITIS

Psoriatic arthritis developing in those younger than 16 years is relatively uncommon, and appears to account for less than 10% of chronic arthritis in childhood[55,56]. In contrast to adult-onset psoriatic arthritis, in juvenile-onset psoriatic arthritis the arthropathy precedes psoriasis in up to

TABLE 31.6 PROPOSED CRITERIA FOR THE DIAGNOSIS OF JUVENILE PSORIATIC ARTHRITIS

Diagnosis	Criteria
Definite psoriatic arthritis	Arthritis onset before age 16 years *and either* Typical psoriasis *or* three minor criteria from: Dactylitis Nail pitting Psoriasis-like rash Family history of psoriasis (first- or second-degree relative)
Probable psoriatic arthritis	Arthritis onset before age 16 years *and* two minor criteria

(After Southwood *et al.*[57] This material is used by permission of Wiley-Liss Inc., a subsidiary of John Wiley & Sons Inc. © 1989.)

50% of cases[55,57]. In view of this, careful attention needs to be paid to examination of the nails and taking an accurate family history in children with arthritis, as reflected in the criteria proposed by Southwood *et al.*[57] (Table 31.6). Juvenile psoriatic arthritis has a female preponderance of 2–3:1[55,57]. It frequently presents as a mono- or oligoarthritis, and the knee is often the first joint affected. As with the adult form, progression toward polyarthritis occurs in a significant proportion of those affected, and involvement of the small joints of the hands and feet occurs commonly during the disease course[55,57,58]. The other typical musculoskeletal features of adult psoriatic arthritis, such as dactylitis, enthesitis and DIP joint involvement, are all recognized. In addition, chronic uveitis is reported in 10–15% of patients, and may be associated with antinuclear antibodies[55,57]. The prognosis of juvenile psoriatic arthritis is good. It can, however, persist into adulthood, and 10–15% of those affected have significant residual disabilities[55,59].

INVESTIGATIONS

Laboratory investigation

There are no diagnostic laboratory tests for psoriatic arthritis. Several studies have shown that the acute-phase reactants display typical inflammatory changes when the disease is active. In particular, anemia of chronic disease, hypoalbuminemia, and increased erythrocyte sedimentation rate (ESR), C-reactive protein and fibrinogen are described[60]. Hypergammaglobulinemia with increased IgG and IgA is observed[16,61]. Increased IgA is especially associated with spondyloarthropathy[34]. Overall, the ESR and C-reactive protein show a good correlation with inflammatory disease activity, particularly in polyarticular disease[31,34,61]. Because, in most series of patients, a positive RF is not taken as an absolute exclusion criteria for the case definition of psoriatic arthritis, an RF-positive status has been reported in 5–10% of patients[16,34]. In a community cohort of patients with recent-onset inflammatory polyarthritis, patients with psoriasis were significantly less likely to be RF-positive compared with those without psoriasis (13% compared with 31%)[10]. Positivity for antinuclear antibody is also found in 10–14% of patients with psoriatic arthritis[16,34]. Hyperuricemia is present in up to 20% of patients with psoriatic arthritis[62]. A prospective study of patients with psoriatic arthritis found that the best predictors of hyperuricemia were renal impairment and increased total cholesterol. There was no correlation with the extent or severity of skin involvement. This suggests that hyperuricemia in the context of psoriatic arthritis is not the result of increased epidermal cell turnover, but rather reflects other relevant metabolic changes[62].

Radiographic changes

Peripheral joint features

Many radiological features reflect the clinical distribution of psoriatic arthritis described above. Therefore, involvement of the DIP joints (Fig. 31.9) and an asymmetric distribution when few joints are affected are well described. In addition, the involvement of entheseal sites can

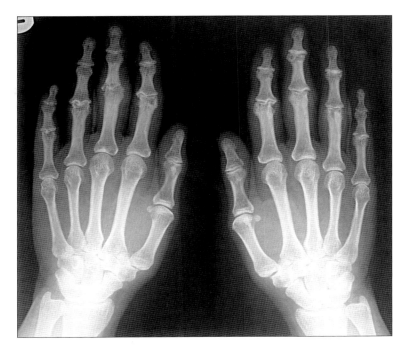

Fig. 31.9 Radiograph of the hands, showing erosive changes at the DIP and PIP joints, with sparing of the MCP joints and wrists. (Copyright Dr R Whitehouse.)

result in proliferative new bone formation in sites of predilection – for example, the plantar fascia and tendo Achillis insertions. With regard to the onset of erosive change in peripheral joints, in a community survey

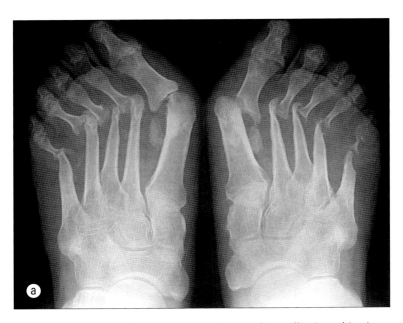

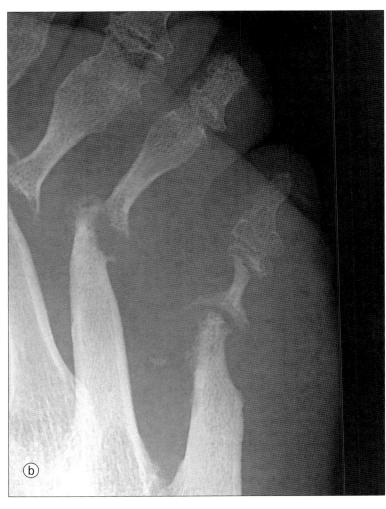

Fig. 31.10 Arthritis mutilans. Marked osteolysis and 'pencilling', resulting in complete disorganization of the metatarsophalangeal (MTP) joints. There is also a 'pencil-in-cup' deformity of the right 5th MTP joint (b). (Copyright Dr R Whitehouse.)

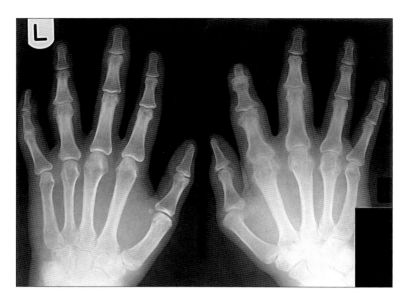

Fig. 31.11 Asymmetric involvement of the hands. Soft tissue swelling and periosteal reaction in the right 2nd and 3rd fingers in the typical 'ray' distribution. (Copyright Dr R Whitehouse.)

of early inflammatory arthritis, patients with psoriasis had a reduced risk of erosions developing at 1 year, compared with patients without psoriasis[10]. This reduced risk was explained by the lower incidence of RF positivity in the psoriasis group. Nevertheless, 22% of patients with psoriasis

and early arthritis had evidence of erosions at 1 year[10]. In more established hospital cohorts, the prevalence of erosions can range from 35% to 70%[16,28,29]. Erosions are most frequent in patients with polyarthritis and in those with longer disease duration[28,29]. As mentioned earlier, there is an association between dactylitis and erosions. With regard to the distribution of erosions, in a case–control study comparing patients with psoriatic arthropathy and patients with seropositive arthritis without psoriasis, erosions were less frequent at the wrist and more common in the DIP joints of those with psoriatic arthritis[63]. In addition to erosions, soft tissue swelling can be seen around sites of active inflammation, although periarticular osteopenia is not a feature in psoriatic arthritis[64]. The other radiographic features of psoriatic arthritis in peripheral joints can be broadly grouped into destructive and proliferative changes.

Destructive changes

- Osteolysis may result in whittling or 'pencilling' of a phalanx. This can occur alone or in association with an erosion at the base of the adjacent phalanx, which causes the classic 'pencil in cup' deformity[65]. Such destruction is typical of the arthritis mutilans pattern of disease (Fig. 31.10).

Proliferative changes[65]

- Periostitis. Proliferative new bone formation can occur along the shaft of the metacarpal and metatarsal bones (Figs 31.11 & 31.12a). When this change occurs adjacent to an erosion, the term 'whiskering' is often used (Fig. 31.12b)

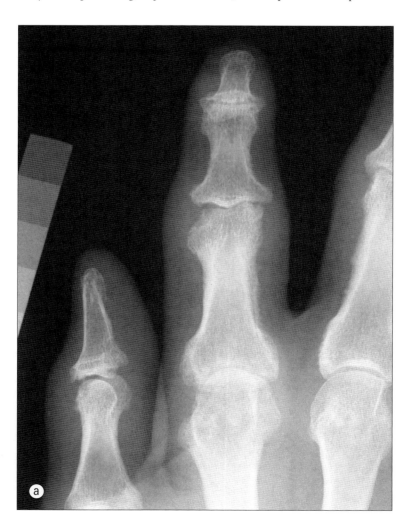

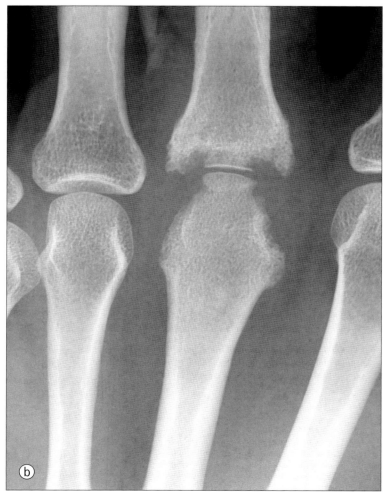

Fig. 31.12 Examples of periosteal reactions. (a) Along the shaft of the proximal phalanx. (b) Adjacent to a large erosion, producing 'whiskering'. (Copyright Dr R Whitehouse.)

- Ivory phalanx (see Psoriatic onycho-pachydermo-periostitis, above)
- Bony ankylosis and joint fusion (Fig. 31.13).

Spinal changes

Radiographic evidence of sacroiliitis in psoriatic arthritis can be symmetric or asymmetric. Asymmetric sacroiliitis is more common in psoriatic arthritis than in ankylosing spondylitis[37] (Fig. 31.14). Many of the classic features of ankylosing spondylitis can be observed in psoriatic arthritis, but patients with psoriatic arthritis tend to have less frequent involvement of the zygapophyseal joint and less severe and extensive involvement of the lumbar spine[37,66]. Overall, the spinal involvement in psoriatic arthritis tends to be more 'spotty' and asymmetric in nature, with frequent involvement of the cervical spine[37,66]. An additional feature in the spine is paravertebral ossification or 'chunky' syndesmophytes[67]. These appear distinct from the classic 'marginal' syndesmophytes observed in ankylosing spondylitis. The chunky syndesmophytes again occur in a patchy and asymmetric fashion throughout the axial spine (Fig. 31.15).

Other imaging modalities

There is increasing interest in the use of MRI and ultrasonography to delineate the clinical manifestation of diseases such as psoriatic arthritis. MRI studies have demonstrated that, in psoriatic arthritis, there is frequent involvement of extra-articular tissue such as ligaments, periarticular soft tissue and tendon sheaths, and bone (Fig. 31.16)[41,68]. In addition to delineating clinical joint involvement, MRI has also demonstrated evidence of 'subclinical' musculoskeletal changes in a significant proportion of patients with apparently uncomplicated psoriasis[69]. Scintigraphy in patients with psoriatic arthritis has also demonstrated more extensive involvement than is appreciated clinically, particularly

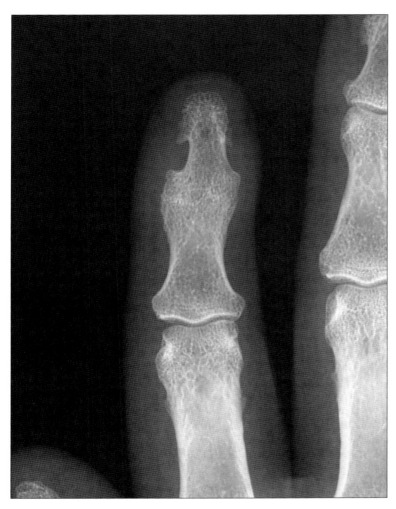

Fig. 31.13 Bony ankylosis of the DIP joint. (Copyright Dr R Whitehouse.)

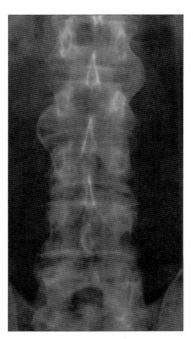

Fig. 31.15 Non-marginal 'chunky' syndesmophytes.

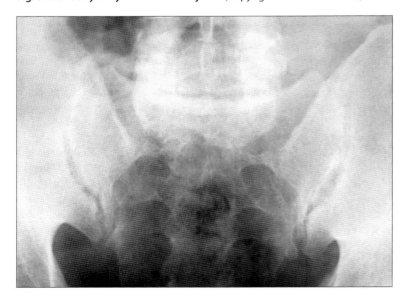

Fig. 31.14 Early asymmetric sacroiliitis, with erosion and sclerosis of the left sacroiliac joint. (Copyright Dr R Whitehouse.)

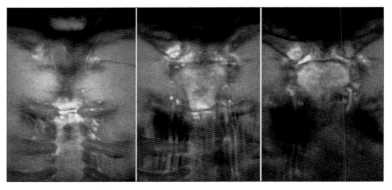

Fig. 31.16 Involvement of extra-articular tissues in psoriatic arthritis. Magnetic resonance images (coronal fat-suppressed proton-density-weighted) showing osteitis and bone edema as high signal in the clavicles, manubrium and upper sternum of a patient with SAPHO. (Copyright Dr R Whitehouse.)

in the anterior chest wall and large peripheral joints[31]. Such techniques can therefore facilitate the clinical evaluation of patients with psoriasis and articular complaints.

DIFFERENTIAL DIAGNOSIS AND CLINICAL EVALUATION

Differential diagnosis

Psoriatic arthritis poses an important diagnostic challenge to the physician. There are no clear diagnostic criteria, and the wide range of clinical presentations from isolated enthesitis or monoarthritis through polyarthritis and spondylitis means that the differential diagnosis is quite extensive. Given the frequency of hyperuricemia, crystal arthropathies also need to be excluded. In this instance, joint fluid analysis may be the only reliable way to exclude this possibility. The distinctions between psoriatic arthritis and RA or psoriatic arthritis and ankylosing spondylitis have been discussed and are summarized in Tables 31.7 and 31.8. In patients in whom

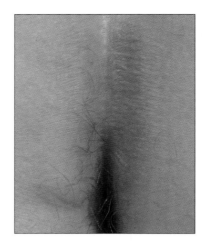

Fig. 31.17 Flexural psoriasis in the natal cleft, a typical 'hidden' site for psoriasis.

there is no clinical evidence of skin or nail disease, distinguishing psoriatic arthritis from other arthropathies is particularly difficult.

Clinical evaluation

When assessing joint involvement in psoriatic arthritis, it is important to bear in mind that patients with this condition can be less tender over affected joints than are patients with RA[70]. In addition, effusions can be more difficult to detect in patients with psoriatic arthritis[71]. For these reasons, it is easy to underestimate the extent of joint involvement in psoriatic arthritis. Examination for other musculoskeletal features such as enthesitis, tenosynovitis and axial spine involvement is also necessary. Limitations in spinal movement may not follow the classic pattern observed in ankylosing spondylitis, and may be confined to the neck or thoracic spine in the absence of lumbar spine or sacroiliac joint involvement. Radiological evaluation complements the clinical examination, particularly when there has been a history of previous joint symptoms, as residual joint damage may be detectable radiologically in the absence of current symptoms. Similarly, previous or current inflammatory back symptoms suggest spondylitis and require radiological examination. Finally, a detailed examination of the skin and nails to include 'hidden areas' such as the scalp, perineum and periumbilical area is important (Fig. 31.17). The choice of therapeutic agent(s) is determined by the extent and severity of the skin *and* joint disease, and by an estimation of the risk of disease progression.

TABLE 31.7 KEY FEATURES THAT HELP DISTINGUISH BETWEEN PSORIATIC ARTHRITIS AND RHEUMATOID ARTHRITIS		
Feature	Psoriatic arthritis	Rheumatoid arthritis
Sex M:F	1:1	1:2
RF	<10%	80%
DIP joints	30–50%	Uncommon
Pattern of joint involvement	Asymmetric 'Ray' pattern	Symmetric 'Row' pattern
Sacroiliac joints/axial spine	35% – any level	Cervical spine in late disease
Other musculoskeletal	Enthesitis Dactylitis Periarticular erythema	
Extra-articular	Skin Nail dystrophy	Nodules Sicca Vasculitis
Radiology	Erosion (DIP joints) Periostitis/bony proliferation	Periarticular osteopenia Erosion (wrists)

TABLE 31.8 KEY FEATURES THAT HELP DISTINGUISH BETWEEN PSORIATIC ARTHRITIS AND ANKYLOSING SPONDYLITIS		
Feature	Psoriatic arthritis	Ankylosing spondylitis
Sex M:F	1:1	9:1
Sacroiliac joints/ axial spine	35%	100%
Spinal movements	↓	↓↓
Peripheral joint involvement	90–95%	40%
Peripheral joint pattern	Upper and lower limbs Large and small joints	Lower limbs Large joints
Dactylitis	Common	Uncommon
HLA-B27	10–25%	90%
Spinal radiology	Random distribution Asymmetric 'Chunky' syndesmophytes	Contiguous involvement Symmetric Classic syndesmophytes

PROGNOSIS

Functional impairment

There have been only a few prospective studies of prognosis in psoriatic arthritis. The general impression is that the condition is associated with less long-term disability than is observed in RA[1]. Several hospital clinic series have, however, shown that between 11% and 42% of patients with psoriatic arthritis have American College of Rheumatology grade III or IV functional impairment at time of study[16,28,29,34]. All studies are agreed that there is an association between polyarthritis and functional disability. With regard to disease progression, studies from the University of Toronto Psoriatic Arthritis Clinic have shown that patients with at least five joint effusions at the time of presentation to the clinic are significantly more likely to develop progressive joint deformity at follow-up. Additional predictive factors include the presence of HLA-B27, -B39 or -DQw3[72,73].

Mortality

With regard to mortality, a community-based study in Olmsted County, Minnesota, USA showed no difference in survival for patients with psoriatic arthritis compared with members of the general population[14]. In contrast, in a hospital cohort an increased mortality rate compared with that in the general population was observed, with standardized mortality ratio values of 1.65 and 1.59 for males and females, respectively[74]; this likely reflects the spectrum of disease under long-term follow-up in hospital clinics. In this series, there was a particular excess of deaths as a result of diseases of the respiratory system such as pneumonia and obstructive airways disease[74]. The most significant pre-

dictive factors for mortality in this study were radiological damage, increased ESR and prior use of disease-modifying drugs, with nail lesions being identified as a 'protective factor'[75]. From these studies, one can conclude that patients with polyarthritis are most likely to have functional impairment and progression of disease. In addition, extensive and progressive disease may also be associated with an excess mortality.

REFERENCES

1. Moll JMH, Wright V. Psoriatic arthritis. Semin Arthritis Rheum 1973; 3: 55–78.
2. Wright V. Rheumatism and psoriasis. A re-evaluation. Am J Med 1959; 27: 454–462.
3. Blumberg BS, Bunim JJ, Calkins E et al. ARA nomenclature and classification of arthritis and rheumatism (tentative). Arthritis Rheum 1964; 7: 93–97.
4. Dawson MH, Tyson TL. Psoriasis arthropathica. With observations on certain features common to psoriasis and rheumatoid arthritis. Trans Assoc Am Physicians 1938; 53: 303–309.
5. Hellgren L. Association between rheumatoid arthritis and psoriasis in total populations. Acta Rheumatol Scand 1969; 15: 316–326.
6. Baker H. Epidemiological aspects of psoriasis and arthritis. Br J Dermatol 1966; 78: 249–261.
7. Mongan ES, Atwater EC. A comparison of patients with seropositive and seronegative rheumatoid arthritis. Med Clin North Am 1968; 52: 533–538.
8. Leczinsky CG. The incidence of arthropathy in a ten-year series of psoriasis cases. Acta Dermatoken 1948; 28: 483–487.
9. van Romunde LKJ, Valkenburg HA, Swart-Bruinsma W et al. Psoriasis and arthritis. I: A population study. Rheumatol Int 1984; 4: 55–60.
10. Harrison BJ, Silman AJ, Barrett EM et al. Presence of psoriasis does not influence the presentation or short term outcome of patients with early inflammatory polyarthritis. J Rheumatol 1997; 24: 1744–1749.
11. Scarpa R, Oriente P, Pucino A et al. Psoriatic arthritis in psoriatic patients. Br J Rheumatol 1984; 23: 246–250.
12. Little H, Harvie JN, Lester RS. Psoriatic arthritis in severe psoriasis. Can Med Assoc J 1975; 112: 317–319.
13. Lomholt G. Psoriasis. Prevalence, spontaneous course and genetics. A census study of the prevalence of skin diseases on the Faroe Islands. GEC GAD; Copenhagen: 1963.
14. Shbeeb M, Uramoto KM, Gibson LE et al. The epidemiology of psoriatic arthritis in Olmsted County, Minnesota, USA, 1982–1991. J Rheumatol 2000; 27: 1247–1250.
15. Kaipiainen-Seppanen O. Incidence of psoriatic arthritis in Finland. Br J Rheumatol 1996; 35: 1289–1291.
16. Gladman DD, Shuckett R, Russell ML et al. Psoriatic arthritis (PSA) – an Analysis of 220 patients. Q J Med 1987; 238: 127–141.
17. Jones SM, Armas J, Cohen M et al. Psoriatic arthritis: outcome of disease subsets and relationship of joint disease to nail and skin disease. Br J Rheumatol 1994; 33: 834–839.
18. Rahman P, Schentag CT, Gladman DD. Immunogenetic profile of patients with psoriatic arthritis varies according to the age at onset of psoriasis. Arthritis Rheum 1999; 42: 822–823.
19. Solinger AM, Hess EV. Rheumatic diseases and AIDS – is the association real? J Rheumatol 1994; 20: 678–683.
20. Mijiyawa M, Oniankitan O, Khan MA. Spondyloarthropathies in sub-Saharan Africa. Curr Opin Rheumatol 2000; 12: 281–286.
21. Njobvu P, McGill P, Kerr H et al. Spondyloarthropathy and human immunodeficiency virus infection in Zambia. J Rheumatol 1998; 25: 1553–1559.
22. Njobvu P, McGill P. Psoriatic arthritis and human immunodeficiency virus infection in Zambia. J Rheumatol 2000; 27: 1699–1702.
23. Calabrese LH, Kelley DM, Myers A et al. Rheumatic symptoms and human immunodeficiency virus infection. The influence of clinical and laboratory variables in a longitudinal cohort study. Arthritis Rheum 1991; 34: 257–263.
24. Berman A, Espinoza LR, Diaz JD et al. Rheumatic manifestations of human immunodeficiency virus infection. Am J Med 1988; 85: 59–64.
25. Espinoza LR, Berman A, Vasey FB et al. Posriatic arthritis and acquired immunodeficiency syndrome. Arthritis Rheum 1988; 31: 1034–1040.
26. Duvic M, Johnson TM, Rapini RP et al. Acquired immunodeficiency syndrome-associated psoriasis and Reiter's syndrome. Arch Dermatol 1987; 123: 1622–1632.
27. Dougados M, Van der Linden S, Juhlin R et al. The European Spondylarthropathy Study Group preliminary criteria for the classification of spondylarthropathy. Arthritis Rheum 1991; 34: 1218–1227.
28. Veale D, Rodgers S, Fitzgerald O. Classification of clinical subsets in psoriatic arthritis. Br J Rheumatol 1994; 33: 133–138.
29. Marsal S, Armadans-Gil L, Martinez M et al. Clinical, radiographic and HLA associations as markers for different patterns of psoriatic arthritis. Br J Rheumatol 1999; 38: 332–337.
30. Gladman DD, Brubacher B, Buskila D et al. Psoriatic spondyloarthropathy in men and women: a clinical, radiographic and HLA study. Clin Invest Med 1992; 15: 371–375.
31. Helliwell P, Marchesoni A, Peters M et al. A re-evaluation of the osteoarticular manifestations of psoriasis. Br J Rheumatol 1991; 30: 339–345.
32. Helliwell P, Hetthen J, Sokoll K et al. Joint symmetry in early and late rheumatoid and psoriatic arthritis. Arthritis Rheum 2000; 43: 865–871.
33. Van Romunde LKJ, Cats A, Hermans J, Valkenburg HA. Psoriasis and arthritis: II. A cross-sectional comparative study of patients with psoriatic arthritis and seronegative and seropositive polyarthritis: clinical aspects. Rheumatol Int 1984; 4: 61–65.
34. Torre Alonso JC, Rodriguez Perez A, Arribas Castrillo JM et al. Psoriatic arthritis (PA): a clinical, immunological and radiological study of 180 patients. Br J Rheumatol 1991; 30: 245–250.
35. Gladman DD, Brubacher B, Buskila D et al. Differences in the expression of spondyloarthropathy: a comparison between ankylosing spondylitis and psoriatic arthritis. Clin Invest Med 1992; 16: 1–7.
36. Hanly JG, Russell ML, Gladman DD. Psoriatic spondyloarthropathy: a long term prospective study. Ann Rheum Dis 1988; 47: 386–393.
37. Helliwell P, Hickling P, Wright V. Do the radiological changes of classic ankylosing spondylitis differ from the changes found in the spondylitis associated with inflammatory bowel disease, psoriasis, and reactive arthritis? Ann Rheum Dis 1998; 57: 135–140.
38. Jenkinson T, Armas J, Evison G et al. The cervical spine in psoriatic arthritis: a clinical and radiological study. Br J Rheumatol 1994; 33: 255–259.
39. Salvarani C, Macchioni P, Cremonesi T et al. The cervical spine in patients with psoriatic arthritis: a clinical, radiological and immunogenetic study. Ann Rheum Dis 1992; 51: 73–77.
40. Brockbank AJ, Stein M, Schentag CT et al. Characteristics of dactylitis in psoriatic arthritis (PsA). Arthritis Rheum 2000; 43(suppl): S105.
41. Olivieri I, Barozzi L, Favaro L et al. Dactylitis in patients with seronegative spondylarthropathy. Assessment by ultrasonography and magnetic resonance imaging. Arthritis Rheum 1996; 39: 1524–1529.
42. Olivieri I, Barozzi L, Pierro A et al. Toe dactylitis in patients with spondyloarthropathy: assessment by magnetic resonance imaging. J Rheumatol 1997; 24: 926–930.
43. McGonagle D, Gibbon W, Emery P. Classification of inflammatory arthritis by enthesitis. Lancet 1998; 352: 1137–1140.
44. Scarpa R. Peripheral enthesopathies in psoriatic arthritis. J Rheumatol 1998; 25: 2259–2290.
45. Cantini F, Salvarani C, Olivieri I et al. Distal extremity swelling with pitting edema in psoriatic arthritis: a case–control study. Clin Exp Rheumatol 2001; 19: 291–296.
46. Mulherin DM, FitzGerald O, Bresnihan B. Lymphedema of the upper limb in patients with psoriatic arthritis. Semin Arthritis Rheum 1993; 22: 350–356.
47. Salvarani C, Cantini F, Olivieri I et al. Distal extremity swelling with pitting edema in psoriatic arthritis: evidence of 2 pathological mechanisms. J Rheumatol 1999; 26: 1831–1834.
48. Hayem G, Bouchaud-Chabot A, Benali K et al. SAPHO syndrome: a long-term follow-up study of 120 cases. Semin Arthritis Rheum 1999; 29: 159–171.
49. Goupille P, Laulan J, Vedere V et al. Psoriatic onycho-periostitis. Scand J Rheumatol 1995; 24: 53–54.
50. Boisseau-Garsaud A-M, Beylot-Barry MD, Doutre M-S et al. Psoriatic onycho-pachydermo-periostitis. Arch Dermatol 1996; 132: 176–180.
51. Resnick D, Broderick TW. Bony proliferation of terminal toe phalanges in psoriasis: the 'ivory' phalanx. J Can Assoc Radiol 1977; 28: 187–189.
52. Stern RS. The epidemiology of joint complaints in patients with psoriasis. J Rheumatol 1985; 12: 315–320.
53. Cohen MR, Reda JD, Clegg DO. Baseline relationship between psoriasis and psoriatic arthritis: analysis of 221 patients with active psoriatic arthritis. J Rheumatol 1999; 28: 1752–1756.
54. Gladman DD. Psoriatic arthritis. Spine 1990; 4: 637–656.
55. Lambert JR, Ansell BM, Stephenson E, Wright V. Psoriatic arthritis in childhood. Clin Rheum Dis 1976; 2: 339–352.
56. Ansell BM. Juvenile psoriatic arthritis. Baillière's Clin Rheumatol 1994; 8: 317–332.
57. Southwood TR, Petty RE, Malleson PN et al. Psoriatic arthritis in children. Arthritis Rheum 1989; 32: 1007–1013.
58. Hamilton ML, Gladman DD, Shore A et al. Juvenile psoriatic arthritis and HLA antigens. Ann Rheum Dis 1990; 49: 694–697.
59. Shore A, Ansell BM. Juvenile psoriatic arthritis: an analysis of 60 cases. J Pediatr 1982; 100: 529–535.
60. Troughton PR, Morgan AW. Laboratory findings and pathology of psoriatic arthritis. Ballière's Clin Rheumatol 1994; 8: 439–463.
61. Laurent MR, Panayi GS, Shepherd P. Circulating immune complexes, serum immuno-globulins and acute phase protein in psoriasis and arthritis. Ann Rheum Dis 1981; 40: 66–69.
62. Bruce IN, Schentag CT, Gladman DD. Hyperuricemia in psoriatic arthritis prevalence and associated features. J Clin Rheumatol 2000; 6: 6–9.
63. Van Romunde LKJ, Cats A, Hermans J et al. Psoriasis and arthrisis. III: A cross-sectional comparative study of patients with psoriatic arthritis and seronegative and seropositive polyarthritis: radiological and HLA aspects. Rheumatol Int 1984; 4: 67–73.
64. Resnick D, Niwayama J. Psoriatic arthritis. In: Diagnosis of bone and joint disorders, 2nd edn. Philadelphia: WB Saunders 1988: 1171–1198.
65. Wright V. Psoriasis and arthritis. A study of the radiographic appearances. Br JRadiol 1957; 30: 113–119.

66. McEwen C, DiTata D, Lingg C *et al.* Ankylosing spondylitis and spondylitis accompanying ulcerative colitis, regional enteritis, psoriasis and Reiter's disease. A comparative study. Arthritis Rheum 1971; 14: 291–318.

67. Bywaters EGL, Dixon AStJ. Paravertebral ossification in psoriatic arthritis. Ann Rheum Dis 1965; 24: 313–331.

68. Jevtic V, Watt I, Rozman B *et al.* Distinctive radiological features of small hand joints in rheumatoid arthritis and seronegative spondyloarthritis demonstrated by contrast-enhanced (Gd-DTPA) magnetic resonance imaging. Skeletal Radiol 1995; 24: 351–355.

69. Offidani A, Cellini A, Valeri G, Giovagnoni A. Subclinical joint involvement in psoriasis: magnetic resonance imaging and X-ray findings. Acta Derm Venereol (Stockh) 1998; 78: 463–465.

70. Buskila D, Langevitz P, Gladman DD *et al.* Patients with rheumatoid arthritis are more tender than those with psoriatic arthritis. J Rheumatol 1992; 19: 1115–1119.

71. Bruce IN, Gladman DD. Psoriatic arthritis. Recognition and management. BioDrugs 1998; 9: 271–278.

72. Gladman DD, Farewell VT, Nadeau C. Clinical indicators of progression in psoriatic arthritis: multivariate relative risk model. J Rheumatol 1995; 22: 675–679.

73. Gladman DD, Farewell VT. The role of HLA antigens as indicators of disease progression in psoriatic arthritis. Arthritis Rheum 1995; 38: 845–850.

74. Wong K, Gladman DD, Husted J *et al.* Mortality studies in psoriatic arthritis. Arthritis Rheum 1997; 40: 1868–1872.

75. Gladman DD, Farewell VT, Wong K, Husted J. Mortality studies in psoriatic arthritis. results from a single outpatient center. II. Prognostic indicators for death. Arthritis Rheum 1998; 41: 1103–1110.

32 Psoriatic arthritis: management

Marta L Cuéllar and Luis R Espinoza

- Management of psoriatic arthritis should be comprehensive and includes non-pharmacological, pharmacological, rehabilitative and surgical reconstructive therapies with concomitant skin management

- Most patients with psoriatic arthritis – particularly those with peripheral joint involvement – exhibit excellent clinical response to traditional or non-selective non-steroidal anti-inflammatory drugs (NSAIDs). Selective cyclo-oxygenase-2 inhibitors also appear to be effective, but prospective controlled studies regarding their efficacy are not yet available

- Disease-modifying agents, including methotrexate and leflunomide alone or in combination, are effective in the management of psoriatic arthritis refractory to NSAIDs

- The use of biological agents (infliximab, etanercept) is being shown to be highly efficacious and their use accompanied by a high remission rate and decreased progression of radiographic damage

TABLE 32.1 THERAPEUTIC MANAGEMENT OF PSORIATIC ARTHRITIS

Patient education	Assistive devices and educational material
Rehabilitation and physical therapy	Early and aggressive active and passive physical therapy Dynamic strengthening exercises Preservation of a normal upright posture Avoidance of contact sports and heavy physical activity
Pharmacologic measures	Non-steroidal anti-inflammatory drugs Selective COX-2 inhibitors Disease-modifying drugs
Dermatologic measures	Photochemotherapy with psoralen Steroids
Surgical measures	Synovectomy Joint arthroplasty

Early institution of an aggressive comprehensive medical management program may prevent the development of serious joint deformity and disability

INTRODUCTION

The introduction, in recent years, of more powerful and specific anti-inflammatory agents with improved efficacy or decreased toxicity, or both, is having a major impact in the way rheumatologists manage patients with chronic arthritis, including rheumatoid arthritis (RA) and psoriatic arthritis. The use of cyclo-oxygenase (COX)-2-selective non-steroidal anti-inflammatory drugs (NSAIDs), leflunomide, and specific tumor necrosis factor (TNF)-α inhibitors has expanded the therapeutic armamentarium for the management of these chronic rheumatic disorders[1-3]. Although it has become quite clear that treatment with methotrexate, sulfasalazine and cyclosporin is efficacious and associated with a fairly acceptable safety profile in patients with psoriatic arthritis[4,5], it is increasingly being demonstrated, particularly in RA, that the use of the newer compounds, especially the biologic agents etanercept and infliximab, is accompanied by a high rate of remission and decreased progression of radiographic damage[6,7].

These major advances in drug development are ameliorating the care provided to patients with psoriatic arthritis. More importantly, the early use of these agents allows better suppression of skin and joint inflammation, maintenance and improvement of musculoskeletal function, prevention of joint deformity and disability, and emotional adjustment to the presence of skin rash and arthritis[8,9]. A multidisciplinary approach involving the close collaboration of rheumatologists, dermatologists, primary care physicians, orthopedists and rehabilitation specialists is needed in order to accomplish these objectives.

The management of psoriatic arthritis should be a comprehensive one, and includes pharmacological, rehabilitative and surgical reconstructive treatments, with concomitant management of skin involvement[10] (Tables 32.1–32.3).

PHARMACOLOGIC MANAGEMENT

Non-steroidal anti-inflammatory treatment

Most patients with psoriatic arthritis exhibit excellent clinical response of their peripheral joint involvement while receiving NSAIDs. With the exception of aspirin, the great majority of traditional or non-selective NSAIDs, given at full doses, have been shown to be beneficial for patients with psoriatic arthritis presenting with the oligoarticular or monoarticular pattern of joint involvement[11]. In contrast, patients with psoriatic

TABLE 32.2 DISEASE-MODIFYING DRUGS IN PSORIATIC ARTHRITIS

- Methotrexate
- Sulfasalazine
- Cyclosporin A
- Azathioprine
- Leflunomide
- Biological agents
  - Etanercept (Enbrel)
  - Infliximab (Remicade)
  - Alefacept
- Gold compounds
- Retinoid treatment
- Corticosteroids
- Colchicine

The most common agents used in treatment of psoriatic arthritis – alone or in combination

TABLE 32.3 MISCELLANEOUS AGENTS USED IN THE TREATMENT OF PSORIATIC ARTHRITIS

- Antimalarials
- Vitamin D derivatives
- D-penicillamine
- Apheresis
- Antibiotics
- Non-selective inhibitors of TNF-α
  - Pamidronate?
  - Thalidomide?
- Alternative treatment?
- Autologous stem cell transplantation

The use of some of these agents and treatment modalities, such as alternative therapy, autologous stem cell transplantation and non-selective inhibitors of TNF-α, requires further investigation

arthritis exhibiting polyarticular, spondylitic or more severe forms of joint involvement usually require a more aggressive form of treatment, including the use of second-line agents alone or in combination.

There is still no great body of evidence regarding the use of celecoxib and rofecoxib, both COX-2-selective inhibitors, in patient with psoriatic arthritis. COX-2-selective inhibitors are replacing non-selective NSAIDs because of their better gastrointestinal safety[12], but their role in the management of psoriatic arthritis is not yet established. There is a need for prospective and controlled studies with selective COX-2 inhibitors in psoriatic arthritis, in order to define their precise role.

Disease-modifying agents

It is well established that psoriatic arthritis may not be benign, but can lead to significant functional limitation and deforming destructive arthropathy in up to 20–30% of patients[13]. Risk factors associated with poor prognosis have been identified (Table 32.4), and early use of more aggressive treatment, including disease-modifying agents, is widespread, with the added advantage that most of these agents also have a beneficial effect on psoriasis. A variety of disease-modifying agents have been used, including sulfasalazine, methotrexate, antimalarials, gold compounds, azathioprine, retinoids and cyclosporin A. More recently, the use of biologic agents such as etanercept and infliximab, and other agents such as leflunomide, has been shown to have an excellent beneficial effect for both skin and joint involvement, accompanied by a good safety profile.

Methotrexate

Methotrexate is the agent of choice for a large proportion of patients with psoriatic arthritis unresponsive to NSAIDs[14]. Its use in early psori-

atic arthritis with or without NSAIDs or in combination with other disease-modifying agents, particularly sulfasalazine or cyclosporin A, has been recommended. The average dose is between 7.5 and 15mg per week, given as a single dose or divided into two doses taken 12h apart on the same day; we prefer the former. The dosage can be increased to 25–30mg per week until improvement occurs, and then it should be tapered down to a maintenance dose, which varies from patient to patient. Methotrexate given at these dosages has been shown to be effective for both skin and joint inflammatory involvement in most studies, both control and uncontrolled. Some studies, however, have failed to demonstrate its efficacy in the treatment of psoriatic arthritis.

Lacaille et al.[15] recently reported on their experience with long-term treatment with intramuscular gold and methotrexate. They reviewed medical records from all patients with psoriatic arthritis attending the gold and methotrexate clinics at the Vancouver Mary Pack Arthritis Centre between 1971 and 1995. The odds of a clinical response (defined as at least 50% reduction in active joint count from initial to last visit or for at least 6 months) and the relative risk of discontinuing treatment (methotrexate or intramuscular gold) were estimated after controlling for significant baseline covariates, using logistic regression and Cox regression analyses, respectively. The frequency of side effects and the reasons for treatment cessation were also compared. Eighty-seven patients received 111 treatment courses, 43 of methotrexate and 68 of intramuscular gold. The likelihood of a clinical response was 8.9 times greater [95% confidence interval (CI) 1.8 to 44.0] with methotrexate than with intramuscular gold. The frequency of side effects was similar for both treatments, but patients were 5 times more likely (95% CI 2.4 to 10.4) to discontinue treatment with intramuscular gold than with methotrexate. No major or severe toxicity occurred. Of interest, patients with psoriatic arthritis with a longer duration of disease before initiation of study treatment were less likely to achieve a clinical response. The authors concluded that methotrexate was well tolerated and superior to intramuscular gold, and that their data supported the notion that earlier treatment may be associated with a better clinical response.

In general, methotrexate is well tolerated and has a very good safety profile. It is necessary, however, to monitor carefully liver and renal function, hematological indexes and other predisposing risk factors, such as low serum albumin, concomitant use of antibiotics, in order to prevent serious toxicity[16]. Serious side effects may occur, but appear to be relatively infrequent, particularly if monitoring is performed every 6–8 weeks (Table 32.5). At present, there are no adequate evidence-based guidelines for monitoring liver toxicity in patients with psoriatic arthritis who are receiving methotrexate treatment. Therefore, it is recommended that each patient's need for liver biopsy should be evaluated individually and that patients should undergo biopsy only if a specific cumulative dose of methotrexate has been reached (>3g) or a persistent significant increase in liver enzymes is present (more than three times the upper limit of normal). The American College of Rheumatology guidelines for monitoring liver toxicity in methotrexate-treated patients with RA recommend that liver biopsies need not be

TABLE 32.4 PSORIATIC ARTHRITIS: RISK FACTORS FOR A POOR PROGNOSIS

- Juvenile onset
- Young adult onset
- Extensive skin involvement
- Polyarticular involvement
- Failed response to non-steroidal anti-inflammatory drugs
- Association with HIV infection
- Association with certain HLA antigens
  - HLA-B27, correlates with spondylotic involvement
  - HLA-B27, -B39 and -DQw3 correlate with progressive disease
  - HLA-DR3, -DR4 correlate with erosive disease.

Recognition of these risk factors associated with disease severity allows better and prompt planning of an early and aggressive therapeutic program

TABLE 32.5 RISK FACTORS ASSOCIATED WITH METHOTREXATE TOXICITY

- Renal insufficiency
- Low serum albumin
- Concomitant use of antibiotics
- Folate deficiency
- Older age
- Cumulative dose

Predisposing factors most commonly associated with methotrexate toxicity

performed before methotrexate administration or routinely thereafter. These suggestions were based on the incidence of clinically significant liver disease, the factors predictive of its occurrence, the cost of the procedure and the complications arising from it[17].

Sulfasalazine

Evidence accumulated over the past several years has provided support for a beneficial effect of sulfasalazine in patients with psoriatic arthritis. Both controlled and uncontrolled studies have demonstrated a good clinical response of the peripheral arthritis in patients with psoriatic arthritis. Its main limiting factor is its well-recognized gastrointestinal intolerance, with up to 40% of patients unable to tolerate full doses because of severe gastrointestinal distress.

Clegg et al.[18] have published their experience with sulfasalazine in the treatment of psoriatic arthritis. Their objective was to determine whether sulfasalazine at a dosage of 2g/day was effective for the treatment of active psoriatic arthritis unresponsive to NSAIDs. They recruited 221 patients with psoriatic arthritis from 15 clinics, allocated them randomly to groups to receive sulfasalazine or placebo, and followed them for 36 weeks. Treatment response was based on joint pain/tenderness and swelling scores, and physician and patient global assessment. Longitudinal analysis revealed a trend favoring sulfasalazine treatment, although this did not reach statistical significance. At the end of treatment, response rates were 58% for sulfasalazine, compared with 45% for placebo ($p = 0.05$). In addition, the Westergren erythrocyte sedimentation rate declined more in the group taking sulfasalazine than in those taking placebo ($p < 0.0001$). Adverse reactions were few and were mainly non-specific gastrointestinal complaints such as dyspepsia, nausea, vomiting and diarrhea.

In a subsequent analysis, Clegg et al.[19] examined the data comparing the effects of sulfasalazine 2g/day and placebo on the axial and peripheral articular manifestations of psoriatic arthritis. Patients were classified as treatment responders on the basis of meeting predefined improvement criteria in four outcome measures: both patient and physician global assessments in all patients, morning stiffness and back pain in patients with axial manifestations, and joint pain/tenderness scores and joint swelling scores in patients with peripheral articular manifestations. Of the patients with axial disease, 40% of the sulfasalazine group and 43% of the placebo group met the predefined response criteria ($p = 0.67$). Of the patients with peripheral arthritis, 59% of the sulfasalazine-treated patients and 43% of the placebo-treated patients showed a response ($p = 0.0007$). Therefore, it appears that the response to sulfasalazine of patients with seronegative spondyloarthropathy including psoriatic arthritis is related to the peripheral articular manifestations of their disease. Axial and peripheral articular manifestations of seronegative spondyloarthropathy appear to respond differently to sulfasalazine. In patients with persistently active peripheral arthritis, sulfasalazine is safe, well tolerated, and effective.

Rahman et al.[20] also published their experience of the use of sulfasalazine in patients with psoriatic arthritis attending their psoriatic arthritis clinic at the University of Toronto. For patients who were able to tolerate sulfasalazine for at least 3 months, a matched control was identified who did not receive sulfasalazine. The primary outcome measures were the tolerability of sulfasalazine, clinical response of the actively inflamed joints at 6 and 12 months, and the change in radiograph score at 24 months. Thirty-six patients received sulfasalazine. Fourteen patients discontinued sulfasalazine because of one or more side effects occurring within 3 months of initiation of treatment. For the remaining 20 patients, a 50% reduction in actively inflamed joint count was seen in seven of 20 patients at 6 months and 11 of 15 patients at 12 months, compared with seven of 19 patients in the control group at 6 months and 10 of 20 at 12 months. No change in radiographic score at 24 months was observed in either group. In this study, sulfasalazine treatment was accompanied by a high frequency of side effects, did not show beneficial effect over the control group, and did not halt radiographic progress in psoriatic arthritis.

There is a high rate of discontinuation of sulfasalazine secondary to gastrointestinal intolerance. In order to minimize this, a 'start low, go slow' approach is recommended. In addition, the use of enteric-coated formulations of sulfasalazine should improve gastrointestinal tolerability and thus patient acceptance. It is recommended to start with 500mg of sulfasalazine twice daily for the first 10–14 days, and then to increase it gradually over, the next 2–3 weeks, to 2g daily. Some patients may require doses up to 3g daily.

Cyclosporin A

The use of cyclosporin A alone or in combination with other disease-modifying antirheumatic drugs (DMARDs), most commonly methotrexate, sulfasalazine, or both, has been shown to be an effective therapeutic agent for the treatment of severe, recalcitrant psoriasis and its related arthritis. Cyclosporin A has also been shown to be effective in patients with palmoplantar pustulosis, and in the presence of certain extra-articular and dermatological complications, including lymphedema[21].

The efficacy of cyclosporin A in the treatment of these disorders has been demonstrated in several placebo-controlled studies[22]. Most recently, Raffayova et al.[23] conducted an open 18-week study with cyclosporin A administered to patients with psoriatic arthritis and confirmed its therapeutic efficacy. A significant improvement in psoriatic symptoms was observed during the study. As early as 2 weeks after administration of an average daily dose of cyclosporin A 4.8mg/kg, skin symptoms improved by 66%. Arthritis also improved after 18 weeks. In this study, the lowest optimal effective maintenance dose was 3.3mg/kg. Improvement was achieved after an average of 10 weeks of administration of cyclosporin A.

In general, the clinical response of both skin and joint involvement is dose related, and may occur with doses of cyclosporin A appreciably lower than those used in transplantation – for example, 2.5–5mg/kg per day – and improvement is seen at 3–4 weeks in most patients. Some concern, however, remains about serious side effects, particularly renal, even with low doses. The exact rate of relapse upon discontinuation of the drug, its long-term side effects, and its high costs are issues that remain unsolved.

Leflunomide

Leflunomide is a relatively new agent in the antirheumatic treatment of RA[24]. The active metabolite, A-77-1726, inhibits the enzyme dihydroorotate dehydrogenase, which has a critical role in de novo production of pyrimidine. It controls mitogen-induced T cell proliferation, as the presence of pyrimidine is needed for this process to proceed. Psoriasis and its related arthritis are believed to be mediated by T cell dependent mechanisms[25,26].

Liang and Barr[27] recently evaluated the efficacy and toxicity of this compound in the treatment of both psoriasis and psoriatic arthritis. Twelve consecutive patients with psoriatic arthritis who had failed to respond to at least one DMARD were started on a regimen of leflunomide alone or in addition to their previous disease-modifying medication. Global assessment of improvement in psoriasis and psoriatic arthritis was scored on a 0–3 scale after 2–3 months of treatment. Modified tender and swollen joint counts, patients' and physicians' global assessments and grip strength before and after treatment were available for analysis in 50% of these patients. Eight patients had combined moderate-to-marked improvement in both psoriasis and psoriatic arthritis. Three patients in whom toxicity necessitated the temporary discontinuation of the drug were able to resume the drug at lower dosage with a good clinical benefit. Three patients discontinued the treatment, but in none of them was this because of toxicity. Effect on radiological progression of the disease was not evaluated. These data suggest that leflunomide alone or in combination with another DMARD may be effective in controlling both skin and joint disease in patients with psoriasis and psoriatic arthritis. Improvement was seen within 4–8 weeks, and arthritis appeared to have a better and more rapid response than skin involvement. There is a need, however, for placebo-controlled trials of leflunomide in psoriatic arthritis.

The correct place of leflunomide in the management of psoriatic arthritis remains to be determined. Extrapolating from the experience seen in RA, it appears that leflunomide may be indicated initially in those patients with psoriatic arthritis who have suboptimal responses to methotrexate, or in combination with methotrexate. This combination – leflunomide and methotrexate – is well tolerated by RA patients and there are no significant pharmacokinetic interactions between the drugs[28]. The potential risk of serious liver damage should be kept in mind, however, when combination treatment with leflunomide and methotrexate is used[29].

Leflunomide is contraindicated during pregnancy and lactation. Contraception is mandatory for women of childbearing age who are receiving this drug. Women receiving leflunomide who are suspected to be pregnant should stop it immediately and be carefully monitored by their physician. A negative pregnancy test before initiation of treatment is recommended. Men receiving leflunomide should also use adequate contraception.

Gold therapy

Chrysotherapy is beneficial in a subset of patients with psoriatic arthritis[30]. Patients with psoriatic arthritis exhibiting polyarticular involvement present a better clinical response to gold compounds than do patients with psoriatic arthritis presenting with the oligoarticular and spondylitic types. It has been shown, however, to be much less effective than methotrexate treatment[15].

Azathioprine

Azathioprine has been shown to be effective in psoriasis for both skin and joint involvement[31]. Doses ranging from 2 to 3mg/kg per day are recommended, with close monitoring of bone marrow function, because of the potential of the drug for serious marrow toxicity. Patients receiving long-term azathioprine treatment should also be screened for underlying malignancy. Azathioprine hypersensitivity reactions may also occur[32].

Retinoid treatment

Retinoid compounds, particularly etritinate, have been shown to be highly effective in the management of psoriasis and psoriatic arthritis[33]. A main limitation in the use of these compounds, however, is the high incidence of side effects. In addition, the teratogenic potential of these compounds remains a serious limitation for their use in women of childbearing age.

Mycophenolate mofetil

Mycophenolate mofetil is widely used as an immunosuppressant in organ transplantation, and also in some autoimmune disorders such as pyroderma gangrenosum, systemic lupus erythematosus and dermatomyositis[34]. It has recently been used with great effectiveness in psoriasis and psoriatic arthritis. Grundman-Kollman et al.[35] reported their experience in five patients with moderate to severe chronic plaque psoriasis and six patients with psoriatic arthritis refractory to conventional systemic or topical antipsoriatic treatment and who were treated with mycophenolate mofetil monotherapy (2g/day) in a 10-week study. Patients with moderate psoriasis and psoriatic arthritis responded well to treatment, whereas those with severe psoriasis did not respond to this

drug. It was well tolerated, and this compound may develop into a therapeutic alternative in patients with psoriatic arthritis.

Meta-analysis of DMARDs

Jones et al.[36] performed a meta-analysis in psoriatic arthritis, with the objective of determining the relative efficacy and toxicity of pharmacological agents in the treatment of the condition. The main outcome measures included individual component variables derived from the Outcome Measures in Rheumatology Clinical Trials Core Set for RA. These include acute-phase reactants, disability, pain, patient global assessment, swollen joint count, tender joint count and radiographic changes of joints in any trial of 1 year or longer, and the change in pooled disease index. Nineteen randomized trials were identified, of which 11 were included in the quantitative analysis with data from 777 individuals. All agents were better than placebo, but only parenteral high-dose methotrexate, salazopyrin, azathioprine and etretinate achieved statistical significance for the global index of disease activity. Analysis of response in individual disease activity markers was more variable, with considerable differences between different medications and responses. In all trials, the placebo group improved over baseline. There were insufficient data to allow examination of toxicity. It was concluded that parenteral high-dose methotrexate and salazopyrin are the only two agents with well-demonstrated published efficacy in psoriatic arthritis. The magnitude of the effect with etretinate, oral low-dose methotrexate and azathioprine suggests that they may be effective, but that further multicenter clinical trials are needed to establish their efficacy.

Biologic agents

Two biologic agents, etanercept and infliximab – both TNF-α inhibitors – have been approved for their use in the treatment of RA[37,38]. Inhibition of the proinflammatory cytokine, TNF, is associated with a marked decrease in the signs and symptoms of RA in the majority of patients.

Both psoriasis and its related arthritis are pathological processes mainly mediated by activated T cells, which appear to be responsible for the epidermal and synovial hyperproliferation seen, and also inflammatory infiltration in the epidermis, dermis and subsynovial space[25,26]. These activated T cells release a variety of cytokines, including TNF-α, interleukin (IL)-6, IL-8, granulocyte-macrophage colony-stimulating factor (GM-CSF), and interferon gamma. The proinflammatory cytokine TNF-α has a major role in this process, and has been detected in increased concentrations in both psoriatic skin and synovial lesions. TNF-α, through activation of nuclear factor (NF) κB, induces synthesis of several cytokines, particularly IL-6, IL-8 and GM-CSF. In addition, TNF-α favors the accumulation of inflammatory cells in both skin and synovium, by upregulating the expression of intracellular adhesion molecule-I on endothelial cells and keratinocytes[39]. Therefore, it is quite logical to assume a potential role for TNF-α in both psoriasis and psoriatic arthritis, and also infer that use of inhibitors of TNF-α may result in amelioration of disease activity in these disorders.

Evidence is rapidly accumulating, from both controlled and uncontrolled trials, that inhibition of TNF-α results in significant clinical response of both psoriasis and psoriatic arthritis.

The first randomized, double-blind, placebo-controlled trial of etanercept, a TNF-α inhibitor, in patients with psoriatic arthritis was a 12-week study undertaken to assess the efficacy and safety of etanercept 25 mg twice weekly by subcutaneous injection or placebo, in 60 patients with psoriasis and psoriatic arthritis[40]. Psoriatic arthritis endpoints included the proportion of patients who met the Psoriatic Arthritis Response Criteria and who met the American College of Rheumatology preliminary criteria for improvement (ACR20). Psoriasis endpoints included improvement in the psoriasis area and severity index (PASI), and improvement in prospectively identified individual target lesions. Most psoriatic arthritis patients (87%) fulfilled the Psoriatic Arthritis Response Criteria, compared with seven (23%) of patients in the placebo-controlled group. The ACR20 was achieved by 22 (73%) of etanercept-treated patients, compared with four (13%) of placebo-treated patients. Of the 19 patients in each treatment group assessed for psoriasis, five (26%) of the etanercept-treated patients achieved a 75% improvement in the PASI, compared with none of the placebo-treated patients ($p = 0.015$). The median improvement in PASI was 46%, compared with 9% in etanercept-treated and placebo-treated patients, respectively; similarly, median target lesion improvements were 50% and 0, respectively. Etanercept was well tolerated.

Several pilot studies have shown similar results[41–43]. In our experience with more than 20 patients with psoriatic arthritis treated in this manner, etanercept has been shown to be highly effective for both skin and nails, and also joint involvement – both peripheral and spinal. Some of our patients with psoriatic arthritis have also experienced a significant radiologic improvement in their erosive involvement, in a manner similar to that described for RA patients. Etanercept has also been shown to be effective in human immunodeficiency virus-associated psoriatic arthritis refractory to DMARDs[44]. Its use in this situation, however, should be carefully monitored, in view of the fatal sepsis that occurred in that particular patient[44].

An open trial of infliximab, the second inhibitor of TNF-α approved for the treatment of RA, has shown this agent to be highly effective in the treatment of severe psoriatic arthritis, and well tolerated over 1 year of use. As already shown with etanercept, skin involvement also responds well[45].

Data on the use of these agents in psoriasis are also relevant for consideration. Chaudhari et al.[46] recently published their experience with infliximab in a group of patients with psoriasis who had moderate to severe plaque psoriasis involving at least 5% of the body surface area. Their objective was to assess the clinical benefit and safety of infliximab monotherapy and to determine the role of TNF-α in the pathogenesis of psoriasis. Thirty-three patients were randomly assigned to receive intravenous placebo ($n = 11$) or infliximab 5mg/kg ($n = 11$) or infliximab 10mg/kg ($n = 11$) at weeks 0, 2 and 6. Patients were assessed at week 10 for the primary endpoint (score on the physician's global assessment). Three patients withdrew from the study. Both groups of infliximab-treated patients experienced significant and similar clinical improvement when compared with those receiving placebo. The median time to response was 4 weeks for patients in both infliximab groups. Infliximab was well tolerated and no serious side effects were noted. These findings confirm the efficacy of inhibition of TNF-α in the treatment of psoriasis, and also provide support for an important role of TNF-α in the pathogenesis of these disorders.

Accumulated evidence strongly suggests that both available inhibitors of TNF-α are powerful anti-inflammatory agents and extremely effective for both psoriasis and psoriatic arthritis. Issues that remain to be defined include whether or not they should be used in patients refractory to other DMARDs, whether they should be used alone or in combination with other DMARDS, and for how long they should be used. Their place in the management of these disorders, however, remains to be defined. There is a need for long-term studies to determine their safety profile, especially given the recent reports of rare but serious infectious complications in patients with RA[47].

A highly promising disease-remitting agent, alefacept, has recently been shown to be effective in the treatment of chronic plaque psoriasis. Alefacept exerts a pronounced inhibitory effect on CD45RO$^+$ T lymphocytes and was shown in a multicenter, randomized, placebo-controlled, double-blind study to be associated with significant and, in some patients, sustained clinical response after the cessation of treatment.

Patients with psoriatic arthritis were not included in the study, however[48].

Other drugs
Corticosteroid treatment
Systemic corticosteroids should be used only in extreme situations such as in patients with severe exacerbation of both skin and joint disease refractory to conventional treatment. Their topical use, however, is recommended for control of skin disease. Their use in children should be avoided because of the high relapse rate, and toxicity upon reduction or discontinuation of their use. Intra-articular corticosteroid use may be of great benefit in patients with mono- or oligoarticular psoriatic arthritis. The use of high-frequency ultrasonography may provide great guidance when approaching small joints[49].

Colchichine treatment
Colchicine at a dose of 1.5 mg/day in divided doses may be of benefit to a subset of patients with psoriatic arthritis, such as those presenting with arthro-osteitis and SAPHO syndrome[50]. It has been reported that colchicine may be beneficial for renal amyloidosis associated with psoriatic arthritis[51].

Miscellaneous agents
A variety of agents, including antimalarials, apheresis, vitamin D derivatives, D-penicillamine and photochemotherapy with methoxypsoralen, have been used to treat patients with psoriatic arthritis[52,53]. The use of these agents, however, has almost been abandoned in favor of methotrexate or newer DMARDs or biologic agents, because of their limited clinical response, or their high frequency of side effects.

It would be of great interest to assess the clinical response of patients with psoriatic arthritis to less selective inhibitors of TNF-α. Both pamidronate – a bisphosphonate synthetic analog of pyrophosphate – and thalidomide have been shown to inhibit the action of TNF-α. To date, clinical experience with these compounds has shown promising clinical responses in patients with ankylosing spondylitis[54,55]. Autologous stem cell transplantation is a promising therapeutic option in some refractory autoimmune disorders. To date, however, there is only limited experience in psoriatic arthritis, and further studies are needed to define its indications and effectiveness in the management of psoriatic arthritis[56].

NON-DRUG TREATMENTS

Balneotherapy
Balneotherapy (mud packs and sulfur baths) at the Dead Sea has been shown to benefit patients with psoriatic arthritis[57]. More recently, Elkayan et al.[58] reported on their experience in a total of 42 patients with psoriatic arthritis treated for 4 weeks. Patients were randomly allocated to two groups. Both groups received daily sun exposure and regular bathing at the Dead Sea; one group was also treated with mud packs and sulfur baths. Patients were assessed 3 days before arrival, at the end of 4 weeks, and at weeks 8, 16 and 28 from the start of treatment. Comparison between groups revealed a similar statistically significant improvement for variables such as PASI, morning stiffness, patient self-assessment, right and left grip, Schober test and distance from finger to floor when bending forward. Improvement in other variables such as number of tender and swollen joints, and inflammatory neck and back pain, was statistically significant only in the group receiving balneotherapy. Thus the addition of balneotherapy to sun exposure and Dead Sea baths appears to prolong beneficial effects and improves inflammatory neck and back pain. Sukenik et al.[59] obtained similar results in patients with psoriatic arthritis and concomitant fibromyalgia.

REHABILITATION

The indications for rehabilitation management follow the same guidelines as those for any other chronic inflammatory articular disorder. Rehabilitation therapy should be considered in every patient with psoriatic arthritis, and should be aimed at maximizing the potential for normal physical and emotional activities.

Most patients with psoriatic arthritis will benefit from a combination of rest, exercise and, when appropriate, selective joint immobilization. The implementation of any of these measures alone or in combination will depend on the degree of active synovitis and the type and size of joint involvement. Early joint mobilization after surgery, particularly of small joints of the hands, is necessary because rapid development of joint/bone fusion is characteristically seen in psoriatic arthritis. Local heat facilitates implementation of exercise therapy in the postoperative phase.

Cryotherapy in the form of ice packs, ethyl chloride or fluromethane sprays, or ice massage is more beneficial and physiologic in the presence of enthesitis and joint inflammation.

In patients with spondylitis, implementation of exercise designed to preserve a normal upright posture is recommended. Treatment to prevent or to treat osteoporosis should be instituted as early as possible and prolonged use of corsets or bed rest should also be avoided. Patients with psoriatic arthritis should be counseled and advised to avoid heavy physical activity and contact sports, but swimming should be encouraged.

The use of orthotic devices including crutches, walkers, canes and splints should be advised in order to improve both ambulation and the functional capacity of a given joint.

SURGICAL MANAGEMENT

Considerable progress in the medical management of psoriasis and psoriatic arthritis has occurred. This is expected to translate into an improved morbidity and other related complications in these disorders. With the advent of newer therapeutic modalities, particularly the use of biologic agents, it is anticipated that there will be a greater rate of remission and, more importantly, preservation of joint function and prevention of joint destruction and deformity, in patients with psoriatic arthritis. Synovectomy may still be used in highly selected cases, and major reconstructive surgery, including joint replacement, is to be performed when necessary.

REFERENCES

1. Dougados M, Behier JM, Jolchine I et al. Efficacy of celecoxib, a COX-2 specific inhibitor in ankylosing spondylitis: a placebo and conventional NSAID controlled study. Arthritis Rheum 2001; 44: 180–185.
2. Weinblatt ME, Kremer JM, Coblyn JS et al. Pharmacokinetics, safety, and efficacy of combination treatment with MTX and leflunomide in patients with active rheumatoid arthritis. Arthritis Rheum 1999; 42: 1322–1328.
3. Jones RE, Moreland LW. Tumor necrosis factor inhibitors for rheumatoid arthritis. Bull Rheum Dis 1999; 48: 1–4.
4. Cuellar ML, Espinoza LR. Management of the spondyloarthropathies. Curr Opinion Rheumatol 1996; 8: 288–295.
5. Salvarani C, Olivieri I, Cantini F et al. Psoriatic arthritis. Curr Opinion Rheumatol 1999; 11: 251–256.
6. Moreland LW, Schiff MH, Baumgartner SW et al. Etanercept therapy in rheumatoid arthritis. A randomized, controlled trial. Ann Intern Med 1999; 130: 478–486.
7. Antoni C, Kalden JR. Combination therapy of the chimeric monoclonal anti-tumor necrosis factor alpha antibody (infliximab) with methotrexate in patients with rheumatoid arthritis. Clin Exp Rheumatol 1999; 17(suppl 18): S73–S77.
8. Cuellar ML, Citera G, Espinoza LR. Treatment of psoriatic arthritis. Baillières Clin Rheumatol 1994; 8: 483–498.
9. Gladman DD. Natural history of psoriatic arthritis. Baillières Clin Rheumatol 1994; 8: 379–394.
10. Cuellar ML, Espinoza LR. Psoriatic arthritis: current development. J Fla Med Assoc 1995; 82: 338–342.
11. Gladman DD, Brockbank J. Psoriatic arthritis. Exp Opinion Invest Drugs 2000; 9: 1511–1522.
12. Lipsky PE, Abramson SB, Breedveld FC et al. Analysis of the effect of COX-2 specific inhibitors and recommendations for their use in clinical practice. J Rheumatol 2000; 27: 1338–1340.
13. Gladman DD, Schuckett R, Russell ML et al. Psoriatic arthritis (PSA) – an analysis of 220 patients. Q J Med 1987; 238: 127–141.
14. Espinoza LR, Zakraoui L, Espinoza CG et al. Psoriatic arthritis: clinical responses and side effects to methotrexate therapy. J Rheumatol 1992; 12: 872–877.
15. Lacaille D, Stein HB, Raboud J, Klinkhoff AV. Longterm therapy of psoriatic arthritis: intramuscular gold or methotrexate? J Rheumatol 2000; 27: 1922–1927.
16. Gutierrez-Urena S, Molina JF, Garcia C et al. Pancytopenia secondary to methotrexate therapy in rheumatoid arthritis. Arthritis Rheum 1996; 39: 272–276.
17. Kremer JM, Alarcon GS, Lightfoot RW Jr et al. Methotrexate for rheumatoid arthritis: suggested guidelines for monitoring liver toxicity. Arthritis Rheum 1994; 37: 316–328.
18. Clegg DO, Reda DJ, Mejias E et al. Comparison of sulfasalazine and placebo in the treatment of psoriatic arthritis. A Department of Veterans Affairs Study. Arthritis Rheum 1996; 39: 2013–2020.
19. Clegg DO, Reda DJ, Abdellatif M. Comparison of sulfasalazine and placebo for the treatment of axial and peripheral articular manifestations of the seronegative spondyloarthropathies: a Department of Veterans Affairs cooperative study. Arthritis Rheum 1999; 42: 2325–2329.
20. Rahman P, Gladman DD, Cook RJ et al. The use of sulfasalazine in psoriatic arthritis: a clinic experience. J Rheumatol 1998; 25: 1957–1961.
21. Vaccaro M, Borgia F, Guarneri F et al. Successful treatment of pustulotic arthro-osteitis (Sonozaki syndrome) with systemic cyclosporin. Clin Exp Dermatol 2001; 26: 45–47.
22. Mahrle G, Schulze HJ, Farber L et al. Low-dose short-term cyclosporine versus etretinate in psoriasis: improvement of skin, nail, and joint involvement. J Am Acad Dermatol 1995; 32: 78–88.
23. Raffayova H, Rovensky J, Malis F. Treatment with cyclosporin in patients with psoriatic arthritis: results of clinical assessment. Int J Clin Pharmacol Res 2000; 20: 1–11.
24. Kremer JM. Methotrexate and leflunomide: biochemical basis for combination therapy in the treatment of rheumatoid arthritis. Semin Arthritis Rheum 1999; 29: 14–26.
25. Gottlieb AB. Immunopathogenesis of psoriasis. Arch Dermatol 1997; 133: 781–782.
26. Espinoza LR, van Solingen R, Cuellar ML, Angulo J. Insights into the pathogenesis of psoriasis and psoriatic arthritis. Am J Med Sci 1998; 316: 271–276.
27. Liang GC, Barr WG. Leflunomide for psoriasis and psoriatic arthritis. J Clin Rheumatol 2001; 7: 366–370.
28. Fox RI. Mechanism of action of leflunomide in rheumatoid arthritis. J Rheumatol 1998; 25: 5306–5326.
29. Mroczkowski PJ, Weinblatt ME, Kremer JM. MTX and leflunomide combination therapy for patients with active rheumatoid arthritis. Clin Exp Rheumatol 1999; 17: S66–S68.
30. Bruckle W, Dexel T, Grasedyck K, Schatten Kirchner M. Treatment of psoriatic arthritis. Clin Rheumatol 1994; 13: 209–216.
31. Levy J, Paulus H, Eugene V et al. A double-blind controlled evaluation of azathioprine treatment in rheumatoid arthritis and psoriatic arthritis. Arthritis Rheum 1992; 15: 116–117.
32. Fields CL, Robinson JW, Roy JM et al. Hypersensitivity reaction to azathioprine. South Med J 1998; 91: 471–474.
33. Klinkhoff AV, Gertner E, Chalmers A et al. Pilot study of etretinate in psoriatic arthritis. J Rheumatol 1989; 16: 789–791.
34. Gelber AC, Nousari HC, Wigley FM. Mycophenolate mofetil in the treatment of severe skin manifestations of DM: a series of 4 cases. J Rheumatol 2000; 27: 1542–1545.
35. Grundman-Kollman M, Mooser G, Schraeder P et al. Treatment of chronic plaque-stage psoriasis and psoriatic arthritis with mycophenolate mofetil. J Am Acad Dermatol 2000; 42: 835–837.
36. Jones G, Crotty M, Brooks P. Psoriatic arthritis: a quantitative overview of therapeutic options. The psoriatic arthritis meta-analysis study group. Br J Rheumatol 1997; 36: 95–99.
37. Moreland LW, Baumgartner SW, Schiff MH et al. Treatment of rheumatoid arthritis with a recombinant human tumor necrosis factor receptor (p75)–Fc fusion protein. N Engl J Med 1997; 337: 141–147.
38. Maini RN, Breedveld FC, Kalden JR et al. Therapeutic efficacy of multiple i.v. infusions of anti-tumor necrosis factor alpha monoclonal antibody combined with low-dose weekly methotrexate in rheumatoid arthritis. Arthritis Rheum 1998; 41: 1552–1563.
39. Ettehadi P, Greaves MW, Wallach D et al. Elevated tumor necrosis-alpha biological activity in psoriatic skin lesions. Clin Exp Immunol 1994; 96: 146–151.
40. Mease PJ, Goffe BS, Metz J et al. Etanercept in the treatment of psoriatic arthritis and psoriasis: a randomized trial. Lancet 2000; 356: 385–390.
41. Elkayam O, Yaron M, Caspi D. From wheels to feet: a dramatic response of severe chronic psoriatic arthritis to etanercept. Ann Rheum Dis 2000; 59: 839.
42. Yazici Y, Erkan D, Lockshin MD. A preliminary study of etanercept in the treatment of severe, resistant psoriatic arthritis. Clin Exp Rheumatol 2000; 18: 732–734.
43. Cuellar ML, Mendez EA, Collins RD et al. Efficacy of etanercept in refractory psoriatic arthritis. Arthritis Rheum 2000; 43:(suppl): S106.
44. Aboulafia DM, Bundow D, Wilkse K, Ochs UI. Etanercept for the treatment of human immunodeficiency virus-associated psoriatic arthritis. Mayo Clin Proc 2000; 75: 1093–1098.

45. Dechant C, Antoni C, Wendler J et al. One year outcome of patients with severe psoriatic arthritis treated with infliximab. Arthritis Rheum 2000; 43 (suppl): S102.

46. Chaudhari U, Romano P, Mulcahy LD et al. Efficacy and safety of infliximab monotherapy for plaque-type psoriasis: a randomized trial. Lancet 2001; 357: 1842–1847.

47. Keane J, Gershon S, Wise RP et al. Tuberculosis associated with infliximab, a tumor necrosis factor α-neutralizing agent. N Engl J Med 2001; 345: 1098–1104.

48. Ellis CN, Krugeger GG. Treatment of chronic plaque psoriasis by selective targeting of memory effector T lymphocytes. N Engl J Med 2001; 345: 248–255.

49. Grassi W, Lamanna G, Farina A, Cervini C. Synovitis of small joints: sonographic guided diagnostic and therapeutic approach. Ann Rheum Dis 1999; 58: 595–597.

50. McKendry RJ, Kraag G, Seigel S, al-Awadhi A. Therapeutic value of colchicines in the treatment of patients with psoriatic arthritis. Ann Rheum Dis 1993; 12: 826–828.

51. Kagan A, Husza'r M, Frunkin A, Rapoport J. Reversal of nephrotic syndrome due to AA amyloidosis in psoriatic patients on longterm colchicine treatment. Case report and review of the literature. Nephron 1999; 82: 348–353.

52. Huckins D, Felson DT, Holick M. Treatment of psoriatic arthritis with oral 1,25-dihydroxyvitamin D_3: a pilot study. Arthritis Rheum 1990; 33: 1723–1727.

53. Jorstad S, Bergh K, Iversen OJ et al. Effects of cascade apheresis in patients with psoriasis and psoriatic arthropathy. Blood Purif 1998; 16: 37–42.

54. Maksymowych WP, Jhangri GS, Leclercq S et al. An open study of pamidronate in the treatment of refractory ankylosing spondylitis. J Rheumatol 1998; 25: 714–717.

55. Moreira AL, Sampaio EP, Zmudzinas A et al. Thalidomide exerts its inhibitory action on tumor necrosis factor alpha by enhancing mRNA degradation. J Exp Med 1993; 177: 1675–1680.

56. Burt RK, Traynor AE, Pope R et al. Treatment of autoimmune disease by intense immunosuppressive conditioning and autologous hematopoietic stem cell transplantation. Blood 1998; 92: 3505–3514.

57. Sukenik S, Giryes H, Halevy S et al. Treatment of psoriatic arthritis at the Dead Sea. J Rheumatol 1994; 21: 1305–1309.

58. Elkayam O, Ophir J, Brener S et al. Immediate and delayed effects of treatment at the Dead Sea in patients with psoriatic arthritis. Rheumatol Int 2000; 19: 77–82.

59. Sukenik S, Baradin R, Codish S et al. Balneotherapy at the Dead Sea area for patients with psoriatic arthritis and concomitant fibromyalgia. Israel Med Assoc J 2001; 3: 147–150.

CONNECTIVE TISSUE DISORDERS
SYSTEMIC LUPUS ERYTHEMATOSUS

33 Clinical features

Dafna D Gladman and Murray B Urowitz

Definition

- An inflammatory multisystem disease of unknown etiology with protean clinical and laboratory manifestations and a variable course and prognosis
- Immunologic aberrations give rise to production of excessive amounts of autoantibodies, some of which cause cytotoxic damage, whereas others participate in immune complex formation resulting in immune inflammation

Clinical features

- Clinical manifestations may be constitutional or result from inflammation in various organ systems, including skin and mucous membranes, joints, kidney, brain, serous membranes, lung, heart and, occasionally, the gastrointestinal tract
- Organ systems may be involved singly or in any combination
- Involvement of vital organs, particularly the kidneys and central nervous system, accounts for significant morbidity and mortality
- Morbidity and mortality result from tissue damage due to the disease process or its treatment

HISTORY

The term 'lupus', Latin for wolf, was used in the 18th century to describe a variety of skin conditions. However, the first historical account of lupus erythematosus was by Biett, in 1833[1]. For a number of decades the disease was considered a chronic dermatologic disorder, but in 1872 Kaposi described the systemic nature of lupus erythematosus. Indeed, many of the manifestations of systemic lupus erythematosus (SLE) were recognized by Kaposi.

Current understanding of SLE has evolved from the clinical descriptions that followed, and was enhanced by the discovery of the LE cell phenomenon by Hargraves et al. in 1948[2]. The subsequent recognition of the antinuclear factor by Friou[3] provided some insight into the pathogenesis of the disease, whereas recognition of the inflammatory and immunologic features of the disease provided insight into therapeutic modalities.

Subsequently, late causes of mortality and morbidity not immediately related to immunologic abnormalities of SLE have been described, such as premature atherosclerosis,[4] neurocognitive dysfunction and avascular necrosis[5].

EPIDEMIOLOGY

Systemic lupus erythematosus is recognized worldwide. Estimates of its prevalence vary widely and range from 15–124/100 000 population in the USA[6,7], 12–24.7/100 000 in Britain[8], and 22.1/100 000[9] in the province of Manitoba, Canada, to 39/100 000 in Sweden[10] (Fig. 33.1). This variation may reflect true differences in the prevalence of the disease in different geographic areas, or differences in case selection in various studies. On the basis of the most recent studies in the USA, it is likely that the true prevalence is close to the often quoted prevalence rate of 1:1000. Incidence rates have also varied, from 1.8/100 000 per year in Rochester to 7.6/100 000 per year in San Francisco[7,10]. In Scandinavia, the incidence rates lie between these extremes at 4.5/100 000 per year[11], whereas the incidence rate in the Nottingham study was 4.0/100 000[8].

Systemic lupus erythematosus is clearly more prevalent in women, particularly in their reproductive years. In most studies of SLE, 90% of patients are women. For the 14–64 years age group, the ratios of age-specific and sex-specific incidence rates show a 6- to 10-fold female excess, which is not noted in patients younger than 14 years, or older than 65 years of age. This effect of age and sex on the incidence and prevalence rates of SLE suggests a role for hormonal factors in its pathogenesis.

In the USA, SLE is three times more common among blacks than whites. A study in Hawaii demonstrated a greater frequency of SLE among Orientals than among whites. Nonetheless, a high frequency of SLE was noted in Sweden in a population that is strictly white. The highest prevalence rates for SLE in Nottingham, England, were noted for Afro-Caribbeans (207/100 000) followed by Asians (48.8/100 000), and whites (20.3/100 000)[8]. The study from Manitoba, Canada, demonstrated a greater frequency of SLE among North American Indians (42.3/100 000) than in the remainder of the population (20.6/100 000)[9].

In addition to their effect on prevalence and incidence, age, sex, race and socioeconomic status have been suggested to have an influence on disease expression. Black patients with SLE have been shown more commonly to have Sm and RNP antibodies, discoid skin lesions, cellular casts and serositis[12]. These were not related to age, sex or socioeconomic status. Conversely, socioeconomic factors have been identified as important prognostic indicators.

Genetic epidemiology

Genetic factors have long been considered to have a role in the etiopathogenesis of SLE. Support for this concept has come from the observation that there is a high prevalence of SLE among monozygotic twins[13]. Further evidence for a hereditary predisposition to SLE comes from family studies. It is estimated that 5–12% of relatives of patients with SLE develop the condition[14,15].

Human leukocyte antigen (HLA) studies have allowed a more detailed analysis of genetic epidemiology in SLE, and the further determination of the mode of inheritance and the number of genes that might contribute to disease susceptibility. In population studies, class II antigens, particularly HLA-DR2 and -DR3, were found to occur more frequently among patients with SLE[16]. Several investigators have identified an association between SLE and the C4A null allele. Although Schur et al.[17] found a significantly increased frequency of the alleles C4AQo and DR3 and the complotype SCo1 only in patients of English/Irish descent, others have shown an association between C4A null alleles in white and black populations in the USA, and in Chinese and Japanese patients[18–21].

Population studies have demonstrated associations between several HLA genes and SLE, but the associations have not been uniform, suggesting that, in this complex condition, different genes are responsible

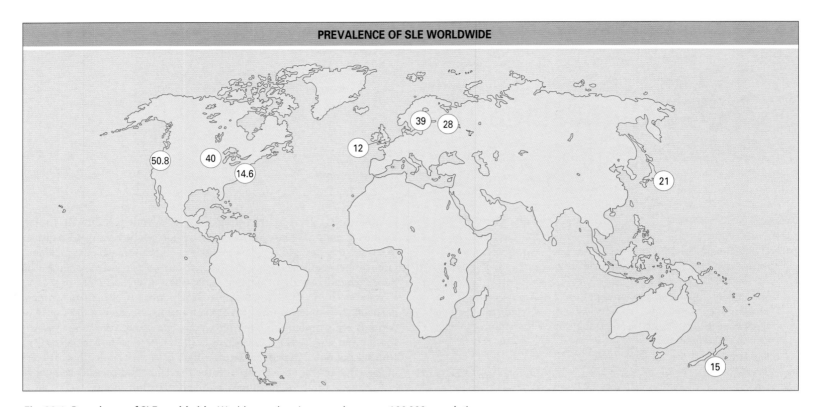

PREVALENCE OF SLE WORLDWIDE

Fig. 33.1 Prevalence of SLE worldwide. World map showing prevalence per 100 000 population.

for the development of a variable disease pattern. For example a study of patients with clinical evidence of lupus nephritis identified an increased frequency of DR2, DQw1, and especially DQb1.AZH, and a decreased frequency of HLA-DR4 in these patients[22]. Another study suggested an interaction between C4A*Q0 and DQA*0501[23]. Associations with other polymorphic genes, including immunoglobulin and T cell receptor genes, have also been reported[24]. Indeed, data from genome scans in families with several members affected with SLE identified a number of genetic loci to be associated with SLE and suggest a multigene theory as an explanation for the inheritance of lupus[25,26].

CLINICAL FEATURES

Clinical manifestations at onset and at any time in the course of the disease in three of the largest reported SLE series in the English literature, the University of Toronto Clinic, the University of Southern

TABLE 33.1 FREQUENCY OF LUPUS MANIFESTATIONS (%)					
Manifestation	**Toronto (n = 994)**		**Europe (n = 1000)**		**USC (n = 464)**
	Onset	**Ever**	**Onset**	**Ever**	**Ever**
Constitutional	53	80	36	52	41
Arthritis	42	64	69	84	91
Skin	66	86	40	58	55
Mucous membranes	21	50	11	24	19
Pleurisy	14	27	17	36	31
Lung	6	14	3	7	7
Pericarditis	11	20	?	?	12
Myocarditis	1	3	?	?	2
Raynaud's	32	61	18	34	24
Thrombophlebitis	1	5	4	14	11
Vasculitis	12	32	?	?	?
Renal	42	73	16	39	28
Nephrotic syndrome	6	13	?	?	14
Azotemia	7	17	?	?	?
CNS	20	49	12	27	11
Cytoid bodies	2	2	?	?	2
Gastrointestinal	15	39	?	?	?
Pancreatitis	1	2	?	?	2
Lymphadenopathy	15	30	7	12	10
Myositis	3	4	4	9	5

CNS, central nervous system; USC, University of Southern California; ?, information not available

Frequencies at onset, and at any time, in three large series of lupus patients.

California at Los Angeles Clinic and the 'Euro-Lupus' project are displayed in Table 33.1[27].

General

Constitutional complaints such as malaise, overwhelming fatigue, fever and weight loss are common presenting features of SLE. The presence of these features does not help the physician in the diagnosis of the disease, or in the identification of a flare, because they are just as likely to represent the development of infection or of fibromyalgia.

Fever in SLE is a challenging clinical problem. Many patients develop fever during the course of their disease as a manifestation of active lupus. However, patients with lupus are highly prone to developing infections, which account for a large proportion of the deaths from the disease. In addition, other causes of fever should be considered, including drug-related or malignancy. A diligent history and physical examination, with particular attention to specific features of SLE or to a source of infection, will help guide the physician, and appropriate laboratory tests and radiographs should be ordered. At times it may be necessary to treat for an infection empirically until results of laboratory cultures have been received.

Although some organ system involvements such as skin disease or arthritis are common in SLE, any system may be involved and present in variable combinations with other organ systems. Thus SLE may have such diverse clinical presentations as rash and arthritis, or pleurisy and proteinuria, or Raynaud's phenomenon and seizures or pyrexia of unknown origin. It is only with a high index of suspicion, a careful history and physical examination, and by obtaining appropriate laboratory confirmation, that the diagnosis will become obvious.

Skin manifestations

The skin lesions seen in patients with lupus can be classified into those that are lupus-specific histologically, and those that are lupus-non-specific[28] (Table 33.2). The lupus-specific lesions may be further divided into those that are acute, subacute and chronic.

Lupus-specific lesions

Acute lesions

The most recognized skin manifestation of SLE is the 'butterfly' rash (Fig. 33.2), which usually presents acutely as an erythematous, elevated

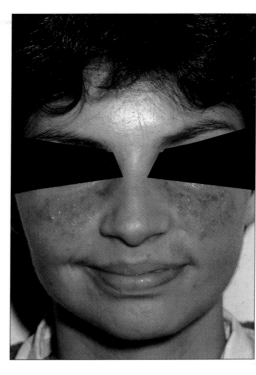

Fig. 33.2 Erythematous malar rash of SLE. Note that the rash does not cross the nasolabial fold.

lesion, pruritic or painful, in a malar distribution, commonly precipitated by exposure to sunlight. The rash may last from days to weeks. Its presence facilitates the diagnosis of SLE and is commonly accompanied by other inflammatory manifestations of the disease. Pathologically, the lesions may show only non-specific inflammation, although by immunofluorescence the classic immune deposits at the dermal–epidermal junction may be seen. The presence of immune deposits in uninvolved skin in patients with SLE has been believed to be helpful in diagnosis[29]. Other acute cutaneous lesions include generalized erythema and bullous lesions. The latter lesions are uncommon cutaneous manifestations of SLE; their histology is characterized by acute inflammation, which may be immune-complex mediated, and which differentiates them from primary vesiculobullous disease[30].

More than 50% of patients with SLE demonstrate photosensitivity. In addition to the skin reaction, patients may develop exacerbations of their systemic disease. The mechanism for the photosensitivity is unknown, but it has been suggested that lymphocytes from patients with SLE are sensitive to 360–400nm light, related to a clastogenic factor in these cells[31]. The damaged chromatin may then provide a substrate for autoantibody production, with the development of a local, or systemic, inflammatory response. Indeed, a recent study showed that ultraviolet B light increased the binding of antibody probes for Ro(SS-A) and La(SS-B) on keratinocytes in a dose-dependent manner[32,33].

Subacute cutaneous lupus erythematosus

Subacute cutaneous lupus erythematosus (SCLE) refers to a distinct cutaneous lesion that is non-fixed, non-scarring, exacerbating and remitting. This lesion is thus intermediate between the evanescent malar rash of active lupus, and the chronic lesions of the disease, which usually cause scarring. These lesions commonly occur in sun-exposed areas and may be generalized. The lesions originate as erythematous papules or small plaques with a slight scale, and may evolve further into a plaque and scale, the papulosquamous variant, which mimics psoriasis or lichen planus, or merge and form polycyclic or annular lesions, which may mimic erythema annulare centrifugum (Fig. 33.3). SCLE may be accompanied by musculoskeletal complaints and serologic abnormalities, the most common of which is the antibody to Ro(SS-A), which has been demonstrated in the lesion. Many patients with antinuclear antibody (ANA)-negative lupus have demonstrated the annular lesions of SCLE.

TABLE 33.2
CLASSIFICATION OF CUTANEOUS LESIONS
Lupus-specific lesions
Acute
Malar 'butterfly' rash
Generalized erythema
Bullous lupus erythematosusL
Subacute cutaneous lupus
Annular – polycyclic
Papulosquamous (psoriasiform)
Chronic lupus
Localized discoid
Generalized discoid
Lupus profundus
Lupus-non-specific lesions
Panniculitis
Urticarial lesions
Vasculitis
Livedo reticularis
Oral lesions
Non-scarring alopecia
Associated skin conditions (psoriasis, lichen planus, porphyria)

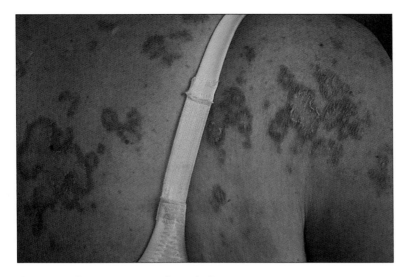

Fig. 33.3 Subacute cutaneous lupus lesions.

The overall prognosis for patients with SCLE is generally better than that for patients with acute cutaneous lesions, although the skin lesions may be more refractory.

Chronic lupus

Discoid lesions are chronic cutaneous lesions that may occur in the absence of any systemic manifestations, as discoid lupus, or may be a manifestation of SLE. These lesions often begin as erythematous papules or plaques, with scaling that may become thick and adherent, with a hypopigmented central area. As the lesion progresses, follicular plugging occurs, with the development of scarring with central atrophy (Fig. 33.4). Discoid lesions may occur in the malar region, or in other sun-exposed areas. Lesions in the scalp lead to extensive, and often permanent, alopecia. Discoid lupus may be localized or generalized, the latter being more likely to be associated with systemic features and serologic abnormalities. Pathologically, the discoid lesion typically demonstrates hyperkeratosis, follicular plugging, edema and mononuclear cell infiltration at the dermal–epidermal junction. On the basis of the pathologic differences between SCLE and discoid skin lesions, different pathogenetic mechanisms contribute to the development of these lesions, such that antibody-mediated cytotoxicity leads to SCLE lesions, whereas chronic cutaneous lesions result from T cell mediated cytotoxicity[28].

Lupus-non-specific lesions

Panniculitis is a rare cutaneous manifestation of SLE. The lesion presents as a deep, firm nodule, with or without a surface change. A biopsy may

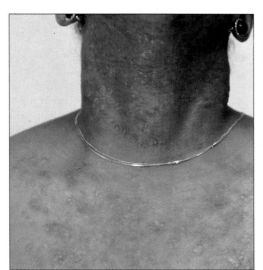

Fig. 33.4 Discoid lupus involving neck and upper chest. The lesions have characteristic central scarring.

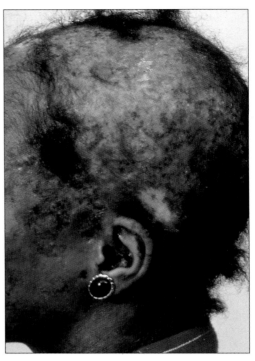

Fig. 33.5 Scarring discoid lupus of the scalp, with permanent alopecia.

show perivascular infiltration of mononuclear cells and fat necrosis. There may be a skin lesion over the nodule, which may demonstrate the perivascular infiltrate without fat necrosis that is known as lupus profundus.

Alopecia is a common feature of SLE. Hair loss may be diffuse or patchy. It may be associated with exacerbations of the disease, in which case it tends to regrow when the disease is under control. Alternatively, it may result from the extensive scarring of discoid lesions, in which case it may be permanent (Fig. 33.5). Alopecia may also be drug-induced, for example by corticosteroids or cytotoxic drugs.

Mucous membrane lesions may result in ulcers of the mouth (Fig. 33.6) or vagina, or produce nasal septal erosions. The latter occasionally lead to nasal septal perforation (Fig. 33.7). Such lesions have been reported to result from vasculitis.

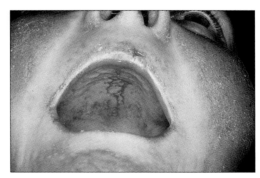

Fig. 33.6 Mouth ulcers in a patient with SLE.

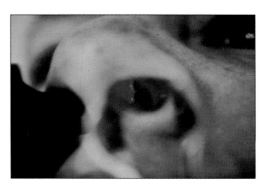

Fig. 33.7 Nasal septal perforation in a patient with SLE.

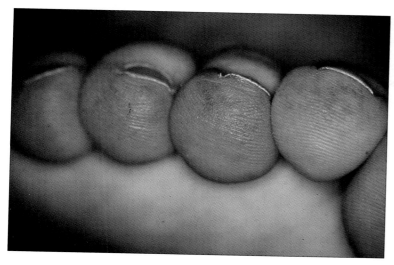

Fig. 33.8 Early vasculitic lesions over the tips of the toes in a patient with active SLE.

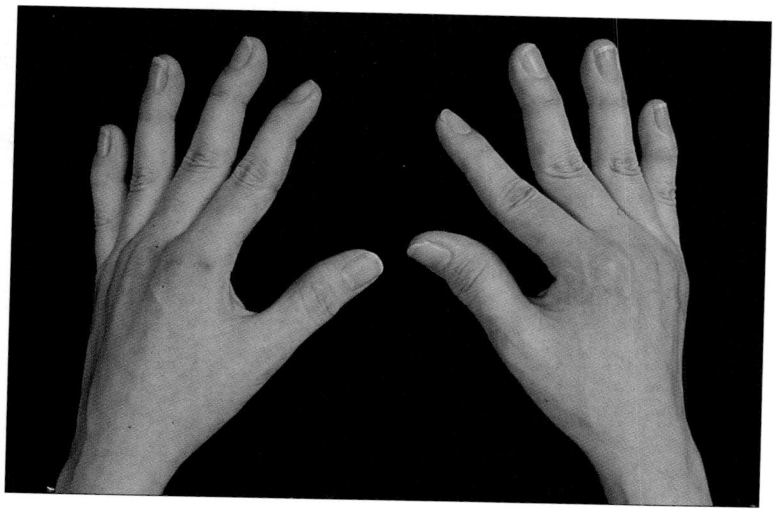

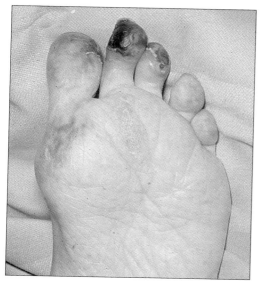

Fig. 33.9 Gangrene of the toe in a patient with SLE and vasculitis.

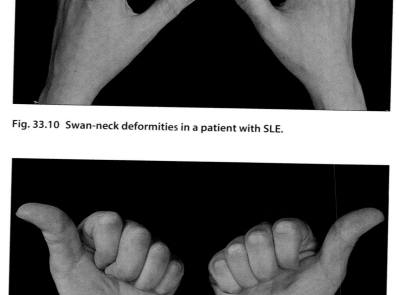

Fig. 33.10 Swan-neck deformities in a patient with SLE.

Fig. 33.11 Fists of the patient in Figure 33.10, showing the deformities reduced.

Urticarial lesions occur in 5–10% of patients, are often chronic and typically represent cutaneous vasculitis. Vasculitic lesions may also manifest as palpable purpura, nailfold or digital ulcerations, subcutaneous nodules, livedo reticularis, splinter hemorrhages, pulp space and palmar or plantar lesions (Fig 33.8), simulating Osler's nodes and Janeway's lesions. Vasculitic lesions at the tip of a digit may result in gangrene (Fig. 33.9). Raynaud's phenomenon occurs in more than 50% of patients. Unlike scleroderma, the Raynaud's phenomenon of lupus is not commonly associated with pulp-space pits or ulcerations.

Musculoskeletal features

Arthritis

Arthralgias or arthritis, or both constitute the most common presenting manifestation of SLE[34]. The acute arthritis may affect any joint but, typically, the small joints of the hands, wrists and knees are involved. Most cases are symmetric, but a significant percentage may have an asymmetric polyarthritis. Swelling is usually soft tissue, with effusions tending to be minimal. The acute inflammation may be migratory in nature or persistent and become chronic. Nodules similar to those found in rheumatoid arthritis (RA) are found in approximately 10% of patients with lupus. Synovial fluid analysis reveals mild inflammatory changes and may reveal LE cells, ANA positivity and diminished complement concentrations.

Unlike RA, the arthritis of systemic lupus is typically not erosive or destructive of bone. However, clinically deforming arthritis does occur, and may take a number of different forms[35]. There may be mild synovial thickening about proximal interphalangeal joints or over tendon sheaths, ulnar deviation of the fingers, and subluxations and contractures. When subluxations occur in the small joints of the hands, they are initially reversible (Figs 33.10 & 33.11), but can become fixed. This pattern of non-erosive but deforming disease has been called Jaccoud's arthritis[34]. Other authors have noted flexion contractures of the elbows[36], and deforming arthropathy of the feet[37]. Often, patients who go on to develop deforming arthropathy have had continuous low-grade active arthritis, sometimes in the absence of other signs of SLE. Histologic examination of synovium in the acute stage reveals mild, usually perivascular inflammatory cell infiltrate, mild synovial cell proliferation and mild fibrinous deposition in synovial lining cells. In the more chronic stage, more synovial cell proliferation may be seen, but not approaching the intensity seen in RA. Radiographic findings in SLE arthritis are usually minimal, but may be found in up to 50% of patients[34,35]. There may be periarticular or diffuse osteoporosis and soft tissue swelling, but, unlike RA, there are no erosions even when severe deformities from subluxations are present. Occasionally, one may see hook-like erosions of the metacarpal heads late in the disease, similar to the erosions described in post-rheumatic fever Jaccoud's syndrome.

These changes are more likely a result of bone trauma, due to misplaced tendon sheaths, rather than to erosions from a proliferative synovitis.

As tenosynovitis is an early manifestation of the synovitis of SLE, it is not surprising that tendon rupture syndromes have been reported in a number of different sites in the body, including the patellar tendons, the long head of the biceps, the triceps and the extensor tendons of the hands. Patients who present with tendon ruptures may give a history of the sudden onset of pain or inability to move a joint. Dramatic traumas are not often a part of the history and most patients have a history of long-standing use of corticosteroids. Histologic examination of the ruptured tendons has revealed inflammation in some instances, but not invariably. Thus one may incriminate either inflammation or corticosteroid-induced tendon degeneration as the mechanism for tendon damage.

Two complications of SLE or its treatment, septic arthritis and osteonecrosis, may confuse the diagnosis of acute synovitis in SLE. Although septic arthritis is not common in SLE, despite the immuno-suppressed state, it should be suspected when one joint is inflamed out of proportion to all others. This state necessitates aspiration and culture of the synovial fluid to rule out infection.

Osteonecrosis

Acute joint pain presenting in the later stages of SLE, especially localized to a very few areas, most commonly the hips, may indicate the development of osteonecrosis. In most large series now, osteonecrosis is recognized as an important cause of disability in late lupus, occurring in about 10% of patients followed over a long period of time[38]. Patients with osteonecrosis are generally in the younger age group and have an interval between diagnosis of lupus and osteonecrosis of about 4 years. The hip is the joint most commonly involved, although most joints in the body have been reported to have been affected. From 50% to 67% of patients with osteonecrosis will have several affected sites and, typically, will have been taking high-dose corticosteroids at some time during the course of their illness.

There is no general agreement as to the predictive role of any specific manifestation of SLE, such as Raynaud's phenomenon or vasculitis, in the subsequent development of osteonecrosis, and there is currently no general consensus on pathogenesis. Findings of a recent nested

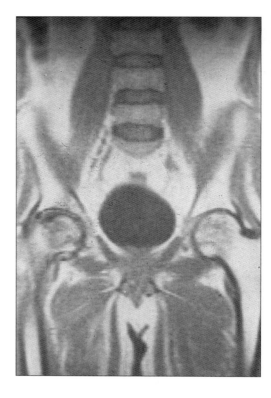

Fig. 33.13
MRI showing advanced changes of osteonecrosis of the right hip and early changes on the left.

case–control study suggests that osteonecrosis is related to previous arthritis, steroid use and treatment with cytotoxic drugs[38].

Diagnosis of osteonecrosis in patients presenting with focal pain can be difficult. Changes in the routine radiographs (Fig. 33.12) are late findings. Earlier diagnosis can be made using radionuclide bone scans or magnetic resonance imaging (MRI) to demonstrate bone abnormality (Fig. 33.13). Although many patients with osteonecrosis have a poor outcome with respect to pain and disability, leading to joint replacement, some patients do respond to decreased weight bearing and the passage of time. These patients may be left with some joint irregularity, but with joint space adequate to avoid surgery. The size and exact location of the avascular area may determine the future necessity for joint replacement. Core decompression with or without bone grafting has not yet been demonstrated to be a useful treatment. Osteonecrosis is not associated with decreased survival, but is associated with physical disability[39].

Myositis

Patients with SLE may complain of muscle pain and weakness. The nature of the myalgia is not always clear. It may be secondary to joint inflammation, in which case the arthritis will be easily demonstrable on physical examination. Patients with SLE may develop a drug-related myopathy, secondary to corticosteroid use or as a complication of anti-malarials. In addition, true muscle inflammation may be seen in patients with SLE. However, the histologic features of myositis in SLE may not be as striking as in idiopathic polymyositis[34]. Finol et al.[40] described the ultrastructural pathology in patients with SLE. Findings included myositis, with muscle atrophy, microtubular inclusions and a mononuclear cell infiltrate and, in one patient with an increased creatine phosphokinase concentration, fiber necrosis. Vacuolar myopathy was found in one patient not treated with antimalarials.

Fibromyalgia

In the differential diagnosis of musculoskeletal complaints in patients with SLE one must consider the possibility of fibromyalgia, which is common in this patient population[41]. Fibromyalgia may be distinguished from true arthritis or myositis by the presence of tender points, and the absence of true inflammatory arthritis or evidence of muscle weakness.

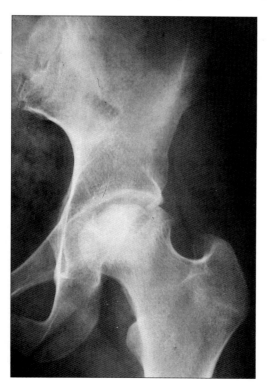

Fig. 33.12
Radiograph demonstrating advanced osteonecrosis of the hip.

On the other hand, fibromyalgia may accompany true arthritis, and its presence needs to be taken into consideration when planning a treatment program for the patient. Fibromyalgia has been shown to contribute to reduced quality of life in patients with SLE[42].

Renal disease

Specific symptoms referable to the kidney are not volunteered by the patient until there is advanced nephrotic syndrome or renal failure. The revised criteria for the classification of SLE recognizes proteinuria of more than 0.5g per 24 hours (or a qualitative dipstick score of >3+ if a quantitative evaluation is not done) or the presence of casts (including red blood cells, heme, granular, tubular or mixed) as evidence of renal disease. In addition, the presence of hematuria (>5 red blood cells/high power field) or pyuria (>5 white blood cells/high power field), or both, in the absence of infection, and the detection of an increased serum creatinine concentration, have been recognized as evidence for clinical renal disease[43]. It is important to appreciate that, in order to identify the presence of renal disease, urine analysis, in addition to a serum creatinine test, must be performed regularly. A renal biopsy may provide a more accurate documentation of renal disease. Most patients with lupus manifest some abnormality on renal biopsy, although in some cases it is possible to document this only with special techniques, such as immunofluorescence or electron microscopy.

The World Health Organization (WHO) has classified lupus nephritis according to the presence of changes on light, immunofluorescence and electron microscopy (Table 33.3)[44]. Mesangial alterations (WHO class II, Fig. 33.14) including mesangial widening or hypercellularity are most common. Proliferative changes may be either focal (WHO class II, Fig. 33.15) or diffuse glomerulonephritis (WHO class IV, Fig. 33.16). Membranous lesions (WHO class V, Fig. 33.17), and glomerulosclerosis (WHO class VI, Fig. 33.18) may also be seen. Renal biopsies may demonstrate hematoxylin bodies, which are the tissue equivalent of the LE cell phenomenon (Fig. 33.19). Most patients with mesangial lesions do not demonstrate clinical renal disease, as might be demonstrated by the presence of an active sediment or increased serum creatinine. However, patients with mesangial lesions may, on occasion, have prominent clini-

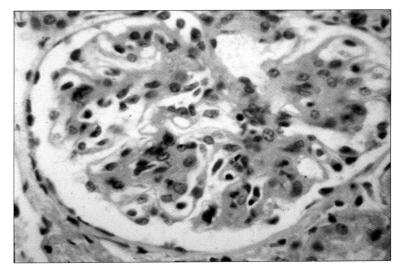

Fig. 33.14 Kidney biopsy specimen showing mesangial lesions (WHO class II).

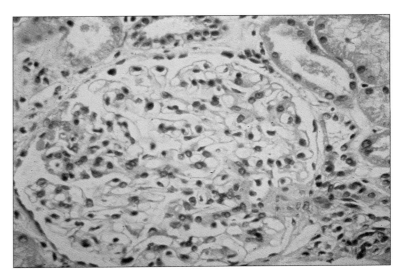

Fig. 33.15 Kidney biopsy showing focal proliferative glomerulonephritis (WHO class III).

cal evidence of renal involvement, and without a biopsy may be treated more aggressively than is perhaps indicated by the lesion itself[45]. Patients with class III and class IV disease tend to have evidence of clinical renal disease and impaired renal function; however, this is not universal. Knowledge of the various morphologic patterns contributes to decisions regarding treatment[44]. Further information may be derived from the renal biopsy with regards to the site of immune deposits, seen by either immunofluorescence (Fig. 33.20) or electron microscopy (Figs 33.21 & 33.22).

The role of kidney biopsy in the assessment of lupus nephritis has been controversial. Several studies have supported the concept that diffuse proliferative lupus nephritis is associated with poor prognosis, both in terms of renal function and in terms of patient survival. Other reports, however, have repudiated the usefulness of renal biopsy in predicting outcome, and claimed that the renal morphology does not add to the clinical information obtained before biopsy[44]. Using a quantitative classification system (Table 33.4), it is clear that these morphologic features seen on kidney biopsies have both prognostic and therapeutic implications[44]. The presence of chronic lesions is clearly associated with lower survival, both for the patient and for the kidney. Moreover, the presence of active lesions would suggest that aggressive anti-inflammatory immunosuppressive treatment, or both, should be considered.

TABLE 33.3 WHO CLASSIFICATION OF LUPUS NEPHRITIS IN 148 BIOPSIES	
I Normal glomeruli	**12**
a) Nil (by all techniques)	3
b) Normal by light but deposits on electron microscopy or immunofluorescence	9
II Pure mesangial alterations (mesangiopathy)	**62**
a) Mesangial widening and/or mild hypercellularity	51
b) Moderate hypercellularity	11
IIIA Focal segmental glomerulonephritis	**19**
a) 'Active' necrotizing lesions	14
b) 'Active' and sclerosing lesions	5
IIIB Focal proliferative glomerulonephritis	**3**
a) 'Active' necrotizing lesions	1
b) 'Active' and sclerosing lesions	2
IV Diffuse glomerulonephritis	**37**
a) Without segmental lesions	9
b) With 'active' necrotizing lesions	13
c) With 'active' and sclerosing lesions	14
d) With sclerosing lesions	1
V Diffuse membranous glomerulonephritis	**11**
a) Pure membranous glomerulonephritis	2
b) Associated with lesions of category II	7
c) Associated with lesions of category III	0
d) Associated with lesions of category IV	2
VI Advanced sclerosing glomerulonephritis	**4**

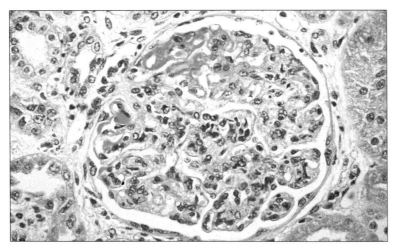

Fig. 33.16 Kidney biopsy showing diffuse proliferative glomerulonephritis (WHO class IV).

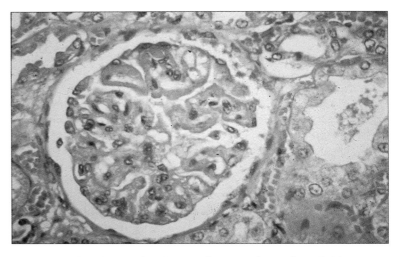

Fig. 33.17 Kidney biopsy showing membranous glomerulonephritis (WHO class V).

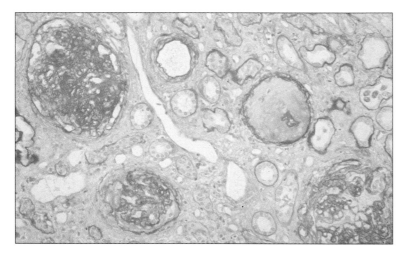

Fig. 33.18 Kidney biopsy showing advanced sclerosis (WHO class VI).

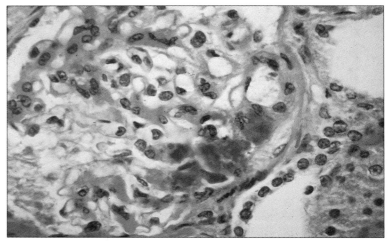

Fig. 33.19 Hematoxylin bodies in a glomerulus of a patient with lupus nephritis.

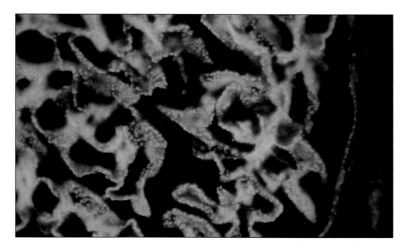

Fig. 33.20 Immunofluorescence showing C3 deposits in a capillary distribution.

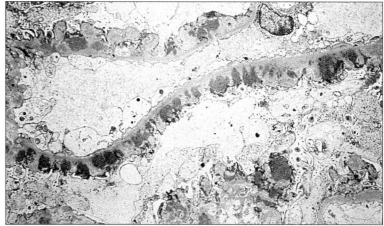

Fig. 33.21 Electron micrograph of a glomerulus showing intramembranous immune deposits.

Several studies have looked at the predictive value of clinical manifestations of renal disease using renal insufficiency as the outcome measure. Austin et al.[46] found increased risk of renal failure to be associated with younger age, male sex and an increased serum creatinine concentration. This model was enhanced by including the renal chronicity index. Nossent et al.[47] concluded that a chronicity index greater than 3

(Table 33.4), especially in young patients, is the most important factor associated with decreased renal survival. Indeed, their findings suggest that, unlike a histologic evaluation, renal function tests alone cannot distinguish between reversible and irreversible renal disease. McLaughlin et al.[48] demonstrated the prognostic value of renal biopsy in patients with normal serum creatinine at the time of the biopsy. In patients with

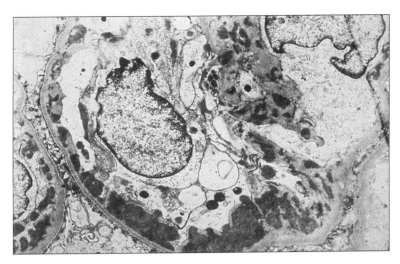

Fig. 33.22 Electron micrograph of a glomerulus showing subendothelial immune deposits.

TABLE 33.4 ACTIVITY AND CHRONICITY INDICES FOR LUPUS NEPHRITIS		
	Activity	Chronicity
Glomerular lesions	1. Proliferation	1. Sclerotic glomeruli
	2. Necrosis/karyorrhexis	2. Fibrous crescents
	3. Hyaline thrombi	
	4. Cellular crescents	
	5. Leukocytic exudation	
Tubulointerstitial lesions	1. Mononuclear cell infiltration	1. Tubular atrophy
		2. Interstitial fibrosis

evidence of diffuse proliferative glomerulonephritis with glomerular thrombosis, there may be improved prognosis through the use of ancrod[49]. Jacobson et al.[50] retrospecively studied 94 patients with normal serum creatinine at the time of biopsy and analyzed the prognostic value of renal biopsy and clincial variables for the development of end-stage renal disease. They found that duration of renal disease of more than 1 year at the time of biopsy, and the presence of WHO class IV glomerulonephritis, hyaline thrombi, leukocyte infiltration and an active urinary sediment were associated with the development of end-stage renal disease.

Repeat renal biopsies also have a role in the management of patients with SLE. Morphological changes have been observed, and the majority of patients have had changes in treatment based on the biopsy results[51].

Several investigators had suggested that patients with lupus nephritis who develop renal insufficiency have decreased lupus disease activity. However, more recent studies refute this notion. Patients with renal insufficiency, whether undergoing dialysis or transplantation, continue to demonstrate current disease activity measured by the SLE disease activity index (SLEDAI)[52,53].

Neuropsychiatric manifestations

The diagnosis of neuropsychiatric involvement in SLE has been difficult. The American College of Rheumatology (ACR) Ad Hoc Committee on Neuropsychiatric Lupus Nomenclature has proposed a standardized nomenclature for the neuropsychiatric syndromes of SLE[54]. The relationship of neuropsychiatric features to the lupus disease process is not always clear[55]. There is a wide spectrum of clinical manifestations (Table 33.5), which may be grouped into neurologic, including the central nervous system (CNS), cranial and peripheral nerves, and

TABLE 33.5 NEUROPSYCHIATRIC MANIFESTATIONS OF SLE
Neurologic
Seizures – grand mal, petit mal, focal, temporal lobe Stroke syndrome Movement disorder Headache Transverse myelitis Cranial neuropathy Peripheral neuropathy
Psychiatric
Organic brain syndrome Psychosis Psychoneurosis Neurocognitive dysfunction

psychiatric, including psychosis and severe depression[56]. Many patients present with mixed neurologic and psychiatric manifestations[55,56]. Furthermore, patients may have more than one manifestation at a time, a fact that makes their classification more difficult.

Neurologic features

Intractable headaches, unresponsive to narcotic analgesics, are the most common feature of neurologic disease in patients with lupus[57]. The headaches may be migrainous in type[58], and may accompany other neuropsychiatric features. Seizure may be either focal or generalized. The occurrence of chorea in SLE has also been recognized. Chorea occurs early in the course of the disease and resembles Sydenham's chorea. Its association with the anticardiolipin antibody has been suggested[55]. Cerebrovascular accidents, including paresis or subarachnoid hemorrhage, may be associated with vasculitis or, like chorea, related to the anticardiolipin syndrome, resulting in vessel occlusion. Cranial neuropathies may present with visual defects, blindness, papilledema, nystagmus or ptosis, tinnitus and vertigo, or facial palsy. By far the most common are those related to the function of the eye. The retinopathy seen in patients with SLE is likely to be secondary to vasculitis[59]. The majority of these patients have cotton-wool spots (cytoid bodies) (Fig. 33.23), hemorrhages or areas of vasculitis (Fig. 33.24). Abnormalities of the optic nerve head manifested by papilledema or optic atrophy may also be seen.

Peripheral neuropathy is uncommon, and may include motor, sensory (stocking glove distribution) or mixed motor and sensory polyneuropathy or mononeuritis multiplex. An acute ascending motor paralysis indistinguishable from Guillain–Barré syndrome has been reported.

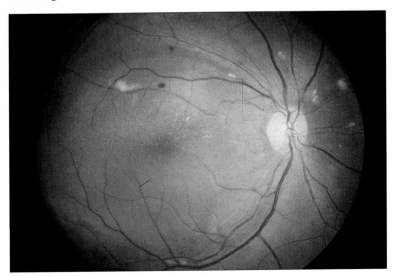

Fig. 33.23 Funduscopic examination in a patient with SLE demonstrating cytoid bodies.

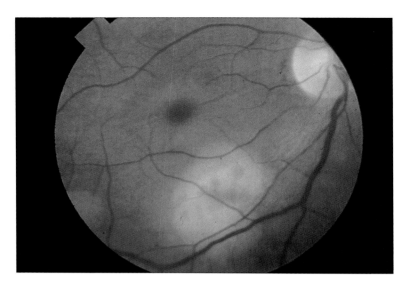

Fig. 33.24 Funduscopic examination in a patient with SLE demonstrating choroidal vasculitis.

Transverse myelitis, presenting with lower extremity paralysis, sensory deficits and loss of sphincter control, has rarely been reported in patients with SLE[55].

Psychiatric features

Frank psychosis has long been recognized as a manifestation of SLE[55,56]. The use of corticosteroids has been implicated in causing psychosis in some patients; however, stopping the drug in these patients and demonstrating that the psychosis gets worse confirms its relationship to the lupus process. The reported association between antiribosomal P protein antibodies and lupus psychosis in some studies, and severe depression in others, suggests a pathogenic relationship, but these findings are not consistent. Therefore the use of antiribosomal P antibody in diagnosis or monitoring patients is not useful, and the exact role of this antibody in SLE remains to be determined[60].

Organic brain syndrome in SLE is defined as a state of disturbed mental function with delirium, emotional inadequacy, and impaired memory or concentration, in the absence of drugs, infection or a metabolic cause. The prevalence of cognitive impairment in SLE is likely to be underestimated. Kremer et al.[61] attempted a systematic definition of the broader range of psychiatric symptoms in patients with lupus, using a combination of a standard psychiatric interview and several well-validated measures, and reported a high prevalence of psychopathology. There was a lack of correlation between the presence of non-organic non-psychotic psychopathology and underlying organic CNS disease or SLE disease activity. No correlation was found with non-organic non-psychotic psychopathology and use of corticosteroids.

In a similar study of neurocognitive function in SLE, it has been found that more than 80% of patients with SLE who had either active or inactive neuropsychiatric involvement, and 42% of patients who had never had neuropsychiatric manifestations, demonstrated significant cognitive impairment, as compared with 17% of patients with RA and 14% of the normal controls. However, a variety of cognitive deficits were present in patients with SLE, without a significant association with emotional disturbances[62].

In a study from São Paulo, Brazil[63], 63% of patients with active SLE were diagnosed with a psychiatric disorder. Patients with a psychiatric disorder were more likely to have neurologic abnormalities and subjective cognitive impairment than patients who did not have psychiatric manifestations. Patients with major psychiatric features (e.g. delirium, dementia, organic hallucinations, delusional syndromes, major depressive episodes) had more severe neurocognitive abnormalities, more

ophthalmologic abnormalities and calcifications on computed tomography (CT) scanning than did patients with mild depressive symptoms or patients without psychiatric manifestations.

Pathogenesis

The pathogenesis of CNS lupus is not well understood, but it is generally believed that more than one mechanism must be postulated, to encompass the wide spectrum of clinical findings. The most common finding in postmortem series is the presence of several microinfarcts[55,56]. Non-inflammatory thickening of small vessels by intimal proliferation is also seen, which may result from the reaction of antibodies with the phospholipids in the vascular endothelial cell membranes. Other pathologic findings include thrombotic occlusion of major vessels, which are the likely cause of some cerebrovascular accidents, whereas others may be related to the anticardiolipin antibody, intracerebral hemorrhage or embolism from mitral valve endocarditis. The pathologic findings do not always correlate with the clinical picture. A true vasculitis with inflammatory cell infiltrate and fibrinoid necrosis has rarely been demonstrated in brain pathology. However, it should be remembered that, unlike skin and renal disease, in which biopsies are readily available, most of the available pathology in the CNS comes from postmortem studies, and therefore vasculitis would be difficult to demonstrate, even if it existed.

Support for vascular inflammation comes from studies showing enhanced cerebral blood flow during episodes of CNS activity[55,59]. Autoantibodies that cross-react with neuronal membrane antigens, and lymphocytotoxic antibodies, have been found in both the serum and cerebrospinal fluid of patients with SLE. These antibodies may be produced locally or pass through an immunologically damaged cerebral circulation or choroid plexus. Changes in antineuronal antibodies frequently parallel concurrent changes in anti-DNA antibodies and overall disease activity, in addition to cognitive dysfunction[56]. These antibodies may exert their effects by binding to molecules on neuronal membranes, preventing signal responses or propagation. Potentially important target molecules on the cell surface include the very late antigens family of integrins and heat shock proteins[64].

An increased incidence of antineurofilament antibody has been found in patients with SLE who have 'diffuse' neuropsychiatric manifestations, and was frequently negative in 'focal' neuropsychiatric disease[65]. Patients with SLE and diffuse neuropsychiatric disease were more likely to have an increased IgG index, oligoclonal bands and antineuronal antibodies in the cerebrospinal fluid than were patients with focal lesions[63]. The association between antiribosomal P protein and psychiatric manifestations of SLE may have a similar mechanism[62,66]. Patients with focal lesions had evidence of peripheral vasculitis, lupus anticoagulant or anticardiolipin antibody, or both, and lesions on cranial MRI, perhaps suggesting immune complex vasculitis with resultant vascular occlusion as the mechanism for these manifestations[66].

Diagnosis

The diagnosis of neuropsychiatric lupus is primarily clinical. Exclusion of possible etiologies such as sepsis, uremia and severe hypertension is mandatory. Evidence of disease activity in other organs is helpful, but not always present. Non-specific cerebrospinal fluid abnormalities such as increased cell count, increased protein or reduced glucose may be present in 33% of the patients. Increases in IgG, IgA or IgM indices have been described in patients with CNS lupus, and proposed as evidence of CNS disease activity[55,65,66]. Electroencephalogram abnormalities are common in patients with neuropsychiatric lupus, but are non-specific[67]. The development of computerized quantitative electroencephalography may be more sensitive in detecting subtle electrophysiologic changes associated with lupus, and requires evaluation. Evoked potentials have been proposed as a sensitive measure of CNS involvement in SLE.

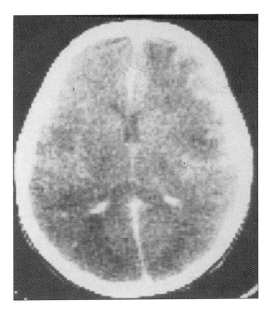

Fig. 33.25
CT scan of the brain, demonstrating microinfarcts.

Radionuclide scans have not uniformly been helpful. However, positron emission tomography, showing areas of low attenuation that may represent areas of disturbed cerebral circulation and metabolism, appears promising[67]. CT findings such as evidence of cerebral infarction (Fig. 33.25) and hemorrhage may reflect specific pathologic processes. Cortical atrophy may be found in SLE, but does not necessarily reflect CNS disease[55,65,66]. Single photon emission computed tomography has been increasingly used to identify abnormalities in patients with neuropsychiatric lupus[68,69]. This technique still requires further study into its sensitivity and specificity in patients whose symptoms are not easily discernible clinically.

Magnetic resonance imaging appears to be superior to conventional CT, and particularly useful in the evaluation of patients with diffuse presentations[67]. Some of the lesions seen on MRI, particularly the small focal areas of increased signal intensity in both the cerebral white matter and the cortical gray matter, tend to disappear after treatment with corticosteroids. These lesions may therefore represent either areas of local edema or inflammatory infiltrates that resolve with treatment. A more advanced technique, magnetic resonance spectroscopy, using either phosphorus-31 or hydrogen-1, may provide better demonstration of brain lesions in neuropsychiatric lupus[67,70]. Further research is clearly indicated before any of these techniques becomes the 'gold standard' for the diagnosis of neuropsychiatric lupus.

Serositis

Serositis in SLE is common and may present as pleurisy, pericarditis or peritonitis. Pleural manifestations have been variously reported in 30–60% of patients with SLE[71,72]. A clinical history of pleuritic pain is more common than radiographic change. Pleural rubs are found less frequently than either clinical pleurisy or radiographic abnormalities. However, autopsy findings of pleural involvement are more common than in clinical diagnoses.

Pleural effusions may occur and are usually small, but can occasionally be massive. They are also frequently bilateral. Pleural effusions are seen more frequently in the aged and in drug-induced lupus. When pleural effusions are significant, other causes of effusion such as infection must be ruled out by thoracocentesis before treatment is initiated. The fluid is usually an exudate and the glucose concentration is usually normal, in contrast to RA in which it is low. The white blood cell count is moderately increased and the differential count commonly reveals neutrophils in the acute stage and lymphocytes in the later stages of the illness. LE cells have been described in the pleural fluid. Some investigators have suggested that ANA positivity in the pleural fluid is the most sensitive test for lupus pleuritis[73], although others have not found this test helpful[74].

Pericarditis is the most common presentation of heart involvement in SLE, but is less frequent than pleurisy as a feature of serositis. Clinical pericarditis has an incidence of 20–30% in most large series, but may be found in more than 60% of patients with lupus, at autopsy[75–77]. The clinical diagnosis is frequently difficult and depends on a constellation of clinical findings, including typical precordial chest pain and a pericardial rub. However, pericarditis may also be painless and clinically silent[76]. Conversely, posterior pericardial effusions may be found on echocardiography in patients who have no suspected history of pericarditis. Pericardial effusions (Fig. 33.26) are seen frequently as a feature of pericarditis in lupus, but cardiac tamponade is rare. However, this complication does occur, and on rare occasions may be the presenting manifestation of SLE[78]. Pericardial fluid has been examined in only a small number of cases. Most samples demonstrated a leukocytosis, with a high percentage of neutrophils. Glucose concentrations are significantly lower than in the serum samples, and several reports have documented reduced complement activity in addition to increased ANA concentrations and positive LE cells, and the presence of immune complexes in the pericardial effusions.

Certain patients may be more predisposed to large pericardial effusions because of concomitant diseases such as uremia. In addition, infectious pericarditis in SLE has been reported both with bacteria and with fungi[79,80] Pericardiocentesis should be performed in patients with cardiac tamponade or in patients in whom infection is suspected. Constrictive pericarditis can occasionally develop in patients with pericardial involvement, although this is very uncommon.

The gastrointestinal syndrome of acute SLE usually manifested by diffuse abdominal pain, anorexia, nausea and occasionally vomiting, and a pseudo-obstruction presentation has a number of possible etiologies,

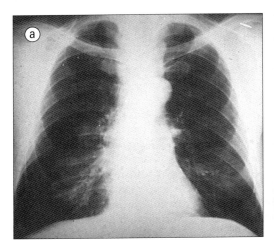
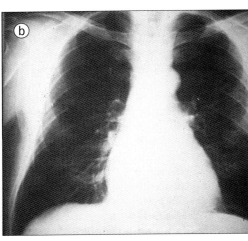

Fig. 33.26 Pericardial effusion. Change in cardiac silhouette from (a) normal baseline in (b) a patient with SLE and acute pericarditis.

including diffuse peritonitis, bowel vasculitis, pancreatitis or inflammatory bowel disease[81]. It is likely that, in the majority of such cases, peritoneal inflammation is the cause of the symptoms. Ascites may be associated with peritonitis in about 11% of cases. However, at autopsy, evidence of peritoneal inflammation may be found in up to 60% of cases[82]. When ascites is present in conjunction with abdominal pain and active lupus elsewhere, it generally follows the course and response to treatment of the other features of lupus. However, in a small number of patients, ascites may become chronic. In those circumstances it may be painless and associated with only minimal or no other manifestations of active lupus. The peritoneum may also be thickened with adhesions.

Acute lupus peritonitis must be differentiated from bowel infarction with perforation, acute pancreatitis or bacterial peritonitis. Chronic lupus peritonitis must be differentiated from congestive heart failure, constrictive pericarditis, nephrotic syndrome, Budd–Chiari syndrome, intra-abdominal malignancy and intra-abdominal sepsis with a chronic infectious agent such as tuberculosis. When infection or malignancy is suspected, aspiration of ascitic fluid is required.

Pulmonary involvement

Pulmonary involvement in SLE may consist of lupus pleuritis, lupus pneumonitis, pulmonary hemorrhage, pulmonary embolism or pulmonary hypertension[56,83].

Pneumonitis

Lupus pneumonitis may present either as an acute or as a chronic illness. The acute illness simulates pneumonia and may present with classic symptoms of fever, dyspnea, cough and occasionally hemoptysis. The pulmonary infiltrates are usually associated with other signs of active SLE. The chronic form of lupus pneumonitis presents as a diffuse interstitial lung disease and is characterized by dyspnea on exertion, non-productive cough and basilar rales. The acute pneumonitis syndrome must be differentiated from infection and, when doubt persists, invasive investigation is indicated, including bronchoalveolar lavage. In chronic lupus pneumonitis, the major clinical question revolves around whether the pulmonary fibrosis has an active component. Gallium scanning of the lung may help differentiate active from inactive disease.

On occasions, lupus pneumonitis may present as a lymphocytic interstitial pneumonia simulating a lymphangitic pulmonary malignancy. Usually, this lesion is associated with active disease and will respond to the treatment of active lupus. Lung involvement in SLE may be more common than may be appreciated by plain radiography. A recent prospective CT study of 48 patients with SLE without previously known lung involvement identified 38% of patients with normal plain radiographs to have abnormal CT findings. These correlated with disease duration and decreased single-breath diffusing capacity for carbon monoxide[84].

Pulmonary hemorrhage

Pulmonary hemorrhage presenting with cough and hemoptysis or as a pulmonary infiltrate is an uncommon but very serious feature of SLE[85]. It is presumed to be due to pulmonary vasculitis. Other causes of hemorrhagic pneumonia, such as some forms of viral pneumonia, must be considered in differential diagnoses.

Pulmonary hypertension

Lupus pulmonary involvement may also give rise to a syndrome of pulmonary hypertension that is similar to idiopathic pulmonary hypertension[86]. In this syndrome, patients present with dyspnea and a normal chest radiograph. They are mildly hypoxic and have a restrictive pattern on pulmonary function testing. Carbon dioxide diffusion capacity is reduced and Raynaud's phenomenon is frequently present. Doppler studies and cardiac catheterization confirm pulmonary hypertension. Pulmonary hypertension was found in 14% of 28 patients enrolled in an

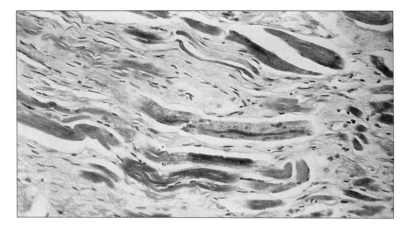

Fig. 33.27 Micrograph of the diaphragm in a patient with a shrinking lung syndrome demonstrating fibrosis.

echocardiographic study in patients with SLE[87]; over a period of 5 years, the prevalence of pulmonary hypertension increased to 43%. An increase in pulmonary artery resistance was documented in patients with SLE compared with controls[87]. Patients are frequently treated with systemic vasodilators, and more recently with epoprostenol[88]; however, the prognosis is generally grave. One must always exclude secondary pulmonary hypertension by searching for sites of deep venous thrombosis and for multiple pulmonary emboli. When there is any doubt, pulmonary angiography should be performed, as a diagnosis of multiple pulmonary emboli might lead to potential life-saving treatment. One must also exclude the antiphospholipid antibody syndrome with intrapulmonary clotting.

Shrinking lung syndrome

Unexplained dyspnea, small lung volumes with restrictive pulmonary function studies and an elevated diaphragm can signal an acute shrinking lung syndrome[89]. The syndrome responds to acute treatment of SLE with corticosteroids.

Patients may present in the late stages of lupus with the symptom of increasing dyspnea in the face of a normal chest examination. Chest radiographs may reveal increased diaphragms, but normal lung fields. Pulmonary function tests will usually reveal small lung volumes and a restrictive pattern. This chronic form of the shrinking lung syndrome is a result of altered respiratory mechanics, on the basis of either impaired respiratory muscle or diaphragmatic function, or problems in the respiratory skeletal apparatus. Some studies have demonstrated specific intercostal muscle weakness or diaphragmatic weakness[90]. One postmortem study revealed the diaphragm in a patient with shrinking lung syndrome in late lupus to be fibrotic and thinned[91] (Fig. 33.27). When shrinking lung syndrome occurs in the face of late stage lupus without other signs of active disease, the prognosis is grave.

Cardiac involvement

Cardiac involvement in SLE may consist of pericarditis, myocarditis, endocarditis and coronary artery disease.

Myocarditis

Myocarditis should be suspected in patients who present with arrhythmias or conduction defects, unexplained cardiomegaly with or without congestive heart failure or an unexplained tachycardia. Such patients usually have associated pericarditis and other features of active SLE. Peripheral myositis may be an associated feature. Congestive heart failure is a less common feature of SLE and is usually secondary to a combination of factors, which may include myocarditis. However, associated hypertension and the use of corticosteroids are usually more important contributing factors.

The myocardial involvement may be subtle in systemic lupus, with abnormalities only being detected with non-invasive testing. Sasson et al.[92], using pulsed Doppler echocardiography, demonstrated impaired left ventricular diastolic dysfunction in 64% of patients with active SLE and 14% of patients with inactive SLE, all of whom did not have any clinical evidence of cardiac disease, had normal electrocardiograms and no evidence for pericardial or valvular disease. Repeat Doppler echocardiographic studies at 7 months showed a trend towards improvement in left ventricular function in patients whose SLE became inactive. Badui et al.[93] found 16 of 100 consecutive patients with SLE to have evidence of ischemic heart disease as judged by electrocardiography, echocardiography, or both. Hosenpud et al.[94] described abnormal thallium scans in 10 of 26 patients with SLE selected randomly. These abnormalities included reversible defects suggesting ischemia, in addition to persistent defects suggesting scarring. These findings may suggest either previous myocarditis or coronary artery disease. In patients with suspected myocarditis, endomyocardial biopsy may help confirm the diagnosis[95].

Endocarditis

The true incidence of endocarditis is very difficult to discern in lupus, because the majority of murmurs heard clinically are not associated with any organic valvular disease on investigation or at autopsy. Non-bacterial verrucous vegetations described by Libman and Sacks[75] are found in 15–60% of patients at autopsy. Vegetations may vary from mere valvular thickening detected by two-dimensional echocardiography, to very large lesions causing significant valvular dysfunction[75,96]. Valvular replacement has been required on occasion, with significant mortality. Acute and subacute bacterial endocarditis may occur on previously involved valves. For this reason, prophylactic antibiotics for certain surgical procedures are advisable in patients with lupus endocarditis.

Coronary heart disease

Coronary artery disease in lupus is primarily a manifestation of generalized atherosclerosis, which is discussed in greater detail in the section on late-stage lupus. Coronary vasculitis, in contrast, is much less common in SLE[97], and when it occurs is usually associated with other features of active disease, in contradistinction to atherosclerotic coronary artery disease, which is usually associated with inactive lupus. Coronary artery occlusion may also occur in association with a circulating anticoagulant.

Gastrointestinal involvement

The gastrointestinal tract may be involved in many different ways in systemic lupus[98]. Many patients complain of a nondescript dyspepsia and nausea associated with active disease, without clear evidence of involvement of the gastrointestinal tract. However, this may represent low-grade peritoneal inflammation or vascular disease of the bowel, or be related to medication. Gastrointestinal involvement may, in addition, present as esophageal disease, mesenteric vasculitis, inflammatory bowel disease, pancreatitis and liver disease. Esophageal complaints, especially dysphagia, are uncommon in systemic lupus, but may be associated with esophageal dysrhythmias seen in those patients who frequently also manifest Raynaud's phenomenon.

Mesenteric vasculitis

The gastrointestinal presentation of greatest significance is that associated with mesenteric vasculitis[99]. Patients generally present with lower abdominal pain, which may be insidious and may be intermittent over a period of weeks or months. Arteriography may reveal the presence of vasculitis. Bleeding per rectum may occur and both small bowel and colonic ulcerations may be seen on colonoscopy. Intestinal perforations from mesenteric vasculitis have been described. Although patients with mesenteric vasculitis often have evidence of vasculitis elsewhere, this is not always the case[100]. Thus, if mesenteric vasculitis is suspected, inten-

sive investigation should be undertaken and treatment instituted to abort perforation. However, if perforation is suspected or does occur, surgical intervention is necessary.

Inflammatory bowel disease

Inflammatory bowel disease has been rarely reported in SLE[101]. Clinically, it may be difficult to distinguish between idiopathic inflammatory bowel disease and lupus enteritis. If it is caused by SLE, other features of that illness are usually present.

Pancreatitis

Acute pancreatitis occurs in about 8% of patients with lupus. Presentation includes the typical symptoms of abdominal pain, nausea and vomiting and an increased serum amylase. Although one may question whether the pancreatitis is due to lupus or corticosteroids, pancreatitis has been described in some patients not receiving corticosteroids[102,103].

Liver involvement

Although hepatomegaly occurs commonly in SLE, overt clinical liver disease is uncommon. The most common abnormality is increased liver enzymes, including aspartate aminotransferase, alanine aminotransferase, lactate dehydrogenase and alkaline phosphatase. These abnormalities have been associated with active SLE and the administration of non-steroidal anti-inflammatory medications, especially salicylates. So striking is this coincidence that, if a young woman presents with a polyarthritis, is treated with aspirin and develops increased liver enzyme, one should suspect SLE. Liver enzyme abnormalities return to normal when the lupus is under control and the anti-inflammatory medications are stopped.

Lupoid hepatitis is a subset of chronic active hepatitis, with an array of immunologic phenomena, both serologically and clinically. However, in that condition the liver is the primary organ of involvement, and this may result in liver damage and its consequences. An association between primary biliary cirrhosis and autoimmune disease has been suggested, and several patients with primary biliary cirrhosis who present with a multisystem disease consistent with SLE have been reported. Whether this is a chance coexistence of the two diseases or a direct relationship is not clear.

Reticuloendothelial system involvement

Periarterial fibrosis, or 'onion-skin lesions' in the spleen, has been considered pathognomonic of SLE. It has been suggested that saturation of the reticuloendothelial system contributes to the prolonged circulation of immune complexes and their subsequent tissue deposition[104]. Indeed, defective Fc receptor function in patients with SLE has been demonstrated and varies with disease activity. Splenic atrophy has been reported in patients with SLE[105] and the occurrence of splenic lymphoma has also been recognized[106].

Lymphadenopathy is a common non-specific feature of SLE. The nodes are usually soft, non-tender and vary in size. In some patients there may be fluctuation of the lymphadenopathy with disease exacerbations. Pathologically, the lymph nodes demonstrate reactive hyperplasia[107].

LABORATORY FEATURES

Hematologic abnormalities

Cytopenias, including anemia, leukopenia or lymphopenia, and thrombocytopenia, are frequent manifestations of SLE, and are included in the revised criteria for classification.

Anemia

Although anemia in SLE may have many different etiologies, including those secondary to chronic inflammatory disease, renal insufficiency, blood loss or drugs, the most significant in acute SLE is the autoimmune hemolytic anemia caused by autoantibodies directed against RBC antigens[108], detected by Coombs' test. Occasionally, the hemolytic anemia in lupus is Coombs' negative. Similarly, one may find a positive Coombs' test in the absence of any evidence of hemolysis.

Leukopenia/lymphopenia

Leukopenia generally ranges between 2500 and 4000/mm³ and is often associated with active disease. One must always consider other causes for leukopenia, such as drugs and infection. When the leukopenia is secondary to active lupus, the bone marrow is usually normal. The white blood count rarely decreases to less than 1500/mm³ in active SLE, unless there is an additional cause. In some instances, when the total white count does reach these values, patients have been noted to have high spiking fevers requiring significant doses of corticosteroids to suppress the active disease. Lymphocytopenia is usually associated with antibodies to lymphocytes and is associated with active SLE.

Thrombocytopenia

As with anemia, other etiologies such as infection or drugs must be ruled out as a cause of thrombocytopenia in patients with lupus. Although antiplatelet antibodies are a frequent finding in SLE, they are not always associated with thrombocytopenia.

Two distinct subsets of patients with thrombocytopenia have been identified in SLE: a subset in whom the thrombocytopenia is one feature of a severely active patient with SLE, and a second subset in whom the thrombocytopenia is an isolated finding. In the former, the thrombocytopenia tends to be refractory and follows the course of the acute lupus and its response to treatment. In the latter subset, patients usually present with a platelet count of less than 50 000/mm³, without serious bleeding. In both groups, patients may present with mild petechiae or purpura[109].

In some instances of refractory thrombocytopenia with SLE, often without platelet antibodies, the antiphospholipid syndrome should be suspected. In addition, thrombocytopenia may be a feature of thrombotic thrombocytopenic purpura (TTP) syndrome, which may complicate SLE[110]. TTP is characterized by thrombocytopenia, microangiopathic hemolytic anemia, CNS deficits, renal dysfunction and fevers. Recognition of this form of microangiopathy in patients with SLE has increased over the past two decades. TTP may occur in either quiescent or active lupus disease states. A high level of suspicion for TTP is appropriate when a patient with SLE presents with multiorgan system deterioration and microangiopathy. Because of similarities in presentation, it is often difficult to distinguish between active SLE and TTP on clinical grounds. As treatment of TTP differs from that of SLE, prompt diagnosis is crucial.

Pancytopenia

Pancytopenia in SLE may result from the effects of drugs, particularly immunosuppressive drugs. It may also complicate infections in patients with SLE. In addition, patients with SLE may develop pancytopenia as a result of the hemophagocytic syndrome[111].

Other findings

A variety of hemostatic abnormalities have been reported in lupus, the most common being the lupus anticoagulant. The most frequent laboratory accompaniments of this syndrome include a prolonged partial prothrombin time, the presence of anticardiolipin antibody, thrombocytopenia, a positive Coombs' test and a false-positive Venereal Disease Research Laboratories (VDRL) test for syphilis. The false-positive VDRL test may precede the onset of the other symptoms of SLE by many years.

The erythrocyte sedimentation rate is frequently increased during the course of active SLE, but it does not mirror the activity of the disease, and in lupus in remission may remain increased for long periods of time. A positive C reactive protein test, at one time purported to measure infection in lupus, has not been proven to be a constant indicator of a superimposed infection. However, C reactive protein has now been associated with a predisposition to coronary artery disease in otherwise healthy individuals, and with a poor prognosis in patients with myocardial infarction[112]. Its role in predicting coronary artery disease in SLE is currently under intensive study.

Serologic abnormalities

Complement concentrations, measured as either total hemolytic complement or complement components C3 and C4, have been shown to be depressed in active SLE, most commonly from consumption by immune complexes. Alternatively, depressed concentrations of serum complement may reflect inherited deficiencies of complement components, decreased production by as yet unidentified mechanisms or protein loss in the urine when there is nephrotic syndrome.

Some of the antibodies seen in SLE are more specific for certain disease states and may therefore be useful in diagnosis. These include anti-Sm, which is seen primarily in systemic lupus, antihistone antibody, which is seen primarily in drug-induced lupus, and anti-Ro and anti-La antibodies, which are seen in Sjögren's syndrome and in systemic lupus. Antibodies to double-stranded (ds)DNA are seen primarily in lupus.

Antibodies such as anti-DNA antibodies were initially believed to reflect disease activity in SLE and therefore to be monitors of treatment in this disease[113]. However, clinical experience indicates that DNA antibodies and depressed concentrations of serum complement are an imperfect predictor of clinical disease activity. Increased concentrations do not appear to correlate consistently with any clinical feature except renal disease. In some patients, these abnormalities may persist for many years, and on occasion return to normal without any intervening flare of disease[114].

Approximately 5% of patients with SLE do not demonstrate the classic antibody systems for SLE, namely ANA and LE cells, and have been referred to as having 'ANA-negative lupus'. These patients have clinical evidence of SLE and tend to have more skin rash, photosensitivity, Raynaud's phenomenon and serositis. Some of these patients have subsequently been shown to have the anti-Ro(SS-A) antibody[115].

Complement deficiency and SLE

In a patient with SLE and possible complement deficiency, such as one in whom the C3 and C4 concentrations are normal but the CH50 is low (or C3 or C4 concentrations are low even in the absence of active disease or high autoantibody levels), results first need to be confirmed with a correctly collected sample before evaluation for a possible complement deficiency is begun. Because complement components are not stable at room temperature for more than a few hours, one cause of spurious low CH50 concentrations in the face of normal C3 and C4 concentrations is improper sample handling.

Complete complement deficiency from a congenital cause is very unusual in patients with SLE – it usually accounts for fewer than 2% of patients in large series. Therefore, the great majority of low complement values that are measured in patients are acquired as part of the disease process. A common genetic deficiency affects the C2 gene. About 1 in 3 C2-deficient individuals have an autoimmune disease, most commonly SLE.

In complete deficiencies of the early classic pathway components (C1, C4 and C2) or C3, the risk of SLE or autoimmune disease is very high (from around 33% for C2 to >90% for C1). In contrast, individuals with deficiencies of later components (C5–C9) generally have far fewer autoimmune manifestations, but a much greater risk of recurrent infection, particularly with *Neisseria* species. Patients with complete complement deficiencies are believed, in general, to have a more benign SLE disease course that is characterized by an earlier age at disease onset, decreased incidence of renal and CNS disease, lower-titer or negative ANA and, usually, no anti-dsDNA antibodies. For example, patients with C2 deficiency typically have prominent cutaneous disease and high-titer SS-A/Ro antibodies, whereas patients with C1q deficiency frequently have severe nephritis with or without CNS disease, even in the face of low-titer ANAs and negative dsDNA antibodies.

THE EVOLVING SPECTRUM OF SLE

Disease patterns

The many different combinations of organ system involvement in SLE have long been known in medicine. Current concepts of pathogenesis implicate an immune complex inflammation in a variety of tissues, giving rise to clinical symptoms. However, patients may present with signs and symptoms loosely tied to SLE, but with a different underlying pathogenesis and natural history, thus requiring different therapeutic approaches. One must be aware of these presentations so that not all patients are painted with the same therapeutic brush. Some of these altered patterns include latent lupus, drug-induced lupus, antiphospholipid antibody syndrome and late-stage lupus (Fig. 33.28).

Latent lupus

The term 'latent lupus' is used to describe a group of patients who present with a constellation of features suggestive of SLE, but who do not qualify by 'criteria' or by a rheumatologist's intuition as having classic SLE[116,117]. These patients usually present with either one or two of the ACR classification criteria for SLE, plus a number of additional and much less specific features suggestive of lupus. These features may include lymphadenopathy, fever, headache, nodules, Sjögren's syndrome, fatigue, neuropathy, few active joints, an increase in partial prothrombin time, hypergammaglobulinemia and an increased erythrocyte sedimentation rate, depressed complement, positive rheumatoid factor or aspirin-induced hepatotoxicity.

Many of these patients will persist with their constellation of signs and symptoms over many years, without ever developing classic lupus. They generally do not respond well to treatment for lupus and are best followed with symptomatic treatment. Although a small number do eventually develop classic lupus, none of the presenting clinical or laboratory features are sufficiently predictive to identify such patients in advance. Patients with latent lupus tend to have a milder form of disease, not presenting with CNS involvement or renal disease.

Drug-induced lupus

Drug-induced lupus may be diagnosed in a patient in whom there is no prior history suggestive of SLE, in whom the clinical and serologic manifestations of lupus appear while they are receiving the drug concerned, and in whom improvement in clinical symptoms occurs quickly on stopping the drug, with a more gradual resolution of the serologic abnormalities[118,119].

The drugs associated with drug-induced lupus can be classified into three categories: those for which proof of the association is definite and for which appropriate, controlled, prospective studies have been performed, those drugs that are only possibly associated and, finally, drugs for which the association is still questionable. Examples of drugs in the first category include chlorpromazine, methyldopa, hydralazine, procainamide and isoniazid. Examples of drugs in the second category include dilantin, penicillamine, minocycline and quinidine; the third category is represented by a wide variety of drugs, including gold salts, a number of antibiotics, and griseofulvin and infliximab[120].

The clinical features of drug-related lupus are usually less severe than those of idiopathic SLE. The most commonly reported clinical features are constitutional symptoms, fever, arthritis and serositis. Central nervous system and renal involvement are distinctly uncommon. Laboratory tests reveal the presence of cytopenias, and positive LE cell preparation, ANA and rheumatoid factor tests. Antibodies to single-stranded DNA are commonly found, but antibodies to dsDNA are not. Complement concentrations are generally not depressed. Antihistone antibodies occur in more than 90% of cases. However, antihistone antibodies are not specific, as they are also found in 20–30% of patients with idiopathic SLE.

An interesting clinical question arises when patients with idiopathic SLE require drugs known to induce drug-induced lupus in other instances. The general practice is to use these drugs in such patients when they are necessary, because, generally, they pose no increased problems in patients with idiopathic lupus.

Late-stage lupus

Although short-term prognosis in lupus has improved dramatically over the past three decades, the mortality rates in patients surviving more than 5 years, and especially more than 10 years, have not shown a similar dramatic improvement. Patients with disease duration of more than 5 years tend to die of causes other than active SLE[121]. In such patients, mortality and morbidity are affected by long-term complications in SLE that are either the result of the previous SLE itself or a consequence of its treatment (Table 33.6).

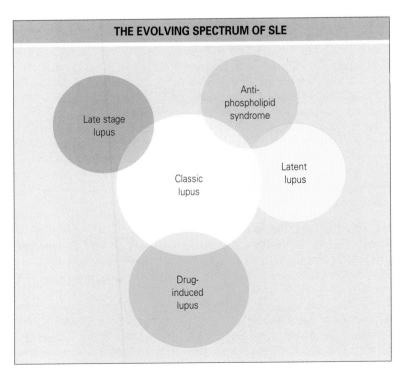

THE EVOLVING SPECTRUM OF SLE

Late stage lupus — Anti-phospholipid syndrome — Classic lupus — Latent lupus — Drug-induced lupus

Fig. 33.28 The evolving spectrum of SLE.

TABLE 33.6 LATE COMPLICATIONS OF SLE	
Acute episodes	**Chronic morbidity**
Glomerulonephritis	End-stage renal disease, dialysis, transplantation
Vasculitis	Atherosclerosis, venous syndromes, pulmonary emboli
Arthritis	Osteonecrosis
Cerebritis	Neuropsychiatric dysfunction
Pneumonitis	Shrinking lung syndrome

Atherosclerosis

Atherosclerosis manifests in patients with SLE as coronary artery disease, cerebral vascular disease and peripheral vascular disease. Patients best studied to date have been those who presented with atherosclerotic heart disease. These patients have usually demonstrated a significantly increased frequency of pericarditis, myocarditis, congestive heart failure and hypertension in their earlier active phase of systemic lupus[122]. Furthermore, metabolic risk factors such as hyperlipidemia, hyperglycemia and frank diabetes are more common among patients who develop atherosclerosis than in lupus patients in general[122]. There has been no reported difference in the use of corticosteroids in patients with or without atherosclerosis, although the average corticosteroid dose and the duration of use have generally been found to be greater. Vasculitis has not been shown to be increased in patients who later present with atherosclerosis, and cigarette smoking has also not been shown to be a clear predisposing factor.

Population and cohort studies have indicated that the prevalence of coronary artery disease and the incidence of myocardial infarction are significantly greater in patients with SLE, even in the face of a lesser number of traditional risk factors, compared with the general population. This suggests that SLE itself is a risk factor for accelerated atherosclerosis[122].

Thrombophlebitis/pulmonary emboli

Approximately 10% of patients with systemic lupus may demonstrate acute thrombophlebitis as a feature of their illness, either as a manifestation of lupus vasculitis or associated with a circulating anticoagulant[123]. In the former instance, there will usually be other signs of active systemic lupus. However, either early or late in the course of the lupus, patients may present with a bland phlebothrombosis (Fig. 33.29), with or without pulmonary emboli. In some patients, multiple pulmonary emboli may be the first indication that there is a venous problem. In such instances, one may presume that previous venous inflammation gave rise to secondary thrombosis, followed by multiple pulmonary emboli. The relationship between clotting and the antiphospholipid syndrome is discussed elsewhere.

Neurologic disorders

Assessments of cognitive function changes in SLE patients have demonstrated unequivocal deterioration in mental function. In the acute illness, both active systemic lupus and corticosteroids have been implicated as causative factors in organic brain dysfunction, as discussed previously. However, in late-stage lupus, when there is no longer any evidence of active disease and the patient is taking little or no corticosteroid, neurocognitive disabilities remain a frequent complaint. Patients often complain of decreased memory, decreased ability to do mathematical chores and increased speech disabilities. When such patients are submitted to a battery of neurocognitive tests, they are indeed shown to have significant impairment.

In addition, patients with systemic lupus undergoing neurologic investigation have been shown to demonstrate significant cortical atrophy on CT scanning. This has been shown both in patients who have had previous CNS disease caused by lupus and in those who have not, in addition to those who have current neurocognitive symptoms and in those who do not. Thus the exact pathogenesis of the neurocognitive disabilities that occur in latent lupus are not clear at present. They may be a feature of SLE in general, CNS disease of SLE in particular, related to the corticosteroids used to treat SLE or a combination of these factors.

CRITERIA FOR THE CLASSIFICATION OF SLE

For a disease with such protean manifestations and variable course as SLE, the need for classification criteria that would allow comparison of patients from different centers is quite clear[124]. The 1997 modification[125] of the 1982 revised ACR criteria for SLE are listed in Table 33.7. The ACR criteria for the classification of SLE help distinguish patients with SLE from patients with other connective tissue diseases, and thus enable this comparison.

Criteria for disease activity in SLE

More than 60 systems to assess clinical disease activity in SLE have been devised, but there have only been a handful of instruments that have been validated[126]. Three of these, the SLE Disease Activity Index, the British Isles Lupus Assessment Group and the SLE Activity Measure all distinguished among patients, and correlate highly with each other[126]. The SLE Disease Activity Index was recently modified and used to define flare[127]. Regardless of the instrument used to score the disease activity, a full history, physical examination and laboratory tests including serologic markers for SLE are required[128].

Criteria for damage in SLE

As patients with SLE live longer, they accumulate organ damage both as a result of previous inflammation and from complications of treatment. The Systemic Lupus International Collaborating Clinics (SLICC) group, in conjunction with the ACR, developed a damage index for SLE. The SLICC/ACR Damage Index describes the accumulation of damage in patients with SLE since disease onset, and includes items that may have resulted from the inflammatory process, disease treatment or intercurrent events without attribution[129]. The SLICC/ACR Damage Index has been validated and used in a number of studies[126]. It has been found to predict mortality[130]. The Damage Index may thus provide an important outcome measure in SLE, both for studies of prognosis, and in the assessment of long-term effects of treatment. It may also be used to stratify patients for therapeutic trials.

Health status criteria in SLE

Measurements of health status include quality-of-life assessments, psychologic and social impact of the disease, and physical disability. The Medical Outcome Survey Short-Form-36 has been recommended as the instrument of choice to assess quality of life in SLE[131,132].

It is clear that some patients with lupus have difficulty keeping a job and are depressed. Most patients note some effect of the disease on their lifestyle. The relationship between impaired quality of life and disease activity and damage is not clear. Several investigators have found no correlation between health status and disease activity or damage, and consider these to be independent domains in the assessment of patients

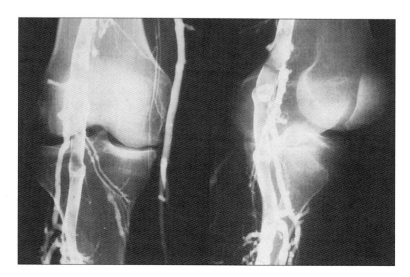

Fig. 33.29 A venogram showing venous thrombosis in a patient with SLE of the right leg and early changes on the left.

TABLE 33.7 THE 1997 REVISED ACR CRITERIA FOR THE CLASSIFICATION OF SLE

Item	Definition
Malar rash	Fixed erythema, flat or raised, over the malar eminences, sparing the nasolabial folds
Discoid rash	Erythematous raised patches with adherent keratotic scaling and follicular plugging: atrophic scarring may occur in older lesions
Photosensitivity	Skin rash as a results of unusual reaction to sunlight, by patient history or physician observation
Oral ulcers	Oral or nasopharyngeal ulceration, usually painless, observed by a physician
Non-erosive arthritis	Involving two or more peripheral joints, characterized by tenderness, swelling, or effusion
Pleuritis or pericarditis	(a) Pleuritis – convincing history of pleuritic pain or rub heard by a physician or evidence of pleural effusion *or* (b) Pericarditis – documented by electrocardiogram or rub or evidence of pericardial effusion
Renal disorder	(a) Persistent proteinuria >0.5g/day or >3+ if quantitative not performed *or* (b) Cellular casts – may be red cell, hemoglobin, granular, tubular or mixed
Seizures or psychosis	(a) Seizures – in the absence of offending drugs or known metabolic derangement: e.g. uremia, ketoacidosis or electrolyte imbalance *or* (b) Psychosis – in the absence of offending drugs or known metabolic derangement: e.g. uremia, ketoacidosis or electrolyte imbalance
Hematologic disorder	(a) Hemolytic anemia with reticulocytosis *or* (b) Leukopenia – less than 4000/mm³ on two occasions *or* (c) Lymphopenia – less than 1500/mm³ on two occasions *or* (d) Thrombocytopenia – less than 100 000/mm³ in the absence of offending drugs
Immunologic disorder	(a) Anti-DNA: antibody to native DNA in abnormal titer *or* (b) Anti-Sm: presence of antibody to Sm nuclear antigen *or* (c) Positive finding of antiphospholipid antibodies based on: (1) an abnormal serum concentration of IgG or IgM anticardiolipin antibodies (2) a positive test for lupus anticoagulant using a standard method *or* (3) a false-positive test for at least 6 months and confirmed by *Treponema pallidum* immobilization or fluorescent treponomal antibody absorption test
Positive ANA	An abnormal titer of ANA by immunofluorescence or an equivalent assay at any point in time in the absence of drug

with SLE, whereas others found that it is related to disease activity and damage[132–134]. The role of formal education in the assessment of health status in patients with SLE was studied by Callahan and Pincus[135]. They administered a clinical status questionnaire to 124 patients with SLE, and found that those with more than 12 years of formal education were more likely to be working full-time than those with 11 years or less of formal education. Moreover, patients with a lower level of education had poorer clinical status on all five self-report scales than did patients with 12 or more years of formal education.

PROGNOSIS

Our understanding of the prospects of recovery from SLE has evolved in the past four decades, both because of better comprehension of the disease process itself, and through the development of methods with which to assess outcome. Survival rates have increased over the past four decades, from less than 50% in 5 years in 1955, to more than 90% survival at 5 years in the 1990s (Table 33.8[136–144]). Recent studies provide survival rates of close to 70% at 20 years[145]. Several reasons have been cited for this improved survival. These include earlier diagnosis, which allows inclusion of milder cases, better therapeutic modalities for lupus, including better use of corticosteroids and immunosuppressive agents,

and advances in medical treatment in general, such as improved antibiotics, antihypertensive agents, availability of renal dialysis and transplantation. However, the pattern of disease in SLE has not changed significantly over the past two decades[146]. A specific study of the reasons for improved survival in SLE also showed that, over a 24-year period, the disease expression did not change, nor did the medications, and yet improved survival in patients with SLE was noticeable above that of the general population. This was believed to reflect more judicious use of currently available medications and better management of the complications of SLE[147].

Despite the improved survival, patients with SLE still die at a rate three times that of the general population[138,147]. The causes of death may be divided into those related to the SLE disease process itself, those related to treatment, and deaths from unrelated causes. The causes related to the SLE include active disease, vasculitis leading to CNS disease or intestinal perforation, intractable bleeding and end-organ failure, such as renal, cardiac or pulmonary. Treatment for SLE may in itself result in fatal complications such as fulminant infection (which may just as likely be associated with active disease), perforation or peptic ulcer disease and, possibly, vascular disease.

In addition to the general principles for improved survival in SLE, there may be specific factors that affect mortality (Table 33.9). These

TABLE 33.8 SURVIVAL RATES IN SLE

Study	No. of patients	Outcome year	Center	Survival (%) 5	10	15	20
Estes and Christian[136]	150	1971	New York	77	60	50	–
Wallace et al.[137]	609	1979	Los Angeles	88	79	74	–
Reveille et al.[138]	389	1990	Alabama	89	83	79	–
Pistiner et al.[139]	570	1990	Los Angeles	97	93	83	–
Ward et al.[140]	408	1991	Durham	82	71	63	–
Massardo et al.[141]	218	1993	Chile	92	77	66	–
Abu-Shakra et al.[121]	665	1993	Toronto	93	85	79	68
Tucker et al.[142]	165	1993	London	93	86	78	–
Blanco et al.[143]	306	1993	Spain	90	85	80	–
Jacobsen et al.[144]	513	1999	Denmark	91	76	64	53

Findings in large series (>100 patients) with data for at least 15 years.

TABLE 33.9 FACTORS THAT AFFECT MORTALITY IN SLE

Study	Year	Time	Age	Race	Sex	SES	Renal	CNS	BP	Plat	DA
Estes and Christian[136]	1955	A	–	–	–	?	+	+	?	?	?
Wallace et al.[137]	1981	D	+	–	–	?	+	–	–	–	?
Reveille et al.[138]	1990	D	+	+	–	–	+	?	+	+	?
Pistiner et al.[139]	1991	D	–	–	+	–	+	?	?	+	?
Ward et al.[140]	1993	A	+	–	–	+	?	?	?	?	?
Massardo et al.[141]	1993	A	–	–	–	–	+	–	–	+	+*
Abu-Shakra et al.[148]	1993	A	+	–	–	–	+	–	–	+	+*
Blanco et al.[143]	1993	A	–	–	+	?	+	+	?	?	?
Jacobsen et al.[144]	1999	A	+	NA	+	?	–	+	?	?	?

A, any time before death; BP, blood pressure; D, at diagnosis; DA, disease activity; NA, not applicable; Plat, platelets; SES, socioeconomic status; –, negative association; +, positive association; ?, not studied; *at study entry

include general features that are unrelated to the disease process itself, such as race, sex, age at onset and socioeconomic status.

Racial differences

Black patients with SLE have been considered to have a poorer prognosis than white patients. Although race did not appear as an important prognostic factor in a logistic regression analysis in the multicenter study published by Ginzler et al.[149], it was found to be a factor adversely affecting survival in SLE when a Cox multivariate analysis was applied to a group of 389 patients studied by Reveille et al.[138]. It has been difficult to separate out the effects of race and socioeconomic status, particularly with reference to differences between white and black patients in the USA. In Reveille's study, white patients with private insurance fared better than black patients with private insurance[138]. However, there was no difference in outcome when black patients with and without private insurance were compared. This supports the notion that there may be racial differences in the expression of this disease and its outcome. However, Ward et al.[140] demonstrated that, although survival was better for whites than for blacks, it was related to socioeconomic status, which was poorer among blacks. In Malaysia, Indian patients were found to fare worse than Chinese[150].

Sex

The relationship between sex and prognosis has been controversial. A higher mortality in females than males with SLE has been suggested by some, whereas others demonstrated a better prognosis for women than for men. Sex did not appear as a significant predictor in the statistical analysis performed by Ginzler et al.[149], or in the University of Toronto cohort[148]. Thus the issue of the effect of sex on prognosis in SLE remains unanswered.

Age at onset

Age at onset of SLE was found to be a significant predictor of survival at both 1 and 5 years in the multicenter study, with better survival in the older patients[149]. In contrast, Reveille et al.[138] found that increasing age of onset adversely affected survival, and Abu-Shakra et al.[148] found age older than 50 years at diagnosis to be a risk for death. Onset of SLE in the pediatric age group has been associated with worse prognosis, but a study of childhood SLE found the 5-year survival to be the same as for the adult populations, at 85.3%[151]. Indeed, a comparison with the estimated survival of the age-matched segment of the US population showed that SLE patients fared worse in all age groups[140].

Socioeconomic status

Patients with better education and higher socioeconomic status seem to fare better than the poorer population. Patients of a lower education level, which may reflect lower socioeconomic status, do less well than those of a higher education level.

Disease factors

The association between specific disease manifestations and outcome in SLE has been well recognized. The presence of CNS disease has been found commonly in patients who die with active lupus[121], and has been found to be associated with decreased survival. Similarly, the presence of nephritis carries a poor prognosis for patients with lupus. The predictive value of serum creatinine concentration for overall mortality in SLE has been recognized for some time. A recent 10-year case–control study demonstrated that, compared with patients with SLE but no nephritis matched for age and sex, patients with lupus nephritis had a greater prevalence of hyperlipidemia (44% compared with 2%, P<0.001), hypertension (44% compared with 9%, P<0.001) and antiphospholipid antibodies (45% compared with 22%, P=0.01) at study onset. More patients with lupus nephritis died (16% compared with 2% P=0.02), the majority from cardiovascular complications[152].

Early studies of the relationship of renal morphology based on light microscopy suggested that advanced lesions, such as diffuse proliferative glomerulonephritis, were associated with greater mortality than was seen with the milder lesions, such as mesangial or minimal lesion. Conversely, several investigators have suggested that, as new predictive information, renal biopsy adds only a limited value to already available clinical variables. McLaughlin et al.[48], using univariate analysis, found a trend for the association of WHO classes with mortality. However, it was the presence of proliferative lesions that was associated with a significantly greater risk of dying. The presence of chronic lesions, such as glomerular sclerosis and interstitial fibrosis, was also significantly associated with reduced survival rates. Moreover, the predictive value of proliferative and chronic

lesions was particularly useful in patients with normal serum creatinine concentrations. Nossent et al.[47] also demonstrated that a high chronicity index was associated with patient mortality in both univariate and multivariate analyses. Thus, although renal biopsy may not be of additional help in patients who already demonstrate clinical evidence of renal damage (increased creatinine), it provides useful information in patients who are studied before damage occurs[153]. Moreover, the presence of proliferative lesions on the biopsy is prognostically significant. Renal damage (increased serum creatinine, dialysis or transplantation) has been found to be a risk factor for mortality[150].

Aside from the association of neuropsychiatric manifestations and renal disease with increased mortality, other disease manifestations have been found to affect prognosis. In the multicenter study[149], anemia from any cause was found to be a predictor for mortality. In the University of Alabama study[138], and in the Toronto cohort[150], thrombocytopenia emerged as an important predictor of mortality. Lung involvement was also found to be a risk factor for mortality. Overall disease activity at presentation measured by the SLEDAI has also been identified as a risk factor for poor outcome[150]. Moreover, a high SLEDAI over follow-up is also associated with death within 6 months[154]. Early damage, within the first year of diagnosis of SLE, is also associated with mortality[130].

REFERENCES

1. Smith CD, Cyr M. The history of lupus erythematosus. From Hippocrates to Osler. Rheum Dis Clin North Am 1988; 14: 1–14.
2. Hargraves MM, Richmond H, Morton R. Presentation of two bone marrow elements. The 'tart' cell and the 'L.E.' cell. Proc Mayo Clin 1948; 23: 25–28.
3. Friou GJ. Identification of the nuclear component of the interaction of lupus erythematosus globulin and nuclei. J Immunol 1958; 80: 476–481.
4. Urowitz MB, Bookman AAM, Koehler BE et al. The bimodal mortality in systemic lupus erythematosus. Am J Med 1976; 60: 221–225.
5. Gladman DD, Urowitz MB. Morbidity in systemic lupus erythematosus. J Rheum 1986; 14(suppl 13): 223–226.
6. Hochberg MC, Perlmutter SL, Medsger TA et al. Prevalence of self-reported physician-diagnosed systemic lupus erythematosus in the USA. Lupus 1995; 4: 454–456.
7. Uramoto KM, Michet CJ, Thumboo J et al. Trends in the incidence and mortality of systemic lupus erythematosus (SLE) 1950–1992. Arthritis Rheum 1999; 42: 46–50.
8. Hopkinson ND, Doherty M, Powell RJ. Clinical features and race-specific incidence/prevalence rates of systemic lupus erythematosus in a geographically complete cohort of patients. Ann Rheum Dis 1994; l53: 675–680.
9. Peschken CA, Esdaile JM. Systemic lupus erythematosus in North American Indians: a population based study. J Rheumatol 2000; 27: 1884–1891.
10. Hochberg MC. Systemic lupus erythematosus. Rheum Dis Clin North Am 1990; 16: 617–639.
11. Stahl-Hallengren C, Jonsen A, Nived O, Sturfelt G. Incidence studies of systemic lupus erythematosus in Southern Sweden: increasing age, decreasing frequency of renal manifestations and good prognosis. J Rheumatol 2000; 27: 685–691.
12. Ward MM, Studenski S. Clinical manifestations of systemic lupus erythematosus. Identification of racial and socioeconomic influence. Arch Intern Med 1990; 150: 849–953.
13. Block SK, Winfield JB, Lockshin MC et al. Studies of twins with systemic lupus erythematosus. A review of the literature and presentation of 12 additional sets. Am J Med 1975; 59: 533–552.
14. Lawrence JS, Martins L, Drake G. A family survey of lupus erythematosus. J Rheumatol 1987; 14: 913–921.
15. Hochberg MC. The application of genetic epidemiology to systemic lupus erythematosus. J Rheumatol 1987; 14: 867–869.
16. Reinersten JL, Klippel JH, Johnson AH et al. B-lymphocyte alloantigens associated with systemic lupus erythematosus. N Engl J Med 1978; 299: 515–518.
17. Schur PH, Marcus-Bagley D, Awdeh Z et al. The effect of ethnicity on major histocompatibility complex complement allotypes and extended haplotypes in patients with systemic lupus erythematosus. Arthritis Rheum 1990; 33: 985–992.
18. Olsen ML, Goldstein R, Arnett FC et al. C4A gene deletion and HLA associations in black Americans with systemic lupus erythematosus. Immunogenetics 1989; 30: 27–33.
19. Petri M, Watson R, Winkelstein HA, McLean RH. Clinical expression of systemic lupus erythematosus in patients with C4A deficiency. Medicine 1993; 72: 236–244.
20. Hartung K, Fontana A, Klar M et al. Association of class I, II, and III MHC gene products with systemic lupus erythematosus. Results of a central European multicenter study. Rheumatol Int 1989; 9: 13–18.
21. Dunckley J, Gatenby PA, Hawkins B et al. Deficiency of C4A is a genetic determinant of systemic lupus erythematosus in three ethnic groups. J Immunogenet 1987; 14: 209–218.
22. Fronek A, Timmerman LA, Alper CA et al. Major histocompatibility complex genes and susceptibility to systemic lupus erythematosus. Arthritis Rheum 1990; 33: 1542–1553.
23. Davies EJ, Steers G, Ollier WER et al. Relative contributions of HLA-SQA and complement C4A loci in determining susceptibility to systemic lupus erythematosus. Br J Rheumatol 1995; 34: 221–225.
24. Huang DF, Siminovitch KA, Liu XY et al. Population and family studies of three disease-related polymorphic genes in systemic lupus erythematosus. J Clin Invest 1995; 95: 1766–1772.
25. Gaffney PM, Kearns GM, Shark KB et al. A genome-wide search for susceptibility genes in human systemic lupus erythematosus sib-pair families. Proc Natl Acad Sci USA 1998; 95: 14875–14879.
26. Moser KL, Neas BR, Salmon JE et al. Genome scan of human systemic lupus erythematosus: evidence for linkage on chromosome 1q in African-American pedigrees. Proc Natl Acad Sci USA 1998; 95: 14869–14874.
27. Cervera R, Khamashta M, Font J et al. Systemic lupus erythematosus: clinical and immunologic patterns of disease expression in a cohort of 1000 patients. Medicine 1993; 72: 113–124.
28. Boumpas DR, Fessler BJ, Austin HA et al. Systemic lupus erythematosus: emerging concepts. Part 2: Dermatologic and joint disease, the antiphospholipid antibody syndrome, pregnancy and hormonal therapy, morbidity and mortality, and pathogenesis. Ann Int Med 1995; 123: 42–53.
29. Cardinali C, Caproni M, Fabbri P. The utility of the lupus band test on sun-protected non-lesional skin for the diagnosis of systemic lupus erythematosus. Clin Exp Rheumatol 1999; 17: 427–432.
30. Gammon RW, Briggaman RA, Inman AO et al. Evidence supporting a role for immune complex-mediated inflammation in the pathogenesis of bullous lesions of systemic lupus erythematosus. J Invest Dermatol 1983; 81: 320–325.
31. Emerit I, Michelson AM. Mechanism of photosensitivity in systemic lupus erythematosus patients. Proc Natl Acad Sci USA 1984; 78: 2537–2540.
32. Furukawa P, Kshihara-Sawami M, Lyons MB, Norris DA. Binding of antibodies to the extractable nuclear antigens SS-A/Ro and SS-B/La is induced on the surface of human keratinocytes by ultraviolet light (UVL): implications for the pathogenesis of photosensitive cutaneous lupus. J Invest Dermatol 1990; 94: 77–85.
33. Nyberg F, Hasan T, Skoglund C, Stephansson E. Early events in ultraviolet light-induced skin lesions in lupus erythematosus: expression patterns of adhesion molecules ICAM-1, VCAM-1 and E-selectin. Acta Dermato-Vener 1999; 79: 431–436.
34. Cronin ME. Musculoskeletal manifestations of systemic lupus erythematosus. Rheum Dis Clin North Am 1988; 14: 99–116.
35. Reilly PA, Evison G, McHugh NJ, Maddison PJ. Arthropathy of hands and feet in systemic lupus erythematosus. J Rheumatol 1990; 17: 777–784.
36. Esdaile JM, Danoff D, Rosenthal L, Gutowsko A. Deforming arthritis in systemic lupus erythematosus. Ann Rheum Dis 1981; 40: 124–126.
37. Morley KD, Leung A, Rynes RI. Lupus foot. BMJ 1982; 284: 557–558.
38. Gladman DD, Urowitz MB, Chaudhry-Ahluwalia V et al. Predictive factors for symptomatic osteonecrosis in systemic lupus erythematosus. J Rheumatol 2001; 28: 761–765.
39. Gladman DD, Urowitz MB, Chaudhry-Ahluwalia V et al. Outcome of symptomatic osteonecrosis in 95 patients with systemic lupus erythematosus. J Rheum 2001; 28: 2226–2269.
40. Finol HR, Montagnani S, Marquez A et al. Ultrastructural pathology of skeletal muscle in systemic lupus erythematosus. J Rheumatol 1990; 17: 210–219.
41. Smythe H, Lee D, Rush P, Buskila D. Tender shins and steroid therapy. J Rheumatol 1991; 18: 1568–1572.
42. Gladman D, Urowitz M, Gough J, MacKinnon A: Fibromyalgia is a major contributor to quality of life in lupus. J Rheumatol 1997; 24: 2145–2149.

43. Rahman P, Gladman DD, Dominique Ibanez, Urowitz MB. Significance of isolated hematuria and isolated pyuria in systemic lupus erythematosus. Lupus 2001; 10: 418–423.

44. Golbus J, McCune WJ. Lupus nephritis. Classification, prognosis, immunopathogenesis and treatment. Rheum Dis Clin North Am 1994; 20: 213–242.

45. Gladman DD, Urowitz MB, Cole E et al. Kidney biopsy in SLE. I. A clinical–morphologic evaluation. Q J Med 1989; 73: 1125–1153.

46. Austin HA, Muenz LR, Joyce KM et al. Prognostic factors in lupus nephritis. Contribution of renal histologic data. Am J Med 1983; 75: 382–3891.

47. Nossent HC, Nenzen-Logmans SC, Vroom TM et al. Contribution of renal biopsy data in predicting outcome in lupus nephritis. Arthritis Rheum 1990; 33: 970–977.

48. McLaughlin J, Gladman DD, Urowitz MB et al. Renal biopsy in SLE. II: Survival analyses according to biopsy results. Arthritis Rheum 1991; 34: 1268–1273.

49. Hariharan S, Pollak VE, Kant KS et al. Diffuse proliferative lupus nephritis: long-term observations in patients treated with ancrod. Clin Nephrol 1990; 34: 61–69.

50. Jacobsen S, Starklint H, Petersen J et al. Prognostic value of renal biopsy and clinical variables in patients with lupus nephritis and normal serum creatinine. Scand J Rheumatol 1999; 28: 288–299.

51. Bajaj S, Albert L, Gladman DD et al. Serial renal biopsy in systemic lupus erythematosus. J Rheumatol 2000; 27: 2822–2826.

52. Bruce IN, Gladman DD, Urowitz MB. Extra-renal disease activity in SLE is not suppressed by chronic renal insufficiency or renal replacement therapy. J Rheumatol 1999; 26: 1490–1494.

53. Krane NK, Burjak K, Archie M, O'Donovan R. Persistent lupus activity in end-stage renal disease. Am J Kid Dis 1999; 33: 872–879.

54. ACR Ad Hoc Committee on Neuropsychiatric Lupus Nomenclature. The American College of Rheumatology nomenclature and case definitions for neuropsychiatric lupus syndromes. Arthritis Rheum 1999; 42: 599–608.

55. Kovacs JAJ, Urowitz MB, Gladman DD. Dilemmas in neuropsychiatric lupus. Rheum Dis Clin North Am 1993; 19: 795–814.

56. Boumpas DT, Austin HA, Fessler BJ et al. Systemic lupus erythematosus: emerging concepts. Part 1: Renal, neuropsychiatric, cardiovascular, pulmonary and hematologic disease. Ann Int Med 1995; 122: 940–950.

57. Amit M, Molad Y, Levy O, Wisenbeek AJ. Headache in systemic lupus erythematosus and its relation to other disease manifestations. Clin Exp Rheumatol 1999; 17: 467–470.

58. Glanz BI, Venkatezan A, Schur PH, Lew RA et al. Prevalence of migraine in patients with systemic lupus erythematosus. Headache 2001; 41: 285–289.

59. Stafford-Brady FJ, Urowitz MB, Gladman DD, Easterbrook M. Lupus retinopathy. Patterns, associations and prognosis. Arthritis Rheum 1988; 31: 1105–1110.

60. Teh L, Isenberg DA. Antiribosomal P protein antibodies in systemic lupus erythematosus. A reappraisal. Arthritis Rheum 1994; 37: 307–315.

61. Kremer JM, Rynes RI, Bartholomew LE et al. Non-organic non-psychotic psychopathology (NONPP) in patients with systemic lupus erythematosus. Semin Arthritis Rheum 1981; 11: 182–189.

62. Denburg SD, Denburg JA, Carbotte RM, Fisk JD et al. Cognitive deficits in systemic lupus erythematosus. Rheum Dis Clin North Am 1993; 19: 815–831.

63. Miguel EC, Rodriques Pereira RM, de Bragança Pereira CA et al. Psychiatric manifestations of systemic lupus erythematosus: clinical features, symptoms, and signs of central nervous system activity in 43 patients. Medicine 1994; 73: 224–232.

64. Minota S, Koyasu S, Yahara I, Winfield J. Autoantibodies to the heat shock protein hsp90 in systemic lupus erythematosus. J Clin Invest 1988; 81: 106–109.

65. Robbins ML, Kornguth SE, Bell CL et al. Antineurofilament antibody evaluation in neuropsychiatric systemic lupus erythematosus. Combination with anticardiolipin antibody assay and magnetic resonance imaging. Arthritis Rheum 1988; 31: 623–631.

66. West SG, Emlen W, Wener MH, Kotzin BL. Neuropsychiatric lupus erythematosus: a 10-year prospective study on the value of diagnostic tests. Am J Med 1995; 99: 153–163.

67. Sibbitt WL Jr, Sibbitt RR, Brooks WM. Neuroimaging in neuropsychiatric systemic lupus erythematosus. Arthritis Rheum 1999; 42: 2026–2038.

68. Kovacs JAJ, Urowitz MB, Gladman DD, Zeman R. The use of SPECT in neuropsychiatric SLE: a pilot study. J Rheumatol 1995; 22: 1247–1253.

69. Kodama K, Okada S, Hino T et al. Single photon emission computed tomography in systemic lupus erythematosus with psychiatric symptoms. J Neurol Neurosurg Psychiatry 1995; 58: 307–311.

70. Griffey RH, Brown MS, Bankhurst AD et al. Depletion of high-energy phosphates in the central nervous system of patients with systemic lupus erythematosus, as determined by phosphorus-31 nuclear magnetic resonance spectroscopy. Arthritis Rheum 1990; 33: 827–833.

71. Segal AM, Calabrese LH, Ahmad M et al. The pulmonary manifestations of systemic lupus erythematosus. Semin Arthritis Rheum 1985; 14: 202–224.

72. Orens JB, Martinez FJ, Lynch III JP. Pleuropulmonary manifestations of systemic lupus erythematosus. Rheum Dis Clin North Am 1994; 20: 159–193.

73. Good Jr JT, King TE, Antony VB, Sahn SA. Lupus pleuritis: clinical features and pleural fluid characteristics with special reference to pleural fluid antinuclear antibodies. Chest 1983; 84: 714–718.

74. Wang DY, Yang PC, Yu WL et al. Serial antinuclear antibodies titre in pleural and pericardial fluid. Eur Resp J 2000; 15: 1106–1110.

75. Leung WH, Wong KL, Lau CP et al. Cardiac abnormalities in systemic lupus erythematosus: a prospective M-mode, cross-sectional and Doppler echocardiographic study. Int J Cardiol 1990; 27: 367–375.

76. Sturfelt G, Eskilsson J, Nived O, Truedsson L et al. Cardiovascular disease in systemic lupus erythematosus. A study of 75 patients from a defined population. Medicine 1992; 71: 216–223.

77. Bulkley BH, Roberts WC. The heart in systemic lupus erythematosus and the changes induced in it by corticosteroid therapy. Am J Med 1975; 58: 243–264.

78. Zashin SJ, Lipsky PE. Pericardial tamponade complicating systemic lupus erythematosus. J Rheumatol 1989; 16: 374–377.

79. Kaufman LD, Seifert FC, Eilbott DJ et al. Candida pericarditis and tamponade in a patient with systemic lupus erythematosus. Arch Intern Med 1988; 148: 715–717.

80. Coe MD, Hamer DH, Levy CS et al. Gonococcal pericarditis with tamponade in a patient with systemic lupus erythematosus. Arthritis Rheum 1990; 33: 1438–1441.

81. Mok MY, Wong RW, Lau CS. Intestinal pseudo-obstruction in systemic lupus erythematosus: an uncommon but important clinical manifestation. Lupus 2000; 9: 11–18.

82. Schoshoe JT, Koch AE, Chang RW. Chronic lupus peritonitis with ascites: review of the literature with a case report. Semin Arthritis Rheum 1988; 18: 121–126.

83. Carette S. Cardiopulmonary manifestations of systemic lupus erythematosus. Rheum Dis Clin North Am 1988; 14: 135–147.

84. Bankier AA, Kiener HP, Wiesmayr MN et al. Discrete lung involvement in systemic lupus erythematosus: CT assessment. Radiology 1995; 196: 835–840.

85. Zamora MR, Warner ML, Tuder R, Schwarz MI. Diffuse alveolar hemorrhage and systemic lupus erythematosus. Clinical presentation, histology, survival, and outcome. Medicine 1997; 76: 192–202.

86. Asherson RA, Oakley CM. Pulmonary hypertension in a lupus clinic: experience with twenty-four patients. J Rheumatol 1990; 17: 1292–1298.

87. Winslow TM, Ossipov MO, Fazio GP et al. Five-year follow-up study of the prevalence and progression of pulmonary hypertension in systemic lupus erythematosus. Am Heart J 1995; 129: 510–515.

88. Robbins IM, Gaine SP, Schilz R et al. Epoprostenol for treatment of pulmonary hypertension in patients with systemic lupus erythematosus. Chest 2000; 117: 14–18.

89. Walz-Leblanc BA, Urowitz MB, Gladman DD, Hanly PJ. The 'shrinking lungs syndrome' in systemic lupus erythematosus – improvement with corticosteroid therapy. J Rheumatol 1992; 19: 1970–1972.

90. Warrington KJ, Moder KG, Brutinel WM. The shrinking lung syndrome in systemic lupus erythematosus. Mayo Clin Proc 2000; 75: 467–472.

91. Rubin LA, Urowitz MB. Shrinking lung syndrome in SLE – a clinical pathologic study. J Rheumatol 1983; 10: 973–976.

92. Sasson Z, Rasooly Y, Chow CW et al. Impairment of left ventricular diastolic function in systemic lupus erythematosus. Am J Cardiol 1992; 69: 1629–1634.

93. Badui E, Garcia-Rubi D, Robles E et al.. Cardiovascular manifestations in systemic lupus erythematosus. Angiology 1985; 36: 431–441.

94. Hosenpud JD, Montanaro A, Hart MV et al. Myocardial perfusion abnormalities in asymptomatic patients with systemic lupus erythematosus. Am J Med 1984; 77: 286–292.

95. Tamburino C, Fiore C, Foti R et al. Endomyocardial biopsy in diagnosis and management of cardiovascular manifestations of systemic lupus erythematosus. Clin Rheumatol 1989; 8: 108–112.

96. Straaton KV, Chatham WW, Reveille JD et al. Clinically significant valvular heart disease in systemic lupus erythematosus. Am J Med 1988; 85: 645–650.

97. Korbet SM, Schwartz MM, Lewis EJ. Immune complex deposition and coronary vasculitis in systemic lupus erythematosus. Am J Med 1984; 77: 141–145.

98. Hallegua DS, Wallace DJ. Gastrointestinal manifestations of systemic lupus erythematosus. Curr Opin Rheumatol 2000; 12: 379–385.

99. Zizic TM, Classen JN, Stevens MB. Acute abdominal complications of systemic lupus erythematosus and polyarteritis nodosa. Am J Med 1982; 73: 525–531.

100. Gladman DD, Ross T, Richardson B, Kulkarni S. Bowel involvement in systemic lupus erythematosus: Crohn's disease or lupus vasculitis. Arthritis Rheum 1985; 28: 466–470.

101. Nagata M, Ogawa Y, Hisano S, Ueda K. Crohn's disease in systemic lupus erythematosus: a case report. Eur J Pediatr 1989; 148: 525–526.

102. Reynolds JC, Inman RD, Kimberly RP et al. Acute pancreatitis in systemic lupus erythematosus: report of twenty cases and a review of the literature. Medicine 1982; 61: 25–32.

103. Saab S, Corr MP, Weisman MH. Corticosteroids and systemic lupus erythematosus pancreatitis: a case series. J Rheumatol 1998; 25: 801–806.

104. Haakenstad AO, Mannik M. Saturation of the reticuloendothelial system with soluble immune complexes. J Immunol 1974; 112: 1939–1948.

105. Dillon AM, Stein HB, English RA. Splenic atrophy in SLE. Ann Intern Med 1982; 96: 40–43.

106. Buskila D, Gladman DD, Hanna W, Kahn HJ. Primary malignant lymphoma of the spleen in systemic lupus erythematosus. J Rheumatol 1989; 16: 993–996.

107. Kojima M, Nakamura S, Morishita Y et al. Reactive follicular hyperplasia in the lymph node lesions from systemic lupus erythematosus patients: a clinicopathological and immunohistological study of 21 cases. Pathol Int 2000; 50: 304–312.

108. Voulgarelis M, Kokori SI, Ioannidis JP et al. Anaemia in systemic lupus erythematosus: aetiological profile and the role of erythropoietin. Ann Rheum Dis 2000; 59: 217–222.

109. Miller MH, Urowitz MB, Gladman DD: The significance of thrombocytopenia in systemic lupus erythematosus. Arthritis Rheum 1983; 26: 1181–1186.

110. Musio F, Bohen EM, Yuan CM, Welch PG. Review of thrombotic thrombocytopenic purpura in the setting of systemic lupus erythematosus. Semin Arthritis Rheum 1998; 28: 1–19.

111. Papo T, Andre MH, Amoura Z et al. The spectrum of reactive hemophagocytic syndrome in systemic lupus erythematosus. J Rheumatol 1999; 26: 927–930.

112. Ridker PM, Hennekens CH, Buring JE, Rifai NC. C-Reactive protein and other markers of inflammation in the prediction of cardiovascular disease in women. N Engl J Med 2000; 342: 836–843.

113. Lloyd W, Schur PH. Immune complexes, complement, and anti-DNA in exacerbations of systemic lupus erythematosus (SLE). Medicine 1981; 60: 208–207.

114. Walz-Leblanc B, Gladman DD, Urowitz MB, Goodman PJ. Serologically active clinically quiescent SLE. J Rheumatol 1994; 21: 2239–2241.

115. Reichlin M. ANA negative systemic lupus erythematosus sera revisited serologically. Lupus 2000; 9: 116–119.

116. Ganczarczyk L, Urowitz MB, Gladman DD. Latent lupus. J Rheumatol 1989; 16: 475–478.
117. Swaak AHG, van de Bring H, Smeenk RJT et al. Incomplete lupus erythematosus: results of a multicentre study under the supervision of EULAR Standing Committee on International Clinical Studies Including Therapeutic Trials (ESCISIT). Rheumatology 2001: 40: 89–94.
118. Hess EV. Drug-related lupus. N Engl J Med 1988; 318: 1460–`1462.
119. Rubin RL. Etiology and mechanisms of drug-induced lupus. Curr Opin Rheumatol 1999; 11: 357–363.
120. Schaible TF. Long term safety of infliximab. Can J Gastroenterol 2000; 14(suppl C): 29–32.
121. Abu-Shakra M, Urowitz MB, Gladman DD, Gough J. Mortality studies in systemic lupus erythematosus. Results from a single centre. I. Causes of death. J Rheumatol 1995; 22: 1259–1264.
122. Bruce IN, Gladman DD, Urowitz MB. Premature atherosclerosis in SLE. Rheum Dis Clin North Am 2000; 26: 257–278.
123. Gladman DD, Urowitz MB. Venous syndromes and pulmonary embolism in systemic lupus erythematosus. Ann Rheum Dis 1980; 39: 340–343.
124. Tan EM, Cohen AS, Fries JF et al. The 1982 revised criteria for the classification of systemic lupus erythematosus. Arthritis Rheum 1982; 25: 1271–1277.
125. Hochberg MC. Updating the American College of Rheumatology revised criteria for the classification of systemic lupus erythematosus [letter]. Arthritis Rheum 1997; 40: 1725.
126. Urowitz MB, Gladman DD. Assessment of disease activity and damage in SLE. Baillière's Clinical Rheumatology 1998; 12: 405–413.
127. Gladman DD, Ibañez D, Urowitz MB. Systemic lupus erythematosus disease activity index 2000. J Rheumatol 2002; 29: 288–291.
128. Gladman DD, Urowitz MB, Esdaile JM et al. American College of Rheumatology Ad Hoc Committee on SLE Guidelines. Guidelines for referral and management of systemic lupus erythematosus in adults. Arthritis Rheum 1999; 42: 1785–1796.
129. Gladman D, Ginzler E, Goldsmith CH et al. The development and initial validation of the SLICC/ACR damage index for SLE. Arthritis Rheum 1996; 39: 363–369.
130. Rahman P, Gladman DD, Urowitz MB et al. Early damage as measured by the SLICC/ACR Damage Index is a predictor of mortality in SLE. Lupus 2001; 10: 93–96.
131. Gladman DD, Urowitz M, Fortin P et al. Workshop Report: Systemic Lupus Erythematosus International Collaborating Clinics (SLICC) Conference on Assessment of Lupus Flare and Quality of Life Measures in SLE. J Rheumatol 1996; 23: 1953–1535.
132. Gordon C, Clarke AE. Quality of life and economic evaluation in SLE clinical trials. Lupus 1999; 8: 645–654.
133. Hanly JG. Disease activity, cumulative damage and quality of life in systematic lupus erythematosus: results of a cross-sectional study. Lupus 1997; 6: 243–247.
134. Wang C, Mayo NE, Fortin PR. The relationship between health related quality of life and disease activity and damage in systemic lupus erythematosus. J Rheumatol 2001; 28: 525–532.
135. Callahan LF, Pincus T. Associations between clinical status questionnaire scores and formal education level in persons with systemic lupus erythematosus. Arthritis Rheum 1990; 33: 407–411.
136. Estes D, Christian CL. The natural history of systemic lupus erythematosus by prospective analysis. Medicine 1971; 50: 85–95.
137. Wallace DJ, Podell T, Weiner J et al. Systemic lupus erythematosus survival patterns. Experience with 609 patients. JAMA 1981; 245: 934–938.
138. Reveille JD, Bartolucci A, Alarcón-Segovia D. Prognosis in systemic lupus erythematosus. Negative impact of increasing age at onset, black race, and thrombocytopenia, as well as causes of death. Arthritis Rheum 1990; 33: 37–48.
139. Pistiner M, Wallace DJ, Nessim S et al. Lupus erythematosus in the 1980s: a survey of 570 patients. Semin Arthritis Rheum 1991; 21: 55–64.
140. Ward MM, Pyun E, Studenski S. Long-term survival in systemic lupus erythematosus. Patient characteristics associated with poorer outcomes. Arthritis Rheum 1995; 38: 274–283.
141. Massardo L, Martinez ME, Jacobelli S et al. Survival of Chilean patients with systemic lupus erythematosus. Semin Arthritis Rheum 1994; 24: 1–11.
142. Tucker LB, Menon S, Schaller JG, Isenberg DA. Adult and childhood onset systemic lupus erythematosus: a comparison of onset, clinical features, serology and outcome. Br J Rheumatol 1995; 34: 866–872.
143. Blanco FJ, Gomez-Reino JJ, de la Mata J et al. Survival analysis of 306 European Spanish patients with systemic lupus erythematosus. Lupus 1998; 7: 159–163.
144. Jacobsen s, Petersen J, Ulman S et al. Mortality and causes of death of 513 Danish patients with systemic lupus erythematosus. Scand J Rheumatol 1999; 28: 75–80.
145. Urowitz MB, Gladman DD. How to improve morbidity and mortality in systemic lupus erythematosus. Rheumatology 2000; 39: 237–243.
146. Swaak AJG, Nieuwenhuis EJ, Smeenk RJT. Changes in clinical features of patients with systemic lupus erythematosus followed prospectively over 2 decades. Rheumatol Int 1992; 12: 71–75.
147. Urowitz MB, Gladman DD, Abu-Shakra M, Farewell VT. Mortality studies in systemic lupus erythematosus. Results from a single centre. III. Improved survival over 24 years. J Rheumatol 1997; 24: 1061–1065.
148. Abu-Shakra M, Urowitz MB, Gladman DD, Gough J. Mortality studies in systemic lupus erythematosus. Results from a single centre. II. Predictor variables for mortality. J Rheumatol 1995; 22: 1265–1270.
149. Ginzler EM, Diamond H, Weiner M et al. A multicenter study of outcome in systemic lupus erythematosus. I. Entry variables as predictors of prognosis. Arthritis Rheum 1982; 25: 601–611.
150. Wang F, Wang CL, Tan CT, Manivasagar M. Systemic lupus erythematosus in Malaysia: a study of 539 patients and comparison of prevalence and disease expression in different racial and gender groups. Lupus 1997; 6: 248–253.
151. Lacks S, White P. Morbidity associated with childhood systemic lupus erythematosus. J Rheumatol 1990; 17: 941–945.
152. Font J, Ramos-Casals M, Cervera R et al. Cardiovascular risk factors and the long-term outcome of lupus nephritis. Q J Med 2001; 94: 19–26.
153. McLaughlin JR, Bombardier CB, Farewell VT et al. Kidney biopsy in systemic lupus erythematosus. III. Survival analysis controlling for clinical and laboratory variables. Arthritis Rheum 1994; 37: 559–567.
154. Cook RJ, Gladman DD, Pericak D, Urowitz MB. Prediction of short-term mortality in SLE with time-dependent measures of disease activity. J Rheumatol 2000; 27: 1892–1895.

34 Treatment of constitutional symptoms, skin, joint, serositis, cardiopulmonary, hematologic and central nervous system manifestations

Cynthia Aranow and Ellen M Ginzler

- The management of patients with systemic lupus erythematosus (SLE) is decided on an individual basis, guided by the degree and severity of specific symptoms and organ system involvement
- Non-steroidal anti-inflammatory drugs are an important first-line therapy for the treatment of constitutional signs, musculoskeletal symptoms and mild serositis
- Antimalarials are frequently effective for chronic constitutional signs and cutaneous and musculoskeletal manifestations, with an excellent therapeutic benefit to toxicity profile
- Most clinical manifestations of SLE respond well to corticosteroids, with a wide dose range depending upon the organ systems involved and the degree of severity. However, short- and long-term corticosteroid toxicities account for substantial morbidity
- Immunosuppressive agents are useful in patients with life- or organ-threatening manifestations, as well as for steroid sparing in patients who are either steroid dependent or refractory

INTRODUCTION

Systemic lupus erythematosus (SLE) is an autoimmune inflammatory multisystem disease with diverse manifestations and a course characterized by flares (increases in disease activity) and remissions. Treatment will vary between patients and from flare to flare even within the same patient, depending upon the severity and the particular manifestation(s) of the increased disease activity (Table 34.1). Although useful for epidemiologic studies of lupus cohorts, disease activity indices such as SLEDAI, SLAM and BILAG may not be useful guides upon which to base therapeutic interventions. Some clinical flares may be life threatening, whereas others consist predominantly of constitutional symptoms. Activity scores may not accurately capture the severity of the flares. For example, using the SLEDAI alopecia and a malar rash will score equivalently to an increase in proteinuria. Disease management after achieving control of the inflammatory features typically includes tapering of the immunosuppression required to suppress disease activity while closely monitoring for evidence of a potential relapse. In many instances long-term maintenance therapy may be required. This chapter reviews the management of the heterogenous (non-renal) features of SLE. Although new interventions have recently become available, the approach to many of these manifestations has changed little. This chapter will not discuss the management of the potential adverse effects associated with corticosteroid treatment or with the use of other anti-inflammatory and immunosuppressive medications. Similarly, treatment of associated medical conditions (i.e. hypertension in lupus nephritis, dialysis, infections) seen by rheumatologists caring for lupus patients will not be covered.

PATIENT EDUCATION

A knowledgeable patient who understands the disease is more likely to be compliant with appointments and medications. There is abundant

	Manifestations of SLE				
Agents	**Constitutional**	**Musculoskeletal**	**Serositis**	**Cutaneous**	**Major organ**
NSAIDs	✓	✓	✓		
Corticosteroids					
Topical				✓	
Low dose (i.e. prednisone <0.5mg/kg/day)	✓	✓	✓	✓	
High dose (i.e. prednisone 1.0mg/kg/day or 1g IV methylprednisolone)					✓ ✓
Antimalarials	✓	✓	✓	✓	
Dapsone				✓	
Thalidomide				✓	
Immunosuppressives					
Azathioprine	✓	✓	✓	✓	✓
Cyclophosphamide					✓
Chlorambucil					✓
Cyclosporin					✓
Methotrexate		✓	✓		
Immunoglobulins					✓
Danazol					✓

TABLE 34.1 DRUGS USED IN THE MANAGEMENT OF SYSTEMIC LUPUS ERYTHEMATOSUS

literature available from sources such as the Lupus Foundation of America and the Arthritis Foundation. Patient support groups are another valuable source of information and are also a forum through which patients may share the skills they have acquired for coping with this chronic disease. Establishing a good doctor–patient relationship is fundamental to the management of any chronic disease.

THERAPEUTIC INTERVENTION: NON-STEROIDAL ANTI-INFLAMMATORY DRUGS (NSAIDs)

Although NSAIDs are not specifically approved by the Food and Drug Administration for use in SLE they are approved for arthritis and soft tissue complaints and are ubiquitously used in lupus. NSAIDs are usually used for mild lupus activity before low-dose corticosteroids are initiated, or with antimalarials. NSAIDs are additionally combined with corticosteroids in an effort to minimize the corticosteroid dose, or to suppress lupus activity when alternate-day corticosteroids are used. They are commonly administered for the symptomatic treatment of musculoskeletal manifestations, mild serositis and systemic features such as fever. NSAIDs prevent the formation of prostaglandins by inhibiting the cyclo-oxgenases COX-1 and COX-2. As with other rheumatic diseases, there seem to be differences in patient responsiveness to individual NSAIDs, and drugs from different chemical classes may need to be tried before settling on the single best drug for a particular patient.

Adverse effects from NSAIDs may occur in lupus patients. Deleterious effects on the kidneys, liver and CNS may pose diagnostic dilemmas, as they may mimic features of active lupus. Renal dysfunction may result from impairment of glomerular filtration, tubular function or renal blood flow. Nephrotic syndrome, interstitial nephritis, acute tubular necrosis and minimal change disease are also reported to occur rarely with NSAID administration[1]. Lupus patients taking NSAIDs who present with renal abnormalities should be taken off the NSAID and monitored before assuming the presence of lupus nephritis. Similarly, NSAID-induced hepatitis must be considered in a patient taking NSAIDs who develops liver enzyme abnormalities before concluding the presence of autoimmune hepatitis. Lupus patients taking NSAIDs, particularly ibuprofen, have an increased susceptibility to developing aseptic meningitis, characterized by headache, meningismus, fever with a lymphocytosis and elevated protein in cerebrospinal fluid[2]. This syndrome may be confused with features of CNS lupus. Rechallenging with ibuprofen may result in a recurrence within 24 hours. Headaches, dizziness, confusion or depression are other neuropsychiatric symptoms that may result from NSAID administration.

Although treatment with the newer COX-2 specific inhibitors has the advantage of less gastrointestinal toxicity, other potential adverse effects of NSAIDs are not limited. Additionally, as the COX-2 specific inhibitors do not affect platelet function, certain subsets of lupus patients, such as those with antiphospholipid antibodies, may be prone to developing thrombosis after exposure to COX-2 inhibition. There is a report of four patients with high-titer anticardiolipin antibodies who experienced thrombotic events after treatment with a COX-2 specific inhibitor[3].

CORTICOSTEROIDS

Corticosteroids are clearly the cornerstone of SLE treatment. Their rapid onset of action reduces inflammation and results in resolution of the inflammatory manifestations of lupus activity. They are typically prescribed orally in low, medium (0.5mg/kg) or high doses (1mg/kg), depending upon the targeted manifestation(s) (Table 34.2). Although usually given as a single morning dose, corticosteroids may be given in split doses (2–4 times a day) for enhanced effectiveness. Pulse steroids (intravenous methylprednisolone 1g, usually given for 3 consecutive days) may be useful for treatment of severe or life- or organ-threatening features of disease. After control of disease activity is achieved, tapering of the prednisone dose is initiated. The rapidity of the dose reduction varies significantly and is dependent upon the initial disease manifestations, the duration of corticosteroid treatment, the responsiveness of the patient's disease (does the disease remain under control, or do new or recurrent symptoms re-emerge as the dose is lowered?) and the patient's tolerance of steroids (do steroid toxicities develop?), as well as the experience and practice patterns of the individual rheumatologist. Typically, the dose is not lowered by more than 25% decrements. Although total discontinuation of corticosteroids is a goal desired by both patients and physicians, many patients require maintenance with low-dose corticosteroids (5–10mg/day) to prevent recurrence. One small retrospective study suggests that continuation of low-dose prednisone may be protective for patients initially treated for major disease activity[4].

As corticosteroids are associated with multiple toxicities, monitoring of blood pressure, cholesterol, glucose, bone density and ocular pressure is an important adjunctive measure taken by most rheumatologists. Maintaining a high index of suspicion for the development of other toxicities, including gastrointestinal ulceration, avascular necrosis, atherosclerosis and steroid myopathy, is also important in the management of patients on corticosteroids.

ANTIMALARIALS

Antimalarial agents are commonly used to treat non-life threatening manifestations of SLE which either do not respond to non-steroidal anti-inflammatory drugs and/or low-dose corticosteroids, or which recur when these agents are tapered or discontinued. Typically these features include constitutional symptoms such as fatigue, musculoskeletal symptoms, skin rashes and pleuritic chest pain (Table 34.3). Hydroxychloroquine, a 4-aminoquinolone derivative, is the most commonly used antimalarial, generally begun at a dose of 400mg daily. Clinical response may be expected within 4–6 weeks, and in some patients this is sustained even with a dose reduction to 200mg daily.

TABLE 34.2 CORTICOSTEROIDS IN SLE		
Indication	**Corticosteroid regimen**	
Rashes	Topical	Short-acting: hydrocortisone (0.125–1.0%) Intermediate-acting: triamcinolone (0.025–0.5%) Long-acting: betamethasone (0.01–0.1%)
	Intralesional (discoid lupus)	Triamcinolone acetonide
Minor disease activity	Oral prednisone (or equivalent) <0.5mg/kg/day in single or divided daily dose	
Major disease activity	Oral prednisone (or equivalent) 1.0mg/kg/day in single or divided daily dose or Intravenous methylprednisolone (1g or 15mg/kg), usually repeated for 3 consecutive days	

TABLE 34.3 ANTIMALARIALS USED IN LUPUS

Drug	Daily dose	
4-Aminoquinolone derivatives	Hydroxychloroquine	200–400mg*
	Chloroquine	250mg*
9-Aminoacridine derivatives	Quinacrine (mepacrine)	100mg*

* In patients weighing less than 45kg, dose reductions are necessary: 5–7mg/kg for hydroxy-chloroquine, 4mg/kg for chloroquine, 1–2mg/kg for quinacrine.

Chloroquine, also an aminoquinolone derivative, is less commonly used than hydroxychloroquine. Patients who do not demonstrate a benefit from an aminoquinolone may respond to the 9-aminoacridine compound quinacrine in a dose of 100mg/day. In some cases in which only a partial response to a single antimalarial agent has been achieved, the combination of two or more of these agents may prove to be synergistic[5,6]. A recent uncontrolled report on six SLE patients suggests that the combination of hydroxychloroquine and quinacrine may be beneficial not only for chronic cutaneous lupus manifestations, but also for maintenance of remission of major organ involvement[7]. It should be noted that the production of Atabrine® was discontinued in the United States in 1992, but quinacrine hydrochloride is available from compounding pharmacies.

Antimalarials were used in the treatment of rheumatic diseases many years before any knowledge of their mechanism of action was available. It is now generally accepted that they have important immunomodulatory effects (Table 34.4), decreasing antigen processing and presentation by both macrophages and lymphoid dendritic cells. This appears to result from an increase in intracytoplasmic pH, which in turn alters the molecular assembly of α-ϵ-peptide complexes of class II MHC molecules. Subsequent decreased stimulation of CD4 T cells ultimately leads to a downregulation of responses, including decreased production of cytokines such as IL-1, IL-2, IL-4, IL-5, IL-6 and tumor necrosis factor[8]. Although a number of potential side effects of antimalarials are well described, in practice toxicity does not significantly limit their usefulness. Antimalarials may induce a hemolytic anemia in individuals (most often those of black race) with glucose-6 phosphate dehydrogenase

TABLE 34.4 IMMUNOMODULATORY EFFECTS OF ANTIMALARIALS

Mechanism	Effect
Accumulation in lysosomes, resulting in increase in intracellular pH	Delays recycling of proteins such as enzymes and surface receptors from lysosomes to the cell surface Disrupts normal assimilation of peptides with class II MHC molecules, resulting in decreased interaction between antigen presenting cells and T cells Decreases cytokine production (eg. IL-1, IL-6, TNF-α)
Inhibits activity of phospholipases A₂ and C	Decreases production of leukotrienes and prostaglandins, resulting in decreased phagocytosis and chemotaxis
Bind to DNA by intercalation between adjacent base pairs	Stabilizes DNA, inhibiting its denaturation Blocks the LE cell phenomenon

deficiency; therefore, it is advisable to screen for the presence of this enzyme prior to instituting therapy. Decreased levels in patients with a heterozygous trait do not appear to trigger hemolysis.

Ocular toxicity is responsible for the most significant concern with regard to antimalarial therapy. Deposition of these agents in the melanin of the pigmented epithelial layer of the retina may damage rods and cones. Early damage is usually reversible but is most often asymptomatic, necessitating regular ophthalmologic examination, including visual acuity, slit-lamp, fundoscopic and visual field testing, usually every 6–12 months. The initial retinal changes are noted in the macula, with edema, increased stippling pigmentation, and loss of the foveal reflex to bright light. Visual field defects are generally associated with more severe retinal changes, including optic disc pallor and atrophy, attenuation of retinal arterioles, fine granular pigmentary changes in the peripheral retina, and prominent choroidal patterns in the advanced stages. The development of retinopathy is generally dose and duration dependent. Chloroquine has been clearly shown to have an increased risk of ocular toxicity compared to hydroxychloroquine; 95% of long-term chloroquine users will develop corneal deposits, compared to less than 10% of hydroxychoroquine users[9]. In a Canadian study of 156 SLE patients receiving antimalarials, one developed retinopathy after 6 years at a dose of 6.5mg/kg/day (0.95 cases/1000 patient years of hydroxychloroquine)[10]. Nevertheless, reports of hydroxychloroquine macular toxicity continue to appear, underscoring the need for careful follow-up and detection of early lesions[11,12].

The toxicity associated with chronic antimalarial therapy should not be confused with early side effects related to deposition of drug in the cornea, occasionally resulting in blurred vision, photophobia or visual halos. These visual problems generally resolve within several weeks.

Other manifestations of antimalarial toxicity are uncommon. Gastrointestinal distress often resolves with continued administration. Other early side effects include headache, malaise, and rarely erythematous pruritic rashes. Long-term antimalarial therapy may be associated with a reversible neuromyopathy which may be confused with symptoms of active lupus; muscle biopsy may be necessary to confirm the diagnosis[13]. A single case report of the institution of hydroxychloroquine in a young SLE patient with a history of complex partial seizure suggests that this agent may have precipitated a tonic–clonic seizure[14]. Case reports of the development of cardiac conduction disorders, including complete heart block, in one instance associated with a hypertrophic cardiomyopathy, have been described in patients receiving both short- and long-term treatment with antimalarials for SLE. Both patients improved with discontinuation of antimalarial therapy[15,16]. Ototoxicity secondary to antimalarials remains a controversial issue, and is generally attributed to chloroquine. Two patients receiving several years of hydroxychloroquine therapy are reported to have suffered irreversible sensorineural hearing loss; however, this is also a well-recognized manifestation of autoimmune disease itself[17].

Antimalarials are generally considered to be contraindicated in pregnancy, and conventional wisdom holds that it is not advisable to institute antimalarial therapy in a woman who intends to become pregnant. Rare cases of congenital defects such as cleft palate, sensorineural hearing loss and posterior column defects have been reported, generally associated with chloroquine or quinacrine. The decision regarding discontinuation of antimalarials in a patient who has had a therapeutic benefit and who is now contemplating pregnancy, is more difficult. The half-life of hydroxychloroquine is about 8 weeks, and it may remain detectable in urine for up to 6 months after discontinuation, so that fetal exposure to the agent is not avoided by discontinuation at the time when pregnancy is confirmed. Many rheumatologists opt to continue antimalarials during pregnancy, considering the danger to the fetus of an exacerbation of disease activity in the mother to be greater than the risk of fetal abnormalities[18]. Several reports have documented series of

16–36 SLE pregnancies in patients receiving 4-aminoquinolones; none were associated with congenital abnormalities[19–21].

In addition to the therapeutic effects of antimalarials on SLE disease manifestations, beneficial effects have been reported with regard to improvement in lipoprotein profiles. This is particularly important in patients treated with corticosteroids or those with nephrotic syndrome and secondary hypercholesterolemia. Chloroquine is known to inhibit cholesterol synthesis through its effect on 2,3-oxidosqualene-lanesterol cyclase[22]. It also stimulates LDL receptor activity in cultured fibroblasts[23] and increases the activity of HMG-CoA reductase[22]. Although a recent study of 44 Chinese patients with mild or inactive disease receiving hydroxychloroquine showed no significant effect of the antimalarial therapy on serum lipid profiles[24], many other investigators have demonstrated significant reductions in total cholesterol, triglycerides and LDL cholesterol in association with antimalarial therapy, whether the patient was receiving concomitant steroid therapy or not[25–28]. In her cohort of 264 lupus patients with repeated measures of serum cholesterol during 3027 visits, Petri[29]demonstrated that hydroxychloroquine was able to counteract the adverse effect of 10mg of prednisone on cholesterol level.

Another potential benefit of antimalarials is in prophylaxis against thromboembolic events. Since the 1970s some British orthopedic surgeons have used hydroxychloroquine immediately prior to and after surgery to prevent deep venous thrombosis and pulmonary emboli, with generally beneficial results reported in both uncontrolled and randomized series. Petri reported in her SLE cohort that hydroxychloroquine was protective against future thrombosis in prospectively ascertained venous and arterial thrombotic events[29]. She suggested that this phenomenon might be due to an inhibitory effect on platelet aggregation, an immunosuppressive effect resulting in the lowering of procoagulant antiphospholipid antibody levels, or secondary to either reduction of SLE activity in general or a decrease in atherosclerotic risk factors such as hypercholesterolemia.

Despite the widespread use of antimalarials in SLE, no randomized controlled studies of their efficacy exist. Similarly, information regarding the appropriate duration of therapy after therapeutic success or even disease remission was lacking, until a 1991 study of the effect of discontinuing hydroxychloroquine therapy was carried out by the Canadian Hydroxychloroquine Study Group[30]. In a 24-week randomized double-blind placebo-controlled study in 47 patients with clinically stable SLE, 25 were assigned to continue their same dose of hydroxychloroquine and 22 were assigned to the placebo group. The relative risk of a disease exacerbation was 2.5 times higher (16 of 22 vs. 9 of 25) in the patients taking placebo than in those continuing to take hydroxychloroquine, and 6.1 times greater for severe exacerbations (5 of 22 vs. 1 of 25); the time to flare was also shorter in the placebo group (p=0.02)[30]. In an additional 3-year follow-up period of the same patients, the primary outcome measure was the time to a major flare, defined as the institution or increase in dose of prednisone of 10mg/day or the institution of an immunosuppressive agent. Overall, hydroxychloroquine discontinuation reduced major disease flares by 57%, suggesting that this antimalarial agent has a long-term protective effect[31].

IMMUNOSUPPRESSIVE DRUGS

Immunosuppressive drugs have been used to treat SLE for at least three decades, often borrowed from the oncology and transplantation experience, and became part of the therapeutic regimen for lupus manifestations long before much was known about their mechanism of action in suppressing autoimmunity. Most of these agents are used acutely primarily for life-threatening lupus manifestations, and will be discussed in more detail in relation to specific organ system involvement. In exchange for their immunosuppressive potency they have many and varied toxicities, but virtually all cause a high frequency of gastro-intestinal complaints. The potential for suppression of both erythroid and myeloid elements of the bone marrow and an increased risk of infection require vigilance when monitoring patients receiving these agents.

Azathioprine

Azathioprine is probably the most common immunosuppressive drug used not specifically for acute treatment of active disease manifestations but as a steroid-sparing agent in SLE patients who are steroid dependent or who have repeated disease exacerbations necessitating reinstitution of steroids[32]. Maintenance treatment with azathioprine in doses of 1.5–2.5mg/kg/day has been shown to be associated with a lower rate of development of severe forms of SLE, such as nephritis, or central nervous system involvement[33]. Azathioprine is a purine analog generated by the attachment of an imidazole group to 6-mercaptopurine. Its immunosuppressive action appears to be derived from a suppression of DNA synthesis by the nucleoprotein metabolites of 6-mercaptopurine which inhibit the enzymatic conversion of inosinic acid to xanthylic acid and of adenylsuccinic acid to adenylic acid.

In addition to its effects on the bone marrow, azathioprine can cause hepatotoxicity, usually when given in doses higher than 2.5g/kg/day. Drug hypersensitivity may also result in an acute hepatitis, with elevated transaminases and hepatocellular necrosis and mild biliary stasis on liver biopsy. This syndrome may be accompanied by fever, abdominal pain and a maculopapular rash. The findings are generally reversible upon discontinuation of the drug[34]. Pancreatitis has also been reported to occur in SLE patients receiving azathioprine, but its occurrence may have been associated with other features of disease activity.

Individual case reports have suggested an association of azathioprine with an increased risk of malignancy. An increase in the development of cervical atypia has been documented in women receiving azathioprine[35], thereby indicating the need for regular follow-up with PAP smears. Although it has been suggested that prolonged treatment with azathioprine results in an increase in hematologic and lymphoproliferative malignancies, a large study documenting a higher than expected rate of such malignancies in SLE patients concluded that none of the affected patients had received azathioprine or other immunosuppressive agents[36].

Potential teratogenic effects on the fetus have limited the use of most immunosuppressive agents in pregnant lupus patients. For many years this prohibition included azathioprine. Nevertheless, uncomplicated pregnancies resulting in normal infants have been reported since the 1970s, and only a single case report of an infant born with preaxial polydactyly to a mother taking azathioprine implicates the drug as teratogenic[37]. It is now widely accepted among rheumatologists and obstetricians that azathioprine can be safely continued during pregnancy in women with lupus[38], and may in fact help to preserve the pregnancy by preventing a disease exacerbation.

TREATMENT OF SPECIFIC DISEASE OR ORGAN SYSTEM MANIFESTATIONS: CONSTITUTIONAL SYMPTOMS

Constitutional symptoms such as fatigue, arthralgia, myalgia, weight loss and low-grade fevers are frequent in patients with SLE and can occur alone or may accompany or herald the onset of a more severe organ flare. As fever, arthralgias and myalgias are also symptoms of infections, the appearance of constitutional symptoms should prompt an investigation for an infectious etiology as well as for features of an active lupus flare. NSAIDs are often effective treatment for constitutional symptoms, particularly arthralgias, myalgias and low-grade fevers. Low-dose steroids may be useful if intervention with NSAIDs is unsuccessful or if their use is contraindicated (e.g. in a patient with renal insufficiency). It is worth noting that secondary fibromyalgia has been reported to occur in up to one-third of lupus patients[39]. Fatigue with aches and pains may be difficult to treat in this subset of non-inflammatory patients, but may respond to low-dose tricyclic antidepressants, muscle relaxants and increased aerobic conditioning.

SKIN RASH

Malar rashes and other mild photosensitive rashes associated with mild to moderate exacerbations of SLE activity usually respond to the avoidance of ultraviolet light, coupled with the use of sunscreens and topical or low-dose oral corticosteroids (doses up to 20mg/day), commonly resolving with no sequelae. Intralesional steroids may be appropriate for isolated lesions, especially in the absence of other systemic manifestations of active disease. More persistent rashes requiring higher doses of steroids, or those that recur when steroids are tapered, including both erythematous inflammatory lesions and discoid lupus lesions, are most often treated with antimalarial agents.

Before a patient is considered to be resistant to antimalarial therapy several other possibilities should be considered, including failure to avoid excessive ultraviolet light exposure, or that the continuing or worsening rash is actually the result of a lichenoid drug reaction secondary to the antimalarial itself[40]. It has also been suggested that smoking decreases the efficacy of antimalarial therapy in cutaneous lupus through the induction of hepatic cytochrome P450, thus altering the metabolism of antimalarials[41]. In a study of 61 patients with discoid lupus or subacute cutaneous lupus rashes, 90% of the non-smokers and only 40% of the smokers ($p<0.0002$) responded to antimalarial therapy[42].

In patients who fail to respond to low- to moderate-dose steroids and antimalarials despite attention to the above caveats, the antilepromatous agent dapsone in oral doses of 25–100mg/day has been beneficial, especially for cutaneous manifestations such as bullous lupus, lupus panniculitis ('lupus profundus'), vasculitic lesions and oral ulcers[43–45]. A positive response is often observed within 1–4 weeks. Some patients with antimalarial-refractory discoid lupus and subacute cutaneous lupus rashes may also respond to dapsone. The most common side effect is hemolytic anemia; however, many other rare toxic manifestations have been described, most notably agranulocytosis and toxic epidermal necrolysis.

For patients with refractory skin manifestations of systemic and isolated discoid lupus there has been a renewed interest in the use of thalidomide, a drug developed as a sedative in the 1950s and subsequently withdrawn from the market in 1961 because of its severe teratogenic effects. Thalidomide has known immunologic effects, which provide the rationale for its use in treating autoimmune disease (Table 34.5).

It reduces TNF-α production by human monocytes, decreases peripheral CD4:CD8 lymphocyte ratios, enhances the production of TH2-dependent cytokines, suppresses in vitro neutrophil function, inhibits angiogenesis (probably the effect responsible for its teratogenicity), and modulates lipopolysaccharide induction of adhesiveness in postcapillary venules[46].

In 1983, a series of 60 patients with refractory discoid lupus treated with high starting doses of thalidomide (400mg/day) was reported[47]. The response rate was 90%, but the development of peripheral neuropathy was common and limited its continued use. Although it has been difficult to obtain in the United States, thalidomide is now being produced in Germany. No controlled studies of thalidomide in lupus skin disease have been reported, but a number of recent uncontrolled low-dose open-label series of 10–22 patients have been described[48–52]. The starting dose is usually 100mg/day, tapering to 25–50mg/day after a clinical response is achieved. A complete response was observed in 44–72% of patients in these series, and a partial response in 18–37%. Discontinuation of thalidomide was reported in 0–14% of patients, predominantly for severe drowsiness or paresthesias and documented peripheral neuropathy. Relapses of skin disease were common (65–75%) upon discontinuation, but reinstitution of therapy generally resulted in a return of benefit. Because of the severe potential for birth defects, women of childbearing age must be carefully counseled before therapy is instituted, and effective contraception must be ensured. In order to prescribe thalidomide, both patient and physician must comply with a program guaranteeing safety, the System for Thalidomide Education and Prescribing Safety (STEPS).

Beneficial effects of other agents have been reported in small series of steroid and antimalarial-resistant cutaneous lupus. These include high-dose intravenous immunoglobulin, immunosuppressive agents (azathioprine, methotrexate, cyclophosphamide, cyclosporine, cytarabine, mycophenolate mofetil), the oral gold agent auranofin, and both topical and oral retinoids[53,54]. Severe disfiguring skin lesions which appear to be irreversible may in fact respond to aggressive immunosuppressive therapy, sometimes initiated for more life-threatening manifestations of lupus activity such as nephritis or cerebritis (Fig. 34.1).

ARTHRITIS

The classic description of the musculoskeletal involvement in SLE is non-erosive, non-deforming arthralgias and/or arthritis in a distribution similar to that of rheumatoid arthritis, primarily affecting the small joints of the hands and the wrists. It may be the presenting symptom of SLE or accompany other manifestations of an active disease exacerbation. Acutely, a response to NSAIDs or low-dose steroids is not uncommon. Antimalarials are frequently the drug of choice for SLE patients whose musculoskeletal symptoms are chronic, particularly if they are associated with palpable synovitis.

In SLE patients whose arthritis is chronic and antimalarial resistant or who develop radiologic evidence of erosive disease, treatment with agents more frequently used in rheumatoid arthritis has become well accepted. Despite its potential for renal toxicity, especially proteinuria, which might be confused with active lupus nephritis, in our own experience parenteral gold injections have been used with beneficial results and an acceptable safety profile. In recent years, as weekly oral methotrexate has become the first-line disease-modifying antirheumatic drug for rheumatoid arthritis, it has been shown to be efficacious for antimalarial resistant lupus arthritis as well. Wilke et al.[55] described methotrexate's steroid-sparing ability as well as its usefulness for lupus arthritis in 17 patients studied retrospectively, but concluded that side effects were more common in SLE than among 87 similarly dosed rheumatoid arthritis patients. Leukopenia, oral ulcers and parenchymal hepatotoxicity were the most common side effects. Rahman et al.

TABLE 34.5 IMMUNOMODULATORY EFFECTS OF THALIDOMIDE	
Mechanism	Action
Suppresses neutrophil function *in vitro*	Decreases chemotaxis and phagocytosis
Suppresses production of Th1-dependent cytokines	Decreases monocyte TNF-α production Inhibits interferon-γ production by cultured peripheral blood mononuclear cells
Enhances production of Th2-dependent cytokines	Enhances production of IL-4 and IL-5
Co-stimulates human T cells *in vitro*	Increases IL-2-mediated T-cell proliferation Greater effect on CD8⁺ cells results in decreased CD4:CD8 ratio
Inhibits basic fibroblast growth factor	Suppresses angiogenesis

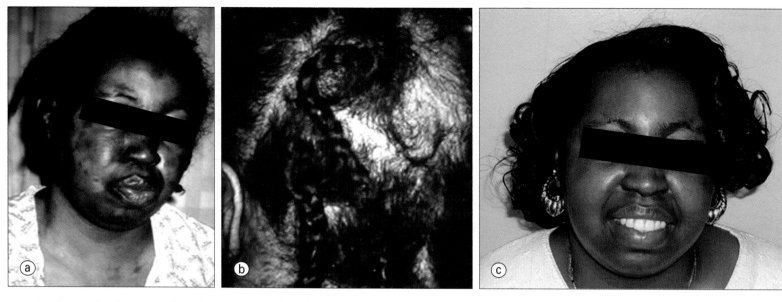

Fig. 34.1 Severe discoid lupus. This patient with severe discoid lupus lesions and cutaneous vasculitis involving her face, trunk and extremities (a) and generalized alopecia (b) failed to respond to moderate doses of corticosteroids (up to 40mg prednisone/day, hydroxychloroquine 400mg/day, and dapsone 100mg/day) over a period of at least 6 months. She subsequently developed central nervous system involvement and nephritis with the nephrotic syndrome and azotemia. Aggressive therapy with pulse methylprednisolone followed by oral steroids in doses up to 120mg prednisone/day and monthly doses of intravenous cyclophosphamide resulted not only in a dramatic improvement in her CNS and renal manifestations but also in complete resolution of her cutaneous manifestations, with no scarring sequelae (c).

subsequently described a series of 17 antimalarial-resistant SLE patients who received methotrexate for persistently active arthritis; during a mean 3.5-year follow-up period, toxicity leading to termination of therapy was infrequent, occurring in only two patients[56]. Compared to a control group, the methotrexate-treated patients had a higher mean joint count at baseline ($p = 0.003$). After 6 months 15 of 17 patients in the methotrexate group showed at least a 60% improvement in joint count compared to only 2 of 17 in the control group ($p < 0.001$). A greater decrease in steroid dose and SLEDAI score were also observed in the methotrexate group. Similarly, in a series of 24 SLE Australian patients treated with 25 courses of methotrexate principally for arthritis over a mean period of 14.4 months, only two terminated therapy because of toxicity[57]. The median initial and peak methotrexate doses were 7.5 and 10mg/week, respectively. A reduction in steroid dose was successful in 36% of patients, but the change was not statistically significant. In the only prospective controlled study reported to date, Sato[58] found a significant improvement in SLEDAI score, steroid requirement and frequency of articular involvement after 6 months of methotrexate therapy. None of these studies have commented on the incidence or progression of radiographic erosions in methotrexate-treated SLE patients with chronic arthritis.

CARDIOPULMONARY

There has been little change in the treatment of serositis over the years in patients with SLE. Many episodes of pleuritis or pericarditis respond to NSAIDs; corticosteroids in moderate doses are useful in refractory cases. Hydroxychloroquine may be added as adjunctive therapy in patients with recurring episodes of serositis. Intravenous immunoglobulin has also been used anecdotally for life-threatening pericarditis[59,60].

Pulmonary hemorrhage requires treatment with high-dose corticosteroids in combination with a cytotoxic agent, typically cyclophosphamide. Plasmapheresis[61] may offer additional benefit in these patients with severe life-threatening disease.

Lupus pneumonitis is an additional manifestation of severe life-threatening disease requiring aggressive therapeutic intervention. Although controlled trials are not available for this clinical feature, high-dose corticosteroid therapy with the addition of azathioprine, cyclophosphamide or intravenous immunoglobulin (IVIG) is warranted and may improve morbidity and mortality[32,61,62].

Pulmonary hypertension is usually treated with a variety of vasodilatory agents and anticoagulants, in addition to immunosuppression with corticosteroids and cytotoxics, in an effort to alleviate clinical symptoms and improve hemodynamic abnormalities. Vasodilatory agents have included calcium channel blockers and prostaglandin analogs, such as intravenous epoprostenol (prostaglandin I_2)[63] and monthly low-dose infusion of iloprost, a prostaglandin I_2 analog[64]. There has been a preliminary report of the effectiveness of continuous infusion of treprostinil, another prostaglandin I_2 analog, in patients with connective tissue disease, including SLE, which demonstrated improved symptoms and hemodynamics in these patients[65]. Bosentan, an oral endothelin-receptor antagonist, has recently become available for the treatment of pulmonary hypertension. It increases exercise capacity and improves hemodynamics in patients with pulmonary hypertension[66]. Its role in SLE remains to be determined. Pulmonary thromboendarterectomy has been reported to be successful in three patients with pulmonary hypertension in association with the antiphospholiplid syndrome[67].

Myocarditis is an uncommon cardiac manifestation of SLE which usually requires high-dose prednisone (1mg/kg/day) for treatment. Cytotoxic intervention with azathioprine or cyclophosphamide has been useful in some patients; intravenous immunoglobulin has also been used successfully for this feature[68–70].

HEMATOLOGIC

Immune-mediated cytopenias occur commonly in SLE and when mild require no treatment. When low counts become clinically significant, corticosteroids in moderate or high doses usually result in a beneficial response. However, there are patients who are either unresponsive to high-dose corticosteroids or in whom high-dose steroids are unable to be tapered; in these circumstances other interventions are necessary.

Other measures used for patients with hemolytic anemia include azathioprine[32,71], danazol[72,73], IVIG[74] and plasmapheresis.[75,76] Splenectomy may be beneficial but its efficacy may not be sustained. Severe neutropenia in the febrile patient is usually responsive to treatment with granulocyte-stimulating factor[77,78]. Lymphopenia per se does not require treatment. Lymphocyte counts usually rise as the patient's overall activity is treated. However, patients with CD4 counts below 200 may be prone to opportunistic infections such as *Pneumocystis carinii*[79] and may require prophylaxis while they are at risk. Adjunctive measures in corticosteroid-resistant or -dependent patients with thrombocytopenia have included IVIG. The effect although prompt, is often only temporary, requiring the administration of other agents. Cyclosporin, danazol, dapsone and cyclophosphamide have been used successfully in anecdotal and case series[80–84]. Newer biologic agents may eventually play a role in this arena; there is a report of refractory thrombocytopenia in a lupus patient responding to interleukin-11[85]. The role of splenectomy in refractory thrombocytopenia in lupus remains unclear, with some series demonstrating long-term effectiveness whereas others show the necessity for continued immunosuppression despite surgical removal of the spleen.

Thrombotic thrombocytopenic purpura (TTP) is a rare feature that may occur with lupus. Treatment of TTP in lupus has been similar to that for primary TTP, i.e. steroids with plasma exchange. There are reports of improved survival in lupus when cyclophosphamide is added to the treatment regimen[86,87].

NEUROPSYCHIATRIC

There are numerous neuropsychiatric symptoms that occur in patients with lupus resulting from a multitude of etiologies. These include adverse events due to medications (e.g. NSAID-induced aseptic meningitis, corticosteroid psychosis or mood swings), infections, and features of the antiphospholipid antibody syndrome, i.e. strokes, seizures and chorea. Management of these symptoms requires the ability to identify the causative factor, followed by appropriate interventions directed at the specific etiology (removal of the offending medication, administration of antibiotics, anticoagulation etc.). Neuropsychiatric symptoms that are believed to respond to anti-inflammatory and immunosuppressive agents include organic brain syndromes, pyschoses, some seizures, some headaches, peripheral neuropathies and myelopathy. These features almost always require high-dose corticosteroids, and often pulse methylprednisolone. Pulse cyclophosphamide administered every 3–6 weeks may be efficacious in steroid-resistant cases[88–90]; intravenous immunoglobulin[91,92] and intrathecal methotrexate[93] are other therapies that have been reported to be of benefit. The outcomes of some neuropsychiatric manifestations such as transverse myelitis have been shown to be favorably affected by the prompt initiation of cyclophosphamide[94].

Despite the lack of a 'gold standard' for diagnosing central nervous system manifestations of SLE, cognitive deficit is easier to identify than to treat. Some patients will demonstrate reversible manifestations of cognitive dysfunction which appear to be associated with other manifestations of disease activity, especially organic brain syndrome, but also in the presence of electrolyte disturbances or azotemia and during episodes of infection. Treatment of the underlying SLE activity or infection should result in improvement of cognitive impairment. Medications such as anticonvulsants may also have side effects that appear as cognitive impairments.

In other lupus patients cognitive impairment appears to be slowly progressive and irreversible, even in the absence of other manifestations of disease activity. This is frequently associated with the presence of antiphospholipid antibodies, even in the absence of other evidence of thromboembolic disease. Long-term anticoagulation may halt the progression of cognitive deficit in such patients. When no inciting factor can be found, therapeutic intervention may be directed at lifestyle changes, including occupational therapy and the involvement of family members in enhancing the patient's daily environment.

HORMONE THERAPY

The safety of hormone (estrogen) therapy in SLE remains an area of controversy. Premenopausal patients could benefit from the positive effects of hormones given as oral contraceptive agents or as estrogen replacement therapy in the perimenopausal and menopausal years. However, there are theoretical concerns that estrogen administration to lupus patients may trigger an increase in disease activity, including the exacerbation of lupus-like disease in animal models and epidemiologic data in humans. Epidemiologic data include the strong female predominance observed in lupus, onset occurring primarily in the childbearing years, and the association between postmenopausal hormone therapy and an increased risk for subsequent development of SLE[95]. There are clearly lupus patients in whom estrogens are contraindicated, i.e. those with antiphospholipid antibodies. However, it is uncertain whether a majority of lupus patients might receive estrogen without potential harm. A case–control study comparing 16 postmenopausal patients on hormone replacement therapy (HRT) with 32 controls not receiving HRT showed no difference in the rate of flares over a follow-up period of 1 year[96]. In another small study of 34 patients, the rate of flare was equivalent in a group of patients given hormonal replacement therapy ($n = 11$) to that in patients ($n = 23$) not receiving replacement; the magnitude of the observed flares was also not significantly different between the two groups[97]. A preliminary report of hormone replacement given to a larger group of postmenopausal lupus patients ($n = 106$) also showed no exacerbation of disease activity in the 52 patients randomized to receive therapy compared to patients receiving placebo[98]. There are no reports of the safety of hormone therapy as oral contraception in premenopausal lupus patients. The results of an ongoing trial assessing the safety of hormone contraception as well as hormone replacement therapy are eagerly anticipated.

INNOVATIVE THERAPIES: AVAILABLE DRUGS NOT APPROVED FOR SLE INDICATIONS

Many of the immunosuppressive agents used to treat SLE in general or specific organ system manifestations have been 'borrowed' from the oncology or transplant experience. In fact, the only class of drugs specifically approved by the Food and Drug Administration (FDA) for the treatment of lupus is the 4-aminoquinolone antimalarials, despite the absence of controlled randomized clinical trials. Given the knowledge that SLE is predominantly a disease of women of childbearing age, it has become clear that a number of hormonal mechanisms may be important in its pathogenesis and hence a potential target for new therapies. Drugs approved and marketed for other indications are being used in uncontrolled series and controlled clinical trials.

Bromocriptine

Prolactin, a peptide hormone synthesized by the pituitary gland, as well as at multiple other sites including lymphocytes, has been found to be elevated in the serum of some women with SLE[99]. As a cytokine, prolactin has many immunologic effects on T cells, B cells, macrophages and natural killer cells, including induction of interleukin (IL)-2 receptors on lymphocytes[99]. Circulating prolactin binds to prolactin receptors distributed throughout the immune system.

Bromocriptine is a dopamine agonist that selectively inhibits secretion of prolactin by the pituitary gland. Bromocriptine therefore has the capacity to inhibit the immune functions stimulated by prolactin, resulting in decreased antibody formation and cell-mediated immune

TABLE 34.6 IMMUNOMODULATORY EFFECTS OF BROMOCRIPTINE

Mechanism	Action
Suppresses prolactin secretion by the pituitary receptors on lymphocytes	Decreases prolactin induction of IL-2 Decreases circulating autoantibody levels (e.g. antipituitary antibodies, anti-dsDNA) in hyperprolactinemic individuals
Direct suppressive effects on T and B cells	Decreases early stages of T-cell activation Inhibits proliferation and immunoglobulin production of mitogen-stimulated human B cells *in vitro*

TABLE 34.7 IMMUNOMODULATORY EFFECTS OF DEHYDROEPIANDROSTERONE

- Enhances IL-2 production by T lymphocytes *in vitro*
- Partially reverses the decreased IL-2 production by SLE T lymphocytes *in vitro*

responses (Table 34.6). It has also been suggested that bromocriptine may act directly to suppress the early phases of human T-cell activation and the proliferation and immunoglobulin production in mitogen-stimulated B lymphocytes[100].

Initial observations suggesting the possible benefit of bromocriptine in SLE occurred during its use in patients with SLE and concomitant prolactinomas, in which the lupus symptoms resolved[101] and subsequently recurred with discontinuation of the drug[102]. Despite the fact that some investigators have failed to show a correlation between prolactin levels and SLE disease activity[103,104], uncontrolled series in patients with both normal and elevated prolactin levels[105], and later randomized controlled double-blind studies, have shown improvement in SLE symptoms and serologic measures of disease activity in prolactin-treated patients[99,105]. Therapeutic benefit was noted for fatigue, headache, arthralgias, skin rash, and anti-dsDNA titers. Steroid-sparing effects, a decreased number of flares and an increased time to flare similar to that achieved with hydroxychloroquine were observed[99]. The dose of bromocriptine in most reported studies was 2.5–3.75mg/day, but doses up to 30mg/day have been used to normalize prolactin levels. Bromocriptine is not teratogenic, has no significant drug interactions, and has been used safely in combination with steroids, antimalarials and other immunosuppressive agents[106].

Dehydroepiandrosterone

Dehydroepiandrosterone (DHEA, prasterone), a naturally occurring weak male androgen, has also shown promise in ameliorating symptoms and serologic abnormalities in SLE. The rationale for its use is based on the known hormonal influence of estrogens and androgens on SLE

activity. Decreased serum levels of DHEA have been demonstrated in some SLE patients, unrelated to levels of disease activity[107]. DHEA has also been shown to have immunomodulatory effects on T lymphocytes (Table 34.7)[108]. An uncontrolled trial of DHEA in 50 lupus patients in doses ranging from 50 to 200mg/day demonstrated improvement in SLEDAI scores and decreased steroid requirement among the 21 patients who completed 12 months of treatment[109]. In a subsequent double-blind, randomized placebo-controlled trial in 191 female patients receiving 10–30mg prednisone/day at onset, treatment with 200mg/day of DHEA was significantly associated with a sustained reduction in prednisone dose <7.5mg/day while maintaining stabilization or improvement in disease activity[110].

In a subset of 37 patients treated in the above controlled study, the effect of DHEA on bone density was examined[111]. Bone mineral density was significantly improved in patients receiving DHEA compared to those on placebo, particularly in the postmenopausal group. As an anabolic steroid, DHEA has also been shown to ameliorate the deleterious effects of glucocorticoids, such as diabetes, amino acid deamination and hypertension[112]. It may have a benefit in diminishing the severity of steroid-induced myopathy and avascular necrosis as well. In fact, Robinzon and Cutolo suggest that as SLE patients with chronic glucocorticoid administration have suppression of ACTH secretion resulting in a further decrease in DHEA levels, DHEA replacement therapy should be considered in order to prevent glucocorticoid side effects. Side effects of DHEA are minimal, most commonly the development or worsening of acne.

Lipid-lowering statins

Premature atherosclerosis is now a well recognized complication of SLE, and recommendations for reducing known risk factors for atherogenesis should be part of the therapeutic regimen for all lupus patients. This includes measures to minimize glucose intolerance, hypertension and hyperlipidemia. Recently, the properties of statins have been shown to extend beyond their lipid-lowering ability to include immunomodulatory activity, probably related to effects on endothelial cell function, which may be beneficial even in lupus patients with normal lipid levels[113]. Controlled trials of statins aimed at assessing their ability to decrease disease activity in lupus are currently in the design phase.

REFERENCES

1. Clive DM, Stoff JS. Renal syndromes associated with nonsteroidal antiinflammatory drugs. N Engl J Med 1984; 310: 563–572.
2. Bouland DL, Specht NL, Hegstad DR. Ibuprofen and aseptic meningitis. Ann Intern Med 1986; 104: 731 [letter].
3. Crofford LJ, Oates JC, McCune WJ et al. Thrombosis in patients with systemic lupus erythematosus treated with specific cyclooxygenase 2 inhibitors. A report of four cases. Arthritis Rheum 2001; 43: 1891–1896.
4. Aranow C, Emy J, Barland P. Reactivation of inactive systemic lupus erythematosus. Scand J Rheumatol 1996; 25: 282–286.
5. Tye MJ, White H, Appel B. Lupus erythematosus treated with a combination of quinacrine, hydroxychoroquine and chloroquine. N Engl J Med 1959; 260: 63–66.
6. Feldmann R, Salomon D, Saurat JH. The association of the two antimalarials chloroquine and quinacrine for treatment-resistant chronic and subacute cutaneous lupus erythematosus. Dermatology 1994; 189: 425–427.
7. Toubi E, Rosner I, Rozenbaum M et al. The benefit of combining hyroxychoroquine with quinacrine in the treatment of SLE patients. Lupus 2000; 9: 92–95.
8. Fox RI, Kang H-I. Mechanism of action of antimalarial drugs: Inhibition of antigen processing and presentation. Lupus 1993; 2 (Suppl 1): S9–S12.
9. Easterbrook M. Is corneal deposition of antimalarial any indication of retinal toxicity? Can J Ophthalmol 1990; 25: 249–225.
10. Wang C, Fortin PR, Li Y et al. Discontinuation of antimalarial drugs in systemic lupus erythematosus. J Rheumatol 199; 26: 808–815.
11. Bienfang D, Coblyn JS, Liang MH. Corzillius M. Hydroxychloroquine retinopathy despite regular ophthalmologic evaluation: a consecutive series. J Rheumatol 2000; 27: 2703–2706.
12. Warner AE. Early hydroxychloroquine macular toxicity. Arthritis Rheum 2001; 44: 1959–1961.
13. Avina-Zubeta JA, Johnson ES, Suarez-Almozar ME, Russell AS. Incidence of myopathy in patients treated with antimalarials. A report of three cases and a review of the literature. Br J Rheumatol 1995; 34: 166–170.
14. Malcangi G, Fraticelli P, Palmieri C et al. Hydroxychloroquine-induced seizure in a patient with systemic lupus erythematosus. Rheumatol Int 2000; 20: 31–33.
15. Baguet JP. Tremel F, Fabre M. Chloroquine cardiomyopathy with conduction disorders. Heart 1999; 81: 221–223.
16. Comin-Colet J, Sanchez-Corral MA, Alegre-Sancho JJ et al. Complete heart block in an adult with systemic lupus erythematosus and recent onset of hydroxychloroquine therapy. Lupus 2001; 10: 59–62.

17. Johansen PB, Grant JT. Ototoxicity due to hydroxychloroquine: report of two cases. Clin Exp Rheumatol 1998; 16: 472–474.
18. Schulzer M, Esdaile JM. The use of antimalarial treatment in lupus pregnancy and lactation. Arthritis Rheum 2000; 43 (Suppl): S272.
19. Parke A, West B. Hydroxychloroquine in pregnant patients with systemic lupus erythematosus. J Rheumatol 1996; 23: 1715–1718.
20. Buchanan NM, Toubi E, Khamashta MA et al. Hydroxychloroquine and lupus pregnancy. Ann Rheum Dis 1996; 55: 486–488.
21. Tincani A, Faden D, Lojacono A et al. Hydroxychloroquine in pregnant patients with rheumatic disease. Gestational and neonatal outcome. Arthritis Rheum 2001; 44 (Suppl): S397.
22. Chen HW, Leonard DA. Chloroquine inhibits cyclization of squalene oxide to lanosterol in mammalian cells. J Biol Chem 1984; 259: 8156–8162.
23. Oram JF, Albers JJ, Cheung MC, Bierman EL. The effects of subfractions of high density lipoprotein on cholesterol efflux from cultured fibroblasts. Regulation of low density lipoprotein receptor activity. J Biol Chem 1981; 256: 8348–8356.
24. Tam LS, Li EK, Lam CW, Tomlinson B. Hydroxychloroquine has no significant effect on lipids and apolipoproteins in Chinese systemic lupus erythematosus patients with mild or inactive disease. Lupus 2000; 9: 413–416.
25. Wallace DJ, Metzger AL, Stecher VJ et al. Cholesterol-lowering effect of hydroxychloroquine in patients with rheumatic disease: reversal of deleterious effects of steroids on lipids. Am J Med 1990; 89: 322–326.
26. Hodis HN, Quismorio FP Jr, Wickham E, Blankenhorn DH. The lipid, lipoprotein and apolipoprotein effects of hydroxychloroquine in patients with systemic lupus erythematosus. J Rheumatol 1993; 20: 661–665.
27. Tam LS, Gladman DD, Hallett DC et al. Effect of antimalarial agents on the fasting lipid profile in systemic lupus erythematosus. J Rheumatol 2000; 27: 2142–2145.
28. Borba EF, Bonfa E. Longterm beneficial effect of chloroquine diphosphate on lipoprotein profile in lupus patients with and without steroid therapy. J Rheumatol 2001; 28: 780–785.
29. Petri M. Hydroxychloroquine use in the Baltimore Lupus Cohort: effects on lipids, glucose and thrombosis. Lupus 1996; 5 (Suppl 1): S16–S22.
30. The Canadian Hydroxychloroquine Study Group. A randomized study of the effect of withdrawing hydroxychloroquine sulfate in systemic lupus erythematosus. N Engl J Med 1991; 324: 150–154.
31. The Canadian Hydroxychloroquine Study Group. A long-term study of hydroxy-chloroquine withdrawal on exacerbations in systemic lupus erythematosus. Lupus 1998; 7: 80–85.
32. Abu-Shakra M, Shoenfeld Y. Azathioprine therapy for patients with systemic lupus erythematosus. Arthritis Rheum 2001; 10: 152–153.
33. Ginzler E, Sharon E, Diamond H, Kaplan D. Long-term maintenance therapy with azathioprine in systemic lupus erythematosus. Arthritis Rheum 1975; 18: 27–34.
34. Jeurissen MEC, Boerbooms AM Th, van de Putte LBA, Kruijsen MWM. Azathioprine induced fever, chills, rash, and hepatotoxicity in rheuamtoid arthritis. Ann Rheum Dis 1990; 49: 25–27.
35. Nyberg G, Eriksson O, Westberg NG. Increased incidence of cervical atypia in women with systemic lupus erythematosus treated with chemotherapy. Arthritis Rheum 1981; 24: 649–650.
36. Abu-Shakra M, Gladman DD, Urowitz MB. Malignancy in SLE. Arthritis Rheum 1996; 39: 1050–1054.
37. Williamson RA, Karp LE. Azathioprine teratogenicity: review of the literature and case report. Obstet Gynecol 1981; 58: 247–250.
38. Ramsey-Goldman R, Schilling E. Immunosuppressive drug use during pregnancy. Rheum Dis Clin North Am 1997; 23: 149–167.
39. Akkasilpa S, Minor M, Goldman D et al. Association of coping responses with fibromyalgia tender points in patients with systemic lupus erythematosus. J Rheumatol 2000; 27: 671–674.
40. Callen JP. Management of antimalarial-refractory cutaneous lupus erythematosus. Lupus 1997; 6: 203–208.
41. Rahman P, Gladman DD, Urowitz MB. Smoking interferes with efficacy of antimalarial therapy in cutaneous lupus. J Rheumatol 1998; 25: 1716–1719.
42. Jewell ML, McCauliffe DP. Patients with cutaneous lupus erythematosus who smoke are less responsive to antimalarial treatment. J Am Acad Dermatol 2000; 42: 983–987.
43. Neri R, Mosca M, Bernacchi E, Bombardieri S. A case of SLE with acute, subacute and chronic cutaneous lesions successfully treated with Dapsone. Lupus 1999; 8: 240–243.
44. Nishijima C, Hatta N, Inaoki M et al. Urticarial vasculitis in systemic lupus erythematosus: fair response to prednisolone/dapsone and persistent hypocomplementemia. Eur J Dermatol 1999; 9: 54–56.
45. Cotell S, Robinson ND, Chan LS. Autoimmune blistering skin diseases. Am J Emerg Med 2000; 18: 288–299.
46. Karim MY, Ruiz-Irastorza G, Khamashta MA, Hughes GRV. Update on therapy – thalidomide in the treatment of lupus. Lupus 2001; 10: 188–192.
47. Knop J, Bonsmann G, Happle R et al.Thalidomide in the treatment of sixty cases of chronic discoid lupus erythematosus. Br J Dermatol 1983; 108: 461–466.
48. Walchner M, Meurer M, Plewig G, Messer G. Clinical and immunologic parameters during thalidomide treatment of lupus erythematosus. Int J Dermatol 2000; 39: 383–388.
49. Ordi-Ros J, Cortes F, Cucurull E et al. Thalidomide in the treatment of cutaneous lupus refractory to conventional therapy. J Rheumatol 2000; 27: 1429–1433.
50. Kyriakos PK, Kontochristopoulos GJ, Panteleos DN. Experience with low-dose thalidomide therapy in chronic discoid lupus erythematosus. Int J Dermatol 2000; 39: 218–222.
51. Duong DJ, Spigel GT, Moxley RT, Gaspari AA. American experience with low-dose thalidomide for severe cutaneous lupus erythematosus. Arch Dermatol 1999; 135: 1079–1087.
52. Stevens RJ, Andujar C, Edwards CJ et al. Thalidomide in the treatment of the cutaneous manifestations of lupus erythematosus: experience in sixteen consecutive patients. Br J Rheumatol 1997; 36: 353–359.
53. Callen JP. New and emerging therapies for collagen-vascular diseases. Dermatol Clin 2000; 18: 139–146.
54. Goyal S, Nousari HC. Treatment of resistant discoid lupus erythematosus of the palms and soles with myophenolate mofetil. J Am Acad Dermatol 2001; 45: 142–144.
55. Wilke WS, Krall PL, Scheetz RJ et al. Methotrexate for systemic lupus erythematosus: a retrospective analysis or 17 unselected cases. Clin Exp Rheumatol 1991; 9: 581–587.
56. Rahman P, Humphrey-Murto S, Gladman DD, Urowitz MB. Efficacy and tolerability of methotrexate in antimalarial resistant lupus arthritis. J Rheumatol 1998; 25: 243–246.
57. Kipen Y, Littlejohn GO, Morand EF. Methotrexate use in systemic lupus erythematosus. Lupus 1997; 6: 385–389.
58. Sato EI. Methotrexate therapy in systemic lupus erythematosus. Lupus 2001; 10: 162–164.
59. Hjortkjoer Petersen H, Nielsen H, Hansen M, Stensgaard-Hansen F, Helin P. High-dose immunoglobulin therapy in pericarditis caused by SLE. Scand J Rheumatol 1990; 19: 91–93.
60. Meissner M, Sherer Y, Levy Y, Chwalinska-Sadowska H, Langevitz P, Shoenfeld Y. Intravenous immunoglobulin therapy in a patient with lupus serositis and nephritis. Rheumatol Int 2000; 19: 199–201.
61. Erickson RW, Franklin WA, Emlen W. Treatment of hemorrhagic lupus pneumonitis with plasmapheresis. Semin Arthritis Rheum 1994; 24: 114–123.
62. Eiser AR, Shanies HM. Treatment of lupus interstitial lung disease with intravenous cyclophosphamide. Arthritis Rheum. 1994; 37: 428–431.
63. Robbins IM, Gaine SP, Schilz R, Tapson VF, Rubin LJ, Loyd JE. Epoprostenol for treatment of pulmonary hypertension in patients with systemic lupus erythematosus. Chest. 2000 ; 117: 14–18.
64. Mok MY, Tse HF, Lau CS. Pulmonary hypertension secondary to systemic lupus erythematosus: prolonged survival following treatment with intermittent low dose iloprost. Lupus. 1999; 8: 328–331.
65. Oudiz RJ, Schilz RJ, Arneson C, Jeffs RA. Treprostinil (Remodulin) in connective tissue disease associated pulmonary hypertension. Presented at the American College of Rheumatology Annual Meeting, "Late Breaking Abstract #4," San Francisco, November, 2001.
66. Channick RN, Simonneau G, Sitbon O et al. Effects of the dual endothelin-receptor antagonist bosentan in patients with pulmonary hypertension: a randomised placebo-controlled study. Lancet. 2001; 358: 1113–1114.
67. Sato N, Kyotani S, Sakamaki F, Nagaya N, Oya H, Nakanishi N. Pulmonary thrombo-endarterectomy for chronic pulmonary thromboembolism in three patients with systemic lupus erythematosus and antiphospholipid syndrome. Nihon Kokyuki Gakkai Zasshi 2000; 38: 958–964.
68. Naarendorp M, Kerr LD, Khan AS, Ornstein MH Dramatic improvement of left ventricular function after cytotoxic therapy in lupus patients with acute cardio-myopathy: report of 6 cases. J Rheumatol 1999; 26: 2257–2260.
69. Fairfax MJ, Osborn TG, Williams GA, Tsai CC, Moore TL Endomyocardial biopsy in patients with systemic lupus erythematosus. J Rheumatol 1988; 15: 593–596.
70. Sherer Y, Levy Y, Shoenfeld Y. Marked improvement of severe cardiac dysfunction after one course of intravenous immunoglobulin in a patient with systemic lupus erythematosus. Clin Rheumatol 1999; 18: 238–240.
71. Pirofsky B. Immune haemolytic disease: the autoimmune haemolytic anaemias. Clin Haematol. 1975; 4: 167–80.
72. Ahn YS, Harrington WJ, Mylvaganam R, Ayub J, Pall LM. Danazol therapy for auto-immune hemolytic anemia. Ann Intern Med. 1985; 102: 298–301.
73. Cervera H, Jara LJ, Pizarro S et al. Danazol for systemic lupus erythematosus with refractory autoimmune thrombocytopenia or Evans' syndrome. J Rheumatol 1995; 22: 1867–1871.
74. Majer RV, Hyde RD. High-dose intravenous immunoglobulin in the treatment of autoimmune haemolytic anaemia. Clin Lab Haematol 1988; 10: 391–395.
75. von Keyserlingk H, Meyer-Sabellek W, Arntz R, Haller H. Plasma exchange treatment in autoimmune hemolytic anemia of the warm antibody type with renal failure. Vox Sang. 1987; 52: 298–300.
76. al-Shahi R, Mason JC, Rao R, Hurd C, Thompson EM, Haskard DO, Davies KA. Systemic lupus erythematosus, thrombocytopenia, microangiopathic haemolytic anaemia and anti-CD36 antibodies. Br J Rheumatol 1997; 36: 794–798.
77. Euler HH, Harten P, Zeuner RA, Schwab UM.Recombinant human granulocyte colony stimulating factor in patients with systemic lupus erythematosus associated neutropenia and refractory infections. J Rheumatol 1997; 24: 2153–2157.
78. Hellmich B, Schnabel A, Gross WL. Treatment of severe neutropenia due to Felty's syndrome or systemic lupus erythematosus with granulocyte colony-stimulating factor. Semin Arthritis Rheum 1999; 29: 82–99.
79. Godeau B, Coutant-Perronne V, Le Thi Huong D et al. Pneumocystis carinii pneumonia in the course of connective tissue disease: report of 34 cases. J Rheumatol. 1994; 21: 246–251.
80. Morton SJ, Powell RJ. An audit of cyclosporin for systemic lupus erythematosus and related overlap syndromes: limitations of its use. Ann Rheum Dis 2000; 59: 487–491.
81. Sugiyama M Ogasawara H, Kaneko H et al. Effect of extremely low dose cyclosporin on the thrombocytopenia in systemic lupus erythematosus. Lupus 1998; 7: 53–56.
82. Blanco R, Martinez-Taboada VM, Rodriguez-Valverde V, Sanchez-Andrade A, Gonzalez-Gay MA. Successful therapy with danazol in refractory autoimmune thrombocytopenia associated with rheumatic diseases. Br J Rheumatol 1997; 36: 1095–1099.
83. Nishina M, Saito E, Kinoshita M. Correction of severe leukocytopenia and thrombocy-topenia in systemic lupus erythematosus by treatment with dapsone. J Rheumatol 1997; 24: 811–812.

84. Boumpas DT, Barez S, Klippel JH, Balow JE. Intermittent cyclophosphamide for the treatment of autoimmune thrombocytopenia in systemic lupus erythematosus. Ann Intern Med 1990; 112: 674–677.

85. Feinglass S, Deodar A. Treatment of lupus-induced thrombocytopenia with recombinant human interleukin-11. Arthritis Rheum 2001; 44: 170–175.

86. Vaidya S, Abul-ezz S, Lipsmeyer E. Thrombotic thrombocytopenic purpura and systemic lupus erythematosus. Scand J Rheumatol 2001; 30: 308–310.

87. Perez-Sanchez I, Anguita J, Pintado T. Use of cyclophosphamide in the treatment of thrombotic thrombocytopenic purpura complicating systemic lupus erythematosus: report of two cases. Ann Hematol 1999; 78: 285-287.

88. Boumpas DT, Yamada H, Patronas NJ, Scott D, Klippel JH, Balow JE. Pulse cyclo-phosphamide for severe neuropsychiatric lupus. QJ Med 1991; 81: 975–984.

89. Neuwelt CM, Lacks S, Kaye BR, Ellman JB, Borenstein DG. Role of intravenous cyclophosphamide in the treatment of severe neuropsychiatric systemic lupus erythematosus. Am J Med 1995; 98: 32–41.

90. Ramos PC, Mendez MJ, Ames PR, Khamashta MA, Hughes GR. Pulse cyclophosphamide in the treatment of neuropsychiatric systemic lupus erythematosus. Clin Exp Rheumatol 1996; 14: 295–299.

91. Viertel A, Weidmann E, Wigand R, Geiger H, Mondorf UF. Treatment of severe systemic lupus erythematosus with immunoadsorption and intravenous immunoglobulins. Intensive Care Med 2000; 26: 823–824.

92. Levy Y, Sherer Y, Ahmed A et al. A study of 20 SLE patients with intravenous immunoglobulin – clinical and serologic response. Lupus 1999; 8: 705–712.

93. Valesini G, Priori R, Francia A et al. Central nervous system involvement in systemic lupus erythematosus: a new therapeutic approach with intrathecal dexamethasone and methotrexate. Springer Semin Immunopathol 1994; 16: 313–321.

94. Harisdangkul V, Doorenbos D, Subramony SH. Lupus transverse myelopathy: better outcome with early recognition and aggressive high-dose intravenous cortico-steroid pulse treatment. J Neurol 1995; 242: 326–331.

95. Sanchez-Guerrero J, Liang MH, Karlson EW, Hunter DJ, Colditz GA. Postmenopausal estrogen therapy and the risk for developing systemic lupus erythematosus. Ann Intern Med 1995; 122: 430–433.

96. Kreidstein S, Urowitz MB, Gladman DD, Gough J. Hormone replacement therapy in systemic lupus erythematosus. J Rheumatol 1997; 24: 2149–2152.

97. Mok CC, Lau CS, Ho CT, Lee KW, Mok MY, Wong RW. Safety of hormonal replacement therapy in postmenopausal patients with systemic lupus erythematosus. Scand J Rheumatol 1998; 27: 342–346.

98. Sanchez-Guerrero J, Gonzalez-Perez M, Durand-Carbajal M, Lara-Reyes P, Bahina-Amezcua S, Cravioto MC. Effect of hormone replacement therapy (HRT) on disease activity in postmenopausal patients with SLE. A two year follow-up clinical trial. Arthritis Rheum 2001; 44 (Suppl): S263.

99. Walker SE. Treatment of systemic lupus erythematosus with bromocriptine. Lupus 2001; 10: 197–202.

100. Morikawa K, Oseko F, Morikawa S. Immunosuppressive property of bromocriptine on human B lymphocyte function in vitro. Clin Exp Immunol 1993; 93: 200–205.

101. McMurray RW, Allen SH, Braun All, Rodriguez F, Walker SE. Longstanding hyperprolactinemia assoicated with systemic lupus erythematosus: possible hormonal stimulation an autoimmune disease. J Rheumatol 1994; 21: 843–850.

102. McMurray RW, Weidensaul D, Allen SH, Walker SE. Efficacy of bromocriptine in an open label therapeutic trial for systemic lupus erythematosus. J Rheumatol 1995; 22: 2084–2091.

103. Buskila D, Lorber M, Neumann L, Flusser D, Shoenfeld Y. No correlation between prolactin levels and clinical activity in patients with systemic lupus erythematosus. J Rheumatol 1996; 23: 629–632.

104. Jimena P, Aguirre MA, Lopez-Curbelo A, de Andres M, Garcia-Courtay C, Cuadrado MD. Prolactin levels in patients with systemic lupus erythematosus: a case controlled study. Lupus 1998; 7: 383–386.

105. Alvarez-Nemegyei J, Cobarrubias-Cobos A, Escalante-Triay F, Sosa-Munoz J, Miranda JM, Jara LJ. Bromocriptine in systemic lupus erythematosus: a double-blind, randomized, placebo-controlled study. Lupus 1998; 7: 414–419.

106. McMurray RW. Bromocriptine in rheumatic and autoimmune diseases. Semin Arthritis Rheum 2001; 31: 21–32.

107. Van Vollenhoven RF, Engleman EF, McGuire JL. An open study of dehydroepiandrosterone in systemic lupus erythematosus. Arthritis Rheum 1994; 37: 1305–1310.

108. Suzuki T, Suzuki N, Daynes RA, Engleman EG. Dehydroepiandrosterone enhances IL-2 production and cytotoxic effector function of human T cells. Clin Immunol Immunopathol 1991; 61: 202–211.

109. Von Vollenhoven RF, Morabito LM, Engleman EG, McGuire JL. Treatment of systemic lupus erythematosus with dehydroepidandrosterone: 50 patients treated up to 12 months. J Rheumatol 1998; 25: 285–289.

110. Petri MA, Lahita RG, van Vollenhoven RF et al. Systemic lupus erythematosus and autoimmunity effects of prasterone on corticosteroid requirements of women with systemic lupus erythematosus: a double-blind, randomized, placebo-controlled trial. Arthritis Rheum 2002; 46: 1820–1829.

111. Mease PJ, Ginzler EM, Gluck OS et al. Improvement in bone mineral density in steroid-treated SLE patients during treatment with GL701 (prasterone, dehydroepiandrosterone). Arthritis Rheum 2000; 43 (Suppl): S271.

112. Robinzon B, Cutolo M. Should dehydroepiandrosterone replacement therapy be provided with glucocorticoids? Rheumatology 1999; 38: 488–495.

113. Wierzbicki AS. Lipid-lowering drugs in lupus: an unexplored therapeutic intervention. Lupus 2001; 10: 233–236.

35 Clinical features of systemic sclerosis

Fredrick M Wigley and Laura K Hummers

Definition

- A generalized disorder of connective tissue affecting skin and internal organs
- Characterized by fibrotic arteriosclerosis of peripheral and visceral vasculature
- Variable degrees of extracellular matrix accumulation (mainly collagen) occur in both skin and viscera
- Associated with specific autoantibodies, most notably anticentromere and anti-Scl-70 (antitopoisomerase)
- Various subsets of disease with specific clinical features and variable involvement of internal organs

Clinical features

- Raynaud's phenomenon
- Tightening and thickening of skin (scleroderma)
- Involvement of internal organs, including gastrointestinal tract, lungs, heart and kidneys, accounts for increased morbidity and mortality
- Risk of internal organ involvement strongly linked to extent and progression of skin thickening

HISTORY

Although there is evidence in the writings of Galen and Hippocrates of scleroderma, the first convincing description was in 1753 by Carlo Curzio. He described a 17-year-old patient as having 'extensive tension and hardness of skin all over her body'. Curzio managed the case with bloodletting, warm milk and 'small doses of quicksilver'[1]. However, it was only in the mid-19th century that scleroderma was established as a clinical entity and given its current name[2]. In reviewing the described cases to date, Gintrac, in 1847, ascribed the name *sclerodermie*[1]. Maurice Raynaud described Raynaud's phenomenon in 1865[3] and Jonathan Hutchinson reported a case with Raynaud's phenomenon who had definite features of scleroderma in 1883[2]. William Osler referred to the systemic nature of the disease in his 1894 textbook of medicine (patients were 'apt to succumb to pulmonary complaints or to nephritis')[4] and Klemperer, Pollack and Baehr, in 1942, proposed that scleroderma should be considered as a 'systemic disease of the connective tissue'[5]. It was not until 1945, however, that Goetz proposed the term progressive systemic sclerosis to emphasize the degree of visceral disease[6]. In 1964, Winterbauer described the CRST syndrome (now the CREST syndrome of calcinosis, Raynaud's phenomenon, esophageal dysmotility, sclerodactyly and telangiectasia)[7], although it was first described in 1910 and originally termed Thiberge–Weissenbach syndrome after the presenting physicians[8]. In 1969 a major pathologic review delineated the widespread fibrotic and vascular disease of scleroderma[9]. Clinical and pathologic surveys of patients with scleroderma followed, giving new insight into the clinical features, risk factors, pathogenesis of fibrosis and associa-

tions of scleroderma with the immune response. In the last decade, there has been remarkable progress in understanding the molecular mechanisms of fibrosis, microvascular injury and the autoimmune process in this rare disease.

EPIDEMIOLOGY

It is estimated that new cases of scleroderma occur at a rate of approximately 18–20 per million of the general population per year[10]. The incidence appears to have increased steadily from the 1940s to the 1970s but according to more recent surveys this trend may have stabilized. The apparent increase in cases may be related to a new awareness of scleroderma created by the introduction of classification criteria in 1980[11]. Surveys that include the full clinical spectrum of scleroderma and the related disorders find the prevalence to be 5–19 times higher than previous reports[12].

The prevalence and severity of scleroderma also vary among different racial and ethnic groups. Estimates of the prevalence in the Japanese suggest 38 per million have scleroderma, while the prevalence is 4690 per million among full-blooded Choctaw Native Americans[13]. A national survey of Iceland reports 71 cases of scleroderma per million, although most of these patients had limited scleroderma[14]. The limited variant of scleroderma is found more commonly in Caucasians[15], while African-American females appear to have an increased risk for diffuse cutaneous scleroderma and a younger age at disease onset[16].

While the incidence of scleroderma is higher in females than in males (3:1), this difference is greater in younger age groups (7:1) and less in patients over 50 years old (2:1)[17]. The average age of onset of disease is approximately 50 years. Scleroderma is uncommon in children. The diagnosis of scleroderma by a physician is often delayed years after symptoms first begin; this is particularly true in patients with the more indolent disease course of the CREST syndrome.

There are several reports suggesting geographic clustering of cases of scleroderma. In some cases environmental etiologies are proposed but definite proof is lacking[18,19]. Typical scleroderma is found among male workers exposed to silica[20] and epidemics of a scleroderma-like illness following exposure to toxins contaminating preparations of tryptophan and rapeseed oil are well described.

Familial aggregation and concordance of disease in twin pairs rarely occurs[21]. This suggests that the genetic influence is probably complex, involving multiple genetic susceptibilities. Among twin pairs with at least one twin with scleroderma, there is a strong concordance rate for antinuclear antibody positivity (100% in monozygous pairs). However, none of the healthy twins had scleroderma-specific antibodies and only 6% have concordance for scleroderma[22]. First-degree relatives of patients with scleroderma also have a significantly higher frequency of antinuclear antibody positivity and other autoimmune diseases, but multiplex families of scleroderma are rare[23]. It is very likely that both genetic susceptibility to autoimmune disease and some environmental factors influence the clinical expression of scleroderma.

CLINICAL FEATURES

Systemic sclerosis (scleroderma) is a disfiguring multisystem disease that may alter every aspect of an individual's life. It includes a broad spectrum of disease with varying degrees of organ involvement. Thus subsets of patients exist with unique clinical features and distinct outcomes. Raynaud's phenomenon, the manifestation of perturbation of the terminal arteries of the circulatory system, is almost universal in scleroderma. This outward manifestation of vascular disease is a marker of tissue ischemia that is linked to a progressive fibrosing process in specific target organs: the skin, lung, heart, gastrointestinal tract and kidney. In the diffuse cutaneous variant of scleroderma, fibrosis of the skin and other organs is widespread and potentially life-threatening. In the limited form of scleroderma the skin fibrosis is restricted to the fingers and/or distal limbs with a more benign and indolent disease course. Limited cutaneous scleroderma is less likely to be associated with serious internal organ involvement.

The term scleroderma, therefore, encompasses many unique phenotypic subsets of disease with varying degrees and severity of organ involvement. In many cases the unique clinical subset is associated with specific autoantibodies. For example, the presence of antibody to topoisomerase associates with diffuse cutaneous scleroderma and severe interstitial lung disease (see later).

In addition, patients may have 'overlap' features, in which scleroderma is coupled with another autoimmune diseases such as systemic lupus erythematosus (SLE), polymyositis, Sjögren's syndrome or autoimmune thyroid disease.

Diagnostic criteria

A subcommittee of the American Rheumatism Association (now the American College of Rheumatology) established criteria by consensus for scleroderma in 1980 after initiating a multicenter prospective study of early scleroderma patients and comparing them to patients with other autoimmune diseases (SLE, polymyositis and Raynaud's phenomenon)[11]. Criteria were chosen for their discriminatory value and to assure diagnostic certainty to allow for consistency in research and other comparative purposes. The criteria include proximal skin thickening as the major criteria and evidence of digital ischemia, sclerodactyly and pulmonary fibrosis as minor criteria. These criteria were found to be 97% sensitive and 98% specific for a diagnosis of scleroderma, but they have been criticized for failing to include many patients with signs of limited scleroderma or CREST syndrome. These criteria also do not take into account cases that have subtle features of the disease and specific serological markers known to be associated with scleroderma.

Classification

Patients with scleroderma are classified into subsets of disease by the degree of clinically involved skin (Table 35.1). Attempting to classify or subdivide patients is useful both in terms of uniformity and for prognostic implications. Patients with more diffuse skin disease (i.e. those with higher skin scores) have more severe organ involvement and a worse survival[24]. Several proposals exist defining subsets of scleroderma patients[25–28]. The most popular classification distinguishes between patients with truncal skin involvement (diffuse) and those with limited skin involvement (distal to elbows and knees). The limited group includes patients with CREST syndrome, whose skin findings are limited to the digits and face. Within these two subsets, there are groups of patients who have distinct clinical phenotypes (i.e. patients with limited disease and late-onset pulmonary hypertension).

In addition, there may be mild expressions of scleroderma that do not meet current diagnostic criteria, such as the presence of Raynaud's phenomenon alone with abnormal nailfold capillary loops and

---

TABLE 35.1 CLASSIFICATION OF SYSTEMIC SCLEROSIS

- **Diffuse scleroderma** – skin thickening present on the trunk in addition to the face, proximal and distal extremities
- **Limited scleroderma** – skin thickening restricted to sites distal to the elbow and knee but also involving the face and neck
  - **CREST syndrome** (C, subcutaneous calcinosis; R, Raynaud's phenomenon; E, esophageal dysmotility; S, sclerodactyly; T, telangiectasia)
- *Sine* **scleroderma** – no clinically apparent skin thickening but with characteristic internal organ changes, vascular and serologic features
- **Overlap syndrome** – criteria fulfilling systemic sclerosis occurring concomitantly with features of SLE, RA or inflammatory muscle disease
- **Undifferentiated connective tissue disease** – Raynaud's phenomenon with clinical and/or laboratory features of systemic sclerosis; these include scleroderma-specific antibodies, abnormal nailfold capillaroscopy, finger edema and ischemic injury

---

autoantibodies associated with scleroderma. Many of these patients are diagnosed as undifferentiated connective tissue disorder with features of scleroderma. Recently, it has been proposed to include patients with Raynaud's phenomenon and specific scleroderma serologies as definite scleroderma[29]. About 5% of patients may have systemic sclerosis without skin thickening (systemic sclerosis *sine* scleroderma)[30].

Scleroderma patients with definite clinical signs and laboratory parameters of another rheumatic disease such as SLE or polymyositis are considered to have an 'overlap syndrome'. Mixed connective tissue disease is considered to be an overlap syndrome with features of scleroderma, myositis and a polyarthritis. Some consider it a distinct disease entity[31]. Longitudinal studies of patients with mixed connective tissue disease suggest that most eventually meet defined criteria for another rheumatic disease such as scleroderma or SLE[32,33].

Natural history of disease

Other autoimmune illnesses such as SLE are characterized by exacerbations or 'flares,' while the course of scleroderma is predominantly monophasic (Fig. 35.1). A re-flare of the cutaneous disease occurs in only

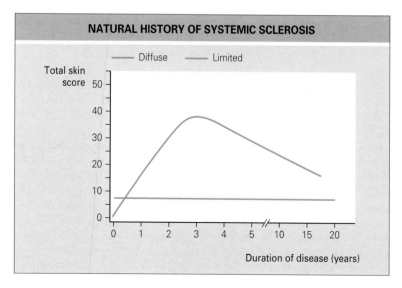

Fig. 35.1 Natural history of systemic sclerosis. Diffuse scleroderma is typified by rapid progression of skin involvement in the early years. New internal organ involvement occurs most frequently during the active early phase of disease. Limited disease slowly increases in severity of skin involvement and internal organ involvement is typically delayed until the second decade of disease.

about 5% of patients. The course of other organ involvement is complex and difficult to define clinically. In general, in the diffuse form of the disease, internal organ involvement tends to progress in concert with cutaneous disease. The clinical course and prognosis vary significantly among the different subsets of disease. Diffuse cutaneous scleroderma has an early rapid phase, usually followed by regression of skin disease after years. In contrast, limited disease has an indolent course, often with years of Raynaud's phenomenon alone before other features of scleroderma become evident.

Diffuse cutaneous scleroderma

In general, patients with diffuse disease have a narrow interval between onset of Raynaud's phenomenon, skin thickening and internal organ involvement. The early stage of scleroderma is usually characterized by inflamed, edematous skin (Fig. 35.2) and significant systemic manifestations such as fatigue, arthralgias, myalgias, diffuse pruritus and an elevated erythrocyte sedimentation rate (ESR). In this initial phase there is early rapid progression of skin thickening over months to years. There is also a significant risk of internal organ involvement, particularly in the first 3 years[34]. The higher the skin score (degree of skin thickening determined by the physician), the greater the risk for renal disease and higher mortality. Approximately 10–20% of patients with diffuse scleroderma will develop severe, life-threatening internal organ disease (heart, renal, pulmonary, gastrointestinal). Further significant internal organ involvement or progression rarely occurs after skin changes have reached a peak or maximal skin score.

The later stages of diffuse cutaneous scleroderma are characterized by gradual softening of the skin[24]. Remission of the skin disease is accompanied by resolution of systemic symptoms and lack of progression (or new development) of internal organ disease. Despite overall improvement in skin thickness, areas of irreversible skin fibrosis, especially in the forearms and hands, often exist. Skin atrophy and deeper tissue fibrosis cause contractures and prolonged disability. A small subset of patients, even in this late stage, will have progressive active disease. Chronic organ dysfunction and failure is also the result of permanent damage caused by prior active disease.

Although patients with scleroderma have a mortality rate four to five times greater than that of the general population, overall mortality for diffuse cutaneous disease has improved over the last 30 years. This is in part because of improved management of scleroderma renal crisis, previously the leading cause of death in scleroderma. Estimates suggest that the 5-year survival has improved from the figure in the 1950s–1970s of 50% to approximately 75% (since 1980)[10,35]. Predictors for higher mortality include higher skin scores (Rodnan score >20), reduced lung diffusion capacity, elevated sedimentation rate and evidence of heart or renal involvement.

Limited scleroderma

The clinical course, survival and clinical features of limited disease are quite different than in the diffuse form (Fig. 35.1). The overall 5-year survival in limited scleroderma is 80–85%, which is significantly better than is seen in diffuse disease[36]. Patients with limited disease often have many years of Raynaud's phenomenon prior to the development of other signs or symptoms of scleroderma. The most common first non-Raynaud's symptom is caused by esophageal dysfunction manifested by dysphagia or gastroesophageal reflux.

The major causes of morbidity and mortality in limited disease are severe Raynaud's phenomenon with occlusive digital vascular disease and pulmonary hypertension. Patients with limited disease, particularly those with anticentromere antibodies, are more likely to have severe digital ischemia and digital loss related to advanced arterial vascular disease (see Figs 35.6–35.8)[37]. Pulmonary hypertension is the leading cause of scleroderma-related mortality among limited disease patients. This complication occurs in approximately 10% of cases with limited scleroderma and often occurs in the absence of interstitial lung disease. In patients who develop pulmonary hypertension, the disease is almost uniformly fatal secondary to progressive right-sided heart failure.

Brief introduction to pathophysiology

The diverse clinical manifestations of scleroderma can be better appreciated by understanding the possible underlying pathophysiological mechanisms involved in this disease. The three key pathologic features are:

- a unique vascular disease
- abnormal accumulation of extracellular matrix components (fibrosis)
- autoimmunity.

It is unclear how and when the immune system is involved, but evidence suggests that it is important early in the disease and probably the immune process initiates and propagates the inflammatory process that causes vascular damage and eventual tissue fibrosis. The vasculopathy of scleroderma is fundamental to the other pathological events. It is characterized by arterial vasospasm, smooth muscle hyperactivity, intimal proliferation and eventual vascular occlusion. The vascular disease is manifested clinically by the presence of nailfold capillary changes, telangiectasias, Raynaud's phenomenon and most strikingly by digital and other tissue ischemia. Associated with the vascular disease is tissue fibrosis that varies in degree but occurs in the skin and other targeted organs. Fibrosis is the most characteristic pathologic finding; however, the cause of organ dysfunction is complex and it can be seen in the absence of severe fibrosis. This is particularly true in the gastrointestinal tract, where smooth muscle atrophy is striking and fibrosis is limited.

Raynaud's phenomenon

Raynaud's phenomenon is vasoconstriction of the digital arteries in response to cold. This manifests with color changes in the skin, corresponding to the stage of the vasospastic process. Initially there is sharply demarcated pallor (Fig. 35.3) and/or cyanosis (Fig. 35.4). This is followed by erythema of the skin, a manifestation of the reactive hyperemia that follows the ischemic episode. Raynaud's is caused by vasoconstriction of the muscular digital arteries, precapillary arterioles and arteriovenous (AV) shunts of the skin in response to colder temperature and to neural signals associated with emotional stress.

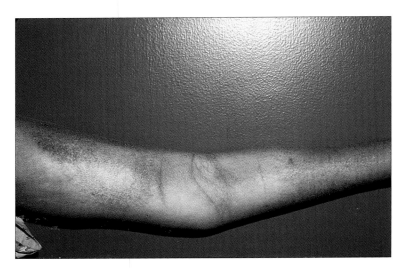

Fig. 35.2 Diffuse scleroderma. Inflamed, indurated skin of the arm in early diffuse scleroderma.

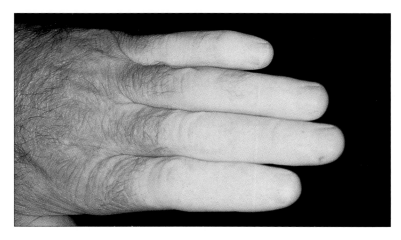

Fig. 35.3 Raynaud's phenomenon. Sharply demarcated pallor of the fingers.

TABLE 35.2 CLINICAL AND LABORATORY FEATURES IN THE DIFFERENTIAL DIAGNOSIS OF RAYNAUD'S PHENOMENON		
Feature	**Primary Raynaud's**	**Systemic sclerosis**
Sex	F:M 4:1	F:M 3:1
Age at onset	Puberty	25 years or older
Frequency	Usually <5 per day	>5–10 attacks per day
Precipitants	Cold, emotional stress	Cold
Ischemic injury	Absent	Present
Other vasomotor phenomena	Yes	Yes
Antinuclear antibodies	Absent	90–95%
Anticentromere antibody	Absent	50–60%
Anti-Scl-70 antibody	Absent	20–30%
Abnormal capillaroscopy	Absent	>95%
In vivo platelet activation	Absent	>75%

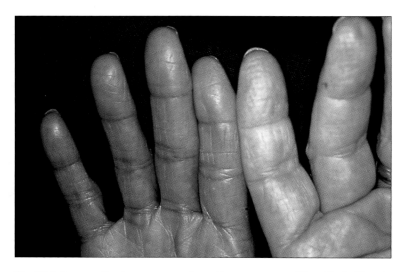

Fig. 35.4 Raynaud's phenomenon. Cyanotic appearance of the affected hand compared with the normal other hand.

Surveys find that 4–15% of the general population have symptoms characteristic of Raynaud's phenomenon[38,39]. In the majority of cases, Raynaud's phenomenon is not associated with either structural vascular changes or ischemic tissue damage (primary Raynaud's phenomenon). Primary Raynaud's typically begins in the teenage years and is more common in women (female:male ratio approximately 4:1). Approximately 30% of the first-degree relatives also have Raynaud's phenomenon. In primary Raynaud's phenomenon, the patients are otherwise healthy, the episodes are symmetric in the fingers and/or toes and they do not lead to tissue ulceration or gangrene. Examination of these patients is unremarkable and laboratory data, including antinuclear antibody and ESR, are normal.

The challenge for the physician is to determine whether the presence of Raynaud's phenomenon is an uncomplicated primary process or the first symptom of a secondary illness such as scleroderma (Table 35.2) or another disease (Table 35.3). Patients who have Raynaud's attacks without digital pitting, ulceration or gangrene and who have normal nailfold capillaries, a normal ESR and a negative antinuclear antibody test, are unlikely to have an underlying disease such as scleroderma[40].

TABLE 35.3 DIFFERENTIAL DIAGNOSIS OF RAYNAUD'S PHENOMENON		
Structural vasculopathies	Large and medium arteries	Thoracic outlet syndrome Brachiocephalic trunk disease (atherosclerosis, Takayasu's arteritis)
	Small artery and arteriolar	Systemic lupus erythematosus Dermatomyositis Overlap syndromes Cold injury Vibration disease Arteriosclerosis (thromboangiitis obliterans) Chemotherapy (bleomycin, vinblastine) Polyvinyl chloride disease
Normal blood vessels	Abnormal blood elements	Cryoglobulinemia Cryofibrinogenemia Paraproteinemia Cold agglutinin disease Polycythemias
	Abnormal vasomotion	Primary (idiopathic) Raynaud's phenomenon Drug-induced (ergots sympathomimetics) Pheochromocytoma Carcinoid syndrome Other vasospastic disorders (migraine, Prinzmetal's angina)

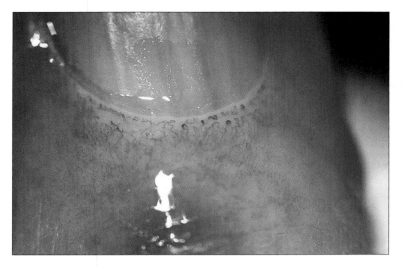

Fig. 35.5 Capillary loop abnormalities. Nailfold capillaroscopy showing the scleroderma pattern with dilated capillary loops and vessel dropout.

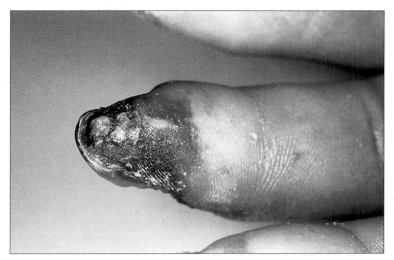

Fig. 35.7 Digital gangrene. Sharply demarcated gangrene of several weeks duration of the fingertip of a woman with CREST syndrome.

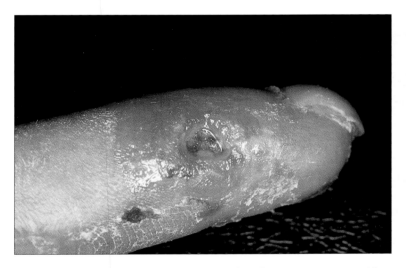

Fig. 35.6 Digital tip ulcer. Typical ulceration of the fingertip in a patient with diffuse scleroderma.

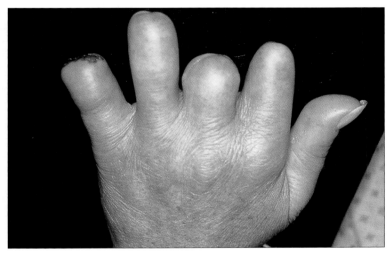

Fig. 35.8 Digital loss. Cumulative loss of multiple digits in a patient with limited scleroderma and anticentromere antibodies.

The presence of nailfold capillaries with enlarged capillary loops and/or the loss of capillaries or avascularity (a scleroderma pattern; Fig. 35.5) suggest that the patient has scleroderma[41,42]. Approximately 13% of patients presenting to a university medical center with Raynaud's phenomenon alone develop a connective tissue disease[43]. Patients with limited scleroderma often have mild or vague symptoms and are initially diagnosed with undifferentiated connective tissue disorder. Predictors of the development of scleroderma among such patients include older age at onset of Raynaud's phenomenon, severe Raynaud's phenomenon, nailfold capillary abnormalities and the presence of antinuclear/scleroderma-specific antibodies[44].

Raynaud's phenomenon and scleroderma

In scleroderma, over 90% of patients have intense Raynaud's phenomenon associated with tissue fibrosis, digital ulceration (Fig. 35.6) and, on occasion, ischemic demarcation and digital amputation (Fig. 35.7). The severity of the Raynaud's attacks is a manifestation of both vasospasm and structural abnormalities of the digital arteries. Compared to normals, scleroderma patients have a more pronounced decrease of both nutritional and thermoregulatory blood flow to the skin in response to cold temperatures. This sensitivity is coupled with long delays in recovery of local blood flow following rewarming and relief of stimulants of vasoconstriction (cold, emotional stress). In addition, reactive hyperemia, which normally follows periods of digital ischemia and is present in patients with primary Raynaud's, is absent in scleroderma, indicating that fixed irreversible structural disease is a significant cause of tissue ischemia[45]. In addition to vasospasm, vascular occlusion occurs secondary to activation of platelets and the intravascular clotting cascade, leading to fibrin deposition and vascular occlusion.

A vascular occlusive event that involves the digital artery or major arteries of the peripheral circulation (palmar arch, ulnar or tibial arteries) can cause deep tissue infarction with gangrene and/or digital amputation (Fig. 35.8). Rarely, major vessel disease may lead to loss of the distal part of a limb. These major vascular events are more likely to occur in patients with limited skin disease who have anticentromere antibody[37].

There is good evidence that a generalized vasospastic disorder exists in scleroderma ('systemic Raynaud's phenomenon') involving the terminal arterial system of the kidney, heart and probably other viscera. The renal crisis of scleroderma is a clear example of reversible vasoconstriction of the cortical blood flow to the kidney[46]. Cold-induced vasospasm of the pulmonary circulation has been more difficult to prove[47,48], in part because irreversible structural changes of the arteries occur very early in the lung. Management of patients with scleroderma must carefully address the systemic vascular disease that is present.

The cutaneous manifestations of scleroderma

The skin disease of scleroderma follows a course characterized by three phases: an inflammatory edematous phase, an indurative phase and an atrophic phase. These stages do not have a distinct beginning and ending and there is a high degree of variability in the duration of inflammatory signs and in the severity and extent of the skin involvement. Evidence also suggests that a subclinical inflammatory process is present even in areas of clinically normal skin.

In the initial edematous stage, the patient experiences puffiness, swelling and a sense of decreased flexibility of the skin, especially in the forearms, hands and digits, as well as in the feet. These symptoms may be accompanied by intense pruritus. The fingers appear puffy (Fig. 35.9) with a moon-like fullness of the fingertip and there is loss of normal digital creases. Reduced sweat and oil production results in drying and scaling of the skin's surface, which may cause small fissures leading to complications such as cellulitis or paronychia. Loss of the finger pad and tapering of the finger due to fingertip ischemia is often seen during this early phase of scleroderma. This inflammatory process may last for months, during which time induration and skin thickening becomes evident.

After the initial intense inflammatory stage has diminished there is a long course of progressive fibrosis of the skin in diffuse cutaneous scleroderma (Fig. 35.10). This is characterized by marked tightening and thickening of the skin that can involve the extremities, chest, neck, face and abdomen. Areas of the midback are usually spared even in severe diffuse disease but the posterior neck and lower flanks of the trunk can have thickened skin. The skin of the abdomen is usually diffusely thickened, or there can be patches of hyperpigmented thick skin that primarily occurs over pressure points such as the belt line. Interestingly, the area around the areola of the breast is spared. In patients with diffuse skin disease, a pulling, tight sensation around the upper chest and shoulder girdle is a common complaint. The anterior neck may develop thick horizontal folds of skin called the scleroderma 'neck sign' (Fig. 35.11). These folds can be present in patients with either limited or diffuse disease.

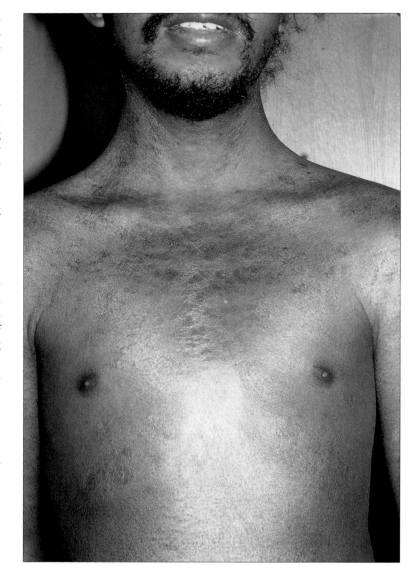

Fig. 35.10 Truncal scleroderma. Skin thickening of the chest and abdomen of a patient with diffuse scleroderma. Both hyperpigmentation and hypopigmentation are demonstrated.

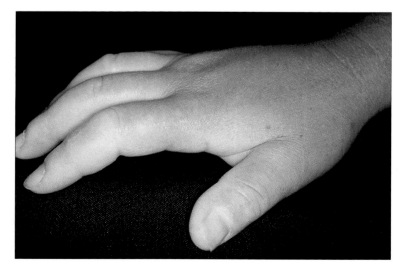

Fig. 35.9 Early puffy scleroderma. Extensive edema of the fingers in a man with several months of preceding Raynaud's phenomenon. Skin was not clinically thickened but became so on follow-up.

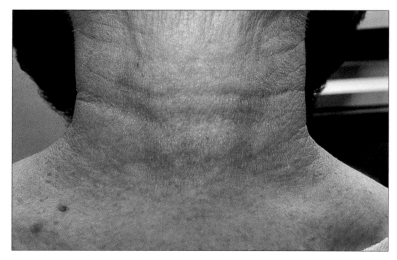

Fig. 35.11 Scleroderma neck sign.

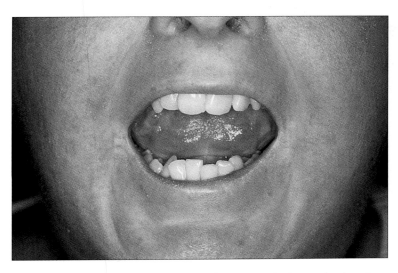

Fig. 35.12 Facial scleroderma. Taut smooth skin over the face and reduced oral aperture of a woman with long-standing disease. Furrowing is present around the mouth, along with some facial telangiectasias.

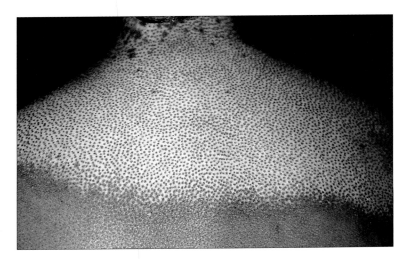

Fig. 35.13 Depigmentation of the skin. 'Salt and pepper' appearance of skin secondary to perifollicular sparing of pigment loss.

The face can appear expressionless because of reduced capacity to smile or move the eyelids or cheeks. The opened mouth becomes circular with a remarkable reduction in the maximum oral aperture. Vertical lines or furrowing of the skin around the lips gives a pursed-lip appearance as though a string had pulled tight the borders of the lips to close the mouth (Fig. 35.12). The tight perioral skin sometimes makes the frontal teeth appear more prominent, especially if there is associated gum retraction caused by local fibrosis and bone resorption. The nose becomes pinched and the facial creases smooth so that the face has a mouse-like appearance (*Mauskopf*).

Pigmentary changes of the skin also occur during the edematous and fibrotic stages of scleroderma but these changes vary in intensity and distribution. Some patients develop areas of depigmentation that is similar to vitiligo, especially in the scalp, eyebrows, upper back and chest and over areas of trauma, such as the dorsum of the hand or shins. This vitiligo pattern gives the skin a 'salt and pepper' appearance because of perifollicular sparing of pigment loss (Fig. 35.13). Some patients develop diffuse tanning of the skin; others have scattered patches of hyperpigmentation, particularly over pressure points. Areas of marked hyperpigmentation can be seen in the skin creases.

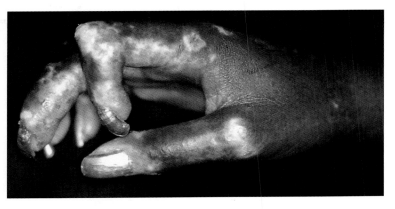

Fig. 35.14 Digital and hand scleroderma. Advanced changes of scleroderma have caused digital contractions and limitation of finger movement.

On average, after 1–3 years of disease activity, the inflammatory and fibrotic process gradually stops. These areas of the skin begin to thin or remodel and return to clinically normal skin (especially the trunk and proximal limbs). The first signs of improvement may be regrowth of hair on the forearms, a decrease in pruritus and a sense of improved flexibility. In the late stage of scleroderma, the skin becomes atrophic (especially over the fingers, hands and distal limbs) and thinned, with tethering secondary to fibrotic tissue binding to underlying structures. Areas of thinned skin can ulcerate with minor trauma, especially in areas such as the tip of the elbow, the medial or lateral ankle or over sites of a flexion contracture. Flexion contractures of the fingers are very common in the diffuse form of scleroderma (Fig. 35.14). These contractures evolve in the setting of intense deep tissue fibrosis and likely reflect stronger flexors, compared to extensors, of the digits. In severe cases, similar contractures can occur in the wrists, elbows, shoulders, knees, ankles and rarely the hip girdle. Thickened skin and fibrosis of deeper tissue of the palm and hand tendons reduce mobility and cause muscle atrophy and loss of function of the hands.

In patients with limited skin disease, the fibrotic skin changes are usually limited to the fingers (sclerodactyly). Sclerodactyly may present as puffy fingers with thickening only of the very distal digits. Facial changes are much less dramatic in limited disease but perioral furrowing can occur. More prominent in limited disease are small and large mat-like telangiectasias that appear on the face, upper chest, palms, fingertips and mucous membranes (Figs 35.15 & 35.16). These telangiectasias are dilated capillaries, which gradually increase in number. In diffuse cutaneous disease they can appear in the later stages on the face, arms and trunk.

Subcutaneous calcinosis, composed of calcium hydroxyapatite deposits at sites of trauma such as the forearms, elbows or fingers (Fig. 35.17), occurs in all subsets of scleroderma but is more prominent in limited scleroderma and patients with anticentromere antibody. The calcinosis can become superficial, ulcerate the skin and lead to secondary infection. More often the deposits remain bothersome subcutaneous lumps that rarely cause recurrent local inflammation due to the release of crystals of hydroxyapatite into the tissue.

Ulceration of the skin can occur for various reasons in scleroderma. Sudden episodes of ischemic ulceration are common and are seen more frequently during the cold temperatures of the winter months. Digital ischemic ulcerations are located on the fingertips (Fig. 35.18) or distal toes and may be either very small and superficial or deep painful lesions that are 1–2cm in size. They may also occur under the fingernail and appear as a painful hazy area of necrotic debris trapped under the nail. Untreated cutaneous ulcers form a thick eschar of

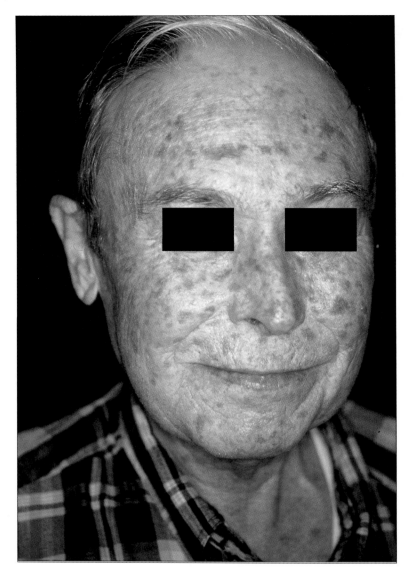

Fig. 35.15 **Facial telangiectasias.** Extensive facial telangiectasias in a man with CREST syndrome.

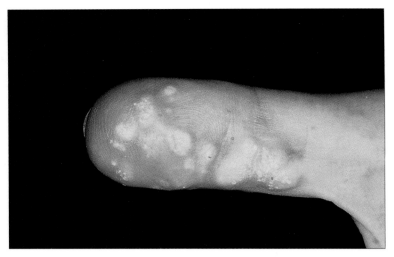

Fig. 35.17 **Subcutaneous calcinosis.** Calcinosis of the finger tip.

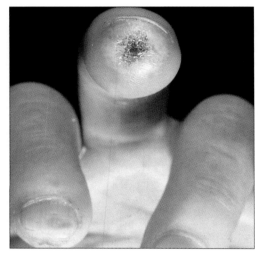

Fig. 35.18
Fingertip ulceration.
Large digital infarction in a patient with limited scleroderma.

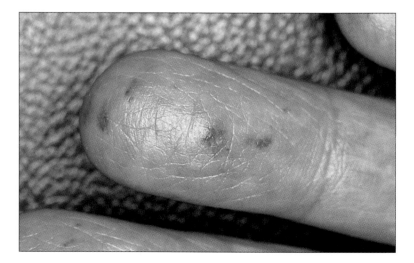

Fig. 35.16 **Telangiectasias of the fingers.**

debris, which can develop secondary infection with cellulitis. With proper management, healing will occur in 6–9 weeks. After healing of an ulcer, a digital 'pit' remains or there is loss of the pulp of the finger pad. Pitting and digital pad atrophy may occur without definite ulceration.

Traumatic ulceration occurs at sites of flexion contractures or areas of repeated minor trauma such as the pinna of the ear or over the proximal interphalangeal joints of the fingers, a common site of severe flexion contractures. Ankle ulcers are usually traumatic or, rarely, secondary to an associated vasculitis. Vasculitis in scleroderma has been reported to be associated with Sjögren's syndrome[49].

Systemic manifestations of scleroderma
Musculoskeletal features

Non-specific musculoskeletal complaints such as arthralgias and myalgias are one of the earliest symptoms of scleroderma. Synovitis similar to rheumatoid arthritis occurs in a small subset of patients and involves multiple joints, including the fingers, wrists, knees or ankles. These patients represent an overlap syndrome with polyarthritis and scleroderma. This inflammatory arthritis is usually responsive to typical therapy used for rheumatoid arthritis. The more common situation is that pain and stiffness are generally greater than objective inflammatory signs would predict. Discomfort from joints often extends along tendons and into the muscles of the arms and legs. Pain on motion of the ankle, wrist, knee or elbow may be accompanied by a coarse 'friction' rub caused by fibrinous deposits on the tendon sheath. These rubs are detected in approximately 30% of patients with diffuse scleroderma[50]. The presence of friction rubs can be used as a clinical predictor of worse disease and is associated with higher skin scores, increased frequency of cardiac and renal involvement and increased mortality[50].

The dominant musculoskeletal problem in late scleroderma is muscle atrophy and loss of joint function secondary to restricted motion, usually caused by the abnormal overlying thickened and non-flexible skin. In diffuse scleroderma this can occur over any articulation but is almost universal over the fingers, wrist and elbows. Radiographs of the bones in scleroderma will frequently show osteopenia. Osseous resorption of the digital tuft, secondary to ischemia, and soft tissue calcinosis may also be seen. Joint space narrowing, erosions or bony ankylosis are seen infrequently.

Muscle weakness is a significant problem in scleroderma and often has more than one cause[51]. In diffuse scleroderma, muscle atrophy and weakness can result from deconditioning secondary to restricted mobility and contractures. A myopathy also occurs from a direct extension of the fibrosis process into the muscle itself. These patients present with weakness and fatigue associated with a mild elevation in serum creatine phosphokinase (CPK) and an abnormal electromyogram (EMG)[52]. An 'overlap' syndrome with typical polymyositis or dermatomyositis is seen in a subset of patients with a high CPK, proximal muscle weakness, abnormal EMG and inflammation on muscle biopsy[51,52]. Myopathy secondary to drugs (e.g. corticosteroids, D-penicillamine) used in the treatment of scleroderma can also mimic polymyositis or scleroderma muscle disease. Global weakness and muscle deconditioning are often present in patients with severe disease and multiple organ dysfunction.

Gastrointestinal involvement

Gastrointestinal tract involvement is found in almost every patient with scleroderma and is characterized by abnormal motility secondary to dysfunctions caused by abnormal innervation, smooth muscle atrophy and tissue fibrosis[53]. Every area of the gastrointestinal tract can be involved, including the oropharynx, esophagus, stomach, small and large bowel and rectum. Many scleroderma patients are without significant symptoms despite measurable abnormalities of gastrointestinal function. Unfortunately, severe disease frequently occurs, causing significant morbidity. Patients with both limited and diffuse variants of scleroderma are at equal risk, with gastrointestinal disease being the most common first non-Raynaud's symptom of scleroderma.

The smooth muscle is the major pathologic site of disease in scleroderma gastrointestinal disease. It is not clear, however, whether the smooth muscle abnormality is primary or secondary to abnormal innervation or a defective vascular supply. Although the autonomic nerves of the gastrointestinal tract appear normal by microscopy, functional studies suggest that a neurogenic process precedes muscle dysfunction[54]. The microvascular abnormalities in scleroderma are also seen in the gastrointestinal tract (i.e. intimal proliferation) but clear evidence of ischemic injury is absent. Whatever the primary insult, smooth muscle atrophy and some degree of fibrosis of the submucosal and muscular layers of the gastrointestinal tract becomes the dominant pathology. Irreversible and severe life-threatening bowel dysfunction can result.

Oropharynx

A small oral aperture and dry mucosal membranes with periodontal disease can lead to problems with chewing foods, loss of teeth and failure of good nutrition. Many patients with scleroderma have a sensation of dry eyes and mouth (the sicca complex). Minor salivary gland biopsies usually show fibrosis without the typical lymphocytic aggregates of Sjögren's syndrome. In addition, the majority of scleroderma patients with sicca complaints usually do not have antibodies against Ro/SSA or La/SSB, suggesting that the mechanism of dry membranes in scleroderma is a secondary process different from that seen in Sjögren's syndrome[55].

Upper pharyngeal function is generally considered to be normal in scleroderma unless there is involvement of striated pharyngeal muscles with an inflammatory myositis or a neuromuscular disease. In this case, movement of food from the mouth to the esophagus is abnormal and the patient may complain of coughing upon swallowing, nasal regurgitation of fluids or a sense of inability to swallow.

Esophagus

Esophageal dysfunction affects almost every scleroderma patient, with dysphagia and dyspepsia being the most common symptom. The dysphagia is usually described as solid foods sticking after normal initiation of swallowing. This sensation is relieved by the intake of extra fluids to clear the esophagus. Substernal burning pain may be coupled with a feeling of indigestion or nausea. These reflux symptoms are typically worse after meals, with exercise and after bedtime. Severe esophageal reflux and esophagitis occur equally in patients with either limited or diffuse scleroderma. However, the degree of symptoms does not directly correlate with objective measurements of acid reflux events documented by 24-hour pH monitoring. Patients with motility problems of the esophagus may also present with early satiety, regurgitation of food, progressive weight loss and malnutrition or with emergency impaction of food.

Atypical manifestations of esophageal disease include aspiration, unexplained coughing, hoarseness, a feeling of excess oral secretions, chest pain and localized *Candida* infection.

Low or absent primary and secondary peristalsis of the distal esophagus and low lower esophageal sphincter pressure in the presence of a normal proximal (striated muscle) esophagus are typical manometric findings in scleroderma[56]. Excessive air in the esophagus is commonly detected on routine chest X-ray. Although symptoms are a poor guide to the degree of esophageal disease, patients who are asymptomatic on or off treatment are unlikely to have significant complications. Esophagitis appears to occur only in patients with impaired peristalsis and delayed acid clearance[57].

Untreated or persistent esophagitis can lead to mucosal erosions and occult bleeding, distal esophageal stricture, Barrett's metaplasia or, rarely, adenocarcinoma. Gastrointestinal bleeding occurs from esophagitis, gastritis or gastrointestinal telangiectasias of the stomach, small bowel or colon.

If there is unexplained weight loss with poor caloric intake or other symptoms of esophageal dysfunction, a barium swallow (Fig. 35.19), endoscopic and/or manometric investigation of the esophagus are warranted. A 24-hour pH probe study is a helpful method to quantify the degree and frequency of acid reflux in difficult-to-manage cases.

Stomach and small bowel

Delayed emptying of the stomach with retention of solid foods aggravates reflux and is a frequent cause of bloating, nausea, vomiting, early satiety and poor appetite. Patients frequently reduce their caloric intake to avoid these symptoms and as a consequence lose weight. Gastric

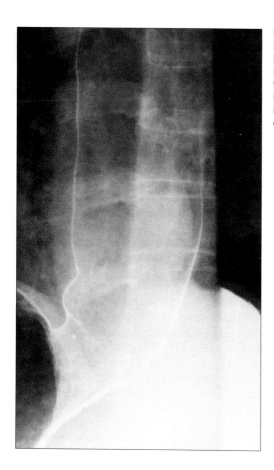

Fig. 35.19 Esophageal involvement. This barium contrast study reveals the characteristic findings of a hypomotile lower esophagus and an incompetent lower esophageal sphincter.

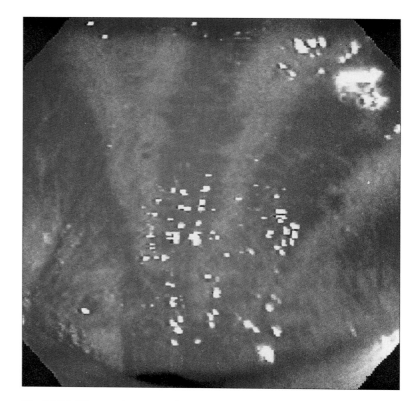

Fig. 35.20 Watermelon stomach. Endoscopy evaluation of a patient with scleroderma with recent gastrointestinal bleeding.

antral vascular ectasia (watermelon stomach) can be a cause of gastrointestinal bleeding in scleroderma patients. Endoscopy of these patients reveals antral gastritis and prominent longitudinal vascular folds that resembles the surface of a watermelon (Fig. 35.20)[58].

Dysmotility of the small intestine may be asymptomatic or it can cause serious intermittent pseudo-obstruction of the intestine presenting with abdominal pain, distention and vomiting that ultimately requires total parenteral nutrition for survival. Motility problems of the small bowel more commonly result in recurrent bouts of mild abdominal pain, diarrhea, weight loss and malnutrition. Malnutrition and diarrhea are usually a consequence of malabsorption caused by bacterial overgrowth in stagnant intestinal fluids. Occasionally, pneumatosis cystoides intestinalis occurs in patients with advanced bowel disease. In this situation, intestinal gas dissects into the bowel wall or, on occasion, into the peritoneal cavity, mimicking a ruptured bowel.

Large bowel

The large intestine and rectum are also affected by scleroderma. Scleroderma patients have decreased distensibility of the colon that does not necessarily correlate with symptoms[59]. Rarely diarrhea, but more frequently constipation, lower abdominal distention or impaction are manifestations of colonic involvement. Because of muscular atrophy of the bowel wall, asymptomatic wide mouthed diverticula unique to scleroderma are commonly found in the transverse and descending colon (Fig. 35.21). Anorectal dysfunction due to reduced capacity, compliance and anal sphincter tone may lead to rectal prolapse and incontinence or alternatively aggravate constipation.

Liver

The liver is rarely involved in scleroderma. An association exists between primary biliary cirrhosis and limited scleroderma[60]. This disease is manifested by cholestatic liver disease with elevations in alkaline phosphatase

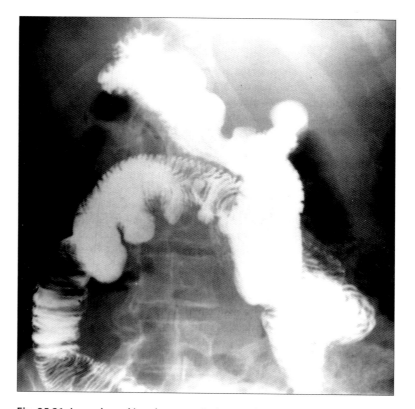

Fig. 35.21 Large bowel involvement. Barium study showing wide-mouthed colonic diverticula.

and jaundice and is associated with antimitochondrial antibodies. Autoimmune hepatitis has been reported in patients with limited scleroderma as well. Transaminase elevations from muscle disease are often mistaken for liver disease in patients with scleroderma.

Pulmonary involvement

Lung involvement in scleroderma is almost universal and now accounts for significant lifetime morbidity and is the leading cause of death. Both interstitial fibrosis and pulmonary arterial vascular disease are present in the lungs of patients with scleroderma but often one pathologic process will be the dominant cause of clinical problems. Pulmonary interstitial fibrosis is more likely to be severe in patients with diffuse skin disease, while pulmonary vascular disease and pulmonary hypertension can be the dominant problem of the lung in patients with the CREST syndrome. Most patients have some degree of both processes and any patient with scleroderma with pulmonary symptoms needs to be evaluated thoroughly for both interstitial lung disease and pulmonary hypertension. Approximately 80% of patients will have abnormal pulmonary function measured by specific and sensitive testing[61]. Yet, the majority of the lung disease will be clinically silent until advanced pulmonary fibrosis or moderate to severe pulmonary arterial hypertension is present.

Patients with interstitial lung disease (ILD) commonly have a rapid decline in pulmonary function that occurs in conjunction with progressive skin disease. Dyspnea on exertion without chest pain is the most common presenting symptom with a dry cough being a late manifestation of ILD. Examination of the patients with ILD reveals 'Velcro-like' crackles at the lung bases in the absence of signs of heart failure. A chest radiograph is relatively insensitive to detect lung disease, but, if abnormal, the fibrosis appears as bilateral reticulonodular changes in the lower lobes of the lung parenchyma (Fig. 35.22).

The most sensitive method for detecting early lung disease in scleroderma is to perform pulmonary function testing. Mild changes in function can be detected before any symptoms develop. The most common changes of pulmonary function testing are either a reduced diffusion capacity ($D_{L}CO$) or a reduction in lung volumes (forced vital capacity, FVC) typical of a restrictive ventilatory defect with associated reduction in gas exchange. A high-resolution computed tomography (HRCT) scan of the chest is a very sensitive technique for detecting changes in the lung parenchyma. Findings of ground-glass opacification of the lung bases on HRCT corresponds with active alveolitis and progressive restrictive lung disease.

Bronchoalveolar lavage (BAL) is used to detect inflammation and active alveolitis. BAL demonstrates an increased total number of cells with an increased percentage of neutrophils, eosinophils or CD8+ T cells. Evidence of active alveolitis by either BAL or HRCT predicts progressive lung disease. Therefore, patients with ground-glass findings on HRCT should be studied with a BAL and, if positive, considered for immunosuppressive therapy. When the disease progresses, fibrosis becomes prominent and is irreversible. In this late stage, there is worsening interstitial fibrosis and 'honeycombing' of the lung parenchyma. When lung fibrosis is present, pulmonary function[62,63] testing will show a restrictive ventilatory defect with reduced lung volumes or a low $D_{L}CO$.

Pulmonary arterial vascular disease with associated pulmonary hypertension is one of the most difficult clinical problems in scleroderma. The pulmonary vascular process can be indolent and remain clinically undetectable until severe irreversible pulmonary hypertension and signs of right-sided heart failure develop. Significant pulmonary hypertension presents clinically with dyspnea on exertion and fatigue. Physical exam findings include a loud pulmonic component of S2, an S3 gallop and other signs of cor pulmonale such as an elevated jugular venous pulse, hepatomegaly and peripheral edema (Fig. 35.23). Electrocardiography shows evidence of right-sided heart strain with right ventricular hypertrophy and right axis deviation. Pulmonary

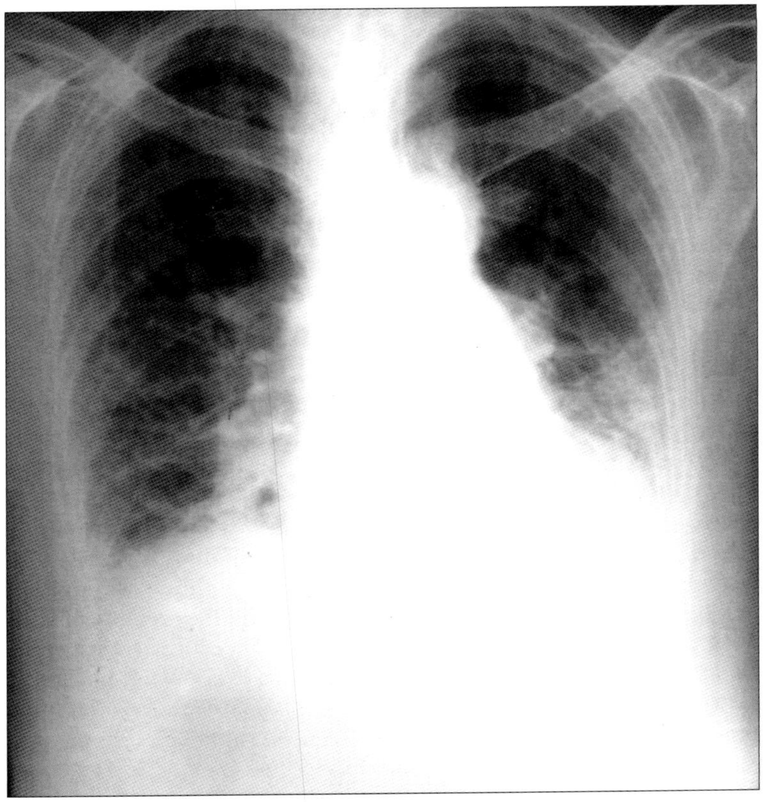

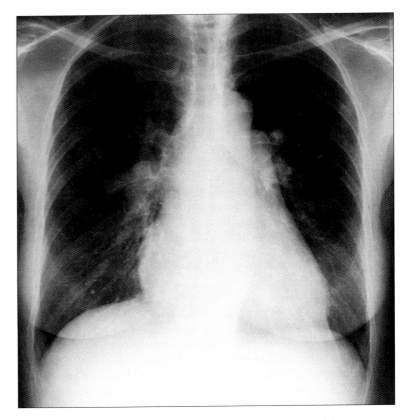

Fig. 35.22 Interstitial lung disease. Chest radiograph in scleroderma showing increased interstitial markings in the lower two-thirds and associated cystic changes.

Fig. 35.23 Pulmonary hypertension. This patient had severe pulmonary hypertension documented on right heart catheterization. The lung fields are clear but the left heart border is straightened from elevation of the pulmonary conus and there is enlargement of the pulmonary arteries. This syndrome is most typical of later years of limited scleroderma.

hypertension can be detected early and non-invasively by measuring the pulmonary artery pressure with two-dimensional Doppler echocardiography. Pulmonary function testing often reveals an isolated decrease in diffusion capacity when pulmonary vascular disease is present.

The natural history of the lung disease in scleroderma is highly variable; the majority of patients will have an early but modest decline in function and then follow a stable course or improve[61]. Approximately a third will have a more severe progressive decline in lung function that continues for 4–5 years and then appears to stabilize. Patients with diffuse skin changes tend to have serious lung involvement in the first 5 years of disease, while patients with CREST syndrome usually do not experience clinical symptoms until more than 5 years after diagnosis. Risk factors for serious restrictive lung disease are African-American or Afro-Caribbean race and antitopoisomerase antibodies[64]. A low diffusing capacity (less than 40% predicted)[65] or rapidly declining D_{LCO} and/or lung volumes predict a high mortality rate.

Less common problems of the lung include aspiration pneumonia (secondary to severe esophageal dysfunction), endobronchial telangiectasias, pulmonary hemorrhage, bronchiolitis obliterans organizing pneumonia, pleural reactions and pneumothorax. Studies are inconclusive about the association between pulmonary function impairment and abnormal esophageal function[66]. There is likely an increased risk of lung cancer in patients with ILD[67]. Chest pain is generally not caused by scleroderma lung disease and if present can usually be explained by another process such as musculoskeletal pain, reflux esophagitis, pleurisy or pericarditis.

Cardiac involvement

The clinical manifestations of scleroderma heart disease are quite variable, usually subtle in expression and often not seen until late in the course of the disease. Frequently, when clinical symptoms are absent, sensitive diagnostic testing can detect the presence of cardiac disease. Overt clinical signs of cardiac disease of any type are a poor prognostic sign and predict shortened survival[68].

Symptoms of scleroderma heart involvement include dyspnea on exertion, palpitations and less frequently chest discomfort. Clinical manifestations of pericarditis, congestive heart failure, pulmonary hypertension and arrhythmias are the main categories of cardiac disease reported in both limited and diffuse scleroderma. The evaluation of the heart can be done with a variety of sensitive methods but it must be remembered that many symptoms of cardiac disease are often linked to pulmonary scleroderma. Dyspnea on exertion is more likely to be secondary to scleroderma lung disease than significant heart problems until late in the course of scleroderma. However, palpitations, atypical chest pain or syncope may be secondary to arrhythmia or pericardial disease. A two-dimensional echocardiogram or ambulatory monitoring of the electrocardiogram is helpful in evaluating patients with symptoms suggesting cardiac disease.

Pericardial disease is found frequently by echocardiography and at autopsy but is usually asymptomatic. The most common finding by echocardiography is a pericardial effusion, although pathological specimens at autopsy also reveal fibrinous pericarditis with adhesions and inflammatory infiltrates[69]. Clinically overt pericarditis is uncommon, although hemodynamic compromise and pericardial tamponade can occur that require acute intervention. Uremic pericardial effusions may also occur in renal failure, a consequence of scleroderma renal crisis.

Ischemic chest pain and myocardial infarction are uncommon clinical problems in scleroderma. Thallium perfusion defects reflecting vascular disease of the endomyocardial vessels (not larger coronary arteries) are seen among scleroderma patients both at rest and with exercise. Because of this, the scleroderma patient with angina-like chest pain may need angiographic studies to rule out coronary arteriosclerosis because thallium scans are likely be abnormal as a result of the microvascular disease of scleroderma heart. In fact, cold provocation of Raynaud's phenomenon can temporarily increase the number of thallium scan defects and induce local abnormalities in ventricular wall motion, supporting the notion that reversible vasospasm of the myocardial microcirculation occurs in scleroderma[70]. Thallium scan perfusion defects predict more severe myocardial disease and poor outcome.

Patchy myocardial fibrosis is a fairly common finding at autopsy in scleroderma patients[70]. This finding is thought to occur secondary to ischemia–reperfusion events in the heart microvasculature causing contraction band necrosis of heart muscle. A decline in left ventricular ejection fraction is a late clinical manifestation, primarily in patients with diffuse skin disease. An abnormal left ventricular ejection fraction is demonstrated by radionucleotide scanning during exercise in approximately 40–50% of all patients, and approximately 15% of diffuse scleroderma patients have abnormalities at rest. Echocardiographic studies suggest that both right and left ventricular dysfunction is common in scleroderma and that diastolic left ventricular dysfunction may occur independent of systolic dysfunction. Diastolic dysfunction may be secondary to hypertension (with or without renal disease) or myocardial fibrosis and may manifest with abnormal left ventricular compliance and pulmonary vascular congestion. Unexplained dyspnea on exertion may be the initial clinical manifestation of unappreciated diastolic dysfunction.

Myocarditis can be associated with inflammatory muscle disease and present as sudden onset of congestive heart failure in a patient with scleroderma and myositis. In fact, patients with skeletal myositis are more likely to develop congestive heart failure or sudden cardiac death than patients without skeletal muscle involvement independent of clear evidence of myocarditis[71]. An endomyocardial biopsy may differentiate myocarditis from the muscle fibrosis seen in scleroderma.

Electrocardiography or Holter monitoring often shows conducting system disease or arrhythmias, which are usually clinically silent. Premature ventricular contractions are the most common arrhythmia; frequently they are in couplets or are multifocal. Premature atrial contractions, supraventricular tachycardia, AV or intraventricular conduction disorders are seen less commonly[72]. The prevalence of arrhythmias and conduction defects is greater among patients with diffuse scleroderma than in those with limited disease. The presence of arrhythmias is associated with a worse overall prognosis.

Renal involvement

The most important clinical manifestation of scleroderma kidney is accelerated hypertension and/or rapidly progressive renal failure: the scleroderma renal crisis[73]. Surveys suggest that only about 10% of all scleroderma patients develop a crisis. The majority of patients who develop renal crisis have diffuse cutaneous disease and approximately 80% of cases of renal crisis occur within 4 years of disease onset[74]. Risk factors for renal crisis include rapidly progressing diffuse skin disease, tendon friction rubs, new unexplained anemia and the presence of anti-RNA polymerase III antibody. Antecedent use of corticosteroids is also associated with a higher risk of developing renal crisis[75]. Non-malignant hypertension, abnormalities on urinalysis, plasma renin level[76] and the presence of anticentromere or antitopoisomerase antibodies are not predictors of a scleroderma renal crisis.

Patients with renal crisis may present with typical signs of malignant hypertension, including headache, altered vision, signs of heart failure and confusion or neurologic signs such as seizures in the setting of an abnormally high blood pressure (>150/90mmHg). However, there may be no specific symptoms and occasionally a normotensive crisis can occur. Laboratory data show normal or high creatinine, proteinuria and/or microscopic hematuria. A microangiopathic hemolytic anemia and thrombocytopenia can be present, especially in normotensive patients with renal crisis. A poorer outcome is seen in males, patients with an older age of onset and those who present with creatinine levels higher than 3mg/dl (230μmol/l)[77].

The typical vasculopathy of scleroderma is present in the renal vessels of patients with or without renal crisis. This suggests that other factors, such as vasospasm, probably contribute to the development of renal crisis. Scleroderma patients may have a reduced creatinine clearance, proteinuria, microscopic hematuria and non-malignant hypertension, but often another cause for these abnormalities is found. For example, an immune complex process may be the cause for glomerulonephritis in patients with an overlap syndrome of SLE and scleroderma. A reversible proteinuria or even a crescentic glomerulonephritis may occur secondary to treatment with D-penicillamine[78].

Other common clinical problems

Nervous system
Although it has been argued that the clinical features of scleroderma could be explained by a diffuse degenerative process in the nervous system, conclusive evidence for a primary nervous system disease is still lacking. Scleroderma spares the central nervous system and therefore signs of central nervous system disease usually have another explanation. The exception is trigeminal neuropathy, which may first present with facial numbness and then later with facial pain. Abnormal neural function, perhaps secondary to microvascular disease, may explain the early manifestation of gastrointestinal disease (see above). Similarly, Raynaud's phenomenon may partially be a manifestation of enhanced adrenergic nerve responses of vascular smooth muscle. Sensitive peripheral nerve testing may disclose abnormal cutaneous sensory thresholds. Entrapment neuropathy occurs from carpal tunnel syndrome or ulnar nerve entrapment at the elbow. A recent survey shows that nearly 50% of patients with scleroderma have symptoms of depression[79]. The severity of depression correlates more with personality traits and the degree of supportive care available than with the severity of the disease. Sexual dysfunction is also common in scleroderma. Impotence among male patients is usually secondary to neurovascular disease, although non-organic dysfunction should be investigated.

Fertility and pregnancy
Investigations thus far do not clarify whether patients with scleroderma have any increased risk for infertility, miscarriage or low-birthweight infants or not. However, it is clear that pregnancy aggravates the gastrointestinal and cardiopulmonary symptoms of scleroderma and adds risk for the patient[80]. There is also evidence that an increased risk for scleroderma renal crisis exists. Therefore, patients should be closely monitored, in conjunction with a high-risk obstetrician, with frequent measurements of blood pressure and urinalyses.

Malignancy in scleroderma
Population-based surveys reveal a higher incidence of malignancy in scleroderma patients[81,82]. The types of cancer reported include lung cancer, non-melanoma skin cancer and liver cancer[81]. Although there has been some controversy over the association of scleroderma with excess breast cancer, there is strong evidence that more lung cancer occurs than would be expected in the general population, probably related to interstitial lung disease[67]. Adenocarcinoma of the esophagus associated with chronic gastroesophageal reflux has also been reported in patients with scleroderma[83].

Endocrinopathy
Hypothyroidism can occur either secondary to thyroid fibrosis or from autoimmune thyroiditis. One study revealed that all patients with hypothyroidism had some degree of fibrosis on microscopic evaluation, although some did have a lymphocytic infiltrate as well[84]. Subclinical thyroid disease was detected in up to 20% of patients by a sensitive evaluation[85]. Other endocrinopathies are no more common in scleroderma patients than in the general population.

INVESTIGATIONS

Measuring disease activity and severity
Ideal clinical and laboratory measurements of disease 'activity' do not exist in scleroderma[86]. The degree of disease activity can be confused with 'severity-damage' or irreversible loss of function of an organ or body system[86]. A variety of laboratory measurements have been proposed as important tools to measure disease, including various cytokines, collagen metabolites, factors signifying vascular perturbation (e.g. von Willebrand factor) and components signifying inflammation or activation of the immune system, although none of these are widely used clinically.

Subjective clinical parameters are also used as measurements of disease activity, although it is unclear what is the best parameter to measure this activity. Popular clinical measurements include skin score, hand extension, oral aperture, finger flexion and global patient and physician assessments of disease activity. Most clinical observations detail the cutaneous manifestations because the skin is directly measurable by observation and palpation. Although the natural course of the skin changes is reasonably well described in diffuse scleroderma, it must be remembered that the cutaneous disease may not be the ideal surrogate for the overall disease activity. For example, significant cardiopulmonary and gastrointestinal disease can emerge later in the course, at a time when the skin may be improving or thinning. In limited scleroderma, the skin fibrosis is minimal and does not parallel the vascular disease such as pulmonary hypertension and digital loss.

Recently, a quantitative measure of disease severity has been developed that documents the degree of severity of involvement of each major organ graded from 0 (normal) to 4 (end-stage)[87] (Table 35.4). This scale has been externally validated on a large group of scleroderma patients and may be helpful in comparing groups of patients in clinical trials and for following disease in individual patients.

Method of measuring skin involvement
Palpation of the skin to detect skin thickening has been shown to be a reliable semiquantitative method that correlates with the weight of a punch biopsy of the skin in the same area[88]. The examiner should attempt to pinch the skin and then assess the thickness of the skinfold between the fingers. Although the thickness is due to an increase in the dermal skin layer, often the skin will be fixed to subdermal tissues. It is important to distinguish thickening of the skin of early disease from 'involved skin' of late disease, which can be thinned (atrophic), tethered or bound down. Late-stage skin is often thinner than normal skin and less flexible.

A simplified total skin score (modified Rodnan skin thickness score) is obtained by the examiner pinching the skin in 17 sites, scoring each area from 0–3 (0 = normal skin; 3 = extreme thickening) and then summing the score of all the palpated sites (Fig. 35.24)[88]. In clinical practice, serial measurements of the skin involvement will help define the stage and course of the skin disease, with higher skin scores suggesting more aggressive internal organ disease.

TABLE 35.4 DISEASE SEVERITY SCALE

System	0 (normal)	1 (mild)	2 (moderate)	3 (severe)	4 (end-stage)
General	Normal	Weight loss of 5.0–9.9kg or hematocrit 33.0–36.9	Weight loss of 10.0–14.9kg or hematocrit 29.0–32.9	Weight loss of 15.0–19.9kg or hematocrit 25.0–28.9	Weight loss of 20+kg or hematocrit <25.0
Raynaud's	Normal	Vasodilator-requiring	Digital pitting scars	Active digital pit ulceration	Digital gangrene
Skin score	0	1–14	15–29	30–39	40+
Finger to palm (cm)	<1	1.0–1.9	2.0–3.9	4.0–4.9	5.0+
Proximal weakness	None	Mild	Moderate	Severe	Cannot walk
GI status	Normal	Requires antireflux medication or abnormal small bowel series	High dose antireflux medication or antibiotics for bacterial overgrowth	Malabsorption syndrome or episodes of pseudo-obstruction	TPN required
Lung	Normal	FVC or $D_L$co 70–80% predicted or rales or fibrosis on chest X-ray	FVC or $D_L$co 50–69% predicted or mild pulmonary hypertension	FVC or $D_L$co 50% predicted or moderate–severe pulmonary hypertension	Oxygen required
Heart	Normal	ECG conduction defect or LVEF 45–49%	Arrhythmia or RVE + LVE or LVEF 40–44%	LVEF <40%	Congestive heart failure or arrhythmia requiring medication
Kidney	Normal	Creatinine 1.3–1.6 or uprot 2+	Creatinine 1.7–2.9 or uprot 3–4+	Creatinine 3.0+	Requires dialysis

LVE, left ventricular enlargement; LVEF, left ventricular ejection fraction, RVE, right ventricular enlargement; TPN, total parenteral nutrition. (Modified from Medsger et al.[87])

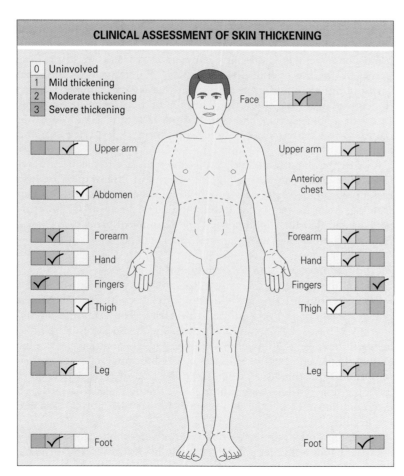

CLINICAL ASSESSMENT OF SKIN THICKENING

0 Uninvolved
1 Mild thickening
2 Moderate thickening
3 Severe thickening

Face

Upper arm   Upper arm

Abdomen   Anterior chest

Forearm   Forearm

Hand   Hand

Fingers   Fingers

Thigh   Thigh

Leg   Leg

Foot   Foot

Fig. 35.24 Total skin score. Semiquantitative estimates by clinical palpation of the extent and severity of scleroderma skin change. In all cases, the initial areas involved are peripheral and are the most severely affected. The mild skin change on the chest permits classification of this subject as diffuse scleroderma.

TABLE 35.5 AUTOANTIBODY ASSOCIATIONS WITH SCLERODERMA

Antibody	Prevalence (%)*	Clinical associations
Anti-topoisomerase 1 (Scl-70)	20–40	Diffuse skin disease Interstitial lung disease Increased mortality Cardiac disease
Anti-centromere	20–40	CREST syndrome Digital loss Pulmonary hypertension Primary biliary cirrhosis
Nucleolar antibodies		
RNA Polymerases	4–20	Renal crisis Cardiac disease Diffuse skin disease Tendon friction rubs Increased mortality
U3snRNP (fibrillarin)	8	African-American males Diffuse skin disease Pulmonary disease
Th	5	Limited skin disease
Nor-90	Rare	Unknown
Pm-Scl	1	Myositis
U1snRNP	5	Mixed connective tissue disease

* Among patients with scleroderma.

Serologic associations

Recent findings suggest that serologic data can help predict clinical features and survival (Table 35.5). Scleroderma patients with anticentromere antibody are more likely to have CREST syndrome and have a relatively good prognosis but may develop pulmonary hypertension, digital amputation or biliary cirrhosis. Patients with anti-RNA polymerase antibody have an increased risk of cardiac or renal disease and a poor prognosis[89], while patients with antitopoisomerase[90] have a higher risk of pulmonary disease. Anti-U3-RNP (antifibrillarin) is seen in approximately 5% of patients, primarily African–American or Afro-Caribbean males with serious pulmonary disease[91]. Anti-PM-Scl and anti-Ku are associated with scleroderma with myositis in Caucasians and Japanese respectively[92].

DIFFERENTIAL DIAGNOSIS

The differential diagnosis of scleroderma includes other disorders associated with Raynaud's phenomenon, toxic exposures, other connective tissue diseases and conditions with cutaneous disease resembling scleroderma (Table 35.6). Silica exposure can cause a disease indistinguishable from idiopathic scleroderma including typical skin changes, Raynaud's phenomenon and antitopoisomerase antibodies in masons, gold and coal miners[93]. Eosinophilia–myalgia syndrome and toxic oil syndrome have skin disease that mimics scleroderma but are distinguished by other manifestations such as cognitive impairment, chronic pain and muscle cramping. Eosinophilic fasciitis causes a widespread deep tissue fibrosis but typically spares the fingers, hands and face. Scleredema also presents with skin thickening, especially in the back, neck and shoulder girdle, and occurs in association with type 1 diabetes and in patients with paraproteinemias. Scleroderma skin changes are seen in a variety of other disorders including chronic graft-versus-host disease, porphyria cutanea tarda, phenylketonuria, progeria-like syndromes, POEMS syndrome, localized lipoatrophies and bleomycin exposure.

TABLE 35.6 DIFFERENTIAL DIAGNOSIS OF SCLERODERMA

Disorders characterized by similar presentations

Systemic lupus erythematosus
Rheumatoid arthritis
Inflammatory myopathy

Disorders characterized by similar visceral features

Primary pulmonary hypertension
Primary biliary cirrhosis
Idiopathic intestinal hypomotility
Collagenous colitis
Idiopathic interstitial pulmonary fibrosis

Disorders characterized by skin thickening

Affecting the fingers
  Diabetic digital sclerosis
  Vinyl chloride disease
  Vibration syndrome
  Bleomycin-induced scleroderma
  Chronic reflex sympathetic dystrophy
  Amyloidosis
  Acrodermatitis
  Scleromyxedema

Sparing the fingers
  Scleredema
  Eosinophilic fasciitis
  Eosinophilia–myalgia syndrome
  Generalized subcutaneous morphea
  Fibrosis associated with augmentative mammoplasty
  Amyloidosis
  Carcinoid syndrome
  Pentazocine-induced scleroderma

REFERENCES

1. Rodnan GP, Benedek TG. An historical account of the study of progressive systemic sclerosis (diffuse scleroderma). Ann Intern Med 1962; 57: 305–319.
2. Barnett AJ. History of scleroderma. In: Clements PJ, Furst DE, eds. Systemic sclerosis. Baltimore, MD: Williams & Wilkins; 1996: 3–22.
3. Raynaud M. On local asphyxia of the extremities, 1864. London: New Sydenham Society; 1888.
4. Osler, W. The principles and practice of medicine. New York: Appleton, 1894: 993.
5. Klemperer P, Pollack AD, Boehr G. Diffuse collagen disease: acute disseminated lupus erythematosus and diffuse scleroderma. JAMA 1942; 119: 331.
6. Goetz RH. Pathology of progressive systemic sclerosis (generalized scleroderma) with special reference to changes in the viscera. Clin Proc (S Afr) 1945; 4: 337–342.
7. Winterbauer RH. Multiple telangiectasia, Raynaud's phenomenon, sclerodactyly, and subcutaneous calcinosis: a syndrome mimicking hereditary hemorrhagic telangiectasia. Bull Johns Hopkins Hosp 1964; 114: 361–383.
8. Meyer O. From Thibierge–Weissenbach syndrome (1910) to anti-centromere antibodies (1980). Clinical and biological features of scleroderma. Ann Med Interne (Paris) 1999; 150: 47–52.
9. D'Angelo WA, Fries JF, Masi AT, Shulman LE. Pathologic observations in systemic sclerosis (scleroderma). A study of fifty-eight autopsy cases and fifty-eight matched controls. Am J Med 1969; 46: 428–440.
10. Medsger TA Jr. Epidemiology of systemic sclerosis. Clin Dermatol 1994; 12: 207–216.
11. Masi AT, Rodnan GP, Medsger TA Jr et al. Preliminary criteria for the classification of systemic sclerosis (scleroderma). Arthritis Rheum 1980; 23: 581–590.
12. Maricq HR, Kel JE, Sith EA et al. Prevalence of scleroderma spectrum disorders in the general population of South Carolina. Arthritis Rheum 1989; 32: 998–1006.
13. Arnett FC, Howard RF, Tan F et al. Increased prevalence of systemic sclerosis in a native American tribe in Oklahoma. Arthritis Rheum 1996; 39: 1362–1370.
14. Geirsson AJ, Steinsson K, Guthmundsson S, Sigurthsson V. Systemic sclerosis in Iceland. A nationwide epidemiological study. Ann Rheum Dis 1994; 53: 502–505.
15. Tan EM, Rodnan GP, Garcia I et al. Diversity of antinuclear antibodies in progressive systemic sclerosis. Anti-centromere antibody and its relationship to CREST syndrome. Arthritis Rheum 1980; 23: 617–615.
16. Laing TL, Gillespie BW, Toth MB et al. Racial differences in scleroderma among women in Michigan. Arthritis Rheum 1997; 40: 734–742.
17. Medsger TA Jr, Masi AT. Epidemiology of systemic sclerosis. Ann Intern Med 1971; 74: 714–721.
18. Silman AJ, Howard Y, Hicklin AJ, Black C. Geographical clustering of scleroderma in south and west London. Br J Rheumatol 1990; 29: 93–96.
19. Maricq HR. Geographic clustering of scleroderma. Br J Rheumatol 1990; 29: 241–243.
20. Haustein UF, Herrmann K. Environmental scleroderma. Clin Dermatol 1994; 12: 467–473.

21. Cook NJ, Silman AJ, Propert J, Cawley MI. Features of systemic sclerosis (scleroderma) in an identical twin pair. Br J Rheumatol 1993; 32: 926–928.
22. Feghali CA, Wright TM. Epidemiologic and clinical study of twins with scleroderma. Arthritis Rheum 1995; 38: S308.
23. Maddison PJ, Stephens C, Briggs D et al. Connective tissue disease and autoantibodies in the kindreds of 63 patients with systemic sclerosis. The United Kingdom Systemic Sclerosis Study Group. Medicine 1993; 72: 103–112.
24. Clements PJ, Hurwitz EL, Wong WK et al. Skin thickness score as a predictor and correlate of outcome in systemic sclerosis. Arthritis Rheum 2000; 43: 2445–2454.
25. Giordano M. Classification of progressive systemic sclerosis (scleroderma). In: Black CM, Myers AR, eds. Systemic sclerosis (scleroderma). New York: Gower; 1985: 21–23.
26. Masi A. Classification of systemic sclerosis (scleroderma). In: Black CM, Myers AR, eds. Systemic sclerosis (scleroderma). New York: Gower; 1985: 7–15.
27. Medsger TA Jr. Classification of systemic sclerosis. In: Jayson MIV, Black CM, eds. Systemic sclerosis: scleroderma. New York: John Wiley & Sons; 1988: 1–6.
28. Barnett AJ. Classification of systemic sclerosis (scleroderma). In: Black CM, Myers AR, eds. Systemic sclerosis (scleroderma). New York: Gower; 1985: 18–20.
29. LeRoy EC, Medsger TA Jr. Criteria for the classification of early systemic sclerosis. J Rheum 2001; 28: 1573–1576.
30. Poormoghim H, Lucas M, Fertig N et al. Systemic sclerosis sine scleroderma: demographic, clinical, and serologic features and survival in forty-eight patients. Arthritis Rheum 2000; 43: 444–451.
31. Alarcon-Segovia D. Mixed connective tissue disease and overlap syndromes. Clin Dermatol 1994; 12: 309–316.
32. Black C, Isenberg DA. Mixed connective tissue disease – goodbye to all that. Br J Rheumatol 1992; 31: 695–700.
33. Van de Hoogen FHJ, Spronk PE, Boerbooms AMT et al. Longterm follow-up of 46 patients with anti-U1snRNP antibodies. Br J Rheumatol 1994; 33: 1117–1120.
34. Steen VD, Medsger TA Jr. Severe organ involvement in systemic sclerosis with diffuse scleroderma. Arthritis Rheum 2000; 43: 2437–2444.
35. Bryan C, Knight C, Black CM et al. Prediction of five-year survival following presentation with scleroderma. Arthritis Rheum 1999; 42: 2660–2665.
36. Jacobsen S, Halberg P, Ullman S. Mortality and causes of death of 344 Danish patients with systemic sclerosis (scleroderma). Br J Rheumatol 1998; 37: 750–755.
37. Wigley FM, Wise RA, Miller R et al. Anti-centromere antibody predicts the ischemic loss of digits in patients with systemic sclerosis. Arthritis Rheum 1992; 35: 688–693.
38. Maricq HR, Carpentier PH, Weinrich MC et al. Geographic variation in the prevalence of Raynaud's phenomenon: Charleston, SC, USA, vs. Tarentaise, Savoie, France. J Rheumatol 1993; 20: 70–76.
39. O'Keeffe ST, Tsapatsaris NP, Beetham WP Jr. Color chart assisted diagnosis of Raynaud's phenomenon in an unselected hospital employee population. J Rheumatol 1992; 19: 1415–1417.
40. LeRoy EC, Medsger TA Jr. Raynaud's phenomenon: a proposal for classification. (Review). Clin Exp Rheumatol 1992; 10: 485–488.
41. Maricq HR, Weinberger AB, LeRoy EC. Early detection of scleroderma-spectrum disorders by in vivo capillary microscopy: a prospective study of patients with Raynaud's phenomenon. J Rheumatol 1982; 9: 289–291.
42. Zufferey P, Depairon M, Chamot AM, Monti M. Prognostic significance of nailfold capillary microscopy in patients with Raynaud's phenomenon and scleroderma-pattern abnormalities. A six-year follow-up study. Clin Rheumatol 1992; 11: 536–541.
43. Spencer-Green G. Outcomes in primary Raynaud phenomenon. Arch Intern Med 1998; 158: 595–600.
44. Kallenberg CG. Early detection of connective tissue disease in patients with Raynaud's phenomenon. Rheum Dis Clin North Am 1990; 16: 11–30.
45. Rodnan GP, Myerowitz RL, Justh GO. Morphologic changes in the digital arteries of patients with progressive systemic sclerosis (scleroderma) and Raynaud phenomenon. Medicine 1980; 59: 393–408.
46. Clements PJ, Lachenbruch PA, Furst DE et al. Abnormalities of renal physiology in systemic sclerosis. A prospective study with 10-year follow-up. Arthritis Rheum 1994; 37: 67–74.
47. Wigley FM, Wise RA, Stevens MB, Newball H. The effect of cold exposure on carbon monoxide diffusing capacity in patients with Raynaud's phenomenon. Chest 1982; 81: 695–698.
48. Shuck JW, Oetgen WJ, Tesar JT. Pulmonary vascular response during Raynaud's phenomenon in progressive systemic sclerosis. Am J Med 1985; 78: 221–227.
49. Oddis CV, Eisenbeis CH, Reidbord HE et al. Vasculitis in systemic sclerosis: association with Sjögren's syndrome and the CREST syndrome variant. J Rheumatol 1987; 14: 942–948.
50. Steen VD, Medsger TA Jr. The palpable tendon friction rub. Arthritis Rheum 1997; 40: 1146–1151.
51. Olsen NJ, King LE, Park JH. Muscle abnormalities in scleroderma. Rheum Dis Clin North Am 1996; 22: 783–796.
52. Clements PJ, Furst DE, Campion DS et al. Muscle disease in progressive systemic sclerosis: diagnostic and therapeutic considerations. Arthritis Rheum 1978; 21: 62–71.
53. Young MA, Rose S, Reynolds JC. Gastrointestinal manifestations of scleroderma. Rheum Dis Clin North Am 1996; 22: 797–823.
54. Cameron AJ, Payne WS. Barrett's esophagus occurring as a complication of scleroderma. Mayo Clin Proc 1978; 53: 612.
55. Clements PJ, Furst DE. Systemic sclerosis. Baltimore, MD: Williams & Wilkins; 1996.
56. Bassotti G, Battaglia E, Debernardi V et al. Esophageal dysfunction in scleroderma. Arthritis Rheum 1997; 40: 2252–2259.
57. Basilisco G, Barbera R, Molgora M et al. Acid clearance and oesophageal sensitivity in patients with progressive systemic sclerosis. Gut 1993; 34: 1487–1491.
58. Watson M, Hally R, McCue P et al. Gastric antral vascular ectasia (watermelon stomach) in patients with systemic sclerosis. Arthritis Rheum 1996; 39: 341–346.
59. Whitehead ME, Taitelbaum G, Wigley FM, Schuster MM. Rectosigmoid motility and myoelectric activity in progressive systemic sclerosis. Gastroenterology 1989; 96: 428–432.
60. Rose S, Young MA, Reynolds JC. Gastrointestinal disorders and systemic disease, Part I. Gastroenterol Clin North Am 1998; 27: 563–594.
61. Schneider P, Hochberg MC, Wise RA, Wigley FM. Serial pulmonary function in patients with systemic sclerosis. Am J Med 1982; 73: 385–394.
62. Steen VD, Conte C, Owens GR, Medsger TA Jr. Severe restrictive lung disease in systemic sclerosis. Arthritis Rheum 1994; 37: 1283–1289.
63. Steen VD, Conte G, Owens GR et al. Isolated diffusing capacity reduction in systemic sclerosis. Arthritis Rheum 1992; 35: 765–770.
64. Greidinger EL, Flaherty KT, White B et al. African-American race and antibodies to topoisomerase I are associated with increased severity of scleroderma lung disease. Chest 1998; 114: 801–807.
65. Peters-Golden M, Wise R, Hochberg M et al. Clinical and demographic predictors of loss of pulmonary function in systemic sclerosis. Medicine 1984; 63: 221–232.
66. Troshinsky MB, Kane GC, Varga J et al. Pulmonary function and gastroesophageal reflux in systemic sclerosis. Ann Intern Med 1994; 121: 6–10.
67. Peters-Golden M, Wise R, Hochberg M et al. Incidence of lung cancer in systemic sclerosis. J Rheumatol 1985; 12: 1136–1139.
68. Clements PJ, Lachenbruch PA, Furst DE et al. Cardiac score. A semiquantitative measure of cardiac involvement that improves prediction of prognosis in systemic sclerosis. Arthritis Rheum 1991; 34: 1371–1380.
69. Byers RJ, Marshall AS, Freemont AJ. Pericardial involvement in systemic sclerosis. Ann Rheum Dis 1997; 56: 393–394.
70. Deswal A, Follansbee WP. Cardiac involvement in scleroderma. Rheum Dis Clin North Am 1996; 22: 841–860.
71. Follansbee WP, Zerbe TR, Medsger TA Jr. Cardiac and skeletal muscle disease in systemic sclerosis (scleroderma): a high risk association. Am Heart J 1993; 125: 194–203.
72. Follansbee WP, Curtiss EI, Rahko PS et al. The electrocardiogram in systemic sclerosis (scleroderma). Study of 102 consecutive cases with functional correlations and review of the literature. Am J Med 1985; 79: 183–192.
73. Steen VD. Renal involvement in systemic sclerosis. Clin Dermatol 1994; 12: 253–258.
74. Traub YM, Shapiro AP, Rodnan GP et al. Hypertension and renal failure (scleroderma renal crisis) in progressive systemic sclerosis. Review of a 25 year experience with 68 cases. Medicine 1983; 62: 335–352.
75. Steen VD, Medsger TA Jr. Case-control study of corticosteroids and other drugs that either precipitate or protect from the development of scleroderma renal crisis. Arthritis Rheum 1998; 41: 1613–1619.
76. Clements PJ, Lachenbruch PA, Furst DE et al. Abnormalities of renal physiology in systemic sclerosis. A prospective study with 10-year follow-up. Arthritis Rheum 1994; 37: 67–74.
77. Steen VD, Medsger TA Jr. Long-term outcomes of scleroderma renal crisis. Ann Intern Med 2000; 133: 600–603.
78. Garcia-Porrua C, Gonzalez-Gay MA, Bouza P. D-Penicillamine-induced crescentic glomerulonephritis in a patient with scleroderma. Nephron 2000; 84: 101–102.
79. Roca RP, Wigley FM, White B. Depressive symptoms in systemic sclerosis (scleroderma). Arthritis Rheum 1996; 39: 1035–1040.
80. Steen VD. Scleroderma and pregnancy. Rheum Dis Clin North Am 1997; 23: 133–147.
81. Abu-Shakra M, Guillemin F, Lee P. Cancer in systemic sclerosis. Arthritis Rheum 1993; 36: 460–464.
82. Rosenthal AK, McLaughlin JK, Gridley G et al. Incidence of cancer among patients with systemic sclerosis. Cancer 1995; 76: 910–914.
83. Heath EI, Limburg PJ, Hawk ET et al. Adenocarcinoma of the esophagus: risk factors and prevention. Oncology 2000; 14: 507–514.
84. Gordon MB, Klein I, Dekker A et al. Thyroid disease in progressive systemic sclerosis: increased frequency of glandular fibrosis and hypothyroidism. Ann Intern Med 1981; 95: 431–435.
85. Kahl LE, Medsger TA Jr, Klein I. Prospective evaluation of thyroid function in patients with systemic sclerosis (scleroderma). J Rheumatol 1986; 13: 103–107.
86. Clements PJ. Measuring disease activity and severity in scleroderma. Curr Opin Rheum 1995; 7: 517–521.
87. Medsger TA Jr, Silman AJ, Steen VD et al. A disease severity scale for systemic sclerosis: development and testing. J Rheumatol 1999; 26: 2159–2167.
88. Clements P, Lachenbruch P, Seibold J, Wigley FM. Inter- and intra-observer variability of total skin thickness score (modified Rodnan) in systemic sclerosis (SSc). J Rheumatol 1995; 22: 1281–1285.
89. Kuwana M, Kaburaki J, Mimori T et al. Autoantibody reactive with three classes of RNA polymerases in sera from patients with systemic sclerosis. J Clin Invest 1993; 91: 1399–1404.

90. Steen VD, Powell DL, Medsger TA Jr. Clinical correlations and prognosis based on serum autoantibodies in patients with systemic sclerosis. Arthritis Rheum 1988; 31: 196–203.
91. Okano Y, Steen VD, Medsger TA Jr. Autoantibody to U3 nucleolar ribonucleoprotein (fibrillarin) in patients with systemic sclerosis. Arthritis Rheum 1992; 35: 95–100.
92. Reichlin M, Maddison PJ, Targoff I et al. Antibodies to a nuclear/nucleolar antigen in patients with polymyositis overlap syndrome. J Clin Immunol 1984; 4: 40–44.
93. Rodnan GP, Benedek TG, Medsger TA Jr et al. The association of progressive systemic sclerosis (scleroderma) with coal miners' pneumoconiosis and other forms of silicosis. Ann Intern Med 1967; 66: 323–334.

36 Raynaud's phenomenon

Abdul-Wahab Al-Allaf and Jill J F Belch

- Raynaud's phenomenon is an episodic reversible peripheral ischemia provoked by cold or emotion
- Classically, constriction of the digital vessels leads to pallor of the digits, followed by cyanosis secondary to static venous blood
- The recovery phase features reactive hyperemia, with resulting erythema

EPIDEMIOLOGY

The terms 'Raynaud's disease' and 'Raynaud's phenomenon' are often used interchangeably to identify two distinct disorders that initially appear with similar symptoms but then have different sequelae or associated conditions. In the UK, 'Raynaud's phenomenon' is the blanket term usually used to describe any form of cold-related vasospasm, which can be further subdivided into Raynaud's syndrome when there is an associated disorder, and Raynaud's disease when there is not. However, in the USA the terminology most used is 'primary Raynaud's phenomenon' and 'secondary Raynaud's phenomenon'. Thus care must be taken with literature comparisons.

Raynaud's phenomenon may affect as many as 20–30% of young women and have an overall prevalence in the population of approximately 10%, with a female:male ratio of 2:1[1]. By far the largest group of patients presenting to their primary care physician are those with a primary Raynaud's disorder, which typically occurs in young women in their teens and 20s, has a familial predisposition and accounts for the vast majority of all cases of Raynaud's phenomenon. In contrast, more than 50% of the patients referred to hospital will have an associated underlying systemic disease. Recent studies have shown that the Raynaud's syndrome may predate systemic illness by up to two decades.

TABLE 36.1 CONDITIONS ASSOCIATED WITH RAYNAUD'S PHENOMENON

Immune-mediated
- Systemic sclerosis (90%)
- Mixed connective tissue disease (85%)
- Sjögren's syndrome (33%)
- Systemic lupus erythematosus (10–44%)
- Polymyositis/dermatomyositis (29%)
- Rheumatoid arthritis (10–15%)
- Cryoglobulinemia and cryofibrinogenemia (10%)
- Arteritis (e.g. giant cell arteritis, Takayasu arteritis)
- Antiphospholipid syndrome
- Primary biliary cirrhosis

Occupation-related
- Cold injury (e.g. frozen-food packers)
- Polyvinyl chloride exposure
- Vibration exposure
- Ammunition workers (outside work)

Obstructive vascular disease
- Atherosclerosis
- Microemboli
- Thromboangiitis obliterans (50%)
- Thoracic outlet syndrome (e.g. cervical rib)
- Walking-crutch pressure
- Diabetic microangiopathy

Metabolic disorders
- Hypothyroidism
- Carcinoid syndrome
- Pheochromocytoma
- Uremia

Drug-induced
- Antimigraine compounds
- β-blockers (particularly non-selective)
- Cytotoxic drugs
- Cyclosporin
- Bromocriptine
- Sulphasalazine
- Minocycline
- Interferon-α
- Interferon-β
- Ergotamine derivatives

Infections
- Chronic viral liver diseases (hepatitis B and C)
- Cytomegalovirus
- Parvovirus B19
- *Helicobacter pylori*

Miscellaneous
- Arteriovenous fistula
- Artificial acrylic nails
- Carpal tunnel syndrome (60%)
- POEMS syndrome
- Neoplasm
- Complex regional pain syndrome type 1
- Toxic oil syndrome
- Fibromyalgia syndrome
- Polycythemia
- Paraproteinemia
- Myalgic encephalitis (postviral fatigue syndrome)

% values are percentage of patients with disease who have Raynaud's phenomenon.

POEMS, polyneuropathy, organomegaly, endocrinopathy, monoclonal proteins and skin changes

ETIOLOGY

There is a wide spectrum of disease associated with Raynaud's syndrome, including connective tissue disorders, both drug-induced and those associated with thromboangiitis obliterans and with occupational exposure to vibration (Table 36.1).

Raynaud's phenomenon occurs in 90% of patients with systemic sclerosis and 85% of patients with mixed connective tissue disease. Between 10% and 45% of patients with systemic lupus erythematosus, 33% of patients with Sjögren's syndrome and 20% of those with dermatomyositis/polymyositis experience Raynaud's phenomenon. Patients with rheumatoid arthritis have a similar overall prevalence of Raynaud's phenomenon as compared with the general population (10%); however, symptomatology tends to be more severe.

It is estimated that about 50% of all workers using vibrating equipment can develop Raynaud's phenomenon, and it is the most common form of occupational Raynaud's phenomenon. This is now called hand–arm vibration syndrome or HAVS (previously known as vibration white finger syndrome or VWF). β-Blockers are a commonly used group of drugs that can induce Raynaud's phenomenon. More recently, prescribing β-blockers for those suffering from Raynaud's phenomenon has been revolutionized by the development of vasodilating β-blockers. This allows safe prescription of these drugs to patients with Raynaud's phenomenon. In the older age group, obstructive vascular disease is the most common cause of Raynaud's phenomenon and it has been reported that 60% of Raynaud's phenomenon occurring in individuals older than 60 years is atherosclerotic in origin. Many other conditions can be associated with Raynaud's phenomenon and are listed in Table 36.1.

PATHOPHYSIOLOGY

The pathophysiology of the triphasic color changes is well recognized: constriction of the digital vessels leads to pallor of the digits, followed by cyanosis secondary to deoxygenation of static venous blood, and then a reactive hyperemic stage with resulting erythema. There are three pathophysiological mechanisms that may mediate these changes and therefore need to be considered in patients with Raynaud's phenomenon: (1) neurogenic mechanisms; (2) blood and blood vessel wall interactions; (3) abnormalities of the inflammatory and immune responses.

Neurogenic mechanisms

Maurice Raynaud believed that hyper-reactivity of the parasympathetic nervous system caused an increase in vasoconstrictor response to cold. The α-adrenergic receptor and β-presynaptic receptor sensitivity, density, or both, are increased in Raynaud's phenomenon. However, the endothelium possesses at least five different adrenoceptor subtypes ($\alpha 2A/D$, $\alpha 2C$, $\beta 1$, $\beta 2$ and $\beta 3$), which either directly or through the release of nitric oxide, actively participate in the regulation of vascular tone. The central sympathetic system has some role in the pathogenesis of Raynaud's phenomenon, as indicated by the fact that local vibration of one hand induces vasoconstriction of the other, which is abolished by proximal nerve blockade.

In patients with systemic sclerosis, of whom 90% have Raynaud's phenomenon, it has been demonstrated that there is a high incidence of peripheral neuropathy, which supports the neurogenic mechanism for Raynaud's phenomenon. The involvement of nerve terminals reduces the vasodilatory endothelial-dependent or -independent potential of the neuropeptides released by sensory nerve endings. It has also been found that Raynaud's phenomenon is significantly more common in patients with carpal tunnel syndrome, and this could be explained by the presence of autonomic dysfunction, which is evident by swelling of the fingers and dry palms, in addition to the Raynaud's phenomenon.

However, other work does not support the neurogenic concept. Infusions of α- and β-adrenergic agonists in patients with Raynaud's phenomenon do not produce any abnormalities in their response to reflex cooling or indirect heating. Thus, although abnormalities in the nervous system may exist, they are, at present, not clearly defined.

Blood and blood vessel wall interactions

The most important cellular element in Raynaud's phenomenon is the endothelium, which is a functioning organ releasing important mediators, such as prostacyclin (PGI_2), which is a potent antiplatelet agent and vasodilator. It has been found that there are abnormal endothelial responses to both endothelium-dependent and endothelium-independent induced vasodilatation in patients with Raynaud's phenomenon; however, in patients with Raynaud's syndrome secondary to systemic sclerosis, this abnormality is limited to the endothelium-dependent vasodilatation. Here it seems that the disease, perhaps through the injury to the endothelium, jeopardizes the endothelium-dependent vascular control. A reduction in nitric oxide, one of the main endothelial vasodilators, is also involved in the genesis of Raynaud's phenomenon in these patients. It could also be extrapolated from different studies that, in patients with Raynaud's phenomenon, there is possibly a decrease in the synthesis of nitric oxide, rather than impaired sensitivity to it, which could be an important factor in the pathogenesis of Raynaud's phenomenon and may have therapeutic value in the future.

The damaged endothelium in Raynaud's phenomenon can also release factor VIII von Willebrand factor antigen, which can have a prothrombotic effect. Another manifestation of endothelial dysfunction is a defect in the lysis of fibrin. Concentrations of endothelin, another endothelial product that causes vasoconstriction, are increased in Raynaud's phenomenon.

Other blood cellular elements may have a pathological role in Raynaud's phenomenon. The platelets exhibit greater aggregation, releasing increased amounts of the vasoconstrictor and platelet aggregant, thromboxane A_2, and other platelet-release products. The red blood cell appears to be more stiff and rigid, and thus can occlude the microcirculation. An important role has also been claimed for the white blood cell which, when activated, releases prothrombotic free radicals and increases cell aggregation, leading to more reduction in blood flow. Some of the above changes are likely to be a consequence of the Raynaud's phenomenon, rather than a cause, but they may augment the symptoms of vasospasm and their attenuation is a potentially important feature in the drug management of Raynaud's phenomenon.

Abnormalities of the inflammatory and immune responses

Disordered immune and inflammatory processes occur in the majority of severe cases of Raynaud's phenomenon via their association with the connective tissue disorders, but also in HAVS, which has no clear immune/inflammatory basis. Tumor necrosis factor and lymphotoxin, phagocyte/macrophage and T cell derived proteins, along with immune complex deposition in the vessel wall, are likely to be activated in vascular damage seen in Raynaud's phenomenon.

It seems that a combination of the above factors will be involved in the development and propagation of Raynaud's phenomenon.

CLINICAL FEATURES

Detailed history and examination are essential in making the diagnosis, in finding any associated underlying causes, in assessing the likelihood of progression to connective tissue disorder, and in deciding about the most appropriate management plan. A detailed occupational history, particularly in men, allows a diagnosis of HAVS to be made. Drug history is equally important, and it should be noted that even the cardioselective β-blockers produce a degree of peripheral vasoconstriction

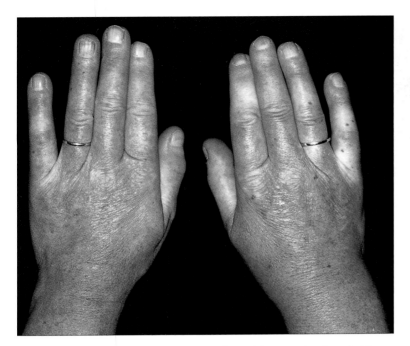

Fig. 36.1 Raynaud's phenomenon in a patient with systemic sclerosis. The white discoloration is an essential clinical finding in Raynaud's phenomenon. The asymmetric involvement and the presence of telangiectasia point to a possibility of a secondary cause for the Raynaud's phenomenon. Digital pitting scarring is one of the main criteria for the diagnosis of systemic sclerosis.

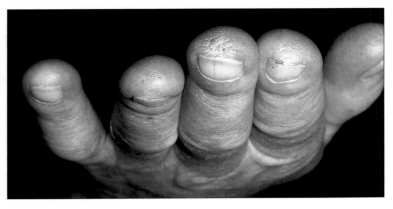

Fig. 36.2 Digital pitting, scarring and sclerodactyly commonly associated with systemic sclerosis. These lesions form two of the three main criteria for systemic sclerosis; the third criterion is pulmonary interstitial fibrosis. A diagnosis of systemic sclerosis requires two of these three findings.

(Table 36.1). Use of the newer vasodilating β-blockers is probably more appropriate in these patients, especially when β-blockade is necessary.

Raynaud's phenomenon is classically manifested by blanching of the affected part (pallor), reflecting vasospasm (Fig. 36.1), followed by cyanosis and then rubor; however, this typical triphasic color change is not necessarily present in all patients. Symptoms associated with Raynaud's phenomenon include numbness, cold and pain, which are secondary to ischemia, which can be severe enough to result in digital ulceration, gangrene and loss of digits. During the reactive hyperemic stage, patients usually experience an unpleasant burning sensation and sweating of the affected parts. The most severely affected patient may experience marked, year-round restrictions in their daily activity. The predictors for the attack rate, severity and pain are the average daily temperature, stress, anxiety, age and sex.

The occurrence of certain clinical features may suggest a greater likelihood of disease progression to connective tissue disorder (Table 36.2). This is important, as we know that, in up to 50% of patients referred to hospital, Raynaud's phenomenon could progress to connective tissue disorder. For instance, sclerodactyly and pitting scars over the finger pulp are associated with later development of connective tissue disorder (Fig. 36.2).

Patients presenting for the first time in their third and fourth decade are at high risk of developing connective tissue disorders, and Raynaud's phenomenon occurring in very young children, although rare, is usually due to an underlying connective tissue disorders. If Raynaud's phenomenon precedes the connective tissue disorder by years, in those who develop systemic sclerosis, the limited form of the disease is more likely to become apparent. Systemic enquiry should concentrate on the presence of migraine (or a family history of migraine), esophageal problems and the presence of vasospastic angina[2].

A full physical examination should be directed to look for any obstructive vascular disease and for signs of associated autoimmune conditions. Simple blood pressure measurement in both arms will help to detect significant occlusive vascular disease above the brachial artery. Looking for evidence of pulmonary hypertension is also important, to point to possible involvement of the pulmonary vascular system. Livedo reticularis could point to cold agglutinin disease or underlying connective tissue disorder. Patients with abnormal nailfold microscopy are more likely to progress to a connective tissue disorder. Patients should also be examined carefully for evidence of carpal tunnel syndrome, as 60% of these patients also have Raynaud's phenomenon.

INVESTIGATIONS

Investigations in patients with Raynaud's phenomenon have three functions: first to confirm the diagnosis of Raynaud's phenomenon, secondly to assess possible disease progression, and thirdly to look for underlying secondary causes or associated conditions[3].

Diagnosis of Raynaud's phenomenon

In the majority of cases the diagnosis of Raynaud's phenomenon can be made from the clinical history. Digital blanching on exposure to cold

TABLE 36.2 FEATURES SUGGESTIVE OF PROGRESSION OF RAYNAUD'S PHENOMENON
Clinical
• Older age at onset (>35 years)
• Recurrence of chilblains as adult
• Vasospasm all year round
• Asymmetric attacks (Fig. 36.1)
• Sclerodactyly
• Digital ulceration
• Finger pulp pitting scars
Laboratory
• Increased inflammatory markers
• Detection of autoantibodies
• Increased von Willebrand factor antigen
Nailfold microscopy
• Abnormal vessels

469

with or without cyanosis or rubor in the absence of clinical evidence of obstructive vascular disease allows the diagnosis of Raynaud's phenomenon to be made. However, in rare situations when the patient is unable to give a clear history, in the presence of occlusive vascular disease when the contribution of vasospasm to the clinical problem needs to be determined, or for medicolegal reasons in HAVS, objective measures of blood flow are needed.

There are many different techniques that can be used to measure blood flow to the digits. However, in clinical practice, measurement of digital systolic blood pressure before and after local cooling of the hands in cool water at a temperature of approximately 15°C is widely used because of its simplicity. A decrease in pressure greater than 30mmHg is usually significant. This technique, however, will give a significant number of false-negative responses unless certain precautions are observed[4]. First, the patient must be warm before the first pressure recordings and, ideally, the starting digital pressure must be as near brachial pressure as can be achieved. Unfortunately, many patients who have cold hands at the start of the tests have been told that they did not have Raynaud's phenomenon when no further pressure decrease was detected after cold challenge. Conversely, on hot days the body itself is too warm, and this will prevent digital vasospasm if digital cooling is used in isolation. Secondly, in premenopausal women, assessment should be avoided in mid-cycle, as poor blood flow before the start of the test can also occur at the time of ovulation. Thirdly, all vasoactive medication should be stopped 24h before the test, as drug-induced vasodilatation can also lead to failure to detect a pressure decrease. For the same reason, the test should be avoided when the patient is in the reactive hyperemic phase. Ideally, patients should not have had a vasospastic attack on the day of the test.

Thermography, radioisotopic clearance and laser Doppler flometry are other methods used to help in the diagnosis of Raynaud's phenomenon. However, these methods have their disadvantages and usually are unnecessary.

Investigations for secondary causes

More than 50% of patients with Raynaud's phenomenon who are referred to hospital will have an associated underlying disease; therefore, once diagnosis of Raynaud's phenomenon is confirmed, it is essential to look carefully for any underlying cause. More importantly, early intervention in these patients could resolve the problem, such as in patients with vibration exposure or those who take vasospastic drugs. Those with an obvious associated disorder will be easily detected, but difficulty arises in diagnosing early connective tissue disorders. Earlier studies had found that progression to connective tissue disorder occurred in 24–50% of patients with Raynaud's phenomenon. However, more recent studies showed that as many as 46–81% of cases of Raynaud's phenomenon have been found to have some underlying secondary condition.

Blood biochemistry, including thyroid function test and full blood count should be carried out. A normochromic, normocytic or microcytic anemia of chronic disease can be found in patients with connective tissue disorders. The inflammatory markers such as erythrocyte sedimentation rate, plasma viscosity or C-reactive protein are usually normal in primary Raynaud's phenomenon, but they may be increased in secondary Raynaud's phenomenon. It should be noted, however, that there might be some impairment of the acute-phase response in patients with systemic sclerosis. Urine analysis will help in detecting early renal disease in patients with connective tissue disorders or diabetes. A chest X-ray will determine whether a bony cervical rib is present, and will show if there is any basal lung fibrosis, which may be seen early in connective tissue disorders. A median nerve conduction study is important in detecting carpal tunnel syndrome when symptoms warrant this.

Immunologic tests will help to detect the immune pathologic origin of the secondary Raynaud's phenomenon. Rheumatoid factor will help in

detection of early rheumatoid arthritis, antinuclear antibody and anti-DNA antibodies in systemic lupus erythematosus, anticentromere antibodies for limited systemic sclerosis, and antitopoisomerase antibody (formerly known as scleroderma 70 antibody) for diffuse systemic sclerosis. Anti-La and anti-Ro antibodies may suggest the diagnosis of Sjögren's syndrome. The presence of these antibodies early on in the history of Raynaud's phenomenon suggests that later progression to connective tissue disorder will occur. Increased von Willebrand factor antigen tends to be seen in patients with the secondary Raynaud's phenomenon. Detection of cold-precipitated proteins will help in the diagnosis of cryoglobulinemia and cryofibrinogenemia. Nailfold microscopy may also help to point to Raynaud's phenomenon of rheumatologic origin, especially when associated with positive serum antibodies.

MANAGEMENT

Not all patients experiencing digital vasospasm require drug treatment. The obvious clinical need for medication in patients with digital gangrene and ulceration does not need to be emphasized, but potential prescribers should also be aware that the severity of the pain produced by vasospastic attack and the degree of interruption that a patient may experience in her or his normal daily routine may be profound, and drug treatment should be instituted in these patients.

General measures

Initial treatment in mild disease is conservative, and drug treatment may be avoided. Patients with Raynaud's phenomenon may be apprehensive about their condition and education is important. From our experience, a specialist rheumatology nurse and occupational therapists can provide useful help for the Raynaud's sufferer. It is important to advise patients on protecting themselves from the cold. Electrically heated gloves and socks and chemical hand warmers are the perfect solution for some patients.

Stopping smoking (including exposure to passive smoking) is beneficial. In the case of HAVS, early diagnosis and early discontinuation of vibration exposure resolve the problem. Withdrawal of vasoconstrictor drugs is essential. Although the contraceptive pill has been linked anecdotally to the development of Raynaud's phenomenon, this has never been conclusively proven in epidemiological studies. It is our policy not to discontinue the contraceptive pill or hormone replacement therapy unless it is clearly related to the patient's Raynaud's phenomenon.

In the management of digital ulceration in patients with severe Raynaud's phenomenon, it is essential to treat any infection as soon as possible, and aggressively. Significant infection can be present even in the absence of increased inflammatory markers, formal erythema and pus formation.

Drug treatment of Raynaud's phenomenon

Patients in whom symptoms are severe enough to cause interference with either their social or work lifestyle should be offered drug treatment (Table 36.3).

Calcium channel blockers

Nifedipine has now become the gold standard of Raynaud's treatment. Its mechanism of action is predominantly through vasodilation, but it also has antiplatelet and possibly other antithrombotic effects. The dose in treating Raynaud's phenomenon ranges from 10mg to 20mg two or three times daily, which should be introduced very gradually – for example, 10mg at night for 2 weeks, then twice a day, etc. It has been found to be useful in decreasing the frequency and severity of vasospastic attacks, and improves the objective measures of blood flow after cold exposure. Furthermore, nifedipine is a good alternative to a β-blocker for patients with concomitant hypertension and migraine. Its use, however, is limited by the vasodilatory side effects to which the Raynaud's phenomenon patients appear very susceptible. These effects usually disappear with continued treatment and so, unless they are intolerable, the patient should persevere for at least 2 weeks before a decision is made to discontinue the treatment. The use of the controlled-release preparation is better tolerated than nifedipine itself. If side effects necessitate discontinuation of the treatment, two options are possible. The first is to try another calcium channel antagonist with less vasodilatory effect, such as diltiazem and isradipine. The second option is to use nifedipine capsule (not the Retard tablet) as a rescue medication during a severe spastic attack, the capsule being crushed by the teeth and placed below the tongue.

Other vasodilators

The use of other vasodilators in patients with Raynaud's phenomenon remains controversial, as most studies have been small or uncontrolled. The use of inositol nicotinate and naftidrofuryl has produced encouraging results in mild to moderate Raynaud's phenomenon. Another role of these medications is to use them as adjuncts to calcium channel blockade when adverse effects from calcium antagonists prevent the achievement of high dosage. These drugs may take up to 3 months to produce their effects, suggesting that their action in Raynaud's phenomenon may be through other mechanisms.

Losartan, the angiotensin II receptor antagonist, has been shown in a randomized controlled trial[5] to be effective in treating Raynaud's phenomenon. In a meta-analysis[6], prazosin, an α-blocker, was found to have modest effects. Accordingly, these medications should be considered for those with concomitant hypertension, or as an extra option in those who cannot tolerate the calcium channel blockers. More recently, a pilot study[7] showed that fluoxetine, a selective serotinin reuptake inhibitor, was found to be effective in treating Raynaud's phenomenon.

Prostaglandin treatment

Prostaglandins are the metabolic products of essential fatty acids and both prostacyclin (PGI_2) and alprostadil (PGE_1) have potent vasodilatory and antiplatelet properties. Treatments with both PGI_2 and PGE_1, however, require intravenous administration and are very unstable. Thus the use of a more stable analog such as iloprost has been evaluated in a number of studies[8–10].

Iloprost

A number of double-blind placebo controlled studies of iloprost infusion given intravenously have shown benefit in Raynaud's phenomenon[11,12]. In addition to its vasodilatory and antiplatelets effects, iloprost has been shown to downregulate lymphocyte adhesion to the endothelium[13]. When compared with nifedipine, it was found to have the same effect on reducing the frequency of the vasospastic attacks, but was more effective in healing digital ulcers and appeared to produce fewer adverse effects. Accordingly, iloprost is the second-choice treatment for patients with severe Raynaud's phenomenon who have not responded to nifedipine, and the first choice for those who have critical ischemia or digital ulceration, or both. It can be infused through a peripheral vein, and can produce benefit lasting for between 6 weeks and 6 months in most patients.

Alprostadil

A recent study confirmed the efficacy of PGE_1 (alprostadil) in the management of Raynaud's phenomenon secondary to systemic sclerosis. Accordingly, alprostadil could be used in patients who have significant side effects and cannot tolerate iloprost infusion. The effectiveness of using $PGE_1\alpha$–cyclodextrin infusions prophylactically to cover the winter has been proved by a recent study[11].

Oral and transdermal prostaglandins

Studies of orally active prostacyclin analogs have given conflicting results. Cicaprost proved disappointing, whereas oral iloprost has shown clinical benefit in some studies, but this was not confirmed in others[14–17]. A pilot study of oral limaprost, an alprostadil analog, was encouraging[18]. Prostaglandin delivery through the skin has also been studied, but to date no transdermally applied prostaglandin has obtained a license for use in Raynaud's phenomenon.

Role of surgery

Operations to remove part of the terminal phalanx and, occasionally, amputation is necessary for severe ischemia, but this is becoming increasingly infrequent. Patients with peripheral arterial disease and Raynaud's phenomenon of the toes may gain benefit from endovascular intervention. In patients with Raynaud's phenomenon secondary to carpel tunnel syndrome, surgical decompression of the carpal tunnel has been shown to improve the Raynaud's phenomenon symptoms significantly.

Conventional upper limb sympathectomy gives a high relapse rate and poor response in patients with Raynaud's syndrome. However, recent studies show that videoscopic sympathectomy may be successful in a number of patients, despite some untoward effects and partial relapses. Localized digital sympathectomy enjoyed some support initially, as earlier results were encouraging; however, further work is required in this area. Although modified upper limb sympathectomy requires further study, sympathectomy still has an important role in the treatment of Raynaud's phenomenon affecting the feet.

CONCLUSION

Raynaud's phenomenon is a common condition and, until recently, its management was difficult. However, with a careful clinical history and examination and with selection of specific investigations, it is now possible to diagnose correctly both Raynaud's phenomenon and its underlying or associated conditions. When it occurs as a primary phenomenon, it is usually mild, with symmetric involvement and no laboratory

TABLE 36.3 DRUGS COMMONLY USED IN RAYNAUD'S PHENOMENON

Drug	Dosage
Oral	
Nifedipine Retard (or other calcium-channel blocker)	10–20mg two or three times a day
Naftidrofuryl	100–200mg three times a day
Inositol nicotinate	500mg three times, or inositol nicotinate forte 750mg twice a day
Thymoxamine	40–80mg four times a day (initial 2 week trial)
Gamolenic acid	12 capsules a day (3 month trial)
Omega-3 marine triglycerides	10 capsules a day (3 month trial)
Losartan	50mg a day
Fluoxetine	20mg a day
Intravenous infusion	
Iloprost	Start infusion (peripheral line) at 1μg/h, increase by 1μg every 30min until reach maximum tolerable dose (maximum dose should not be greater than 3μg/h) given over 6h each day over 3–7 days on each occasion
Prostaglandin E1	60μg in 250ml physiological infusion over 3h daily for 5–6 days. This could be repeated every 6 weeks to cover the cold weather in severe cases, specially if associated with critical ischemia or digital ulceration

abnormalities, and often needs no drug treatment. Features suggesting secondary Raynaud's syndrome include painful attacks, ischemic digital ulcers, asymmetric attacks, a positive autoantibody test result, and increased inflammatory markers. Vasodilatory treatment is the mainstay of medical management, and calcium channel blockers are usually the drugs of choice. Surgical treatment nowadays is very rarely needed. Lastly, the better evaluation and understanding of the pathophysiology of Raynaud's phenomenon and increasing knowledge on the involvement of vascular adrenoceptors in the condition will contribute to new and better therapeutic approaches. The future of oral and transdermal vasodilators, including prostaglandin analogs, and improvement in the delivery systems still need further study.

ACKNOWLEDGMENT

Professor J J F Belch receives funding from the Raynaud's and Scleroderma Association, UK.

REFERENCES

1. Cooke ED, Nicolaides AN, Porter JM. Raynaud's syndrome. London: Med-Orion Publishing Company; 1991.
2. Belch JJF. Temperature related disorders. In: Tooke J, Lowe GDO, eds. Textbook of vascular medicine. London: Edward Arnold; 1995: 329–352.
3. Bolster MB, Maricq HR, Leff RL. Office evaluation and treatment of Raynaud's phenomenon. Cleve Clin J Med 1995; 62: 51–61.
4. Belch JJF, Zurier RB. Connective tissue diseases, 1E. London: Chapman and Hall Medical; 1995.
5. Dziadzio M, Denton CP, Smith R et al. Losartan therapy for Raynaud's phenomenon and scleroderma: clinical and biochemical findings in a fifteen-week, randomized, parallel-group, controlled trial. Arthritis Rheum 1999; 42: 2646–2655.
6. Pope J, Fenlon D, Thompson A et al. Prazosin for Raynaud's phenomenon in progressive systemic sclerosis. (Cochrane Review). In: The Cochrane Library, Issue 3, 2001. Oxford: Update Software.
7. Coleiro B, Marshall SE, Denton CP et al. Treatment of Raynaud's phenomenon with the selective serotonin reuptake inhibitor fluoxetine. Rheumatology 2001; 40: 1038–1043.
8. Belch JJF, Greer IA, McLaren M et al. The effects of intravenous infusion of ZK36374, a synthetic prostacyclin derivative, on normal volunteers. Prostaglandins 1984; 28: 67–78.
9. Martin MFR, Dowd PM, Ring EFJ et al. Prostaglandin E$_1$ infusions for vascular insufficiency in progressive systemic sclerosis. Ann Rheum Dis 1981; 40: 350–354.
10. Belch JJF, Drury JK, Capell H et al. Intermittent epoprostenol (prostacyclin) infusion in patients with Raynaud's syndrome – a double-blind controlled trial. Lancet 1983; I: 313–315.
11. Rademaker M, Thomas RHM, Provost G et al. Prolonged increase in digital blood flow following iloprost infusion in patients with systemic sclerosis. Postgrad Med J 1987; 63: 617–620.
12. Wigley FM, Wise RA, Seibold JR et al. Intravenous iloprost infusion in patients with Raynaud phenomenon secondary to systemic sclerosis. Ann Intern Med 1994; 120: 199–206.
13. Della Bella S, Molteni M, Mocellin C et al. Novel mode of action of iloprost: in vitro down-regulation of endothelial cell adhesion molecules. Prostaglandins Other Lipid Mediat 2001; 65: 73–83.
14. Gardinali M, Pozzi MR, Bernareggi M et al. Treatment of Raynaud's phenomenon with intravenous prostaglandin E1alpha-cyclodextrin improves endothelial cell injury in systemic sclerosis. J Rheumatol 2001; 28: 786–794.
15. Lau CS, McLaren M, Saniabadi A et al. The pharmacological effects of cicaprost, an oral prostacyclin analogue, in patients with Raynaud's syndrome secondary to systemic sclerosis – a preliminary study. Clin Exp Rheumatol 1991; 9: 271–273.
16. Pope J, Fenlon D, Thompson A et al. Iloprost and cisaprost for Raynaud's phenomenon in progressive systemic sclerosis. (Cochrane Review). In: The Cochrane Library, Issue 3, 2001. Oxford: Update Software.
17. Belch JJF, Capell HA, Cooke ED et al. Oral iloprost as a treatment for Raynaud's syndrome: a double-blind multi-centre placebo controlled study. Ann Rheum Dis 1995; 54: 197–200.
18. Murai C, Sasaki T, Osaki H et al. Oral limaprost for Raynaud's phenomenon. Lancet 1989; I: 1218.

37 Inflammatory muscle disease: clinical features

Chester V Oddis and Thomas A Medsger Jr

Definition

- Characterized by chronic inflammation of striated muscle (myositis), distinguishable cutaneous features (rash of dermatomyositis), and a variety of systemic complications
- Cellular and humoral immunologic features including serum autoantibodies that are associated with clinical syndromes with myositis as a major manifestation
- A member of the connective tissue disease family, as indicated by other autoimmune disease associations

Clinical and laboratory features

- Painless symmetric proximal muscle weakness with or without rash
- Increase in serum muscle enzymes, most notably creatine kinase
- Abnormal electromyogram and biopsy showing myositis
- Involvement of other organ systems including the lung, heart, gastrointestinal tract and joints
- Association of dermatomyositis with malignancy in middle-aged and elderly population

HISTORY

The characteristic 'heliotrope' rash of dermatomyositis was recognized before the disease itself in 1875, in a 17-year-old waiter in Paris, France, who presented with fatigue, pain in the extremities and erythema of the eyelids[1]. Eleven years later, in 1886, Wagner coined the term 'polymyositis' to describe a woman presenting with muscle weakness and diffuse muscle and joint pain who developed swelling of the extremities and forearm erythema[2]. In 1888, the first American case of polymyositis documented by muscle biopsy was reported in New York[3]. Because trichinosis was common at that time and could cause periorbital edema and diffuse myalgias, it was necessary that polymyositis or dermatomyositis be a diagnosis of exclusion, requiring an incompatible dietary history and a muscle biopsy lacking *Trichinella spiralis* cysts. In 1891, Unverricht described a 39-year-old pregnant woman with facial erythema and tense, swollen and erythematous legs and thighs, who later delivered a healthy infant. She subsequently developed myalgias with muscle weakness and atrophy and Unverricht introduced the term 'dermatomyositis' to describe her condition[4]. In 1930, Gottron reported on the skin lesions of dermatomyositis that bear his name, describing 'rounded foci of tense atrophy over carpo-metacarpal joints'[5]. The first published cases of dermatomyositis associated with carcinoma were independently reported in 1916[6,7], but Beczeny, a Prague dermatologist, suggested a more definitive relationship between dermatomyositis and cancer in 1935[8]. More recently, in 1967, the pathology of inclusion body myositis was described[9], and it was named a short time later, in 1971[10].

EPIDEMIOLOGY

Classification criteria

The purposes of disease classification are to separate the disease of interest from others in order to determine incidence and prevalence, to describe the occurrence of disease in large populations, to compare one patient group with others, and to identify clinically homogeneous subsets of patients. Classification facilitates clinical studies of natural history and response to treatment, in addition to laboratory investigations of pathogenesis and etiology. With no knowledge of cause, and with inadequate understanding of pathogenesis, classifications are necessarily preliminary and must ultimately be revised as appropriate. Classification criteria differ from diagnostic criteria, which pertain to confirming the suspected diagnosis in individual cases[11].

In polymyositis–dermatomyositis, many classification systems have been proposed. For purposes of defining patient groups for clinical research and to aid in the diagnosis of the individual patient, the 1975 Bohan and Peter criteria have served extremely well for more than two decades (Table 37.1)[12]. The essential elements are proximal muscle weakness on physical examination, increased serum muscle enzymes, abnormal electromyogram (EMG), muscle biopsy consistent with myositis and the characteristic rash of dermatomyositis. Definite, probable (most likely diagnosis) and possible (consistent with) disease have been defined. The sensitivity of the Bohan and Peter criteria in a number of

---

TABLE 37. 1 BOHAN AND PETER CRITERIA FOR DIAGNOSIS OF POLYMYOSITIS AND DERMATOMYOSITIS

Individual criteria

1. Symmetric proximal muscle weakness
2. Muscle biopsy evidence of myositis
3. Increase in serum skeletal muscle enzymes
4. Characteristic electromyographic pattern
5. Typical rash of dermatomyositis

Diagnostic criteria

Polymyositis:
Definite:	all of 1–4
Probable:	any 3 of 1–4
Possible:	any 2 of 1–4

Dermatomyositis:
Definite:	5 plus any 3 of 1–4
Probable:	5 plus any 2 of 1–4
Possible:	5 plus any 1 of 1–4

(Modified with permission from Bohan and Peter[12].)

TABLE 37.2 INCIDENCE RATES OF POLYMYOSITIS–DERMATOMYOSITIS IN DIFFERENT POPULATIONS

Source	Geographic area	Inclusive dates of study	Annual incidence (per million)	Pertinent features
Rose and Walton (1966)[26]	Northeast England	1954–1964	2.25	
Kurland et al. (1969)[27]	Rochester, MN, USA	1951–1967	6.0	Almost exclusively white population
Findlay et al. (1969)[28]	Transvaal, South Africa	1960–1967	7.5	Includes dermatomyositis only
Medsger et al. (1970)[29]	Memphis and Shelby County, TN, USA	1947–1968	5.0	Hospital-diagnosed cases only; 40% population was African-American
Benbassat et al. (1980)[30]	Israel	1960–1976	2.2	Hospital diagnosed cases only; Bohan and Peter criteria used for diagnosis
Oddis et al. (1990)[31]	Allegheny County, PA, USA	1963–1982	5.5	Hospital diagnosed cases only; predominantly white population (91%); incidence rate 10.2 million during 1978–1982
Weitoft (1997)[32]	Gälveborg, County, Sweden	1984–1993	7.6	Medical center records and biopsy sources
Patrick et al. (1999)[33]	Victoria, Australia	1989–1991	7.4	Hospital diagnosis and muscle biopsy sources

published studies averaged 70% for definite and 20% for probable myositis. Most probable and possible cases result, not from uncertainty about diagnosis, but instead because one or more of the diagnostic laboratory tests (enzymes, EMG, biopsy) were not performed. The specificity of the Bohan and Peter criteria against 436 patients with systemic lupus erythematosus (SLE) or systemic sclerosis combined was 93%[13]. The addition of myositis-specific serum autoantibodies and magnetic resonance imaging (MRI) to supplement the Bohan and Peter criteria has been recently proposed[14,15]. None of the classification systems mention inclusion body myositis, a more recently recognized entity with distinctive clinical and pathologic features, or amyopathic dermatomyositis, in which patients have the rash of dermatomyositis but no overt muscle weakness.

Association with other disorders

Polymyositis–dermatomyositis frequently occurs in overlap with systemic sclerosis, usually associated with one of several serum autoantibodies, including anti-U1-RNP, anti-PM-Scl or anti-U3-RNP[16,17]. Myositis has been described complicating rheumatoid arthritis[18], SLE[19], Sjögren's syndrome[20], Churg–Strauss vasculitis[21], localized forms of scleroderma[22,23], thrombotic thrombocytopenic purpura[24] and antiphospholipid antibody syndrome[25].

Incidence by age, race and sex

The reported overall annual incidence of polymyositis–dermatomyositis ranges from 2 to 10 new cases per million persons at risk in various populations (Table 37.2)[26–33]. These rates are likely to be underestimates, because not all possible sources of ascertainment were examined. For example, in most instances only hospital-diagnosed cases were sought, and patients with potential misdiagnoses (e.g. muscular dystrophy) were not reviewed. There is a trend towards increasing incidence in several communities over time[29,31], probably because of increased physician awareness, rather than a true increase in disease occurrence. A

nationwide study of inclusion body myositis in The Netherlands revealed a prevalence of 4.9 cases/million per year[34].

Although inflammatory myopathy can occur at any age, the observed pattern of incidence includes childhood and adult peaks and a paucity of patients with onset in the adolescent and young adult years[29,31]. This finding supports the concept of separating childhood from adult forms of the disease. As expected, the mean age of myositis onset is increased when there is an associated malignancy. The overall female:male incidence ratio is 2.5:1. This ratio is lower (nearly 1:1) in childhood disease and with associated malignancy, but is very high (10:1) when there is a coexisting connective tissue disease. Polymyositis–dermatomyositis has a 3–4:1 Afro-American to white ratio of incidence. There is a younger adult-onset peak among Afro-Americans, which is also true of SLE and systemic sclerosis.

The epidemiologic characteristics of the commonly recognized classification subsets are summarized in Table 37.3.

Environmental factors

No striking associations with environmental factors have been identified. Spatial clustering was found in one series[33], but neither spatial nor temporal clustering was detected in another[29]. The relative prevalence of polymyositis–dermatomyositis in Europe increases significantly (sevenfold) with latitude, from the north (Iceland) to the south (Greece), which could have either an environmental or a genetic explanation[35].

Disease onset is more frequent in the winter and spring months, especially in childhood cases, consistent with precipitation by viral and bacterial infections[29]. Serum antibodies to Coxsackie B viruses are more frequent in patients with dermatomyositis in childhood compared with controls with juvenile rheumatoid arthritis[36]. A patient with dermatomyositis and Lyme disease had *Borrelia burgdorferi* organisms detected in his dermatomyositis skin and muscle lesions[37]. Human T cell leukemia/lymphoma virus type-1 infection has been associated with polymyositis, including the identification of viral particles in affected

TABLE 37.3 EPIDEMIOLOGIC CHARACTERISTICS OF POLYMYOSITIS–DERMATOMYOSITIS CLINICAL CLASSIFICATION SUBSETS

	Adult polymyositis	Adult dermatomyositis	Childhood myositis	Myositis/connective tissue disease overlap	Myositis with malignancy	Inclusion body myositis	All patients
Proportion of all patients (%)	50	20	10	10	10	<5	
Mean age at diagnosis (years)	45	40	10	35	60	>65	45
Incidence sex ratio (F:M)	2:1	2:1	1:1	10:1	1:1	1:2	2.5:1
Incidence race ratio (B:W)	5:1	3:1	1:1	3:1	2:1	Unknown	3:1

B:W, black: white; F:M, female:male.

skeletal muscle[38]. Dermatomyositis has occurred in an individual infected with human immunodeficiency virus[39], and polymyositis caused by both a muspiceoid nematode[40] and mycoplasma pneumoniae infection[41] have been reported. In one study, patients with polymyositis–dermatomyositis reported excessive physical exercise and emotional stress antedating the onset of their illness significantly more frequently than did sex-matched unaffected sibling controls[42], but these associations have not been confirmed. Drug-induced myositis occurs with D-penicillamine[43] and the statin agents (see below, section on Drug-induced Myopathy). Despite many case reports, an association between polymyositis–dermatomyositis and bovine collagen injections has not been found in epidemiologic studies[42,44].

Genetic factors

The occurrence of polymyositis–dermatomyositis in monozygotic twins[45] and first-degree relatives of cases[46,47] supports a genetic predisposition, at least in some families. Homozygosity at the human leukocyte antigen *HLA-DQA1* locus has been shown to be associated with familial inflammatory myopathy[48]. Other autoimmune diseases occur four times more frequently in first-degree relatives of patients with polymyositis–dermatomyositis (21.9%) than in first-degree relatives of control probands (4.9%)[49].

The genetics of polymyositis–dermatomyositis has recently been reviewed[50]. Juvenile dermatomyositis has been found to be associated with *HLA-DQA1*0501*[51]. The closely linked *DRB1*0301* allele is also a risk factor for polymyositis–dermatomyositis in white populations[52]. Different *HLA* alleles appear to be important in either conferring risk for or protection from myositis in distinct ethnic, serologic and environmental exposure groups. Certain non-*HLA* genetic risk factors, such as genes regulating cytokines and their receptors – for example, interleukin (IL)-1[53] and tumor necrosis factor α[54] – appear to have a role in the development of myositis.

PRESENTATION

At presentation, the different clinical syndromes vary considerably from patient to patient (Table 37.4). The most frequent problem is insidious, progressive painless symmetric proximal muscle weakness over the course of 3–6 months before the first visit to a physician. Some patients, especially children and young adults with dermatomyositis, have a more acute onset of disease, with muscle pain and weakness developing rapidly over the course of several weeks. In the latter case, constitutional features such as fever and fatigue are more common. A few patients complain only of proximal myalgias. There is also a subset of patients with very slowly evolving weakness over the course of 1–10 years before diagnosis; they are typically older men with weakness of the pelvic girdle and muscles of the distal extremities who have pathologic features of inclusion body myositis on muscle biopsy.

Other presenting features may be attributable to muscle weakness. Several such findings, each occurring in approximately 5% of patients,

TABLE 37.4 TYPES AND FREQUENCIES OF PRESENTING CLINICAL SYNDROMES IN POLYMYOSITIS–DERMATOMYOSITIS

Syndrome	Estimated frequency (%)
Painless proximal weakness (over 3–6 months)	55
Acute or subacute proximal pain and weakness (over weeks to 2 months)	30
Insidious proximal and distal weakness (over 1–10 years)	10
Proximal myalgia alone	5
Dermatomyositis rash alone; extremity edema	<1

are pitting edema of the extremities as a result of lack of muscle tone needed to promote central venous return, hoarseness or dysphagia as a result of bulbar muscle weakness, nasal regurgitation of liquids or aspiration pneumonia, also because of pharyngeal dysphagia, and dyspnea resulting from either ventilatory muscle weakness or interstitial lung disease (ILD).

Presenting features often 'cluster' together, resulting in distinct clinical syndromes. For example, patients with serum anti-aminoacyl tRNA synthetase antibodies such as anti-Jo-1 antibody often have a constellation of findings, including fever, polyarthritis and ILD, in addition to myositis. When polymyositis or dermatomyositis overlap with another connective tissue disease, certain combinations of features tend to occur. When the overlap is with systemic sclerosis, one often finds Raynaud's phenomenon, puffy fingers, sclerodactyly and distal esophageal (smooth muscle) hypomotility. Lupus overlap features include photosensitive and malar rash, alopecia, polyarthralgias, pleurisy and leukopenia. These syndromes are discussed in greater detail below (see section on Clinical Features).

Finally, certain presenting manifestations tend to be mutually exclusive, depending on the patient subset. Of particular note are the rarity of Raynaud's phenomenon and arthralgias in pure (non-synthetase) polymyositis, the absence of calcinosis except in dermatomyositis (typically a late finding) and the unusual condition termed 'amyopathic dermatomyositis' in which the typical dermatomyositis skin rash occurs without objective evidence of myopathy.

CLINICAL FEATURES

Constitutional

Fatigue is a prominent complaint in patients with polymyositis–dermatomyositis and may persist well after adequate treatment with corticosteroids or other immunosuppressive agents. Fever is more commonly observed with childhood dermatomyositis, but adults with the antisynthetase syndrome may have fever accompanying or heralding active disease. Weight loss may occur with any systemic illness, but if it is persistent and severe in a myositis patient, malignancy should be considered. Weight loss also may result from poor caloric intake associated with pharyngeal striated muscle dysfunction or esophageal dysmotility.

Skeletal muscle

Patients complain of difficulty in performing activities requiring normal upper or lower limb strength. Involvement is insidious, bilateral, symmetric, usually painless and proximal greater than distal. An exception is inclusion body myositis, in which asymmetric distal weakness and atrophy are prominent, often accompanied by similar proximal muscle findings. In polymyositis and dermatomyositis, the lower extremity (pelvic girdle) is usually affected initially with difficulty walking up steps or arising from a chair or toilet seat. Walking may become clumsy, with a 'waddling' gait. The patient may fall and be unable to arise without assistance. Upper extremity (shoulder girdle) symptoms follow, with patients experiencing difficulty raising their arms overhead or combing their hair. Neck flexor weakness is manifested by the inability to raise the head from a pillow. Muscle pain may occur and is more common in dermatomyositis, particularly with exercise. Proximal dysphagia, with nasal regurgitation of liquids and pulmonary aspiration reflects pharyngeal striated muscle involvement and is a poor prognostic sign seen with severe disease. Pharyngeal weakness also results in hoarseness or a change in voice, giving it a nasal quality. Ocular or facial muscle weakness is very uncommon[55] in polymyositis–dermatomyositis, and their presence should prompt consideration of another diagnosis.

Physical examination using manual muscle testing is necessary to confirm weakness of individual muscles or groups of muscles, and many such measures are in current use. A standardized grading system for

TABLE 37.5 GRADING OF MUSCLE WEAKNESS IN POLYMYOSITIS–DERMATOMYOSITIS
1. No abnormality on examination
2. No abnormality on examination, but easy fatiguability and decreased exercise tolerance
3. Minimal degree of atrophy of one or more muscle groups, without functional impairment
4. Waddling gait; unable to run, but able to climb stairs without needing arm support
5. Marked waddling gait; accentuated lordosis; unable to climb stairs or rise from a standard chair without arm support
6. Unable to walk without assistance

(Modified with permission of Oxford University Press from Rose and Walton[26].)

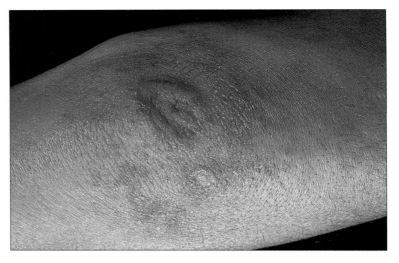

Fig. 37.2 Gottron's sign. Scaling, macular erythema over the extensor surface of the elbow in a patient with dermatomyositis.

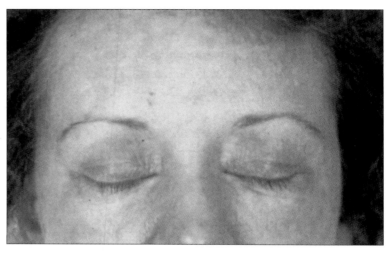

Fig. 37.3 Heliotrope rash of dermatomyositis. The erythematous or violaceous rash over the eyelids of this patient with dermatomyositis and breast cancer is a characteristic cutaneous feature.

muscle weakness has been proposed (Table 37.5). The severity of weakness should be serially assessed and recorded. Quantitative assessment of muscle strength is important, because laboratory tests may not accurately reflect disease activity. However, a more complete assessment should combine muscle strength testing with functional ability. Other means of assessing and quantifying strength include an age- and sex-standardized lower extremity measure[56], a modified sphygmomanometer to quantitate shoulder abductor strength[57] and a hand-held pull gauge to measure isometric strength in different muscle groups[58]. Muscle hypertrophy is seen with muscular dystrophy, not with polymyositis or dermatomyositis. Muscle atrophy and joint contractures are late findings in chronic myositis, as a result of fibrous replacement of muscle or in inclusion body myositis.

Skin

The presence of a characteristic skin rash indicates the clinical subset of dermatomyositis; the rash may precede, develop simultaneously with, or follow muscle symptoms. Gottron's papules and the heliotrope rash are considered pathognomonic cutaneous features of dermatomyositis. Gottron's papules (Fig. 37.1) are scaly, erythematous or violaceous plaques located over bony prominences, particularly the metacarpophalangeal and proximal and distal interphalangeal joints of the hands. Gottron's sign (Fig. 37.2) is a macular erythema that generally occurs in the same distribution, and over other extensor areas such as the elbows, knees and ankles. Either of these rashes is seen in 60–80% of patients

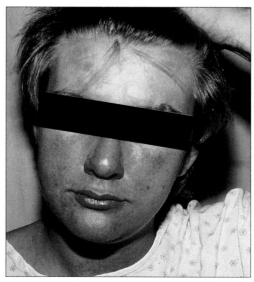

Fig. 37.4 The facial rash of dermatomyositis. Note the malar-like rash of dermatomyositis, which involves the nasolabial area (an area often spared in SLE). Patchy involvement of the forehead and chin is also present.

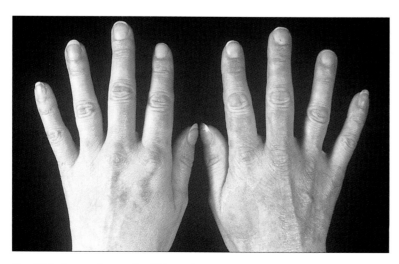

Fig. 37.1 Gottron's papules. This erythematous, scaling rash over the knuckles and dorsum of the hand is a common early sign in dermatomyositis. It can be distinguished from the rash of SLE, which usually affects the phalanges and spares the knuckles.

with dermatomyositis. Later in the disease course, the affected skin lesions may become shiny, atrophic and hypopigmented. The heliotrope rash, seen in fewer than 50% of patients with dermatomyositis, is purplish in color, may be edematous and is located in the periorbital area, especially over the upper eyelids (Fig. 37.3). Cutaneous photosensitivity, with facial erythema (Fig. 37.4) or a 'V sign' over the anterior chest, is more common than reported in dermatomyositis. Pruritus of affected areas is more severe than that seen with the rash of SLE and is particularly common when dermatomyositis involves the scalp (Fig. 37.5)[59]. Another distinguishing feature of the dermatomyositis rash compared with SLE is involvement of the nasolabial area and the forehead with dermatomyositis. The 'shawl sign' refers to a rash located over the upper back and across both shoulders in a shawl-like distribution. Cuticular hypertrophy and hemorrhage with periungual erythema, telangiectasia, infarcts and capillary dilatation are seen in some patients with dermatomyositis and in patients with myositis in overlap with another connective tissue disease. Cracking, fissuring, or both, of the lateral and palmar digital skin pads is termed 'mechanic's hands' (Fig. 37.6), and is most frequently seen in patients with polymyositis who have autoantibodies directed against a tRNA synthetase or the PM-Scl autoantigen[60].

Other cutaneous findings seen in patients with inflammatory myopathy are listed in Table 37.6[61–73]. Panniculitis (with membranocystic changes on biopsy) is being increasingly reported in association with myositis, and may be the presenting feature in some cases[61–65]. In fact, a recent report noted occult MRI abnormalities in the subcutaneous tissue of children with dermatomyositis, indicating active panniculitis, which progressed later to clinically evident calcinosis[65]. 'Centripetal flagellate erythema' consists of non-pruritic linear streaks on the trunk and proximal extremities demonstrating an interface dermatitis on biopsy[66]; it may be a marker of disease activity in dermatomyositis[67]. Hyperkeratotic skin lesions, including pityriasis rubra pilaris, have been reported[68,69].

Some patients may present with the classic biopsy-confirmed rash(es) of dermatomyositis and no muscle weakness, normal muscle enzymes or even a normal EMG. These patients are said to have 'amyopathic dermatomyositis' (ADM) if these findings have been present for 2 years or longer[74]. There are no population-based data that describe the prevalence of adult or childhood ADM, but these patients are more frequently observed in dermatology practices. Many such patients have a favorable outcome, but some may develop malignancy[75,76].

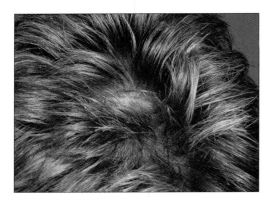

Fig. 37.5 Scalp rash of dermatomyositis. Note the scaling erythema of the scalp in this patient with dermatomyositis.

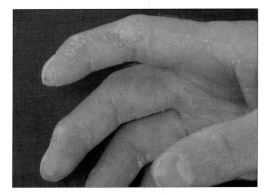

Fig. 37.6 'Mechanic's hands'. Note the hyperkeratotic changes and cracking of the skin on the lateral aspects of the fingers in this patient with the anti-PM-Scl autoantibody.

TABLE 37.6 CUTANEOUS FEATURES OF THE IDIOPATHIC INFLAMMATORY MYOPATHIES
Pathognomonic signs in dermatomyositis
Gottron's papules/sign (60–80% of patients)
Heliotrope rash (50% or fewer)
Less specific signs in dermatomyositis
Photosensitivity
'V sign'
Scalp involvement
'Shawl sign'
Nailfold capillary changes with cuticular overgrowth
Other skin findings in polymyositis or dermatomyositis
Calcinosis
'Mechanic's hands'
Panniculitis[61–65]
'Centripetal flagellate erythema' (linear streaks)[66,67]
Pityriasis rubra pilaris (palmar plantar hyperkeratoses)[68,69]
Facial seborrhea[70]
Papular mucinosis (scleromyxedema)[71]
Acquired ichthyosis[72]
Vesiculobullous disorders[73]
Urticarial (lymphocytic) vasculitis
Acanthosis nigricans
Vitiligo
Multifocal lipoatrophy
Poikiloderma

Calcinosis

Soft tissue calcification, which can be a disabling late problem, occurs most commonly in chronic dermatomyositis, especially with onset in childhood, and is uncommon in adult-onset disease. Myositis may be well controlled when calcinosis appears, but patients most often previously have had chronic, active disease or a delay in the initiation of corticosteroid treatment. Recent findings suggest that childhood dermatomyositis may be mediated by activated macrophages, IL-6, IL-1 and tumor necrosis factor, which are found in calcinotic fluid[77]. Calcinosis may be intracutaneous, subcutaneous, fascial or intramuscular in location, with a predilection for sites of repeated microtrauma (elbows, knees, flexor surfaces of fingers and buttocks). Troubling complications of calcinosis include cutaneous ulceration with drainage of calcareous material and secondary infection, and joint contractures that interfere with physical therapy intervention.

Articular

Polyarthralgias or polyarthritis, if they occur, are early in the disease course, rheumatoid-like in distribution and relatively mild. Joint involvement is more common, with overlap syndromes and the antisynthetases, but is frequently encountered in childhood dermatomyositis also[78]. The arthropathy associated with the anti-Jo-1 autoantibody, in addition to other antisynthetases[79], can be chronic and deforming[80], with interphalangeal thumb joint instability ('floppy thumb sign') and erosive[79], with periarticular calcifications[81]. Such 'pseudorheumatoid' changes in a Jo-1-positive patient are depicted radiographically and clinically in Figure 37.7. Other unusual anti-Jo-1 antibody-associated articular features have been described[82,83].

Pulmonary

Lung involvement is common in polymyositis–dermatomyositis, and dyspnea in the patient with myositis warrants an aggressive diagnostic approach (Table 37.7). Pulmonary disease may overshadow

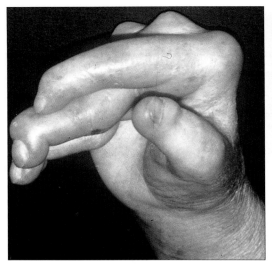
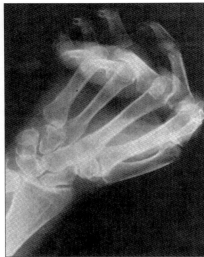

Fig. 37.7 Deforming arthropathy of polymyositis.
(a) Rheumatoid-like deformities of the hand in a patient with the anti-Jo-1 autoantibody. (b) Radiograph of this patient's hand, showing numerous subluxations, but minimal bony erosive changes.

TABLE 37.7 CAUSES OF DYSPNEA IN THE PATIENT WITH IDIOPATHIC INFLAMMATORY MYOPATHY

Non-pulmonary etiology

Respiratory muscle weakness[86–88]
Cardiac involvement (see text)

Pulmonary etiology

Diffuse alveolitis
Adult respiratory distress syndrome[89]
Slowly progressive interstitial lung disease
Pulmonary hypertension
Alveolar hemorrhage[90,91]
Bronchiolitis obliterans organizing pneumonia[92,93]
Pneumomediastinum[94–97]
Pleural effusion
Infection (with or without aspiration due to pharyngeal myopathy)[98,99]
Drug-induced (e.g. methotrexate)

---

the features of myositis and may be observed in patients without overt myositis or with ADM[84,85]. Dyspnea may result from non-parenchymal problems such as ventilatory (diaphragmatic and intercostal) muscle weakness or cardiac dysfunction (see below). Ventilatory muscle weakness leading to ventilatory failure is uncommon, but four patients have been reported who developed ventilator-dependent respiratory failure with diaphragmatic involvement, and one had myositis of the diaphragm at autopsy[86,87]. Hypercapnia is likely in polymyositis when the vital capacity is less than 55% of predicted normal[88].

In general, the presence of alveolitis with a 'ground glass' appearance on high resolution computed tomography (CT), as opposed to fibrosis characterized by 'honeycombing', indicates a potentially treatment-responsive condition with a more favorable prognosis. Arterial hypoxemia with exercise desaturation is common, and pulmonary function testing reveals restrictive physiology, with a decrease in the diffusion capacity. This type of pulmonary involvement is commonly seen in association with anti-Jo-1 or another antiaminoacyl-tRNA synthetase autoantibody, as part of the 'antisynthetase' syndrome. Interstitial disease may be slowly progressive or even asymptomatic (usually bibasilar) in some patients with polymyositis–dermatomyositis with or without an associated antisynthetase autoantibody. The most ominous intrinsic lung complication is rapidly progressive diffuse alveolitis. This

form of pulmonary involvement may be fatal in weeks to months, often terminating with adult respiratory distress syndrome[89].

Patients with myositis-associated progressive pulmonary fibrosis can develop pulmonary hypertension secondary to pulmonary vasoconstriction as a result of chronic hypoxemia. Diffuse alveolar hemorrhage with pulmonary capillaritis is uncommon[90,91], but bronchiolitis obliterans with organizing pneumonia (BOOP) is increasingly observed as the initial manifestation of polymyositis[92,93]. Pneumomediastinum with subcutaneous emphysema is associated with rapidly progressive ILD and dermatomyositis with cutaneous vasculitis[94–97]. Fulminant *Pneumocystis carinii* pneumonia has been reported in four patients with human immunodeficiency virus-negative dermatomyositis who were lymphopenic before initiation of corticosteroids[98], and *Nocardia* pleural empyema complicated the disease in a Jo-1-positive polymyositis patient during treatment with intravenous immunoglobulin and corticosteroids[99].

Cardiac

Although heart involvement may be common in polymyositis–dermatomyositis, it is seldom symptomatic; the frequency of cardiac abnormalities reported is dependent on the aggressiveness of detection measures[100]. The most common finding is a rhythm disturbance, presumably from inflammatory or fibrotic alteration of the conducting system. More severe forms of cardiac involvement, such as congestive heart failure or pericardial tamponade, may occur on presentation, but are very unusual[101,102]. Congestive heart failure is typically caused by myocarditis or myocardial fibrosis[103,104]. Patients complain of palpitations or dyspnea on exertion and on physical examination have tachycardia and other features of congestive heart failure. Myocardial infarction may result from coronary vasospasm, accelerated atherosclerosis associated with prolonged corticosteroid use or arteritis that may be seen with coronary angiography[105,106].

Gastrointestinal tract

The pharyngeal musculature is striated and thus can become inflamed and weak like striated muscle in other locations. Swallowing problems (upper dysphagia) manifest as difficulty in the initiation of deglutition or nasal regurgitation of liquids, with dysphonia. If severe, aspiration of oral contents leads to chemical pneumonitis, sometimes complicated by secondary bacterial infection. Cricopharyngeal muscle dysfunction also can result in dysphagia, with the complaint of a 'blocking' sensation with swallowing; it is more common in inclusion body myositis[107].

Involvement of the smooth muscle of any portion of the intestinal tract is possible in both overlap disorders or pure polymyositis and dermatomyositis. Patients note a retrosternal 'sticking' sensation on swallowing bread or meat and heartburn (reflux) with esophageal body and gastroesophageal sphincter involvement, respectively. In rare cases, esophageal dysmotility is complicated by megaesophagus or rupture[108]. Postprandial symptoms of bloating, pain and distention (pseudo-obstruction) in addition to watery diarrhea with weight loss (malabsorption syndrome) indicate small bowel involvement. Pneumatosis cystoides intestinalis has been reported[109].

Childhood-onset dermatomyositis is most commonly associated with gastrointestinal ulceration and hemorrhage as a result of vasculitis. Adult-onset dermatomyositis also may have severe gastrointestinal manifestations[110]. Active and quiescent myositis are increasingly reported in conjunction with inflammatory bowel disease[111,112], as are primary biliary cirrhosis, sclerosing cholangitis and celiac disease in adults and children[113–116].

Peripheral vascular system

Raynaud's phenomenon is observed in all subsets of the inflammatory myopathies except for malignancy-associated forms. Systemic vasculitis is common in childhood dermatomyositis, but uncommon in adults[117]. The inflammatory vascular lesions of dermatomyositis include tender dermal and or subcutaneous nodules, periungual infarcts and digital ulcerations.

Kidney

Renal disease is rare in myositis, but an occasional patient has proteinuria and, less commonly, nephrotic syndrome. Patients with overlap syndromes may develop kidney problems from the non-myositis components of their disorders. Polymyositis-induced myoglobuinuric acute renal failure can occur, but is rare[118].

Miscellaneous

Visual complications have been increasingly reported in association with polymyositis–dermatomyositis, including visual blurring and loss as a result of retinopathy or retinal vasculitis[119,120]. Two patients with dermatomyositis developed acute abdominal pain as a result of spontaneous hemorrhage leading to abdominal hematomas[121]. Central nervous system features of polymyositis or dermatomyositis are rare, but progressive multifocal leukoencephalopathy and central nervous system vasculitis have been seen in association with dermatomyositis[122,123].

DIFFERENTIAL DIAGNOSIS

History and physical examination

Among patients with impaired muscle function, only 50% voluntarily complain about 'weakness'. Other frequent symptoms are 'tiredness' and 'fatigue'. The examining physician must differentiate between difficulty in performing a motor task (muscle weakness) or its repetitive performance (fatigue of muscle) and difficulty doing activities of daily living that require more endurance than muscle strength.

Muscle weakness and muscle fatigue imply primary disease of muscle or the neuromuscular unit, whereas inability to perform normal activities may include or be solely caused by cardiovascular, metabolic, endocrine or psychiatric disorders. The patient's complaint of fatigue may refer to a variety of problems that have the common feature of loss of sense of well-being. Fatigue may include indifference to tasks at hand, preoccupation with unimportant activities or difficulty initiating or sustaining an activity. The patient often does not separate physical from mental function. For example, disinclination to interact with one's family members and friends during leisure hours may be termed 'fatigue' by the patient, but be interpreted as a symptoms of depression by the discerning physician. Some of these non-neuromuscular causes of weakness, separated into conditions causing episodic or persistent symptoms, are listed in Table 37.8.

TABLE 37.8 NON-NEUROMUSCULAR CAUSES OF WEAKNESS

Episodic weakness (acute attacks with recurrence)

Hypotension, cardiac arrhythmias
Hypoxia, hypercapnia
Hyperventilation
Hypoglycemia
Cerebrovascular insufficiency
Emotional states (hyperventilation, anxiety)

Persistent weakness

Anemia
Chronic or acute infection
Malignancy
Malnutrition
Advanced organ system failure (lung, heart, liver, kidney)
Metabolic disorders (hyperthyroidism, hyperparathyroidism, hypophosphatemia)

If true muscle weakness is suspected, other medical history features should be elicited because of their usefulness in differential diagnosis. Some complaints are distinctly unusual in polymyositis–dermatomyositis and should suggest alternative diagnoses. A family history of primary myopathy is common in heritable forms of muscle disease. Episodic weakness, especially after exercise or prolonged use of the affected muscles, occurs in myasthenia gravis and metabolic myopathies. Asymmetric or unilateral weakness, muscle cramps and fasciculations suggest a primary neurologic disorder. Facial and ocular muscle weakness rarely occur in myositis, but are frequent in myasthenia gravis. Finally, a list of the patient's medications may uncover an agent recognized to cause skeletal muscle dysfunction.

Non-inflammatory myopathies

The differential diagnosis of adult polymyositis–dermatomyositis is broad and includes numerous conditions capable of affecting skeletal muscle (Table 37.9). History, physical examination and differences in laboratory test results serve as the primary features distinguishing between these conditions. However, even the muscle biopsy may not be diagnostic in some patients with inflammatory myopathy.

Primary diseases of nerve include the spinal muscular atrophies, autosomal recessive disorders leading to slowly progressive degeneration of spinal anterior horn cells (weakness, wasting) and amyotrophic lateral sclerosis, which results in more rapid degeneration of both lower and upper motor neurons (bulbar or pseudobulbar palsy).

Myasthenia gravis is the prototypical disorder of the neuromusclar junction, in which weakness often affects the extraocular and bulbar muscles and becomes worse with prolonged or repetitive use. A similar pattern of activity-increased weakness is found in Eaton–Lambert syndrome. Both of these diseases can cause proximal muscle weakness. They are distinguished from polymyositis–dermatomyositis by their characteristic patterns on the EMG, in addition to absence of increases in serum muscle enzymes, but some patients with myasthenia gravis have been discovered to have myositis on muscle biopsy[124].

The congenital myopathies, including the various forms of muscular dystrophy and nemaline myopathy, are hereditary conditions with onset of symptoms primarily in infancy or childhood, but occasionally in adulthood, with slow but steady progression. Their genetic patterns of occurrence and clinical features have been well described. Some congenital myopathy cases are difficult to differentiate from inflammatory myopathy but have a slowly progressive downhill course unaffected by corticosteroid or immunosuppressive treatment.

Metabolic and mitochondrial myopathies occur because of genetic defects that cause abnormal energy metabolism[125]. Glycogen storage

TABLE 37.9 DIFFERENTIAL DIAGNOSIS OF MUSCLE WEAKNESS

Denervating conditions	Spinal muscular atrophies*, amyotrophic lateral sclerosis*
Neuromuscular junction disorders	Eaton–Lambert syndrome*, myasthenia gravis*
The genetic muscular dystrophies	Duchenne's facioscapulohumeral, limb girdle*, Becker's, Emery–Dreifuss type*, distal, ocular
Myotonic diseases	Dystrophia myotonica*, myotonia congenita
Congenital myopathies	Nemaline, mitochondrial, centronuclear, central core
Glycogen storage diseases	Adult-onset acid maltase deficiency*, McArdle's disease
Lipid storage myopathies	Carnitine deficiency*, carnitine palmityltransferase deficiency*
The periodic paralyses	
Myositis ossificans*	Generalized and local
Endocrine myopoathies*	Hypothyroidism, hyperthyroidism, acromegaly, Cushing's disease, Addison's disease, hyperparathyroidism, hypoparathyroidism, vitamin D deficiency myopathy, hypokalemia, hypocalcemia
Metabolic myopoathies*	Uremia, hepatic failure
Toxic myopathies*	Acute and chronic alcoholism, drugs including penicillamine*, clofibrate*, chloroquine, emetine
Nutritional myopathies	vitamin E deficiency*, malabsorption*
Carcinomatous neuromyopathy*	carcinomatous cachexia
Acute rhabdomyolysis*	
Proximal neuropathies	Guillain–Barré syndrome*, acute intermittent porphyria*, diabetic lower-limb chronic plexopathies*, chronic autoimmune polyneuropathy
Microembolization by atheroma or carcinoma	
Polymyalgia rheumatica*	
Other collagen vascular diseases	Rheumatoid arthritis, scleroderma, systemic lupus erythematosus, polyarteritis nodosa
Infections	Acute viral, including influenza, mononucleosis, rickettsia, coxsackievirus, rubella and rubella vaccination, acute bacterial including typhoid
Parasites	Including *Toxoplasma*, *Trichinella*, *Schistosoma*, *Cysticercus*, *Sarcosporidia*
Septic myositis	Including *Staphylococcus*, *Streptococcus*, *Clostridium perfringens* (*welchii*) and leprosy

* Indicates the conditions that are most commonly confused with muscle weakness.

diseases result from enzyme deficiencies involving the glycolytic pathway. McArdle's disease, or myophosphorylase deficiency, is caused by failure to degrade glycogen for energy under anerobic conditions. It is characterized by acute episodes of pain, weakness and swelling of voluntary muscles, which are contracted frequently or for a prolonged period of time. On occasion, a late proximal myopathy occurs that can simulate polymyositis. Ischemic exercise testing results in failure to produce lactate and muscle biopsy shows glycogen accumulation and absence of myophosphorylase. Acid maltase deficiency, a metabolic disorder known to mimic polymyositis, results in excessive accumulation of glycogen in membrane-bound lysosomes. Progressive proximal weakness, myotonic changes on the EMG and glycogen deposition on muscle biopsy are observed. Carnitine deficiency results in inability to transport long-chain fatty acids into mitochondria for oxidation, leading to lipid accumulation in muscle fibers and a chronic proximal myopathy. The enzyme carnitine palmityltransferase may also be lacking, resulting in a syndrome resembling McArdle's disease, with exertional pain and weakness as a result of inadequte production of adenosine triphosphate from lipids. A similar symptom complex can occur with myoadenylate deaminase deficiency, in which the ischemic exercise test results in the failure to increase ammonia production.

An increasingly recognized form of weakness that occurs in the seriously ill patient includes both 'critical illness polyneuropathy' and 'acute myopathy of intensive care'[126,127]. The latter is associated with the use of high-dose intravenous corticosteroids and non-depolarizing neuromuscular blocking agents, and is a frequent cause of failure to wean tracheally intubated patients from a respirator. Increased serum creatine kinase (CK) concentrations in the first 10 days of the illness, myopathic EMG changes and myofiber necrosis on biopsy are characteristic, and partial or complete recovery is the rule, but may take months[127].

Other causes of non-inflammatory proximal myopathy include vitamin D deficiency, calciphylaxis, adrenal insufficiency, hypophosphatemia, hyperthyroidism, carcinomatous neuropathy and exposures to certain toxic substances.

Other inflammatory myopathies

Infectious agents are capable of producing polymyositis. Viruses reported to cause widespread, but generally mild and self-limited myositis include influenza A and B, hepatitis B, coxsackie, rubella (both natural infection and after immunization with live attenuated virus), echovirus and human immunodeficiency virus. In such cases, the myositis is self-limited and recovery is almost always complete. Echovirus has been associated with myositis in patients with X-linked hypogammaglobulinemia.

Bacterial infection (pyomyositis) caused by staphylococcal or streptococcal organisms is characterized by the insidious onset of fever and myalgias, progressing to acute focal suppuration of skeletal muscle, with abscess formation. Children and young adults or persons with predisposing comorbid conditions such as human immunodeficiency virus infection are most often affected[128]. Although initially reported to occur primarily in persons residing in tropical areas, pyomyositis has been more frequently diagnosed recently in temperate climates. This disorder is potentially fatal if unrecognized, and disabling if foci of osteomyelitis develop.

One parasitic infection capable of causing acute myositis is trichinosis, which also frequently causes conjunctivitis, eosinophilia and increased serum antibody titers. Toxoplasmosis may also cause a polymyositis-like illness in which the organisms are identified in muscle biopsies and an antibody response develops.

Focal nodular myositis, presenting with tumor-like masses and curiously limited to one or several extremities, has been described[129]. Although not an inflammatory condition, diabetic muscle infarction presents with abrupt onset of thigh pain, tenderness, a palpable mass and increased serum CK concentration[130]. Giant cell myositis is rare, but can be encountered in sarcoidosis. Regenerating muscle in other conditions may result in cells having a multinucleate appearance on light microscopy that must be distinguished from true giant cells in a typical granuloma.

Myositis with an eosinophilic inflammatory infiltrate includes a heterogeneous group of rare conditions[131]. A recently proposed classification system divides patients into groups on the basis of whether they have focal eosinophilic myositis, eosinophilic polymyositis (systemic features including myocardial involvement) or eosinophilic perimyositis[132]. These conditions must be distinguished from eosinophilic fasciitis and eosinophilia–myalgia syndrome. In the last two disorders, true myofiber necrosis, with weakness and increased CK are unusual.

Amyloidosis can mimic polymyositis clinically and histologically; the only clue might be other features typical of amyloidosis, failure to respond to corticosteroid treatment and positive Congo red staining of muscle tissue, with immunohistochemical analysis confirming vascular amyloid deposition[133]. For this reason, some recommend routine serum and urine immunoelectrophoresis in all cases of polymyositis–dermatomyositis.

During recent years, a number of patients in France whose symptoms resembled polymyositis or polymyalgia rheumatica have been reported to have subcutaneous and epimysial, perimysial and perifascicular/endomysial infiltration, with large numbers of periodic acid Schiff-positive macrophages[134]. The term 'macrophagic myofasciitis' has been used to describe such patients. Myofibril damage has been minimal, and the symptoms have responded readily to corticosteroid treatment.

Malignancy and myositis

There has been considerable controversy regarding the validity and magnitude of the relationship between malignancy and inflammatory myopathy. Several clinically pertinent questions should be addressed regarding this purported association:

1. Is there an increased risk of cancer in patients with polymyositis–dermatomyositis?
2. If such an association exists, what types of malignancies are increased?
3. Are there clinical findings that identify patients with myositis who are at risk for malignancy?
4. Who should be screened and what is a reasonable screening evaluation for malignancy?
5. What is the pathogenesis of malignancy-associated myositis?

Recent reports strongly support an increased risk of cancer in patients with polymyositis–dermatomyositis. They include consecutive-patient series, hospital-based analyses, national registries and population-based cohort studies of biopsy-proven cases[135–139]. Standardized incidence ratios (SIRs), computed as ratios of observed to expected cases of cancer, have clearly demonstrated the greatest risk of malignancy in patients with dermatomyositis in whom SIR values range from 3.0 to 12.6[136–138]. In a pooled analysis of published national data from Sweden, Denmark and Finland, 618 cases of dermatomyositis were identified, 198 of whom had cancer (SIR 3.0)[137]. Of these, 115 (59%) developed a malignancy after the diagnosis of dermatomyositis was made. Dermatomyositis was strongly associated with ovarian, lung, pancreatic, stomach and colorectal cancer and non-Hodgkin lymphoma. This same study identified a lower but statistically significant increase in cancer associated with polymyositis in 137 of 914 cases (15%), with an increased risk of non-Hodgkin lymphoma and both lung and bladder cancer. In an effort to address several methodologic issues in earlier reports, an Australian study utilizing a cancer registry and a strict definition of myositis based on histologic criteria also demonstrated an increased risk of malignancy in both polymyositis–dermatomyositis and inclusion body myositis (SIR 2.4)[139]. The overall risk of cancer is greatest in the first 3 years after the diagnosis of myositis[139], but a greater risk of malignancy persists through all years of follow-up, emphasizing the importance of continued surveillance[137,139]. Although older individuals with dermatomyositis are at greater risk, the likelihood of malignancy is increased even in dermatomyositis patients younger than 45 years[137].

The sites of origin of malignancy are typical for the age of the patient, but several points are noteworthy. Ovarian cancer is over-represented in some series[137,140], but screening with pelvic examination rarely detects this cancer before the development of metastatic disease. Serum CA-125 screening proved useful in a case–control study of 14 women with dermatomyositis (four of whom subsequently developed ovarian cancer) in which the sensitivity was 50% and specificity 100%[141]. Prospective studies are needed to determine the effect of screening on the stage of ovarian cancer and long-term survival. Asian and Chinese patients with dermatomyositis have a clear increase in nasopharyngeal carcinoma[138,142]. Many other types of cancer occur coincidentally with myositis, including genitourinary malignancies and melanoma.

Clinical and histologic features that may predict the presence of a malignancy in a patient with dermatomyositis include epidermal necrosis, cutaneous leukocytoclastic vasculitis and the presence of amyopathic dermatomyositis[135,143,144]. In a series of 11 patients with adult dermatomyositis, six had malignancy and both clinical and histologic evidence of epidermal necrosis was present in all six, whereas cutaneous necrosis was absent in the five patients with dermatomyositis without cancer[143]. Similarly, in a retrospective study, vasculitis of lesional skin in dermatomyositis predicted concurrent malignancy[144]. Cancer was diagnosed in four of 12 (25%) with ADM followed for an average of 4.3 years after the patient's diagnosis[135]. The presence of pulmonary fibrosis, myositis-associated or specific serum autoantibodies or a clinically confirmed associated connective tissue disease decreases the likelihood of cancer[138].

A cancer evaluation of high-risk patients could reduce mortality. Recommendations vary widely from careful history and physical examination (including gynecologic examination in women) with routine laboratory screening to age-specific studies with extensive invasive investigations. Given the distribution of tumors noted above, it seems prudent also to include chest, abdominal and pelvic CT, along with fecal blood testing and mammography. As the risk of malignant disease continues to be increased long after the development of dermatomyositis, one needs to follow the patient with myositis carefully for a number of years[137].

The etiology of the link between malignancy and the inflammatory myopathies remains obscure. Speculations include the presence of common environmental factors serving as both carcinogens and triggers of inflammation, paraneoplastic phenomena in which tumor antigens generate an inflammatory response against muscle, or the occurrence of malignant transformation by immunosuppressive agents used to treat patients with polymyositis–dermatomyositis. The last of these seems unlikely, given the close temporal association of myositis with malignancy and the lack of increased risk of malignancy in patients with dermatomyositis treated with cytotoxic drugs[145]. The paraneoplastic theory appears most plausible, given the complete resolution of myositis with cancer resection or chemotherapy-induced remission and the recrudescence of muscle symptoms with tumor recurrence. New onset of dermatomyositis in the setting of tumor recurrence also supports this hypothesis.

Drug-induced myopathy

The frequency of toxic myopathy caused by drugs is unknown, but this condition is likely common and certainly under-diagnosed. Many agents

TABLE 37.10 DRUGS ASSOCIATED WITH MYOPATHY

Amiodarone	Fibric acid derivatives	Phenylbutazone
Amphetamines	Heroin	Phenytoin
Chloroquine	Hydralazine	Procainamide
Cimetidine	Hydroxychloroquine	Rifampin
Cocaine	Hydroxyurea	Statin drugs
Colchicine	Ipecac (emetine)	Sulfonamides
Corticosteroids	Levodopa	Tiopronin
Cyclosporin	Nicotinic acid	Vecuronium bromide
Danazol	Pancuronium	Vincristine
Epsilon amino-caproic acid	Penicillamine	Zidovudine (AZT)
Ethanol	Pentazocine	

are myotoxic, including both prescription medicines and drugs with high abuse potential. Table 37.10 lists many drugs associated with myotoxicity. The text below describes those most likely to cause myositis-like disorders, including rhabdomyolysis.

All types of cholesterol-decreasing agents have been shown to be toxic to muscles, and the frequency of myopathy increases with combined lipid-decreasing treatment. The hydroxymethyl glutaryl-coenzyme A reductase inhibitors (the statin drugs) utilize the cytochrome P450 (CYP) system (specifically CYP3A4) in their metabolism, and drug interactions may result in an increased concentration of the myotoxic statin when agents that inhibit CYP3A4 are administered concomitantly. Inhibitors of CYP3A4 include erythromycin, clarithromycin, fluconazole, cyclosporine, some calcium channel blockers and even grapefruit juice. The resulting toxic myopathy is characterized by severe myalgias, myositis with weakness and increased CK concentrations, or even rhabdomyolysis[146,147]. Pravastatin alone has been associated with a polymyositis-like illness[148] and caused rhabdomyolysis in a patient with mixed connective tissue disease[149]. Lovastatin led to a muscle and cutaneous syndrome consistent with dermatomyositis[150] and simvastatin to isolated polymyositis and dermatomyositis with lung involvement[151,152]. Cerivastatin has been withdrawn from the US market because of reports of fatal rhabdomyolysis, occurring most frequently with higher doses, in elderly patients or in combination with another lipid-decreasing agent. The fibric acid derivatives (benzofibrate, clofibrate, gemfibrozil) and niacin also cause myopathy and the risk is increased when one of these drugs is used with a statin.

Although muscle symptoms may occur within days of beginning cholesterol-decreasing drugs, myotoxic reactions have been reported up to 2 years after the commencement of this form of treatment. The frequency of myopathy is dose-dependent and is increased with renal or hepatic impairment, electrolyte disturbances, defective lipid metabolism, hypothyroidism, drugs of abuse and viral infections. Electromyography reveals myopathic changes with prominent spontaneous potentials and muscle biopsy is characterized by necrosis with or without regenerative fibers or myositis. Recognition is crucial, as most syndromes are reversible on discontinuation of the drug. Persistence of myopathy in some patients treated with statins is poorly understood.

Corticosteroid myopathy is the most common drug-induced muscle problem seen in patients with rheumatic disease. It is characterized by slowly progressive, painless proximal weakness that is worse in the hip girdle. Asthmatic individuals may develop diaphragmatic weakness with an excessive dose of inhaled corticosteroids. Steroid myopathy is clearly dose- and duration-dependent and patients who show prominent Cushingoid features seem more prone to its development. The serum CK concentration is normal and the EMG may be normal or only mildly myopathic. The muscle biopsy demonstrates type II myofiber atrophy, without degeneration, regeneration or inflammatory infiltrates. The treatment is withdrawal or tapering of the drug. Colchicine has well-known adverse neuromuscular effects including muscle weakness and polyneuropathy. The CK concentration is often increased and electromyography demonstrates fibrillations, positive sharp waves and polyphasic myopathic potentials. A vacuolar myopathy with accumulation of lysosomes and autophagic vacuoles without necrosis is seen on muscle biopsy. Renal impairment increases the risk of myotoxicity. Recently, colchicine-induced rhabdomyolysis has been reported, also in a patient with impaired renal function[153].

First described in 1963, antimalarial neuromyopathy is an uncommon side effect of chloroquine or hydroxychloroquine. Toxicity does not appear to be dose- or duration-dependent. Patients note the insidious onset of painless symmetric muscle weakness predominantly affecting the lower extremities. Cardiomyopathy has been reported. The muscle biopsy has classic changes of a vacuolar myopathy and electron microscopy shows characteristic curvilinear bodies adjacent to large complex secondary lysosomes[154]. In contrast, the myopathy of SLE (for which antimalarial drugs are frequently prescribed) rarely demonstrates vacuolar change and has no curvilinear bodies[154]. In a retrospective chart review of 214 patients begun on antimalarial treatment over a period of 6 years for various rheumatic disorders, three patients with rheumatoid arthritis (all receiving chloroquine) were identified as having a myopathy, giving an incidence of 1 per 100 patient-years (95% confidence interval 0.2 to 3)[155]. All patients improved within 2 months of discontinuing the drug.

Hydroxyurea is a chemotherapeutic agent that is commonly used in the treatment of myeloproliferative disorders, particularly chronic myelogenous leukemia. Cutaneous lesions resembling dermatomyositis without myositis have been reported with this agent up to 7 years after initiation of treatment[156] and the course is usually benign. D-Penicillamine is known to cause an inflammatory myopathy and myasthenia gravis. Pentazocine, an injectable analgesic agent, causes a fibrous myopathy adjacent to injection sites, but has recently been shown to produce features of polymyositis in a patient after 13 months of treatment[157]. Reversible polymyositis occurred during psoralen and ultraviolet A treatment in a patient with vitiligo[158], and other connective tissue diseases have been reported after psoralen and ultraviolet A treatment. IL-2[159], interferon-alpha[160] and other cytokines have been used to treat malignancies and are known to be associated with the development of autoantibodies and other immunologic perturbations, including polymyositis. Vinyl chloride, a known carcinogenic agent that is also associated with the development of a systemic sclerosis-like illness, was recently implicated in the development of anti-Jo-1 antibody-positive polymyositis in a middle-aged man[161].

INVESTIGATIONS

General concepts

The assessment of patients with inflammatory myopathy must take into consideration elements of disease activity as opposed to disease damage[162]. Weakness may be the result of myositis, but also of irreparable damage to muscle in the form of atrophy, fatty replacement and fibrosis; the last will not respond to corticosteroids or other immunosuppressive agents. Similarly, alveolitis in the lung may be reversible but fibrosis, at least today, is not. Polyarthritis, dermatitis and vasculitis are active disease manifestations. Measures of disease activity and damage are currently being developed and validated for the cross-sectional and longitudinal assessment of patients with polymyositis–dermatomyositis[163]. The lack of such indices hampers the practitioner, who must develop an individualized plan to treat his/her patient, and the researcher, who must gauge treatment response in patients enrolled in therapeutic trials.

Routine tests

Low-grade anemia of chronic disease may be found in patients with inflammatory myopathy. However, anemia should always be thoroughly evaluated at diagnosis, particularly in patients with dermatomyositis, in whom an occult malignancy may be present. The erythrocyte sedimentation rate is a poor indicator of disease activity, but it and the C-reactive protein may be mildly increased (erythrocyte sedimentation rate 30–50mm/h by the Westergren method).

Serum muscle enzymes

Enzymes that leak from injured skeletal muscle into the serum are valuable aids in detecting active muscle injury. In order of sensitivity, they are CK, aldolase, aspartate and alanine aminotransferases and lactate dehydrogenase. The finding of increased serum transaminases in a patient with fatigue and muscle weakness often leads to an erroneous diagnosis of hepatitis, and an unnecessary liver biopsy.

The serum CK is believed to be the most reliable enzyme test to use in routine patient care. During a flare of disease, the serum CK will usually increase weeks before overt muscle weakness develops. Conversely, with treatment-induced remission, concentrations of this enzyme decrease to normal before objective improvement in strength. The CK is therefore predictive in the management of patients with myositis. However, there are exceptions, as some patients with active biopsy-proven myositis (dermatomyositis > polymyositis and children > adults) have a normal CK and others have circulating inhibitors of CK activity[164]. There is considerable racial variation in CK concentrations, and one cannot apply reference values from white populations to patients of Afro-Caribbean descent, in whom the upper limit of normal CK is increased[165].

Myoglobin is also released from damaged skeletal muscle and cleared by the kidney. Myoglobinemia may be more sensitive than the serum CK concentration in some patients, but the test is cumbersome and not uniformly available; it can be used as an adjunct to routine measurements of serum muscle enzymes in diagnosis and follow-up. Myoglobinuria is less frequent in patients with myositis, but may be followed by acute tubular necrosis of the kidney, with renal failure[166].

Electromyography

Electrical testing is a sensitive but non-specific method of evaluating inflammatory myopathy. Typical findings include irritability of myofibrils on needle insertion and at rest (fibrillation potentials, complex repetitive discharges, positive sharp waves) and short duration, low-amplitude, complex (polyphasic) potentials on contraction. More than 90% of patients with active myositis will have an abnormal EMG, and a normal EMG is a strong point against active disease. Electromyography continues to be helpful in the selection of a muscle for biopsy and it should be performed unilaterally and a contralateral muscle chosen for biopsy, to avoid the confusion of inflammation artifact as a result of injury from the needle itself.

Later in the course of polymyositis–dermatomyositis, EMG examination may be useful for the detection of low-grade disease activity in the setting of chronic damage from fibrosis or fatty infiltration. Unlike biopsy or MRI studies, EMG enables several muscles to be examined.

The EMG may also be useful in the circumstance of normal serum enzyme concentrations and a physical examination of muscle strength that is difficult to interpret. Corticosteroid myopathy causes some electromyographic changes, but the presence of fibrillation potentials suggests another (inflammatory) process.

Muscle biopsy

Biopsy remains the gold standard with which to confirm the diagnosis of inflammatory myopathy. Chronic inflammatory cells in the perivascular and interstitial areas surrounding myofibrils are present in 80% of cases, and lymphocytic invasion of non-necrotic fibers is considered pathognomonic of polymyositis (Fig. 37.8). Besides lymphocytes, other cells – including histiocytes, plasma cells, eosinophils and polymorphonuclear leukocytes – are often present.

More common than inflammatory infiltrates are degeneration and regeneration of myofibrils, with phagocytosis of necrotic fibers and myofibril regeneration (90% of cases). In chronic myositis, fibrous connective tissue or fat replaces necrotic myofibers.

There are important differences noted between polymyositis, inclusion body myositis and dermatomyositis. In dermatomyositis, B cells and the late component of complement (C5–C9, membrane attack complex) predominate in the perivascular area. T cells are mostly CD8$^+$ and cytotoxic, but CD4$^+$ cells are found also. Perifascicular myofibril atrophy (Fig. 37.9), endothelial cell hyperplasia of blood vessels, deposition of immune complexes in the vasculature and frank vasculitis are noted. On quantitative morphologic analysis, muscle capillary depletion and dropout are early findings and myofibril damage results from an ischemic microangiopathy. In contrast, polymyositis and inclusion body myositis feature cytotoxic T cell invasion of myofibrils, with relative sparing of the vasculature. T helper cells may also be found in the perivascular and perimysial areas but, unlike the findings in dermatomyositis, B cells are rarely observed.

Eight of 34 patients with polymyositis in one study had increased numbers of eosinophils in their muscle biopsy specimens (>0.3 eosinophils/mm^2), but no concomitant blood eosinophilia[167]. These patients had frequent myalgias, myoglobinuria and greater concentrations of serum muscle enzymes, and responded well to corticosteroid treatment, with a relatively benign clinical course compared with the 26 other myositis patients without tissue eosinophilia. These patients did not have the eosinophilia-myalgia syndrome. Whether or not they represent a separate subset of myositis is not yet certain.

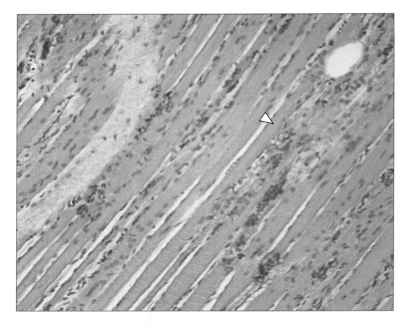

Fig. 37.8 Longitudinal section of fresh-frozen muscle from a patient with polymyositis. Several areas of interstitial involvement, with myofiber destruction, are seen. The arrow indicates an area of degeneration and necrosis of myofibers in association with interstitial lymphocytic and histiocytic cellular infiltration. (Hematoxylin and eosin, medium power.)

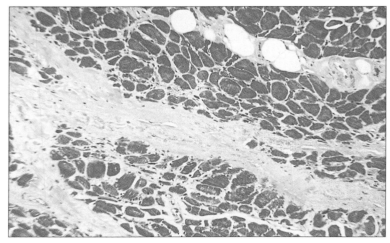

Fig. 37.9 Transverse fresh-frozen section of muscle from a patient with chronic dermatomyositis. Note the atrophic, small fibers in the periphery of the fascicles (perifascicular atrophy) and the increase in fibrous tissue separating bundles of myofibers. (Trichrome stain, low power.)

Despite the characteristic features described above, some patients with active myositis have a normal biopsy, for several reasons. First, the disease is patchy and sampling error precludes 100% sensitivity. Secondly, the wrong muscle may be chosen for biopsy. A weak but not end-stage proximal muscle with EMG abnormalities on the opposite side is the best choice. Open surgical biopsy is the current standard, but percutaneous needle muscle biopsy is a convenient and relatively inexpensive method with a high diagnostic yield in polymyositis–dermatomyositis[168]. Although direct comparison with open techniques is lacking, needle biopsy allows sampling of several muscles with EMG changes, to increase diagnostic sensitivity, and also is useful for detecting other myopathic conditions.

Magnetic resonance imaging

The application of MRI techniques adds an important dimension to our understanding of myositis[169]. MRI is non-invasive and thus has obvious advantages over electromyography and muscle biopsy, particularly in children. Also, large areas of muscle such as both thighs can be visualized, and choosing the most abnormal site can increase the diagnostic yield of biopsy. The T1-weighted image provides excellent anatomic detail, with clear delineation of various muscle groups. Normal tissue is homogeneously dark with a low signal, whereas fat (subcutaneous area and marrow) appears bright, corresponding to a high signal. Muscle is darker on T2-weighted images. Inflammation is bright on both T1 and T2 images. Adding fat suppression in the form of short time inversion recovery (STIR) sequences to the T2 technique improves the detection of muscle inflammation by enhancing the bright signal of inflammation and decreasing the fat signal (dark) (Fig. 37.10). Thus T1-MRI demonstrates damage and chronicity, whereas STIR-MRI shows disease activity. Utilizing these concepts, indications for MRI include (1) documentation of myositis or a disease flare in a patient with a normal CK, EMG or biopsy; (2) confirmation of 'amyopathic dermatomyositis'; (3) distinguishing chronic active from chronic inactive myositis; (4) directing the site of biopsy[170]. Limitations in usefulness remain its expense and focal assessment. Also edema (inflammation on STIR images) is not specific for polymyositis or dermatomyositis, as other inflammatory or even metabolic myopathies may demonstrate similar changes.

Magnetic resonance spectroscopy may provide useful data in conjunction with MRI in children and adults[171]. For example, phosphorus-31 magnetic resonance spectroscopy demonstrated significant differences between patients with amyopathic dermatomyositis and normal controls, indicating inefficient metabolic utilization of ATP and phosphocreatine in the patients dermatomyositis, who had been believed to have no muscle involvement using other objective measures[172].

Other muscle imaging techniques such as ultrasound and CT may have utility in patients with myositis. Ultrasound is commonly available and can image blood flow, but it has a small field of view and cannot provide images deep within muscle. CT provides a larger viewing area and can detect calcification and quantify atrophy, but it cannot detect inflammation in the way that MRI can, and it exposes patients to radiation[169].

Skin

The characteristic cutaneous histopathologic findings of dermatomyositis include focal epidermal atrophy, liquefaction and degeneration of the basal cell layer, and a perivascular or upper dermal mononuclear or lymphocytic infiltrate. Vasculitis or vasculopathy is found in the small vessels of the skin and other organs. Microvascular injury mediated by the terminal components of complement (C_{5b-9}) in the form of the membrane attack complex is well recognized. However, the presence of positive immunofluorescence with immunoglobin or complement staining at the dermal–epidermal junction (i.e. positive lupus band test [LBT]) has been debated. One study noted a positive LBT in only six of 29 patients with dermatomyositis[173], and another found that the presence of a positive LBT correlated strongly with SLE; a negative LBT was seen in dermatomyositis, with a sensitivity of nearly 96%[174]. The latter study emphasized the importance of combining histologic and serologic features to improve sensitivity and specificity; statistically the most powerful predictor of dermatomyositis compared with SLE was the combination of a negative LBT, cutaneous vascular deposition of C_{5b-9} and negative serologic tests for anti-SSA and anti-SSB and anti-U1-RNP antibodies. The variance between the two studies may be the result of the use of different criteria for a positive LBT; lack of standardized criteria will continue to plague interpretation of the literature.

Lung

Reduced ventilatory muscle strength is determined by measuring inspiratory pressures at the mouth. Impaired function results in a weak cough, with an increased risk of aspiration pneumonia. A vital capacity of less than 55% of normal predicts carbon dioxide retention as a result of compromise of the ventilatory musculature. ILD is manifested by restrictive physiology on pulmonary function testing, in addition to reduction in the diffusing capacity for carbon monoxide. The chest radiograph is an insensitive measure of pulmonary interstitial involvement, whereas high-resolution CT can provide greater sensitivity and valuable longitudinal information. High-resolution CT findings include ground-glass opacities (alveolitis), consolidation, subpleural lines or bands, traction bronchiectasis and honeycombing (fibrosis) (Fig. 37.11)[175]. The limiting feature of high-resolution CT is the lack of pathologic correlation in published studies. Radionucleotide gallium scans demonstrate increased radiotracer, and may correlate with active alveolitis and response to treatment, but their sensitivity varies widely among readers.

In an effort to correlate the histologic features of ILD in patients with polymyositis–dermatomyositis with the clinical and radiographic variables, 15 patients with three pathologic patterns were studied: BOOP, interstitial pneumonia and diffuse alveolar damage. Patients with BOOP did well, but all three patients with alveolar damage died[176]. A CD8+ lymphocytic infiltrate is seen in biopsy specimens from patients with ILD who are anti-Jo-1 antibody-positive[177] and CD8+ and DR+ cytotoxic lymphocytes were noted in the bronchoalveolar lavage fluid of eight patients with polymyositis or dermatomyositis and ILD[178].

Other markers are being increasingly reported as indicators of lung involvement in patients with polymyositis–dermatomyositis. Anti-

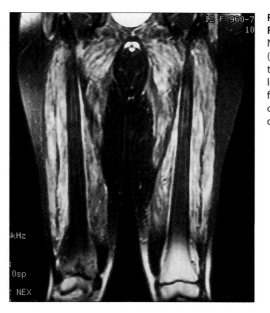

Fig. 37.10
Fat-suppressed MRI.
Note the inflammation (white) in the muscles of the thigh in this longitudinal fat-suppressed MRI of a child with active dermatomyositis.

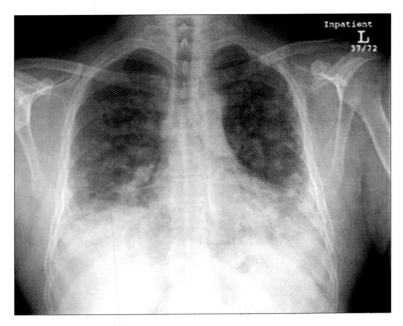

Fig. 37.11 Interstitial lung disease of polymyositis. Chest radiograph of an anti-Jo-1 antibody-positive patient with polymyositis and interstitial lung disease, demonstrating basilar fibrosis and diffuse bilateral interstitial and alveolar infiltrates.

endothelial antibodies were found in 20 of 56 patients with myositis and in 10 of 15 with ILD[179]. Their presence did not correlate with antisynthetase antibodies or any particular polymyositis–dermatomyositis subset, but perhaps they relate to pulmonary endothelial damage from a pathogenetic standpoint[179]. KL-6 is a mucinous glycoprotein expressed on type II pneumocytes and bronchiolar epithelial cells. Its concentration is increased non-specifically in the serum of patients with various connective tissue diseases and pneumonitis[180], and decreases over time after treatment for ILD[181]. Cytokeratin 19 fragment (CK19), a cytoskeletal structural protein of bronchial epithelial cells, was measured in 15 patients with myositis, 10 of whom had pulmonary involvement[182]. The CK19 concentrations were significantly greater in individuals with lung disease, and changed as expected with progression or improvement of ILD.

Heart

Cardiac findings are unusual at disease onset in polymyositis–dermatomyositis, but functional heart problems often develop later. Electrocardiographic abnormalities are common, including non-specific ST–T segment changes and various conduction block disturbances. Holter monitoring can detect arrhythmias and cardiac scintigraphy

using technitium-99m pyrophosphate or indium-labeled antimyosin may be more sensitive in detecting cardiac abnormalities than electrocardiography or gated blood pool studies[183,184]. The use of endomyocardial biopsy is invasive and subject to sampling error.

The myocardial (MB) fraction of CK (CKMB) is increased in patients with myositis, as a result of the release of this isoenzyme from regenerating myoblasts in damaged skeletal muscle. Search for a more specific enzyme marker of cardiac disease led to the use of cardiac troponin T, but a recent study[185] noted that CKMB was increased in 51% and cardiac troponin T in 41% of patients with myositis who had no clinical evidence of cardiac involvement. Cardiac troponin T has also been shown to be expressed in regenerating skeletal muscle in polymyositis and Duchenne muscular dystrophy, and in normal, non-regenerating skeletal muscle[186]. However, cardiac troponin I was increased in only one of 39 patients with polymyositis or dermatomyositis and now appears to be the most cardiac-specific marker in patients with polymyositis–dermatomyositis[185].

Intestine

In patients with pharyngeal (proximal) dysphagia, the barium swallow shows cricopharyngeal muscle spasm, poorly coordinated motion of the pharyngeal musculature and vallecular pooling of the dye and, occasionally, aspiration of barium into the trachea. Oropharyngeal ultrasound may also aid in serial assessment[187]. Distal dysphagia is most frequently accompanied by esophageal hypomotility demonstrated by cinesophagram or manometry, and may occur in patients with non-overlap myositis. Delayed gastric emptying and small bowel dilatation with hypomotility also are documented by barium studies.

Serum autoantibodies

Serum autoantibodies are commonly found in polymyositis–dermatomyositis and are useful in defining clinically homogeneous subsets of patients. The clinical associations of these autoantibodies are reviewed here. Antinuclear autoantibodies or antibodies to cytoplasmic antigens are detected in more than 90% of patients with myositis. Some of these antibodies are termed myositis-specific autoantibodies (MSAs), as they have been previously reported to occur only in patients with features of an inflammatory myopathy. However, the specificity of MSAs is coming under closer scrutiny as more patients without myopathies but having these antibodies are reported[188]. The targets of the MSAs are intracellular antigens (found in all cells) that are commonly involved in protein synthesis, specifically translation. Their role in the pathogenesis of polymyositis–dermatomyositis is unclear; there is no direct evidence that they participate in muscle damage. Autoantibodies typically associated with other connective tissue diseases may also be found in patients with myositis and are termed myositis-associated autoantibodies. Both MSAs and myositis-associated autoantibodies and their clinical

| Autoantibody | Frequency (%) | | | | Clinical features |
	Adult polymyositis	Adult dermatomyositis	Childhood myositis	Overlap	
Jo-1	20–30	5	<5	10	Antisynthetase syndrome
PM-Scl	10	<5	5–10	10	Predominantly overlap with systemic sclerosis
U1-RNP	10	5	5–10	30–40	Predominantly overlap with SLE; MCTD
Mi-2		10	5		Classic rash of DM; good response to treatment
SRP	<5		<1%		Severe muscle weakness; no DM rash
PL-7, PL-12, EJ, OJ, KS	<5				Antisynthetase syndrome
PMS-1[194]	8				No unique features
Ku				5	Polymyositis-scleroderma overlap

TABLE 37.11 SERUM AUTOANTIBODIES IN SUBSETS OF PATIENTS WITH POLYMYOSITIS AND DERMATOMYOSITIS

DM, dermatomyositis; MCTD, mixed connective tissue disease.

TABLE 37.12 ANTIAMINOACYL-tRNA SYNTHETASE ANTIBODIES AND THEIR ASSOCIATED ANTIGENS IN POLYMYOSITIS–DERMATOMYOSITIS

Antibody	Antigen	PM–DM patients with antibody (%)
Anti-Jo-1	Histidyl-tRNA synthetase	20
Anti-PL-7	Threonyl-tRNA synthetase	2
Anti-PL-12	Alanyl-tRNA synthetase	1
Anti-OJ	Isoleucyl-tRNA synthetase	1
Anti-EJ	Glycyl-tRNA synthetase	1
Anti-KS	Asparaginyl-tRNA synthetase	<1

PM–DM, polymyositis–dermatomyositis.

associations are outlined in Table 37.11. Although some patients have more than one autoantibody in their serum, several MSAs are rarely detected in the same patient[189,190]. The frequency of antibody positivity is lower in some myositis subsets such as inclusion body myositis and malignancy-associated myositis, but a negative antinuclear antibody test does not imply that an MSA is absent, as the latter antigens are cytoplasmic in location and the immunofluorescence staining pattern may be subtle. Testing for serum autoantibodies can both solidify the diagnosis of myositis in patients with atypical clinical features and provide prognostic information regarding the likelihood of future clinical complications.

The MSAs are relatively insensitive markers for myositis. Anti-Jo-1 is the most common MSA and is one of a group of anti-aminoacyl-tRNA synthetases (Table 37.12). Anti-Jo-1 is directed against histidyl-tRNA synthetase, an enzyme that binds histidine to its cognate transfer RNA (tRNA^his) so that the amino acid can be incorporated into a growing polypeptide chain. The clinical associations of the various antisynthetase antibodies are similar, and have been described previously as comprising the 'antisynthetase syndrome'. The myositis component of antisynthetase antibody-positive patients is often severe with multiple flares, requiring immunosuppressive agents in addition to corticosteroids. Not all patients with an antisynthetase will manifest all features of the syndrome and some will never develop myositis[84]. For example, anti-PL-12 antibody-positive patients are more likely to have ILD without myositis. Other extramuscular features include fever, inflammatory arthritis, Raynaud's phenomenon and mechanic's hands (see earlier sections and Fig. 37.6). The anti-aminocyl-tRNA autoantibody, anti-WS, binds the L-shaped tertiary structure of tRNA and is therefore different from the other antisynthetases, but patients with this antibody also have recurrent fever, polyarthritis and Raynaud's phenomenon without myositis[191], similar to patients with anti-tRNA synthetases. Antibodies against tRNA or tRNA-associated proteins may also be associated with SLE and Sjögren's syndrome[192]

Antibodies to signal recognition particle (anti-SRP) comprise a separate subgroup of MSAs targeting a ribonucleoprotein involved in translocation. To date, all reported patients with this antibody have pure polymyositis, which is generally refractory to treatment, and progressive. There are no pulmonary, articular or systemic manifestations, but the frequency of cardiomyopathy with congestive heart failure is increased. Anti-Mi-2 is an antinuclear antibody directed against a presumed helicase[193], is strongly associated with the rash of dermatomyositis and has been detected in childhood dermatomyositis and in some patients with malignancy. In general, patients positive for anti-Mi-2 have a favorable response to treatment, but the rash can be severe. A recently described antibody to the DNA mismatch repair enzyme, PMS1, was found in 7.5% of a series of 153 myositis sera and has been proposed as a new MSA[194]. No unique or distinguishing clinical features were identified.

Anti-PM-Scl is an antinucleolar antibody that identifies a subset of patients with myositis who also often have features of systemic sclerosis. It has been seen in patients with polymyositis, dermatomyositis or systemic sclerosis alone, and in patients without evidence of either myositis or scleroderma[195]. Anti-U1-RNP antibodies result in a high-titer speckled antinuclear antibody profile and occur in patients with the so-called 'mixed connective tissue disease'; they may have clinical findings of Raynaud's disease, SLE, polymyositis or dermatomyositis or systemic sclerosis, or any combination thereof.

NATURAL HISTORY OF DISEASE

In some patients, dermatomyositis (but seldom polymyositis) is an illness of brief duration followed by remission that does not require continued treatment. The majority of patients, however, have several exacerbations and remissions or persistent disease activity necessitating chronic use of corticosteroids or immunosuppressive drugs. The frequency of clinical and biochemical relapse was found to be 60% in a series of 50 patients with polymyositis, dermatomyositis and overlap syndrome followed closely for a mean of 13 years[196]. The rates of relapse were similar in each of these patient groups and no features predisposing to relapse were identified. Milder, more easily controlled myositis is reported in community studies as compared with series based on medical centers[197].

With each episode of myositis, there is the potential for absolute loss of muscle mass. The rate of progression and amount of muscle loss differ according to clinical classification and serum autoantibody subtype. The best functional outcome occurs in dermatomyositis, whereas the worst is in inclusion body myositis and polymyositis with anti-SRP antibody. Another poor prognostic feature may be an excess of muscle fibers with absent cytochrome oxidase staining and mitochondrial DNA deletions, but clinically these patients resemble individuals with inclusion body myositis[198].

In childhood-onset dermatomyositis, several predictors of chronic active myositis have been identified, including failure to achieve normal muscle strength after 4 months of corticosteroid treatment, continued increased serum muscle enzyme beyond 3 months and increased plasma von-Willebrand factor antigen over 10 months[199]. Anasarca with hypoalbuminemia has been reported to be an indicator of severe disease in this subset of patients[200].

PROGNOSIS

Assessment of prognosis in polymyositis–dermatomyositis is difficult, for several reasons[201]. First, the disease is relatively uncommon. Some studies involve single referral centers reporting retrospectively on small numbers of patients followed for brief periods of time. Secondly, many reports are cross-sectional in design and combine patients with early and late-stage disease. Thirdly, a classification system with disease subsets based on meaningful pathophysiologic and serologic data has not been developed. Finally, objective criteria for improvement (or deterioration) are not standardized. Today, we lack long-term prospective follow-up of well-defined incident cohorts of patients with myositis that have utilized validated outcome measures[201].

Survival

Studies published before the availability of corticosteroids reveal that a high proportion (up to 50%) of untreated patients with polymyositis–dermatomyositis seen at major medical centers died of its complications[201] (Table 37.13). Although there is no double-blind placebo-controlled documentation of their effect, virtually all investigators agree, and mortality rates demonstrate (Table 37.13), that corticosteroids have improved both muscle weakness and survival during the past 30 years[202–213]. Because of this nearly universal acceptance, for ethical

TABLE 37.13 MORTALITY STATISTICS AND PROGNOSTIC FEATURES OF SEVERAL POLYMYOSITIS–DERMATOMYOSITIS SERIES STRATIFIED BY TREATMENT AND DECADE OF PATIENT ENTRY

Author (year)	Dates of patient entry	No. of patients	Mean follow-up from entry (years)	Mortality rate (%)	Comments
Non-corticosteroid-treated patients					
O'Leary and Waisman[202] (1940)	1926–1939	38	Not stated	50	36/38 with dermatomyositis
Sheard[203] (1951)	1927–1950	25	5.0	52	22/25 with dermatomyositis; 5/7 younger than 20 years died
Winkelmann[204] (1968)	Before 1959	122	3.0	29	(See below)
Corticosteroid-treated patients					**Poor prognostic features**
Rose[26] (1966)	1954–1964	89	6.1	30	Malignancy, other connective tissue disease, acute course
Winkelmann et al.[204] (1968)	Before 1959	157	3.0	35	Malignancy, scleroderma, rapid progression
Medsger et al.[205] (1971)	1947–1968	124	2.5 (median)	36	Pulmonary infiltrates, dysphagia, severe weakness, age >50 years, black race
Carpenter et al.[206] (1977)	1947–1971	62	Not stated	45	Dysphagia, severe weakness
Bohan et al.[207] (1977)	1956–1971	153	4.3	14	Malignancy, older age, delayed treatment
Benbassat et al.[208] (1985)	1956–1976	92	1.8	32	Dysphagia, older age, leukocytosis, fever, failure to induce remission, shorter disease remission
Riddoch and Morgan-Hughes[209] (1975)	1960–1970	20	5.0	40	Study excluded children and patients with cancer and connective tissue disease
Henriksson and Sandstedt[210] (1982)	1967–1978	107	5.0	23	Malignancy, older age, delayed treatment, cardiac involvement
Hochberg et al.[211] (1986)	1970–1981	76	Not stated	17	Age >45 years, cardiac involvement
Tymms and Webb[212] (1985)	1970–1982	105	4.0	18	Older age, delayed treatment
Maugars et al.[213] (1996)	1973–1984	69	11.6	33 (at 5 years)	DM: older age, cancer, interstitial lung disease, asthenia-anorexia; PM: older age, failure to improve muscle strength after 1 month of treatment; absence of myalgia at onset

DM, dermatomyositis; PM, polymyositis.
(Modified from Oddis & Medsger with kind permission of Kluwer Academic Publishers.[201])

reasons, corticosteroids cannot be withheld in today's controlled prospective trials.

During the 1960s, three large series described 265 patients followed for 1.8–5.0 years, with mortality rates varying from 14% to 40%[207–209]. A similar three-study composite of 288 patients reported during the 1970s had only 56 (19%) deaths[210–212]. At the present time, the expected mortality in incident cases of polymyositis–dermatomyositis, excluding those associated with malignancy, is less than 10% at 5 years after initial diagnosis. The reasons for improved survival in recent years are unclear, but may include earlier diagnosis, detection of milder cases, better general medical care and more judicious use of immunosuppressive drugs.

Factors associated with poor survival in these reports include older age, malignancy, delayed initiation of corticosteroid treatment, pharyngeal dysphagia with aspiration pneumonia, ILD, myocardial involvement and complications of corticosteroid or immunosuppressive treatment. Additional adverse risk factors for survival among patients with childhood dermatomyositis are gastrointestinal vasculitis and sepsis[214].

The 5-year cumulative survival rate from the time of first physician diagnosis is worst for cancer-associated myositis (55%) and dermatomyositis (80%) and best for connective tissue disease related myositis (85%) and inclusion body myositis (95%). Among the serum autoantibodies, anti-SRP is the worst prognostic marker (5-year survival 30%), followed by the antisynthetase group (65%). The best survival is among patients with anti-PM-Scl (95%) and anti-Mi-2 (95%).

Disability

The determinants of functional status in polymyositis–dermatomyositis are quite different from those of survival. For example, inclusion body myositis has the worst functional outlook, but a good survival because of the lack of visceral involvement. For all types of myositis, each major exacerbation results in a reduction in muscle strength, but treatment almost never improves the patient to the preceding level of total body muscle mass or strength. Fortunately, minor residual atrophy and weakness in one or more muscle groups most often do not translate into functional impairment.

In one 20-year follow-up study of 118 patients, 67% of the 82 survivors had no functional disability[215]. In another report, 87% of 107 patients who improved initially with medical treatment had minimal or no disability after a mean follow-up of 5 years[210]. In a prospective longitudinal study, the patient-completed Health Assessment Questionnaire was used to follow a national cohort of 257 patients with polymyositis–dermatomyositis during years 3–7 after disease diagnosis[216]. Disability (judged by the Health Assessment Questionnaire disability index) increased with disease duration. In individuals with increased disability early in disease, the disability index was highly correlated with the corticosteroid treatment-related complications of osteonecrosis and osteoporotic compression fractures of the lumbar spine.

A childhood Health Assessment Questionnaire for measuring disability in juvenile dermatomyositis has been validated[217]. Children with dermatomyositis have been shown to have decreased calcium absorption, especially while receiving corticosteroids[218], and may thus be at much greater risk for osteoporosis when they become adults. Other disease-related sequelae include calcinosis (especially in juvenile dermatomyositis), arthropathy, Raynaud's phenomenon, respiratory insufficiency as a result of pulmonary interstitial fibrosis or diaphragmatic muscle involvement, and myocardial involvement with congestive heart failure or ventricular arrhythmias.

The contribution of corticosteroid and immunosuppressive drug toxicity to long-term disability has not been adequately addressed, but the frequency of serious adverse reactions has been reported to be 20–40%[12,197,210,212]. The most commonly encountered disabling side effects include osteoporotic bone fractures, osteonecrosis, serious bacterial and fungal infections, and cataracts. Problems that are inconvenient and require frequent physician visits, expensive medications and toxicity monitoring are diabetes mellitus, hypertension and peptic ulcer disease. Early cytopenias, with complications including septicemia, and late hematologic malignancies are serious concerns in patients with myositis requiring immunosuppressive drugs.

REFERENCES

1. Potain. Morve chronique de formed anomale. Bull Soc Méd Paris 1875; 12: 314–318.
2. Wagner EL. Erin Fall von Polymyositis. Dtsch Arch Klin Med 1886; 40: 241–266.
3. Jacoby GW. Subacute progressive polymyositis. J Nerv Ment Dis 1888; 13: 697–726.
4. Unverricht H. Dermatomyositis acuta. Dtsch Med Wochenschr 1891; 17: 41–44.
5. Gottron H. In: Proceedings of the Berlin Dermatologic Society. Dermatol Z 1930; 61: 415–418.
6. Stertz. Polymyositis. Berl Klin Wochenschr 1916; 53: 489.
7. Kankeleit. Über primäre nichteitrige Polymyositis. Dtsch Arch Klin Med 1916; 120: 335–349.
8. Becezny R. Dermatomyositis. Arch Derm Syph 1935; 171: 242–251.
9. Chou SM. Myxovirus-like structures in a case of human chronic polymyositis. Science 1967; 158: 1453–1455.
10. Yunis EJ, Samaha FJ. Inclusion body myositis. Lab Invest 1971; 25: 240–248.
11. Medsger TA Jr, Oddis CV. Classification and diagnostic criteria for PM and DM [editorial]. J Rheumatol 1995; 22: 581–585.
12. Bohan A, Peter JB. Polymyositis and dermatomyositis. N Engl J Med 1975; 292: 344–347, 403–407.
13. Medsger TA Jr. Polymyositis and dermatomyositis. In: Lawrence RC, Shulman LE, eds. Epidemiology of the rheumatic diseases. New York: Gower Medical Publishing; 1984: 176–180.
14. Targoff IN, Miller FW, Medsger TA Jr et al. Classification criteria for the idiopathic inflammatory myopathies. Curr Opin Rheumatol 1997; 9: 527–535.
15. Hausmanowa-Petruseqicz I, Kowalska-Oledzka E, Miller FW et al. Clinical, serologic, and immunogenetic features in Polish patients with idiopathic inflammatory myopathies. Arthritis Rheum 1997; 40: 1257–1266.
16. Okano Y, Steen VD, Medsger TA Jr. Autoantibody to U3 nucleolar ribonucleoprotein (fibrillarin) in patients with systemic sclerosis. Arthritis Rheum 1992; 35: 95–100.
17. Ioannou Y, Sultan S, Isenberg DA. Myositis overlap syndromes. Curr Opin Rheumatol 1999; 11: 468–474.
18. Miro' O, Pedrol EN, Casademont J et al. Muscle involvement in rheumatoid arthritis: clinicopathological study of 21 symptomatic cases. Semin Arthritis Rheum 1996; 25: 421–428.
19. Garton MJ, Isenberg DA. Clinical features of lupus myositis versus idiopathic myositis: a review of 30 cases. Br J Rheumatol 1997; 36: 1067–1074.
20. Gran JT, Myklebust G. The concomitant occurrence of Sjögren's syndrome and polymyositis. Scan J Rheumatol 1992, 21: 150–154.
21. De Vlam K, De Keyser F, Goemaere S et al. Churg–Strauss syndrome presenting as polymyositis. Clin Exp Rheumatol 1995; 13: 505–507.
22. Al Attia HM, Ezzeddin H, Khader T et al. A localised morphoea/idiopathic polymyositis overlap. Clin Rheumatol 1996; 15: 307–309.
23. Dunne JW, Heye N, Edis RH et al. Necrotizing inflammatory myopathy associated with localized scleroderma. Muscle Nerve 1996; 19: 1040–1042.
24. Miyaoka Y, Urano Y, Nameda Y et al. A case of dermatomyositis complicated by thrombotic thrombocytopenic purpura. Dermatology 1997; 194: 68–71.
25. Sherer Y, Livneh A, Levy Y et al. Dermatomyositis and polymyositis associated with the antiphospholipid syndrome – a novel overlap syndrome. Lupus 2000; 9: 42–46.
26. Rose AL, Walton JN. Polymyositis. A survey of 89 cases with particular reference to treatment and prognosis. Brain 1966; 89: 747–768.
27. Kurland LT, Hauser WA, Ferguson RH et al. Epidemiologic features of diffuse connective tissue disorders in Rochester, Minnesota, 1951–1967, with special reference to systemic lupus erythematosus. Mayo Clin Proc 1969; 44: 649–663.
28. Findlay GH, Whiting DA, Simson IW. Dermatomyositis in the Transvaal and its occurrence in the Bantu. S Afr Med J 1969; 43: 694–697.
29. Medsger TA, Dawson WN, Masi AT. The epidemiology of polymyositis. Am J Med 1970; 48: 715–723.
30. Benbassat J, Geffel D, Zlotnick A. Epidemiology of polymyositis–dermatomyositis in Israel, 1960–76. Isr J Med Sci 1980; 16: 197–200.
31. Oddis CV, Conte CG, Steen VD et al. Incidence of PM-DM. A 20-year study of hospital diagnosed cases in Allegheny County, PA 1963–1982. J Rheumatol 1990; 17: 1329–1334.
32. Weitoft T. Occurrence of polymyositis in the country of Gavleborg, Sweden. Scand J Rheumatol 1997; 26: 104–106.
33. Patrick M, Buchbinder R, Jolley D et al. Incidence of inflammatory myopathies in Victoria, Australia, and evidence of spatial clustering. J Rheumatol 1999; 26: 1094–1100.
34. Badrising UA, Maat-Schieman M, van Duninen SG et al. Epidemiology of inclusion body myositis in the Netherlands: a nationwide study. Neurology 2000; 55: 1385–1387.
35. Hengstman GJD, van Venrooij WJ, Vencovsky J et al. The relative prevalence of dermatomyositis and polymyositis in Europe exhibits a latitudinal gradient. Ann Rheum Dis 2000; 59: 141–142.
36. Christensen ML, Pachman LM, Schneiderman R et al. Prevalence of Coxsackie B virus antibodies in patients with juvenile dermatomyositis. Arthritis Rheum 1986; 29: 1365–1370.
37. Hoffman JC, Stichtenoth DO, Zeidler H et al. Lyme disease in a 74-year-old forest owner with symptoms of dermatomyositis. Arthritis Rheum 1995; 38: 1157–1160.
38. Sherman MP, Amin RM, Rodgers-Johnson PEB et al. Identification of human T cell leukemia/lymphoma virus type I antibodies, DNA, and protein in patients with polymyositis. Arthritis Rheum 1995; 38: 690–698.
39. Baguley E, Wolfe C, Hughes GRV. Dermatomyositis in HIV infection [letter]. Br J Rheumatol 1988; 27: 493–494.
40. Dennett X, Siejka SJ, Andrews JRH et al. Polymyositis caused by a new genus of nematode. Med J Aust 1998; 168: 226–227.
41. Perez C, Gurtubay I, Martinez-Ibanex F et al. More on polymyositis associated with mycoplasma pneumoniae infection. Scan J Rheumatol 1999; 28: 125.
42. Lyon ME, Bloch DA, Hollak B et al. Predisposing factors in PM–DM: results of a nationwide survey. J Rheumatol 1989; 16: 1218–1224.
43. Fernandes L, Swinson DR, Hamilton EBD. Dermatomyositis complicating penicillamine treatment. Ann Rheum Dis 1977; 36: 94–95.
44. Hanke CW, Thomas JA, Lee EW-T et al. Risk assessment of polymyositis/dermatomyositis after treatment with injectable bovine collagen implants. J Am Acad Dermatol 1996; 34: 450–454.
45. Harati Y, Niakan E, Bergman EW. Childhood dermatomyositis in monozygotic twins. Neurology 1986; 36: 721–723.
46. Leonhardt T. Familial occurrence of collagen diseases. II. Progressive systemic sclerosis and dermatomyositis. Acta Med Scand 1961; 169: 735–742.
47. Davies MG, Hickling P. Familial adult dermatomyositis. Br J Dermatol 2001; 144: 415–448.
48. Rider LG, Gurley RC, Pandey JP et al. Clinical, serologic, and immunogenetic features of familial idiopathic inflammatory myopathy. Arthritis Rheum 1998; 41: 710–719.
49. Ginn LR, Lin J-P, Plotz PH et al. Familial autoimmunity in pedigrees of idiopathic inflammatory myopathy patients suggests common genetic risk factors for many autoimmune diseases. Arthritis Rheum 1998; 41: 400–405.
50. Shamim EA, Rider LG, Miller FW. Update on the genetics of the idiopathic inflammatory myopathies. Curr Opin Rheum 2000; 12: 482–491.
51. Reed AM, Pachman LM, Hayford J et al. Immunogenetic studies in families of children with juvenile dermatomyositis. J Rheumatol 1998; 25: 1000–1002.
52. West JE, Reed AM. Analysis of HLA-DM polymorphism in juvenile dermatomyositis (JDM) patients. Hum Immunol 1999; 60: 255–258.
53. Rider LG, Artlett CM, Foster CB et al: Polymorphisms in the IL-1 receptor antagonist gene VNTR are possible risk factors for juvenile idiopathic inflammatory myopathies. Clin Exp Immunol 2000; 120: 1–7.
54. Pachman LM, Liotta-Davis M, Hong D, et al. TNF alpha-308A allele in juvenile dermatomyositis: associations with increased production of tumor necrosis factor alpha, disease duration, and pathologic calcifications. Arthritis Rheum 2000; 43: 2368–2377.
55. Bogousslavsky JE, Perentes E, Regli F, Deruaz JP. Polymyositis with severe facial involvement. J Neurol 1982; 228: 277–281.
56. Csuka ME, McCarty DJ. A rapid method for measurement of lower extremity muscle strength. Am J Med 1985; 78: 77–81.
57. Helewa A, Goldsmith CH, Smythe HA. Patient, observer and instrument variation in the measurement of strength of shoulder abductor muscles in patients with rheumatoid arthritis using a modified sphygmomanometer. J Rheumatol 1986; 6: 1044–1049.
58. Stoll T, Bruehlmann P, Stucki G et al. Muscle strength assessment in polymyositis and dermatomyositis: evaluation of the reliability and clinical use of a new, quantitative, easily applicable method. J Rheumatol 1995; 22: 473–477.
59. Kasteler JS, Callen JP. Scalp involvement in dermatomyositis. JAMA 1994; 272: 1939–1941.
60. Oddis CV, Okano Y, Rudert WA et al. Serum autoantibody to the nucleolar antigen PM-Scl. Arthritis Rheum 1992; 35: 1211–1217.
61. Sabroe RA, Wallington TB, Kennedy CTC. Dermatomyositis treated with high-dose intravenous immunoglobulins and associated with panniculitis. Clin Exp Dermatol 1995; 20: 164–167.
62. Chao Y-Y, Yang L-J. Dermatomyositis presenting as panniculitis. Int J Dermatol 2000; 39: 141–144.
63. Molnar K, Kemeny L, Korom I et al. Panniculitis in dermatomyositis: report of two cases. Br J Dermatol 1998; 139: 161–163.
64. Ishikawa O, Tamura A, Ryuzaki K et al. Membranocystic changes in the panniculitis of dermatomyositis. Br J Dermatol 1996; 134: 773–776.
65. Kimball AB, Summers RM, Turner M et al. Magnetic resonance imaging detection of occult skin and subcutaneous abnormalities in juvenile dermatomyositis. Arthritis Rheum 2000; 43: 1866–1873.
66. Nousari HC, Ha VT, Laman SD et al. 'Centripetal flagellate erythema': a cutaneous manifestation associated with dermatomyositis. J Rheumatol 1999; 26: 692–695.
67. Ferrer M, Herranz P, Manzano R et al. Dermatomyositis with linear lesions. Br J Dermatol 1996; 134: 600–601.

68. Requena L, Grilli R, Soriano L et al. Dermatomyositis with a pityriasis rubra pilaris-like eruption: a little-known distinctive cutaneous manifestation of dermatomyositis. Br J Dermatol 1997; 136: 768–771.

69. See Y, Rooney M, Woo P. Palmar plantar hyperkeratosis – a previously undescribed skin manifestation of juvenile dermatomyositis. Br J Rheumatol 1997; 36: 917–919.

70. Katayama I, Sawada Y, Nishioka K. The seborrhoeic pattern of dermatomyositis. Br J Dermatol 1999; 140: 978–979.

71. Del Pozo J, Almagro M, Martinez W et al. Dermatomyositis and mucinosis. Int J Dermatol 2001; 40: 120–124.

72. Inuzuka M, Tomita K, Tokura Y et al. Acquired ichthyosis associated with dermatomyositis in a patient with hepatocellular carcinoma. Br J Dermatol 2001; 14: 416–417.

73. McCollough ML, Cockrell CJ. Vesiculo-bullous dermatomyositis. Am J Dermatopathol 1998; 20: 170–174.

74. Sontheimer RD. Cutaneous features of classic dermatomyositis and amyopathic dermatomyositis. Cur Opin Rheumatol 1999; 11: 475–482.

75. Osman Y, Narita M, Kishi K et al. Case report: amyopathic dermatomyositis associated with transformed malignant lymphoma. Am J Med Sci 1996; 311: 240–242.

76. Whitmore SE, Watson R, Rosenshein NB et al. Dermatomyositis sine myositis: association with malignancy. J Rheumatol 1996; 23: 1010–1015.

77. Mukamel M, Horev G, Mimouni M. New insight into calcinosis of juvenile dermatomyositis: a study of composition and treatment. J Pediatr 2001; 138: 763–766.

78. Tse S, Lubelsky S, Gordon M et al. The arthritis of inflammatory childhood myositis syndromes. J Rheumatol 2001; 28: 192–197.

79. Wasko MC, Carlson GW, Tomaino MM et al. Dermatomyositis with erosive arthropathy: association with the anti-PL-7 antibody. J Rheumatol 1999; 26: 2693–2694.

80. Oddis CV, Medsger TA Jr, Cooperstein LA. A subluxing arthropathy associated with the anti Jo-1 antibody in polymyositis/dermatomyositis. Arthritis Rheum 1990; 33: 1640–1645.

81. Citera G, Lazaro MA, Cocco JAM et al. Apatite deposition in polymyositis subluxing arthropathy. J Rheumatol 1996; 23: 551–553.

82. Brennan MT, Patronas NJ, Brahim J. Bilateral condylar resorption in dermatomyositis: a case report. Oral Surg Oral Med Oral Pathol 1999; 87: 446–451.

83. Queiro-Silva R, Banegil I, deDios-Jimenez de Aberassturi JR et al. Periarticular calcinosis associated with anti-Jo-1 antibodies sine myositis. Expanding the clinical spectrum of the antisynthetase syndrome. J Rheumatol 2001; 28: 1401–1404.

84. Friedman AW, Targoff IN, Arnett FC. Interstitial lung disease with autoantibodies against aminoacyl-tRNA synthetases in the absence of clinically apparent myositis. Semin Arthritis Rheum 1996; 26: 459–467.

85. Chow SK, Yeap SS. Amyopathic dermatomyositis and pulmonary fibrosis. Clin Rheumatol 2001; 19: 484–485.

86. Selva-O'Callaghan A, Sanchez-Sitjes L, Munoz-Gall X et al. Respiratory failure due to muscle weakness in inflammatory myopathies: maintenance therapy with home mechanical ventilation. Br J Rheumatol 2000; 39: 914–916.

87. Rini BI, Gajewski TF. Polymyositis with respiratory muscle weakness requiring mechanical ventilation in a patient with metastatic thymoma treated with octreotide. Ann Oncol 1999; 10: 913–919.

88. Braun NMT, Aroyan S, Rochester DF. Respiratory muscle and pulmonary function in polymyositis and other proximal myopathies. Thorax 1983; 38: 616–623.

89. Clawson K, Oddis CV. Adult respiratory distress syndrome in polymyositis patients with the anti-Jo-1 antibody. Arthritis Rheum 1995; 38: 1519–1523.

90. Schwarz MI, Sutarik JM, Nick JA et al. Pulmonary capillaritis and diffuse alveolar hemorrhage. A primary manifestation of polymyositis. J Respir Crit Care Med 1995; 151: 2037–2040.

91. Horiki T, Fuyuno G, Ishii M et al. Fatal alveolar hemorrhage in a patient with mixed connective tissue disease presenting polymyositis features. Intern Med 1998; 37: 554–560.

92. Fata F, Rathore R, Schiff C et al. Bronchiolitis obliterans organizing pneumonia as the first manifestation of polymyositis. South Med J 1997; 90: 227–230.

93. Knoell KA, Hook M, Grice DP et al. Dermatomyositis associated with bronchiolitis obliterans organizing pneumonia (BOOP). J Am Acad Dermatol 1999; 40: 328–330.

94. Jansen TLTA, Barrera P, van Engelen BGM et al. Dermatomyositis with subclinical myositis and spontaneous pneumomediastinum with pneumothorax: case report and review of the literature. Clin Exp Rheumatol 1998; 16: 733–735.

95. Yamanishi Y, Maeda H, Konishi F et al. Dermatomyositis associated with rapidly progressive fatal interstitial pneumonitis and pneumomediastinum. Scand J Rheumatol 1999; 28: 58–61.

96. Kono H, Inokuma S, Nakayama H et al. Pneumomediastinum in dermatomyositis: association with cutaneous vasculopathy. Ann Rheum Dis 2000; 59: 372–376.

97. Korkmaz C, Ozkan R, Akay M et al. Pneumomediastinum and subcutaneous emphysema associated with dermatomyositis. Rheumatology 2001; 40: 476–478.

98. Bachelez H, Schremmer B, Cadranel J et al. Fulminant Pneumocystis carinii pneumonia in patients with dermatomyositis. Arch Intern Med 1997; 157: 1501–1503.

99. LaCivita L, Battiloro R, Celano M. Nocardia pleural empyema complicating anti-Jo-1 positive polymyositis during immunoglobulin and steroid therapy. J Rheumatol 2001; 28: 215–216.

100. Gonzalez-Lopez L, Gamez-Nava JI, Sanchez L et al. Cardiac manifestations in dermato–polymyositis. Clin Exp Rheumatol 1996; 14: 373–379.

101. Gordon M-M, Madhok R. Fatal myocardial necrosis. Ann Rheum Dis 1999; 58: 198–199.

102. Chraibi S, Ibnabdeljalil H, Habbal R et al. Pericardial tamponade as the first manifestation of dermatopolymyositis. Ann Med Intern 1998; 149: 464–466.

103. Lie JT. Cardiac manifestations in polymyositis/dermatomyositis: how to get to the heart of the matter. J Rheumatol 1995; 22: 809–811.

104. Anders H-J, Wandes A, Rihl M et al. Myocardial fibrosis in polymyositis. J Rheumatol 1999; 26: 1840–1842.

105. Badui EI, Valdespino A, Lepe L et al. Acute myocardial infarction with normal coronary arteries in a patient with dermatomyositis. Angiology 1996; 47: 815–818.

106. Riemekasten G , Optiz C, Audring H et al. Beware of the heart: the multiple picture of cardiac involvement in myositis. Br J Rheumatol 1999; 38: 1153–1157.

107. Shapiro J, DeGirolami U, Martin S et al. Inflammatory myopathy causing pharyngeal dysphagia: a new entity. Ann Otol Rhinol Laryngol 1996; 105: 331–335.

108. Caramaschi P, Biasi D, Carletto A et al. Megaesophagus in a patient affected by dermatomyositis. Clin Rheumatol 1997; 16: 106–107.

109. Kuroda T, Ohfuchi Y, Hirose S et al. Pneumatosis cystoides intestinalis in a patient with polymyositis. Clin Rheumatol 2001; 20: 49–52.

110. Eshraghi N, Farahmand M, Maerz LL et al. Adult-onset dermatomyositis with severe gastrointestinal manifestations: case report and review of the literature. Surgery 1998; 123: 356–358.

111. Braun-Moscovici Y, Schapira D, Balbir-Gurman A et al. Inflammatory bowel disease and myositis. Clin Rheumatol 1999; 18: 261–263.

112. Voigt E, Griga T, Tromm A et al. Polymyositis of the skeletal muscles as an extraintestinal complication in quiescent ulcerative colitis. Int J Colorectal Dis 1999; 14: 304–307.

113. Bondeson J, Veress B, Lindroth Y et al. Polymyositis associated with asymptomatic primary biliary cirrhosis. Clin Exp Rheumatol 1998; 16: 172–174.

114. Seibold F, Klein R, Jakob F. Polymyositis, alopecia universalis, and primary sclerosing cholangitis in a patient with Crohn's disease. J Clin Gastroenterol 1996; 22: 121–124.

115. Russo RAG, Katsicas MM, Davila M et al. Cholestasis in juvenile dermatomyositis. Arthritis Rheum 2001; 44: 1139–1142.

116. Evron E, Abarbanel JM, Branski D et al. Polymyositis, arthritis, and proteinuria in a patient with adult celiac disease. J Rheumatol 1996; 23: 782–783.

117. Oddis CV. Inflammatory diseases of blood vessels. Hoffman GS, Weyand CM, eds. New York: Marcel Dekker, Inc.; 2001: 665–674.

118. Thakur V, DeSalvo J, McGrath J Jr et al. Case report: polymyositis-induced myoglobinuric acute renal failure. Am J Med Sci 1996; 312: 85–87.

119. Yeo LMW, Swaby DSA, Situnayake RD et al. Irreversible visual loss in dermatomyositis. Br J Rheumatol 1995; 34: 1179–1181.

120. Backhouse O, Griffiths B, Henderson T et al. Ophthalmic manifestations of dermatomyositis. Ann Rheum Dis 1998; 57: 447–449.

121. Orrell RW, Johnston HM, Gibson C et al. Spontaneous abdominal hematoma in dermatomyositis. Muscle Nerve 1998; 21: 1800–1803.

122. Tubridy N, Wells C, Lewis D et al. Unsuccessful treatment with cidofovir and cytarabine in progressive multifocal leukoencephalopathy associated with dermatomyositis. J R Soc Med 2000; 93: 374–375.

123. Regan M, Haque U, Pomper M et al. Central nervous system vasculitis as a complication of refractory dermatomyositis. J Rheumatol 2001; 28: 207–211.

124. Aarli JA. Inflammatory myopathy in myasthenia gravis. Curr Opin Neurol 1998; 11: 233–234.

125. Wortmann RL. Metabolic and mitochondrial myopathies. Curr Opin Rheumatol 1999; 11: 462–467.

126. Bolton CF. Critical illness polyneuropathy and myopathy. Crit Care Med 2001; 29: 2388–2390.

127. Lacomis D, Giuliani MJ, Cott AV et al. Acute myopathy of intensive care: clinical, electromyographic, and pathological aspects. Ann Neurol 1996; 40: 645–654.

128. Patel SR, Olenginski TP, Perruquet JL et al. Pyomyositis: clinical features and predisposing conditions. J Rheumatol 1997; 24: 1734–1738.

129. Heffner RR, Armbrustmacher WV, Earle KM. Focal myositis. Cancer 1977; 40: 302–306.

130. Umpierrez GE, Stiles RG, Kleinbart J et al. Diabetic muscle infarction. Am J Med 1996; 101: 245–250.

131. Pickering MC, Walport MJ. Eosinophilic myopathic syndromes. Curr Opin Rheumatol 1998; 10: 504–510.

132. Hall FC, Krausz T, Walport MJ. Idiopathic eosinophilic myositis. Q J Med 1995; 88: 581–586.

133. Mandl LA, Folkerth RD, Pick MA et al. Amyloid myopathy masquerading as polymyositis. J Rheumatol 2000; 27: 949–952.

134. Cherin P, Gherardi RK. Macrophagic myofasciitis. Curr Rheum Reports 2000; 2: 196–200.

135. Whitmore SE, Watson R, Rosenshein NB et al. Dermatomyositis sine myositis: association with malignancy. J Rheumatol 1996; 23: 101–105.

136. Maoz CR, Langevitz P, Livneh A et al. High incidence of malignancies in patients with dermatomyositis and polymyositis: an 11-year analysis. Semin Arthritis Rheum 1998; 27: 319–324.

137. Hill CL, Zhang Y, Sigurgeirsson B et al. Frequency of specific cancer types in dermatomyositis and polymyositis: a population-based study. Lancet 2001; 357: 96–100.

138. Chen Y-J, Wu C-Y, Shen J-L. Predicting factors of malignancy in dermatomyositis and polymyositis: a case–control study. Br J Dermatol 2001; 144: 825–831.

139. Buchbinder R, Forbes A, Hall S et al. Incidence of malignant disease in biopsy-proven inflammatory myopathy. Ann Intern Med 2001; 134: 1087–1095.

140. Whitmore SE, Rosenshein NB, Provost TT. Ovarian cancer in patients with dermatomyositis. Medicine 1994; 73: 153–160.

141. Whitmore SE, Anhalt FJ, Provost TT et al. Serum Ca-125 screening for ovarian cancer in patients with dermatomyositis. Gynecol Oncol 1997; 65: 241–244.

142. Hu W, Chen D, Min H. Study of 45 cases of nasopharyngeal carcinoma with dermatomyositis. Am J Clin Oncol 1996; 19: 35–38.

143. Mautner GH, Grossman ME, Silvers DN et al. Epidermal necrosis as a predictive sign of malignancy in adult dermatomyositis. Cutis 1998; 61: 190–194.

144. Hunger RE, Durr C, Brand CU. Cutaneous leukocytoclastic vasculitis in dermatomyositis suggests malignancy. Dermatology 2001; 202: 123–126.

145. Airio A, Pukkala E, Isomaki H. Elevated cancer incidence in patients with dermatomyositis: a population based study. J Rheumatol 1995; 22: 1300–1303.

146. Lee AJ, Maddix DS. Rhabdomyolysis secondary to a drug interaction between simvastatin and clarithromycin. Ann Pharmacother 2001; 35: 26–31.

147. Renders L, Mayer-Kadner I, Koch C et al. Efficacy and drug interactions of the new HMG-Co-A reductase inhibitors cerivastatin and atorvastatin in CsA-treated renal transplant recipients. Nephrol Dial Transplant 2001; 16: 141–146.

148. Schalke BB, Schmidt B, Toyka K et al. Pravastatin-associated inflammatory myopathy. N Eng J Med 1992; 327: 649–650.

149. Hino I, Akama H, Furuya T et al. Pravastatin-induced rhabdomyolysis in a patient with mixed connective tissue disease. Arthritis Rheum 1996; 39: 1259–1261.

150. Rodriguez-Garcia JL, Serrano Commino M. Lovastatin-associated dermatomyositis. Postgrad Med J 1996; 72: 694.

151. Giordano N, Senesi M, Mattii, G et al. Polymyositis associated with simvastatin. Lancet 1997; 349: 1600–1601.

152. Hill C, Zeitz C, Kirkham B. Dermatomyositis with lung involvement in a patient treated with simvastatin. Aust NZ J Med 1995; 25: 745–746.

153. Dawson TM, Starkebaum G. Colchicine induced rhabdomyolysis. J Rheumatol 1997; 24: 2045–2046.

154. Estes ML, Ewing-Wilson D, Chou SM et al. Chloroquine neuromyotoxicity: clinical and pathologic perspective. Am J Med 1987; 82: 447–455.

155. Avina-Zubieta JA, Johnson ES, Suarez-Almazor ME et al. Incidence of myopathy in patients treated with antimalarials. A report of three cases and a review of the literature. Br J Rheumatol 1995; 34: 166–170.

156. Marie I, Joly P, Levesque H et al. Pseudo-dermatomyositis as a complication of hydroxyurea therapy. Clin Exp Rheumatol 2000; 18: 536–537.

157. Kim HA, Song YW. Polymyositis developing after prolonged injections of pentazocine. J Rheumatol 1996; 2: 1644–1646.

158. Kivanc MT, Klaus MV, Nashel DJ. Reversible polymyositis occurring during psoralen and ultraviolet A (PUVA) therapy. J Rheumatol 2000; 27: 1823–1824.

159. Esteva-Lorenzo FJ, Janik JE, Fenton RG et al. Myositis associated with interleukin-2 therapy in a patient with metastatic renal cell carcinoma. Cancer 1995; 76: 1219–1223.

160. Kalkner K-M, Ronnblom L, Parra AK et al. Antibodies against double-stranded DNA and development of polymyositis during treatment with interferon. Q J Med 1998; 91: 393–399.

161. Serratrice J, Granel B, Pache X et al. A case of polymyositis with anti-histidyl-t-RNA synthetase (Jo-1) antibody syndrome following extensive vinyl chloride exposure. Clin Rheumatol 2001; 20: 379–382.

162. Rider LG. Assessment of disease activity and its sequelae in children and adults with myositis. Curr Opin Rheumatol 1996; 8: 495–506.

163. Miller FW, Rider LG, Churg Y-L et al. Proposed preliminary core set measures for disease outcome assessment in adult and juvenile idiopathic inflammatory myopathies. Rheumatology 2001; 40: 1262–1273.

164. Kagen LJ, Aram S. Creatine kinase activity inhibitor in serum from patients with muscle disease. Arthritis Rheum 1987; 30: 213–217.

165. Johnston JD, Lloyd M, Mathews J et al. Racial variation in serum creatine kinase levels. J Roy Soc Med 1996; 89: 462–464.

166. Rose MR, Kissel JT, Bickley LS et al. Sustained myoglobinuria: the presenting manifestation of dermatomyositis. Neurology 1996; 47: 119–123.

167. Kumamoto T, Ueyama H, Fujimoto S et al. Clinicopathologic characteristics of polymyositis patients with numerous tissue eosinophils. Acta Neurol Scand 1996; 94: 110–114.

168. Campellone JV, Lacomis D, Giuliani MJ et al. Percutaneous needle muscle biopsy in the evaluation of patients with suspected inflammatory myopathy. Arthritis Rheum 1997; 40: 1886–1891.

169. Park JH, Olsen NJ. Utility of magnetic resonance imaging in the evaluation of patients with inflammatory myopathies. Curr Rheum Reports 2001; 3: 334–345.

170. Lampa J, Nennesmo I, Einarsdottir H et al. MRI guided muscle biopsy confirmed polymyositis diagnosis in a patient with interstitial lung disease. Ann Rheum Dis 2001; 60: 423–426.

171. Park JH, Niermann KJ, Ryder NM et al. Muscle abnormalities in juvenile dermatomyositis patients. Arthritis Rheum 2000; 43: 2359–2367.

172. Park JH, Olsen NJ, King LE et al. MRI and P-31 magnetic resonance spectroscopy detect and quantify muscle dysfunction in the amyopathic and myopathic variants of dermatomyositis. Arthritis Rheum 1995; 38: 68–77.

173. Vaughan Jones SA, Black MM. The value of direct immunofluorescence as a diagnostic aid in dermatomyositis – a study of 35 cases. Clin Exp Dermatol 1997; 22: 77–81.

174. Magro CM, Crowson AN. The immunofluorescent profile of dermatomyositis: a comparative study with lupus erythematosus. J Cutan Pathol 1997; 24: 543–552.

175. Akira M, Hara H, Sakatani M. Interstitial lung disease in association with polymyositis-dermatomyositis: long-term follow-up CT evaluation in seven patients. Radiology 1999; 210: 333–338.

176. Tazelaar HD, Viggiano W, Pickersgill J et al. Interstitial lung disease in polymyositis and dermatomyositis. Clinical features and prognosis as correlated with histologic findings. Am Rev Respir Dis 1990; 141: 727–733.

177. Sauty A, Rochat TH, Schoch OD et al. Pulmonary fibrosis with predominant CD8 lymphocytic alveolitis and anti-Jo-1 antibodies. Eur Respir J 1997; 10: 2907–2912.

178. Kourakata H, Takada T, Suzuki E et al. Flow cytomeric analysis of bronchoalveolar lavage fluid cells in polymyositis/dermatomyositis with interstitial pneumonia. Respirology 1999; 4: 223–228.

179. D'Cruz D, Keser G, Khamashta MA et al. Antiendothelial cell antibodies in inflammatory myopathies: distribution among clinical and serologic groups and association with interstitial lung disease. J Rheumatol 2000; 27: 161–164.

180. Nakajima H, Harigai M, Hara M et al. KL-6 as a novel serum marker for interstitial pneumonia associated with collagen diseases. J Rheumatol 2000; 7: 1164–1170.

181. Bandoh S, Fujita J, Ohtsuki Y et al. Sequential changes of KL-6 in sera of patients with interstitial pneumonia associated with polymyositis/dermatomyositis. Ann Rheum Dis 2000; 59: 257–262.

182. Fujita J, Dobashi N, Tokuda M et al. Elevation of cytokeratin 19 fragment in patients with interstitial pneumonia associated with polymyositis/dermatomyositis. J Rheumatol 1999; 26: 2377–2382.

183. Buchpiguel CA, Roizemblatt S, Pastor EH et al. Cardiac and skeletal muscle scintigraphy in dermato- and polymyositis: clinical implications. Eur J Nucl Med 1996; 23: 199–203.

184. Sarda L, Assayag P, Palazzo E et al. Indium antimyosin antibody imaging of primary myocardial involvement in systemic diseases. Ann Rheum Dis 1999; 58: 90–95.

185. Erlacher P, Lercher A, Falkensammer J et al. Cardiac troponin and β-type myosin heavy chain concentrations in patients with polymyositis or dermatomyositis. Clin Chim Acta 2001; 306: 27–33.

186. Bodor GS, Survant L, Voss EM et al. Cardiac troponin T composition in normal and regenerating human skeletal muscle. Clin Chem 1997; 43: 476–484.

187. Sonies BC. Evaluation and treatment of speech and swallowing disorders associated with myopathies. Curr Opin Rheumatol 1997; 9: 486–495.

188. Mierau R, Dick T, Genth E. Less specific myositis autoantibodies? Ann Rheum Dis 2001; 60: 810.

189. Gelpi C, Kanterewicz E, Gratacos J et al. Coexistence of two antisynthetases in a patient with the antisynthetase syndrome. Arthritis Rheum 1996; 39: 692–697.

190. Brouwer R, Hengstman GJD, Vree Eberts W et al. Autoantibody profiles in the sera of European patients with myositis. Ann Rheum Dis 2001; 60: 116–123.

191. Ohosone Y, Matsumura M, Chiba J et al. Anti-transfer RNA antibodies in two patients with pulmonary fibrosis, Raynaud's phenomenon and polyarthritis. Clin Rheumatol 1998; 17: 144–147.

192. Ohosone Y, Ishida M, Takahashi Y et al. Spectrum and clinical significance of auto-antibodies against transfer RNA. Arthritis Rheum 1998; 41: 1625–1631.

193. Seelig HP, Moosbrugger I, Ehrfeld H et al. The major dermatomyositis-specific Mi-2 autoantigen is a presumed helicase involved in transcriptional activation. Arthritis Rheum 1995; 38: 1389–1399.

194. Casciola-Rosen LA, Pluta AF, Plotz PH et al. The DNA mismatch repair enzyme PMS1 is a myositis specific autoantigen. Arthritis Rheum 2001; 44: 389–396.

195. Schnitz W, Taylor-Albert E, Targoff IN et al. Anti-PM/Scl autoantibodies in patients without clinical polymyositis or scleroderma. J Rheumatol 1996; 23: 1729–1733.

196. Phillips BA, Zilko P, Garlepp MJ, Mastaglia FL. Frequency of relapses in patients with polymyositis and dermatomyositis. Muscle Nerve 1998; 21: 1668–1672.

197. Hoffman GS, Franck WA, Raddatz DA, Stallones L. Presentation, treatment and prognosis of idiopathic inflammatory muscle disease in a rural hospital. Am J Med 1983; 75: 433–438.

198. Blume G, Pestronk A, Frank B, Johns DR. Polymyositis with cytochrome oxidase negative muscle fibres: early quadriceps weakness and poor response to immunosuppressive therapy. Brain 1997; 120: 39–45.

199. Huang J-L. Long-term prognosis of patients with juvenile dermatomyositis initially treated with intravenous methylprednisolone pulse therapy. Clin Exp Rheumatol 1999; 17: 621–624.

200. Mitchell JP, Dennis GJ, Rider LG. Juvenile dermatomyositis presenting with anasarca: a possible indicator of severe disease activity. J Pediatr 2001; 138: 942–945.

201. Oddis CV, Medsger TA Jr. Polymyositis–dermatomyositis. In: Bellamy N, ed. Prognosis in the rheumatic diseases. Lancaster: Kluwer Academic Publishers; 1991: 233–249.

202. O'Leary PA, Waisman M. Dermatomyositis. Arch Derm Syph 1940; 41: 1001–1019.

203. Sheard C Jr. Dermatomyositis. Arch Intern Med 1951; 88: 640–658.

204. Winkelmann RK, Mulder DW, Lambert EH. Course of dermatomyositis–polymyositis: comparison of untreated and cortisone-treated patients. Mayo Clin Proc 1968; 43: 545–556.

205. Medsger TA Jr, Robinson H, Masi AT. Factors affecting survivorship in polymyositis: a life-table tudy of 124 patients. Arthritis Rheum 1971; 14: 249–258.

206. Carpenter JR, Bunch TW, Engel AG, O'Brien PC. Survival in polymyositis: corticosteroids and risk factors. J Rheumatol 1977' 4: 208–214.

207. Bohan A, Peter JB, Bowman RI et al. A computer-assisted analysis of 153 patients with polymyositis and dermatomyositis. Medicine 1976; 55: 89–104.

208. Benbassat J, Gefel D, Larholt K et al. Prognostic factors in PM-DM: a computer assisted analysis of 92 cases. Arthritis Rheum 1985; 28: 249–555.

209. Riddoch D, Morgan-Hughes JA. Prognosis in adult polymyositis. J Neurol Sci 1975; 26: 71–80.

210. Henriksson KG, Sandstedt P. Polymyositis – treatment and prognosis: a study of 107 patients. Acta Neurol Scand 1982; 65: 280–300.

211. Hochberg MC, Feldman D, Stevens MB. Adult onset polymyositis/dermatomyositis: an analysis of clinical and laboratory features and survival in 76 patients with a review of the literature. Semin Arthritis Rheum 1986; 15: 168–178.

212. Tymms KE, Webb J. Dermatopolymyositis and other connective tissue diseases. A review of 105 cases. J Rheumatol 1986; 12: 1140–1148.

213. Maugars YM, Berthelot J-MM, Abbas AA et al. Long-term prognosis of 69 patients with dermatomyositis or polymyositis. Clin Exp Rheum 1996; 14: 263–274.

214. Miller LC, Michael AF, Kim Y. Childhood dermatomyositis: clinical course and long-term follow-up. Clin Pediatr 1987; 26: 561–566.

215. DeVere R, Bradley WG. Polymyositis: its presentation, morbidity and mortality. Brain 1975; 98: 637–666.

216. Clarke AE, Bloch DA, Medsger TA Jr, Oddis CV. A longitudinal study of functional disability in a national cohort of polymyositis–dermatomyositis patients. Arthritis Rheum 1995; 38: 1218–1224.

217. Feldman BM, Ayling-Campos A, Luy L et al. Measuring disability in juvenile dermatomyositis: validity of the childhood health assessment questionnaire. J Rheumatol 1995; 22: 326–331.

218. Perez MD, Abrams SA, Koenning G et al. Mineral metabolism in children with dermatomyositis. J Rheumatol 1994; 21: 2364–2369.

SECTION

10

THE VASCULITIDES

38 Polymyalgia rheumatica and giant cell arteritis

Brian L Hazleman

Definitions

Polymyalgia rheumatica

- A clinical syndrome of the middle-aged and elderly, characterized by pain and stiffness in the neck, shoulder and pelvic girdles
- The clinical response to small doses of corticosteroids can be dramatic

Giant cell arteritis

- A vasculitis commonly accompanying polymyalgia rheumatica. Other terms used include temporal arteritis, cranial arteritis and granulomatous arteritis
- Early recognition and treatment can prevent blindness and other complications resulting from occlusion or rupture of involved arteries

Clinical features

Polymyalgia rheumatica

- The musculoskeletal symptoms are usually bilateral and symmetric
- Stiffness is the predominant feature; it is particularly severe after rest and may prevent the patient getting out of bed in the morning
- Muscular pain is often diffuse and is accentuated by movement; pain at night is common
- Corticosteroid treatment is usually required for at least 2 years. Most patients should be able to stop taking corticosteroids after 4–5 years
- Systemic features include low-grade fever, fatigue, weight loss and an increased erythrocyte sedimentation rate

Giant cell arteritis

- There are a wide range of symptoms, but most patients have clinical findings related to involved arteries
- Frequent features include fatigue, headaches, jaw claudication, loss of vision, scalp tenderness, polymyalgia rheumatica and aortic arch syndrome

HISTORY

The earliest description of giant cell arteritis may have been in the 10th century in the *Tadkwat* of Ali Iba Isu, where removal of the temporal artery was recommended as treatment. Dequeker describes two paintings – Jan Van Eyck's work in the Municipal Museum, Bruges, depicting the Holy Virgin with Canon Van der Paele (1436) and Pieri di Cosimo's portrait of Francesco Gamberti (1505), now in the Rijksmuseum, Amsterdam[1]. Both show signs of prominent temporal arteries and contemporary accounts document rheumatic pains, difficulty attending morning service with possible stiffness and general ill health.

Recognizable descriptions of polymyalgia rheumatica and giant cell arteritis were recorded throughout the 19th and 20th centuries. Jonathan Hutchinson in 1890 described 'a peculiar form of thrombotic arteritis of the aged, which is sometimes productive of gangrene'[2]. Horton *et al.*[3] described the typical histologic appearances at temporal artery biopsy.

The first description of polymyalgia rheumatica was probably made by Bruce in 1888[4], and Barber[5] suggested the present name in 1957. In 1960, Paulley and Hughes reported on 67 patients, emphasizing the occurrence of 'an arthritic rheumatism' in giant cell arteritis, providing more solid clinical evidence for the relationship between polymyalgia rheumatica and giant cell arteritis[6]. Histologic support came from the work of Alestig and Barr[7], and Hamlin *et al.*[8] confirmed the coexistence of the two conditions.

EPIDEMIOLOGY

Giant cell arteritis affects the white population almost exclusively. Most reports originate from Northern Europe[9] and parts of the northern USA. However, the disease is recognizable worldwide and there have been several reports of its occurrence in American blacks. In Tennessee, there is a lower incidence in the southern white population.

In Europe, studies from Southern Europe (Italy, Spain and France) have consistently reported lower incidence rates than those from Scandinavia. Multiple regression analysis correcting for the effect of increasing incidence with time suggests that there is a significant trend towards increasing incidence with more northerly latitude[10]. O'Brien and Regan[11] proposed that long-term exposure to sunlight (including both infrared and ultraviolet radiation could alter the structure of the internal elastic lamina of superficial arteries, making them antigenic (actinic degeneration). Recently, actinic changes have been demonstrated in the posterior ciliary arteries of patients.

Both polymyalgia rheumatica and giant cell arteritis affect elderly people and are seldom diagnosed in those younger than 50 years. A

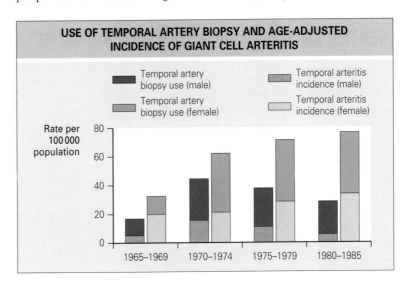

Fig. 38.1 **Use of temporal artery biopsy and sex-adjusted incidence of giant cell arteritis.** Data for residents of Olmsted County, Minnesota, from 1965 to 1985, per 100 000 population aged 50 years or more. Incidence was also age-adjusted to the 1980 white population of the USA.

study of biopsy-proven giant cell arteritis diagnosed from 1950 through to 1985 in Olmsted County, Minnesota, demonstrated an average annual incidence and prevalence of 17 and 223, respectively, per 100 000 inhabitants aged 50 years or more. The age-adjusted incidence rates were approximately three times greater in women than in men. In addition, the incidence increased in both sexes with old age. The incidence also increased significantly during the period 1950–1985 for females, but decreased in males over the same period (Fig. 38.1)[12]. In Olmsted County, there has been a steady increase of polymyalgia rheumatica, from 7.3 per 100 000 to 19.1 per 100 000 inhabitants aged more than 50 years[13]. The predicted rate of increase was 2.6% every 5 years. Similar increases have been reported from Spain[14] and Scandinavia[15]. The Olmsted County study identified peaks occurring every 7 years, a finding that could be consistent with an infectious etiology[13] (see section on Pathogenesis, below).

The incidence rates reported from Olmsted County are similar to those in Göteborg, Sweden. In a study of 284 biopsy-proven cases of giant cell arteritis collected over a 10-year period (1977–1986) in Göteborg, Nordborg and Bengtsson[16] observed an incidence rate among those aged 50 years or more of 18.3 per 100 000; for women the rate was 25 per 100 000 and for men it was 9.4 per 100 000. The temporal arteries and aorta of all adults who died in Malmö throughout 1 year were examined by Ostberg[17], and although active temporal arteritis was not found, evidence of previous arteritis was found in 1.7% of the 889 cases. It was found that in 75% of these individuals there had been either biopsy evidence or a clinical history suggestive of temporal arteritis.

The epidemiology of polymyalgia rheumatica has been less well defined. Silman and Currey[18] found three cases of polymyalgia among 247 persons older than 65 years who were resident in old peoples' homes and/or attending day centers. Only one case had been previously diagnosed. Kyle et al.[19], using a similar questionnaire in 656 patients older than 65 years, found a prevalence of arteritis/polymyalgia of 3300 per 100 000.

Familial aggregation of polymyalgia rheumatica and giant cell arteritis has been reported by several workers. Liang et al. in 1974[20] described four pairs of first-degree relatives, and they noted a further six pairs in the world literature. Clustering of cases in time and space was seen in Liang's study and suggested that, in addition to a genetic predisposition, environmental factors may be important. Rhodes[21] noted that nine of 11 cases seen over 6 years in a practice of 3000 lived in one small part of the same village, and of these, two lived in the same house, two were neighbors and two others were close friends.

IMMUNOGENETICS

The increased prevalence of cases of polymyalgia rheumatica and giant cell arteritis in individuals of European background, compared with other populations, has suggested a genetic relationship. In polymyalgia rheumatica, most genetic studies have involved human leukocyte antigen (HLA) typing using serologic methods. Class I antigens have shown variable results, which suggests that a significant relationship is unlikely.

Human leukocyte antigens in susceptibility to giant cell arteritis and polymyalgia rheumatica

Giant cell arteritis is the best example of an association between vasculitis and genes that lie within the HLA class II region[22]. Most studies have shown an association with *HLA-DRB1*04* alleles[14]. In addition, the severity and risk of visual complications is also associated with *HLA-DRB1*04* alleles.

Polymyalgia rheumatica is associated with *HLA* class II genes, but this varies from one population to another[23]. Relapses of polymyalgia rheumatica, however, have been found to be significantly more common in patients who have the *HLA-DRB1*04* allele, and particularly

in those carrying the *HLA-DRB1*0401* allele[14]. A lack of homozygosity of the shared epitope in giant cell arteritis has been reported; this contrasts with observations in rheumatoid arthritis, in which homozygosity of the shared epitope is associated with more severe disease. It has been suggested that the pathology seen in giant cell arteritis may be due to antigenic cross-reactivity after exposure to an infectious agent.

Clonal expansion of T lymphocytes with identical T cell antigen receptor β chains in distinct inflammatory foci within the same temporal artery has been demonstrated in giant cell arteritis, consistent with T-cell activation within the arterial wall in response to disease-specific antigen. This concept gains support by sequence analysis of the *HLA-DRB1* allelic variants, which shows that *DR4*-positive and *DR4*-negative patients share a 'disease associated' sequence of the same four amino acids (DRYF). This 'motif' maps to the second hypervariable region located in the antigen-binding groove of the *HLA-DR* molecule[24]. Patients rarely suffer from both giant cell arteritis and rheumatoid arthritis, consistent with the view that different and distinct domains of the *HLA-DR* molecule are important in determining susceptibility to the two diseases.

Role of tumor necrosis factor in susceptibility to giant cell arteritis and polymyalgia rheumatica

It is likely that other genetic factors may contribute to the susceptibility to these conditions. However, concentrations of tumour necrosis factor (TNF)-α have not been found to be increased in either condition. In Northwestern Spain[25], giant cell arteritis and polymyalgia rheumatica are associated with different TNF microsatellite polymorphisms. Giant cell arteritis is associated with the allele encoding the TNF-α2 microsatellite; this is largely independent of the association of giant cell arteritis with *HLA* class II genes. In contrast, patients with polymyalgia rheumatica have a positive association with TNF-β3, which is also independent of the *HLA* class II genes. Therefore TNF and HLA associations appear to be able to influence susceptibility to these conditions independently of each other[26]. In addition, genetic polymorphisms in endothelial cell adhesion molecules have also been considered to be important candidate susceptibility factors for giant cell arteritis and polymyalgia rheumatica. Recently, Boiardi and colleagues[27] reported a significant association between susceptibility to polymyalgia rheumatica and the interleukin (IL)-1 *RN*2* allele, particularly in the homozygous state.

CLINICAL FEATURES

The mean age at onset of giant cell arteritis and polymyalgia rheumatica is approximately 70 years, with a range of about 50 to more than 90 years of age. Women are twice as likely to be affected as men. The onset of the disease can be dramatic, and some patients can give the date and hour of their first symptom. Equally, the onset can be insidious. In most instances, the symptoms have been present for weeks or months before the diagnosis is established.

Constitutional symptoms, including fever, fatigue, anorexia and weight loss, and depression, are present in the majority of patients. Patients may present with pyrexia/fever of unknown origin and subjected to many investigations. Giant cell arteritis accounts for about 15% of patients older than 65 years presenting with fever of unknown origin. A hidden malignancy can mimic the symptoms of polymyalgia rheumatica. Although, at present, there is no evidence to suggest that malignancy is more common in patients with polymyalgia than in other people, deterioration in health or a poor initial response to corticosteroids must always be taken seriously and a search for an occult neoplasm made. In some cases, onset is associated with recent bereavement.

Polymyalgia rheumatica
Musculoskeletal involvement
Patients usually locate the source of their pain and stiffness to the muscles. The onset is most common in the shoulder region and neck, with eventual

involvement of the shoulder and pelvic girdles and the corresponding proximal muscle groups. Involvement of distal limb muscles is unusual. The symptoms are usually bilateral and symmetric. Stiffness is usually the predominant feature, is particularly severe after rest, and may prevent the patient from getting out of bed in the morning. The muscular pain is often diffuse and movement accentuates the pain; pain at night is common. Muscle strength is usually unimpaired, although the pain makes interpretation of muscle testing difficult. There is tenderness of involved structures, including periarticular structures such as bursae, tendons and joint capsules. In late stages, muscle atrophy may develop, with restriction of shoulder movement that rapidly improves with corticosteroid treatment. Occasionally, the painful arc sign of subacromial bursitis is present; this is important to recognize, as a local injection of corticosteroid will give relief and save the patient from an increase in systemic corticosteroid dosage.

Synovitis

Inflammatory synovitis and effusions have been noted by several authors, the reported incidence varying from 0 to 100% in various series[28]. Synovitis of the knees, wrists and sternoclavicular joints is most common, but involvement is transient and mild. An association between carpal tunnel syndrome and polymyalgia has been noted by several authors. Erosive changes in joints or sclerosis of the sacroiliac joints, or both, have been reported, although they are difficult to demonstrate in the sternoclavicular joints other than by tomography. Abnormal technetium pertechnetate scintigrams have shown widespread uptake over joints, particularly shoulders, knees, wrists and hands.

The synovial tissue shows non-specific inflammatory changes and the synovial fluid has the appearance of a mild inflammatory exudate. The synovitis of polymyalgia differs from that of rheumatoid arthritis in that it does not cause typical juxta-articular osteoporosis and erosions. The discrepancies in frequency of synovitis reported in various studies may be due to differing diagnostic criteria, the definition of synovitis and difficulty in interpretation of scans and radiographs because of coexisting degenerative disease.

Inflammation of synovial cavities and bursae is a common feature of shoulders in polymyalgia rheumatica on histology[29], magnetic resonance imaging and ultrasound assessment[30]. These findings rapidly improve after a few days of corticosteroid treatment. These findings are also seen in patients with symptoms of polymyalgia rheumatica with a normal erythrocyte sedimentation rate (ESR). It has been suggested that this is the basis for the diffuse symptoms in polymyalgia rheumatica. Nevertheless the symptomatology of polymyalgia rheumatica is difficult to explain on the basis of synovitis alone. McGonagle and colleagues[31] have recently demonstrated extracapsular abnormalities in the shoulder of early polymyalgia rheumatica by magnetic resonance imaging. This could explain the diffuse nature of the symptoms.

Salvarani and Hunder[24] have also described peripheral synovitis, distal extremity swelling with pitting edema, and tenosynovitis and carpal tunnel compression in patients with polymyalgia rheumatica and giant cell arteritis.

Kassimos et al.[32] examined the hypothesis that cytidine deaminase may be useful in the differentiation of polymyalgia rheumatica and RA. The mean serum cytidine deaminase concentrations were significantly greater in patients with rheumatoid arthritis compared with those with polymyalgia rheumatica and giant cell arteritis, suggesting that measurement of cytidine deaminase may be a useful laboratory parameter to help distinguish between the two conditions.

Giant cell arteritis

Giant cell arteritis causes a wide range of symptoms, but most patients have clinical features related to affected arteries. Common features include fatigue, headache and tenderness of the scalp, particularly around the temporal and occipital arteries.

Headache

Headache is the most common symptom and is present in 67% or more of patients. It usually begins early in the course of the disease and may be the presenting symptom. The pain is severe and localized to the temple. However, it may be occipital or be less defined and precipitated by brushing the hair. It can be severe even when the arteries are clinically normal and, conversely, may subside even though the disease remains active. The nature of the pain varies; it is described by some patients as shooting and by others as a more steady ache. Scalp tenderness is common, particularly around the temporal and occipital arteries, and may disturb sleep. Tender spots or nodules, or even small skin infarcts, may be present (Fig. 38.2). The vessels are thickened, tender and nodular, with absent or reduced pulsation (Fig. 38.3). Occasionally, they are red and clearly visible.

Ophthalmic features

Visual disturbances have been described in 25–50% of cases of giant cell arteritis. The incidence of visual loss is now regarded as much lower, about 6–10% in most series, probably because of earlier recognition and treatment.

There are a variety of ocular lesions that are essentially caused by occlusion of the various orbital or ocular arteries (Table 38.1 &

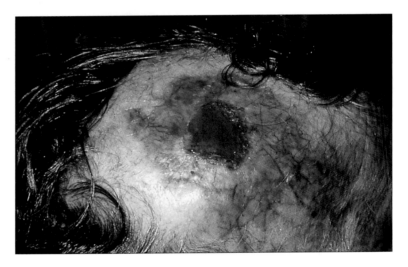

Fig. 38.2 Scalp necrosis in giant cell arteritis.

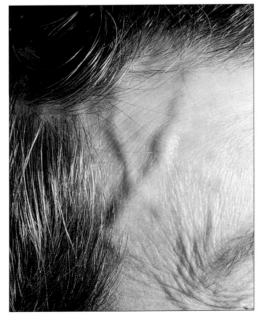

Fig. 38.3 Dilated temporal arteries in a patient with giant cell arteritis.

TABLE 38.1 OCULAR LESIONS IN GIANT CELL ARTERITIS

Lesions	Feature
Optic nerve ischemic lesions:	
Anterior ischemic optic neuropathy	The most common lesion and associated with partial or, more frequently, complete visual loss
Posterior ischemic optic neuropathy	Less common and may cause partial or complete visual loss
Retinal ischemic lesions:	
Central retinal artery occlusion	Leads to severe visual loss
Cilioretinal artery occlusion	Seen occasionally and associated with anterior ischemic optic neuropathy
Choroidal infarcts	Seen rarely
Extraocular motility disorders	Seen rarely and not usually associated with visual loss
Anterior segment ischemic lesions	Seen rarely and not usually associated with visual loss
Pupillary abnormalities	Usually secondary to visual loss
Cerebral ischemic lesions	Associated visual loss is rare

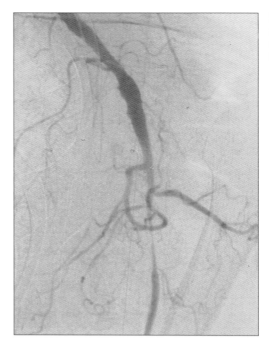

Fig. 38.5 Arteriogram showing narrowing of axillary artery in giant cell arteritis.

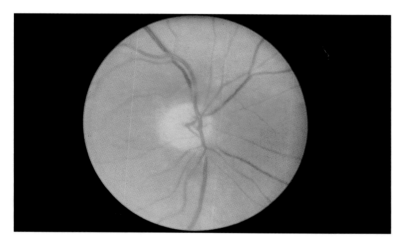

Fig. 38.4 Fundus photograph showing optic atrophy secondary to giant cell arteritis.

Fig. 38.4). Blindness is the most serious and irreversible feature. The visual loss is usually sudden, painless and permanent; it may vary from mistiness of vision, or involvement of a part of the visual field, to complete blindness. There is a risk of the second eye being involved if the patient is not treated aggressively. Blindness may be the initial presentation of giant cell arteritis, but tends to follow other symptoms by several weeks or months[33], premonitory symptoms including blurring of vision or amaurosis fugax or visual hallucinations. Visual symptoms are an ophthalmic emergency; if they are identified and treated urgently, blindness is almost entirely preventable.

The most common ocular lesion resulting from occlusion of orbital or ocular arteries is anterior ischemic optic neuropathy (AION) which usually leads to complete visual loss. In a series of 800 patients with this condition, 12% were found to have the arteritic form[34]. Features suggesting arteritic anterior ischemic optic neuropathy included systemic symptoms, an increased ESR, amaurosis fugax and early visual loss. A chalky white disc was highly suggestive of the arteritic form. Optic disc edema was associated with cilioretinal occlusion and was caused by arteritis. Early non-filling of the choroid on angiography was also associated with arteritis.

Extraocular motility disorders are usually transient and not associated with visual loss. Pupillary abnormalities can be seen secondary to visual

loss. Cerebral ischemic lesions producing visual loss are rare, as are anterior segment ischemic lesions and choroidal infarcts. Retinal ischemic lesions can affect the central retinal artery; this is associated with severe visual loss.

Other symptoms

Pain on chewing, resulting from claudication of the jaw muscles, occurs in up to 67% of patients. Tingling in the tongue, loss of taste, and pain in the mouth and throat can also occur, presumably because of vascular insufficiency.

Less common features of giant cell arteritis include hemiparesis, peripheral neuropathy, deafness, depression and confusion. Involvement of the coronary arteries may lead to myocardial infarction. Aortic regurgitation and congestive cardiac failure may also occur. Abnormalities of thyroid and liver function are well described.

Clinical evidence of large artery involvement is present in 10–15% of cases (Fig. 38.5), and in some instances aortic dissection and rupture occur. Bruits are often present over large arteries and there may be tenderness, particularly over the subclavian artery. An early sign of arteritis

TABLE 38.2 ACR CRITERIA FOR THE CLASSIFICATION OF GIANT CELL ARTERITIS

Criterion	Definition
1. Age at onset >50 years	Development of symptoms or findings beginning aged 50 years or older
2. New headache	New onset of, or new type of, localized pains in the head
3. Temporal artery abnormality	Temporal artery tenderness to palpation or decreased pulsation, unrelated to atherosclerosis of cervical arteries
4. Increased ESR	ESR >50mm/h by Westergren method
5. Abnormal artery biopsy	Biopsy specimen with artery showing vasculitis characterized by a predominance of mononuclear cell infiltration or granulomatous inflammation

A classification of giant cell arteritis requires three of the five criteria.

(From Hunder et al.[35] The material is used by permission of Wiley-Liss Inc., a subsidiary of John Wiley & Sons Inc. © 1996.)

is increased sensitivity of the carotid sinus. Light pressure will often lead to transient asystole for two or more beats, so it is advisable for the patient to be lying down when examined.

CLASSIFICATION/DIAGNOSTIC CRITERIA FOR GIANT CELL ARTERITIS/POLYMYALGIA RHEUMATICA

The cause of giant cell arteritis and polymyalgia rheumatic is unknown, and in neither is there a single diagnostic test. As a result, a combination of findings is needed for their diagnosis. The American College of Rheumatology has established criteria for the classification of giant cell arteritis[35] (Table 38.2). Their criteria are best used in research studies involving patients with a diagnosis of vasculitis.

As polymyalgia can mimic a number of different clinical conditions, there should ideally be clear criteria that enable the diagnosis to be made. Currently, there are a number of different criteria sets, all of which differ slightly. The attraction of the criteria proposed by Bird and colleagues[36] (Table 38.3) lies in its practical application in clinical practice. A diagnosis requires three of the seven listed features; the presence of just three features confirms a sensitivity of 92% and a specificity of 80%.

The differential diagnosis between polymyalgia rheumatica and elderly-onset rheumatoid arthritis can be difficult because these conditions may have similar clinical presentations. At present there are no clinical or routine laboratory features allowing early differentiation between polymyalgia rheumatica and rheumatoid arthritis with a polymyalgia rheumatica-like onset. After a 1-year study, 20% of patients presenting with an initial diagnosis of polymyalgia rheumatica developed rheumatoid arthritis[37].

RELATIONSHIP BETWEEN POLYMYALGIA RHEUMATICA AND GIANT CELL ARTERITIS

In recent years, giant cell arteritis and polymyalgia rheumatica have been considered as closely related conditions that form a spectrum of diseases. The conditions may occur independently or may occur in the same patient, either together or separated by time. Certainly, it is difficult to maintain a practical distinction between them by clinical or histologic criteria. Some patients originally suffering from polymyalgia rheumatica have later had symptoms of cranial arteritis, and in a number of patients with typical myalgia and no symptoms from the temporal region, biopsies have shown arteritic changes. Systemic involvement is similar in groups with or without clinical or biopsy evidence of arteritis.

Among patients with polymyalgia rheumatica who have no symptoms or signs of arteritis, positive temporal biopsies are found in 10–15%. There are many similarities between the two conditions. The age and sex distribution is similar, the biopsy findings show an identical pattern and the laboratory features are similar, even though many are non-specific inflammatory changes. In addition, there is similarity in the myalgia, the associated systemic features and in the response to corticosteroid treatment.

The onset of myalgic symptoms may precede, coincide with or follow that of the arteritic symptoms. No difference has been found between the characteristics of those myalgic patients with a positive biopsy and those with no histologic evidence of arteritis. Mild aching and stiffness may persist for months after other features of giant cell arteritis have remitted. There is little evidence to suggest that the musculoskeletal symptoms are related to vasculitis. Many patients with giant cell arteritis do not have polymyalgia rheumatica, even when large vessels are involved.

MALIGNANCY IN ASSOCIATION WITH POLYMYALGIA RHEUMATICA AND GIANT CELL ARTERITIS

A syndrome resembling giant cell arteritis or polymyalgia rheumatica may occasionally present as a paraneoplastic phenomenon, with a close relationship between the onset of symptoms and the appearance of malignancy. However, several studies have failed to demonstrate that patients with giant cell arteritis or polymyalgia rheumatica appear susceptible to cancer[38]. None of the studies compared the patient population with matched controls, and studies suffered from small numbers and short follow up. Haga and colleagues, who carried out a prospective study using matched controls in the early 1990s[39], showed that patients with a positive biopsy had an increased risk of cancer compared with matched controls. The onset of malignancy was a mean of 6.5 years from diagnosis of giant cell arteritis.

INVESTIGATIONS

The ESR is usually greatly increased in polymyalgia rheumatica/giant cell arteritis and provides a useful means of monitoring treatment, although it must be appreciated that some increase in the ESR may occur in otherwise healthy elderly people. A normal ESR is occasionally found in patients with active biopsy-proven disease[40], and patients with a low ESR at diagnosis had similar clinical characteristics and course of disease as patients with a high ESR at diagnosis[41]. Some investigators have reported varying percentages (7–20%) of patients with polymyalgia rheumatica who had a normal ESR (<40mm/h) at diagnosis.

Anemia, usually of a mild hypochromic type, is common and resolves without specific treatment, but a more marked normochromic anemia occasionally occurs and may be a presenting symptom. Leukocyte and differential counts are generally normal; platelet counts are also usually normal, but may be increased. Protein electrophoresis may show a non-specific increase in α_2-globulin, with less frequent increase in α_1-globulin and gammaglobulin. Quantification of the acute-phase proteins and α_1-antitrypsin, orosomucoid, haptoglobin and C-reactive protein are no more helpful than ESR in the assessment of disease activity[42]. Measurement of α_1-antichymotrypsin concentrations may help in management[43].

Abnormalities of thyroid and liver function have also been well described. In patients with hyperthyroidism, arteritis follows the thyrotoxicosis by intervals of 4–15 years. Individual cases of hypothyroidism have also been reported.

Increased serum values for alkaline phosphatase are commonly found in polymyalgia rheumatica. Sulfobromophthalein retention is also often abnormal and transaminases may be mildly increased. Liver biopsies have shown portal and intralobular inflammation, with focal liver cell necrosis and small epithelioid cell granuloma. Abnormal liver scans may also occur. In patients presenting with non-specific features, the findings of abnormal liver function tests and abnormal scans may be misleading and prompt investigations for malignancy.

A significant number of patients with polymyalgia rheumatica or giant cell arteritis, or both, have increased concentrations of anticardiolipin

TABLE 38.3 BIRD AND COWORKERS' CRITERIA FOR THE DIAGNOSIS OF PMR/GCA[36]
• Age >65 years
• ESR >40mm/h
• Bilateral upper arm tenderness
• Morning stiffness >1 hour
• Onset of illness within 2 weeks
• Depression or weight loss, or both
Diagnosis requires three of the seven listed features. Presence of just three features confirms a sensitivity of 92% and a specificity of 80%.
GCA, giant cell arteritis; PMR, polymyalgia rheumatica.

antibody at presentation[44]. These patients appear to be at increased risk of developing giant cell arteritis or other major vascular complications. It is possible that anticardiolipin may be an independent prognostic marker for future vascular complications with polymyalgia rheumatica or giant cell arteritis. Other studies have shown that anticardiolipin concentrations are greater in patients with active arteritis and decrease rapidly after corticosteroid treatment.

Temporal artery biopsy

Clinicians vary greatly in their approach to temporal artery biopsy. Some emphasize the value of a positive histologic diagnosis, especially months or years later, when side effects of the corticosteroid treatment have developed. Others feel that a high false-negative rate diminishes the value of the procedure. In most instances, the high false-negative rate can be attributed to the focal nature and involvement of the superficial temporal artery by the inflammatory process. A pragmatic policy would include the following:

● Perform biopsy if diagnosis is in doubt, particularly if systemic symptoms predominate
● Biopsy is most useful within 24 hours of starting treatment, but do not delay treatment for sake of biopsy. The artery biopsy will still show inflammatory changes for several days after corticosteroids have been started
● A negative biopsy does not exclude giant cell arteritis
● A positive result helps to prevent later doubts about diagnosis, particularly if treatment causes complications.

A third of patients with signs and symptoms of cranial arteritis may have a negative temporal artery biopsy, which may be the result of localized involvement of arteries in the head and neck. 'Skip' lessons are evident in about 67% of biopsies; some segments showing active disease are as short as 350μm[45]. The rate of false-negative biopsies depends on many variables, including the size of the biopsy, the number of levels examined, whether biopsies were taken from one or both sides of the scalp, and the duration of corticosteroid treatment before the procedure.

Involvement of the temporal arteries occasionally occurs in vasculitides other than giant cell arteritis, among which polyarteritis nodosa appears to be the most common[46]. There have also been sporadic reports of temporal artery involvement in Churg–Strauss syndrome, Wegener's granulomatosis, microscopic polyangiitis, cryoglobulinemia or rheumatoid vasculitis[47].

Occasionally, a temporal artery biopsy reveals small-vessel vasculitis surrounding a spared temporal artery. Esteban and colleagues performed a clinical and histological study of 28 patients with small-vessel vasculitis surrounding a spared temporal artery[48]. The diagnosis of giant cell arteritis can be reasonably established in most of these patients when there is no apparent evidence of additional organ involvement. However, when fibrinoid necrosis is observed or the temporal artery vasa vasorum are not involved, then systemic necrotizing vasculitis must be excluded.

Color Doppler ultrasonography can be used to examine the superficial arteries and is a new, non-invasive method for the diagnosis of giant cell arteritis. Findings include a hypoechoic wall thickening (halo) caused by edema. It disappears within 16 days of corticosteroid treatment in giant cell arteritis[49]. Color Doppler can detect stenosis and occlusion, and is confirmed by simultaneous pulsed-wave Doppler ultrasound. In the cases with abnormal findings, biopsy can be performed to confirm the diagnosis of giant cell arteritis.

Magnetic resonance imaging can demonstrate large-vessel vasculitis in giant cell arteritis, and preliminary positron emission tomography scanning reports support the concept that large-vessel vasculitis may be common in polymyalgia rheumatica[50].

DIFFERENTIAL DIAGNOSIS

The diagnosis of polymyalgia rheumatica is initially one of exclusion. The differential diagnosis (Table 38.4) in an elderly patient with muscle pain, stiffness and an increased ESR is wide, because the prodromal phases of several serious conditions can mimic it. Despite a typical pattern of musculoskeletal symptoms and the presence, in many, of significant systemic features, there is often a considerable delay of several months before diagnosis. Polymyalgia rheumatica can usually be differentiated from late-onset rheumatoid arthritis by the absence of prominent peripheral joint pain and swelling. In patients with polymyositis, the muscular weakness is the predominant factor limiting movement, whereas in polymyalgia rheumatica, pain causes limited function.

The diagnosis of giant cell arteritis should be considered in any patient over the age of 50 years who has recent onset of headache, transient or sudden loss of vision, myalgia, unexplained fever or anemia or an increased ESR. Because the symptoms and signs may vary in severity and be transient, patients must be questioned carefully about recent and current symptoms. The arteries of the head, neck and limbs should be examined for tenderness, enlargement, thrombosis and bruits. Angiography of the temporal arteries is not usually helpful – there is no characteristic abnormality, and false-positives (usually attributable to atheroma) are not uncommon. An angiographic examination of the aortic arch and its branches may prove helpful in patients with symptoms of large-artery involvement. There is usually little difficulty in separating giant cell arteritis from other forms of arteritis, because of the different distribution of lesions, histopathology and organ involvement.

PATHOLOGY

The histologic appearance of giant cell arteritis is one of the most distinctive of vascular disorders. The dense granulomatous inflammatory infiltrates that characterize the acute stages of the disease resemble those of Takayasu's arteritis, but the clinicopathologic features in patients with positive temporal artery biopsies are diagnostic. The arteritis is histologically a panarteritis with giant cell granuloma formation, often in close proximity to a disrupted internal elastic lamina. Large and medium-sized arteries are affected, the involvement is patchy and skip lesions are often found. There is preferential involvement of muscular arteries with well developed internal and external elastic laminae.

The gross features are not characteristic. The vessels are enlarged and nodular and have little or no lumen. Thrombosis often develops at sites of active inflammation. Later, these areas may recanalize. The lumen is narrowed by intimal proliferation (Fig. 38.6). This is a common finding in arteries and may result from advancing age, nearby chronic

TABLE 38.4 DIFFERENTIAL DIAGNOSIS OF POLYMYALGIA RHEUMATICA	
Neoplastic disease	Muscle disease
Joint disease	Polymyositis
Osteoarthritis, particularly of cervical spine	Myopathy
Rheumatoid arthritis	Infections, e.g. bacterial endocarditis
Connective tissue disease	Bone disease, particularly osteomyelitis
Multiple myeloma	Hypothyroidism
Leukemia	Parkinsonism
Lymphoma	Functional

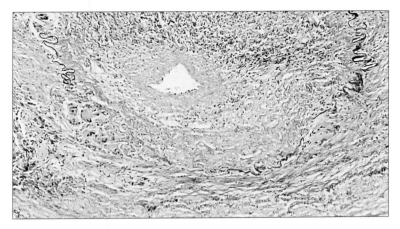

Fig. 38.6 Elastic stain of temporal artery, showing disruption of elastic lamina in giant cell arteritis, and narrowing of the lumen.

inflammation or low blood flow. The adventitia is usually invaded by mononuclear, and occasionally polymorphonuclear, inflammatory cells. There is cuffing of the vasa vasorum and fibrous proliferation is frequent. The changes in the media are dominated by the giant cells, which vary from small cells with two to three nuclei up to masses of $100\mu m$ containing many nuclei. There is invasion by mononuclear cells resembling histiocytes. Fibrinoid necrosis is infrequent. Giant cells are not seen in all sections, and therefore are not required for the diagnosis if other features are compatible; however, the more sections that are examined in the area of arteritis, the more likely it is that giant cells will be found.

A progression of changes can be demonstrated, from the active infiltrative phase to the scarred artery with little cellular infiltrate. At first, the most severe changes are centered on the internal elastic lamina, which becomes swollen and fragmented. Fragments of elastic tissue can be demonstrated within giant cells, which are surrounded with plasma cell and lymphocytic infiltration (Fig. 38.7). The findings of electron microscopy studies have suggested that altered or damaged smooth muscle cells are critical in the pathogenesis.

Histologic changes also occur in temporal arteries with advancing age; they differ only in degree with those encountered in giant cell arteritis and it can sometimes be difficult to distinguish between them. However, an inflammatory cell infiltrate does not occur, except in relationship to large plaques of atherosclerosis. The degree of intimal thickening in arteritis is usually greater, a well-developed smooth muscle layer is seen by the lumen, and loss of the internal elastic lamina is considerable. The histologic changes of healed arteritis include medial chronic inflammation with ingrowth of new blood vessels, focal medial scarring and a bizarre pattern of intimal fibrosis; the last is the most important change. The biopsy finding of healed vasculitis by no means excludes the possibility of active lesions elsewhere. Not infrequently, episodes of vasculitis are recurrent. The widespread nature of the vasculitis has been well documented, and occasionally veins are affected.

Involvement of the aorta and its branches, the abdominal vessels and the coronary arteries have all been described. Giant cell arteritis as a cause of aortic dissection has been recorded rarely at autopsy, and most exceptionally during life. Most patients had a history of hypertension in life or other features of hypertensive disease at autopsy. In addition, the majority of patients described in the literature are women[51].

Although there is a high incidence of involvement of the head and neck vessels in giant cell arteritis, it is interesting that the intracranial vessels are seldom involved. Wilkinson and Russell[52] studied the head and neck vessels and demonstrated a close correlation between susceptibility to arteritis and the amount of elastic tissue present in the arterial wall. The greatest incidence of severe involvement was noted in the superficial temporal arteries, vertebral arteries and ophthalmic and posterior ciliary arteries. The internal carotid, external carotid and central retinal arteries were affected less frequently (Fig. 38.8). In some instances, follow-up biopsy or autopsy surveys showed persistence of mild chronic inflammation even though symptoms had resolved.

There has been little to support a concept of primary muscle disease in polymyalgia rheumatica. Serum aldolase and creatine phosphokinase are normal, and there is no abnormality on electromyography. Muscle biopsy has shown type II atrophy alone and there is no evidence of inflammatory changes[53]. Recently there have been reports of focal changes in muscle ultrastructure and abnormalities of mitochondrial form and function, similar to those associated with inherited mitochondrial myopathies. These abnormalities are not caused by gene deletions or mutations associated with mitochondrial myopathy, and persist even after successful treatment. Arteritis in skeletal muscle appears to be uncommon.

Liver biopsy can show non-specific inflammatory changes or focal liver cell necrosis. There are occasional reports of granulomata and

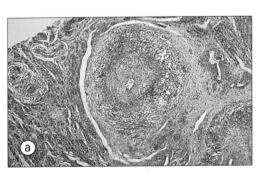
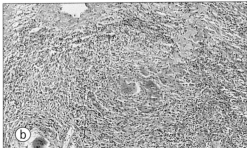

Fig. 38.7 Histology of giant cell arteritis.
(a) Low-powered view of arterial wall, showing infiltration by lymphocytes and plasma cells. (b) High-powered view showing giant cells in close relationship to elastic lamina.

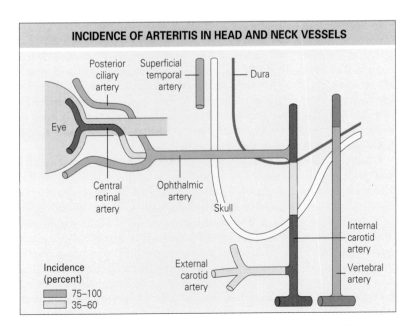

Fig. 38.8 Incidence of arteritis in pathologic study of head and neck vessels.

hepatic arteritis. Synovial biopsy has shown non-specific inflammatory changes with lymphocytic infiltration of knees, sternoclavicular joints and shoulders.

ETIOLOGY AND PATHOGENESIS

At present it is impossible to define the underlying pathologic abnormality in polymyalgia and, indeed, it may well be that there are several different mechanisms responsible for a largely similar pattern of pain. The relative homogeneity of groups of patients and the apparent rapid clinical response to corticosteroids do not exclude this possibility. Although the increasing incidence of giant cell arteritis and polymyalgia rheumatica after the age of 50 years implies a relationship with aging, the significance of this observation is not understood.

A distinct prodromal event resembling influenza or viral pneumonia is often noted by patients. However, viral studies have generally produced negative results. In studies by Bacon et al.[54], hepatitis antigen was not found in any of 12 patients with polymyalgia, although hepatitis B surface antibody was found in nine patients.

Parvovirus B19 infection occurs in epidemic cycles similar to those seen in giant cell arteritis. Salvarani and colleagues[55] have recently used the polymerase chain reaction technique to demonstrate the presence of parvovirus B19 DNA in temporal artery biopsy specimens.

Cimmino and colleagues[56] reported an increase in antibody to respiratory syncytial virus and adenovirus and Duhaut et al.[57] performed a large case–control study suggesting that reinfection with human parainfluenza virus (a virus known to induce human multinucleated giant cells) is associated with the onset of giant cell arteritis, particularly in those with a positive biopsy. No association was seen with other viruses that induce multinucleated giant cells, such as measles, herpes simplex, Epstein–Barr and respiratory syncytial viruses.

In Denmark, peak incidences were correlated with occurrences of Mycoplasma pneumoniae infection[58]. Using a matched case–control method, Russo et al.[59] showed a correlation between infection and onset of giant cell arteritis, but could not identify a specific infection. In addition to cyclic peaks, occasional clusters have been reported; in Jerusalem, Sonnenblick and colleagues[60] observed five cases in a 7-week period when the expected background rate was one case per year. A seasonal pattern of onset has been reported in several studies, but the precise season of maximum occurrence has not been consistent and some studies have failed to document a seasonal effect.

In summary, despite large studies looking for an infectious etiology, no unifying hypothesis has emerged. Cimmino[61] has proposed that infrared and solar radiation damage the internal elastic lamina of superficial arteries, and that this facilitates the localization of an unknown antigen (possibly viral protein), which is then presented in the context of class II major histocompatibility complex molecules. Macrophages and CD4+ lymphocytes are stimulated, producing cytokines that lead to giant cell arteritis or polymyalgia rheumatica, depending on the pattern. This process is accentuated in elderly females with specific HLA-DRB1 alleles.

Giant cell arteritis is limited to vessels with an internal elastic lamina, and electron microscopy shows fragmentation of this with mononuclear cell accumulation compatible with cell-mediated injury. Fragments of elastic tissue can be demonstrated within giant cells. Immunofluorescence studies have also demonstrated the presence of immunoglobulins and complement in the vessel wall of patients with arteritis. Both intra- and extracellularly, deposits of all immunoglobulin classes plus complement (C3) have been noted, adjacent to the internal elastic lamina in many cases. The presence of immunoglobulin or complement within a lesion does not prove that it has been caused by hypersensitivity; rather, it may reflect non-specific immune complex deposition at the site of vascular injury of different cause. Using an immunoperoxidase method, Gallagher and Jones[62] found only intracellular deposits and did not detect extracellular complement. This pattern of intracytoplasmic staining for immunoglobulins would be anticipated in any chronic inflammatory reaction. It is possible that the changes reflect a non-specific reaction to injury. Immunoglobulin and complement deposition may occur in the synovium in polymyalgia rheumatica, but there are few systematic studies. Dasgupta et al.[63] have reported antibodies against intermediate filaments in 67% of patients at the onset of giant cell arteritis. Antibodies against intermediate filaments are found in viral infections and autoimmune diseases.

Increased numbers of circulating lymphoblasts are seen in patients with active polymyalgia rheumatica, and immunoglobulins are also increased. These observations have led to the suggestion that these diseases may have an immunologic basis, perhaps an age-related autoimmune process directed against arterial wall constituents. The cells from patients with active untreated giant cell arteritis or polymyalgia rheumatica show no difference from normal controls with respect to in vitro lymphocytotoxicity to arterial smooth muscle. The lymphocytes in the arteritic lesions express the T cell phenotype and only a few B cells are found[64].

Lesional T cells are predominately of the CD4 subtype, and produce interferon-γ and IL-2, together with the macrophage products IL-1β, IL-6 and transforming growth factor-β, leading to local and systemic inflammation. They are also the likely source of matrix metalloproteinase 2, and a growth factor for smooth muscle cells, platelet-derived growth factor, which have been implicated in the narrowing and constriction of affected blood vessels[65]. In an animal model of giant cell arteritis in which temporal arteries are implanted onto severe combined immunodeficient mice, arterial T cells are vital to the occurrence of inflammation[66]. T cell clonotypes with identical T cell receptor molecules have been isolated from separate vascular lesions[67]. Immunogenetic studies indicate an association with HLA-DR4[68] and more specifically with HLA DRB*0401[23]. These findings suggest that inflammation in giant cell arteritis is an antigen-driven T-cell-mediated immune process, but the nature of the antigen remains unknown.

Macrophages, epithelioid cells and giant cells are seen in the arterial wall and the majority express HLA-DR antigen, in addition to the adhesion molecules lymphocyte function-associated antigens (LFA)-1 and -3 and intercellular adhesion molecule (ICAM)-1. About 25% of the infiltrating T cells express the HLA-DR antigen and the integrin receptor, vascular leucocyte antigen (VLA)-1, which suggests that these cells are immunologically activated. Further support for a local activation of the T cells is the finding of IL-2 receptors on the lymphocytes from biopsy specimens[69]. The expression of IL-2 receptors on lymphocytes is not as frequent as that of HLA-DR. The reason for this discrepancy is not known, but is seen in other inflammatory lesions. Roche et al.[69] also reported interdigitating reticulum cells in 40% of patients with biopsy-proven giant cell arteritis; these were seen in patients with a shorter disease duration. It has been suggested that interdigitating reticulum cells are seen in lesions in which a local stimulus for an immune response is suspected, but not in diseases caused by immune complexes or degenerative processes. Both IL-2 and interferon-γ are produced by cells located in the inflamed arterial wall. Circulating concentrations of IL-6 are increased, with normal concentrations of TNF-α both in patients with an arteritic presentation of giant cell arteritis and in those presenting with polymyalgia rheumatica. A selective depletion of circulating CD8 T lymphocytes in patients with giant cell arteritis has been observed in most studies. No increase in expression of HLA-DR has been found on circulatory CD4+ T cells; this contrasts with the high incidence on the T lymphocytes in the arterial wall. The surface expression of ICAM-1 by smooth muscle cells within granulomata in the arterial wall in giant cell arteritis might be exposing these cells to LFA-1-mediated macrophage and cytotoxic T cell attack, and suggests that smooth muscle may be an important immune target in giant cell arteritis.

It has been proposed that a serum toxic factor leads to endothelial breakdown and then to disruption of the internal elastic lamina. Elastin fragments are chemotactic to monocytes that have elastolytic potential; this is increased in giant cell arteritis. Also, linear deposits of leukocyte elastase are found along the fragmented internal elastic lamina.

Aging of the immune and neuroendocrine systems may be important factors in the late onset of giant cell arteritis. Breakdown in tolerance, increased susceptibility to infectious triggers or perpetuation of inflammation as a result of relative cortisol deficiency are possible mechanisms. Basal cortisol concentrations are increased in the elderly, but the release of cortisol in response to stress is attenuated.

MANAGEMENT

Corticosteroids are mandatory in the treatment of giant cell arteritis; they reduce the incidence of complications such as blindness and rapidly relieve symptoms. Non-steroidal anti-inflammatory drugs (NSAIDs) will lessen the painful symptoms, but they do not prevent arteritic complications. The response to corticosteroids is usually dramatic, and occurs within days. Corticosteroid treatment has improved the quality of life for patients, although there is no evidence that treatment reduces the duration of the disease. A fear of vascular complications in those patients with a positive biopsy often leads to the use of high doses of corticosteroids. Recent studies have emphasized the importance of adopting a cautious and individual treatment schedule, and have highlighted the efficacy of lower doses of prednisolone.

Initially, the corticosteroids should be given in a dosage sufficient to control the disease; subsequently, they should be maintained at the lowest dose that will control the symptoms and decrease the ESR. In giant cell arteritis, corticosteroids should preferably be given after the diagnosis has been confirmed histologically. However, when giant cell arteritis is strongly suspected, there should be no delay in starting treatment, as the artery biopsy will still show inflammatory changes for several days after corticosteroids have been started, and the result is unlikely to alter therapeutic decisions. If the temporal (or other) artery biopsy shows no arteritis, but the suspicion of disease is strong, corticosteroid treatment should be started. The great danger is delaying treatment, as blindness may occur at any time.

In practice, most studies report using 10–20mg prednisolone daily to treat polymyalgia and 40–60mg for giant cell arteritis, because of the greater risk of arteritic complications in giant cell arteritis. Some ophthalmologists suggest an initial dose of at least 60mg, as they have seen blindness occur in those treated with a lower dose. However, this has to be balanced against the potential complication of high dosage in this older age group. Intravenous corticosteroids are occasionally used if there are visual complications. Patients should be advised that, while they are taking a maintenance dose of corticosteroids, any sudden exacerbation of symptoms, particularly sudden visual deterioration, requires an immediate increase in dose. The initial corticosteroid dose and rate of corticosteroid tapering have been evaluated prospectively by Kyle and Hazleman[70]. They found that patients with polymyalgia relapsed frequently when taking an initial dose of 10mg prednisolone daily, but in those taking 20mg for the first month the disease was well controlled.

Reducing the dosage from 7.5mg to 5mg in the second month was also associated with some relapses. Patients with giant cell arteritis were treated with 40mg for 5 days and then either continued to take 40mg or had their dosage reduced to 20mg for the first month. An initial dose of 40mg controlled symptoms in most cases, whereas giving 20mg and then reducing to 15mg/day after 4 weeks led to more relapses. There is little information on the rate of reduction of corticosteroid dosage once initial symptoms are controlled. Weekly decrements of not more than 5mg have been proposed. The reduction is more gradual when a daily dose of 10mg is reached. It is suggested that 1mg every 2–4 weeks is

sufficient. These dosages are suggestions only, and are not to be interpreted rigidly, as individual cases vary greatly.

Rapid reduction or withdrawal of corticosteroids has been reported to contribute to deaths in patients with giant cell arteritis[71]. Of 17 deaths, 13 were believed to be due to an inadequate dose of corticosteroids or too rapid reduction of the dose. Fortunately, complications are rare, and the activity of the disease seems to decline steadily. Relapses are more likely within 1 year of withdrawal of corticosteroids. There is no reliable method of predicting those most at risk, but arteritic relapses in patients who presented with pure polymyalgia rheumatica are unusual. Temporal artery biopsy does not seem helpful in predicting outcome.

Methylprednisolone has a 20% greater glucocorticoid potency (and a lower mineral corticoid effect) than oral prednisolone. In a prospective study of 60 patients with polymyalgia rheumatica, it has been shown that intramuscular methylprednisolone can confer a remission rate similar to that achieved with oral prednisolone, but with a superior side-effect profile. However, the study excluded patients with giant cell arteritis[72].

Controversy exists as to the expected duration of the disease. Most European studies report that between 33% and 50% of the patients are able to discontinue corticosteroids after 2 years of treatment. Studies from the USA have reported a shorter duration of disease for both polymyalgia rheumatica (75% of patients discontinue corticosteroids by 2 years) and giant cell arteritis (most patients had stopped corticosteroids within 2 years). However, a Mayo Clinic study has substantially confirmed the European view[73]. Both patients with polymyalgia rheumatica and those with giant cell arteritis needed a median duration of treatment of 1.8 years (mean 2.4 years). Most importantly, the median cumulative dose of prednisolone during the treatment period was between 4.5g and 5.4g and with such doses several important side effects were seen. Compared with age matched controls, patients with polymyalgia rheumatica who received corticosteroid treatment were found to have a two to five times greater risk of developing diabetes and vertebral, femoral neck and hip fractures[73]. The consensus view seems to be that stopping treatment is feasible from 2 years onwards.

Dasgupta et al.[74] measured serum T cell subsets before and during treatment in patients with polymyalgia rheumatica and giant cell arteritis, and found a profound and selective reduction of CD8+ suppressor/cytotoxic cells that persisted for up to 1 year, despite satisfactory symptomatic control and a normal ESR and C-reactive protein concentration. After 2 years of treatment, CD8+ cell counts had returned to the values found in normal controls.

Concentrations of IL-6 in combination with the ESR may be of value in determining disease severity and in predicting outcome in subgroups of patients with polymyalgia rheumatica.

Patients who are unable to reduce the dosage of prednisolone because of recurring symptoms, or who develop serious corticosteroid-related side effects, pose particular problems. Azathioprine has been shown to exert a modest corticosteroid-sparing effect. There have been reports of the value of methotrexate in corticosteroid resistant cases of polymyalgia rheumatica or giant cell arteritis, but the overall consensus is that methotrexate, azathioprine and cyclosporin are not effective. Most of the published studies have a relatively small number of patients, with a short duration of follow-up and high numbers withdrawing from treatment.

Relapses

Relapses are most likely in the first 18 months of treatment, but they can occur after apparently successful treatment when corticosteroids have been discontinued. At present, there is no way of predicting those patients most at risk. Diagnosis of relapse should be made on the basis of clinical features, because the ESR and C-reactive protein concentration are often not increased during relapses, or may be increased as a result of other causes. During relapses, the dose of prednisolone should be increased to that given before relapse, or more, depending on the severity of symptoms. The risks of relapse, particularly with arteritic complications, have to be balanced against the risks of corticosteroid-associated side effects.

Complications

Between 20% and 50% of patients may experience serious side effects. Serious side effects are significantly related to high initial doses, maintenance doses, cumulative doses and increased duration of treatment[75]. Side effects can be minimized by using low doses of prednisolone whenever possible, and giving corticosteroid-sparing drugs such as azathioprine and methotrexate when necessary.

TABLE 38.5 TREATMENT OF POLYMYALGIA RHEUMATICA AND GIANT CELL ARTERITIS	
For polymyalgia rheumatica*	**Initial dosage** Prednisolone 10–20mg initially for 1 month, reduced by 2.5mg every 2–4 weeks to 10mg daily, then 1mg daily every 4–6 weeks (or until symptoms return). **Maintenance dosage** Maintenance dose 5–7mg daily for 6–12 months. Final reduction, 1mg every 6–8 weeks. Most patients require treatment for 3–4 years, but withdrawal after 2 years is worth attempting. **Special points** In patients who cannot reduce prednisolone dosage because of recurring symptoms or who develop serious corticosteroid-related side effects, azathioprine has been shown to have a modest corticosteroid sparing effect, and methotrexate may be more effective. **Main side effects** Weight gain, skin atrophy, edema, increased intraocular pressure, cataracts, gastrointestinal disturbances, diabetes, osteoporosis. **Risk of side effects** Increased risk with high initial doses (>30mg) of prednisolone, maintenance doses of 10mg and high cumulative doses. Maintenance doses of 5mg are relatively safe.
Giant cell arteritis without visual symptoms	Prednisolone 20–40mg daily initially for 8 weeks reduced by 5mg every 3–4 weeks until dose is 10mg daily; then as for polymyalgia rheumatica.
Giant cell arteritis with possible or definite ocular involvement	Prednisolone 40–80mg daily initially for 8 weeks reduced to 20mg daily over next 4 weeks; then as for uncomplicated giant cell arteritis.
*Recurrence of symptoms requires an increase in prednisolone dose.	

Corticosteroid treatment carries the risk of increasing osteoporosis, especially in older patients. It cannot be overly stressed that patients with polymyalgia rheumatica should be given advice and be assessed for the risk of osteoporosis before beginning treatment, and should, as a minimum, be placed on calcium and vitamin D supplements. In this context, deflazacort, or the methyloxazoline derivative of prednisolone, failed to show a significant difference in bone density changes as compared with conventional oral prednisolone[76].

Conclusions

Some conclusions can be drawn (Table 38.5). The overall strategy should be to use an adequate dose of prednisolone for the first month to obtain good symptomatic control, with a decrease in ESR, then to aim for maintenance doses of less than 10mg after 6 months. The exact doses will need to be adjusted to the needs of the individual patient. A possible schedule is 15mg prednisolone/day for polymyalgia rheumatica, reducing the dose to about 7.5–10mg by 6–8 weeks. Patients with giant cell arteritis should be treated with 40mg daily for the first month unless visual symptoms persist, when higher doses (60–80mg) may be needed. A suitable dose reduction would be to 20mg at about 8 weeks. For both conditions, gradual reduction by 1mg every 2–3 months can be attempted, with possible withdrawal of corticosteroids after 2 years. Reduction of doses of prednisolone on alternate days once doses of less than 5mg are reached makes withdrawal easier, and the addition of a non-steroidal anti-inflammatory drug at this stage may reduce some of the minor muscular symptoms that patients develop as corticosteroids are reduced. Some patients, however, find it impossible to stop taking the final 2–3mg, and this level of maintenance dose is probably safe.

Summary

In summary, patients should be warned to expect treatment for at least 2 years, and most should be able to stop taking corticosteroids after 4–5 years. Monitoring for relapse should continue for 6 months to 1 year after discontinuation of corticosteroids; thereafter patients should be asked to report back urgently if arteritic symptoms occur. The risk of this happening is small and unpredictable. A few patients may need low-dose treatment indefinitely. Polymyalgia rheumatica and giant cell arteritis are amongst the more satisfying diseases for clinicians to diagnose and treat, because the unpleasant effects and serious consequences of these conditions can be almost entirely prevented by corticosteroid treatment. Unfortunately, there is no objective means of determining the prognosis in the individual, and decisions concerning duration of treatment remain empirical.

REFERENCES

1. Dequeker JV. Polymyalgia rheumatica with temporal arteritis as painted by Jan Van Eyck in 1436. Can Med Assoc J 1981; 124: 1597–1598.
2. Hutchinson J. A peculiar form of neurotic arteritis of the aged which is sometimes productive of gangrene. Arch Surg 1890; 1: 323–327.
3. Horton BT, Magath TB, Brown GE. An undescribed form of arteritis of the temporal vessels. Mayo Clin Proc 1932; 7: 700–701.
4. Bruce W. Senile rheumatic gout. BMJ 1888; 2: 811–813.
5. Barber HS. Myalgic syndrome with constitutional effects. Polymyalgia rheumatica. Ann Rheum Dis 1957; 16: 230–237.
6. Paulley JW, Hughes JP. Giant cell arteritis or arthritis of the aged. BMJ 1960; 2: 1562–1567.
7. Alestig K, Barr J. Giant cell arteritis: biopsy study of polymyalgia rheumatica, including one case of Takayasu's disease. Lancet 1963; i: 1228–1230.
8. Hamlin B, Jonsson N, Landberg T. Involvement of large vessels in polymyalgia arteritica. Lancet 1965; 1: 1193–1196.
9. Gran JT, Myklebust G. The incidence of polymyalgia rheumatica and temporal arteritis in the county of Aust Agder, South Norway: a prospective study 1987–94. J Rheumatol 1997; 24: 1739–1743.
10. Watts RA, Lane S, Bentham G, Scott DGI. Is there a latitudinal variation in the incidence of giant cell arteritis? Proceedings of the American College of Rheumatology, Philadelphia, October 2000. Arthritis Rheum 2000; 43(suppl): S137.

11. O'Brien JP, Regan W. Actinically degenerate elastic tissue: the prime antigen in the giant cell (temporal) arteritis syndrome? New data from the posterior ciliary arteries. Clin Exp Rheumatol 1998; 16: 39–48.
12. Machedo EBV, Michet CJ, Ballard DJ et al. Trends in incidence and clinical presentation of temporal arteritis in Olmsted County, Minnesota 1950–1985. Arthritis Rheum 1988; 31: 745–749.
13. Salvarani C, Gabriel S, O'Fallon W et al. Epidemiology of polymyalgia rheumatica in Olmstead County, Minnesota 1970–1991. Arthritis Rheum 1995; 38: 369–373.
14. González-Gay M, Garcia-Porrua C, Rivas M et al. Epidemiology of biopsy proven giant cell arteritis in North Western Spain: trend over an 18 year period. Ann Rheum Dis 2001; 60: 367–371.
15. Petursdottir V, Johansson H, Nordborg E, Nordborg C. The epidemiology of biopsy-positive giant cell arteritis: special reference to cyclic fluctuations. Rheumatology (Oxford) 1999; 38: 1208–1212.
16. Nordberg E, Bengtsson BA. Epidemiology of biopsy proven giant cell arteritis. J Intern Med 1990; 227: 233–236.
17. Ostberg G. On arteritis with special reference to polymyalgia arteritica. Acta Path Microb Scand 1973; 237(suppl.): 1–59.
18. Silman AJ, Currey HLF. Polymyalgia rheumatica in a defined elderly community. Rheumatol Rehabil 1982; 21: 235–237.
19. Kyle V, Silverman B, Silman A et al. Polymyalgia rheumatica/giant cell arteritis in general practice. BMJ 1985; 13: 385–388.

20. Liang M, Simkin PA, Hunder GG *et al*. Familial aggregation of polymyalgia rheumatica and giant cell arteritis. Arthritis Rheum 1974; 17: 19–24.
21. Rhodes DJ. Giant cell arteritis in general practice. J R Coll Gen Pract 1976; 26: 237–246.
22. Weyand CM, Hunder NH, Hicok K *et al*. HLA-DRB1 alleles in polymyalgia rheumatica, giant cell arteritis and rheumatoid arthritis. Arthritis Rheum 1994; 37: 514–520.
23. Dababneh A, Gonzalez-Gay MA, Garcia-Porrua C *et al*. Giant cell arteritis and polymyalgia rheumatica can be differentiated by distinct patterns of HLA class II association. J Rheumatol 1998; 25: 2140–2145.
24. Salvarani C, Hunder G. Musculoskeletal manifestations in a population-based cohort of patients with giant cell arteritis. Arthritis Rheum 1999; 42: 1259–1266.
25. Gonzalez-Gay M, Garcia-Porrus C, Vazguez-Caruncho M *et al*. The spectrum of polymyalgia rheumatica in Northern Spain: incidence and analysis of variables associated with relapse in ten year study. J Rheumatol 1999; 26: 1326–1332.
26. Matley D, Hajeer A, Dababneh A *et al*. Association of giant cell arteritis and polymyalgia rheumatica with different tumour necrosis factor microsatellite polymorphisms. Arthritis Rheum 2000; 43: 1749–1755.
27. Boiardi L, Salvarani C, Timms J *et al*. Interleukin-1 cluster and tumour necrosis factor-α gene polymorphisms in polymyalgia rheumatica. Clin Exp Rheumatol 2000; 18: 675–681.
28. Meliconi R, Pulsatelli L, Uguccioni M *et al*. Leukocyte infiltration in synovial tissue from the shoulder of patients with polymyalgia rheumatica. Quantitative analysis and influence of corticosteroid treatment. Arthritis Rheum 1996; 39: 1199–1207.
29. Salvarani C, Canitini F, Olivieri I *et al*. Proximal bursitis in active polymyalgia rheumatic. Ann Intern Med 1997; 127: 27–31.
30. Lange V, Teichmann J, Strucke H *et al*. Elderly onset rheumatoid arthritis and polymyalgia rheumatica: ultrasonographic study of the glenohumeral joints. Rheumatol Int 1998; 17: 229–232.
31. McGonagle D, Pease C, Mazo-Ortega H *et al*. Comparison of extracapsular changes by magnetic resonance imaging in patients with rheumatoid arthritis and polymyalgia rheumatica. J Rheumatol 2001; 28: 1837–1840.
32. Kassimos D, Kirwan J, Kyle V *et al*. Cytidine deaminase may be a useful marker in differentiating elderly onset rheumatoid arthritis from polymyalgia rheumatica/giant cell arteritis. Clin Exp Rheumatol 1995; 13: 641–644.
33. Hayreh S, Podhajsky Zimmerman B. Ocular manifestations of giant cell arteritis. Am J Opthalmol 1998; 125: 509–220.
34. Hayreh SS. Anterior ischaemic optic neuropathy. Differentiation of arteritis from non arteritic type and its management. Eye 1990; 4: 25–41.
35. Hunder C, Bloch D, Michel B *et al*. The American College of Rheumatology 1990 criteria for the classification of giant cell (temporal) arteritis. Arthritis Rheum 1990; 33: 1122–1128.
36. Bird HA, Esselinckx W, Dixon AS *et al*. An evaluation of criteria for polymyalgia rheumatica. Ann Rheum Dis 1979; 38: 434–439.
37. Caporali R, Montecncco C, Epis O *et al*. Presenting features of PMR and RA with PMR-like onset: a prospective study. Ann Rheum Dis 2001; 60: 1021–1024.
38. von Knorring J, Somer T. Malignancy in association with polymyalgia rheumatica and temporal arteritis. Scand J Rheumatol 1974; 3: 129–135.
39. Haga H, Eide G, Brun J *et al*. Cancer in association with polymyalgia rheumatica and temporal arteritis. J Rheumatol 1993; 20: 1335–1339.
40. Wise M, Agudelo GA, Chimelewski W, McKnight K. Temporal arteritis with low erythrocyte sedimentation rate: a review of 5 cases. Arthritis Rheum 1991; 34: 1571–1574.
41. Proven A, Gabriel S, O'Fallon W, Hunder G. Polymyalgia rheumatica with low erythrocyte sedimentation rate at diagnosis. J Rheumatol 1999; 26: 1333–1337.
42. Kyle V, Cawston TE, Hazleman BL. ESR and C-reactive protein in the assessment of polymyalgia rheumatica/giant cell arteritis on presentation and during follow up. Ann Rheum Dis 1989; 48: 408–409.
43. Pountain GD, Calvin J, Hazleman BL. α_1-Antichymotrypsin C-reactive protein and erythrocyte sedimentation rate in PMR/GCA. Br J Rheumatol 1994; 33: 550–554.
44. Chakravarty K, Pountain G, Merry P *et al*. A longitudinal study of anticardiolipin antibody in polymyalgia rheumatica and giant cell arteritis. J Rheumatol 1995; 22: 1694–1697.
45. Klein GE, Campbell RJ, Hunder GG, Carney JA. Skip lesions in temporal arteritis. Mayo Clin Proc 1976; 51: 504–508.
46. Généreau T, Lortholary O, Pottier M-A *et al*. Temporal artery biopsy : a diagnostic tool for systemic necrotizing vasculitis. Arthritis Rheum 1999; 42: 2674–2681.
47. Lie JT. When is arteritis of the temporal arteries not temporal arteritis? J Rheumatol 1994; 21: 186–189.
48. Estebann M, Font C, Hernandez-Rodriguez J *et al*. Small-vessel vasculitis surrounding a spared temporal artery. Clinical and pathological findings in a series of 28 patients. Arthritis Rheum 2001; 44: 1387–1395.
49. Schmidt W, Kraft H, Völker L *et al*. Colour Doppler sonography to diagnose temporal arteritis. Lancet 1995; 345: 866.
50. Blockmans D, Maes A, Stoobants S *et al*. New arguments for a vasculitic nature of polymyalgia rheumatica using positron emission tomography. Rheumatology (Oxford) 1999; 38: 444–447.
51. Richardson MP, Lever AML, Fink AM *et al*. Survival after aortic dissection in giant cell arteritis. Ann Rheum Dis 1996; 55: 332–333.
52. Wilkinson IMS, Russell RWR. Arteries of the head and neck in giant cell arteritis. A pathological study to show the pattern of arterial involvement. Arch Neurol 1972; 27: 378–387.
53. Kojima S, Tajagi A, Ida M, Shiozawa R. Muscle pathology in polymyalgia rheumatica: a histochemical and immunohistochemical study. Jpn J Med 1991; 30: 516–523.
54. Bacon PA, Doherty S, Zuckerman AJ. Hepatitis B antibody in polymyalgia rheumatica. Lancet 1975; ii: 476–478.
55. Salvarani C, Casali B, Cantini F *et al*. Detection of parvovirus B19 in temporal arteritis/polymyalgia rheumatic. Arthritis Rheum 2001; 44(suppl): S342.
56. Cimmino M, Grazi G, Balistreri M, Accardo S. Increased prevalence of antibodies to adenovirus and respiratory syncytial virus in polymyalgia rheumatica. Clin Exp Rheumatol 1993; 11: 309–313.
57. Duhaut P, Bosshard S, Calvert A *et al*. Giant cell arteritis, polymyalgia rheumatica, and viral hypothesis: a multicenter, prospective case control study. J Rheumatol 1999; 26: 361–369.
58. Elling P, Olsson AT, Elling H. Synchronous variations of the incidence of temporal arteritis and polymyalgia rheumatica in different regions of Denmark, association with epidemics of *Mycoplasma pneumoniae* infection. J Rheumatol 1996; 23: 112–119.
59. Russo MG, Waxman J, Abdoh AA, Serebro LH. Correlation between infection and the onset of the giant cell arteritis (temporal) arteritis syndrome. Arthritis Rheum 1995; 38: 374–380.
60. Sonnenblick M, Nesher G, Friedlande Y *et al*. Giant cell arteritis in Jerusalem: a 12 year epidemiological study. Br J Rheumatol 1994; 33: 938–941.
61. Cimmino MA. Genetic and environmental factors in polymyalgia rheumatica. Ann Rheum Dis 1997; 56: 576–577.
62. Gallagher PJ, Jones K. Immunohistochemical findings in cranial arteritis. Arthritis Rheum 1982; 25: 75–79.
63. Dasgupta B, Duke O, Kyle V *et al*. Antibodies to intermediate filaments in polymyalgia rheumatica and giant cell arteritis: a sequential study. Ann Rheum Dis 1987; 46: 746–749.
64. Cid MC, Campo E, Ercilla G *et al*. Immunohistochemical analysis of lymphoid and macrophage cell subsets and their immunologic activation markers in temporal arteritis. Influence of corticosteroid treatment. Arthritis Rheum 1989; 32: 884–893.
65. Kaiser M, Weyand C, Bjornsson J, Goronzy J. Platelet derived growth factor, intimal hyperplasia and ischaemic complications in GCA. Arthritis Rheum 1998; 41: 623–633.
66. Brack A, Geisler A, Martinez-Taboada *et al*. Giant cell arteritis is a T cell dependent disease. J Mol Med 1997; 8: 29–55.
67. Weyand CM, Schonberger J, Oppitz U *et al*. Distinct vascular lesions in giant cell arteritis share identical T cell clonotypes. J Exp Med 1994; 179: 951–960.
68. Bignon JD, Ferec C, Barrier J *et al*. HLA class II genes polymorphism in DR4 giant cell arteritis patients. Tissue Antigens 1988; 32: 254–258.
69. Roche N, Fulbright J, Wagner A *et al*. Correlation of interleukin 6 production and disease activity in polymyalgia rheumatica and giant cell arteritis. Arthritis Rheum 1993; 36: 1286–1294.
70. Kyle V, Hazleman BL. Treatment of polymyalgia rheumatica and giant cell arteritis. I. Steroid regimes in the first 2 months. Ann Rheum Dis 1989; 48: 658–661.
71. Nordberg E, Bengtsson BA. Death rates and causes of deaths in 284 consecutive patients with giant cell arteritis confirmed by biopsy. BMJ 1989; 299: 549–550.
72. Dasgupta B, Dolan AL, Panayi GS, Fernandes L. An initially double-blinded controlled 96 week trial of depot methylprednisolone against oral prednisolone in the treatment of PMR. Br J Rheumatol 1998; 37: 189–195.
73. Gabriel S, Sunku J, Salvarani C *et al*. Adverse outcomes of anti-inflammatory therapy among patients with polymyalgia rheumatica. Arthritis Rheum 1997; 40: 1873–1878.
74. Dasgupta B, Duke O, Timms A *et al*. Selective depletion and activation of CD8 lymphocytes from peripheral blood of patients with PMR and GCA. Ann Rheum Dis 1989; 48: 307–311.
75. Kyle V, Hazleman BL. Treatment of polymyalgia rheumatica and giant cell arteritis. II. The relationship between steroid dose and steroid associated side effects. Ann Rheum Dis 1989; 48: 662–666.
76. Krogsgaard M, Thamsborg G, Lund B. Changes in bone mass during low dose corticosteroid treatment in patients with PMR: a double-blind, prospective comparison between prednisolone and deflazocort. Ann Rheum Dis 1996; 55: 143–146.

OSTEOARTHRITIS AND RELATED DISORDERS

39 Clinical features

Roy D Altman and Carlos J Lozada

- Osteoarthritis is the most common articular disease
- About 50% of those with radiographic osteoarthritis have symptoms
- Pain is the most common reason the patient consults the physician
- Pain in osteoarthritis has many potential sources. There is no direct pain from cartilage, synovial fluid or the inner two-thirds of menisci. Pain fibers are present in the remaining tissues surrounding the joint
- A variety of other symptoms can result from osteoarthritis that impact on function and quality of life
- Signs of osteoarthritis can be absent, subtle or severe
- Although osteoarthritis can involve virtually any joint in the body, the most commonly involved joints are hands and feet, hips and knees

TABLE 39.1 SYMPTOMS AND SIGNS OF OSTEOARTHRITIS

Symptoms	Signs
Pain	Altered gait
Stiffness	Tenderness
Swelling	Enlargement
Altered function	Crepitus
Weakness	Limitation of motion
Deformity	Deformity
Grinding or clicking	Instability
Instability	

INTRODUCTION

Osteoarthritis (OA) is the most common form of arthritis, accounting for 30% of physician visits[1]. It may be defined as a 'heterogeneous group of conditions that lead to joint symptoms and signs which are associated with defective integrity of articular cartilage, in addition to related changes in the underlying bone and at the joint margins'[2]. It is usually classified as either primary (idiopathic) or secondary (associated with a known condition). Although OA is present by histologic or radiographic criteria in nearly 80% of people by the age of 80 years, only half have symptoms[3], and these are often variable and intermittent. It affects as many as 12% in the US population between the ages of 25 and 74 years[4]. There is a modest correlation between the presence of symptoms and the severity of anatomic changes.

Although variable in its presentation and course, OA often carries significant morbidity. In addition to the effects on the individual, the cost of OA to society is significant[1], related to its high prevalence, the reduced ability of those affected to perform both occupational and non-occupational activities, the occasional loss of a patient's ability to undertake self-care, and the related drain on health-care resources[5].

Osteoarthritis is no longer considered a 'degenerative' or 'wear and tear' arthritis, but rather involves dynamic biomechanical, biochemical and cellular processes[6]. Indeed, the joint damage that occurs in OA is, at least in part, the result of active remodeling involving all the joint structures. Although articular cartilage is at the center of change, OA is currently viewed as a disease of the entire joint and, therefore, the failure of the joint as an organ[7].

Although symptoms are often unilateral, evidence of OA is almost always present bilaterally. However, even when symptoms are bilateral, there is a tendency for one side to be more symptomatic than the other. The symptomatic side may also alternate over time. Unilateral disease may suggest OA secondary to trauma. However, despite the presence of continuing trauma, progression is more common with bilateral disease. In contrast to systemic inflammatory arthritides, OA lacks constitutional symptoms.

When OA is symptomatic, the most prominent complaint is pain. It remains unclear why fewer than 50% of persons with severe radiographic OA (Kellgren and Lawrence grade III and IV[8]) report pain[9]. Most often, the onset of OA symptomatology is insidious. Symptoms and signs of OA are listed in Table 39.1.

SYMPTOMS

Pain

Pain is most often the reason a patient with OA seeks the help of a physician[10]. When pain is present, its cause is often not clear, as the stimulus for pain in OA has many potential mechanisms (Table 39.2)[11]. Pain can be difficult to localize to an area within the joint. In knee OA, patients will commonly describe their pain as involving the entire joint. In one study, medial knee pain was reported in 34% of patients with OA of the knee, as compared with 52% reporting 'generalized' knee pain[12]. Joint pain may be referred proximally, but is more commonly referred distally, for example hip pain referred into the thigh and knee pain referred to the anterior or medial upper tibia. Anterior knee pain may represent patellofemoral (anterior compartment) OA. Patients often ascribe increasing pain and stiffness to changes in weather. Investigation in this area has been inconclusive. Some have suggested that changes in any two of temperature, humidity and barometric pressure may lead to changes in OA symptomatology.

The severity of pain should be noted and, ideally, measured at each visit. The two most commonly used pain scales are the five-point Likert scale (0 = none; 1 = mild; 2 = moderate; 3 = severe; 4 = very severe) or a 100mm visual analog scale (from 0mm = no pain to 100mm = the most pain possible). An alternative to the visual analog scale is a 10-point Numerical Rating Scale (from 0 = no pain to 10 = the most pain possible).

Pain can also be quantified through standardized testing. The Western Ontario McMaster Universities (WOMAC) Osteoarthritis Index pain subscale quantifies five measures of pain. It also measures stiffness and function in separate subscales. The algofunctional scale of Lequesne is

TABLE 39.2 RELATIONSHIP BETWEEN ANATOMIC SITE AND POSSIBLE PHYSIOLOGIC MECHANISM FOR PAIN IN OA

Anatomic site	Mechanism
Cartilage (defective or loss)	*Synovial*: inflammation induced by cartilage 'char' fragments, cartilage crystal shedding, cartilage release of cytokines (e.g. interleukin-1), enzymes (e.g. metalloproteinases). *Subchondral bone*: mechanical stress (see below) *Instability*: stress on capsule
Menisci	Tear or degeneration: stretch at insertion to the joint capsule, catch between surfaces
Synovial cavity	Stretch of joint capsule, transport of inflammatory mediators between synovium and cartilage
Synovium	Inflammation
Subchondral bone	Ischemia with increased pressure, decreased oxygen tension and increased pH Avascular necrosis Regeneration or repair of infarcted bone
Osteophytes	Periosteal elevation Neural impingement
Joint capsule	Stretch from joint distention Stress at insertion to periosteum and bone
Ligaments	Stress at insertion to periosteum and bone
Bursae	Inflammation, with or without calcification
Muscle	Spasm Nocturnal myoclonus
Central nervous system	Dysthymia, cyclothymia, fibromyalgia Ethnic, cultural, coping skills

also a reliable and validated instrument that combines pain and function.

The quality of the pain may hint as to its pathological origin. Pain that occurs after exercise is often caused by subchondral ischemia – so called 'bone angina'. This pain is often aching and deep seated. Pain along the joint margin, with tenderness at the site may indicate periosteal pain from stretching of the capsule or ligaments or overgrowing osteophytes. The sudden onset of pain with a catching sensation of the knee may be associated with a torn meniscus.

A thorough history and physical examination may help direct symptomatic treatment by revealing the source of the pain, which may be categorized by anatomic site (Table 39.2). This then allows the physician to target his therapeutic intervention. The contribution of the different tissues to pain are discussed below.

Articular cartilage

Damage to *articular cartilage* is the hallmark of osteoarthritis, yet articular cartilage is not a direct source of pain, because it lacks nerve endings[13,14]. *Menisci*, similarly, do not contain nerves in their weight-bearing surfaces (i.e. the inner two-thirds), and cannot directly account for pain. Teleologically, it makes evolutionary sense that compressive or shear forces on cartilage would not elicit pain, as pain would make ambulation problematic. Nevertheless, abnormalities in *articular cartilage*, *menisci*, and even *synovial fluid* can indirectly cause pain in OA.

Damaged *articular cartilage* causes symptoms that derive from loss of its structural integrity, cartilage debris and absence of cartilage. Structurally damaged cartilage loses the ability to allow the even gliding that usually occurs across smooth cartilage surfaces. Movement across

uneven surfaces results in a grinding or clicking sensation to the patient and crepitus on examination. These sensations can be accompanied by pain.

When damaged cartilage 'char' fragments are released into the synovial cavity, an attempt is made at clearing them, precipitating an inflammatory synovial response. Other microscopic and submicroscopic particulate material released from damaged articular cartilage – such as collagen, proteoglycans, crystals, proteolytic enzymes and cytokines – trigger a synovial inflammatory response to varying degrees. Although inflammation of the synovium in joints affected by OA is most often less severe than in the traditional 'inflammatory' arthritides (e.g. rheumatoid arthritis and gout), activation of inflammatory responses always occurs in OA joints, at both the synoviocyte and chondrocyte level (justifying the terminology 'osteo*arthritis*')[15,16].

Abnormal cartilage may contain a variety of calcium crystals, including calcium pyrophosphate dihydrate, hydroxyapatite and basic calcium phosphate. Surface disruption may allow 'crystal shedding' into the joint cavity, stimulating varying degrees of inflammation[17]. In cases in which cartilage is fissured and the subchondral bone is exposed, hydroxyapatite crystals from bone or cartilage may leach or be sheared into the synovial cavity. These crystals stimulate intracellular mechanisms of inflammation. In addition, the absence of articular cartilage allows loosening and instability of the joint, with resultant changes in the periarticular structures.

Other loose bodies in the joint, such as 'joint mice' or osteochondromatosis are potential indirect causes of pain. The disrupted portion of torn *menisci* can be displaced and inserted between normally smooth, gliding articular surfaces, stretching the joint capsule. Pain can sometimes be elicited on examination when the torn meniscus is stressed at its outer one-third or when partially torn menisci 'catch' between cartilage surfaces. Horizontal fissures do not usually cause symptoms, but fragments of the defective menisci may elicit an inflammatory response or act as loose bodies in the joint cavity.

Synovium

Synovial fluid can indirectly cause pain by serving as a transport medium, distending the joint capsule or limiting joint function. The synovial fluid shuttles inflammatory mediators between cartilage and synovium. Synovial fluid also serves as a reservoir for inflammatory cytokines, cells and crystals. Furthermore, synovial fluid distends the joint, potentially compressing synovial blood vessels and stimulating pressure receptors in the capsule[18–20]. A distended joint compromises the normal transport of nutrition and gases by synovial fluid between cartilage and synovium. The residual waste products linger in the synovial space and perpetuate inflammation.

The *synovium* contains nerve fibers. These include Aβ (large myelinated mechanoreceptors), Aδ (small myelinated nociceptors) and C (small non-myelinated nociceptors). The latter nociceptors can release both substance P and calcitonin gene-related peptide. Substance P stimulates both the pain response and inflammation[21]. These pain receptors may also be activated through peripheral mechanical, thermal and noxious stimuli. These noxious stimuli include bradykinin, histamine, prostaglandins and leukotrienes[22].

Bone

The *subchondral bone* is directly related to pain in OA[23]. When subchondral ischemia or increased venous pressure occur, peptides such as substance P and calcitonin gene-related peptide are released from the nerve endings in bone[24]. The pain of ischemic bone is aching and deep-seated. When bone death occurs (osteonecrosis), there is a pain-free period. Pain recurs with bone repair and remodeling. In OA, subchondral cysts and sclerosis are the eventual radiographic evidence that localized osteonecrosis has taken place. Providing relief from the pain of ischemic bone has not been specifically studied. It is uncertain whether there is a neurogenic pain component to the bone pain of OA.

Osteophytes are the most consistent pathologic and radiographic finding associated with the presence of pain[25]. The mechanisms are not clear, but osteophytes may cause pain directly by distending the periosteum; pain can sometimes be elicited by applying pressure over an osteophyte of knee or hand. Pain from osteophytes may be due to concomitant inflammation. Osteophytes in the spinal facets are often an indirect cause of pain and other symptoms by compressing nerves as they traverse the spinal foramina (e.g. cervical, lumbar lateral recess) or within the spinal canal (e.g. lumbar spinal stenosis).

Capsule and related tissues

The *joint capsule* and periarticular *ligaments* are stretched by synovial effusions or instability, and may cause pain through mechanoreceptors and nociceptors. Stress at the ligamentous insertion on the *periosteum* stimulates nociceptors. When the joint periarticular tissues are distorted, the ligaments may be abnormally stressed or may be understressed (e.g. varus deformity of the knee stresses the lateral ligaments and fully relaxes the medial ligaments). These phenomena, labeled 'stress enhancement' and 'stress deprivation'[26], result in contractures of the capsule and ligaments. Contractures result in decreasing function and increasing pain from stress at ligamentous insertions, and periarticular muscle spasm.

Periarticular *bursae* may become inflamed and, hence, be a source of pain. Bursal inflammation is sometimes associated with calcium formation (e.g. calcific bursitis).

Muscle

Muscle spasm is probably a common source of pain in OA. Muscle spasm may occur in the form of nocturnal myoclonus, altering sleep patterns and resulting in fibromyalgia-like symptoms[27]. In a study of 429 patients older than 65 years with OA of the knee, there were problems with sleep onset (31%), sleep maintenance (81%) and early morning awakening (51%)[28]. This was influenced by additional psychosocial and medical comorbidities. Muscle spasm of the lower extremities must be differentiated from pain of vascular (e.g. night cramps) or spinal radicular origin. Joint contractures in OA can cause pain upon stretching of the periarticular muscles.

Psychological factors and pain

Joint pain is modulated by the individuals' perception of pain and unique ethnic, cultural and personal circumstances. It tends to be more severe in evenings, at weekends and early in the work week[29]. Pain is complicated by the presence of dysthymia, other forms of depression, cyclothymia and secondary gains. Psychologic evaluation may be needed to determine the overlying psychologic and coping influences on the pain response. In knee OA, a passive coping style that led to resting was found to predict a higher level of disability within 36 weeks[30]. Self-efficacy beliefs appear to relate to functional decline when associated with lower extremity muscular weakness[31].

Stiffness

Stiffness may be defined as a sensation of a 'gelling' or tightening of the involved joint that usually occurs after inactivity, such as in the morning or when arising after sitting for a prolonged period. In contrast to inflammatory arthritides (e.g. rheumatoid arthritis), stiffness in OA usually lasts only a few minutes, almost always less than 30 minutes. However, the duration of stiffness has been found to be of less use than the character of the stiffness, in distinguishing OA from rheumatoid arthritis (Silman A, personal communication). In contrast to the diffuse stiffness of rheumatoid arthritis, that of OA is usually confined to the involved joints.

Other symptoms

The patient may have a sensation of fullness and swelling about the joint. There may be associated warmth and loss of function.

Weight-bearing joints that are inflamed or contracted, or both, are associated with gait disturbance, increased muscle spasm and reduced quality of life. A contracted knee or hip can produce a prominent limp (see below). Aids to ambulation may reduce the severity of altered function.

Impaired function of a weight-bearing joint places stress on the contralateral weight-bearing joints. It is not uncommon for the patient with impaired right knee function (perhaps with pain) to have difficulty with the left hip.

Hypertrophic bone formation in interphalangeal joint OA may contribute to reduced dexterity and difficulty performing fine movements, such as knitting, sewing or playing a musical instrument. OA of the 1st carpometacarpal (CMC) joint may make it difficult to hold a pen.

Inactivity secondary to pain may lead to significant weakness, and can be compounded by periarticular muscle atrophy.

Patients may complain of enlargement of the joints of the hands or knee. They may also complain of increasing deformity of the knees, such as 'knock knees' (valgus) or 'bowing' (varus).

Patients may complain of a click or grinding sensation with joint motion. The grinding may be associated with pain.

Finally, the sensation of instability may cause the patient to seek assistance in ambulation, such as a cane or crutch. In the knee, instability is often associated with a feeling that the knee is 'giving out.'

SIGNS

Gait

Osteoarthritis of weight-bearing joints leads to altered gait patterns, mostly by a conscious or subconscious attempt to protect the joint. Hip, knee, ankle and foot arthritis provide distinctive gait patterns. One should note the patient's gait pattern and make appropriate use of aids to ambulation.

Tenderness

There may be tenderness of soft tissues (e.g. synovium, capsule, bursae, periarticular muscles) or periosteum at the insertion of capsule or ligaments.

Joint swelling

There may be enlargement of the joint from synovitis, synovial effusion, bony enlargement, joint mice or osteochondromatosis. Effusions are usually cool or slightly warm to palpation. The distal interphalangeal joint (DIP) swelling may present as a cystic herniation (Fig. 39.1); aspiration often reveals a jelly-like material reminiscent of a ganglion cyst. Swelling of the joint from an effusion frequently leads to loss of extension. This is in contrast to a periarticular bursitis or tendinitis, in which the joint is splinted, often in full extension.

Crepitus

Crepitus over a joint with OA may be of soft tissue or bony origin. It may be localized (e.g. chondromalacia patella and anterior compartment crepitus of the knee). Grinding, crunching or cracking may be present over a joint with OA. This represents uneven surfaces moving across each other. Although present with passive joint motion, it is most often best demonstrated with active motion of the joint. This should be contrasted with the benign 'cracking' of the metacarpophalangeal (MCP) joints that occurs when smooth cartilage surfaces are separated, creating a vacuum sound.

Needle arthroscopy has been used to define the origin of crepitus of the knee[32]. Transmitted bony crepitus was a specific finding for bone-

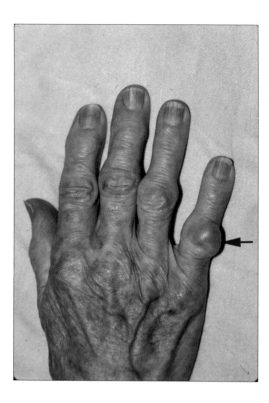

Fig. 39.1 Interphalangeal osteoarthritis of the hand, with cystic herniation of the 5th proximal interphalangeal joint.

on-bone in the compartment being assessed. Added tibiofemoral stress was 65% sensitive and 94% specific for cartilage disruption in the compartment assessed.

Limitation of motion

There may be loss of function with reduced motion as a result of synovitis/effusion or periarticular soft tissue contractures. When there is limitation of motion of a weight-bearing joint, it places additional stress on ipsilateral and contralateral weight-bearing joints.

As above, performance measures can be assessed on examination[32]. The WOMAC physical function subscale score correlates with several performance measures such as walking, stair climb, rising from a chair and range of motion in OA of the knee and hip[33].

Deformity

Deformity may be present in any of the peripheral joints with OA. However, it is most notable in the interphalangeal joints with enlarge-

ment and subluxation, the 1st CMC joint, the knees (varus/valgus) or the hips (shortened extremity). Bony enlargement is a form of deformity. Deformity may be associated with joint fusion or instability.

Instability

Taking joints through their arc of movement may reveal instability in various planes of motion. For example, instability of the knee may be demonstrated in anterior-posterior planes (cruciate ligament laxity or deficiency) or in mediolateral planes (collateral ligament laxity, loss of medial compartment bony stock).

CLINICAL PRESENTATIONS

Osteoarthritis may involve virtually any joint in the body. As it usually has an insidious onset of symptoms, an acute presentation suggests a concomitant inflammatory component (e.g. crystalline synovitis). OA is most often monarticular in presentation, slowly evolving to the contralateral side.

There are patterns to joint involvement. In general, OA of the knees and of the hips occur in different patient populations. OA of the hands and feet are generally present in the same individual, to varying degrees. There appears to be a subset of patients that have osteoarthritis of both central and peripheral joints, which is known as 'generalized' OA[34]. The characteristics of OA at individual sites are discussed below.

Shoulder

Shoulder pain is sometimes related to glenohumeral OA. Pain is typically aching in nature, and associated with the extremes of motion or after activity of the shoulder. There is not usually much loss of function, but crepitus can be found on examination. OA of the shoulder usually coexists with, and is difficult to differentiate from, other abnormalities of the shoulder, e.g. rotator cuff abnormalities, adhesive capsulitis, bursitis.

A peculiar destructive arthropathy (Milwaukee shoulder) is associated with persistent shoulder pain, large synovial effusions and demonstration of a variety of calcium crystals (Fig. 39.2) (see Chapter 43).

Acromioclavicular joint OA can produce pain that can be aggravated by weight bearing or other stressful activities. Painless enlargement of the acromioclavicular joint is common and may be associated with reduced shoulder motion.

Hands

Patients often present for unsightly enlargement of digits or pain at the base of the thumb. Examination demonstrates bony enlargement and

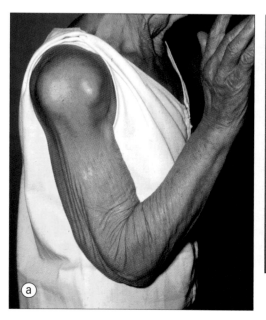

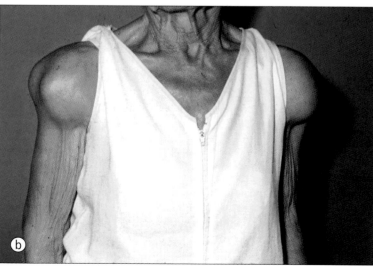

Fig. 39.2 Destructive arthropathy (Milwaukee) of the shoulder. A large synovial effusion is apparent (a) over the lateral aspect of the humerus or (b) anteriorly in front of the glenohumeral joint.

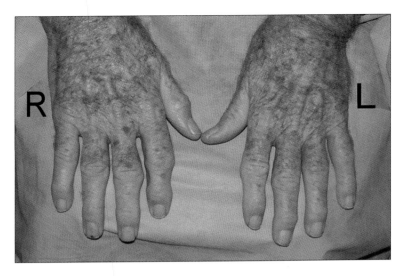

Fig. 39.3 Interphalangeal osteoarthritis of the hands. Knobby, hard tissue changes of the DIP joints. Hard and soft tissue changes of the proximal interphalangeal joints, with deformity. The MCP joints and wrists are spared. There is knobby deformity at the base of the left thumb, reflecting radial subluxation of the 1st proximal metacarpal at the 1st CMC joint.

deformities of the interphalangeal joints. There may be tenderness, and occasionally other signs of inflammation. There is often a partial loss of range of motion.

Distal interphalangeal joints are typically involved, with slow bony enlargement over a period of years (Heberden's nodes) (Fig. 39.3). These nodes are more common in women, and are often present in more than one family member. They often appear around the time of the menopause, but a clear relation to reduced estrogen concentrations has

not been established. The enlargement is not confined to any one aspect of the joint, although there is a predilection for the radio- and ulnodorsal aspects of the joints. Involvement of the 2nd and 3rd DIPs is particularly common. Enlargements are often more severe in the dominant hand. There is often associated deformity, with radial, ulnar or palmar deviations; these are unsightly rather than painful. A predominant palmar subluxation may have the appearance of a 'mallet' finger. There may be some loss of dexterity. OA of the DIPs may result in vertical ridges on the adjacent fingernails. There may be an acute swelling of the DIP, with cystic herniation of the capsule (Fig. 39.1). Aspiration of these cysts yields a jelly-like material. Microscopic examination reveals large polymorphonuclear leukocytes, with several refractile inclusion cysts that stain for fat (reminiscent of the fluid extracted from a wrist ganglion).

There are often associated hard or soft tissue changes in the proximal interphalangeal (PIP) joints (Bouchard's nodes) and erosive changes radiographically. Deformities of the PIPs are particularly common (Fig. 39.3). The 2nd and 3rd PIPs are most commonly involved. Involvement of the MCP joints is uncommon.

The 1st CMC (trapezioscaphoid) joints are commonly involved, particularly in women with hypermobility[35]. There is a tendency for osteophytes to develop on the distal ulnar surface of the trapezoid, associated with subluxation and radial deviation of the proximal head of the 1st metacarpal. This gives the base of the thumb a 'knobby' clinical appearance (Fig. 39.3). In contrast to PIP and DIP involvement, this deviation is commonly associated not only with pain, but also with disability.

Although the course is usually insidious and not very inflammatory, in a subset of these patients the disease may have an aggressive and destructive course. This has suggested classification into a nodal (non-inflammatory) and non-nodal (inflammatory) or erosive interphalangeal OA. On occasion, the evolution of interphalangeal OA may be

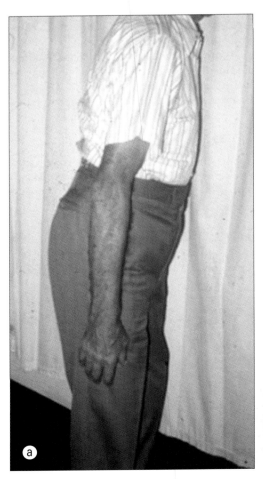

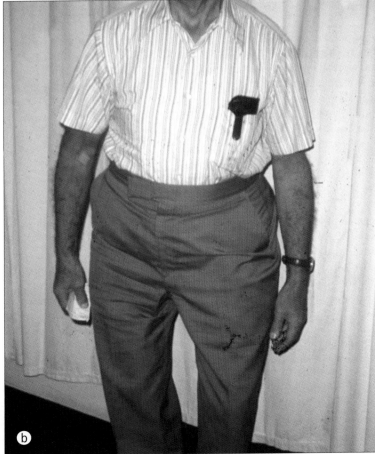

Fig. 39.4 Osteoarthritis of the hips. Severe osteoarthritis secondary to pelvic Paget's disease causes medial migration of the femoral heads into the acetabuli, resulting in hip flexion contractures. The patient stands with a bent forward posture apparent from a lateral (a) or anterior (b) view.

indistinguishable from early-onset rheumatoid arthritis or a spondylo-arthropathy, particularly psoriatic arthritis.

Hips

Patients most often present with groin or anterior hip pain that radiates into the thigh. Pain is associated with weight bearing and is relieved by rest. Examination most often reveals difficulty rising from a seated position, altered gait favoring the arthritic hip and reduced range of motion on examination, with pain on motion.

Hip OA is most commonly associated with an insidious onset of pain (*malum coxae senilis*, coxarthropathy). Pain is noted on weight-bearing activity and must be distinguished from referred lumbar pain. In contrast to hip pain, low back pain is most often aggravated by prolonged sitting and improves with ambulation. Both lumbar and hip OA may be painful when the patient rises from a seated or reclined position and during early ambulation. Pain from lumbar stenosis often has its onset after ambulating for a distance, and is more suggestive of claudication (pseudoclaudication). More symptomatic hip OA may be painful at all times, even at rest. Pain is usually localized to the groin or medial thigh, but may be lateral, suggesting (and associated with) trochanteric bursitis. Hip pain may also be referred posteriorly or toward the knee.

Hip OA is associated with a particular gait – one in which the patient overshifts their weight while walking, to reduce the pain (antalgic gait). There is loss of extension that often goes unnoticed. Loss of hip flexion/rotation is noticed by the patient, because of difficulty while attempting to put on socks or shoes. When severe, flexion contracture is associated with a prominent limp (Fig. 39.4). Significant OA of the hip is associated with a loss of internal rotation (less than 15°) on examination[36]. The severely involved hip is flexed, externally rotated and adducted. The Trendelenburg sign may be present – standing on the involved extremity leads to a drop in the contralateral hip from weakening of the ipsilateral hip abductors. Another late sign is shortening of the extremity as the femoral head migrates into the acetabulum, in association with a flexion contracture of the hip.

Most hip OA is slowly progressive. However, there is a subset of patients with a rapidly progressive form of hip OA, evolving over a few months. Unfortunately, at this time, there is no particular clinical characteristic or set of characteristics that can separate those with rapidly progressive OA from the less aggressive forms.

Hip pain must be distinguished from referred lumbar spine pain, trochanteric bursitis, avascular necrosis, and hip fractures that can be difficult to detect on routine radiography. Additional differential considerations include transient osteoporosis of the hip, non-displaced fracture (e.g. femoral neck or intertrochanteric) and osteonecrosis.

Knee

Patients often present with an insidious onset of pain about the knee, particularly with weight bearing and climbing stairs. They may have noticed enlargement, swelling, varus/valgus deformity. Examination sometimes reveals swelling with loss of the usual crease in the skin over the inner (null) facet between the patella and the condyle, in addition to a bulging suprapatellar sac. When present, the effusions are usually cool to palpation. There may be tenderness, but redness is uncommon. Reduced function may be seen with a flexion contracture (unable to extend to 0°) and sometimes an extension contracture (unable to flex to 115°). There is often tenderness of the anserine bursa and crepitus on active motion of the knee.

Knee OA is also associated with pain on weight bearing (gonarthritis). There is often pain when rising from a seated position. It may be aggravated with climbing stairs or bending. The most common form of symptomatic OA of the knee is from medial tibiofemoral compartment involvement. Pain is often along the medial joint margin and associated

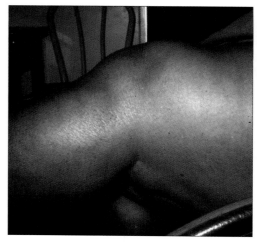

Fig. 39.5
Osteoarthritis of the knee. This morbidly obese woman has an enlarged knee with a flexion contracture. Lack of mobility is reflected by her use of a wheelchair. Synovial effusion of the knee is difficult to detect by inspection or palpation in a knee distal to a thigh of this size.

with tenderness, and may radiate along the upper medial leg. Pain may also be felt distally along the anterior proximal tibia. A knee limp may be present. The knee may be unsteady on weight bearing, causing the patient to complain of a feeling that the knee is buckling or 'giving out.' A flexion contracture may be demonstrated (Fig. 39.5).

There is often crepitus on motion that is best detected on active joint motion. A usually cool, palpable effusion may be present. Occasional distention of the popliteal semitendinosus bursa (Baker's cyst) may be present. There may also be herniation or rupture of the bursa into the thigh or leg (herniated or ruptured popliteal cyst), reminiscent of thrombophlebitis (pseudothrombophlebitis syndrome). Marginal osteophytes, intrasynovial loose bodies (joint mice) or moveable bodies (osteochondromas) may be palpable. There may be a loss of full extension, aggravating the limp. Medial joint space narrowing may lead to a varus deformity, whereas lateral joint space narrowing may lead to a valgus deformity. Varus deformity with valgus deformity of the contralateral knee gives the patient a 'wind-swept' appearance. There is often associated quadriceps weakness and atrophy.

Knee OA may be associated with pain at the distal medial joint margin (anserine bursitis at the insertion on the pes anserinus of the tibia). This is particularly common in the elderly with significant varus deformity. Both varus alignment and standing balance correlate with the severity of knee OA[37]. Thus knee OA has been associated with quadriceps weakness, reduced knee proprioception and increased postural sway[38]. When present, reduced proprioception was present in the contralateral knee[39]. It was felt that both pain and muscle weakness influenced postural sway. Although quadriceps strength was significantly lower in patients with OA of the medial compartment of the knee, the hip adductor muscles were actually stronger, perhaps compensating for the varus deformity[40].

Meniscal tears may be difficult to determine on physical examination of patients with knee OA. A positive McMurray test is the only true predictor of an unstable meniscal tear[41]. A history of swelling and synovial effusion are not helpful.

Patellofemoral OA is not commonly symptomatic, except in young women (chondromalacia patella). Anterior compartment pain is aggravated by sitting in low chairs (e.g. movie theaters) and can be precipitated by pressure and mediolateral movement of the patella in the intercondylar groove. Symptoms from patellofemoral OA are usually self-limiting, resolving in a period of several months.

Osteoarthritis of the knee may be associated with varying degrees of subchondral osteonecrosis. This is suspected in patients with a rather abrupt onset of particularly severe pain refractory to the usual therapy. In early phases, it is best detected by magnetic resonance imaging. Uncommonly, there is a destructive arthropathy associated with a variety of calcium crystals.

Ankle

Talonavicular and subtalar joint osteoarthritis is often secondary, for example to trauma with or without ligamentous damage. Patients complain of ankle pain on weight bearing. Examination reveals synovitis of the ankle that must be distinguished from a variety of conditions, such as Achilles bursitis, plantar fasciitis, talocalcaneal coalition, post-traumatic osteoarthritis (e.g. after calcaneal fracture), painful os trigonum, talonavicular osteoarthritis, posterior tibial tendinitis and pedal edema.

Feet

Patients most often present with pain and enlargement of the 1st metatarsophalangeal (MTP) joint, particularly with walking. Examination commonly reveals an enlarged joint, with medial subluxation and lateral deviation of the big toe. There are sometimes signs of inflammation over the involved joint, with tenderness and loss of dorsiflexion. There are commonly abnormalities of additional toes.

The same processes that occur in the hands can occur concomitantly in the feet. Different members of the same family may have predominant hands or feet involvement.

The typical pattern of involvement of the feet includes the 1st MTP joint, commonly called the 'bunion' joint (hallux valgus) (Fig. 39.6). The joint enlarges medially, with a lateral drift of the 1st toe.

There may be loss of function of the 1st MTP (hallux rigidus), usually occurring without drifting of the great toe, but limiting 'toe off' with ambulation. In this condition, the enlargement is usually dorsal.

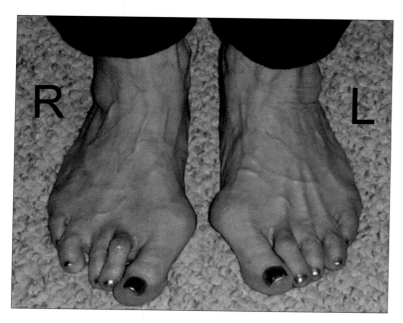

Fig. 39.6 MTP and interphalangeal osteoarthritis of the feet. There is bilateral enlargement of the 1st MTP joint, with medial subluxation of the phalanx. Flexion contraction of toes (particularly of the right 2nd digit) with subluxation of the MTP, has an associated callus over the dorsum of the PIP joint. The right 3rd digit is subluxed under the 2nd digit. There is relaxation of the transtarsal ligament, with medial subluxation of the MTP and bony enlargement of the 5th MTP joints (Tailor bunion, bunionette).

There is often painful and tender swelling of foot joints. Associated contractures of additional (cock-up) toes with loss of plantar fat pads are often seen. Disabling painful ambulation may ensue. Pes planus, with relaxation of the transtarsal ligament and a pronator forefoot deformity, aggravates the symptoms. The patient may find it difficult to wear certain types of shoes, particularly those with high heels.

Temporomandibular

Temporomandibular OA is often associated with hyperextensibility, perhaps with recurrent subluxations. However, most temporomandibular OA is associated with meniscal tears or malalignment between mandible and maxilla.

EVALUATION

Laboratory tests

There are no laboratory tests that are diagnostic of OA. Low-grade inflammation in OA can be detected by measurement of serum acute-phase reactants. Increases in erythrocyte sedimentation rate are more often attributable to age rather than to OA. Subtle, but definite increases in C-reactive protein are present in patients with active OA, and appear to predict disease progression[42].

Synovial fluid and serum markers of OA are being investigated as tools to detect the presence of OA or to predict disease progression. To date, no individual marker has accomplished either of these goals, and a combination of markers may be needed.

Synovial fluid from patients with OA is usually clear and colorless, and the polymorphonuclear leukocyte content is less than 2000/ml. More inflammatory synovitis in OA may demonstrate inflammatory synovial effusions, particularly in the presence of calcium crystals. Synovial fluid from a DIP cyst is often jelly-like and contains large polymorphonuclear leukocytes with several refractile inclusion cysts. Synovial fluid from a joint with osteochondromatosis is often very viscous and relatively acellular.

Crystals may be present in as many as 70% of synovial fluid specimens from patients with OA[43]. Although all calcium crystals have been shown to precipitate inflammation, the relationship between hydroxyapatite and several forms of basic calcium phosphate to the synovitis that is present in patients is not well established.

SUMMARY

Symptomatic OA of the extremities is common, and affects a large segment of the population, particularly those older than 50 years. Although OA can affect nearly any joint in the body, OA of the weight-bearing joints leads to the most disabling symptoms. Hip and knee OA can cause significant morbidity, disability and impairment. Pain is the most common complaint that brings the patient to seek a physician's assistance. Examination often reveals loss of function and may reveal signs of inflammation. The findings on careful history and physical examination should lead to the formulation of an individualized program of therapy.

REFERENCES

1. Kramer JS, Yelin EH, Epstein WV. Social and economic impacts of four musculoskeletal conditions: a study using national community-based data. J Rheumatol 1983; 26: 901–907.

2. Altman RD, Asch E, Bloch D et al. Development of criteria for the classification and reporting of osteoarthritis: classification of osteoarthritis of the knee. Arthritis Rheum 1986; 29: 1039–1049.

3. Hochberg MC, Lawrence RC, Everett DF, Cornoni-Huntley J. Epidemiologic associations of pain in osteoarthritis of the knee: data from the National Health and Nutrition Examination Survey and the National Health and Nutrituion Examination. I: epidemiologic follow-up survey. Semin Arthritis Rheum 1989; 18(suppl 2): 4–9.

4. Lawrence RC, Hochberg MC, Kelsey JL et al. Estimates of the prevalence of selected arthritic and musculoskeletal diseases in the United States. J Rheumatol 1989; 16: 427–441.

5. Levy E, Ferme A, Perocheau D, Bono I. Socioeconomic costs of osteoarthritis in France. Rev Rhum 1993; 60: 63S–67S.

6. Kuettner KE, Goldberg VM. Introduction. In: Kuettner KE, Goldberg VM, eds. Osteoartritic disorders. Rosemont, IL: American Academy of Orthopaedic Surgeons; 1995: xxi–xxv.

7. Lozada CJ, Altman RD. Chondroprotection in osteoarthritis. Bull Rheum Dis 1997; 46: 5–7.

8. Kellgren JH, Lawrence RC. Radiological assessment of osteoarthrosis. Ann Rheum Dis 1957; 16: 494–501.

9. Lethbridge-Cejku M, Scott WW, Reichle R et al. Association of radiographic features of osteoarthritis of the knee with knee pain: data from the Baltimore Longitudinal Study of Aging. Arthritis Care Res 1995; 8: 182–188.

10. Brandt KD. Pain, synovitis, and articular cartilage changes in osteoarthritis. Semin Arthritis Rheum 1989; 18(suppl 2): 77–80.

11. Altman R, Dean D. Introduction and overview: pain in osteoarthritis. Semin Arthritis Rheum 1989; 18(suppl 2): 1–3.

12. Creamer P, Lethbridge-Cejku M, Hochberg MC. Where does it hurt? Pain localization in osteoarthritis of the knee. Osteoarthritis Cartilage 1998; 6: 318–323.

13. Harkness IAL, Higgs ER, Dieppe PA. Osteoarthritis. In Wall PD, Melzadk R, eds. Textbook of pain. London: Churchill Livingstone; 1984: 215–224.

14. Wyke B. The neurology of joints: a review of general principles. Clin Rheum Dis 1981; 7: 223–239.

15. Lindblad S, Hedfors E. Arthroscopic and immunohistologic characterization of knee joint synovitis in osteoarthritis. Arthritis Rheum 1987; 30: 1081–1088.

16. Lindblad S, Hedfors E. Arthroscopic and synovial correlates of pain in osteoarthritis. Semin Arthritis Rheum 1989; 18(suppl 2): 91–93.

17. Schumacher HR. The role of inflammation and crystals in the pain of osteoarthritis. Semin Arthritis Rheum 1989; 18(suppl 2): 81–85.

18. Schaible H-G, Schmidt RF. Effects of an experimental arthritis on the sensory properties of fine articular afferent units. J Neurophysiol 1985; 54: 1109–1122.

19. Grigg P, Schaible H-G, Schmidt RF. Mechanical sensitivity of group III and IV afferents from posterior articular nerve in normal and inflamed cat knee. J Neurophysiol 1986; 55: 635–643.

20. Schaible H-G, Neugebauer V, Schmidt RF. Osteoarthritis and pain. Semin Arthritis Rheum 1989; 18: 30–34.

21. Kolasinski SL, Haines KA, Siegel EL et al. Neuropeptides and inflammation. A somatostatin analog as a selective antagonist of neutrophil activation by substance P. Arthritis Rheum 1992; 35: 369–375.

22. Kantor TG. Concepts in pain control. Semin Arthritis Rheum1989; 18(suppl 2): 94–99.

23. Badalamente MA, Cherney SB. Periosteal and vascular innervation of the human patella in degenerative joint disease. Semin Arthritis Rheum 1989; 18(suppl 2): 61–66.

24. Kiaer T, Gronlund J, Sorensen KH. Intraosseous pressure and partial pressures of oxygen and carbon dioxide in osteoarthritis. Semin Arthritis Rheum 1989; 18(suppl 2): 57–60.

25. Altman RD, Asch E, Bloch D et al. Development of criteria for the classification and reporting of osteoarthritis: classification of osteoarthritis of the knee. Arthritis Rheum 1986; 29: 1039–1049.

26. Akeson WH, Garfin S, Amiel D et al. Para-articular connective tissue in osteoarthritis. Semin Arthritis Rheum 1989; 18(suppl 2): 41–50.

27. Moldofsky H. Sleep influences on regional and diffuse pain syndromes associated with osteoarthritis. Semin Arthritis Rheum 1989; 18(suppl 2): 18–21.

28. Wilcox S, Brenes GA, Levine D et al. Factors related to sleep disturbance in older adults experiencing knee pain or knee pain with radiographic evidence of knee osteoarthritis. J Am Geriatr Soc 2000; 10: 1241–1251.

29. Bellamy N, Sothern RB, Campbell J et al. Circadian and circaseptan variation in pain perception in osteoarthritis of the knee. J Rheumatol 1990; 17: 364–372.

30. Steultjens MP, Dekker J, Bijlsma JW. Coping, pain, and disability in osteoarthritis: a longitudinal study. J Rheumatol 2001; 28: 1068–1072.

31. Rejeski WJ, Miller ME, Foy C et al. Self-efficacy and the progression of functional limitations and self-reported disability in older adults with knee pain. J Gerontol B Psychol Sci Soc Sci 2001; 56: S261–265.

32. Ike R, O'Rourke KS. Compartment-directed physical examination of the knee can predict articular abnormalities disclosed by needle arthroscopy. Arthritis Rheum 1995; 38: 917–925.

33. Lin YC, Davey RC, Cochrane T. Tests for physical function of the elderly with knee and hip osteoarthritis. Scand J Med Sci Sports 2001; 11: 280–286.

34. Kellgren JH, Moore R. Generalized osteoarthritis and Heberden's nodes. BMJ 1952; 1: 181–187.

35. Jonsson H, Valtysdottir ST. Hypermobility features in patients with hand osteoarthritis. Osteoarthritis Cartilage 1995; 3: 1–5.

36. Altman RD, Chairman, for the ACR Subcommittee on Classification Criteria of Osteoarthritis. The American College of Rheumatology criteria for the classification and reporting of osteoarthritis of the hip. Arthritis Rheum 1991; 34: 505–514.

37. Birmingham TB, Kramer JF, Kirkley A et al. Arch Phys Med Rehabil 2001; 82: 1115–1118.

38. Hassan BS, Mockett S, Doherty M. Static postural sway, proprioception, and maximal voluntary quadriceps contraction in patients with knee osteoarthritis and normal control subjects. Ann Rheum Dis 2001; 60: 612–618.

39. Koralewixz LM, Engh GA. Comparison of proprioception in arthritic and age-matched normal knees. J Bone Joint Surg Am 2000; 82A: 1582–1588.

40. Yamada H, Koshino T, Sakai N, Saito T. Hip adductor muscle strength in patients with varus deformed knee. Clin Orthop 2001; 386: 179–185.

41. Dervin GF, Stiell IG, Wells GA et al. Physician's accuracy and interrator reliability for the diagnosis of unstable meniscal tears in patients having osteoarthritis of the knee. Can J Surg 2001; 44: 267–274.

42. Spector TD, Hart DJ, Nandra D et al. Low-level increases in serum C-reactive protein are present in early osteoarthritis of the knee and predict progressive disease. Arthritis Rheum 1997; 40: 723–727.

43. Olmez N, Schumacher HR Jr. Crystal deposition and osteoarthritis. Curr Rheumatol Rep 1999; 1: 107–111.

40 Management of limb joint osteoarthritis

Carlos J Lozada and Roy D Altman

- Osteoarthritis (OA) is the most common form of arthritis and pain is the patient's major symptom

- Distinguishing articular from periarticular sources of pain is important in designing an appropriate therapeutic intervention

- Currently, the aims of treatment are to reduce pain and minimize disability

- The management of OA should be individualized and should include both non-pharmacologic and pharmacologic intervention

- Patient education, weight control and exercise are the cornerstones of the successful management of OA

- Systemic pharmacologic therapies often effectively relieve pain and include non-steroidal anti-inflammatory drugs, cyclo-oxygenase-2 specific inhibitors, non-opioid analgesics and opioid analgesics

- Intra-articular agents include corticosteroids and hyaluronate products, which may be useful in the symptomatic treatment of knee joint OA

- The adverse event profile of the therapeutic plan should be minimized whenever possible

- Pharmacologic structure-modifying interventions are currently under active investigation

- Surgical interventions are available for those that fail to respond to the non-pharmacologic and pharmacologic interventions

INTRODUCTION

Osteoarthritis (OA) is the most common articular rheumatologic disorder[1]. It is characterized by articular cartilage deterioration, subchondral bone remodeling and osteophyte formation. Risk factors include (among others) increasing age, weight, genetic factors and prior trauma. Traditionally, OA has been viewed as an inevitable degenerative condition of the cartilage. It is now viewed as a biomechanical and biochemical inflammatory disease of the entire joint[2]. New insights into pathogenesis have revealed a role for inflammatory pathways in the natural history of the disease[3]. This understanding of inflammation in OA has led to a new focus on the potential for structure modification[4]. Some new investigational approaches include: enzyme inhibitors, cytokines/cytokine blockers and nutritional supplements[5].

The goals of therapy for OA of the perieral joints are summarized in Table 40.1. The patient must know and understand their disease. Because there is no single program that is effective for everyone, the program needs to be individualized. Although alteration of the course of OA is desirable, present programs improve function and reduce disability by treating symptoms. It is felt that the future will identify and prove that it is possible to alter the course of OA with disease/structure modification.

Therapeutic approaches are generally geared to symptom relief and include non-pharmacologic therapy (e.g. exercise and weight loss), pharmacologic therapies (e.g. topical preparations, intra-articular drugs,

systemic pharmacologic agents) and surgery (Table 40.2)[6]. Guidelines for the management of OA at specific sites have been developed and reported by such bodies as the American College of Rheumatology (ACR)[7] and the European League of Associations of Rheumatology[8].

TABLE 40.1 GOALS IN MANAGEMENT OF OA

- Patient education
- Individualize therapeutic regimen (patient specific morbidities)
- Treat symptoms (e.g. reduce pain)
- Minimize disability
- Slow structural change/disease progression

TABLE 40.2 THERAPEUTIC MODALITIES FOR OA

Non-pharmacologic

Patient education
Disease process and prognosis
Management issues
Patient geared literature
Support groups

Psychosocial measures
Identify and treat depression
Identify and treat sleep disturbances
Weight management (if overweight)

Physical modalities
Thermal modalities
Exercise: isotonic, isometric
- range of motion
- passive
- active
Exercise: aerobic
Supportive devices
- canes
- orthotics
Modifications in activities of daily living

Pharmacologic (drug based) therapy

Topical agents
Intra-articular agents
Oral (systemic) agents
Adjunct therapies
Nutraceuticals
Investigational therapies

Surgical interventions

OA involves both axial and peripheral joints. Peripheral limb joint involvement is common, particularly the proximal interphalangeal (PIP), distal interphalangeal (DIP) and first carpometacarpal (CMC) joints of the hand, and the hip and knee.

Pain is the most frequent symptom of OA and is the symptom that most often brings the patient to see the physician. Pain has multiple potential causes, and a careful assessment of the patient may reveal the source of pain, helping to tailor a therapeutic plan. Potential sources include raised intraosseous pressure, peri-articular muscle and ligament strain, capsular stretching, periosteal elevation at joint margins and synovitis[9]. 'Gelling' of involved joints after prolonged immobility is characteristic. Morning stiffness with OA is rarely more than 30 minutes.

Psychosocial factors, like social isolation, anxiety and depression, contribute to the experience of pain and degree of disability in patients with OA[10,11]. The variety of factors influencing the pain experience in OA emphasize the need for careful assessment and determination of appropriate therapy on an individual basis.

Until a structure (disease) modifying agent is available, the objectives in managing the patient with OA are: reducing/eliminating pain and optimizing function, hence minimizing disability. Fortunately, new basic and clinical research suggests a variety of agents that may alter the course of OA, making the potential for disease (or structure) modification more of a reality (Table 40.3).

Guidelines for the conduct of clinical trials in OA have been developed[12,13]. The principal variable for evaluating the efficacy of symptom modifying therapy is pain relief, usually measured with a visual analog scale (VAS). Other tools for measuring symptomatic relief in OA include the Lequesne 'algofunctional index' and the Western Ontario and McMaster Universities (WOMAC) Osteoarthritis Index. For studies of structure modifying drugs the primary outcome measure has been the radiographic joint space assessment in semiflexed, AP radiographs of the knee and weight-bearing views of the hip. It is expected that magnetic resonance imaging (MRI) will be validated in prospective trials and may replace the radiograph as the surrogate for progression. Biochemical markers and arthroscopy are other potential tools for measuring disease modification in OA[14].

NON-PHARMACOLOGIC THERAPIES

Optimal use of non-pharmacologic modalities improves patient outcomes. Non-pharmacologic approaches include: patient education, psychosocial measures, exercise, support devices, thermal modalities and others and should constitute the base on which all other therapeutic interventions are added. Non-pharmacologic therapies also include potentially disease modifying interventions such as weight loss.

Patient education
Patients should be educated on their diagnosis. Misconceptions often exist about OA. Patients are concerned about possible rapid progres-

sion to disability. There should be an emphasis on the natural history of OA and its typically slow progression. Therapeutic options need to be discussed that emphasize lifestyle changes such as exercise and weight control that might be helpful. Lifestyle changes should be individualized, minimizing limitations in activities of daily living.

'Alternative' or 'unproven' therapies and remedies should be openly and objectively discussed. There is a tendency for patients to not advise their physician about 'alternative' pharmaceuticals and nutraceuticals, creating a suboptimal management environment. Educational pamphlets, for example available in the USA through the Arthritis Foundation, may help.

Psychosocial measures
Older age, ethnic background, gender, lower educational level, lower income and unmarried status have been linked to the tendency to become disabled in patients with musculoskeletal complaints[15]. In addition there are a variety of psychosocial factors that modulate the perception of pain and associated disability, including family relationships and secondary gains. Depression needs to be identified and treated; the overall therapeutic program will rarely be effective if depression is not addressed. Continuing emotional support is important, but need not be achieved through frequent doctor visits. Telephone contact with the patient between visits, even by non-professionals, may improve outcomes[16].

Reassurance, counseling and education may minimize the influence of psychosocial factors. Patients must participate in their care, understand their disease and take responsibility for their therapeutic program[17,18]. With a variety of techniques aimed at coping, education and psychosocial factors, one can better achieve patient acceptance, adaptation, compliance and an improved outcome.

A potential application of psychosocial intervention is with the obese patient; weight loss 'groups' and a stable social support system are more effective than simple instructions to diet.

Weight management
There is an epidemiological association between obesity and OA, which is strongest in women with OA of the knee[19–22]. A link between weight and OA of the hands has been proposed as well[23,24]. The mechanisms have not been clearly elucidated and may include increase in body mass, altered biodynamics of gait[25], genetic predisposition (genetically obese mice get more OA), and/or altered metabolism (e.g. estrogens). Pharmacologic approaches to achieving weight loss have been traditionally difficult to achieve. By contrast, through a combination of nutritional consultation, exercise and general lifestyle modifications, patients may be able to succeed. Modest weight loss has been accompanied by a decrease in joint symptoms[26], and perhaps reduced radiographic progression. It may be that a reduction in percentage of body fat, rather than weight itself, may be significant in reducing pain from OA of the knee[27].

Physical measures
There are a variety of physical modalities available for the relief of pain, reducing stiffness, and limiting muscle spasm. These include strengthening the peri-articular structures to provide improved joint support and improve balance. Physical measures make up an integral part of any successful therapeutic program for OA. They can be subdivided into exercise, supportive devices, alterations in activities of daily living, and thermal modalities.

Exercise
Patients with OA should exercise in order to maintain good muscle tone and to help in weight control[28]. Exercise programs have been linked to reduced pain and improved function in OA[29]. In theory, improved muscle support of the joint may retard the progression of OA through improved biomechanics. Care should be taken to choose exercises that maximize muscle strengthening while minimizing stress on the affected

---

TABLE 40.3 POSSIBLE STRUCTURE/DISEASE MODIFYING AGENTS IN OA*

Glucosamine
Degradative enzyme inhibitors, e.g. tetracyclines, specific metalloproteinase
  inhibitors
Bisphosphonates
Diacerein
Cytokine inhibitors
Cartilage repair

*Agents in which clinical trials have been initiated

joints. In general, the onset of pain in the involved joint indicates that exercise tolerance has been reached. Peri-articular strengthening exercises can also be recommended depending on the joints involved. An example of this is quadriceps strengthening exercise in managing OA of the knee. Clinically, quadriceps strengthening appears to help with joint stability and provide symptomatic relief. However, in patients with significant varus or valgus deformity, quadriceps strength may accelerate disease progression[30].

Low impact aerobic exercise such as walking or swimming should be recommended in most patients, unless contraindicated because of concurrent illness. Swimming is particularly effective in that it exercises multiple muscle groups and is useful in nearly all forms of OA. In most instances, exercises can be performed by the patient after basic instruction. Some particular sports or activities, however, may need to be curtailed. There are exceptions where specific exercises may actually worsen symptoms: e.g. chondromalacia patella may be worsened by bicycle riding.

A supervised program of fitness walking and education improves functional status without worsening OA of the knee[31]. The intensity of the exercise program should be graded. If the regimen is advanced too quickly, symptoms may worsen. The patient should be advised that worsening pain during exercise is a warning sign that exercise tolerance has been reached and the exercise should be discontinued.

There should be a commitment from the patient to continue an exercise program. If a program is discontinued, benefit is lost. The benefits of a formal exercise program can be lost 9 months after discontinuation[32].

Support devices

Supportive devices can significantly unload a joint and reduce pain from OA[33]. They include canes (walking sticks), crutches, walking frames, and orthotics for shoes. These various supports are intended to improve patient activity, increase compliance, and allow the patient to retain functional independence.

Canes, when properly used, can increase the base of support, decrease loading, and demands on the lower limb and its joints[34]. A cane can unload an affected hip by as much as 60%[33]. They should be used in the contralateral hand and moved together with the limb with the affected joint(s) and height measured to produce about 20 degrees of flexion at the elbow. The total length of a properly measured cane should be equal to the distance between the upper border of the greater trochanter of the femur and the bottom of the heel of the shoe. In general, a single posted cane is preferred unless there is neurologic impairment. The healthier limb should precede the affected limb when climbing up stairs. However, when climbing down stairs, the cane and the affected limb should be advanced first.

Proper footwear is often of great potential value. An orthotic device, or shoe insert, may help the patient with subluxed metatarsophalangeal joints[35]. Trainers may mitigate pain of walking in firm leather shoes. Trainers are generally lighter than leather shoes and have good arch support. A running trainer has a slightly higher heel than a walking trainer and may be of additional help with forefoot abnormalities. Walking ability and pain from medial compartment OA of the knee may be lessened by the use of a lateral heel wedged insole[36,37]. Athletic shoes can be helpful if attention is paid to selecting ones that have good mediolateral support, good medial arch, and calcaneal cushion.

A knee cage or brace may be of use in patients with tibiofemoral disease, especially those with lateral instability or those with a tendency for the knee to 'give out'[38,39]. The knee cage is not helpful and may worsen symptoms when significant valgus or varus deformity is present. Medial taping of the patella has been advocated by some in order to relieve the symptoms of OA of the knee and particularly in those with chondromalacia patella[40].

The use of the devices should be monitored to insure proper use. For example, cane/crutch tips should be changed when worn, in order to avoid slipping on smooth or wet surfaces.

Thermal modalities

Heat or cold applications are potentially helpful to patients with OA. The use of heat, cold, or alternating heat and cold are based on patient preference and not on any scientific superiority[41]. For chronic pain, most patients prefer the symptomatic relief obtained from heat applications to that obtained from cold. Traditionally, the more acute the process, the more likely cold applications will be of benefit (reduction in blood flow and reduction in pain). Sources of heat include: warm packs, heating pads, paraffin baths, ultrasound and others. The use of heat can be subdivided into superficial and deep, with no proven advantage of one over the other. The therapeutic value of applying heat includes decreasing joint stiffness, alleviating pain, relieving muscle spasm, and preventing contractures. Because of the risk of burns, heat modalities should be used with caution in anesthetized, somnolent or obtunded patients. The use of heat is contraindicated over tissues with inadequate vascular supply, bleeding, or cancer. Heat should also be avoided in areas close to the testicles or near developing fetuses. The range of temperatures used is from 40–45°C (104–113°F)[42] for 3–30 minutes. Dehydration is a risk from prolonged hot baths, particularly in the elderly. Cold is mostly applied through cold packs. Cold can relieve muscle spasm, decrease swelling in acute trauma, and relieve pain from inflammation. There have been no studies demonstrating superiority of spas over home applications in providing heat/cold applications.

Activities of daily living

Alteration in activities of daily living may improve symptoms. For example, raising the height of a chair or toilet seat can be helpful since the hip and knee are subjected to the highest pressures during the initial phase of rising from the seated position.

Miscellaneous

There are several miscellaneous physical modalities that may warrant additional study, such as massage, yoga therapy, acupressure, magnets, pulsed electromagnetic fields and transcutaneous neural stimulation (TENS). In a meta-analysis of seven published trials of OA of the knee acupuncture reduced pain but did not alter function[43].

PHARMACOLOGIC MODALITIES

Since no one agent is uniformly effective in treating the symptoms of OA, there are many pharmacologic agents that are presently in use (Table 40.4). Pharmacologic modalities could potentially be divided into topical, intra-articular and oral (systemic) agents. Furthermore, systemic therapies can be divided into those that relieve symptoms and agents that have the potential of structure (disease) modification[44]. Furthermore, those that relieve symptoms may have a rapid or slow onset of effect.

Topical agents

Capsaicin ointments applied to the skin without rubbing have been formally tested in OA of hand joints[45,46]. Clinically, they are potentially helpful in relieving pain in other joints such as the knees. Capsaicin products are derived from the common hot pepper plant and are usually in concentrations of 0.025 or 0.075%. Capsaicin is also available in a 'roll on' form. The proposed mechanism of action is depletion of the neurotransmitter substance P[47].

The patient feels heat in the area where these are applied. If the patient uses them regularly (e.g. 3–4 times a day), the heat sensation lessens and there is persistent relief of pain. Care should be taken to avoid contact with the eyes as capsaicin can be quite irritating.

TABLE 40.4 PHARMACOLOGIC THERAPY FOR OA

Topical agents

Capsaicin preparations
Salicylate preparations
Topical non-steroidal anti-inflammatory agents

Intra-articular agents

Corticosteroids
Hyaluronan

Systemic agents – rapid onset of effect

Non-narcotic analgesics
Acetaminophen
Opioid related analgesics
Tramadol
Propoxyphene
Codeine
Opioid analgesics (may be topical)
Non-steroidal anti-inflammatory drugs
Non-selective inhibitors
COX-2 specific inhibitors

Systemic agents – slow onset of effect

e.g. glucosamine, chondroitin sulfate, unsoponafiable oils, diacerein

Adjuvants

Antidepressants
Muscle relaxants

There are a variety of non-steroidal anti-inflammatory drug (NSAID) preparations that are available for topical application. Most, but not all, published trials have shown superiority over placebo[48,49].

Intra-articular therapy

Depot corticosteroids have been widely used as intra-articular agents for treatment of peripheral joints with OA[50]. Depot corticosteroids presumably relieve symptoms through an anti-inflammatory effect. The duration of effect of intra-articular depot corticosteroids is usually for more than 1 month and is not related to several risk factors examined[51]. This therapy can be particularly helpful in allowing a patient to participate in physical therapy. There may be a benefit in reducing the reaccumulation of joint effusions. The patient should be warned, however, not to overuse the joint as this may result in paradoxical increase in symptoms. Depot corticosteroids may also be useful in the management of peri-articular disease, such as anserine bursitis, that commonly accompanies OA. Because of concerns over deleterious effects on cartilage[52], it is generally not recommended that a joint be injected with depocorticosteroids more than four times per year[53].

The amount of depot corticosteroid injected varies depending on the joint and the volume to be injected. Infection is the major risk of intra-articular depocorticosteroids injections, though this is fortunately uncommon. In addition, depot corticosteroids are prepared as crystals for their prolonged effect; they may induce a crystalline synovitis[54]. This 'flare' typically occurs within hours of the injection. This is in contrast to infection, which most often happens 24–72 hours after the procedure. The application of cold compresses often reduces the pain of a crystalline flare until symptoms resolve spontaneously within several hours. There is no role for systemic corticosteroids in the management of OA.

Intra-articular hyaluronate (HA) may reduce the symptoms of OA of the knee. HA is administered as 3–5 intra-articular weekly injections[55].

HA is a normal component of synovial joints[56]. Preparations vary widely in molecular weight from 0.5 to over 6 million kDa, with no proven advantage of size or viscosity. Because of a limited half life in the joint, intra-articular HA exerts a short term lubricant and biomechanical effect. The HA long term effects may be due to an anti-inflammatory effect, reduced neuroreceptor activity, altered cartilage metabolism, and/or altering synoviocyte behavior. HA preparations may reduce pain for prolonged periods of time and potentially improve mobility[57]. A problem in studying these and other intra-articular compounds for OA has been a high placebo group response rate[58]. An intra-articular HA (Hyalgan®) derivative was compared to oral naproxen or placebo in a 14 week double blind study. Pain relief was prolonged with the HA, and at 6 months over 60% of the completers had at least a 20% reduction of pain, with half of that group pain free. Even though 40% of the placebo group improved, there was significant improvement in the HA injected group when compared to placebo. The benefit compared favorably to naproxen with significantly fewer adverse effects (fewer gastrointestinal complaints). In another study, three weekly intra-articular injections of HA (Synvisc®) were compared to their combination with an NSAID, and to the NSAID alone. At week 12 and a telephone follow up after 26 weeks, the groups receiving the HA were better in terms of rest pain and lateral joint tenderness[59]. The major adverse effect is a local transient painful reaction in the joint or at the injection site.

Formal use for knee OA has been approved in the USA and trials are underway studying use in other joints such as the shoulders, ankles and hips.

Oral (systemic) pharmacologic agents
Symptom modifying agents
This group of agents includes analgesics such as non-opioid analgesics [e.g. acetaminophen (paracetamol) and tramadol] and opioid analgesics, or anti-inflammatory agents such as NSAIDs. Analgesia may be potentiated by adjuvant agents, such as agents intended to reduce muscle spasm and low dose antidepressant medications, particularly tricyclic antidepressants.

Non-opioid analgesics
For many patients with OA, relief of mild to moderate joint pain can be achieved with acetaminophen (paracetamol). Oral acetaminophen 1g four times daily has a benefit equivalent to ibuprofen 2.4g/day in treating the pain of OA by most measured parameters[60]. However, in several trials, NSAIDs have been more efficacious, particularly in those with moderate to severe symptoms from their OA[61,62]. The revised ACR recommendations for the medical management of OA allow for selection of an NSAID or a COX-2 selective inhibitor as initial therapy in those with more symptomatic OA[63].

There is concern for hepatotoxicity with acetaminophen when taken at doses above the recommended maximum (4g/day). Care should be taken to avoid other acetaminophen containing compounds, such as cold remedies, if the patient is already consuming full OA doses of acetaminophen.

Opioid analgesics
Although there is limited published clinical research, weak opioid analgesics such as propoxyphene and codeine have been commonly administered for OA.

Tramadol has a dual mechanism of action: inhibition of the μ opioid receptor and inhibition of serotonin uptake. It does not have significant addiction potential[64]. Starting doses of less than 50mg daily minimize nausea and other central nervous system adverse effects. High doses have been associated with seizures and allergic reactions[65]. The dose can be titrated to a maximum of 100mg four times daily. Tramadol can be added to medication regimens that use NSAIDs as base therapy and may have NSAID-sparing properties[66]. Tramadol can also be combined with acetaminophen for an added analgesic effect[67].

Stronger narcotics or narcotic derivatives are also useful in selected patients with OA. The World Health Organization stepladder guidelines for the use of narcotic analgesics should be followed. Additional guidelines have been published[68]. Dependence is always of concern, but is less common in patients with OA. Narcotics are used most often as rescue medications for severe pain. Constipation should be anticipated as it is an often encountered adverse effect. Although tablet forms are most often prescribed, alternative dosing regimens such as slow release patches are available.

Non-steroidal anti-inflammatory drugs

Non-steroidal anti-inflammatory drugs continue to be the most commonly used agents in the therapy of OA. NSAIDs are available in both prescription and over-the-counter dose forms. NSAIDs are analgesic, anti-inflammatory and antipyretic, exerting their therapeutic effect by blocking cyclooxygenase (COX) at sites of pain and/or inflammation. Their effects are mostly at peripheral sites of inflammation, but have some central analgesic effects.

Even though non-selective NSAIDs are effective in OA, potential adverse events, particularly gastrointestinal, are of concern. These include gastroduodenal ulcers that can result in pain, bleeding, perforation or obstruction. Some estimates are that, in the USA, NSAID use is linked to 16 000 deaths and over 100 000 hospitalizations a year from gastrointestinal bleeding. Although most major gastrointestinal events occur without warning, there are risk factors that predispose patients to these events. They include: older age, higher dose of NSAIDs, prior history of peptic ulcer disease or of gastrointestinal bleeding, comorbid conditions such as heart disease and concurrent use of systemic corticosteroids and oral anticoagulants.

Various strategies have been utilized to reduce this risk of NSAID-associated gastrointestinal toxicity. The addition of a proton pump inhibitor to the medication regimen has been proven to reduce the incidence of endoscopic peptic ulcers in those on NSAIDs[69]. Misoprostol, a prostaglandin analog, reduces the incidence of clinical GI adverse events when used at a dose of 200μg four times daily[70]. Diarrhea is a potential side effect. Over the counter doses of H-2 blockers and antacids have not been shown to reduce either endoscopic or clinical gastrointestinal events.

Two distinct cyclooxygenase isoenzymes, COX-1 and COX-2, have been identified. COX-1 is constitutive and appears to protect the gastric mucosa from the acidic environment of the stomach. In contrast, COX-2 is mostly inducible and commonly expressed at sites of inflammation such as joints.

COX-2 selective inhibitors have been developed for use in OA[71]. Although no more effective than aspirin or non-selective NSAIDs, there is considerable evidence that they have less gastrointestinal toxicity[72,73]. Platelet aggregation and bleeding time are not significantly affected by COX-2 selective inhibition[74]. The use of daily aspirin for cardiovascular or cerebrovascular prophylaxis reduces, but does not eliminate, COX-2 selective inhibitor derived gastrointestinal protection. The various issues of aspirin/NSAID-COX-2 interactions remain an active area of investigation[75]. Like non-selective NSAIDs, some patients will have increased hypertension and/or peripheral edema with COX-2 selective inhibitors. Both COX-1 and COX-2 are present in the kidney and COX-2 selective inhibitors can precipitate renal insufficiency. As with traditional NSAIDs, they should be used with caution in the presence of even mild renal insufficiency.

Celecoxib, rofecoxib, and valdecoxib are the first available COX-2-selective inhibitors. Recent trials have attempted to compare their efficacy, and that of acetaminophen, in OA[76]. Meloxicam has COX-2 selective inhibition at the recommended doses[77]. More highly selective COX-2 agents are under development (e.g. etoricoxib); the increased selectivity has uncertain additional clinical benefit at this time[78].

Adjunct therapies

Any analgesic program can be supplemented with tricyclic antidepressant medication[79,80]; the antidepressants appear to potentiate the analgesic effects of the other agents. In addition, they may exert part of their benefit by improving sleep patterns altered by nocturnal myoclonus and fibromyalgia-like complaints.

Oral *anti-spasmodics* are purported to reduce muscle pain and spasm in OA[81]. The value of oral medications in relieving the pain of muscle spasm is controversial. However, centrally acting agents may be helpful for improving sleep patterns through their sedating qualities and potential for disrupting neurologic transmission of the pain sensation. Pain associated with muscle spasm may be reduced with a local injection of lidocaine with or without a depot corticosteroid.

'Nutraceuticals'

'Nutraceuticals' are nutritional supplements that appear to have medicinal properties[82]. For a variety of reasons nutraceuticals have gained in popularity. There are increasing attempts to subject nutraceuticals to rigorous clinical research. Some are being tested in double-blind, randomized clinical trials.

Glucosamine sulfate 1500mg/day, has been tested in several clinical trials comparing it to placebo and other NSAIDs. In small European trials it has shown pain relief comparable to that of ibuprofen 1200mg/day in OA of the knee but with a slower onset of action (3–4 weeks)[83,84]. Structure modification with reduced progression of joint space narrowing of the knee was demonstrated in two 3-year, double blind, randomized trials when compared to placebo[85,86]. Serial radiographs of the knee (in full extension) assessed joint space width. Very small joint space benefit has been seen favoring the glucosamine groups.

Oral *chondroitin sulfate*, a glycosaminoglycan with a molecular mass of around 14 000, is composed of repeating units of N-acetyl galactosamine and glucuronic acid. Chondroitin sulfate 800–1600mg/day reduced pain in OA of the knee[87]. There is a relatively slow onset of benefit; NSAIDs have more rapid pain relief.

There is little information on the combination of glucosamine and chondroitin.

A National Institutes of Health sponsored study is currently examining glucosamine hydrochloride, chondroitin sulfate, the combination, a COX-2 selective inhibitor, and placebo in patients with knee OA.

S-adenosylmethionine (SAM-e), a methyl group donor and oxygen radical scavenger, has been used by intravenous loading and oral maintenance[88]. Limited information is available.

MSM (methylsulfonylmethane) has been touted as a 'sulfate donor' (especially through the internet). This 'natural' product is actually chemically manufactured. It is related to DMSO, a solvent that has also been proposed as a remedy for several different conditions. There is minimal information on MSM's efficacy and/or toxicity available in the peer-reviewed scientific literature.

A ginger extract was recently reported to be superior to placebo in a randomized clinical trial of OA of the knee[89].

Other nutraceuticals are entrenched in popular culture. These include compounds such as 'cat's claw' and shark cartilage that are being used with increasing frequency and being sold over the counter in pharmacies and health food stores. There are no carefully performed trials to support their use.

Miscellaneous agents

Although research continues into symptom-modifying medications for OA, there is a new emphasis on the development of structure modifying

515

agents. Structure modifying medications are intended to retard, prevent or reverse the progression of OA.

Since there is no direct measure of progression of OA, imaging studies are used as a surrogate measure of structure modification by measuring the joint space[90]. Several groups of agents are under investigation, mostly directed at cartilage repair:

- growth factors and cytokines
- sulfated and non-sulfated sugars
- hormones and other steroids
- enzyme inhibitors
- chondrocyte/stem cell transplantation.

Tetracyclines, apart from any antimicrobial effect, are inhibitors of tissue metalloproteinases[91] and may have effects on nitric oxide synthase[92]. Doxycycline has reduced the severity of OA in canine models[93] and is currently being evaluated in a multi-center, double blind, placebo controlled trial for 'structure-modification' in obese women with OA of the knee.

Specific metalloproteinase inhibitors are also under investigation for structure modification in OA.

Diacerein[94] and its active metabolite rhein are anthraquinones related to senna compounds. They inhibit the synthesis of interleukin-1 (IL-1) beta in human OA synovium in vitro as well as the expression of IL-1 receptors on chondrocytes[95]. No effects have been reported on TNF or its receptors. Collagenase production and articular damage have been reduced in animal models[96–98]. Early human clinical trials have shown improved pain scores as compared to placebo and comparable efficacy to NSAIDs but slower onset of action[99]. Diarrhea is the main adverse effect[100]. It is usually self-limited. One trial suggested disease/structure modification in OA of the hip joint. Unfortunately, the study had a dropout rate that approached 50%[100]. Furthermore, symptomatic benefit couldn't be confirmed. On the strength of these trials, diacerein has been proposed as a slow acting symptom-modifying and perhaps disease/structure modifying drug for OA.

Oral preparations of *avocado and soya unsaponifiables* (ASU) have been studied in OA of the knee and hand. The unsaponifiable residues of avocado and soya oils are mixed in a 1:2 ratio. *In vitro* studies on cultured chondrocyte have shown partial reversal of IL-1β effects. IL-1β roles in OA are thought to include inhibition of prostaglandin synthesis by chondrocytes and stimulation of MMP and nitric oxide (NO) production. Metalloproteinases and nitric oxide can degrade cartilage matrix and cause chondrocyte apoptosis. Use of ASU also results in inhibited production of IL-6, IL-8, matrix metalloproteases and stimulation of collagen synthesis. The mechanism through which these effects occur is unknown as is the active ingredient in ASU[101]. Symptomatic benefit in double-blind human trials in OA of the hip and knee has also been reported[102]. Some abstract presentations have suggested structure/disease modification in human hip OA[103].

MANAGEMENT OF OA AT SPECIFIC SITES

The hand

Hand joints commonly affected in OA include the first carpometacarpal (CMC) joints, distal interphalangeal joints (DIP) and proximal interphalangeal (PIP) joints. Topical agents such as capsaicin have been tested in OA of these joints and are helpful. Involvement of the CMC joint at the base of the thumb can be particularly disabling. The patient often benefits from intra-articular injection of a corticosteroid preparation. Orthoses, such as a thumb splint, can help a patient that is having difficulty with vocational or avocational chores. Surgery may be needed if the patient cannot be helped with conservative interventions[104].

The knee

Knee crepitus, pain on activity and gelling after prolonged inactivity are characteristic. In some, effusions are evident. A careful assessment as to the cause of the pain should be made. Tendinitis/bursitis components, particularly anserine bursitis should be identified.

Quadriceps strengthening exercises should be taught and the patient should perform them at least every other day. General exercise, such as walking or swimming will help and will also contribute to limb strength. High impact activities such as stair climbing and jogging should be discouraged. When exercising, if pain ensues in the affected joint, it is an indication that exercise tolerance has been reached and the patient should rest. Weight loss is important in overweight individuals but is very difficult to achieve.

In more severe cases, a cane may help unload the joint. It should be held in the contralateral hand and may not only reduce pain, but perhaps increase exercise tolerance. Heel and forefoot wedges may help those with varus deformities[105]. Medial taping of the patella can be useful in those with patellofemoral OA.

Topical agents and systemic therapies such as acetaminophen, NSAIDs or COX-2 selective inhibitors are often used in these patients. Joint aspiration and infiltration with depot corticosteroids or hyaluronate preparations may be helpful in relieving the symptoms of those with knee OA[106]. Tidal lavage with 0.5–1 liter of saline has been tried with some success[107].

Surgical intervention is effective in those refractory to more conservative management. There are no firm guidelines for surgery; however, surgery may be indicated for joint pain due to the OA that is not relieved with the other interventions; particularly if it interferes with the patient's ability to perform his daily activities. Arthroscopic intervention should be limited to patients in whom an additional diagnosis of internal derangement is suspected. Surgical arthroscopy is useful for repair and for partial removal of damaged menisci in some patients; benefit decreases with increasing age. The value of synovectomy and debridement has not been established in OA. Abrasion chondroplasty leads to partial cartilage repair and provides the same symptomatic improvement as irrigation and debridement alone[108]. Arthroscopic lavage has also been tried, with some success. Large-bore needle lavage with saline may be of value in selected patients[109]. It has been shown to be effective in the relief of pain in OA of the knees for up to 6 months[110].

Osteotomies and arthroplasties appear cost effective when the improved quality of life and the alternatives are considered. Osteotomies may serve as alternatives to arthroplasty, in younger, overweight patients, and in unicompartmental disease of the knee. This may delay progression of disease (hence the need for total joint replacement). However, only 50% of patients with knee osteotomies have satisfactory results at 10 years[111].

Total knee arthroplasties have improved the morbidity and probably the indirect mortality of OA. Most series report good to excellent long-term results in over 90% of patients undergoing knee replacement. Overweight patients, along with those with marked varus or valgus deformities and those with flexion contractures offer particular challenges to the orthopedic surgeon. Knee fusions are not recommended because of the poor resulting function. They are only employed in those who have failed arthroplasty.

A particular presentation in younger adults with patellar (anterior knee) pain is chondromalacia patellae. In chondromalacia, there is damage to the patellar cartilage and pain is most notable when walking uphill or upstairs. Avoidance of these activities and quadriceps strengthening exercises should be recommended.

The hip

Symptomatic hip OA is usually insidious in onset. Diminished internal rotation, a limp and groin pain are characteristic. Complaints of pain in

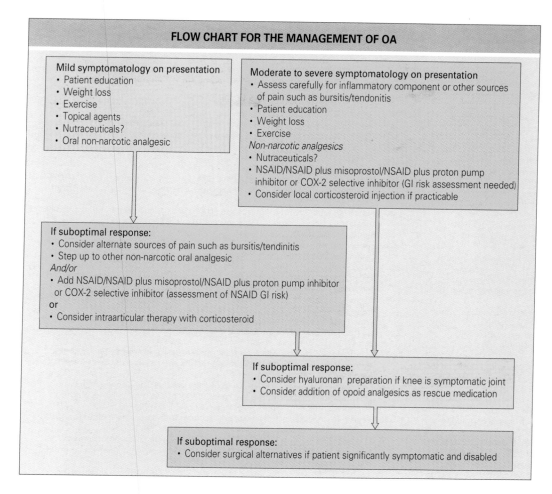

Fig. 40.1 Flow chart for the management of OA.

FLOW CHART FOR THE MANAGEMENT OF OA

Mild symptomatology on presentation
- Patient education
- Weight loss
- Exercise
- Topical agents
- Nutraceuticals?
- Oral non-narcotic analgesic

Moderate to severe symptomatology on presentation
- Assess carefully for inflammatory component or other sources of pain such as bursitis/tendonitis
- Patient education
- Weight loss
- Exercise

Non-narcotic analgesics
- Nutraceuticals?
- NSAID/NSAID plus misoprostol/NSAID plus proton pump inhibitor or COX-2 selective inhibitor (GI risk assessment needed)
- Consider local corticosteroid injection if practicable

If suboptimal response:
- Consider alternate sources of pain such as bursitis/tendinitis
- Step up to other non-narcotic oral analgesic

And/or
- Add NSAID/NSAID plus misoprostol/NSAID plus proton pump inhibitor or COX-2 selective inhibitor (assessment of NSAID GI risk)

or
- Consider intraarticular therapy with corticosteroid

If suboptimal response:
- Consider hyaluronan preparation if knee is symptomatic joint
- Consider addition of opioid analgesics as rescue medication

If suboptimal response:
- Consider surgical alternatives if patient significantly symptomatic and disabled

the buttocks, sciatic region or even knee are not uncommon. Pain in the lateral aspect of the upper thigh that is reproducible on palpation most often represents trochanteric bursitis. Local depocorticosteroid infiltration is particularly effective in managing the bursitis.

The initial management is similar to that for knee OA. Weight loss and exercise are important. Both range of motion and strengthening exercises are important. Formal referral for physical therapy may be necessary in some, particularly in older, debilitated patients. Unloading with a cane should be recommended to significantly symptomatic patients. Use of a cane can reduce stress on the joint by about 20–30%[23].

Systemic pharmacologic therapy is often needed if pain interferes with adequate ambulation. Acetaminophen, NSAIDs or COX-2 selective inhibitors can be used. Opioid analgesics should be used with caution but may be necessary in some and can delay the need for operative therapy. Intra-articular corticosteroid infiltration is not generally advisable but, if performed, fluoroscopic guidance is often needed.

Osteotomy and arthroplasty are the surgical methods employed in those with more severe involvement. The choice of procedure generally depends on the patient's circumstances. Osteotomies are less useful than for knee OA. Arthroplasty provides excellent pain relief and superior function. The need for revision arthroplasty later on in life because of heavier loading, greater duration of usage, and prosthesis deterioration and/or loosening is of concern in younger patients. There has

been an 85% success rates at 20 years followup of the Charnley total hip prosthesis.

Materials used for prostheses include polyethylene and stainless steel. The polyethylene components can 'wear' with time. Loosening of either the acetabular or femoral component is another potential clinical issue. There has been some controversy regarding the use of cemented (polymethylmethacrylate) versus uncemented prostheses and the rates of complications such as loosening. A combination used widely is an uncemented acetabular component with a cemented femoral component. Some have tended to try uncemented femoral components in younger, more active patients. Hip fusion provides more restricted function and is mostly used for failed arthroplasties.

SUMMARY

The therapy of OA involves establishing the diagnosis of OA and trying to determine the cause of the patients symptoms and signs. An algorithm is proposed (Fig. 40.1) that includes a combination of non-pharmacologic therapy, pharmacologic therapy and surgery. As with any chronic disease, therapy is not curative and a stepwise approach is needed that is guided by the severity and impact of OA on the patient. The future therapies of OA will involve attempts at altering the course of OA, either by prevention, stabilization or reversal of the pathogenic mechanisms involved.

REFERENCES

1. Kramer JS, Yelin EH, Epstein WV. Social and economic impacts of four musculoskeletal conditions: a study using national community-based data. J Rheumatol 1983; 26: 901–907.
2. Liang MH, Fortin P. Management of osteoarthritis of the hip and knee. Editorial. N Eng J Med 1991; 325: 125–127.
3. Poole AR, Howell DS. Etiopathogenesis of osteoarthritis. In: Moskowitz R, Howell D, Altman R et al., eds. Osteoarthritis: diagnosis and management, 3rd edn. Saunders: Philadelphia; 2001: 29–47.
4. Lozada CJ and Altman RD. Chondroprotection in osteoarthritis. Bull Rheum Dis 1997; 46: 5–7.

5. Lozada CJ and Altman RD. New and investigational therapies for osteoarthritis. In: Moskowitz R, Howell D, Altman R et al., eds. Osteoarthritis: diagnosis and management, 3rd edn. Saunders: Philadelphia; 2001: 447–448.

6. Lozada CJ and Altman RD. Osteoarthritis: A comprehensive approach to management. J Musculoskeletal Med 1997; 14: 26–38.

7. ACR Subcommittee on osteoarthritis guidelines. Recommendations for the medical management of osteoarthritis of the hip and knee: 2000 update. Arthritis Rheum 2000; 43: 1905–1915.

8. Pendleton A, Arden N, Dougados M et al. EULAR recommendations for the management of knee osteoarthritis. Ann Rheum Dis. 2000; 59: 936–944.

9. Felson DT, Chaisson CE, Hill CL, Totterman SMS et al. The association of bone marrow lesions and pain in knee osteoarthritis. Ann Intern Med 2001; 134: 541–549.

10. Summers MN, Haley WE, Reveille JE, Alarcon GS. Radiographic assessment and psychological variables as predictors of pain and functional impairment in osteoarthritis of the hip or knee. Arthritis Rheum 1988; 31: 204–209.

11. Salaffi F, Cavalieri F, Nolli M et al. Analysis of disability in knee osteoarthritis: relationship with age and psychological variables but not with radiographic score. J Rheumatol 1991; 18: 1581–1586.

12. Altman R, Brandt K., Hochberg M. et al. Design and conduct of clinical trials in patients with osteoarthritis: recommendations from a task force of the Osteoarthritis Research Society. Osteoarthritis Cart 1996; 4: 217–243.

13. Lequesne M, Brandt K, Bellamy N et al. Guidelines for testing slow acting drugs in osteoarthritis. J Rheumatol 1994; 21(suppl 41): 65–73.

14. Altman R. and Lozada CJ. Laboratory findings in osteoarthritis. In: Moskowitz R, Howell D, Altman R et al., eds. Osteoarthritis: diagnosis and management, 3rd edn. Saunders: Philadelphia; 2001: 273–91.

15. Cunningham,LS and Kelsy, JL. Epidemiology of musculoskeletal impairments and associated disability. AJPH 1984; 74: 574–579.

16. Weinberger M, Tierney WM, Cowper PA et al. Cost-effectiveness of increased telephone contact for patients with osteoarthritis. Arthritis Rheum 1993; 36: 243–246.

17. Lorig KR, Mazonson PD, Holman HR. Evidence suggesting that health education for self-management in patients with chronic arthritis has sustained health benefits while reducing health care costs. Arthritis Rheum 1993; 36: 439–446.

18. Hampson SE, Glasgow RE, Zeiss AM et al. Self-management of osteoarthritis. Arthritis Care Res 1993; 6: 17–22.

19. Felson DT. The epidemiology of knee osteoarthritis: results from the Framingham Osteoarthritis Study. Semin Arthritis Rheum 1990; 20: 42–50.

20. Hubert HB, Bloch DA, Fries JF. Risk factors for physical disability in an aging cohort: The NHANES 1 epidemiologic followup study. J Rheumatol 1993; 20: 480–488.

21. Hochberg MC, Lethbridge-Cejku M, Scott WW Jr et al. The association of body weight, body fatness and body fat distribution with osteoarthritis of the knee: data from the Baltimore Longitudinal Study of Aging. J Rheumatol 1995; 22: 488–493.

22. Spector TD, Hart DJ. Incidence and progression of osteoarthritis in women with unilateral knee disease in the general population: the effect of obesity. Ann Rheum Dis 1994; 53: 565–568.

23. Oliveira SA, Felson DT, Cirillo PA, Reed JI. Body weight, body mass index, and incident symptomatic osteoarthritis of the hand, hip, and knee. Epidemiology 1999; 10: 161–166.

24. Carman WJ, Sowers M, Hawthorne VM, Weissfeld LA. Obesity as a risk factor for osteoarthritis of the hand and wrist: a prospective study. Am Med J Epidemiol 1994; 139: 119–129.

25. Leach RE, Baumgard S, Broom J. Obesity: its relationship to osteoarthritis of the knee. Clin Orthop 1973; 93: 271–273.

26. Felson DT., Zhang Y, Anthony JM et al. Weight loss reduces the risk for symptomatic knee osteoarthritis in women. Ann Intern Med 1992; 116: 535–539.

27. Toda Y, Toda T, Takemura S et al. Change in body fat, but not body weight or metabolic correlates of obesity, is related to symptomatic relief of obese patients with knee osteoarthritis after a weight control program. J Rheumatol 1998; 25: 2181–2186.

28. Minor MA. Exercise in the management of osteoarthritis of the knee and hip. Arthritis Care Res. 1994; 7: 198–204.

29. van Baar ME, Dekker J, Oostendorp RA, Bijl D. The effectiveness of exercise therapy in patients with osteoarthritis of the hip or knee: a randomized clinical trial. J Rheumatol 1998; 25: 2432–2439.

30. Sharma L, Song J, Felson DT et al. The role of knee alignment in disease progression and functional decline in knee osteoarthritis. J Am Med Assoc 2001; 286: 188–195.

31. Kovar PA, Allegrante JP, Mackenzie R et al. Supervised fitness walking in patients with osteoarthritis of the knee. Ann Intern Med 1992; 16: 529–534.

32. van Baar ME, Dekker J, Oostendorp RAB et al. Effectiveness of exercise in patients with osteoarthritis of hip or knee: nine months' followup. Ann Rh Dis 2001; 60: 1123–1130.

33. Brand SA, Crowninshield RD. The effect of cane use on hip contact force. Clin Orthop 1980; 147: 181–184.

34. Blount WP. Don't throw away the cane. J Bone Joint Surg 1956; 38-A: 695–708.

35. Thompson JA, Jennings MB, Hodge W. Orthotic therapy in the management of osteoarthritis. Med Assoc 1992; 82: 136–139.

36. Keating EM, Faris PM, Ritter MA, Kane J. Use of lateral heel and sole wedges in the treatment of medial osteoarthritis of the knee. Orthop Rev 1993; 22: 921–924.

37. Sasaki T, Yasuda K. Clinical evaluation and treatment of osteoarthritis of the knee using designed wedge insoles. Clin Orthop 1987; 221: 181–187.

38. Rubin G, Dixon M, and Danisi M. prescription procedures for knee orthosis and knee-ankle–foot orthosis. Orthot Prosthet 1977; 31: 15–25.

39. Marks R, Quinney AH, Wessel J. Reliability and validity of the measurement of position sense in women with osteoarthritis of the knee. J Rheumatol 1993; 20: 1919–1924.

40. Cushnagan J, McCarthy C, Dieppe PA. Taping the patella medially: a new treatment for osteoarthritis of the knee joint? Br Med J 1988; 308: 753–755.

41. Swezey RL. Essentials of physical management and rehabilitation in arthritis. Semin Arthritis Rheum 1974; 3: 349–368.

42. Basford JR. Physical agents and biofeedback. In: DeLisa JA et al. eds. Rehabilitation medicine – principles and practice. Philadelphia: Lippincott; 1988: 257–275.

43. Ezzo J, Hadhazy V, Birch S et al. Acupuncture for osteoarthritis of the knee: a systematic review. Arthritis Rheum 2001; 44: 819–825.44.

44. Dougados M, Devougelaer MP, Annerfeldt M et al. Recommendations for the registration of drugs used in the treatment of osteoarthritis. Ann Rheum Dis 1996; 55: 552–557.

45. McCarthy GM, McCarthy DJ. Effect of topical capsaicin in the therapy of painful osteoarthritis of the hands. J Rheumatol 1992; 19: 604–607.

46. Altman RD, Aven A, Holmburg CE et al. Efficacy of topical capsaicin cream 0.025% as monotherapy in patients with osteoarthritis: a double-blind study. Sem Arthrit Rheum 1994; 23(suppl 3): 25–33.

47. Virus RM, Gebhart GF. Pharmacologic actions of capsaicin: apparent involvement of substance P and serotonin. Life Science 1979; 25: 1273–1284.

48. Moore RA, Tramer MR, Carroll D et al. Quantitative systematic review of topically applied non-steroidal anti-inflammatory drugs. Brit Med J 1998; 316: 333–338.49.

49. Ottilinger B, Gomort B, Michel A et al. Efficacy and safety of eltenac gel in the treatment of knee osteoarthritis. Osteoarthritis Cartilage 2001; 9: 273–280.

50. Miller JH, White J, Norton TH. he value of intra-articular injections in osteoarthritis of the knee. J. Bone Joint Surg 1958; 40A: 636–643.

51. Jones A, Doherty M. Intra-articular corticosteroids are effective in osteoarthritis but there are no clinical predictors of response. Ann Rh Dis 1996; 55: 829.52.

52. Wada J, Koshino T, Morii T, Sugimoto K. Natural course of osteoarthritis of the knee treated with or without intraarticular corticosteroid injections. Bulletin – Hospital for Joint Diseases 1993; 53: 45–48.

53. Schnitzer TJ. Osteoarthritis treatment update. Postgrad Med 1993; 93: 89–93.

54. Altman RD. Osteoarthritis: aggravating factors and therapeutic measures. Postgrad Med 1986; 80: 150–163.

55. Lohmander L, Dalen N, Englund G et al. Intra-articular hyaluronan injections in the treatment of osteoarthritis of the knee: a randomized double-blind, placebo controlled multicentre trial. Ann Rheum Dis 1996; 55: 424–431.

56. Peyron JG. Intraarticular hyaluronan injections in the treatment of osteoarthritis: state-of-the art review. J Rheumatol 1993; 20(suppl 39): 10–15.

57. Dougados M, Nguyen M, Listrat V, Amor B. High molecular weight sodium hyaluronate (hyalectin) in osteoarthritis of the knee: a 1 year placebo-controlled trial. Osteoarthritis and Cartilage 1993; 1: 97–103.

58. Altman RD, Moskowitz R. Intraarticular sodium hyaluronate (Hyalgan) in the treatment of osteoarthritis of the knee: a randomized clinical trial. Hyalgan Study Group. J Rheumatol 1998; 25: 2203–2212.

59. Adams MF, Atkinson M, Lussler AJ et al. Comparison of intra-articular Hyalgan G-F (Synvisc), a viscoelastic derivative of hyaluronan and continuous NSAID therapy in patients with osteoarthritis of the knee. Arthritis Rheum 1993; 37: S165.

60. Bradley JD, Brandt KD, Katz BP et al. Comparison of an antiinflammatory dose of ibuprofen, an analgesic dose of ibuprofen, and acetaminophen in the treatment of patients with osteoarthritis of the knee. N Eng J Med 1991; 325: 87–91.

61. Pincus T, Koch GG, Sokka T et al. A randomized, double-blind crossover clinical trial of diclofenac plus misoprostol versus acetaminophen in paients with osteoarthritis of the hip or knee. Arthritis Rheum 2001; 44: 1587–1598.

62. Altman, RD and the IAP Study Group: Ibuprofen, acetaminophen and placebo in osteoarthritis of the knee: a six-day double-blind study. Arthritis Rheum 1999; 42(suppl): S403.

63. ACR Subcommittee on osteoarthritis guidelines. Recommendations for the medical management of osteoarthritis of the hip and knee: 2000 update. Arthritis Rheum 2000; 43: 1905–1915.

64. Raffa, RB, Friederichs E, Reimann W et al. Opioid and non opioid components independently contribute to the mechanism of action of tramadol, an 'atypical' opioid analgestic. J Pharmacol Exp Ther 1992; 260: 275–285.

65. Goeringer KE, Logan BK, Christian GD. Identification of tramadol and its metabolites in blood from drug-related deaths and drug-impaired drivers. J Anal Toxicol 1997; 21: 529–537.

66. Schnitzer TJ, Kamin M, Olson WH. Tramadol allows reduction of naproxen dose among patients with naproxen-responsive osteoarthritis pain: a randomized, double-blind, placebo-controlled study. Arthritis Rheum 1999; 42: 1370–1377.

67. Mullican WS, Lacy JR Tramadol/acetaminophen combination tablets and codeine/acetaminophen combination capsules for the management of chronic pain: a comparative trial. Clin Ther 2001; 23: 1429–1445.

68. AGS Panel on Chronic Pain in Older Persons. The management of chronic pain in older persons. J Amer Geriatric Soc 1998; 46: 635–651.

69. Hawkey CJ, Karrasch JA, Szczepanski L et al. Omeprazole compared with misoprostol for ulcers associated with nonsteroidal antiinflammatory drugs. Omeprazole versus misoprostol for NSAID-induced ulcer management (OMINUM) study group. N Engl J Med 1998; 338: 727–734.

70. Graham DY, Agrawal NM, Roth SH. Prevention of NSAID-induced gastric ulcer with misoprostol: multicenter, double-blind, placebo-controlled trial. Lancet. 1988; 2: 1277–1280.

71. Schnitzer TJ, Hochberg MC. Cox-2 selective inhibitors in the treatment of arthritis. Cleve Clin J Med 2002; 69(suppl 1): SI 20–30.

72. Silvestein FE, Faich G, Goldstein JL et al. Gastrointestinal toxicity with celecoxib vs. nonsteroidal antiinflammatory drugs for osteoarthritis and rheumatoid arthritis: the CLASS study: a randomized controlled trial. Celecoxib Long-term Arthritis Safety Study. J Am Med Assoc 2000; 284: 1247–1255.

73. Bombardier C, Laine L, Reicin A *et al.* Comparison of upper gastrointestinal toxicity of rofecoxib and naproxen in patients with rheumatoid arthritis. VIGOR Study Group. N Engl J Med. 2000; 343: 1520–1528.

74. Leese PT, Hubbard RC, Karim A *et al.* Effects of celecoxib, a novel cyclooxygenase-2 inhibitor, on platelet function in healthy adults: a randomized, controlled trial. J Clin Pharmacol 2000; 40: 124–132.

75. Ouellet M, Riendeau D, Percival MD. A high level of cyclooxygenase-2 inhibitor selectivity is associated with a reduced interference of platelet cyclooxygenase-1 inactivation by aspirin. Proc Natl Acad Sci USA 2001; 98: 14583–14588.

76. Geba GP, Weaver AL, Polis AB *et al.* Vioxx, acetaminophen, celecoxib trial (VACT) Group. Efficacy of rofecoxib, celecoxib, and acetaminophen in osteoarthritis of the knee: a randomized trial. J Am Med Assoc 2002; 287: 64–71.

77. Yocum D, Fleischmann R, Dalgin P *et al.* Safety and efficacy of meloxicam in the treatment of osteoarthritis: a 12-week, double-blind, multiple-dose, placebo-controlled trial. Arch Intern Med 2000; 23: 2947–2954.

78. Camu F, Beecher T, Recker DP, Verburg KM. Valdecoxib, a COX-2-specific inhibitor, is an efficacious, opioid-sparing analgesic in patients undergoing hip arthroplasty. Am J Ther 2002 ; 9: 43–51.

79. Riendeau D, Percival MD, Brideau C *et al.* Etoricoxib (MK-0663): preclinical profile and comparison with other agents that selectively inhibit cyclooxygenase-2. J Pharmacol Exp Ther 2001; 296: 558–566.

80. Kantor TG. The pharmacological control of musculoskeletal pain. Can J Physiol Pharmacol 1991; 69: 713–718.

81. Curatolo M, Bogduk N. Pharmacologic pain treatment of musculoskeletal disorders: current perspectives and future prospects. Clin J Pain 2001; 17: 25–32.

82. Deal CL, Moskowitz RW. Nutraceuticals as therapeutic agents in osteoarthritis. The role of glucosamine, chondroitin sulfate, and collagen hydrolysate. Rheum Dis Clin North Am 1999; 25: 379–395.

83. Qiu GX, Gao SN, Giacovelli G, Rovati L. Efficacy and safety of glucosamine sulfate versus ibuprofen in patients with knee osteoarthritis. Arzneimittelforschung 1998; 48: 469–474.

84. Muller-Fabender H, Bach GL, Haase W *et al.* Glucosamine sulfate compared to ibuprofen in osteoarthritis of the knee. Osteoarthritis and Cartilage 1994; 2: 61–69.

85. Reginster J-Y, Deroisy R, Rovati LC *et al.* Long term effects of glucosamine sulphate on osteoarthritis progression: a randomized, placebo-controlled clinical trial. Lancet 2001; 357: 251–256.

86. Pavelka K, Gatterova J, Olejarova M *et al.* Glucosamine sulfate decreases progression of knee osteoarthritis in a long-term, randomized, placebo-controlled, independent, confirmatory trial. Arthritis Rheum 2000; 43(suppl): S384.

87. Leeb BF, Schweitzer H, Montag K, Smolen JS. A metaanalysis of chondroitin sulfate in the treatment of osteoarthritis. Rheum 2000; 27: 205–211.

88. Bradley JD, Flusser D, Katz BP *et al.* A randomized, double blind, placebo controlled trial of intravenous loading with S-adenosylmethionine (SAM) followed by oral SAM therapy in patients with knee osteoarthritis. J Rheumatology 1994; 21: 905–911.

89. Altman RD, Marcussen KK. Effects of a ginger extract on knee pain in patients with osteoarthritis. Arthritis Rheum 2000; 44: 2531–2538.

90. Lozada CJ and Altman RD. Chondroprotection in osteoarthritis. Bull Rheum Dis 1997; 46: 5–7.

91. Yu LP Jr., Smith GN Jr, Hasty KA, Brandt KD. Doxycycline inhibits type XI collagenolytic activity of extracts from human osteoarthritic cartilage and of gelatinase. J Rheumatol 1991; 18: 1450–1452.

92. Amin AR, Attur MG, Thakker GD *et al.* A novel mechanism of action of tetracyclines: Effects on nitric oxide synthases. Proc Natl Acad Sci USA 1996; 93: 14014–14019.

93. Brandt KD, Yu LP, Amith G *et al.* Therapeutic effect of doxycycline (doxy) in canine osteoarthritis (OA). Osteoarthritis and Cartilage 1993; 1: 14.

94. Spencer CM and Wilde MI. Diacerein. Drugs 1997; 53: 98–108.

95. Martel-Pelletier J, Mineau F, Jolicoeur FC *et al.* In vitro effects of diacerhein and rhein on interleukin 1 and tumor necrosis factor-alpha systems in human osteoarthritic synovium and chondrocytes. J Rheumatol 1998; 25: 753–762.

96. Carney SL, Hicks CA, Tree B, Broadmore RJ. An in vivo investigation of the effect of anthraquinones on the turnover of aggrecans in spontaneous osteoarthritis in the guinea pig. Inflamm Res 1995; 44: 182–186.

97. Brun PH. Effect of diacetylrhein on the development of experimental osteoarthritis. A biochemical investigation (letter). Osteoarthritis Cartilage 1997; 5: 289–291.

98. Brandt K, Smith G, Kang SY *et al.* Effects of diacerhein in an accelerated canine model of osteoarthritis. Osteoarthritis Cartilage 1997; 5: 438–449.

99. Pelletier JP, Yaron M, Haraoui B *et al.* Efficacy and safety of diacerein in osteoarthritis of the knee. Arthritis Rheum 2000; 43: 2339–2348.

100. Dougados M, Nguyen M, Berdah L *et al.* Evaluation of the structure-modifying effects of diacerein in hip osteoarthritis: ECHODIAH, a three-year, placebo-controlled trial. Evaluation of the chondromodulating effect of diacerein in OA of the hip. Arthritis Rheum 2001; 44: 2539–2547.

101. Henroitin YE, Labasse AH, Jaspar JM *et al.* Effects of three avocado/soybean unsaponifiable mixtures on metalloproteinases, cytokines and prostaglandin E2 production by human articular chondrocytes. Clin Rheumatol 1998; 17: 31–39.

102. Maheu E, Mazieres B, Valat JP *et al.* Symptomatic efficacy of avocado/soybean unsaponifiables in the treatment of osteoarthritis of the knee and hip. A prospective, randomized, double-blind, placebo-controlled, multicenter clinical trial with six-month treatment period and two-month followup demonstrating a persistent effect. Arthritis Rheum 1998; 41: 81–91.

103. Lequesne M, Maheu E, Cadet C *et al.* Effect of avocado/soya unsaponifiables (ASU) on joint space loss in hip osteoarthritis (HOA) over 2 years. A placebo controlled trial. Arthritis Rheum 1996; 39(suppl 9): S227.

104. Pellegrini VD. Osteoarthritis at the base of the thumb. Orthop Clin N Am 1992; 23: 83–102.

105. Keating EM, Faris PM, Ritter MA, Kane J. Use of lateral heel and sole wedges in the treatment of medial osteoarthritis of the knee. Orthop Rev 1993; 22: 921–924.

106. Gaffney K, Ledingham J, Perry J. Intra-articular triamcinolone hexacetonide in knee osteoarthritis: factors influencing the clinical response. Ann Rheum Dis 1995; 54: 379–381.

107. Chang RW, Falconer J, Stulberg SD *et al.* Randomized controlled trial of arthroscopic surgery versus closed needle joint lavage for patients with osteoarthritis of the knee. Arthritis Rheum 1993; 36: 289–296.

108. Gibson JNA, White MD, Chapman VM *et al.* Arthroscopic lavage and debridement for osteoarthritis of the knee. J Bone Joint Surg 1992; 74-b: 534–537.

109. Liveseley PJ, Doherty M, Needoff M *et al.* Arthroscopic lavage of osteoarthritic knees. J Bone Joint Surg 1991; 73-B: 922–926.

110. Ravaud P, Moulinier L, Giraudeau B *et al.* Effects of joint lavage and steroid injection in patients with osteoarthritis of the knee. Arthritis Rheum 1999; 42: 475–482.

111. Oldenbring S, Egund N, Knutson K *et al.* Revision after osteotomy for gonarthrosis: a 10–19 year follow-up of 314 cases. Acta Orthop Scand 1990; 61: 128–130.

CRYSTAL-RELATED ARTHROPATHIES

CRYSTAL-RELATED ARTHROPATHIES

41 Clinical features of gout

Terry Gibson

Clinical features

- Abrupt initial onset involving, most commonly, big toe, ankle or other joints of foot
- Upper limbs are affected in chronic tophaceous or recurrent acute gout, especially the distal interphalangeal joint
- Men in middle life who are obese and drink alcohol regularly are the most susceptible
- Women when affected are most commonly on diuretics or heavy alcohol drinkers
- There are associations with hypertension, hypertriglyceridemia and mild renal impairment
- HPRT deficiency, PRPP synthetase overactivity or hereditable renal disease should be suspected in children, adolescents or young adults with gout

HISTORICAL BACKGROUND

The common concept of gout comprises an image of a stout, portly gentleman of substance with his foot elevated on a stool and a glass of alcoholic beverage and a table heavy with food near at hand. In 19th century England, this image of 'aldermanic' gout was perpetuated by satirical and political illustrators who wished to lampoon royalty and politicians. The picture of male predominance and an indirect association with excess of wine was recognized much earlier by Hippocrates in his aphorisms. The nature of gout and tophi was discussed in the first and second centuries by Celsus, Galen and Aretaeus the Cappadocian. Pliny and Seneca noted the absence of gout in the early period of the Roman republic, viewing it as a sign of decadence and debauchery in the empire of the first century. A succession of authorities over several subsequent centuries attested to the consistent pattern of the arthritis and its association with plenty. Sydenham himself was a sufferer and added a commentary on the distinctive nature of gout and a first-hand description of tophaceous material.

The picture of unmistakable classical tophaceous gout was described vividly in 16th century Spanish manuscripts. However, the separate recognition of chronic gout from rheumatoid arthritis and other forms of rheumatism was a discussion point until the early 19th century, when Landre Beavais and then Heberden in his commentaries, clarified that gout was indeed a separate condition. The clinical distinction of gout was further emphasized by Sir Alfred Garrod in the same century and to a much smaller extent by his son Sir Archibald at the close of the century.

A galaxy of 20th century clinicians, including Talbott, Scott and Emmerson, wrote extensively on the clinical and biochemical features of gout. The role of the kidney in the pathogenesis of gout and its sequential impairment were pursued relentlessly by Guttman and Yu.

The underlying purine metabolic defects of gout and their clinical expression received impetus from yet more 20th century figures of stature such as Seegmiller, Kelley, Holmes, Simmonds and Wyngaarden.

Meanwhile, the importance of the monosodium urate to the initiation of acute gout was confirmed and consolidated by McCarty, Phelps and Schumacher. By contrast to acute gout the clinical picture of the chronic disease is still poorly appreciated. Even less well remarked upon are the acute and chronic manifestations affecting the axial skeleton, the bizarre displays of subcutaneous tophi, the compressive effects of tophi on nerves, spinal column and bone and the associated non-articular features of hypertension, renal dysfunction, alcoholism and hypertriglyceridemia. This chapter attempts to extend the clinical spectrum beyond the stereotypical image and also to describe the rare causes of juvenile gout and the clinical picture associated with women and older people.

ACUTE GOUT

Risk factors

The archetypical patient is male, age 40–50, overweight and with a proclivity for regular alcohol consumption. No race or social class is excluded. There are plentiful exceptions to this picture and these are also described in this chapter. A family history of gout may be evident. Acute episodes seem to occur more commonly in the spring but this does not seem to be associated with variations of serum uric acid levels or with diet[1,2]. An episode of acute gout is more likely to occur during an infectious or other illness or during a period of hospital in-patient care or following trauma. Withdrawal from alcohol during such an illness may cause a consequent fall in serum uric acid level[3] and disturbance of urate homeostasis. This may in turn induce any microtophi within the joint to fragment, releasing urate crystals which excite local inflammation. There may be other explanations for the relationship between incidental illness, hospital admission and precipitation of gout but these are unknown.

Clinical features

The sudden onset of pain and swelling is often preceded by a period of irritability or the premonition of an attack. The first indication of pain is

TABLE 41.1 DISTRIBUTION OF INDIVIDUAL ACUTE AND CHRONIC JOINT INVOLVEMENT IN 354 PATIENTS WITH RECURRENT ACUTE GOUT

Joint	Cumulative frequency (%)
Big toe	76
Ankle or foot	50
Knee	32
Finger	25
Elbow	10
Wrist	10
Other joint	4
Bursitis	3
More than one site simultaneously	11

Half the patients had experienced gout for more than 10 years[5].

often at night. Usually a single joint is affected and the initial episode involves the first metatarsophalangeal joint (podagra) in most cases. Next in frequency are the mid tarsal and hind foot joints including the ankle. The foot is involved in nearly all cases at some time and if not affected in the first episode, is very likely to become so in subsequent acute events. The susceptibility of the foot and its pre-eminence in gout has no known explanation. With the passage of time, recurrent acute arthritis may involve multiple sites including the knee and the joints of the upper limbs. The shoulders are usually spared but may be involved. Not only does acute gout seem to spread upward from the feet with the cumulative frequency of episodes but the number of joints involved is also increased so that polyarticular acute gout tends to be a later feature, thus departing from the classical monarticular description and expanding the differential diagnosis. Acute gout affecting more than four sites simultaneously is an uncommon initial presentation but two to three joints may be affected during the first episode in a third of cases[4]. Involvement of the wrist and elbow has a clear relationship to disease duration[5] (Table 41.1). Bursae which are near to or communicate with joints may also be the site of acute inflammation. Olecranon and pre-patellar bursitis are the most common of these[6].

The pain of acute gout is often extreme, especially in the first few episodes. This regularly interrupts sleep, prevents walking and interferes with work and leisure. The severity of disability ranges from complete prostration to a slight limp. The experience of recurrent acute episodes and the development of chronic tophaceous gout are associated with increased tolerance of the symptoms. Patients adapt in other ways. They may amend their footwear by cutting holes in shoes or wear slippers or sandals in inappropriate circumstances, visible evidence of their diagnosis and their desperation (Fig. 41.1). The involved joint becomes red, shiny and very tender especially when the big toe is affected. There may be surrounding cellulitis especially when the ankle or a bursa is involved. This may be extensive and suggestive of local infection. These symptoms and signs develop over a period of hours. The intense inflammation is often accompanied by fever which when associated with a neutrophilia and a pronounced acute phase response is highly suggestive of septic arthritis or infective cellulitis of surrounding soft tissues. Fever is more common in polyarticular acute gout[7] but the degree of fever and of leukocytosis does not correlate with the number of affected joints[4]. The natural history of acute gout is of resolution over a period of several days or when multiple joints are affected simultaneously, over a few weeks. As the inflammation recedes, the red apple shine is replaced by a purple plum hue associated with exfoliation of overlying skin.

Some patients experience a single isolated episode without recurrence. For some of those who do not receive appropriate advice and prophylaxis, there may be recurrent sporadic episodes of acute pain and swelling affecting one or more joints at variable intervals.

Differential diagnosis

Alternatives to the diagnosis of acute gout need to be considered in all situations except a recurring, painful swelling of the big toe in a middle age, overweight male. The likelihood of an alternative diagnosis in this context is improbable. Any history of acute, intermittent painful swelling and discoloration of the foot in males should be considered to be gout until proved otherwise. When a joint or joints other than the ankle or foot is inflamed and when multiple sites are involved, the diagnostic options are increased. When acute arthritis affects one or a few joints the possible diagnoses include pseudogout, septic arthritis and reactive arthritis. This is especially problematic when a knee joint is inexplicably hot and swollen without a preceding history of articular symptoms. A likely clinical diagnosis in an elderly, slender woman not receiving diuretics is probably that of pseudogout but in an obese male who drinks a lot of beer, gout is the more likely. A patient with quiescent rheumatoid arthritis, an infected leg ulcer and an acute hot swollen knee very likely has septic arthritis. In a slender young man or woman with a recent history of diarrhea or urethritis, reactive arthritis is probable. The presence of fever does not distinguish between them. The ruddy facial flush of alcohol excess, the clinical features of alcoholic liver disease or of alcoholic peripheral neuropathy and the presence of chalk like tophi on the ears or fingers and tophaceous nodules on the elbows, knees or Achilles tendons may provide corroborative evidence of gout (Figs 41.2 & 41.3). A prosthetic joint which becomes hot and swollen is most likely due to sepsis but gout, especially when a previous history is noted, could be the cause[8]. Patients with systemic lupus erythematosus (SLE) with worsening joint pain, especially in the context of renal failure and when the fingers and toes are affected may have gout rather than lupus arthri-

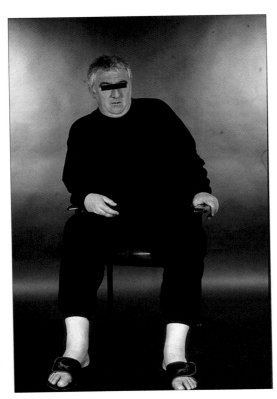

Fig. 41.1 This patient presented complaining of painful big toes. His body habitus and the shoes he was wearing on a cold morning suggested a diagnosis of gout. This was supported by the tophi visible on his fingers.

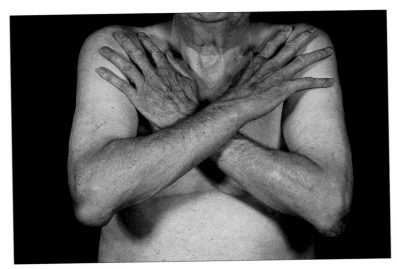

Fig. 41.2 Tophi on the elbows in a patient with chronic polyarthritis affecting the fingers. He was thought to have nodular rheumatoid arthritis and was treated with sodium aurothiomalate injections despite a negative test for rheumatoid factor.

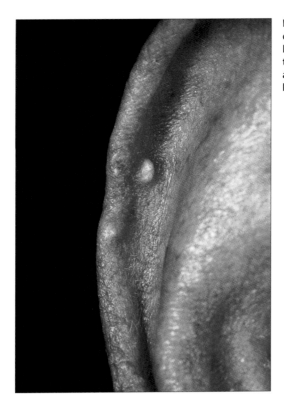

Fig. 41.3 The true diagnosis of gout became evident when the patient developed a chalk-like tophus on his right ear.

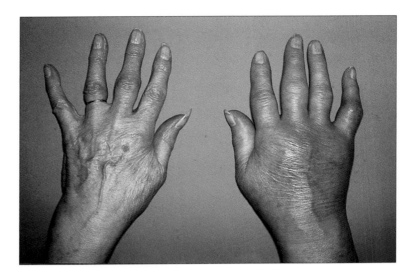

Fig. 41.4 Chronic tophaceous gout affecting the small joint of the fingers reminiscent of rheumatoid arthritis.

tis. In some of the described cases, large tophi have developed over the fingers and toes helping to simplify the diagnosis[9,10]. The chronic renal failure of SLE together with the prescription of diuretics in this illness explain the occasional concurrence with tophaceous gout. The co-existence of gout and other chronic peripheral joint diseases has been rarely documented but may be underestimated. Gout arising in a patient with rheumatoid arthritis has been described[11]. The theoretical risk of hyperuricemia and gout co-existing with rheumatoid arthritis is increased among those receiving cyclosporine as a disease modifying agent. The crucial investigation to discriminate between these possibilities is the examination of synovial fluid or nodules for the presence of monosodium urate crystals. Even when the clinical diagnosis of gout seems secure, the immediate satisfaction of diagnostic confirmation by synovial fluid analysis and the documented diagnostic clarification make it worthwhile.

CHRONIC TOPHACEOUS GOUT

When recurrent acute gout and hyperuricemia go untreated and when there is a failure to eradicate causative factors such as alcohol excess, obesity or diuretic therapy, the condition may evolve from a picture of sporadic acute mono and oligoarthritis through recurrent polyarthritis to persistent low grade joint inflammation, joint deformity and deposition of urate crystals to form visible tophi. Tophaceous deposits develop within the same joints affected by acute gout and especially the first metatarsophalangeal joint. The relatively mild discomfort of chronic gout may be punctuated by episodes of acute arthritis. About one third of chronic gout patients develop visible tophi[12]. Within the joints, tophi contribute to the development of bone erosions especially in the big toe but also elsewhere. Tophi are classically found on the pinnae, the elbows and Achilles tendons but they may be distributed more widely, occurring within and around the finger joints, in the finger tip pulp, around the knee and within olecranon and pre-patellar bursae. Swelling and deformity become the characteristic signs, but without the intense inflammation (Fig. 41.4) associated with acute gout. No diarthrodial joint is immune to this process and although the joints of the feet are

notoriously involved in the acute illness it is the hands where evidence of chronic gout is more evident. Swelling of the distal, and proximal interphalangeal and metacarpophalangeal joints are often due to articular and periarticular tophi. Swan neck, Boutonniere and flexion deformities may develop resembling rheumatoid arthritis. The diagnosis is sometimes suggested by the pallor of tophaceous material beneath the skin which is stretched over an involved joint. Toes, ankles, elbows and wrists may all be similarly affected. Careful inspection of tophi may reveal a white subcutaneous granular appearance due to the accumulation of monosodium urate crystals. Tophi may emerge at unexpected sites becoming suddenly visible and discharging uric acid crystals as a paste or pus like material, especially during hypouricemic treatment.

Differential diagnosis

The swelling and deformity of fingers and toes may affect the metacarpophalangeal and proximal interphalangeal joints symmetrically. Typical rheumatoid-like deformities may add to the confusion and when tophi are confined to the elbows they may be so suggestive of rheumatoid nodules that the diagnosis is followed by antirheumatoid treatment. This clinical pitfall may be compounded by radiological joint erosions reminiscent of rheumatoid arthritis. A perceptive clinician would seek further information if such a patient had negative tests for rheumatoid factor since positive tests would be the normal expectation in a patient with nodular rheumatoid disease. Involvement of the distal interphalangeal joints and fusiform swelling of fingers indicative of dactylitis may suggest psoriatic arthritis or chronic reactive arthritis (Fig. 41.5). Only the diligent search for tophi or the examination of synovial aspirates for urate crystals may establish the true diagnosis. Widespread, visible tophi over the fingers, especially when these ulcerate, can resemble the calcium hydroxyapatite deposits of scleroderma. The converse is also true. The radiolucency of tophi and the demonstration of urate crystals in aspirate or exudate will resolve this dilemma. Localized subcutaneous or dermal tophi may also suggest infection with pus formation. Many tophi which discharge their contents are treated mistakenly with antibiotics (Fig. 41.6).

Atypical clinical features

In acute gout, unusual presentations departing from the classical description are on close inspection usually atypical episodes of established but sporadic gout. Recognition of acute gout affecting the manubriosternal, acromioclavicular and cervical spine joints is usually on a background of previous more typical and sometimes forgotten gouty arthritis affecting

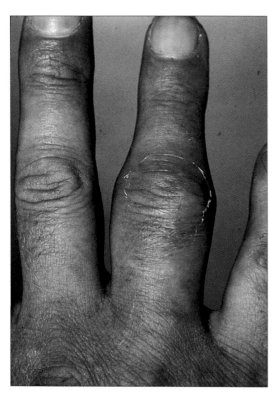

Fig. 41.5 Gouty dactylitis of a finger. This appearance is indistinguishable from other rheumatic diseases such as psoriatic or reactive arthritis. Cutaneous exfoliation indicates the resolving of a recent episode of acute gout affecting the interphalangeal joint.

the foot[13,14,15]. Acute involvement of the knee may be associated with popliteal cyst formation, leakage of synovial fluid and lower limb cellulitis or swelling simulating a deep vein thrombosis[16].

It is chronic tophaceous gout which provides more opportunity for anecdotal reports of uncommon manifestations. Tophi within the flexor tendons of the hand and wrist may cause discrete palmar or extensor swelling and carpal tunnel syndrome[17]. These tumorous swellings may also compress the spinal cord as well as peripheral nerves. Tophi and acute gout within the cervical and lumbar spine have been well documented causing acute and chronic spinal pain, cord compression and paralysis. Fever, a raised acute phase response and suggestive X-ray or MRI scans may confuse these complications with an infective discitis or an epidural abscess[18,19]. Spinal involvement may occur without visible tophi and reportedly as an initial manifestation of gout[20]. In addition to subcutaneous tophi which arise within or around the joints, the skin itself may contain intradermal deposits which may appear as widespread pustules mainly on the legs and forearms[21,22]. These are seen in severe tophaceous gout, often in association with renal failure and diuretic treatment.

INVESTIGATIONS

The concurrence of hyperuricemia with acute or chronic joint symptoms and signs is not sufficient to establish a diagnosis of gout. Both musculoskeletal pain and unrelated hyperuricemia are common in all communities and for a variety of environmental reasons. Furthermore, acute gout may occur in the presence of normouricemia and although the presumption is that such patients have been hyperuricemic in the past, an anecdotal case has been made for gout developing despite consistently normal blood uric acid levels[23].

Demonstration of urate crystals

Metatarsophalangeal joint aspiration is rarely justifiable in a patient with podagra and obvious susceptibility features. The certain diagnosis of both acute and chronic gout, however, requires the demonstration of monosodium urate crystals in samples of synovial fluid, tophaceous material, synovial or other tissue. It is most often required when an isolated joint and especially a knee is hot and swollen without previous history or other diagnostic distinguishing features. The synovial fluid is usually turbid because of large numbers of polymorphs. It may be sufficiently purulent to suggest sepsis and is occasionally milky in appearance[24]. So called 'urate milk' tends to contain few leukocytes and comprises a dense sediment of monosodium urate crystals presumably from intra-articular or bursal tophi[23]. In the acute synovitis of gout the urate crystals can usually be identified lying within phagocytic cells

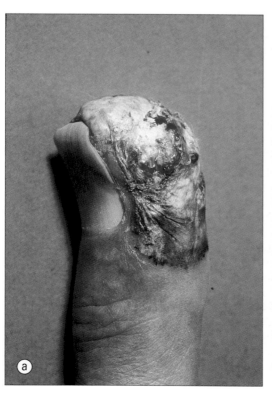

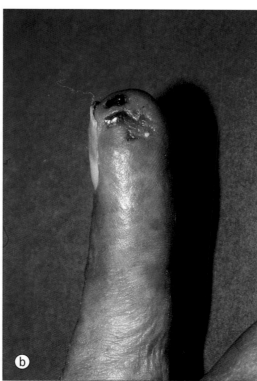

Fig. 41.6 Tophus on a finger tip. (a) During antibiotic treatment for a presumed mistaken diagnosis of local infection; (b) after treatment with allopurinol for 6 months.

which often contain several crystals of different sizes. Visualization and morphological recognition of these slender often pointed crystals is easily achievable with an ordinary light microscope but compensated polarizing microscopy is useful in distinguishing monosodium urate from calcium pyrophosphate dihydrate crystals on the basis of their birefringent properties as well as allowing an esthetic appreciation of their appearance. Urate crystals tend to be more numerous than calcium pyrophosphate crystals and are much brighter under polarizing microscopy. Their number is not related to the severity of the arthritis but they do diminish in both number and size as the attack recedes. It is important to recognize that occasionally gout and sepsis or pseudogout may co-exist so bacteriological examination is a pre-requisite for every turbid sample[26,27]. When gout is suspected but a joint effusion is not detectable, needle aspiration is still worth attempting because a drop of aspirate may contain crystals even when it appears to be blood. In effusions which persist after the signs of inflammation have resolved, the clinical picture of so called inter-critical gout, urate crystals may still be apparent[27]. This can be helpful confirmation of the diagnosis in patients who have an arthritis of unknown cause and whose most recent episode of pain appears to have resolved. By contrast there are occasions when crystals are not demonstrable in synovial fluid. Such fluid is probably from sympathetic joint effusions which have arisen adjacent to periarticular inflammation due to gouty bursitis[28]. Diagnostic scraping or needle probing of tophi or biopsy of synovium and suspect lumps, may yield sheets of monosodium crystals sometimes serendipitously. These specimens are often dramatic under compensated polarizing microscopy but contain no cells.

Blood tests and urine

As stated above, the reliance on a high serum uric acid level for the diagnosis of acute gout is misplaced. A period of sustained hyperuricemia is required before accretions of uric acid accumulate on the cartilage and synovial surfaces but the blood level may normalize before crystals are liberated into the joint cavity. It is a fall in serum uric acid which so often precipitates acute episodes by encouraging tophus dissolution. It has been estimated that about one third of patients are normouricemic during episodes of acute gout and the majority of such cases are not taking hypouricemic drugs[29]. However, hyperuricemia is the most common biochemical abnormality in acute and chronic gout and the higher the level, the more predictive of gout does it become, either as a diagnostic aid or a guide to the future development of gout[30].

There is no requirement to estimate urine uric acid excretion as a routine practice except in children and young adults with gout who are not taking diuretics, low dose aspirin, pyrazinamide or cyclosporine. All of these agents will cause hyperuricemia by reducing uric acid renal clearance. In the rare and exceptional cases of juvenile gout a high excretion of uric acid may denote deficiency of the hypoxanthine-guanine phosphoribosyltransferase (HPRT) or an increase in activity of the phosphoribosylpyrophosphate synthetase (PP-rib-P) enzyme. A very low urate clearance, in a young woman especially, may be evidence of familial nephropathy with hyperuricemia[31]. The overwhelming majority of patients with gout have impaired urate clearance[32].

During an acute episode of gout a modest neutrophilia is common but usually does not exceed 15.0×10^{-9}/l. A rise of erythrocyte sedimentation rate (ESR) and c-reactive protein (CRP) is usual in both acute and chronic gout but in the former, the acute phase response is striking, the ESR frequently exceeding 50mm/h. This often leads investigators to consider more sinister pathology including malignancy and sepsis. An ESR of more than 80mm/h would not be exceptional in the context of acute gout and the search for myeloma or polymyalgia rheumatica is predictably fruitless in such cases.

In chronic gout, a fall in hemoglobin to levels as low as 9.0g/dl reflects chronic low grade inflammation although use of non-steroidal anti-

inflammatory drugs (NSAIDs) may contribute an element of iron deficiency. The etiology of gout in an individual case is often suggested by the macrocytosis of alcohol abuse. Sometimes this is accompanied by alcohol induced thrombocytopenia or neutropenia. Alcoholic liver dysfunction is a common accompaniment with elevation of serum transaminases, alkaline phosphatase or bilirubin.

Imaging

Standard radiology contributes little to the diagnosis of acute gout in the absence of an antecedent history. Plain films may simply confirm soft tissue swelling. However, radiographs of the feet may occasionally show evidence of first metatarsophalangeal joint erosion despite the absence of previous symptoms, attestation of tophaceous development within the joint over a period (Fig. 41.7). The appearance of bone erosions due to tophi is characterized by well demarcated round or oval shaped deficits with sclerotic margins, sometimes with an overhanging margin of bone (Fig. 41.8). The erosions and cysts in the big toe may precede any clinical evidence of tophaceous deposits and in chronic gout, radiographic evidence may be apparent in almost half of those without visible tophi[12,33]. More extensive erosive damage resembling rheumatoid and psoriatic arthritis may develop in the toes, ankles, fingers, wrists and elsewhere in chronic tophaceous gout.

On MR scanning, tophi appear of intermediate signal intensity on T1-weighted images and as heterogeneous signal intensity on T2-weighted images. These views may demonstrate spread of tophaceous material along fascial planes and show early bone damage not visible on standard radiographs[34,35].

DISORDERS ASSOCIATED WITH GOUT

In primary gout there is often a constellation of other health problems including obesity, alcohol abuse, hypertension, renal dysfunction and hypertriglyceridemia. Their cause and effect relationships are complex. In diverse populations there is a striking positive correlation between blood uric acid levels and both body weight and alcohol consumption[36,30]. These traits are even more striking among those with gout. The rise in serum urate following alcohol consumption is higher in gouty compared with normouricemic subjects[37]. Almost half of gout patients

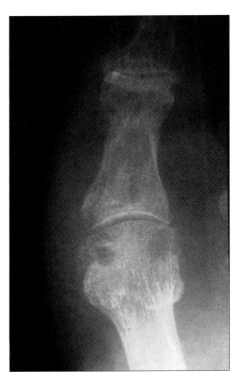

Fig. 41.7 X-ray of big toe showing round erosions due to tophi in the first metatarsophalangeal joint.

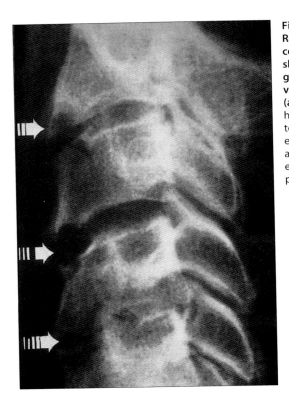

Fig. 41.8 Radiograph of cervical spine showing probable gouty erosions of vertebral bodies (arrows). The patient had severe, disabling tophaceous gout with episodes of neck pain associated with episodic acute peripheral gout.

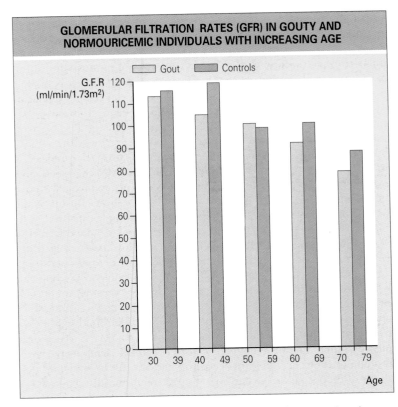

GLOMERULAR FILTRATION RATES (GFR) IN GOUTY AND NORMOURICEMIC INDIVIDUALS WITH INCREASING AGE

Fig. 41.9 Glomerular filtration rates (GFR) in gouty and normouricemic individuals with increasing age. There is a steady decline in both groups but the GFR in the gouty patient is always less than that of the control population.

drink 60g of alcohol or more a day[38]. Such a heavy intake is inevitably associated with an increased prevalence of alcohol dependence, liver dysfunction, depression and the central and peripheral nerve sequelae of alcoholism. Alcohol may cause a rise in blood pressure and together with obesity accounts for some of the increased prevalence of hypertension in gout. This has been reported in as many as 50% of cases in one series[5]. Among hypertensive patients there is a similar frequency of hyperuricemia[39]. Whether it is principally the adverse impact of hypertension on renal function or whether it is an effect of impaired kidneys on blood pressure, the association is real and the cause and effect mechanisms may operate in both directions. Hypertensive patients with gout do have renal dysfunction and lower urate clearance than normal people. The possibility that the renal impairment is the primary phenomenon and causes both the hyperuricemia and the hypertension has been suggested[40]. However, the demographic data strongly implicate environmental factors as well as a relative reduced urate clearance in the development of gout and it is likely that in most patients, hypertension and renal failure are partly if not wholly co-morbid features. Among Polynesian peoples, a relative impairment of urate clearance accounts for their susceptibility to hyperuricemia and in general, they do not develop renal failure although renal function may show a modest decline among those who develop gout[41]. Among Caucasians with gout there is a reduction of glomerular filtration rates, urine concentrating ability and renal disposal of hydrogen ion at all ages[32] (Fig. 41.9).

The question of whether gout itself can cause renal failure is moot. Hyperuricemia in a non-gouty population does not seem deleterious to the kidneys but prior to the availability of effective treatments, there were plentiful descriptions of renal failure, death and urate deposits within the renal parenchyma[42]. This is now a rare event but persistent hyperuricemia among those with gout does seem to cause a slow decline of kidney function[43]. Improvements in renal function have been recorded after treatment of hyperuricemia in gout but this may be partly an effect of a reduced requirement for NSAIDs[44]. Renal failure, whatever the etiology, will cause hyperuricemia but there is no convincing evidence beyond anecdote that the presence of uremia suppresses the acute inflammation of gout and reduces its incidence in chronic renal failure. Some patterns of renal disease, particularly that of familial inter-

stitial nephritis may cause pronounced hyperuricemia and precocious gout as a first manifestation[45]. Other renal disorders preferentially involving tubular function and urate clearance include Bartter's syndrome, Alport's syndrome and saturnine gout due to chronic lead ingestion. These may all cause acute and chronic gout in advance of renal failure. The overproduction and increased excretion of uric acid in HPRT or PP-rib-P synthetase abnormalities tend to produce gout, kidney stones and renal failure whereas the sudden, massive rise in urine uric acid seen during treatment of some malignant disorders is more likely to precipitate acute renal failure due to crystal obstructive nephropathy than gout.

Allied to obesity and alcohol excess is dyslipidemia. This is mostly due to raised serum triglyceride levels which correlate with degrees of obesity[46]. The levels are even higher among those who drink a lot of alcohol. Both serum uric acid and triglyceride can be lowered independently by reducing body weight or alcohol intake[3,47]. There are conflicting reports about a link between high serum cholesterol levels and gout but a strong association has not been demonstrated[48]. Of those with both gout and hypertriglyceridemia, almost three quarters have impaired glucose tolerance and about ten per cent of gouty individuals have or will develop non-insulin-dependent diabetes mellitus[49,50]. The common factor is obesity. It is surprising that cardiovascular disease does not feature more prominently in surveys of gout given the frequency of obesity, hypertension and impaired glucose tolerance. There are population data which support an indirect relationship between hyperuricemia and the risk of coronary artery disease[51,52] but in clinical practice this translates into a recognition that gout may signal the presence of additional health problems.

GOUT IN YOUNG PEOPLE

The possibility of gout needs to be considered in all children, adolescents and young adults of either gender who develop spontaneous pain and swelling of the first metatarsophalangeal joint, the hind foot or the ankle and for which no other explanation is apparent. None of the classical predisposing factors such as obesity, diuretic therapy and alcohol is likely to be present. A family history of gout or renal failure should arouse curiosity and prompt measurement of the blood uric acid level, but no such clues may be available. Such instances are rare and many rheumatologists will not encounter a case of juvenile or adolescent gout within their professional lives.

Diagnosis

If a diagnosis of gout is proven by demonstration of monosodium urate crystals in a joint or by persistent hyperuricemia then further investigation must include an estimate of renal function including creatinine or clearance especially if the serum creatinine and urea are normal or only slightly elevated. The next essential investigation is measurement of 24 hour urine uric acid excretion and calculation of the urate clearance and its expression as a percentage of glomerular filtration (fractional urate clearance). Further investigation of purine metabolism may need to be undertaken if the patient is found to be excreting increased amounts of uric acid. These can be performed at several well known world centres and include measurement of the excretion of other purines and assay of purine enzymes using skin fibroblasts, lymphocytes or red cells. A diagnosis may then be pursued and confirmed by genetic mutation detection techniques.

The diagnosis may be suggested by other features including a personal or family history of renal failure, kidney stones, gout itself or neurological abnormalities.

Purine enzyme abnormalities

There are two purine enzyme abnormalities which result in overproduction of uric acid, precocious gout and increased uric acid excretion in the urine. This results in tubular obstruction by urate crystals, the formation of renal interstitial tophi and uric acid urolithiasis.

HRPT deficiency

One of the enzyme aberrations is a deficiency of hypoxanthine guanine phosphoribosyl transferase (HPRT), a vital enzyme in the purine salvage pathway. The HPRT gene resides on the X chromosome and of the almost 300 reported cases, only five have been female. The defect in females arises as a result of mutations in the maternal or paternal allele with non-random inactivation of the other allele[53]. A spectrum of disease is seen depending on the severity of enzyme deficiency. In the devastating childhood disease known as Lesch–Nyhan syndrome, the enzyme is entirely absent. This is a syndrome of severe neurological illness with cognitive impairment, spasticity, extra-pyramidal motor dysfunction and a propensity to self mutilation by biting. These features are allied to hyperuricosuria and kidney failure. Gout and tophi may develop depending on survival and the duration of disease. The illness usually causes death within the first decade of life. Lesser deficiencies of the enzyme are associated with a longer life expectation and may cause gout, renal dysfunction and varying degrees of pyramidal and extrapyramidal disease but without self-mutilation. The mildest phenotype may be associated with gout and kidney stones only. Cases with residual enzyme activity are sometimes referred to as the Kelley–Seegmiller syndrome. The gene for HPRT possesses nine exons. The many described mutations associated with HPRT deficiency are spread throughout the gene and neither specific locations nor particular base substitutions and deletions can predict the phenotype except in a very limited fashion.

PP-rib-P synthetase superactivity

The second enzyme aberration involves superactivity of phosphoribosylpyrophosphate synthetase (PP-rib-P synthetase). This is a substrate for nucleotide synthesis and like the HPRT gene, it is found on the X chromosome. Gout may occur mainly in male children and young adults but two major phenotypes have been described. When the more serious of these affects heterozygous males, there is neurological impairment, severe sensorineural deafness and death in childhood. In heterozygous females the disease expression of this phenotype is milder but they may also have deafness as well as overproduction of uric acid and gout[54,55]. The other phenotype is not associated with deafness and presents in adolescence or adulthood as gout or urolithiasis. The PP-rib-P synthetase genes (PRPS1 and PRPS2) map to different regions of the X chromosome. Both contain seven exons. The genetic basis of the illness appears to be due to point mutations of the PRPS1 gene.

Familial juvenile hyperuricemic nephropathy

In patients with the rare disorder, familial juvenile hyperuricemic nephropathy there may be a childhood presentation with pain in the big toe due to gout[31]. There is not always a family history of either gout or kidney failure but in affected patients there is usually early evidence of renal impairment as measured by glomerular filtration and tubular function studies. In some families, females are more susceptible. Reduced urate clearance is more pronounced than is anticipated from the degree of renal impairment. The disease is characterized by gout, progressive renal dysfunction, hypertension, reduced kidney size and the histopathological changes of tubulointerstitial nephritis and ischemic damage, fibrosis and tubular atrophy. There is still a debate about whether the hyperuricemia has a renal pathogenetic role but the same familial clinical and pathological picture may occur in the absence of hyperuricemia indicating that the renal disease causes the gout and not vice versa. The condition is transmitted as an autosomal dominant gene which has been localized on chromosome 16p11.2. There is evidence of heterogeneity and reduced penetrance[56,57]. Another pattern of interstitial nephropathy associated with precocious gout and hyperuricemia is autosomal dominant medullary cystic kidney disease (ADMCKD). This typically causes a defect of urine concentrating ability and has clinical and pathological similarity to the recessive disorder, inherited juvenile nephronophthisis which is another renal cystic disease. However, their genetic loci appear to be different. Two loci have been inferred for ADMCKD. One of these is on chromosome 16p12[58].

Glycogen storage diseases

Hyperuricemia is also a feature of some glycogen storage diseases. These are largely autosomal recessive hereditary disorders of glycogen metabolism comprising hepatic and muscular forms of illness. In type 1A (von Gierke's disease) children are short in stature and have large livers. This hepatic form of disease is further characterized by multiple xanthomata, fasting hypoglycemia, elevated serum triglyceride and hyperuricemia leading in adolescence to acute and chronic gout. Liver biopsy reveals deficient glucose-6-phosphatase. There is accelerated ATP turnover causing increased degradation of adenine nucleotides to inosine, hypoxanthine, xanthine and uric acid. Other hepatic forms are not consistently associated with hyperuricemia. Of the muscular forms of glycogen storage disease it is type V (McCardle's disease) and type VII which have been both firmly associated with gout. In type V disease, a deficiency of muscle phosphorylase may be detected on muscle biopsy but the mechanism of the muscle breakdown and fatigue remain uncertain[59]. Patients may remain asymptomatic until adolescence when fatigue and muscle cramps occur after exercise, sometimes followed by myoglobinuria and rhabdomyolysis with renal failure. Exercise may not be followed by the normal rise of venous serum lactate. However, there is a demonstrable increase in blood levels of hypoxanthine, xanthine and uric acid after exercise accounting for the sporadic reports of associated gout[60]. In the type VII disease the clinical picture is similar to type V except that there is associated hemolysis. The disease is caused by muscle phosphofructokinase deficiency. These observations suggest that the hyperuricemia is caused by an increase of purine nucleotide turnover.

Treatment

In all of the disorders which can cause hyperuricemia and gout in young people, allopurinol is effective at reducing the level of blood uric acid. In the two enzyme abnormalities, HPRT deficiency and PP-rib-P synthetase overactivity, the impact of uric acid overproduction on renal function may be obviated but successful treatment does not influence the neurological features of these disorders. In the interstitial kidney diseases associated with precocious gout hypouricemic treatment has no influence on the progression of the renal disease, management of which usually entails dialysis and kidney transplantation in the course of time. Gout associated with glycogen storage disease can also be treated by conventional hypouricemic drugs.

GOUT IN WOMEN

Population surveys have consistently demonstrated higher serum uric acid levels in men than in women. Although female values rise around the menopause and approximate those of males, a disparity persists[61,62,63]. This phenomenon may not be the result of the menopause *per se* since pre and post menopausal subjects of the same age have similar serum uric acid levels[64]. The prevalence of hyperuricemia among females varies between 1–15% depending on the survey population and the definition of hyperuricemia[65]. It is therefore not surprising that of large series of gout patients, women represent a quarter or less of the total[5,66]. As anticipated, most women who develop gout are postmenopausal and a majority are receiving diuretics. The relationship of gout with obesity and alcohol excess is not as apparent in women. There is a stronger association in women of gout with hypertension and renal dysfunction[67]. A growing number of females with gout are renal transplant recipients treated with cyclosporine[68]. A rare familial juvenile hyperuricemic nephropathy may in some families afflict only the females, presenting in childhood or more likely young adulthood as gout or renal failure[31,45]. The pattern of acute and chronic arthritis in women is similar to that of men. Podagra is the most common initial manifestation but polyarticular features are more common than in men at the time of presentation. A predilection for Heberden and Bouchard nodes to be affected by acute and chronic gouty arthritis and as sites for the development of tophaceous deposits are features described mainly in women on diuretics[69,70] (Fig. 41.10). Whether this is due to their older age at presentation and the greater frequency of nodal osteoarthritis among women of this age group is not clear but it is the one clinical characteristic that tends to distinguish women from men with gout

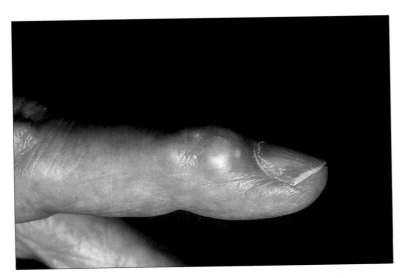

Fig. 41.10 Tophus overlying a Heberden's node in a woman on a diuretic.

although not exclusively. The presence of previous cartilage damage may predispose the osteoarthritic finger joints to urate crystal deposition. The same mechanism has been proposed to explain the susceptibility of the first metatarsophalangeal joint in podagra[71].

GOUT IN OLDER PEOPLE

There is a widely held view that when gout presents in old age, acute arthritis is less common than a polyarticular, deforming arthritis. This impression is partly due to the cumulative impact of chronic gout on the joints with aging and time. The description of elderly women on diuretics with tophaceous deposits over the fingers and elsewhere is firmly established and many of these appear to have no history of acute symptoms[72]. This syndrome is not confined to women but the gender distribution of gout in the elderly approximates parity. Large tophi especially at atypical sites and a chronic polyarthritis in the absence of any history of acute mono- or oligoarticular arthritis can be puzzling. The tophi within joints can cause considerable malformation[73].

Co-morbidity is common and the high percentage of diuretic induced gout and the small contribution of low dose aspirin to the hyperuricemia in this age group reflect the frequency of heart disease. Other concurrent diseases may include hypertension, renal failure and diabetes mellitus. The accentuated risks of gastrointestinal (GI) bleeding and of acute renal failure in the elderly together with the occasional need for anticoagulation in this age group, prohibit the standard NSAIDs traditionally used in acute gout. It is far better to prescribe a short course of oral corticosteroids in reducing dose over 10 days than take the risk of using NSAID in gouty patients over the age of 75 years. Alternatively, joint aspiration and intra-articular injection or intra-muscular injection of a long acting corticosteroid are effective. When NSAIDs are the preferred option of clinicians and their patients, selective Cox II inhibitors will lessen the risk of GI bleeding but not of renal impairment. Colchicine for acute episodes is not recommended because it is reportedly poorly tolerated in the elderly[74]. It retains its value when used in small doses in the early phase of hypouricemic drug treatment as a prophylaxis against recurrent acute gout. The choice of blood uric acid lowering agent in the elderly is allopurinol. Relative kidney impairment which is so common at this age lessens the effectiveness of uricosuric drugs. By the same token, renal impairment reduces the elimination of allopurinol metabolites and increases the risk of associated side effects such as rash and serious vasculitis[75]. Doses of 50–100mg daily are safer and usually adequate.

ASYMPTOMATIC HYPERURICEMIA

Within large population samples the prevalence of hyperuricemia varies depending on the definition of hyperuricemia and the population itself. In a survey of English people the frequency was about 4% in men and in women 0.4% before and about 2% after the menopause[61]. Multiple studies have corroborated the correlation of serum uric acid levels with body weight[63,76] and it is therefore likely that in many areas of the world, the frequency of hyperuricemia is increasing. Average blood uric acid levels vary between populations and are higher in native Taiwanese[77] and most famously among Polynesian people[41]. The gender difference and the association of hyperuricemia with obesity and alcohol excess still pertain to these communities and have been consistently observed over several decades and in all ethnic groups.

The fact that primates convert purines to uric acid and eliminate it through the kidneys is almost unique among mammals. Given the evolutionary standing of the human animal it could be assumed that there is a developmental advantage in the absence of uricase in human tissue and the apparent preference for urate rather than urea excretion. Historically, gout and hyperuricemia have been associated with the upper echelons of society. This observation together with a social class gradient of blood uric acid levels and the recording of gout among worthy and intellectually profound men such as Goethe, Darwin and Newton led to the hypothesis that gout is a correlate of intelligence. As recently as 1963, the documentation of higher blood uric acid levels among executives compared with craftsmen gave support to this notion[78]. The explanation is probably more prosaic. The financial rewards of talent and endeavor together with inherited affluence were until recent times the best guarantees of plentiful food and drink. Hyperuricemia is a condition of affluence and gout does not occur among the malnourished. In western cultures, obesity was until recently a measure of prosperity. The widespread availability of inexpensive food and a decline in levels of physical activity have seen a reversal in the social scale of fatness. No contemporary population data exist but in all likelihood, western affluence and egalitarianism have dissipated the socioeconomic clustering of hyperuricemia and make untenable the always improbable correlation of hyperuricemia with intellectual capacity. This removes the only evolutionary advantage so far proposed for the essential human need to synthesize and excrete uric acid rather than urea and water as the end products of purine turnover.

If hyperuricemia is not to the good in what way is it to the bad? The occurrence of gout is the main risk of asymptomatic hyperuricemia and over a five year period there was a cumulative incidence of gout in 18% of one series of subjects[30]. However, within a given population, the majority with hyperuricemia will not develop gout and a small number of normouricemic individuals will do so[79]. Treating hyperuricemia to prevent gout is not justifiable. The demonstration of hyperuricemia in individuals may be an important health indicator of serious pathology such as alcoholism and hypertension[36,30]. There are no data which support a deleterious affect of hyperuricemia on kidney function despite the association of gout with mild renal impairment[80,81]. Hyperuricemia in chronic renal failure is common and is an effect rather than the cause of the kidney impairment. In renal, liver and cardiac transplant patients receiving cyclosporine, hyperuricemia is a regular finding because of the reduction of urate clearance caused by this agent.

Hyperuricemia has been associated with a panoply of disorders, some real, some contested and others dubious[82]. The serious hyperuricosuria and occasional mild hyperuricemia which occur with myeloproliferative diseases and myelomatosis are accentuated by their treatment unless deflected by allopurinol. The transient impairment of renal urate secretion in diabetic ketoacidosis and starvation will cause a rise of blood uric acid as will renal failure. Gout will not be precipitated by these events alone. Psoriasis has been linked to hyperuricemia in some studies[83] but not in others[84,85]. The evidence so far linking hyperuricemia directly with hypothyroidism, Paget's disease, hyperparathyroidism, sickle cell disease and sarcoidosis is not impressive and is reliant on small series of subjects and anecdotal reports.

There is no convincing evidence that hyperuricemia is by itself an independent risk factor for cardiovascular disease[51,86] although it is associated with an increased relative risk of death from all causes including coronary heart disease, stroke and hepatic disease[52]. It is likely that any association of hyperuricemia with the risk of ischemic heart disease is mediated mainly through the impact of obesity[87]. In any population survey this is compounded by the common prescription of low dose aspirin and diuretics in heart disease. Both drugs may cause hyperuricemia by reducing renal urate clearance. An association of non-diuretic-induced hyperuricemia with both right and left heart failure has been observed but the cause and effect relationships await explanation[88]. There are no benefits from treating asymptomatic hyperuricemia by drugs alone. Incidental reduction of blood uric acid levels consequent on weight reduction and alcohol restriction may be associated with less risk of liver and cardiovascular disease. Hypouricemic drugs do not improve renal impairment which may coincidentally accompany asymptomatic hyperuricemia.

REFERENCES

1. Schlesinger N, Gowin K, Baker DG, Bentler A. Acute gouty arthritic is seasonal. J Rheumatol 1998; 25: 342–344.
2. Gallerani M, Govoni M, Mucinelli M et al. Seasonal variation in the onset of acute microcrystalline arthritis. Rheumatology 1999; 38: 1003–1006.
3. Gibson T, Kilbourn K, Horner I, Simmonds HA. Mechanism and treatment of hypertriglyceridaemia in gout. Ann Rheum Dis 1979; 38: 31–35.
4. Hadler NM, Franck WA, Bress NM, Robinson DR. Acute polyarticular gout. Am J Med 1974; 56: 717–719.
5. Grahame R, Scott JT. Clinical survey of 354 patients with gout. Ann Rheum Dis 1970; 29: 461–468.
6. Dawn B, Williams JK, Walker SE. Prepatellar bursitis: a unique presentation of tophaceous gout in a normouricemic patient. J Rheumatol 1999; 24: 976–978.
7. Ho G, De Nuccio M. Gout and pseudogout in hospitalized patients. Arch Int Med 1993; 153: 2787–9270.
8. Beutler AM, Epstein AL, Policastro D. Acute gouty arthritis involving a prosthetic knee joint. J Clin Rheumatol 2000; 6: 291–293.
9. Helliwell M, Crisp AJ, Grahame R. Co-existent tophaceous gout and systemic lupus erythematosus. Rheum Rehab 1982; 21: 161–163.
10. Veerapen K, Schumacher HR, van Linthoudt D et al. Tophaceous gout in young patients with systemic lupus erythematosus. J Rheumatol 1993; 20: 721–724.
11. Owen DS, Toone E, Irby R. Co-existent rheumatoid arthritis and chronic tophaceous gout. J Am Med Assoc 1966; 197: 953–956.
12. Nakayama DY, Barthelemy C, Carrera G et al. Tophaceous gout: a clinical and radiographic assessment. Arthritis Rheum 1984; 27: 468–470.
13. Kernodle GW, Allen NB. Acute gout presenting in the manubrio-sternal joint. Arthritis Rheum 1986; 29: 570–572.
14. Musgrave DS, Ziran BH. Monarticular acromioclavicular joint gout: a case report. Am J Orthop 2000; 29: 544–547.
15. Sabharwal S, Gibson T. Cervical gout. Br J Rheumatol 1988; 27: 412–413.
16. Nelson C, Haines JD, Harper CA. Gout presenting as a popliteal cyst. A case of pseudothrombophlebitis. Postgrad Med 1987; 82: 73–74.
17. Chen CK, Chung CB, Yeh L et al. Carpal tunnel syndrome caused by tophaceous gout: CT and MR imaging features in 20 patients. Am J Roentgenol 2000; 175: 655–659.
18. St George E, Hillier CE, Hatfield R. Spinal cord compression: an unusual neurological complication of gout. Rheumatology 2001; 40: 712–714.
19. Barett K, Miller ML, Wilson JT. Tophaceous gout of the spine mimicking epidural infection: case report and review of the literature. Neurosurgery 2001; 48: 1170–1173.
20. Varga J, Gianpolo C, Goldenberg DL. Tophaceous gout of the spine in a patient with no peripheral tophi: case report and review of the literature. Arthritis Rheum 1985; 28: 1312–1315.
21. Fam AG, Assaad D. Intradermal urate tophi. J Rheumatol 1997; 24: 1126–1131.
22. Vazquez-Mellado J, Cuan A, Magana M et al. Intradermal tophi in gout: a case-control study. J Rheumatol 1999; 26: 136–140.
23. McCarty DJ. Gout without hyperuricemia. J Am Med Assoc 1994; 271: 302–303.
24. Horowitz M, Abbey L, Sirota DK, Spiera H. Intra-articular non-inflammatory free urate suspension (urate milk) in three patients with painful joints. J Rheumatol 1990; 17: 712–714.
25. Fam AG, Reis MD, Szalai JP. Acute gouty synovitis associated with urate milk. J Rheumatol 1998; 25: 2285–2286.
26. Hamilton ME, Parris TM, Gibson RS, Davis JS. Simultaneous gout and pyarthrosis. Arch Intern Med 1980; 140: 917–919.
27. Pascual E, Batlle-Gualda E, Martinez A et al. Synovial fluid analysis for diagnosis of intercritical gout. Ann Intern Med 1999; 131: 756–759.
28. Schumacher HR, Jimenez SA, Gibson T et al. Acute gouty arthritis without urate crystals identified on initial examination of synovial fluid. Arthritis Rheum 1975; 18: 603–612.
29. Snaith ML, Coomes EN. Gout with normal serum urate concentration. Brit Med J 1977; 1: 685–686.
30. Lin KC, Lin HY, Chou P. The interaction between uric acid level and other risk factors on the development of gout among asymptomatic hyperuricemic men in a prospective study. J Rheumatol 2000; 27: 1501–1505.
31. Warren DJ, Simmonds HA, Gibson T, Naik RB. Familial gout and renal failure. Arch Dis Child 1981; 56: 699–704.
32. Gibson T, Highton J, Potter C, Simmonds HA. Renal impairment and gout. Ann Rheum Dis 1980; 39: 417–423.
33. Barthelemy CR, Nakayama DA, Carrera GF et al. Gouty arthritis: a prospective radiographic evaluation of sixty patients. Skeletal Radiol 1984: 11: 1–8.
34. Popp JD, Bridgood WD, Edwards NL. Magnetic resonance imaging of tophaceous gout in the hands and wrists. Sem Arthritis Rheum 1996; 25: 282–289.

35. Yu JS, Chung C, Recht M *et al*. MR Imaging of tophaceous gout. Am J Roentgenol 1997; 168: 523–527.
36. Yano K, Rhoads GG, Kagan A. Epidemiology of serum uric acid among 8000 Japanese–American men in Hawaii. J Chron Dis 1977; 30: 171–184.
37. Gibson T, Rodgers AV, Simmonds HA, Toseland P. Beer drinking and its effect on uric acid. Br J Rheumatol 1984; 23: 203–209.
38. Gibson T, Rodgers AV, Simmonds HA *et al*. A controlled study of diet in patients with gout. Ann Rheum Dis 1983; 42: 123–127.
39. Garrick R, Bauer GE, Ewan CE, Neale FC. Serum uric acid in normal and hypertensive Australian subjects. Aust NZ J Med 1972; 4: 351–356.
40. Gibson T, Highton J, Simmonds HA, Potter CF. Hypertension, renal function and gout. Postgrad Med J 1979; 55(suppl. 3): 21–25.
41. Gibson T, Waterworth R, Hatfield P *et al*. Hyperuricaemia, gout and kidney function in New Zealand Maori men. Br J Rheumatol 1984; 23: 276–282.
42. Brown J, Mallory GK. Renal changes in gout. N Engl J Med 1950; 243: 325–329.
43. Gibson T, Rodgers V, Potter C, Simmonds HA. Allopurinol treatment and its effect on renal function in gout: a controlled study. Ann Rheum Dis 1982; 41: 59–65.
44. Perez-Ruiz F, Calabozo M, Herrero-Beites AM *et al*. Improvement of renal function in patients with chronic gout after proper control of hyperuricaemia and gouty bouts. Nephron 2000; 86: 287–291.
45. Puig JG, Miranda ME, Mateos FA *et al*. Hereditary nephropathy associated with hyperuricemia and gout. Arch Intern Med 1993; 153: 357–365.
46. Gibson T, Grahame R. Gout and hyperlipidemia. Ann Rheum Dis 1974; 33: 298–303.
47. Dessein PH, Shipton EA, Stanwix AE *et al*. Beneficial effects of weight loss associated with moderate calorie/carbohydrate restriction, and increased proportional intake of protein and unsaturated fat on serum urate and lipoprotein levels in gout: a pilot study. Ann Rheum Dis 2000; 59: 539–543.
48. Darlington LG, Scott JT. Plasma lipid levels in gout. Ann Rheum Dis 1972; 31: 487–489.
49. Berkowitz D. Gout, hyperlipidemia and diabetes inter-relationships. J Am Med Assoc 1966; 197: 117–120.
50. Whitehouse FW, Cleary WJ. Diabetes mellitus in patients with gout. J Am Med Assoc 1966; 197: 113–116.
51. The Coronary Drug Project Research Group. Serum uric acid: its association with other risk factors and with mortality in coronary heart disease. J Chronic Dis 1976; 29: 557–569.
52. Tomita M, Mizuno S, Yamanaka H *et al*. Does hyperuricemia affect mortality? A prospective cohort study of Japanese male workers. J Epidemiol 2000; 10: 403–409.
53. Jinnah HA, De Gregorio L, Harris JC *et al*. The spectrum of inherited mutations causing HPRT deficiency: 75 new cases and a review of 196 previously reported cases. Mut Res 2000; 463: 309–336.
54. Simmonds HA, Webster D, Wilson J, Lingham S. An X-linked syndrome characterised by hyperuricemia, deafness and neurodevelopmental abnormalities. Lancet 1982; 2: 68–70.
55. Becker MA, Mateos FA, Jimenez ML *et al*. Inherited superactivity of phosphoribosyl pyrophosphate synthetase: association of uric acid overproduction and sensorineural deafness. Am J Med 1988; 85: 383–390.
56. Stiburkova B, Majewski J, Sebesta I *et al*. Familial juvenile hyperuricemic nephropathy: localization of the gene on chromosome 16p11.2 and evidence for genetic heterogeneity. Am J Hum Genet 2000; 66: 1989–1994.
57. Kamatani N, Moritani M, Yamanaka H *et al*. Localization of a gene for familial juvenile hyperuricemic nephropathy causing underexcretion-type gout to 16p12 by genome-wide linkage analysis of a large family. Arthritis Rheum 2000; 43: 925–929.
58. Kroiss S, Huck K, Berthold S *et al*. Evidence of further genetic heterogeneity in autosomal dominant medullary cystic kidney disease. Nephrol Dial Transplant 2000; 15: 818–821.
59. DiMauro S, Lamperti C. Muscle glycogenoses. Muscle Nerve 2001; 24: 984–999.
60. Jinnai K, Kono N, Yamamato Y *et al*. Glycogenosis type V (McCardle's disease) with hyperuricemia: report and clinical investigation. Eur Neurol 1993; 33: 204–207.
61. Popert AJ, Hewitt JV. Gout and hyperuricemia in renal and urban populations. Ann Rheum Dis 1962; 21: 154–163.
62. Mikkelsen WM, Dodge HJ, Valkenburg H. The distribution of serum uric acid values in a population unselected as to gout or hyperuricemia. Am J Med 1965; 39: 242–251.
63. Munan L, Kelly A, Petitclerc C. Population serum urate levels and their correlates. The Sherbrooke regional study. Am J Epidemiol 1976; 103: 369–382.
64. Bengtsson C, Tibblin E. Serum uric acid levels in women. Acta Med Scand 1974; 196: 93–102.
65. Lin KC, Lin HY, Chou P. Community based epidemiological study on hyperuricemia and gout in Kn Hu, Kinmen. J Rheumatol 2000; 27: 1045–1050.
66. Kuzell WC, Schaffarzick RW, Naugler WE *et al*. Some observations on 520 gouty patients. J Chron Dis 1955; 2: 645–669.
67. Lally EV, Ho G, Kaplan SR. The clinical spectrum of gouty arthritis in women. Arch Intern Med 1986; 146: 2221–2225.
68. Park YB, Park YS, Song J *et al*. Clinical manifestations of Korean female gouty patients. Clin Rheumatol 2000; 19: 142–146.
69. Macfarlane D, Dieppe PA. Diuretic induced gout in elderly women. Br J Rheumatol 1985; 24: 155–157.
70. Simkin PA, Campbell PM, Larsen EB. Gout in Heberden's nodes. Arthritis Rheum 1983; 26: 94–97.
71. Simkin PA. The pathogenesis of podagra. Ann Intern Med 1977; 86: 230–233.
72. Doherty M, Dieppe PA. Crystal deposition disease in the elderly. Clin Rheum Dis 1986; 12: 97–116.
73. van der Klooster, Peters R, Burgmans JP, Grootendorst AF. Chronic tophaceous gout in the elderly. Neth J Med 1998; 53: 69–75.
74. Fam AG. Gout in the elderly. Clinical presentation and treatment. Drugs and Aging 1998; 13: 229–243.
75. Dieppe PA. Investigation and management of gout in the young and elderly. Ann Rheum Dis 1991; 50: 263–266.
76. Gertler MM, Garn SM, Levine SA. Serum uric acid in relation to age and physique in health and coronary heart disease. Ann Intern Med 1951; 34: 1421–1431.
77. Chou CT, Lai JS. The epidemiology of hyperuricaemia and gout in Taiwan Aborigines. Br J Rheumatol 1998; 37: 258–262.
78. Dunn JP, Brooks GW, Mausner J *et al*. Social class gradient of serum uric acid levels in males. J Am Med Assoc 1963; 185: 431–436.
79. Rigby A, Wood PH. Serum uric acid levels and gout: what does this herald for the population? Clin Exp Rheumatol 1994; 12: 395–400.
80. Fessel WJ, Siegelaub AB, Johnson ES. Correlates and consequences of asymptomatic hyperuricemia. Arch Intern Med 1973; 132: 44–54.
81. Campion EW, Glynn RJ, DeLabry LO. Asymptomatic hyperuricemia: risks and consequences in the normative aging study. Am J Med 1987; 82: 421–426.
82. Smyth CJ. Disorders associated with hyperuricemia. Arthritis Rheum 1975; 18: 713–719.
83. Goldman M. Uric acid in the etiology of psoriasis. Am J Dermatopathol 1981; 3: 397–404.
84. Scott JT, Stodell MA. Serum uric acid levels in psoriasis. Adv Exp Med Biol 1984; 165: 283–285.
85. Lambert JR, Wright V. Serum uric acid levels in psoriatic arthritis. Ann Rheum Dis 1977; 264–267.
86. Myers AR, Epstein FH, Dodge HJ, Mikkelsen WM. The relationship of serum uric acid to risk factors in coronary heart disease. Am J Med 1968; 45: 520–528.
87. Klein R, Klein BE, Cornoni JC *et al*. Serum uric acid. Its relationship to coronary heart disease risk factors and cardiovascular disease, Evans County, Georgia. Arch Intern Med 1973; 132: 401–410.
88. Hoeper MM, Hohlfeld JM, Fabel H. Hyperuricaemia in patients with right or left heart failure. Eur Respir J 1999; 13: 682–685.

CRYSTAL-RELATED ARTHROPATHIES

42

The management of gout

Bryan T Emmerson

Principal goals of treatment

- Treating acute attacks early and effectively
- In some cases, correcting hyperuricemia either by determining a correctable cause or by using drugs

Acute gout

- Choose either non-steroidal anti-inflammatory agents (NSAIDs), colchicine or corticosteroids
- Use colchicine prophylaxis between attacks

Prevention and correction of hyperuricemia

- Seek and correct factors contributing to hyperuricemia, e.g. regular alcohol, high purine intake, obesity, diuretic therapy, suboptimal urine flow, hypertension, or
- Use a urate lowering drug regularly and permanently.

Therapy in gout is directed primarily towards the treatment of acute attacks and secondarily towards the correction of the hyperuricemia, which is the basic cause of these attacks (Fig. 42.1). Treatment should also aim to reverse any complications that may have arisen and attention should also be given to any concomitant or etiologically related conditions such as renal impairment, hypertension or factors promoting vascular disease.

When considering therapy for gout, it is important to distinguish clearly between therapy for reducing inflammation in acute gout and that for managing hyperuricemia. Rarely does any agent offer clinically useful control of both factors. Indeed, the inappropriate use of anti-hyperuricemic agents during acute gout can cause severe exacerbations of the joint inflammation. An outline of the general principles used in the management of gouty arthritis is given in Table 42.1.

ACUTE GOUT

The management of the acute attack of gout is the same, whatever its underlying cause. There are three effective treatments, the particular

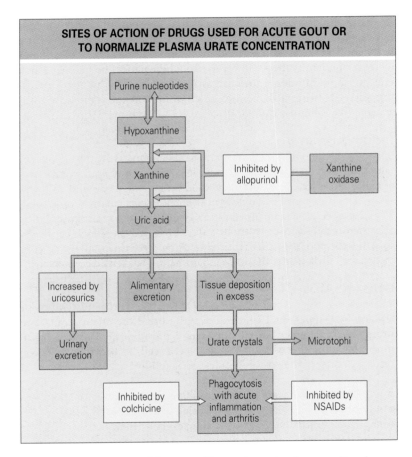

Fig. 42.1 Sites of action of drugs used for acute gout or to normalize plasma urate concentration.

choice depending upon what other diseases are affecting the patient or to which the patient is predisposed. These are colchicine[1,2], non-steroidal anti-inflammatory drugs (NSAIDs)[3,4] and corticosteroids. NSAIDs are superior to colchicine in terms of speed of onset of action but are relatively contraindicated in some patients, particularly those with renal insufficiency, hypertension, peptic ulceration or congestive heart failure. Despite having been used for centuries, colchicine is now usually reserved for those patients in whom NSAIDs are contraindicated. Corticosteroids, often administered as an intra-articular injection, are usually effective and, indeed, joint aspiration alone will often ease the pain. Oral corticosteroids may be chosen if colchicine or NSAIDs are not desired, and parenteral corticosteroids may be used if the gastro-intestinal route is not feasible. Whichever drug is chosen in acute gout, the earlier the therapy is instituted the quicker the resolution of the attack. Patients who have had previous attacks of gout should be advised, and soon learn, to have therapy readily available and to take it at the first indication of an attack. Taken so early, only one or two doses may be sufficient to abort an attack of gout.

TABLE 42.1 GENERAL APPROACHES TO THE MANAGEMENT OF GOUT	
Acute gout	Nonsteroidal anti-inflammatory drugs Colchicine Corticosteroids Do not attempt to modify plasma urate concentrations
Recurrent gout or chronic gout	Reverse factors promoting hyperuricemia Maintain urine output . 1400ml/day When asymptomatic, add agent to lower plasma urate concentration (e.g. probenecid or allopurinol) Continue prophylactic doses of colchicine for at least 12 months after normalization of the plasma urate concentration

Among the various NSAIDs, indomethacin has been the most widely used but most other NSAIDs, if they are used in appropriate doses, have been shown to be effective in the treatment of an acute attack of gout[5]. The newer COX-2 selective inhibitors, celecoxib and rofecoxib, have not yet been assessed in the management of an intense inflammatory arthritis such as occurs in gout, but it is likely that they would be effective if given in appropriate anti-inflammatory dosage[6].

Numerous regimens exist for the use of these drugs in the acute attack and these recommendations provide a guide which may be altered depending upon the severity of the attack and the response to therapy. Nonetheless, it must be noted that the commonest cause of difficulty in controlling an attack is the simultaneous administration (or withdrawal) of drugs that alter the plasma urate concentration. Both increases and decreases in the plasma urate concentration may precipitate or prolong an attack of gout. Therefore, therapy aimed at reducing urate concentrations should be delayed until the complete resolution of all signs of inflammation. However, should the patient be stabilized on a constant dose of a urate-lowering drug at the time of an acute attack, the urate-lowering drug should be continued at the same dose until specific treatment has caused the acute gout to subside.

Indomethacin

Patients will often notice that the pain has begun to ease within 2 hours of taking the first dose. Generally, 50mg four times a day is an average and effective dose schedule, although mild attacks may respond to lower doses. This dose may be doubled with benefit in particularly severe cases[7]. The dose should be maintained for 2 days or until the severe pain settles, and then reduced to three times a day. Provided the attack continues to settle, the dose is further reduced to 25mg three times a day and continued for 1–2 days after the acute inflammation has settled completely.

Other NSAIDs

The doses of the several other NSAIDs used to treat gout tend to be towards the upper limit of, or above, the usual therapeutic range. In most cases, a higher initial dose has been advocated and, as with indomethacin, the dose is generally reduced as the inflammation resolves. Some of the dose schedules are as follows:

- ibuprofen 800mg every 8 hours reducing to 400mg every 6 hours[8]
- diclofenac 50mg every 8 hours reducing to 25mg every 8 hours
- naproxen 750mg initially, then 250mg every 8 hours
- piroxicam 40mg daily for 5 days[9]
- sulindac 200mg initially, then 100mg every 6 hours[10].

Several of the NSAIDs available in suppository or injectable form may be useful in patients unable to take oral medications.

Corticosteroids

Intra-articular administration of corticosteroids is a particularly effective means of terminating an attack of gout[11]. Resolution is typically complete within 12–24 hours. This form of treatment is of particular value in some patients with monoarticular gout associated with renal impairment and other conditions where the use of full doses of other drugs may be relatively contraindicated. A good response without rebound has been reported with either oral prednisone 30–50mg/day tapering over 7–9 days, with intramuscular adrenocorticotropic hormone (ACTH) (40IU)[12] or triamcinolone acetonide (60mg)[13] or betamethasone (7mg), or with intravenous methylprednisolone (125mg)[14].

Colchicine

Colchicine is an alkaloid derived from the autumn crocus, *Colchicum autumnale*. It has an anti-inflammatory action in acute attacks of gout and a prophylactic effect against recurrent attacks. It has no effect on the serum urate concentration or on urate metabolism[15].

TABLE 42.2 MECHANISMS OF ACTION OF COLCHICINE

- Inhibits phagocytosis by the formation of a tubulin–colchicine dimer which caps the assembly ends of the microtubules
- Alters the motility and adhesion of the neutrophil leukocyte by an effect on the membrane
- Reduces the release of the eicosanoids PGE_2 and LTB_4 by monocytes and neutrophil leukocytes by inhibiting phospholipase A_2
- Affects chemotaxis

The effect of colchicine is principally mediated by changes to the neutrophil leukocyte population. Its effects on this cell are multiple and there is controversy as to which effect is the dominant one determining its effectiveness in the treatment of gout[16]. However, by a combination of these mechanisms, colchicine interrupts the inflammatory response to the tissue deposition of urate crystals (Table 42.2).

Pharmacokinetics

Because of its lipid solubility, colchicine rapidly passes into all tissues of the body. After intravenous (i.v.) administration, it has a half-life in plasma of less than 1 hour and is distributed throughout a volume greater than the extracellular water. After oral administration, it is absorbed through the upper small bowel, has a peak plasma concentration in 1–2 hours[17] and a half-life of about 4 hours. It is not bound to plasma protein and does not displace protein-bound drugs. However the drug persists in leukocytes, where it may be detected for up to 10 days following administration. It also appears to be concentrated in the liver, kidney, spleen and intestine. It is extensively metabolized within the liver and is excreted principally in the bile and intestinal secretions. There may be some enterohepatic recirculation. A total of 20% is excreted unchanged in the urine, so that, during chronic administration, the dose should be reduced in the presence of pre-existing renal disease. Traces of the drug can still be found in the urine 10 days after its last administration.

Dosage

Colchicine is usually available in 0.5mg tablets and is most effective in acute gouty arthritis if given early in the acute attack. The therapeutic dose, however, is close to the toxic dose, so that when given orally the dose needs to be graduated to the individual response. The initial dose is usually given as 1mg, with 0.5mg being repeated every 2 hours until the patient develops diarrhea or vomiting, the gout begins to settle or the maximum dose is reached. This maximum dose can range up to 6mg, and caution and close supervision need to be exercised in the use of doses larger than this. Acute gouty arthritis usually subsides within 24 hours of administration of an effective dose of colchicine. The tablets are sensitive to light and may deteriorate.

In some countries, an intravenous preparation is available. If so, it can be given in a dose of 1–2mg initially, with a further 1mg dose in 6 hours if there has been no relief. However, the total dose should not exceed 4mg and this should be reduced in the presence of hepatic or renal disease, in an older patient or if there has been previous dosing with colchicine[18]. The intravenous route has fewer gastrointestinal side effects but it may take 6 hours to be fully effective and the potential for serious systemic toxicity is much greater than by the oral route, particularly in patients with renal insufficiency, volume depletion and underlying cytopenia. It should be administered by intravenous line, well diluted with considerable care to avoid extravasation.

Colchicine is often thought to be specific for gout, and certainly three-quarters of patients with uncomplicated acute gout will respond to a course of colchicine. However, it is not completely specific to gout and will also cause subsidence of sarcoid and psoriatic arthritis and some crystal arthropathies due to hydroxyapatite or pyrophosphate crystals.

Adverse reactions

Most of the adverse effects of colchicine are dose-related and will disappear if a sufficiently low dose is taken. The principal adverse effects are gastrointestinal and usually consist of diarrhea or vomiting. Prolonged high dosage can lead to a malabsorption syndrome and, if sufficiently severe, a hemorrhagic gastroenteritis. Although it is recognized to have an antimitotic effect, bone marrow suppression has been extremely rare. Ovarian and testicular function have generally remained normal during prolonged prophylactic treatment.

More importantly, however, a myoneuropathy has been reported in some patients taking a prophylactic dose of colchicine who were suffering from minor degrees of renal insufficiency[19,20]. Most of these patients presented with proximal muscle weakness or showed elevation of the serum creatine kinase concentrations. An axonal polyneuropathy could be demonstrated, together with disruption of the cytoskeleton in the muscle cells. This report suggests that the prophylactic dose should not exceed 0.5mg per day in the presence of renal insufficiency[21]. Poisoning from colchicine, usually with suicidal intent, causes severe damage to most tissues and presents clinically with severe diarrhea and vomiting with dehydration, hyponatremia, shock and disseminated intravascular coagulation. It has been treated successfully with colchicine-specific Fab fragments[22] but these are not readily available.

Drug prophylaxis of acute gout

Whatever the serum urate concentration, acute attacks of gout may be inhibited by small regular doses of either colchicine or NSAID. Such drug prophylaxis is particularly important because of the increased risk of acute attacks of gout both prior to and during the introduction of urate-lowering drugs and other therapy designed to correct hyperuricemia, at which time there may be considerable fluctuations in the serum urate concentration. Colchicine prophylaxis was totally effective in 82% of such patients and satisfactory in a further 12%[23].

The prophylactic dose of colchicine is usually 0.5mg twice a day but some patients will tolerate only 0.5mg once daily. The prophylactic dose should be adjusted so as not to produce any gastrointestinal symptoms and it should be continued until the patient has been normouricemic and has had no attacks of gout for 1–2 years[23]. The lowest dose should be used in the presence of hepatic or renal disease.

Practical prescribing tips

- Colchicine prophylaxis is of special value in patients with recurrent attacks of gout in whom acute attacks are precipitated by drugs or procedures to normalize the plasma urate concentration.
- Colchicine prophylaxis should be continued until the patient has had no symptoms of gout for about 12 months and the serum urate concentration has remained normal for that time.
- An acute attack of gout in a patient on prophylactic colchicine is usually best treated with an NSAID, although there is no specific reason why a course of oral colchicine should not be used if not contraindicated.
- No controlled comparison between the prophylactic efficacy of low doses of colchicine and NSAID has been carried out. However, their side-effect profile would suggest that colchicine is the preferable agent and should be used on a regular basis, with NSAID being added if colchicine alone is inadequate[24].
- The prophylactic use of these drugs over many years should be undertaken in association with measures to optimize urate concentrations.

TABLE 42.3 CORRECTABLE FACTORS CONTRIBUTING TO HYPERURICEMIA

- Obesity
- Hypertriglyceridemia
- Regular alcohol consumption
- Diuretic therapy
- Inadequately controlled hypertension
- High dietary purine consumption
- Suboptimal urine flow (<1ml/min)

CORRECTION OF THE CAUSES OF HYPERURICEMIA

Prevention of gout is directed at restoring the plasma urate concentration to normal (Fig. 42.1). Many factors contributing to an elevation of the urate concentration have been recognized and a number of these factors can be identified in individual patients with gout. In addition, some of these may be correctable leading to a fall in the serum urate level[25]. Sometimes the resultant plasma urate concentration may be sufficiently low that it is no longer associated with gout. Thus, long-term drug treatment may be avoided and other complications secondary to these contributing factors may not occur (Table 42.3).

Factors already identified as contributing to hyperuricemia include the syndrome of obesity, hypertriglyceridemia, hypertension and insulin resistance, which is an increasing public health and nutritional problem in western societies[26]. Correction of obesity can cause a remission of hyperuricemia[27,28] and even a moderate loss of weight can facilitate the renal excretion of urate. However, the necessary changes in lifestyle and diet are rarely maintained long term, although increasing community recognition of the need to maintain a healthy lifestyle may help this in the future. In addition, diuretic therapy or inadequately treated hypertension will contribute to hyperuricemia[29,30].

A high purine intake will also contribute. Whereas high purine foods are well-recognized contributors, it is less commonly appreciated that a large helping of a food with a medium concentration of purines may provide a much larger purine load than a small helping of a food high in purines. A low purine diet is not a practical solution in the management of hyperuricemia, but rather that moderation of purine intake and avoidance of high purine foods is desirable in most patients with gout, particularly if there is any difficulty in achieving a normal plasma urate. A urine flow rate of less than 1ml/min is also suboptimal for renal elimination of urate[31].

Dietary restriction of purines rarely causes a fall in the plasma urate concentration of more than 1.0mg/dl (0.06mmol/l) unless the diet has had a large purine content. Moreover, such dietary restriction can rarely be sustained for long and is only occasionally clinically useful.

In contrast, alcohol restriction can have a much greater effect on the plasma urate concentration, depending upon the amount previously consumed[32]. Consequently, permanent modification of excessive alcohol consumption should contribute significantly to lowering the plasma urate concentration. Maintaining a urine volume of at least 1400ml/day will also facilitate urate excretion, although this will in itself have only a small impact on plasma urate concentrations.

Effective management of gout requires the patient to understand the nature of his underlying disease and the factors which contribute to it. Such an education needs to be provided by the physician and reinforced by printed material providing a guide to management and prevention[33].

CORRECTION OF HYPERURICEMIA BY DRUG THERAPY

The decision to introduce drugs to normalize hyperuricemia depends in part on the number of previous attacks of acute gout, the degree of hyperuricemia, the presence of reversible factors and the presence of tophi. Urate-lowering drugs will not normally be used after only a single attack of gout but should be considered after the second or third attacks. They should always be used for tophaceous gout. The patient needs to be aware that the decision to commence antihyperuricemic therapy usually implies life-long treatment and the patient, as well as the physician, needs to be committed to this policy.

The goal should be a sustained level of plasma urate of less than 6mg/dl (0.36mmol/l). Lower levels are necessary for the resorption of tophi[34]. This can occur from their surface when an adequately reduced plasma urate concentration [desirably below 5mg/dl (0.30mmol/l)] is maintained for many years. Once a satisfactory urate level is achieved, regular monitoring is desirable to ensure it continues to be maintained.

Antihyperuricemic drugs must not be commenced until an acute attack of gout has settled completely, since this may delay subsidence of the inflammation. In addition, prophylactic doses of colchicine (usually 0.5mg twice daily) should be administered concomitantly to minimize the risk of inducing an attack of acute gout.

Choice of drug

Drugs to correct hyperuricemia act either by promoting the renal excretion of urate (uricosuric agents) or by decreasing urate production by inhibiting xanthine oxidase (allopurinol) (Table 42.4). Although it would be logical to use a uricosuric agent when there is primary urate underexcretion and a xanthine oxidase inhibitor when there is urate overproduction, many patients show features of both overproduction and underexcretion of urate. Thus, the choice between uricosuric agents and allopurinol for an individual with hyperuricemia will depend more upon associated diseases. A uricosuric would be less favored if there had been a history of renal colic or there was coexistent renal disease (creatinine clearance less than 60ml/min), whereas allopurinol would be less favored if there was a history of drug sensitivity. Similarly, a high urine urate excretion would favor the use of allopurinol and a low urinary urate excretion would favor the use of a uricosuric agent (Table 42.5).

Uricosuric agents

A uricosuric agent is one which lowers the serum urate concentration by increasing the excretion of uric acid by the kidney (Fig. 42.2). This will be associated with an increase in the uric acid concentration in the urine

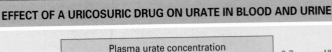

EFFECT OF A URICOSURIC DRUG ON URATE IN BLOOD AND URINE

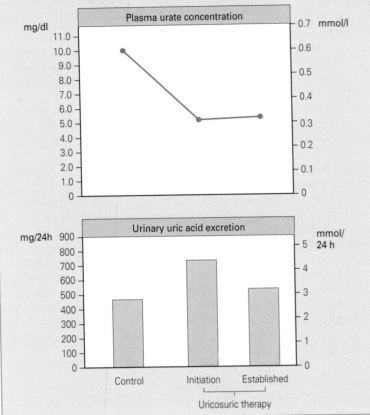

Fig. 42.2 Effect of a uricosuric drug on urate in blood and urine.

unless there is a corresponding increase in the urine flow rate. The tendency for uric acid crystal formation would also be reduced by alkalinization of the urine. Like uric acid, most uricosuric agents are weak organic acids.

Pharmacokinetics and pharmacodynamics

Aspirin or salicylate in high dosage (5g/24h) is uricosuric, whereas low dosage (1–2g/24h) may retain urate. The uricosuric effect depends upon the concentration of salicylate in the tubular fluid, which can be increased by alkalinization of the urine. Thus, a daily dose of 5g of aspirin and 5g of sodium bicarbonate functions as an effective uricosuric agent. However, such doses are not a practical option for long-term therapy. Diflunisal is a fluorinated salicylate which retains the uricosuric effect, and which can usefully lower the serum urate concentration during long-term therapy[35]. Azapropazone is another NSAID with a uricosuric action that can result in modest serum urate-lowering effects[36].

Probenecid was the first modern drug able to produce lowering of the serum urate by a uricosuric action[37]. The drug is well absorbed from the gastrointestinal tract and has a half-life of 6–12 hours, the actual value being dose dependent. It is moderately protein bound (90%) and is thus confined to extracellular fluid. Its metabolism is rapid, with its major metabolite being an acylmonoglucuronide, in which form 40% of the drug is excreted within 48 hours[38]. There are several other active metabolites. Availability of particular uricosuric drugs may vary from country to country.

Sulfinpyrazone, a derivative of phenylbutazone, is a more potent uricosuric agent. It is rapidly absorbed, reaching a peak within an hour and is strongly (98%) bound to plasma proteins. Its metabolites are also actively uricosuric and are rapidly excreted with 20–40% of the drug being excreted unchanged within 24 hours[39].

TABLE 42.4 DRUG MECHANISMS TO NORMALIZE HYPERURICEMIA
Uricosuric drugs
Facilitate urate excretion by the kidney with an increase in the urate clearance and the fractional excretion of filtered urate. Especially useful in urate underexcretion.
Xanthine oxidase inhibiting drugs
Reduce urate production by inhibiting the final enzyme in its pathway. Especially useful in patients with urate overproduction, both primary and secondary.

TABLE 42.5 INDICATIONS FOR ALLOPURINOL WHEN AN ANTIHYPERURICEMIC AGENT IS REQUIRED
Urate overproduction, primary or secondary
Acute uric acid nephropathy
— tumor lysis syndrome
Nephrolithiasis of any type
Renal impairment (dose 100mg/day per 30ml/min glomerular filtration rate)
Low urine volume
24 hour urinary uric acid > 0.42g (2.5mmol) (an arbitrary value on a low purine diet)
Intolerance or allergy to uricosuric agents

Benzbromarone is also an active uricosuric agent. It is not as readily available as probenecid or sulfinpyrazone and has no special benefit except its potency.

Indications and clinical use

Uricosuric drugs are indicated to correct hyperuricemia and gout when there is defective renal excretion of urate and the patient is persuaded that long-term drug therapy is necessary. These drugs are contraindicated if there is a history of renal calculi or if there is a poor urine volume (< 1ml/min). They are relatively ineffective in the presence of renal disease with a glomerular filtration rate (GFR) of less than 60ml/min.

Initial doses should be small with gradual increments to minimize side effects, particularly any potential adverse effects from the increased urinary concentration of uric acid which results. Because of the increased amount of uric acid excreted in the urine during the first few weeks of treatment or after a dose increment, the urine should be alkalinized during this time to minimize the risk of uric acid crystal deposition in the renal tubules and collecting ducts of the kidney. When drug dosage is stable, the alkalinization could be stopped but a good urine volume (always greater than 1500ml/day) should be maintained permanently.

Probenecid in a dose of 1–3g/day in two to three divided doses is usually well tolerated. The starting dose should not be greater than 0.5g/day in order to minimize the risk of a flare-up of acute gout. The usual dose is 0.5g two or three times a day.

Sulfinpyrazone is three to six times as potent as probenecid on a weight for weight basis and more effective than probenecid in patients with renal disease. The initial dose should be 50mg twice a day, increasing to 100mg, then 200mg twice daily. Occasionally, up to 800mg/day may be used.

Efficacy and variability in response

The ultimate effectiveness of these drugs is judged by the degree of fall in the serum urate concentration. This may be affected by many other non-drug factors such as alcohol consumption, diet and hypertension. Despite this, up to 75% of patients receiving 1.5g probenecid daily will develop a serum urate of less than 6.7mg/dl (0.4mmol/l). If the initial fall in the serum urate is inadequate, the dose should be increased to the maximum but should not be increased beyond this until all other factors promoting hyperuricemia have been corrected. The uricosuric response is reduced when there is any impairment of glomerular function.

Adverse reactions

Probenecid blocks the tubular excretion of salicylate, the penicillins and some other uricosuric agents. Its uricosuric effect is blocked by concomitant administration of salicylate. It has numerous effects upon membrane transport, particularly within the kidney. It increases the serum furosemide concentration and augments its diuretic effect[40]. It reduces the renal excretion of indomethacin[41] and dapsone, and prolongs the metabolism of heparin. It is still used to prolong the effects of many other drugs excreted by the kidney, particularly the penicillins and zidovudine.

Fluctuations in the serum urate concentration, whether resulting in an increase or a reduction in the concentration, will often induce a flare-up of an acute attack of gout. Thus, any drug treatment which lowers the serum urate may precipitate an acute attack of gout. This is minimized by starting with a low dose and increasing to full dosage very gradually. Probenecid can cause upper gastrointestinal side effects in 3–8% of patients and a hypersensitivity rash in 2–5% of patients. Nonetheless, serious side effects are rare and the drug is acceptable in 95% of patients.

An important potential complication from all uricosuric agents is uric acid crystalluria in either the renal tubules or the urinary tract. This is a particular risk in the early stages of uricosuric treatment when the urinary urate concentration is high[42]. During this time it is important to alkalinize the urine and keep the urine dilute by means of water diuresis. Once the initial uricosuria has passed and the serum urate has fallen, the increase in urinary urate excretion will be relatively small and the risk of urate crystal formation within the renal tract reduced (see Fig. 42.2).

Sulfinpyrazone is also well tolerated and, although its uricosuric effect is also neutralized by concurrent salicylates, it has an additional specific effect of reducing platelet adhesiveness. It also prolongs platelet survival and reduces the tendency to thrombosis in arteriovenous (AV) shunts and mechanical intravascular devices.

Practical prescribing tips

When instituting uricosuric therapy it is important to:

- use concurrent colchicine prophylaxis (0.5mg once or twice daily)
- use an initial low dose and increase the dose gradually to an effective level over several weeks
- maintain an alkaline diuresis by water loading and the addition of oral sodium bicarbonate 0.5g four times a day (or more) to achieve an alkaline urine
- not use uricosuric agents in patients whose urine volume is less than 1400ml/24h
- ensure the patient always maintains a good urine volume whenever uricosuric agents are being taken. This must be continued even through hot weather when the urine volume may fall despite the maintenance of a usually adequate fluid intake.

The biggest problem in any therapy to lower the serum urate in a gouty patient is the patient's realization that the treatment must be continued even throughout the asymptomatic years. To achieve this it is important that urate-lowering therapy is not started too early, that is before the patient is persuaded of the need to take life-long therapy. If a uricosuric agent is to be used to lower the serum urate concentration in a patient with significant renal disease, the most potent uricosuric agent will probably be needed.

Allopurinol

Allopurinol, a hydroxypyrazolopyrimidine, is an isomer of hypoxanthine which lowers the urate concentration by inhibition of xanthine

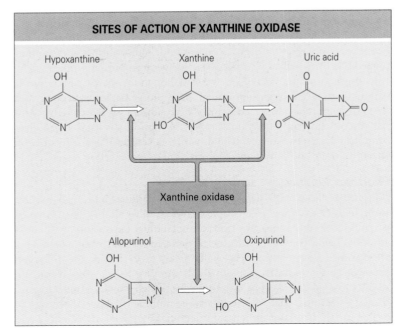

Fig. 42.3 Sites of action of xanthine oxidase.

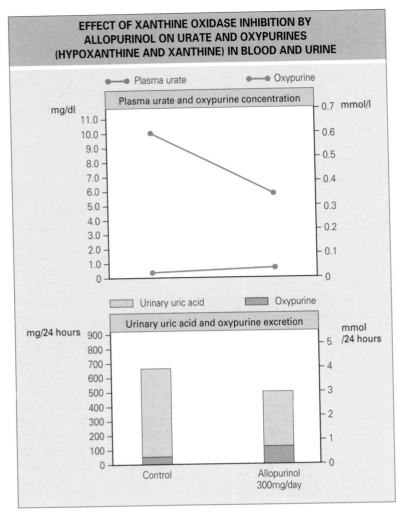

Fig. 42.4 **Effect of xanthine oxidase inhibition by allopurinol on urate and oxypurines (hypoxanthine and xanthine) in blood and urine.**

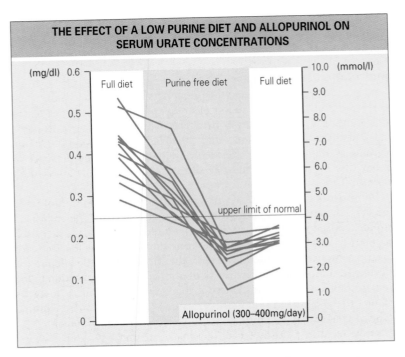

Fig. 42.5 **The effect of a low purine diet and allopurinol on serum urate concentrations.** There is a consistent but usually small fall in serum urate concentrations with low purine diet alone. The addition of allopurinol reliably normalizes the serum urate concentrations an effect which is largely maintained when the patients return to a full diet. (Adapted from Emmerson BT. Aust Ann Med 1969; 16: 205–214.)

oxidase (Fig. 42.3). It reduces the concentration of urate in blood and urine and increases the concentration of the urate precursors xanthine and hypoxanthine[43] (see Fig. 42.4). Except in patients with hypoxanthine phosphoribosyltransferase (HGPRT) enzyme deficiency, allopurinol also reduces total purine production. This is probably because allopurinol utilizes the high energy phosphate compound, phosphoribosyl pyrophosphate (PRPP), which is also necessary for *de novo* purine synthesis. This reaction requires the HGPRT enzyme. Although the increased amount of xanthine produced is less soluble than urate, problems do not arise because the purine excretion is spread among three substances, which reduces the risk of crystallization of any one of these. Allopurinol is itself metabolized by xanthine oxidase to oxypurinol, which is responsible for most of its effects on urate and purine metabolism.

Pharmacokinetics

Allopurinol has a short half-life of about 40 minutes, although this can sometimes be extended to a couple of hours. Most allopurinol, however, is rapidly converted into its principal metabolite, oxypurinol, with small amounts being converted into the ribonucleoside and ribonucleotide of allopurinol. Oxypurinol has a half-life of 14–28 hours and is largely excreted by the kidney, although small amounts are converted into the ribonucleoside. It is oxypurinol, therefore, which is principally responsible for the clinical effect of inhibition of xanthine oxidase. Allopurinol is well absorbed from the alimentary tract but oxypurinol in ordinary tablet form is poorly absorbed, which is why oxypurinol is not a useful therapeutic agent. However, a rapid release preparation of oxypurinol sodium

is available in some countries and appears to be clinically effective[44]. It is noteworthy that uricosuric drugs increase the excretion of oxypurinol whereas renal insufficiency reduces the excretion of oxypurinol. Both allopurinol and oxypurinol are distributed throughout body water and neither is significantly bound to the plasma protein.

Pharmacodynamics

Allopurinol and its metabolite oxypurinol are responsible for the fall in the concentration of urate in serum and urine (Fig. 42.5). The maximum effect is seen between 4–14 days and results in a stable fall of the serum urate. These two compounds deplete cells of PRPP, which is most readily observed with red cell PRPP concentrations. The increased concentrations of hypoxanthine and xanthine in serum and urine rarely cause problems because they are usually well below their solubility limits. After the drug is withdrawn, its effect on urate metabolism mostly disappears in 3–4 days, although some of the more complex metabolic effects may last considerably longer. The concentration of oxypurinol needed to completely inhibit xanthine oxidase activity is well within the therapeutic range usually achieved in clinical practice[45].

Interactions

The main interaction is with 6-mercaptopurine and azathioprine, or with any other drug whose oxidation is inhibited by allopurinol. Their co-administration with allopurinol greatly potentiates all their effects, both beneficial and toxic, and necessitates a reduction in their dose to 25% of normal. The co-administration of ampicillin with allopurinol results in a three-fold increase in the risk of a skin rash. Allopurinol also potentiates the toxic effects of cyclophosphamide, although the mechanism is not clear. It also inhibits several hepatic drug metabolizing enzymes but there is little resultant implication for therapy.

Dosage

Allopurinol is available in 100mg and 300mg tablets. The requisite dose needs to be given once daily and should be adjusted to bring the serum urate concentration to less than 6.0mg/dl (0.36mmol/l). Usually, 300mg per day will be necessary to achieve this, but occasionally 200mg, 400mg or even 600mg per day may be needed. However, should a dose of 400mg not restore the serum urate to this level, it is wise to seek and correct additional factors promoting the hyperuricemia rather than increase the dose further. Since oxypurinol is excreted principally by the kidney, the dose should be reduced in the presence of renal insufficiency. Whereas the dose might be 300mg per day for a GFR or creatinine clearance of 100ml/minute, the dose should be reduced to 200mg/day when the creatinine clearance is 50–60ml/min and to 100mg per day when the GFR is 20–30ml/min[46].

Indications

Allopurinol is immediately indicated in the presence of urate overproduction, either of endogenous origin or of dietary origin, or because of increased marrow cell turnover due to myeloproliferative disorders (so-called secondary gout). It is also used prophylactically against the tumor lysis syndrome when a large initial loading dose should be used to produce a rapid effect. It is effective in HGPRT deficiency and in other varieties of acute uric acid nephropathy. It is also of special value in the presence of renal calculi, either of uric acid or of calcium oxalate[47].

When given in combination with uricosuric agents, such as probenecid, allopurinol prolongs the half-life of the uricosuric agent and the uricosuric agent promotes excretion of oxypurinol, thereby reducing the inhibitory effect on xanthine oxidase. It is therefore better to avoid the simultaneous use of uricosuric agents and allopurinol if possible.

Variability in response and efficacy

There appears to be a moderate degree of variability in the effect of a 300mg dose of allopurinol on the serum urate in different individuals. However, some of this variability may be due to differences of body size and metabolism. Plasma oxypurinol concentrations are of considerable value when patients remain hyperuricemic despite the usual doses of allopurinol. Plasma oxypurinol concentrations between 0.46–1.52mg/dl (30–100μmol/l) are usually effective in maintaining a normal serum urate concentration[46]. However, these readily increase in renal insufficiency unless the dose of allopurinol is reduced in proportion to renal function. Because of inhibition of xanthine oxidase, plasma xanthine concentrations rise significantly, which provides an index of the metabolic effect.

Adverse reactions

Up to 5% of patients are unable to tolerate allopurinol because of adverse reactions. Minor gastrointestinal intolerance is common but can usually be minimized by administering the tablets with food. The major adverse effect is a sensitivity reaction which may range from an erythematous skin rash through to a life-endangering illness which requires corticosteroid therapy. Most commonly it is seen after 3 weeks of therapy. If the reaction is confined to the skin, the rash usually settles after withdrawal of the allopurinol, but may require local or systemic steroids. The more serious allopurinol hypersensitivity reaction involves fever and rash with systemic features of eosinophilia, acute interstitial nephritis[48] (including renal insufficiency) and hepatitis. The severity ranges through an acute interstitial nephritis to a Stevens-Johnson syndrome, to a toxic epidermal necrolysis requiring prolonged steroid therapy and intensive care. There is a 25% mortality. The risk of allopurinol hypersensitivity increases considerably in the presence of renal insufficiency and sometimes appears to be related to the use of higher doses of allopurinol than are indicated. It is therefore important that the dose of allopurinol be lowered in proportion to the GFR and that the three-fold increased risk of sensitivity in the presence of renal insufficiency be avoided.

In some of the less severe cases where the only manifestation of allopurinol sensitivity is cutaneous, slow oral desensitization has been pos-

sible with doses of allopurinol beginning at 50μg and increasing very gradually over a 4 week period to 100 mg/day or sometimes more[49, 50, 51]. In a recent study[52], over 70% of such patients were able to continue to take allopurinol, although sometimes late adjustment of the dose was needed. Even relatively small doses of allopurinol may be very effective in controlling hyperuricemia in some patients with gout and renal disease who do not respond to uricosurics. There is some evidence that the lymphocyte response in these patients is a reaction to oxypurinol rather than to allopurinol itself[53, 54].

Practical prescribing tips

- Allopurinol therapy should be initiated only after the acute attack of gout has entirely resolved. Administration to a patient with subsiding gout can cause severe exacerbation of the gout.
- It is wise to increase the dose of allopurinol slowly so that the full proposed dosage is reached only after 2–4 weeks. This considerably minimizes the risk of an acute exacerbation of gout.
- Concurrent colchicine prophylaxis (0.5mg twice daily) is also of value in preventing acute flare-ups during the institution of urate-lowering therapy. The dose should be adjusted in the presence of renal insufficiency in proportion.
- If no adequate fall occurs in the serum urate concentration, seek an alternative factor which might be maintaining the hyperuricemia. If none can be found and if the patient is still hyperuricemic despite an apparently adequate dose of allopurinol, it would be wise to measure plasma oxypurinol concentrations[46].

Hyperuricemia not responding to drugs

Associated conditions such as renal insufficiency, hypertension, abdominal obesity, hyperlipidemia and regular increased alcohol intake are commonly seen in patients with gout. Each of these conditions needs to be managed at the same time as the hyperuricemia and together they are often more threatening to longevity. In occasional patients, full dosage of allopurinol (300–400mg/day) will not cause the urate concentration to be reduced sufficiently and, in such a case, another factor (e.g. regular alcohol consumption or diuretic therapy) is usually operating[55]. Rarely, patients may need to be treated with the combination of a uricosuric drug and a xanthine oxidase inhibitor but this should be avoided if at all possible because the uricosuric agents alter the pharmacokinetics of oxypurinol. Another uncommon situation is the patient who has a history of renal calculi as well as being intolerant of allopurinol. If urate-lowering therapy is required in such a patient, a uricosuric agent may be cautiously begun with strict attention to maintaining an alkaline urine and a high urine volume. In extreme situations other therapy, including parenteral uricase, may be considered[56].

Asymptomatic hyperuricemia

Whereas the treatment of hyperuricemia is certainly of value in patients with recurrent attacks of gout, there is currently no evidence of benefit to be obtained from treating sustained asymptomatic hyperuricemia unless this is severe [urate > 12mg/dl (0.7mmol/l)] or in situations where there may be acute urate overproduction (as with tumor lysis). Although, as documented earlier, hyperuricemia is associated with a significant risk for the development of gout and a smaller risk of nephrolithiasis and possible renal impairment, it is usually many years between the detection or the development of hyperuricemia and the presentation of any of these problems, if they arise at all[57]. Only when acute severe overproduction of urate can be anticipated should prophylactic therapy with a xanthine oxidase inhibitor be considered. In patients with asymptomatic hyperuricemia, long-term urate-lowering drug therapy cannot be justified either in terms of the risks of drug complications or cost effectiveness.

GOUT IN THE ELDERLY

Gout may develop in the elderly with prolonged hyperuricemia such as that due to diuretics, hypertension or renal insufficiency[58]. Acute attacks may be few, but they may be polyarticular and involve the upper limbs and tophi may develop at a relatively early stage[59]. Although the same principles of management apply, there is a greater frequency of side effects from therapy and NSAID and colchicine are often poorly tolerated. Steroids may be useful for acute attacks. Therapy to normalize the serum urate may need to be considered and this follows the choices as enumerated. One must be particularly alert to the increased risk of side effects, particularly sensitivity to allopurinol. With the age dependent decline in renal function, the renal elimination of the allopurinol metabolite oxypurinol is reduced and its dose needs to be reduced in proportion to renal glomerular function (see previous page). The lowest dose possible to achieve the desired effect on the plasma urate should be used[60].

SURGERY

Surgery is rarely indicated for tophi except in unusual presentations where tophi exert pressure on an important structure (e.g. spinal cord). In other less vital situations, control of the hyperuricemia will cause resorption of the tophi provided there is no urgency to have them removed. Infected tophi can usually be managed with antibiotics and local measures, but debridement may be needed, particularly when there is associated vascular disease.

REFERENCES

1. Ahern MJ, Reid C, Gordon TP et al. Does colchicine work? The results of the first controlled study in acute gout. Aust NZ J Med 1987; 17: 301–304.
2. Roberts WN, Liang MH, Stern SH. Colchicine in acute gout: reassessment of risks and benefits. J Am Med Assoc 1987; 257: 1920–1922.
3. Griffin MR, Piper JM, Daugherty JR et al. Nonsteroidal anti-inflammatory drug use and increased risk for peptic ulcer disease in elderly persons. Ann Intern Med 1991; 114: 257–263.
4. Unsworth J, Sturman S, Lunec J, Blake DR. Renal impairment associated with non-steroidal anti-inflammatory drugs. Ann Rheum Dis 1987; 46: 233–236.
5. Arnold MH, Preston SJ, Buchanan WW. Comparison of the natural history of untreated acute gouty arthritis vs acute gouty arthritis treated with non-steroidal anti-inflammatory drugs. Br J Clin Pharmacol 1988; 26: 488–489.
6. Boutsen Y, Esselinckx W. Novel nonsteroidal anti-inflammatory drugs. Acta Gastroenterol Belg 1999; 62: 421–424.
7. Emmerson BT. Regimen of indomethacin therapy in acute gouty arthritis. Br Med J 1967; 2: 272–274.
8. Schweitz MC, Nashel DJ, Alepa FP. Ibuprofen in the treatment of acute gouty arthritis. J Am Med Assoc1978; 239: 34–35.
9. Widmark PH. Piroxicam: its safety and efficacy in the treatment of acute gout. Am J Med 1982; 72: 63–65.
10. Calabro JJ, Khoury MI, Symth CJ. Clinoril in acute gout. Acta Reuma Port 1974; 8: 163–166.
11. Gray RG, Tenenbaum J, Gottlieb NL. Local corticosteroid injection treatment in rheumatic disorders. Semin Arthritis Rheum 1981; 10: 231–254.
12. Axelrod D, Preston S. Comparison of parenteral adrenocorticotropic hormone with oral indomethacin in the treatment of acute gout. Arthritis Rheum 1988; 31: 803–805.
13. Alloway JA, Moriarty MJ, Hoogland YT, Nashel DJ. Comparison of triamcinolone acetonide with indomethacin in the treatment of acute gouty arthritis. J Rheumatol 1993; 20: 111–113.
14. Werlen D, Gabay C, Vischer TL. Corticosteroid therapy for the treatment of acute attacks of crystal-induced arthritis: an effective alternative to nonsteroidal antiinflammatory drugs. Rev Rhum Engl Ed 1996; 63: 248–254.
15. Wallace SL. Colchicine. Semin Arthritis Rheum 1974; 3: 369–381.
16. Spilberg I, Mandell B, Mehta J et al. Mechanism of action of colchicine in acute urate crystal-induced arthritis. J Clin Invest 1979; 64: 775–780.
17. Ferron GM, Rochdi M, Jusko WJ, Scherrmann JM. Oral absorption characteristics and pharmacokinetics of colchicine in healthy volunteers after single and multiple doses. J Clin Pharmacol 1996; 36: 874–883.
18. Wallace SL, Singer JZ. Review: systemic toxicity associated with the intravenous administration of colchicine – guidelines for use. J Rheumatol 1988; 15: 495–499.
19. Kuncl RW, Duncan G, Watson D et al. Colchicine myopathy and neuropathy. N Engl J Med 1987; 316: 1562–1568.
20. Tapal MF. Colchicine myopathy. Scand J Rheumatol 1996; 25: 105–106.
21. Wallace SL, Singer JZ, Duncan GJ et al. Renal function predicts colchicine toxicity: guidelines for the prophylactic use of colchicine in gout. J Rheumatol 1991; 18: 264–269.
22. Baud FJ, Sabouraud A et al. Brief report: treatment of severe colchicine overdose with colchicine-specific Fab fragments. N Engl J Med 1995; 332: 642–645.
23. Yu TF. The efficacy of colchicine prophylaxis in articular gout – a reappraisal after 20 years. Semin Arthritis Rheum 1982; 12: 256–263.
24. Kot TV, Day RO, Brooks PM. Preventing acute gout when starting allopurinol therapy. Colchicine or NSAID? Med J Aust 1993; 159: 182–184.
25. Emmerson BT. Identification of the causes of persistent hyperuricaemia. Lancet 1991; 337: 1461–1463.
26. Emmerson, BT. Hyperlipidaemia in hyperuricaemia and gout. Ann Rheum Dis 1998; 57: 509–510.
27. Facchini F, Chen Y-DI, Hollenbeck CB, Reaven GM. Relationship between resistance to insulin-mediated glucose uptake, urinary uric acid clearance and plasma uric acid concentration. J Am Med Assoc 1991; 266: 3008–3011.
28. Yamashita S, Matsuzawa Y, Tokunaga K et al. Studies on the impaired metabolism of uric acid in obese subjects: marked reduction of renal urate excretion and its improvement by a low-calorie diet. Int J Obesity 1986; 10: 255–264.
29. Macfarlane DG, Dieppe PA. Diuretic induced gout in elderly women. Br J Rheumatol 1985; 24: 155–157.
30. Scott JT, Higgens CS. Diuretic induced gout: a multifactorial condition. Ann Rheum Dis 1992; 51: 259–261.
31. Brøchner-Mortensen K. Uric acid in blood and urine. Acta Med Scand 1937; 84(suppl): 127–153.
32. Eastmond CJ, Garton M, Robins S, Riddoch S. The effects of alcoholic beverages on urate metabolism in gout sufferers. Br J Rheumatol 1995; 34: 756–759.
33. Emmerson BT. Getting rid of gout – a guide to management and prevention. Melbourne: Oxford University Press; 1996.
34. McCarthy GM, Barthelemy CR, Veum JA, Wortmann RL. Influence of antihyperuricemic therapy on the clinical and radiographic progression of gout. Arthritis Rheum 1991; 34: 1489–1494.
35. Emmerson BT, Hazelton RA, Whyte IM. Comparison of the urate lowering effect of allopurinol and diflunisal. J Rheumatol 1987; 14: 335–337.
36. Gibson T, Simmonds HA, Armstrong RD et al. Azapropazone – a treatment for hyperuricaemia and gout? Br J Rheumatol 1984; 23: 44–51.
37. Bishop C, Rand R, Talbot JH. Effect of benemid (p-[di-n-propyl sulfanyl]-benzoic acid) on uric acid metabolism in one normal and one gouty subject. J Clin Invest 1951; 30: 889–905.
38. Dayton PG, Perel JM. The metabolism of probenecid in man. Ann NY Acad Sci 1971; 179: 399–402.
39. Dieterle W, Faigle JW, Mory H et al. Biotransformation and pharmacokinetics of sulfinpyrazone (Anturan) in man. Eur J Clin Pharmacol 1975; 9: 135–145.
40. Chennavasin P, Seiwell R, Brater DC, Liang WM. Pharmacodynamic analysis of the furosemide–probenecid interaction in man. Kidney Int 1979; 16: 187–195.
41. Brooks PM, Bell MA, Sturrock RD et al. The clinical significance of indomethacin–probenecid interaction. Br J Clin Pharmacol 1974; 1: 287–290.
42. Kovalchik MT. Sulfinpyrazone induced uric acid urolithiasis with acute renal failure. Connecticut Med 1981; 45: 423–424.
43. Rundles RW, Metz EN, Silberman HR. Allopurinol in the treatment of gout. Ann Intern Med 1966; 64: 229–258.
44. Walter-Sack I, de Vries JX et al. Disposition and uric acid lowering effect of oxipurinol: comparison of different oxipurinol formulations and allopurinol in healthy individuals. Eur J Clin Pharmacol 1995; 49: 215–220.
45. Graham S, Day RO et al. Pharmacodynamics of oxypurinol after administration of allopurinol to healthy subjects. Br J Clin Pharmacol 1996; 41: 299–304.
46. Emmerson BT, Gordon RB, Cross M, Thomson DB. Plasma oxipurinol concentrations during allopurinol therapy. Br J Rheumatol 1987; 26: 445–449.
47. Ettinger B, Tang A, Citron JT et al. Randomized trial of allopurinol in the prevention of calcium oxalate calculi. N Engl J Med 1986; 315: 1386–1389.
48. Hande KR, Noone RM, Stone WJ. Severe allopurinol toxicity – description and guidelines for prevention in patients with renal insufficiency. Am J Med 1984; 76: 47–56.
49. Meyrier A. Desensitization in a patient with chronic renal disease and severe allergy to allopurinol. Br Med J 1976; 2: 458.
50. Fam AG, Lewtas J et al. Desensitization to allopurinol in patients with gout and cutaneous reactions. Am J Med 1992; 93: 299–307.
51. Kelso JM, Keating RM. Successful desensitization for treatment of a fixed drug eruption to allopurinol. J Allergy Clin Immunol 1996; 97: 1171–1172.
52. Fam AG, Dunne SM et al. Efficacy and safety of desensitization to allopurinol following cutaneous reactions. Arthritis Rheum 2001; 44: 231–238.
53. Emmerson BT, Hazelton RA, Frazer IH. Some adverse reactions to allopurinol may be mediated by lymphocyte reactivity to oxypurinol. Arthritis Rheum 1988; 31: 436–440.
54. Hamanaka H, Mizutani H et al. Allopurinol hypersensitivity syndrome: hypersensitivity to oxypurinol but not allopurinol. Clin Exp Dermatol 1998; 23: 32–34.
55. Emmerson BT. The management of gout. N Engl J Med 1996; 334: 445–451.
56. Rozenberg S, Roche B, Koeger AC et al. Repeated administration of urate oxidase: treatment for heart transplant gouty arthritis. Arthritis Rheum 1994; 37(suppl): 414.
57. Campion EW, Glynn RJ, De Labry LO. Asymptomatic hyperuricemia: risks and consequences in the normative ageing study. Am J Med 1987; 82: 421–426.
58. Scott JT, Higgins CS. Diuretic induced gout – a multifactorial condition. Ann Rheum Dis 1992; 51: 259–261.
59. Fam AG. Gout in the elderly. Clinical presentation and treatment. Drugs and Aging 1998; 13: 229–243.
60. Turnheim K, Krivanek P, Oberbauer R. Pharmacokinetics and pharmacodynamics of allopurinol in elderly and young subjects. Br J Clin Pharmacol 1999; 48: 501–509.

43

Basic calcium phosphate crystal deposition disease

Geraldine M McCarthy

Definition

Calcific periarthritis

- Periarticular deposits of calcific material (hydroxyapatite)
- May result in calcific periarthritis, tendinitis or bursitis

Intra-articular deposition

- Intra-articular deposits of basic calcium phosphate (BCP) crystals may be found in joint fluid as well as in articular cartilage and synovium

Clinical features

Calcific periarthritis

- The shoulder is the main site affected but deposits have been described near many other joints
- Deposits are often inert and asymptomatic
- Deposits can rupture, causing a local acute, crystal-induced inflammation
- Deposits may also be associated with local chronic pain and functional impairment

Intra-articular deposition

- Deposits are often inert and asymptomatic
- Deposits often occur in patients with osteoarthritis
- Crystals can occasionally be shed into the joint, resulting in an acute synovitis resembling gout
- BCP crystals are also found in abundance in the joints of older patients with large joint destructive arthropathies, such as the 'Milwaukee shoulder' syndrome

HISTORY

Calcific periarthritis

Calcific scapulohumeral periarthritis was first described in 1870 and radiographic demonstration of periarticular shoulder calcifications was accomplished by 1907[1]. These calcifications were initially regarded as having arisen in the subdeltoid bursa but were subsequently demonstrated to occur chiefly in the supraspinatus tendon or the shoulder joint capsule. Thirty years later, renewed interest in periarthritis of the shoulder led to further descriptions of the phenomenon and also the recognition of periarticular calcifications at other sites[2]. After another 30 years, it was recognized that the calcific material consisted of hydroxyapatite[3], and the pathophysiologic theory of primary tendon necrosis leading to secondary calcification followed[4]. Subsequently, aggregates of basic calcium phosphate (BCP) crystals with their various crystalline structures and chemical compositions have been further defined using ultrastructural and physical microanalysis techniques, including analytical electron microscopy, X-ray diffraction and Fourier transformation infrared spectroscopy[5]. The term BCP includes crystals of partially carbonate substituted hydroxyapatite, octacalcium phosphate, and rarely found tricalcium phosphate.

Intra-articular BCP crystal deposition

The earliest description of the pathoanatomical features of the consequences of intra-articular BCP crystal deposition appears to have been by Robert Adams in 1857 and called 'chronic rheumatic arthritis of the shoulder'[6]. In his 1934 monograph, Codman reported the case of a 51-year-old woman who had what he called subacromial space hygroma. He described recurrent swelling of the shoulder, absent rotator cuff, cartilaginous bodies attached to the synovial tissue and severe destructive glenohumeral arthritis[7]. These clinical descriptions were made without the benefit of modern diagnostic tests. The condition has subsequently been known by many different names. In the French literature, the terms 'les caries séniles hémorragique de l'épaule' and 'l'arthropathie destructrice rapide de l'épaule' have been used[8], and in the English literature terms such as 'cuff-tear arthropathy' appear[9]. All early descriptions stress the involvement of older females and the localization to the shoulder joint[10].

The association of intra-articular deposits of BCP crystals with joint disease is much more recent. The presence of solid deposits of BCP crystals in the menisci of postmortem knees was noted in 1966[11], but it was not until 1976 that the first description of BCP crystals in degenerative joint diseases was recorded. Clumps of BCP crystals were discovered in the synovial fluid of patients with osteoarthritis (OA) using analytical electron microscopy[12], a finding which was confirmed by others[13,14]. In 1981, McCarty's group described a similar large joint destructive arthropathy, seen most commonly in the shoulder joints of elderly women, called it 'Milwaukee shoulder', and noted the presence of large quantities of BCP crystals associated with collagenase in the synovial fluid. They hypothesized that the BCP crystals caused the associated joint destruction[15]. Subsequently, others noted that many large joints could be involved, and terms such as 'apatite-associated destructive arthritis' and 'idiopathic destructive arthritis of the shoulder' were added to the list of names. BCP crystals were also described in the joint fluids of a few patients with acute synovitis and other forms of arthropathy[14].

EPIDEMIOLOGY

Calcific periarthritis

There have been very few systematic studies of the incidence or prevalence of juxta-articular deposits of BCP crystals. These deposits are often asymptomatic and are most commonly noted by chance on a radiograph taken for other reasons (Fig. 43.1). In a unique, very large study of office workers published in 1941, a 2.7% prevalence of shoulder deposits was noted in a North American, predominantly Caucasian population, 34–45% of which were associated with clinical problems[16]. Females were affected more commonly than males and the prevalence was highest in those aged between 31 and 40 years (19.5%). No comparable

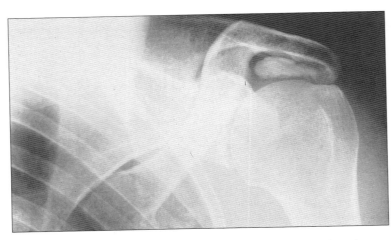

Fig. 43.1 Anteroposterior radiograph of the shoulder joint showing a large calcific deposit in the supraspinatus tendon. The deposit is dense, homogenous and well defined, findings characteristic of inert periarticular deposits of calcific material.

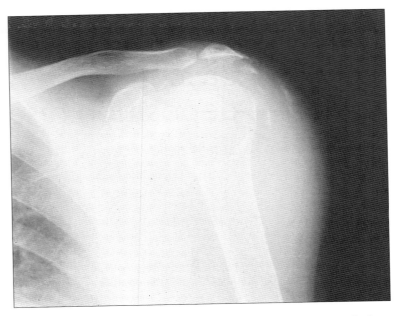

Fig. 43.2 Anteroposterior radiograph of the shoulder during an attack of severe acute calcific periarthritis. The deposit has become indistinct and ill defined as the crystals are shed into the surrounding tissues. In this elderly patient the communication between the shoulder joint and the subacromial bursa led to a large effusion of the glenohumoral joint and a huge extension of the bursa into the upper arm, as shown by the soft tissue swelling seen in the radiograph.

epidemiologic data have been reported subsequently, although a number of smaller pathologic or radiographic studies have documented the relatively high frequency of periarticular calcification. Calcific periarthritis has been reported in children as young as 3 years old, but appears to be relatively uncommon in the elderly. This suggests that many of the deposits seen in young adults must disappear spontaneously.

Articular calcification

The prevalence of intra-articular BCP crystal deposition has not been established. Apatite crystals are found in up to 60% of synovial fluid samples from patients with knee OA[17,18]. The prevalence of BCP crystals in approximately 50% of 53 preoperative OA knees has been noted recently[19]. The prevalence in normal joints at different ages is not known. The 'Milwaukee shoulder' syndrome and related BCP crystal-associated destructive arthropathies are uncommon, tend to occur in elderly individuals and are of unknown prevalence.

CLINICAL FEATURES

Calcific periarthritis

Periarticular calcific deposits are often asymptomatic. However, they are also associated with a number of clinical syndromes (Table 43.1). The most striking clinical presentation is acute calcific periarthritis, which

most commonly involves the shoulder but can occur in association with almost any joint. The episode may be preceded by mild trauma or overuse, but most cases present with a spontaneous onset.

Patients present with sudden onset of severe pain, and within hours the affected part is usually swollen, with redness and warmth of the overlying skin. There is extreme local tenderness and associated loss of function. At the shoulder the pain is most marked around the subacromial region, radiating down the outside of the arm. Glenohumoral movement is usually severely restricted. Severe pain may last for several days, but symptoms then usually resolve slowly over a period of 2–3 weeks. A 'frozen shoulder' may result.

Calcific periarthritis is thought to result from rupture of a calcific deposit into an adjacent soft tissue space or bursa, initiating an acute inflammatory reaction. In the shoulder the crystals may induce intense inflammation in the subacromial bursa (Fig. 43.2). Radiographically, calcium deposits appear dense, with well-defined borders, prior to an attack. With the onset of an attack, however, these calcific deposits appear fluffy, with poorly defined margins. Ultimately, there is a reduction in the size of the deposit seen radiographically, and it may disappear completely.

Calcific deposits in the periarticular tissues are also associated with chronic pain syndromes. However, in the shoulder it is difficult to define what contribution, if any, the deposits themselves make to the clinical findings. This is for two reasons: both chronic shoulder pain and calcification are common; and prior damage to tendons may predispose to the calcification. Moderate to severe pain is described, with varying degrees of tenderness and restriction of motion. Pain usually radiates to the insertion of the deltoid and sometimes beyond, to the forearm. Lying on the affected shoulder is painful and may interfere with sleep. In some patients recurrent acute attacks around the shoulder, separated by pain-free periods of months or years, are followed by the development of chronic pain. Damage to the tendons and muscles of the rotator cuff may result and may lead to total disruption of the cuff apparatus.

The shoulder is the most commonly affected site, followed by the hip, knee, elbow, wrist and ankle joints. The joints of the feet and toes are

TABLE 43.1 SYNDROMES ASSOCIATED WITH BCP CRYSTALS	
Subcutaneous deposits (e.g. calcification of hands in scleroderma)	Asymptomatic chance finding Acute and chronic inflammation Skin ulceration Secondary infection Pressing necrosis of surrounding tissues Mechanical interference with function
Periarticular deposits (e.g. calcification of supraspinatus tendon)	Asymptomatic chance finding Acute calcific periarthritis Chronic periarticular pain and/or dysfunction
Intra-articular deposits (e.g. synovial and cartilage deposits in damaged joints)	Asymptomatic chance finding Acute synovitis Severe osteoarthritis Destructive arthropathies of older people
Clinical syndromes that can be associated with the deposition of BCP crystals in and around joints.	

less commonly involved (less than 1% of all reported cases), as are those of the hands and fingers[20]. Hydroxyapatite pseudopodagra is a term used to describe acute calcific arthritis at the first metatarsal phalangeal joint, usually in young women[21]. Acute neck pain attributed to calcifications surrounding the odontoid process has been described and called the 'crowned dens' syndrome. Calcifications appear to be composed of apatite or calcium pyrophosphate dihydrate, or a combination of both[22].

Some patients with multifocal deposits develop symptoms at several sites, suggesting a more generalized condition rather than a chance localized process with resultant calcification. This manifestation can cause diagnostic confusion and may even mimic a seronegative polyarthritis. Several reports describe familial occurrences of calcific periarthritis[23].

INTRA-ARTICULAR BCP CRYSTALS

Our understanding of the exact relationship between intra-articular BCP crystals and joint pathology is incomplete, especially as special techniques are required to identify the crystals. None the less, current data support the pathogenic role of BCP crystals in articular tissue degeneration (Fig. 43.3). BCP crystals have been linked with several different diseases.

Acute synovitis

Acute attacks of arthritis associated with intra-articular BCP crystals in relatively young individuals have been described in the knee as well as other sites. Pain, swelling and erythema resembled gout[24]. These attacks appear to be rare and the diagnosis is difficult to establish. Occasionally, crystals from a periarticular deposit can rupture into the joint itself, causing acute synovitis. This can occur in some older individuals who have a direct communication between the subacromial bursa and the glenohumoral joint.

Chronic monoarthritis, with or without erosions

A chronic, sometimes erosive monoarthritis has been linked with intra-articular BCP crystals. BCP crystals have been particularly implicated in finger joint arthropathies, including erosive or inflammatory forms of OA[25]. However, this also appears to be a rare phenomenon and the direct contribution of BCP crystals to the observed pathology remains to be established.

Osteoarthritis

The concurrence of BCP crystals and OA is well established. It has been suggested that many OA joint fluids contain clusters of BCP crystals, which are too small or too few in number to be identified by conventional techniques[26]. Ample data support the role of BCP crystals in cartilage degeneration, as their presence correlates strongly with the severity of radiographic OA[27], and larger joint effusions are seen in affected knee joints when compared with joint fluid from OA knees without crystals[28]. Although the basis of cartilage damage by BCP crystals has been the subject of numerous investigations, there are ongoing controversies concerning the direction of the relationship between calcium-containing crystals and OA, i.e. do the crystals cause cartilage damage or are they present as a result of joint damage?

Large joint destructive arthropathies

A distinctive type of destructive arthropathy has been described in elderly individuals and is associated with rotator cuff defects and numerous aggregates of BCP crystals in the fluids of affected joints[15].

The clinical picture is characteristic (Fig. 43.4a). Patients are nearly always over 70 years old, and approximately 90% are females. They usually present with a history (months or years) of increasing pain, swelling and loss of function of the affected joint, usually the shoulder. The dominant side is usually involved initially, although 60% have bilateral involvement[29]. The pain may be mild but is usually most apparent at night and on joint use. Examination reflects extensive damage to the periarticular soft tissues as well as to cartilage and subchondral bone on both sides of the joint. There is a reduced active range of motion in all affected joints, sometimes associated with pronounced joint instability. Crepitation and pain may be noted, especially when the humerus is grated passively against the glenoid. The rotator cuff is generally

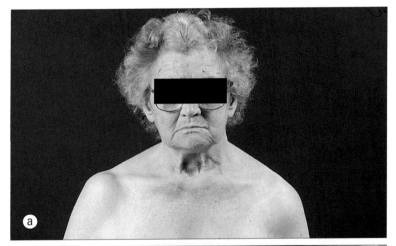
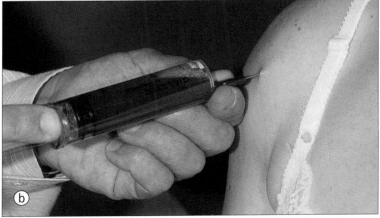

Fig. 43.4 BCP crystal-associated destructive arthritis ('Milwaukee shoulder').
(a) This elderly patient has visible swellings of both shoulders.
(b) Aspiration revealed a large amount of bloodstained fluid which contained numerous particles of basic calcium phosphates.

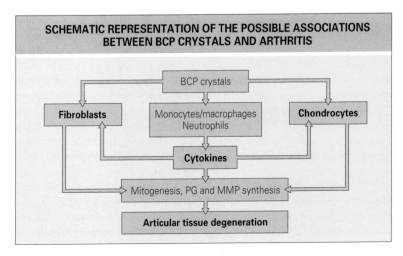

Fig. 43.3 Schematic representation of the possible associations between BCP crystals and arthritis. PG, prostaglandins; MMP, matrix metalloproteases.

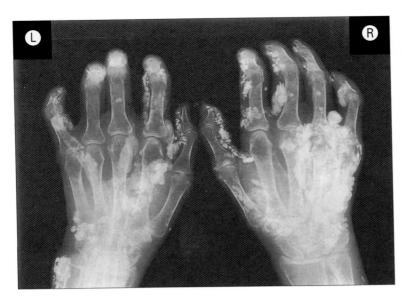

Fig. 43.5 Anteroposterior radiograph of the hands of a patient with severe subcutaneous calcification associated with mild scleroderma.

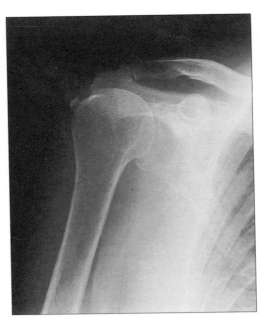

Fig. 43.6 Anteroposterior radiograph of the shoulder joint showing a small periarticular calcific deposit. Other views may be needed to identify small deposits and the site of deposition.

completely destroyed. Joint effusion is typically present and may be massive, extending into the subdeltoid region. Aspiration of affected shoulder joints routinely yields blood-tinged synovial fluid that has a low, predominantly mononuclear, cell count (Fig. 43.4b). Rupture of the effusion can lead to a massive extravasation of blood and synovial fluid into the surrounding tissues[30]. Although the shoulder predominates, knees, hips, elbows and other joints may be involved[31].

The natural history of the condition is unclear, but many cases seem to stabilize after a year or two, with reduction of symptoms, joint effusions and no further radiographic changes.

ASSOCIATED DISEASES AND OTHER CLINICAL PRESENTATIONS

A number of secondary forms of BCP crystal-associated arthropathies have been described. BCP crystal deposits have been reported in the joints and periarticular tissues of renal failure patients, mostly when undergoing dialysis. Renal failure also predisposes to calcium oxalate, monosodium urate, calcium pyrophosphate dihydrate (CPPD) and aluminum phosphate crystal deposition[32]. Intra-articular injection of triamcinolone hexacetonide has been associated with the formation of periarticular calcifications along the injection tract, which may become apparent months after the injection. Such calcification may gradually be resorbed over a period of months to years. Occasionally, severe neurologic damage has been followed by heterotopic ossification in periarticular tissues that may mimic arthritis.

BCP deposition is also associated with the connective tissue diseases, particularly scleroderma and dermatomyositis. Following dermatomyositis in childhood, massive sheets of fascial calcification can occur. In scleroderma the deposits are usually subcutaneous. They are associated with the CREST syndrome, but in some patients there is extensive calcification with very little in the way of other features of the disease (calcinosis cutis) (Fig. 43.5). Occasionally the hand calcification occurs on its own. 'Tumoral calcinosis' is a rare condition in which calcification of bursae, such as the olecranon bursa, occurs in the absence of other problems.

INVESTIGATIONS

Imaging

The plain radiograph is the easiest method with which to detect and describe the calcific material of calcific periarthritis (Fig. 43.6).

Anteroposterior and lateral radiographs are usually sufficient, but special views, with internal or external rotation of the shoulder, may be necessary to visualize retrohumeral deposits. The deposits are usually visualized in the rotator cuff, particularly the supraspinatus tendon a few centimeters from its insertion, but may also be seen in the subacromial bursa. Various appearances have been described, with size varying from a few millimeters to several centimeters across. Other imaging investigations are rarely helpful in calcific periarthritis, although arthrography can be used to confirm cuff rupture, and techniques such as computed tomography (CT) or magnetic resonance imaging (MRI) may help demonstrate small deposits or other changes in the tissues around the lesion. Because bilateral calcification is common, a radiograph of the contralateral side (usually the shoulder) may be warranted. Radiographs of other sites (pelvis, knees, wrists and hands), even if asymptomatic, will sometimes reveal multiple deposits. During acute attacks of periarthritis the deposits may change and disappear, only to reappear subsequently.

Calcification around joints is sometimes mistaken for ossification, although the presence of trabeculae in the latter should permit differentiation. The only other differential diagnosis on the images is with the very rare formation of periarticular deposits of CPPD. These occasionally occur in periarticular tendons but, as in joints, they usually appear as linear rather than nummular shadows.

Intra-articular BCP deposits are rarely visible with any of the conventional imaging procedures. Occasionally, articular calcifications of a nummular sort are seen, contrasting with the linear deposits of chondrocalcinosis due to CPPD crystals. However, pathologic studies indicate that individual aggregates of crystals in cartilage synovium or synovial fluid are generally tiny and well below the size that gives any chance of their being visible on a radiograph.

Radiographs in Milwaukee shoulder syndrome are striking (Fig. 43.7), showing upward subluxation of the humeral head or arthrographic evidence of rotator cuff defects in the majority of patients. Other findings may include cystic degeneration of the humeral tuberosities, erosions of cortical bone at the site of insertion of the rotator cuff, degenerative changes of the humeral head and/or glenoid of the scapula, degenerative changes of the acromioclavicular joint and calcification of the tendinous rotator cuff. Pseudarthrosis formation between the humeral head and the acromion and clavicle is common.

MRI can be used to further define the anatomical changes associated with Milwaukee shoulder syndrome, including loss of cartilage, peri-

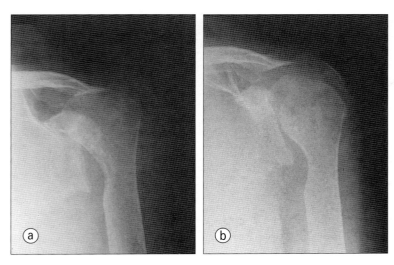

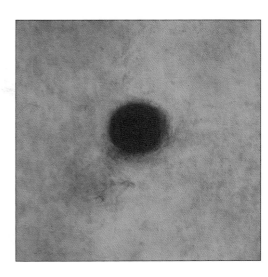

Fig. 43.7 Anteroposterior radiographs of a shoulder joint affected by BCP crystal-associated destructive arthritis ('Milwaukee shoulder'). The extensive destruction of periarticular tissues, including the rotator cuff, has led to instability of the shoulder. The upward subluxation (a) of the humerus can be overcome by traction on the shoulder (b). Note the extensive atrophic destruction and loss of bone of both the acromion and the glenohumeral joint.

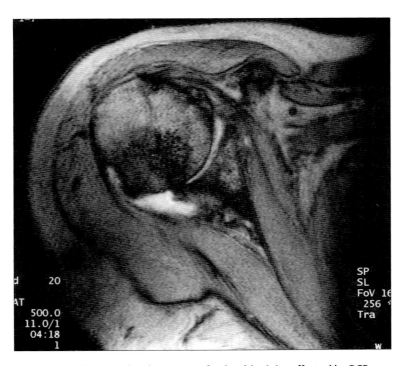

Fig. 43.8 Axial T2-weighted MRI scan of a shoulder joint affected by BCP crystal-associated destructive arthritis ('Milwaukee shoulder'). There is advanced glenohumeral joint degeneration with loss of articular cartilage, truncation of the anterior and posterior labrum, narrowing of the joint space, osteophyte formation, muscle atrophy and joint effusion.

articular bone marrow edema, rupture of the rotator cuff, synovial hypertrophy and joint effusion (Fig. 43.8).

Metabolic

Apatite deposition usually occurs in the absence of any detectable metabolic abnormality. However, if multiple deposits are detected, or if the deposits are unusually large or in unusual sites, the calcium and phosphate levels, as well as renal function, should be checked. High serum phosphate levels seem more likely to predispose to deposition than abnormalities of calcium alone.

Synovial or bursal fluid

In acute calcific periarthritis it is sometimes possible to aspirate a mixture of calcium deposits and inflammatory matter from the bursa or periarticular tissues. This may look like toothpaste, or be a creamy fluid obviously full of 'chalk'. In cases of intra-articular BCP deposition the synovial fluid findings vary. Usually the fluids that contain BCP have a low cell count, are viscous, and are very much the same as fluids from any patient with OA. In the destructive arthropathies of the elderly there is frequent bloodstaining of the fluid. In addition, there may be numerous cartilage fragments and other debris, although the cell count is low.

Identification and characterization of BCP crystals

The study of BCP crystal-associated arthritis has been relatively difficult because of the lack of a simple, easily accessible, reliable diagnostic test[5]. BCP crystals are not birefringent[33]. Therefore, polarized light microscopy is not useful for their detection. This is because individual BCP crystals, which are usually needle-shaped and less than 0.1 μm long, cannot be resolved by light microscopy and are randomly oriented in the much larger aggregates (2–19 μm) in which they are usually found. Plain and polarized light microscopy of samples containing apatite may show globular clumps of crystals, which can look like shiny coins, but the usual appearance of these crystals is nondescript.

Calcium stains such as Alizarin red S have been used by some investigators to identify BCP crystals. Clumps of crystals show up with a 'halo' of stain (Fig. 43.9). Alizarin red S is highly sensitive, but frequent false positive results suggest that it lacks sufficient specificity to qualify for the routine identification of BCP crystals without some other type of confirmatory testing.

A semiquantitative binding assay for BCP crystals has been described which uses [^{14}C]ethane-1-hydroxy-1,1-diphosphonate (EHDP)[13]. Diphosphonates are analogs of inorganic pyrophosphate that adsorb to the surface of BCP crystals but not to monosodium urate, CPPD, cartilage fragments or any other known particulates in joint fluid. This method is performed on a synovial fluid pellet resuspended in phosphate-buffered saline and the results are expressed as μg/ml of hydroxyapatite standard. The limit of sensitivity is approximately 2 μg/ml standard hydroxyapatite.

Electron microscopy can be used to visualize the crystals in synovial fluid pellets, and if elemental analysis or electron diffraction is possible their identity can be confirmed (Fig. 43.10). If sufficient material is available, for example from surgical specimens, other analytical techniques, such as X-ray powder diffraction or Fourier transformation infrared spectroscopy (FTIR), can be used to identify the material. The latter has shown that BCP crystal deposits consist of mixtures of

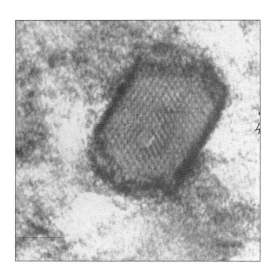

Fig. 43.10 High magnification transmission electron micrographs of BCP crystals. The crystal lattice structure as well as the morphology of the crystals is apparent.

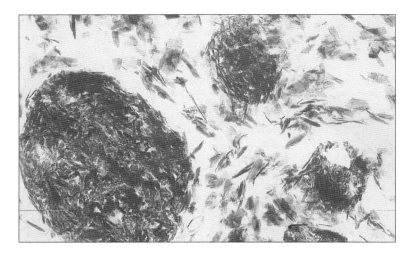

Fig. 43.11 Transmission electron micrograph of BCP crystals from a tendon deposit. This shows the clumps of crystals, dense globular structures of various sizes, and isolated crystals.

hydroxyapatite, octacalcium phosphate and, rarely, tricalcium phosphate crystals. Combinations of BCP and CPPD are not infrequent.

Atomic force microscopy has been applied recently to the identification of synovial fluid microcrystals. This technique is capable of achieving subnanometer resolution of crystal surface topology and measurement of lattice unit cell dimensions[34].

The ability to identify apatite is less crucial from a clinical perspective than the identification of monosodium urate or calcium pyrophosphate dihydrate crystals, as no drug has as yet been identified that specifically inhibits the pathologic effects of BCP crystals *in vivo*.

DIFFERENTIAL DIAGNOSIS

Acute calcific periarthritis
The differential diagnosis of acute calcific periarthritis should include gout, pseudogout and sepsis. However, the distribution of the lesions and the acute onset are often characteristic. Radiographs showing the evolution of the calcific deposit are virtually pathognomonic. The diagnosis can be confirmed if material can be aspirated from the area.

Chronic periarticular syndromes
The usual features are those of a tendonitis, and the only way of implicating crystal deposition in the diagnosis is through visualizing the deposit on the radiograph. Other causes of tendonitis, such as trauma, impingement and inflammatory arthritis, are possible differential diagnoses.

Acute and chronic arthritis
Acute inflammatory arthritis which may mimic gout, pseudogout or other systemic inflammatory rheumatic disease has been attributed to BCP crystals[12,24]. BCP crystals are often detected in osteoarthritic joints and appear to promote the degenerative process, as their presence is associated with more advanced radiographic change and larger joint effusions than in joints without BCP crystals[27,28]. Erosive arthritis with recurrent episodes of pain and swelling involving the wrists and the finger joints has been associated with BCP crystal deposition[25].

Destructive arthropathies of the elderly
The main differential diagnoses include neuropathic or Charcot joints, chronic sepsis, advanced rheumatoid disease, osteonecrosis and CPPD deposition disease. Radiographic involvement of both sides of the joint helps differentiate this condition from osteonecrosis. The absence of any neurologic deficit distinguishes it from Charcot's arthropathy. Synovial fluid examination and culture will aid the differentiation from CPPD deposition disease and sepsis.

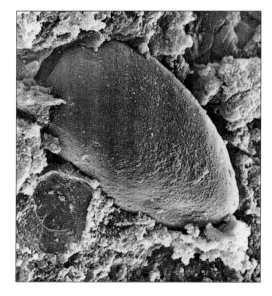

Fig. 43.12 Scanning electron micrograph of a calcific deposit isolated from a tendon.

STRUCTURE AND FUNCTION

Nature of the crystals
Hydroxypatite is a form of calcium phosphate represented by the formula $Ca_5(PO_4)_3OH2H_2O$ and is usually found in partially substituted carbonated form. In periarticular calcific deposits, light microscopy usually shows multifocal aggregates of crystals separated by fibrocollagenous tissue. On transmission electron microscopy the deposits appear as rounded aggregates with isolated crystals in a matrix of fragmented collagen fibers (Fig. 43.11). On scanning electron microscopy they look like rocky bulks embedded in mortar (Fig. 43.12). The crystals are very heterogeneous, both within the sample and in different patients. Typically, they include compounds of varying crystallinities, ranging from amorphous BCP to well-structured stable elements similar to those of bone and tooth, but with a larger crystal size than most of those seen in bone. In bone, poorly crystalline partially carbonated crystals of hydroxyapatite, each of about 500 Å in length, are the main mineral phase. The crystals of periarticular deposits are often more carbonated than bone crystals, and high-resolution electron microscopy suggests that some of them are coated with electron-dense material.

In synovial fluid samples mixed populations of BCP crystals have been reported, including partially carbonate-substituted hydroxyapatite, octacalcium phosphate ($Ca_8H_2(PO_4)_6{\cdot}5H_2O$) and, rarely, tricalcium phosphate ($Ca_3(PO_4)_2$). They frequently coexist with CPPD crystals and are associated with particulate collagens[35]. One recent report suggested that crystals extracted from the synovial fluid were more like those found in periarticular calcific deposits than in bone crystals, suggesting that they were derived from newly formed deposits and not from subchondral bone[36].

Another form of BCP, magnesium whitlockite, has been identified in the superficial region of articular cartilage. Recent studies suggest that it may be a frequent finding in normal as well as diseased hyaline cartilage[37]. This observation, coupled with the identification of some hydroxyapatite crystals in normal cartilage, has led to speculation that some BCP minerals may have a physiologic, rather than a pathologic, role in cartilage homeostasis. However, whitlockite crystals elicit biologic cellular responses, including mitogenesis and matrix metalloprotease production *in vitro* which suggest potential pathogenicity in arthritis[38].

ETIOLOGY

The mechanism of periarticular calcification is largely unknown, although periarticular intratendinous deposits have been thought to be due to ectopic calcification of damaged tendons. In most patients no obvious local, metabolic or genetic cause for the calcification is found. The frequent occurrence of bilateral and multifocal deposits suggests the operation of a generalized predisposition as well as local factors. This is supported by the fact that the sites of deposition in sporadic cases of calcific periarthritis are the same as those associated with a known systemic predisposition, such as diabetes mellitus, hyperthyroidism or parathyroid disorders. The classic description of a relationship between repetitive shoulder use and the formation of calcific deposits has not been established. There is no known relationship with any HLA specificity or other genetic marker, in spite of the known occurrence of familial cases.

PATHOGENESIS

Calcific periarthritis

Pathologic assessments have shown that the calcific deposits are located in tendons, peritendinous tissues, bursae or ligaments. Original studies suggested that 'dystrophic' tendon calcification occurs as a consequence of local trauma, ischemia and necrosis of tendons. Calcific periarthritis frequently localizes to the supraspinatus tendon in a poorly vascularized area of the tendon sheath known as the 'critical zone', at a distance of a few millimeters from the bone insertion. Similarly, calcification in other tendons seems to occur preferentially in hypovascular segments, suggesting local necrosis followed by ectopic calcification.

Some evidence has indicated that calcifying tendinitis is an active cell-mediated process in which local vascular and mechanical changes result in focal transformation of tendinous tissues into fibrocartilaginous material containing chondrocytes. This is followed by local deposition of hydroxyapatite crystals within extracellular matrix vesicle-like structures derived from these chondrocytes[39].

No good animal or *in vitro* model is available to study the formation of periarticular or intra-articular deposits. Aging and the degeneration of collagen fibers do not seem to be sufficient explanation for the phenomenon.

The frequent tolerance of deposits without any apparent inflammation or other response is difficult to explain. The absence of any phagocytic cells in the calcified area may be significant, although the formation of granuloma-like reactions has been reported.

Acute calcific periarthritis appears to be induced by rupture of the deposit and the shedding of crystals into more cellular vascular areas. BCP crystals have been shown to be intrinsically phlogistic. They are phagocytosed *in vitro*, resulting in the release of inflammatory media-

tors[40]. Similarly, *in vivo* models of inflammation show a brisk inflammatory reaction to apatite, and injection into the tissues of human volunteers results in an inflammatory response[41]. Phagocytosis may be one of the main ways in which the crystals are removed.

There is evidence that coating of the crystals, which have highly adsorptive surfaces, can either stimulate or suppress the inflammatory response, depending on the nature of the proteins that attach to the crystals[42]. Immunoglobulins, for example, may activate inflammatory responses, whereas coating of apolipoproteins on the crystal surfaces will suppress it.

RELATIONSHIP WITH OSTEOARTHRITIS AND DESTRUCTIVE ARTHROPATHIES

Crystals of BCP are frequently found in OA cartilage, synovium and synovial fluid. Evidence suggests that human articular cartilage contains matrix vesicles which are capable of progressive mineralization and can generate either BCP or CPPD *in vitro*[43]. However, more than one source of formation is likely. For example, the ANK gene product, a cell membrane protein which regulates extracellular inorganic pyrophosphate (ePPi), has recently been identified. ePPi is an important inhibitor of the nucleation and growth of BCP. This investigation has led to the concept of ANK-mediated control of ePPi levels as a possible mechanism of regulation of tissue calcification[44].

The degree of damage that can occur in apatite-associated destructive arthropathies is marked (Fig. 43.13). The basis of cartilage damage by calcium-containing crystals is still somewhat speculative. Theoretically, crystals in cartilage may directly injure chondrocytes. However, in pathologic specimens crystals are rarely seen in immediate contact with chondrocytes, and even less frequently found engulfed by chondrocytes.

It is more likely that cartilage damage ultimately results from the effects of the crystals on synovial lining. *In vitro* properties of BCP crystals have been observed which emphasize their pathogenic potential. The first is their ability to induce mitogenesis, a characteristic which presumably leads to synovial proliferation, characteristic of both 'Milwaukee shoulder' syndrome and apatite-associated OA[45,46]. Increased cell numbers in the synovial lining enhance the capacity for secretion of cytokines, which may promote chondrolysis. The second is their ability to induce the secretion of proteolytic enzymes, leading to degradation of intra-articular collagenous structures, an observation which correlates with the detection of collagenase and neutral protease activities in synovial fluid from patients with Milwaukee shoulder syndrome[47]. BCP crystals induce production of collagenase 1, stromelysin and 92 kDa gelatinase from human fibroblasts and collagenases 1 and 3 from porcine chondrocytes[46]. Lastly, BCP crystals induce cyclooxygenases-1 and -2, followed by increased prostaglandin E_2 in human fibroblasts[48].

Despite the association of BCP crystals with OA and joint destruction and the biological effects noted *in vitro*, the specific role of the crystals in joint degeneration is controversial. Some hypothesize that BCP crystal aggregates found in association with destructive arthropathies actually originate from damaged subchondral bone and are merely an epiphenomenon. More studies will be necessary to further differentiate between crystals as a cause of cartilage damage and crystals as a result of cartilage damage. An improved understanding of the biological effects of BCP crystals is essential to the ultimate prevention or reversal of the consequences of deposition.

MANAGEMENT

Calcific periarthritis

Asymptomatic deposits require no treatment. Acute attacks of calcific periarthritis have been treated successfully with immobilization and

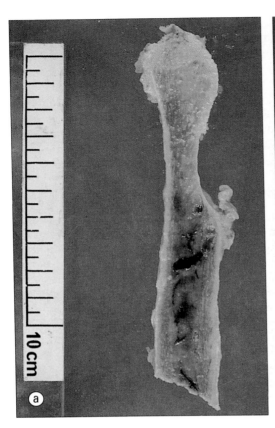

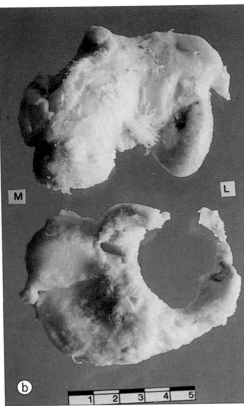

Fig. 43.13 Bones from a patient with advanced BCP crystal-associated destructive arthritis. (a) The humerus shows extensive bony attrition characteristic of this condition. (b) The tibial condyles show the characteristic destruction of the lateral tibiofemoral joint, with extensive loss of subchondral bone.

a variety of non-steroidal anti-inflammatory drugs (NSAIDs) or colchicine. Most patients have markedly reduced symptoms within 5 days and virtual complete resolution within 1–3 weeks. Untreated attacks may last several weeks. Needle aspiration of the paste-like calcific deposits, with or without irrigation, may be helpful. The use of corticosteroids is controversial: local corticosteroid injections will help the acute attacks to resolve but may possibly make further calcification and recurrent attacks more likely.

For patients with chronic periarticular syndromes the treatment is in general much the same as it would be whether the deposit was there or not. There is no known medical way of dispersing or dissolving the deposit. In chronic calcific tendinitis ultrasound treatment helps resolve calcifications and is associated with short-term clinical improvement[49].

If the problem persists and large calcific deposits are present, other treatments can be considered. Local corticosteroid therapy should be used with caution because of the risk of disrupting the deposit or seeding further calcification. Needle aspiration is usually difficult in chronic cases, but arthroscopic or surgical removal may provide permanent symptomatic relief in refractory cases.

Articular BCP crystals

Currently, patients with OA complicated by BCP crystal deposition should be treated in the same manner as if they had simple OA.

Hopefully, ongoing research endeavors will ultimately lead to the development of more specific treatment for apatite deposition. For example, phosphocitrate, a potent inhibitor of hydroxyapatite crystal formation and a relatively non-toxic compound, inhibits BCP crystal-induced cell activation *in vitro*[50,51]. This compound may ultimately prove useful in protecting articular tissues from the harmful biological effects of BCP crystals.

At the time of diagnosis of BCP crystal-associated destructive arthropathies, such as Milwaukee shoulder syndrome, advanced destructive changes are usually present and may even be asymptomatic. The treatment of symptomatic disease is generally unsatisfactory. A conservative approach, including analgesics and NSAIDs, repeated shoulder aspirations and decreased joint use, has sometimes controlled symptoms satisfactorily. Surgical therapy is sometimes successful for the relief of pain and restoration of function, but may be difficult because of the extent of damage to the joint and periarticular tissues. Surgical procedures include arthroscopic lavage and/or debridement, humeral tuberoplasty, arthrodesis, arthroplasty or hemiarthroplasty[7]. Some patients have responded to closed needle tidal-joint irrigation followed by the injection of methylprednisolone acetate (40 mg) and tranexamic acid (0.5g)[52]. Other pain-relieving measures, such as suprascapular nerve blocks for shoulder disease, or transcutaneous nerve stimulation, have been used with some success. Pain may subside with time alone.

REFERENCES

1. Painter CF. Subdeltoid bursitis. Boston Med Surg J 1907; 156: 345–349.
2. Sandstrom C. Peritendinitis calcarea. A common disease of middle life: Its diagnosis, pathology and treatment. Am J Radiol 1938; 40: 1–21.
3. McCarty DJ, Gatter RA. Recurrent acute inflammation associated with focal apatite crystal deposition. Arthritis Rheum 1966; 9: 804–819.
4. Uhthoff HK, Sarker K, Maynard JA. Calcifying tendonitis. A new concept of its pathogenesis. Clin Orthop 1976; 118: 164–168.
5. Rosenthal A, Mandel N. Identification of crystals in synovial fluids and joint tissues. Curr Rheumatol Rep 2001; 3: 11–16.
6. McCarty DJ. Robert Adams' rheumatic arthritis of the shoulder: "Milwaukee Shoulder" revisited. J Rheumatol 1989; 16: 668–670.
7. Jensen K, Williams G, Russell I, Rockwood C. Rotator cuff tear arthropathy. J Bone Joint Surg Am 1999; 81–A(9): 1312–1324.
8. Lequesne M, Fallut M, Couloumb R. L'arthropathie destructice rapide de l'epaule. Rev Rhum 1982; 49: 427–437.
9. Neer CS, Craig EV, Fakuda H. Cuff-tear arthropathy. J Bone Joint Surg 1983; 65A: 1232–1244.
10. Campion GV, McCrae F, Alwan W *et al.* Idiopathic destructive arthritis of the shoulder. Semin Arthritis Rheum 1988; 17: 232–245.
11. McCarty DJ, Hogan JM, Gatter RA, Grossman M. Studies on pathological calcifications in human cartilage. J Bone Joint Surg 1966; 48: 309–325.

12. Dieppe PA, Huskisson EC, Crocker P, Willoughby DA. Apatite deposition disease: a new arthropathy. Lancet 1976; 1: 266–269.

13. Halverson PB, McCarty DJ. Identification of hydroxyapatite crystals in synovial fluid. Arthritis Rheum 1979; 22: 389–395.

14. Schumacher HR, Cherian PV, Reginato AJ et al. Intra-articular apatite crystal deposition. Ann Rheum Dis 1983; 42(Suppl 1): 54–59.

15. McCarty DJ, Halverson PB, Carrera GF et al. Milwaukee shoulder: association of microspheroids containing hydroxyapatite crystals, active collagenase, and neutral protease with rotator cuff defects. i: Clinical aspects. Arthritis Rheum 1981; 24: 464–473.

16. Bosworth BM. Calcium deposits in the shoulder and subacromial bursitis. A survey of 12,222 shoulders. JAMA 1941; 116: 2477–2482.

17. Dieppe PA, Crocker PR, Corke CF et al. Synovial fluid crystals. Q J Med 1979; 192: 533–553.

18. Gibilisco PA, Schumacher HR, Hollander JL, Soper KA. Synovial fluid crystals in osteoarthritis. Arthritis Rheum 1985; 28: 511–515.

19. Kurian J, Daft L, Carrera G, Derfus B. The high prevalence of pathologic calcium crystals in pre-operative joints. Arthritis Rheum 1999; 42: S145.

20. McCarthy GM, Carrera GF, Ryan LM. Acute calcific periarthritis of the finger joints: a syndrome of women. J Rheumatol 1993; 20: 1077–1080.

21. Fam AG, Rubenstein J. Hydroxyapatite pseudopodagra. A syndrome of young women. Arthritis Rheum 1989; 32: 741–747.

22. Bouvet J-P, le Parc J-M, Michalski B et al. Acute neck pain due to calcifications surrounding the odontoid process: the crowned dens syndrome. Arthritis Rheum 1985; 28: 1417–1420.

23. Hajeroussan VJ, Short CL. Familial calcific periarthritis. Ann Rheum Dis 1983; 42: 469–470.

24. Schumacher HR, Smolyo AP, Tse RL, Maurer K. Arthritis associated with apatite crystals. Ann Intern Med 1977; 87: 411–416.

25. Schumacher HR, Miller JL, Ludivico C, Jessar RA. Erosive arthritis associated with apatite crystal deposition. Arthritis Rheum 1981; 24: 31–37.

26. Swan A, Chapman B, Heap P et al. Submicroscopic crystals in osteoarthritic synovial fluids. Ann Rheum Dis 1994; 53: 467–470.

27. Halverson PB, McCarty DJ. Patterns of radiographic abnormalities associated with basic calcium phosphate and calcium pyrophosphate crystal deposition in the knee. Ann Rheum Dis 1986; 45: 603–605.

28. Carroll GJ, Stuart RA, Armstrong JA et al. Hydroxyapatite crystals are a frequent finding in osteoarthritic synovial fluid, but are not related to increased concentrations of keratan sulfate or interleukin 1b. J Rheumatol 1991; 18: 861–866.

29. Halverson PB, Carrera GF, McCarty DJ. Milwaukee shoulder syndrome: Fifteen additional cases and a description of contributing factors. Arch Intern Med 1990; 150: 677–682.

30. McCarty D, Swanson A, Ehrhart R. Hemorrhagic rupture of the shoulder. J Rheumatol 1994; 21: 1134–1137.

31. Dieppe PA, Doherty M, Macfarlane DG et al. Apatite associated destructive arthritis. Br J Rheumatol 1984; 23: 84–91.

32. Halverson PB. Arthropathies associated with basic calcium phosphate crystals. Scanning Microscopy 1992; 6: 791–797.

33. Paul H, Reginato AJ, Schumacher HR. Alizarin red S staining as a screening test to detect calcium compounds in synovial fluid. Arthritis Rheum 1983; 26: 191–200.

34. Blair JM, Sorensen LB, Arnsdorf MF, Ratneshwar L. The application of atomic force microscopy for the detection of microcrystals in synovial fluid from patients with recurrent synovitis. Semin Arthritis Rheum 1995; 24: 259–269.

35. McCarty DJ, Lehr JR, Halverson PB. Crystal populations in human synovial fluid. Identification of apatite, octacalcium phosphate and tricalcium phosphate. Arthritis Rheum 1983; 26: 247–251.

36. Heywood BR, Swan A, Dieppe PA. Chemical, structural and morphological analyses of mineral deposits in synovial fluid. Br J Rheumatol 1991; 30(Suppl 2): 129.

37. Scotchford CA, Ali SY. Magnesium whitlockite deposition in articular cartilage: a study of 80 specimens from 70 patients. Ann Rheum Dis 1995; 54: 339–344.

38. Ryan L, Cheung H, LeGeros R et al. Cellular responses to whitlockite. Calcif Tiss Int 1999; 65: 374–377.

39. Sarker K, Uhthoff HK. Ultrastructural localization of calcium in calcifying tendinitis. Arch Pathol Lab Med 1978; 102: 266–269.

40. Dayer J-M, Evequoz V, Zavadil-Grob C et al. Effect of synthetic calcium pyrophosphate and hydroxyapatite crystals on the interaction of human blood mononuclear cells with chondrocytes, synovial cells and fibroblasts. Arthritis Rheum 1987; 30: 1372–1381.

41. Dieppe P, Doherty M, Papadimitriou GM. Inflammatory responses to intradermal crystals in healthy volunteers and patients with rheumatic diseases. Rheumatol Int 1982; 2: 55–58.

42. Terkeltaub RA, Ginsberg MH. The inflammatory reaction to crystals. Rheum Dis Clin North Am 1988; 14: 353–364.

43. Kranendonk S, Ryan L, Buday M et al. Human osteoarthritic vesicles generate both monoclinic calcium pyrophosphate dihydrate and apatite crystals in vitro. J Bone Joint Surg 1994; 18: 502–503.

44. Ho A, Johnson M, Kingsley D. Role of the mouse ank gene in control of tissue calcification and arthritis. Science 2000; 289: 265–269.

45. Cheung HS, Story MT, McCarty DJ. Mitogenic effects of hydroxyapatite and calcium pyrophosphate dihydrate crystals on cultured mammalian cells. Arthritis Rheum 1984; 27: 668–674.

46. McCarthy G, Westfall P, Masuda I et al. Basic calcium phosphate crystals activate human osteoarthritis synovial fibroblasts and induce matrix metalloproteinase-13 (collagenase-3) in adult porcine articular chondrocytes. Ann Rheum Dis 2001; 60: 399–406.

47. McCarthy GM, Mitchell PG, Struve JS, Cheung HS. Basic calcium phosphate crystals cause co-ordinate induction and secretion of collagenase and stromelysin. J Cell Physiol 1992; 153: 140–146.

48. Morgan M, Fitzgerald D, McCarthy C, McCarthy G. Basic calcium phosphate crystals cause increased production of prostaglandin E2 by induction of both cyclooxygenase-1 and cyclooxygenase-2 in human fibroblasts. Arthritis Rheum 2000; 43: S281.

49. Ebenbichler G, Erdogmus C, Resch K et al. Ultrasound therapy for calcific tendinitis of the shoulder. N Engl J Med 1999; 340: 1533–1538.

50. Cheung H, Sallis J, Mitchell P, Struve J. Inhibition of basic calcium phosphate crystal-induced mitogenesis by phosphocitrate. Biochem Biophys Res Commun 1990; 171: 20–25.

51. Cheung H, Sallis J, Struve J. Specific inhibition of basic calcium phosphate and calcium pyrophosphate crystal-induction of metalloproteinase synthesis by phosphocitrate. Biochim Biophys Acta 1996; 1315: 105–111.

52. Caporali R, Rossi S, Montecucco C. Tidal irrigation in Milwaukee shoulder syndrome. J Rheumatol 1994; 21: 1781–1782.

METABOLIC BONE DISEASES

METABOLIC BONE DISEASES

44 Osteoporosis: clinical features

Piet Geusens

- Osteoporosis is the most common disease that affects bone, and is associated with increased risk of fragility fractures
- The most frequent osteoporotic fractures are those in the spine, hip, and wrist, but fractures related to osteoporosis also occur at many other skeletal sites
- Short- and long-term consequences of osteoporosis fractures include increased mortality, pain, physical impairment, increased costs of medical care, decreased quality of life, and increased risk for new fractures
- Osteoporosis is a multifactorial disease. Clinical features evident before the first fracture has occurred include a number of clinical risk factors, many of which can be readily recognized clinically (e.g. age, gender, low body weight, history of fracture, familial history of fracture, immobilization, and use of glucocorticoids)
- Osteoporosis is more common in women than in men, but the problem in men is by no means insignificant

INTRODUCTION

Osteoporosis is a disease characterized by decreased bone mass and a deterioration of bone architecture. These changes result in weaker, more fragile bone and, therefore, a higher risk of fractures. For the purpose of determining the prevalence of disease, osteoporosis has been defined as having a bone density T-score lower than −2.5. The condition is considered to be severe (symptomatic) if a fragility fracture is present in addition to low bone density[1].

In this chapter we will review the clinical features of osteoporosis. These features include the clinical consequences of fractures (clinical outcome) (Table 44.1) and the clinical predisposition (clinical risk factors) for osteoporosis and fractures (Table 44.2, Fig. 44.1). The clinical features of osteoporosis in men will be discussed separately from those in women.

Osteoporosis increases the risk of fractures, just as hypertension increases the risk of stroke. The estimated lifetime risk of fracture is 40% in 50-year-old white women and 13% in 50-year-old men

TABLE 44.2 RISK FACTORS FOR HIP FRACTURE

Bone		Falls
Bone mass	Age	Neuromuscular function
	Gender	Cognitive functions
	Hyperthyroidism	Vision
Architecture	Genetics	Medication
Micro	Familial fractures	Fall mechanisms
Macro	Previous fracture	Energy absorption
Secondary mineralization	Length	Balance
Bone turnover	Weight	Gait
	Smoking	
	Mobility	
	Glucocorticoids	
	General health	
	Calcium intake	
	Vitamin D	

Risk factors that can be directly evaluated by clinical examination are indicated in bold[94,108,109].

TABLE 44.1 CLINICAL CONSEQUENCES OF HIP, VERTEBRAL AND WRIST FRACTURES

	Hip	Vertebrae Clinical	Vertebrae Radiographic	Wrist
Excess mortality	++	+	+	−
Increased fracture risk	+	+	+	+
Pain				
Acute	+	+	+ or −	+
Chronic	−	+	+ or −	+
Functional decline				
Short-term	+++	+	+	+
Long-term	++	+	+	+
Psychosocial decline	++	+	+	−
Quality of life	+++	++	+	+

+, Yes; −, No.

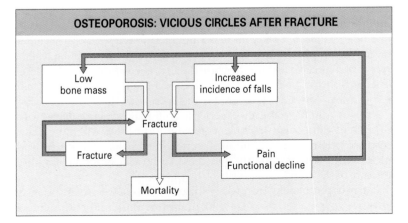

OSTEOPOROSIS: VICIOUS CIRCLES AFTER FRACTURE

Fig. 44.1 Clinical features of osteoporosis include the clinical consequences of fractures (clinical outcome) and the clinical predisposition (clinical risk factors) for osteoporosis and fractures. The clinical consequences of fractures in survivors include physical and functional limitations, reduced quality of life and an increased risk for subsequent fractures, resulting in a vicious circle of new fractures and increasing morbidity[11].

(Chapter 45). In principal, fractures should be easily diagnosed because they usually present as an acute pain episode after trauma, with clinical signs of a fracture. Nevertheless, the clinical picture can be overlooked or hidden, especially in the case of vertebral fractures, which are the most frequent fractures in postmenopausal women[2].

Fractures of long bones commonly result in acute pain with one or more clinical signs of fracture (swelling, hematoma, deformation, local crepitations, localized pain on pressure), and are easily confirmed radiographically. Some fractures, such as stress fractures, are difficult to diagnose, and local clinical signs can be confounded by arthritis or tendinitis[3]. The clinical symptoms of vertebral fractures are variable. Only about one third of all people with radiographic vertebral fractures are diagnosed clinically[2,4]. Although as many as half of people with vertebral fractures seen on radiographs in population surveys do not report having had an episode of acute pain, such fractures are associated with morbidity such as chronic back pain and loss of function[5].

The clinical consequences of fractures are related to the short- and long-term outcomes and differ according to fracture location (Table 44.1) and patient characteristics. Although individual fractures often resolve without severe long-term complications, many studies indicate that, overall, fractures are associated with increased morbidity and mortality. Fractures of the hip and clinical vertebral fractures are associated with increased mortality[6,7]. After a mean time of 7 years, patients with any osteoporosis-related fracture have a doubling of the risk for physical limitations in movement and an even higher risk for functional limitations in daily activities[8]. The clinical consequences of fractures in survivors include physical and functional limitations, reduced quality of life (QoL)[8,9], and an increased risk for subsequent fractures[10], resulting in a vicious cycle of new fractures and increasing morbidity (Fig. 44.1)[11].

Before the first fracture occurs, bone loss is asymptomatic; this fact has led to the description of osteoporosis as a 'silent thief'[12]. This asymptomatic nature of bone loss suggests that osteoporosis cannot be detected clinically before the first fragility fracture occurs, unless bone density is measured. Bone densitometry is considered the gold standard for diagnosis of osteoporosis[1]. The clinical question, then, is how to identify patients at risk for osteoporosis before the first fracture has occurred, in order to select the right patients for bone densitometry and treatment[13,14]. Clinical signs and symptoms, together with anthropometric characteristics of the patient, have limited value for estimating women's actual bone density and need for treatment[13,14]. However, clinical risk factors such as age and weight can be used to help decide which patients are more likely to have osteoporosis, and who should have bone density measurements to confirm the diagnosis or rule out disease[15,16]. Furthermore, clinical risk factors for fracture can be useful in identifying women at high risk of fracture (case finding)[13,14]. Indeed, osteoporosis is a multifactorial disease that includes several risk factors, such as age, sex, and body weight, that can be readily recognized in clinical practice before the first fracture occurs. Therefore, osteoporosis can be rather described as a clinically 'hidden' – but still recognizable – disease before the first fracture occurs.

Patients who have already experienced a fragility fracture have twice the risk of subsequent fractures compared with those without a prior fracture[10]. However, osteoporosis often remains undiagnosed and untreated, even in patients that have sustained a clinical fragility fracture of the vertebrae or hip[17].

Patients can benefit from early diagnosis of osteoporosis, because effective therapies are available for the prevention and treatment of osteoporosis and associated fragility fractures[13,14]. For example, the risk of additional fractures can be reduced in patients with a prevalent vertebral fracture (Chapter 45). In addition, treatment can prevent the occurrence of a first fracture in patients with low bone density (Chapter 45). Furthermore, fracture prevention is associated with preservation of quality of life[18].

CLINICAL FEATURES OF FRACTURES: SHORT- AND LONG-TERM OUTCOMES

Wrist fractures

Wrist fractures occur after a fall. In women, the incidence of wrist fracture increases from approximately 0.1% per year below age 45 to approximately 0.7% per year at ages 65 and older[19]. Functional outcome after fracture has been studied in clinical case studies ranging in duration from weeks up to a decade[20–23]. Persisting hand pain (29–44% of patients), weakness (36–40%), and algodystrophy are the most commonly reported consequences[20–23]. Mortality is not increased after wrist fracture[6].

Impairment of activities of daily living (ADL) is reported in one population-based cohort[8]. Seven years after a wrist fracture, women with fracture were three times more likely than women without fracture to report difficulty in shopping for groceries or clothing[8]. They were nine times more likely to report difficulty cooking and 2–3 times more likely to report difficulty getting in and out a car or descending stairs than women who had never fractured their wrist[8]. The true frequency of reported algodystrophy is unknown with reports varying from 0.1–47%. This high variability is due to differences in diagnostic criteria, patient selection, and measures[24]. Prospective studies indicate that several symptoms of algodystrophy still persist after 10 years[21,23].

Patients with a wrist fracture have an increased risk of having osteoporosis and approximately twice the risk for sustaining other fractures compared with patients without wrist fractures[10]. However, only a small proportion of women with a wrist fracture currently receive osteoporosis follow-up care or treatment[25].

Hip fractures

Hip fractures are the most serious consequence of osteoporosis in terms of disability, mortality, and use of hospital and institutional care[26]. Hip fractures usually occur after a fall to the side or straight down[27], but only 1% of falls among the elderly result in a hip fracture. The frequency of spontaneous insufficiency hip fractures is low (0.27% in a survey in nursing homes)[28]. Clinical signs of hip fracture include severe, acute functional restriction resulting in immobilization and hospitalization. Typically, the leg is shortened and in exorotation. Almost all hip fractures require urgent surgical intervention for optimal recovery[29].

The immediate clinical consequences of hip fracture can be dramatic. Many patients are unable to move or summon help after falling, and may be hypothermic when found. Hospital complications are common (occurring in more than 30% of patients)[30,31] and are often related to the implants used (dislocation, fixation failure, infection) or to anesthetic stress.

Patients with hip fracture are particularly prone to complications. General complications (cardiovascular, pulmonary and cerebral problems, and infections) and local complications (wound and prosthetic problems) also occur in the post-fracture period. These complications have been reported to affect more than 30% of patients 4 months after hip fracture and more than 10% of patients 1 year after hip fracture[30]. Similar data are available from a 2-year follow-up study[31].

Mortality

In-hospital mortality ranges between 1 and 9%[32,33] but can be as high as 55% in patients with end-stage dementia or pneumonia[34]. Approximately 20–25% of hip fracture patients die within the first year[32] and 19% more hip fracture patients than controls die within 5 years[6]. After adjustment for many other predictors of hip fracture, women with a hip fracture are still 2.4 times more likely to die than women without fracture[6].

Hospitalization and institutionalization

The number of hospital bed days for patients with hip fracture is higher than that for patients with stroke, diabetes, or myocardial infarction in at least one survey[35] (Fig. 44.2). The combined costs of hospitalization and medical care during the 12 months after a hip fracture are approximately three times higher than for patients without hip fractures[36].

The wide variation in practice patterns and availability of services make it difficult to estimate the proportions of patients who are transferred to nursing homes[32]. The duration of stay in nursing homes after hip fracture was 1 month in 24% of patients, 6 months in 10%, and more than 1 year in 34%[37].

Morbidity

Substantial short- and long-term morbidity has been documented in survivors of a hip fracture, both in terms of suffering and cost. Functional competence and physical functioning markedly diminish after hip fracture[30,32,33,38–44]. After 3 months, physical performance had decreased by 51%, vitality by 24% and social function by 26% compared with pre-fracture levels[44]. After 6 months, only 24% of patients had returned to prefracture walking competence, and only 43% had returned to prefracture basic ADL[38]. Little further improvement occurred after 1 year[30,41].

Of the women who could dress independently before fracture, only 60% were able to do so after hip fracture, and only two thirds were able to resume independent transferring (from bed to chair or standing from chair) (Fig. 44.3)[39]. The proportion of women that could walk across a room independently dropped from 75% before the hip fracture to 15% 6 months after the fracture. Similarly, the proportions of women able to walk one half mile dropped from 41% before fracture to 6% 6 months after fracture, while the proportion of women able to climb stairs dropped from 63% to 8%[39]. Only 38% of women reporting independence in several ADL and basic mobility measures (including transfer from bed to chair and toilet, putting on socks and shoes, and indoor walking) recovered independence in all functions after a hip fracture[40]. Further limitations were found in cooking, performance of housework, use of transportation, grocery shopping, carrying bundles, taking medication, visiting friends, managing money, and engaging in community activities[32,41].

Indirect evidence for morbidity comes from a prospective case-controlled study of survivors of hip fracture[36]. The medical and non-medical needs were significantly higher in fracture patients than in age- and sex-matched controls. These needs were reflected in an increased number of physician contacts, increased use of physiotherapy, more days of new hospitalizations and home care, and a longer stay in nursing homes (Fig. 44.4)[36].

Fracture risk

Patients with a hip fracture have approximately twice the risk for further fractures, including a second hip fracture, compared with patients without a fracture[10].

Predictors of mortality and morbidity after hip fracture

Many of the predictors of death and long-term physical disability after hip fracture include clinical features related to the patient's health before the fracture occurs.

The elderly tend to have co-morbid conditions (such as other diseases and functional limitations); thus, hip fracture is not the sole factor leading to mortality and functional decline[32]. Indeed, outcome depends largely on the prior condition of individuals who suffer the fracture. Mortality is higher in patients who are living in an institution[31] than in other patients. Most studies evaluate physical function or mortality separately, but it appears that prefracture level of function may influence both outcomes. In a study adjusting for known risk factors, mortality at 6 months after fracture was significantly associated with pre-fracture locomotion, a score of health evaluation, and the use of paid help at home prior to fracture[33]. Furthermore, mortality and functional recovery differed between hospitals, probably because of differences in the type of care provided to patients[33]. Men have more complications than women, on average[31,32]. Longer hospital stay is associated with older age, male sex,

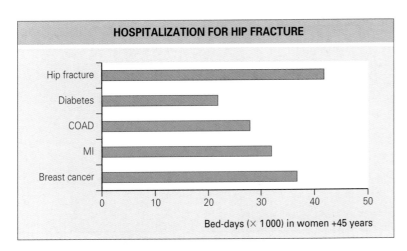

Fig. 44.2 Hospitalization for hip fracture. Number of bed-days for hip fracture or other diseases in women older than 40 years[35].

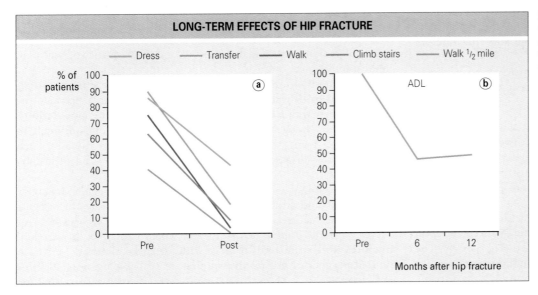

Fig. 44.3 Long-term effects of hip fracture. (a) Proportion of subjects able to perform each activity independently before hip fracture and at 6 months after sustaining a hip fracture[39]. (b) ADL during 1 year[41].

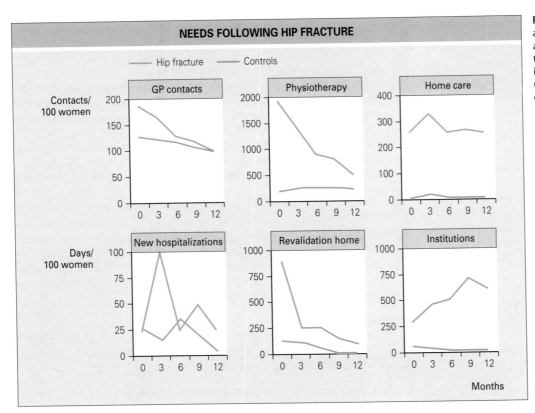

Fig. 44.4 Needs following hip fracture. The medical and non-medical needs during 12 months following a hip fracture in women were significantly higher than in age matched controls. These needs included increased number of physician contacts, increased use of physiotherapy and home care, and more days of new hospitalizations and stay in nursing homes[36].

and poorer general health[32]. Patients living in an institution have a higher risk for pressure sores, surgical complications, and pulmonary and urinary infections than patients living independently before the fracture[31]. Morbidity after hip fracture is higher after an intertrochanteric fracture than after a fracture of the femoral neck but the reason for this is uncertain[32]. Although the level of prefracture condition of the patient is a major determinant for recovery, even patients with good prefracture functioning often recover only partially[39].

Other appendicular fractures

With the exception of fractures in patients with metastatic bone disease, almost all fragility fractures occurring after the age of 40 years are associated with the presence of osteoporosis[4]. Apart from fractures of the vertebrae, wrist, and hip, the most frequent other fractures are those of the ribs, proximal humerus, pelvis, and legs[8]. No data are available concerning the risk of mortality after these fractures. Morbidity, however, can be substantial in the elderly and is associated with complications of the fracture, such as soft tissue lesions and incomplete recovery of adjacent joint function (e.g. in the shoulder after fracture of the proximal humerus)[29].

Furthermore, the risk for new fractures is approximately twice as high in patients with these fractures than in patients without a history of fracture[10].

VERTEBRAL FRACTURES

Hippocrates discussed the diagnosis and treatment of vertebral fractures approximately 2000 years ago, but the fractures he described presumably occurred after severe trauma[45,46]. It was only recently that Albright *et al.* reported that the majority of vertebral fractures in postmenopausal women are a result of relatively minor trauma[46,47].

The clinical features of osteoporotic vertebral fractures are quite different from other osteoporotic fractures. Only one in three vertebral fractures comes to clinical attention and is diagnosed (Fig. 44.5)[4,46]. The reasons for this low rate of diagnosis are not fully understood, but may be related to the variable degree of preceding trauma[47,48], the variable

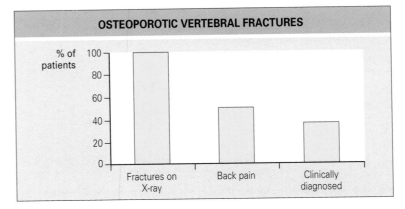

Fig. 44.5 Osteoporotic vertebral fractures. In population-based studies of patients with radiographically identified vertebral fractures, 50% have back pain and only one in three come to clinical attention and diagnosis[2].

degree of pain intensity and duration[49,50], and the frequency of back pain in the population[2].

An evaluation of the clinical outcomes of vertebral fracture is further complicated by differences in the criteria for defining a prevalent or incident vertebral fracture and differences in study populations. Furthermore, 'wedge' vertebral fractures are sometimes difficult to differentiate from wedging associated with other diseases such Scheuermann's disease, remodeling in osteoarthritis[51], and metastatic bone disease[4].

The consequences of vertebral fracture have been extensively reviewed[52–55] and studied from two perspectives: studies in patients with clinical fractures with or without controls (clinical cases)[4,56–64] or surveys of radiographic deformities in which patients with vertebral fractures were compared to those without such fractures[5,18,50,65–72]. A limited number of prospective studies are available using serial spine radiographs[5,18,69,71]. Many studies used a variety of measures that are not specific for evaluation of the outcomes of vertebral fractures. Recently, however, more uniform evaluation of outcomes was introduced with the development of osteoporosis-specific measures of quality of life (QoL; see Table 44.3).

Mortality

Mortality is increased after vertebral fractures by 19% compared with the general population[6], and by 23–60% compared with people without vertebral fractures in other studies[7,73–75]. The age-adjusted relative risk for dying after vertebral fracture is as high as 8.6[7]. Increased mortality is observed shortly after the fracture and has been attributed to poor physical condition and acute medical consequences[6,46]. However, an increased risk of death compared with people without vertebral fracture persists for at least 5 years after a vertebral fracture[46]. In one study, the increased risk of death was associated with clinical problems such as pulmonary disease and cancer[73]. The rate of death among vertebral fracture cases is highest in patients with multiple vertebral fractures[73] and in patients who required hospitalization because of vertebral fracture[76].

Fracture risk

Patients with a prevalent (pre-existing) vertebral fracture have approximately 4 times greater risk for new vertebral fracture[77,78], and twice the risk of hip and other non-vertebral fractures as patients without prevalent fracture[10,75,79,80]. This relationship is independent of bone density; patients who have both low bone density and an existing vertebral fracture have a higher risk of subsequent fractures than those with only low bone density or only an existing vertebral fracture, who in turn have a higher risk than those without either low BMD or prevalent vertebral fracture[10,77]. The risk of additional vertebral fracture is extremely high among those patients with multiple past vertebral fractures[18,77]. For example, the risk of an additional vertebral fracture is 12 times higher among those with two or more vertebral fractures at baseline, compared to women without existing vertebral fracture[77]. More than half of women with five or more vertebral fractures at baseline experienced additional fractures within the subsequent 3.8 years of observation[18]. Importantly, after experiencing an initial vertebral fracture, additional vertebral fractures will occur within 1 year in one in five postmenopausal women with osteoporosis (Fig. 44.6)[78]. Osteoporosis is, therefore, a quickly progressive disease in many postmenopausal women. The clinical message is that vertebral fracture should be recognized and treated early in order to prevent future vertebral fractures.

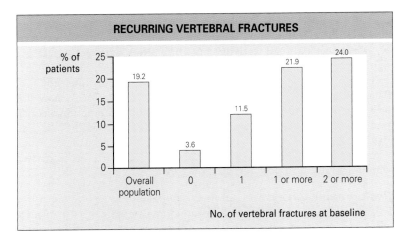

RECURRING VERTEBRAL FRACTURES

Fig. 44.6 Recurring vertebral fractures. Incidence of new vertebral fractures in the year following vertebral fracture. After experiencing an initial vertebral fracture, additional vertebral fractures will occur within one year in one in five postmenopausal women with osteoporosis[78].

Back pain in clinically diagnosed (symptomatic) cases

In patients with severe osteoporosis, vertebral fractures often occur after minimal trauma. In patients with clinically diagnosed vertebral fractures, 14% followed severe trauma, 83% followed moderate or no trauma, and 3% were pathologic[4]. In another study, pain onset was sudden in 73% of women with vertebral fracture, compared with 21% in women with chronic low back pain without fractures[56]. The vertebral fracture occurred after an accident at home (such as a fall or stumble) in 13% of cases, after lifting a heavy load in 24% of cases, and without any evident reason in 44% of cases. A total of 19% of women reported a more gradual beginning of complaints[56]. Severe back pain (71%) and height reduction (10%) were the most common events that triggered further investigation[56]. The mean duration of symptoms before fracture diagnosis was 7 days, but 25% of fractures were diagnosed clinically after more than 1 month[4].

Acute back pain episode

As noted above, not all vertebral fracture patients report having acute pain, and the severity of back pain varies substantially among patients who do experience pain. Symptoms of an acute clinical vertebral fracture include sudden moderate to severe lancing back pain, which worsens on movement and is often relieved by rest[48]. The pain can be sufficiently severe to cause breathlessness, pallor, nausea, and vomiting, and is exacerbated by coughing or sneezing. The pain often radiates laterally following the dermatomal distribution and is often accompanied by spasms of the paraspinal muscles. On clinical examination, tenderness can be elicited over the affected vertebrae and paraspinal muscles and mobility of the spine is restricted and painful. However, pain is sometimes diffuse and not localized to the fractured vertebra. Variable degrees of kyphosis of the thoracic spine can be found in the case of a thoracic vertebral fracture, and flattened (reduced) lumbar lordosis in the case of a lumbar vertebral fracture. This acute, severe pain episode gradually subsides within 2–6 weeks.

Chronic back pain

Restoration of normal spinal anatomy is not possible following vertebral fracture. Therefore, even vertebral fractures without acute symptoms contribute to chronic morbidity[81]. Patients with clinical vertebral fracture are at increased risk for chronic back pain[65]. Pain is most commonly reported as deeply localized and bone- or muscle-related[48]. It is described variously as tearing, burning, piercing, drilling, dull, convulsive, or dragging[48].

The most frequent triggers for pain are sitting, standing, staying in the same position for a long time, bending, walking, and sudden movements[48]. In many patients, pain is relieved by lying, sitting, changing position, application of warmth, gymnastics, drugs, or aversion[48]. Compared with patients with chronic low back pain without fractures, chronic back pain after a vertebral fracture is more effectively relieved by lying down, is more aggravated by doing housework, and is more frequently only present during physical activity[48]. No specific circadian rhythm of pain is found. The frequency of pain is variable (several times per week or per day, permanent, or dependent on physical stress)[48].

Back pain after an acute pain episode can last for many years and decreases over time[48,69]. One study surveyed patients with chronic back pain 4 years after an acute painful fracture; back pain was mild in 27%, moderate in 44% and severe in 29% of these patients[62]. In another study, half of the patients with symptomatic clinically-diagnosed vertebral fracture reported slight to moderate chronic pain after 4 years, the other half reported severe to intolerable pain[48].

In clinical cases, chronic back pain is related to the number and severity of vertebral fractures[48,59,63], but not to small reductions in vertebral height (minor vertebral deformities)[62]. In some studies, pain was related to the degree of kyphosis[59] and height loss[82,83].

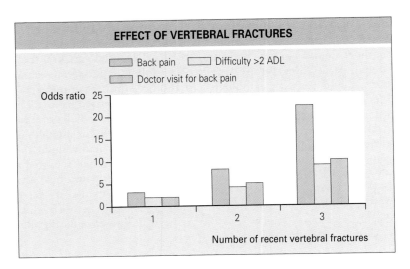

Fig. 44.7 Effect of vertebral fractures. Odds ratio for pain and disability increase by number of recent vertebral fractures[70,71].

Back pain in fractures derived from radiographic surveys

In cross-sectional population studies measuring vertebral dimensions on radiographs, chronic back pain was related to the number and severity of vertebral fractures in some studies[50,65,68]. Other studies failed to detect an association, perhaps because of methodologic problems such as less stringent morphometric vertebral fracture criteria[66], or a relatively small number of women with severe deformities[83].

In prospective studies using serial radiographs to detect new vertebral fractures, a single new vertebral fracture increased the odds for back pain (reported at the end of the study, not at the time of the vertebral fracture) threefold, whereas two and three fractures increased the odds of back pain by eight and 22 times, respectively[70,71] (Fig. 44.7). The pain frequency index increased approximately threefold relative to prefracture levels and pain was long lasting (twofold increase of pain frequency index after 3.5 years)[65]. New vertebral fractures, even those not recognized clinically, are associated with substantial increases in back pain in older women (Fig. 44.8)[5].

In contrast to these studies in which radiographic deformities were meticulously documented, radiographic vertebral fractures are often overlooked in daily clinical practice. A survey of 934 hospitalized older women with an available chest radiograph was used to evaluate the frequency with which vertebral fractures were identified and treated by clinicians[84]. Moderate-to-severe vertebral fractures were identified in 132 (14.1%) of the study subjects, but only 1.7% had a discharge diagnosis of vertebral fracture[84]. Of these, 50% were recorded in the radiology reports and only 17% had a fracture noted in the medical record or discharge summary[84].

Physical and functional outcomes of vertebral fractures

Pain, hyperkyphosis, and loss of spinal mobility result in multiple forms of disability[32]. Pain and disabilities cause a spiralling decline in function, mobility, and muscle strength[58,64,85]. This decline in function, in turn, contributes to pain and to an increased risk of falls[86], bone loss[87], fractures[10], and loss of independence[48,56] (Fig. 44.1).

Clinical cases

Vertebral fractures were associated with increased kyphosis in several studies[56,88-90], but not in one study that analyzed only severe vertebral fractures[50]. Hyperkyphosis results in the typical clinical presentation of a 'dowager's hump' (Fig. 44.9).

Vertebral fractures are associated with height loss[54,56]. During a follow-up period of 8 years, standing height decreased by approximately 1cm with each new wedge or crush vertebral fracture, but not with endplate fractures[72]. Significant height loss has also been described in women with

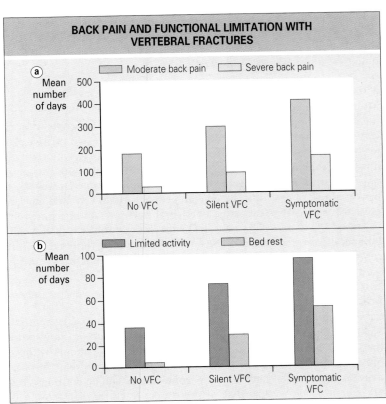

Fig. 44.8 Back pain and functional limitation with vertebral fractures. New vertebral fractures (VFC), even those not recognized clinically, are associated with substantial increases in (a) back pain and (b) functional limitation due to back pain in older women[5].

postmenopausal osteoporosis in control groups of clinical trials and was three times greater (4.6mm/year) in women with new vertebral fractures than in women without vertebral fracture (1.8mm/year)[91].

Hyperkyphosis and height loss also reduce the distance between the iliac crest and ribs[48], resulting in problems with digestion and a protruding abdomen that makes fitting clothes difficult and detracts from appearance[54]. Loss of spinal mobility due to vertebral fracture has been associated with difficulty in dressing, fixing hair, standing, laying down, moving in bed, doing housework, walking, climbing stairs, washing, bathing, using the toilet, and getting to the floor[48,54,59]. Lung function progressively decreases with increasing number of vertebral fractures and the degree of kyphosis, perhaps as a result of increased abdominal pressure[92,93].

Functional disability was higher in patients with two or more vertebral fractures and was related to height reduction, kyphosis, and distance between ribs and iliac crest[48]. Functional performance measures (level of assistance, pain on activity and difficulties with activities) are significantly reduced in patients with vertebral fracture[58].

General measures of health and ADL are significantly affected[48,56-58]. Balance capability, an important risk factor for hip fracture[94], may also be affected[54]. Physical performance measures such as functional reach, mobility skills, and 6 minute walk[58] and muscle strength[58] are also significantly decreased.

Increased dependency with need for help in self-care was associated with moderate and severe vertebral fractures[56,57].

Radiographic surveys

In general, the same physical and functional outcomes as in clinical cases are reported in population and case-controlled radiographic surveys[50,54,59,65,95]. In the Study of Osteoporotic Fractures (SOF), the odds of impaired function (difficulty with more than two ADL) was 2.3 times higher among elderly women with a history of clinically diagnosed vertebral fracture[95]. New vertebral fractures, even those not recognized

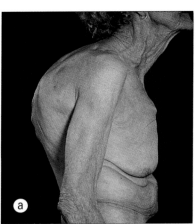

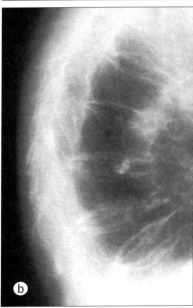

Fig. 44.9 Dowager's hump.
(a) Marked thoracic kyphosis due to multiple osteoporotic fractures in an elderly woman with (b) corresponding radiograph.

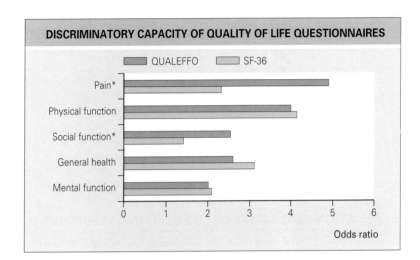

DISCRIMINATORY CAPACITY OF QUALITY OF LIFE QUESTIONNAIRES

Fig. 44.10 Discriminatory capacity of quality of life questionnaires (disease targeted QUALEFFO and generic SF-36) in a radiographic survey comparing patients with and without vertebral fracture[96]. *$p < 0.05$ between QUALEFFO and SF-36.

clinically, are associated with substantial increases in functional limitation due to back pain in older women (Fig. 44.8)[5].

A multidimensional and validated osteoporosis-targeted quality of life questionnaire (QUALEFFO) has been used in another population study to assess the impact of vertebral fractures[68]. Patients with vertebral fracture had a higher QUALEFFO score than patients with low BMD without a vertebral fracture indicating more. The total score and its subdomains (pain, physical function, general health and physical mobility) correlated with the number of vertebral fractures (Fig. 44.10)[68]. Lumbar vertebral fractures led to greater impairment of physical function than thoracic vertebral fractures, and were associated with lower physical function, lower general health, and a lower total QUALEFFO score[68].

Effect of pharmacologic treatment on quality of life (QoL) related to vertebral fracture

One of the earliest clinical observations in the prevention of osteoporosis is a cross-sectional study that found that hormone replacement therapy protected against height loss in postmenopausal women (Chapter 45). More convincing evidence of fracture efficacy comes from several prospective, randomized, placebo-controlled studies using raloxifene or bisphosphonates (Chapter 45).

In a preliminary study with raloxifene, the occurrence of new vertebral fracture was associated with significant deterioration in QUALEFFO score[96].

In patients of the Fracture Intervention Trial, the number of days with limited activity or bed rest rose immediately and sharply after an incident vertebral fracture, most prominently in patients with clinical vertebral fracture but also in patients with morphometric vertebral fracture without acute pain (Fig. 44.8)[18]. Treatment with alendronate significantly reduced the number of days of bedrest and disability; during 3 years of follow up, there were more than 3000 additional days affected by back pain among the 1005 women randomized to placebo compared with the 1022 women in the alendronate group[18]. These findings indicate that effective fracture prevention using bone-specific treatments helps to prevent reductions in QoL associated with osteoporotic fractures.

Psychosocial outcomes of vertebral fractures

Psychosocial consequences may not be evident clinically or may be excluded from the medical history because patients themselves are reluctant to discuss or complain about them[32]. Psychosocial outcome has been studied using a variety of measures, including individual questions, general measures, or osteoporosis-specific measures of psychosocial status[32]. Unfortunately, many studies did not include a control group.

Psychiatric symptoms were significantly worse after vertebral fracture in one study[58], but no effect of vertebral fracture on social and mental function was found in another study[68]. As is the case for pain symptoms, psychosocial outcomes vary with the time after vertebral fracture. Social extroversion and well-being were significantly decreased during the first 2 years after a new vertebral fracture than later on, in spite of similar spine deformity index and height reduction[64]. Even patients with a diagnosis of osteoporosis before fracture have a higher incidence of fear of falling (38% versus 2% in controls) and a higher proportion of patients said that they limited their activities in an attempt to avoid falling (24% versus 2%) following vertebral fracture[98].

Vertebral fractures are associated with depression[32]. Depression is the most prevalent mental health problem of older adults and can be a major problem in osteoporosis[32,99]. Depression is associated with low bone mass throughout the skeleton[100]. Some patients feel angry or depressed because the physical deformity from hyperkyphosis detracts from their appearance. Women with osteoporosis have a score three

TABLE 44.3 EVALUATION OF QUALITY OF LIFE

Instrument	No. of questions	Time (min)	Reliability to clinical	Longitudinal correlation
OFDQ[63]	56	25	yes	NA
OPAQ[102]	71	30	yes	NA
QUALEFFO[103]	54	20	yes	Yes
OPTOQOL[60,62]	26	NA	yes	NA

NA, Not available.

Disease-targeted questionnaires for clinical evaluation of quality of life in osteoporosis.

times higher and prevalence of depression compared to those without osteoporosis[100]. Depression score is related to the number and severity of vertebral fractures[63], and parameters of mood are related to the severity of vertebral fracture[48]. Loss of self-esteem can occur, presumably as a result of deformity, disability, and pain, but no studies are available on the prevalence and relation of self-esteem to vertebral fracture[99]. Many patients with vertebral fractures reported emotional problems, but no comparison with a control group was reported[57].

EVALUATION OF QUALITY OF LIFE (QoL) IN OSTEOPOROSIS

Emphasis on the number of fractures provides an incomplete accounting of the clinical consequences of osteoporosis, given the many non-skeletal consequences of fracture. As discussed above, common physical and social outcomes, such as loss of height, kyphosis, chronic back pain, digestive problems, decreased mobility, loss of independence and depression lead to a chronic decrease in QoL. QoL measures can therefore be helpful in clinical studies, and are applicable in daily clinical practice[101].

QoL includes the functioning and performance of individuals in their daily lives and their subjective perception of well-being[102]. These aspects can be assessed by performance measures and questionnaires (self-reporting or by interview).

Examples of generic (not disease-targeted) questionnaires used in osteoporosis are the SF-36, the AIMS2, the Nottingham Health Profile (NHP), the Sickness Impact Profile (SIP), and the Health Assessment Questionnaire (HAQ)[102]. Generic measures may, however, be unresponsive to changes in a specific disease.

Several disease-targeted measures of QoL in osteoporosis are available (Table 44.3). These include the Osteoporosis Functional Disability Questionnaire (OFDQ)[63], the QoL Questionnaire for Osteoporosis (OPTOQLQ)[60,62], the Osteoporosis Assessment Questionnaire (OPAQ)[102], and the QoL Questionnaire of the European Foundation for Osteoporosis (QUALEFFO)[103]. The use of QoL measures in osteoporosis was reviewed by a working group of the Outcome Measures in Rheumatology Clinical Trials (OMERACT)[104–106]. Several of these QoL measures have been shown to have discriminant value (Table 44.4). Studies on minimal clinically important differences (MCID) of these measures are in progress[106]. Only limited prospective data are available on validated multidimensional QoL measures in the natural course and during therapy of osteoporosis[102,104–106]. Studies are, at the time being, underway[96,105].

QUALEFFO was shown to be more discriminative than SF-36 for pain and social function, indicating that this questionnaire is useful in osteoporosis patients with vertebral fracture (Fig. 44.10)[103]. Postal administration of the QUALEFFO has been shown to be reliable, and comparable to nurse-supported administration[107].

CLINICAL FEATURES BEFORE THE FIRST FRACTURE: CLINICAL RISK FACTORS

A fracture is the result of an overload of the mechanical competence of the skeleton. The risk for fractures is therefore related to the degree of osteo-

TABLE 44.4 CLINICAL RISK FACTORS INCLUDED IN QUESTIONNAIRES

	SCORE[60]	OST[15]	SOFSURF[111]	ORAI[110]
Age	X	X	X	X
Weight	X	X	X	X
History of fracture	X	–	X	–
Smoking	–	–	–	X
Race	X	–	–	–
Rheumatoid arthritis	X	–	–	–
Estrogen intake	X	–	–	X

X, Evaluated; –, Not evaluated.

These are the risk factors included in various questionnaires for the clinical diagnosis of osteoporosis.

porosis and to the risk of trauma, most commonly a fall. The etiology of osteoporotic fragility fractures is thus multifactorial, including a number of clinical risk factors. This fact is best illustrated in studies of risk factors for hip fracture[94,108,109]. These studies have shown that some risk factors are associated with low bone density, others to trauma, and others to both. Furthermore, it has been demonstrated that the number of clinical risk factors is associated with hip fracture risk, independent of and in addition to bone density (Fig. 44.11)[108]. In clinical studies of the effects of bisphosphonates in glucocorticoid-induced osteoporosis, the incidence of vertebral fractures was substantially higher in elderly postmenopausal women than in premenopausal women (Chapter 45).

Clinical risk factors of osteoporosis (e.g. low body weight, age) can be present long before the first fracture occurs, but some risk factors (e.g. use of high-dose glucocorticoids) have dramatic effects within a short time. Some risk factors have a high prevalence (e.g. hip fracture in the mother) but are associated with moderate fracture risk; others are rather rare (e.g. glucocorticoid use after transplantation) but are associated with a high risk for fractures. Among the most common clinical risk factors are the menopause (type I, postmenopausal osteoporosis), age (type II, senile osteoporosis), and the use of glucocorticoids or other drugs known to be associated with bone loss (type III, secondary osteoporosis). Additional common and strong risk factors are history of previous fracture, low body weight, and family history of fractures. Less common risk factors for osteoporosis are primary hypogonadism, anorexia nervosa, mal-absorption, primary hyperparathyroidism, gastrectomy, Cushing's syndrome, organ transplantation, rheumatoid arthritis, epilepsy, Parkinson's disease, dementia, and previous cardiovascular accident.

Clinical evaluation of risk factors

Bone densitometry is the golden standard for the diagnosis of osteoporosis[1]. However, there is no justification for screening the whole population using densitometry[13,14]. Clinical case finding of patients at risk for osteoporosis is therefore advocated[13,14].

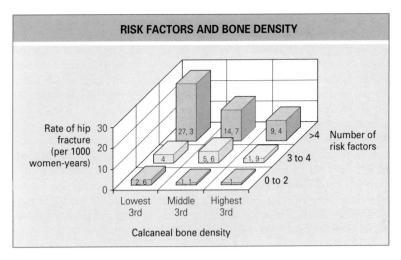

RISK FACTORS AND BONE DENSITY

Fig. 44.11 Risk factors and bone density. Annual risk of hip fracture according to the number of risk factors and the age-specific calcaneal bone density. The number of clinical risk factors is associated with hip fracture risk, independent and additive to bone density[108].

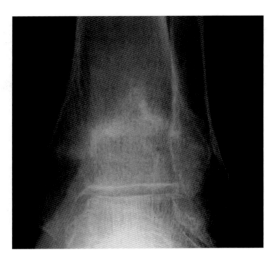

Fig. 44.12 Stress fractures of the distal tibia in a patient with rheumatoid arthritis during methotrexate therapy.

Several questionnaires focusing on the clinical recognition of risk factors for osteoporosis have been studied (Table 44.4). The purpose of these indices is not to diagnose osteoporosis or low BMD, but rather to identify women who are more likely to have low BMD, for the purpose of identifying individuals who could then undergo BMD measurement for a definitive assessment. The simplest questionnaire is the Osteoporosis Self-assessment Tool (OST), which is based on age and weight[15]. Other indices, such as the Simple Calculated Osteoporosis Risk Estimation (SCORE)[60], the Osteoporosis Risk Assessment Index (ORAI)[110], and SOFSURF (derived using data from the Study of Osteoporotic Fractures, SOF)[111], involve 1–4 other risk factors in addition to age and weight. They are based on a combination of risk factors, selected on the basis of the available evidence of their relationhip to osteoporosis and fracture risk.

It is important for the rheumatologist to be aware of the common risk factors and those that may be rare in the general population but more common among patients seen in the rheumatological practice. Indeed, recent data indicate that many patients with metabolic bone disease consult a rheumatologist[112], and that rheumatologists thus are in a favorable position to identify patients with primary and secondary osteoporosis. In a survey of 669 patients with osteoporotic vertebral fractures diagnosed in a rheumatology department over a period of 10 years, one in five women and one in two men had secondary osteoporosis[113]. The conditions most commonly associated with secondary osteoporosis in this setting were glucocorticoid use, chronic obstructive lung disease, and rheumatoid arthritis.

Evaluation of clinical risk factors (with the exception of a history of a fragility fracture) is no substitute for measuring bone density when bone-directed therapy is started. Indeed, in the absence of a prevalent vertebral fracture, a proven low bone density is a prerequisite for patient selection for therapy with bisphosphonates such as alendronate and risedronate (Chapter 16)[114,115]. Risedronate was shown to decrease the risk of hip fracture in elderly postmenopausal women known to have osteoporosis, but no effect could be found in elderly postmenopausal women with mainly fall-related clinical risk factors for hip fracture without proven low bone density in the hip[115].

CLINICAL FEATURES OF OSTEOPOROSIS IN MEN

Osteoporosis is less frequent in men than in women because men develop a higher peak bone mass and lose less bone during later life than women.

However, osteoporotic fractures in men are far from uncommon. The clinical features of osteoporosis in men are less well documented than those in women. The available data indicate that osteoporosis in men has some specific features that are different from osteoporosis in women.

Vertebral fractures

The prevalence of vertebral fractures in men is as high as in women at the age of 50 years[116]. In radiographic surveys, however, these radiographic fractures have not been related to back pain[116]. In contrast, in men with clinical vertebral fracture, back pain can last more than 5 years[113] and height loss of more than 2.5cm is common (more than 50%)[117]. Many men with clinical vertebral fracture have decreased QoL, as measured by NHP, a score that assesses energy, pain, emotion, sleep, social function, and mobility[117].

In contrast to women, half of men with clinical vertebral fractures have secondary osteoporosis[113,118]. Men with symptomatic vertebral fracture are usually younger than women[113]. Therefore, causes of secondary osteoporosis should always be evaluated in men with vertebral fracture (Table 44.5).

Hip fractures

As in women, hip fracture risk in men is associated with reduced bone mass and trauma[119]. In a population survey, an increased risk for hip fracture in men was associated with metabolic disease and disorders of movement or balance[120]. The risk for hip fracture was higher in individuals with a history of thyroidectomy, gastric resection, pernicious anemia, chronic bronchitis, or emphysema[120]. Movement and balance disorders associated with an increased risk for hip fracture include neurological disorders (hemiplegia, Parkinsonism, dementia), vertigo, alcoholism, anemia, blindness and use of a cane or walker[120]. The prognosis of men with hip fracture is worse than in women and mortality is higher[31].

STRESS FRACTURES

Stress fractures (also called fatigue fractures) are a particular presentation of fractures related to fatigue damage of bone[3] (Fig. 44.12). Stress fractures have multifactorial causes, including activity level and intensity, bone geometry and bone density. There are two types of stress fracture. *Insufficiency fractures* occur in diseased bone that is involved in routine activity. There are several reports of these fractures in rheumatoid arthritis, some of which are associated with the use of methotrexate[121]. *Fatigue fractures* occur in normal healthy bone repeatedly subjected to high-level stress. Fatigue fractures typically occur after repetitive strain, such as walking, jogging and jumping, especially in young healthy persons involved in new activities, e.g. military recruits[3].

TABLE 44.5 CAUSES OF OSTEOPOROSIS IN MEN

Endocrine diseases	Hypogonadism*
	Cushing's syndrome
	Hyperthyroidism
	Primary hyperparathyroidism
	Hyperprolactinemia
	Idiopathic renal hypercalciuria*
Accompanying osteomalacia	
Neoplastic disease	Multiple myeloma
	Myelo- and lymphoproliferative disease
	Systemic mastocytosis
	Diffuse bony metastases*
	Vertebral metastasis
Drugs/toxins	Glucocorticoids*
	Alcohol abuse*
	Excessive thyroid hormone replacement
	Heparin
	Anticonvulsants*
Genetic collagen disorders	Osteogenesis imperfecta
	Ehlers–Danlos syndrome
	Marfan's syndrome
	Homocystinuria
	Hemochromatosis
Other disorders	Skeletal sarcoidosis
	Gaucher's disease
	Adult hypophosphatasia
	Hemoglobinopathies
Other factors	Chronic illness (rheumatoid arthritis, liver/renal disease)
	Prolonged immobilization
	Malnutrition (including calcium deficiency and scurvy)
	Gastrectomy*
	Aging*
Idiopathic	Juvenile
	Adult*

* Most frequent causes.

Clinical recognition of stress fractures is often difficult, as they can occur in skeletal sites that are unexpected for classical osteoporosis. They often are difficult to diagnose clinically and not readily recognizable on plain radiographs. Other imaging techniques, such as bone scintigraphy, computer tomography or magnetic resonance imaging, may be needed to identify stress fractures.

DIFFERENTIAL DIAGNOSIS OF VERTEBRAL FRACTURES

Only one in three vertebral fractures comes to clinical attention and diagnosis (Fig. 44.5)[4,46]. Clinical symptoms of vertebral fractures are highly variable. Some vertebral fractures are readily recognizable because of an acute pain episode, with typical irradiating pain and localized pain on pressure. Other patients may have no or mild symptoms and can be overlooked[2]. In contrast to most non-vertebral fractures, many vertebral fractures do not occur as a result of a specific trauma such as a fall, but occur spontaneously or after trivial activities such as bending or lifting[47,48]. Vertebral fractures are common among elderly women, but are often overlooked – perhaps because patients and physicians may accept symptoms of back pain as a normal phenomenon of age and osteoarthritis[2]. Back pain is common in the population, and symptoms of different back conditions are non-specific, making it difficult to distinguish osteoporotic vertebral fracture from other underlying causes of pain[2]. Moreover, an individual can suffer from more than one type of back problem, either at different times or simultaneously[2]. Some patients with acute back pain can be diagnosed erroneously as having an acute fracture, when in fact the deformity had been present on earlier films. Indeed, the duration of pain is difficult to establish, and additional fractures or a progression of an exisiting vertebral deformity can occur, leading to new episodes of pain[49]. In cross-sectional studies, vertebral deformities probably have developed years before the examination, so that acute back pain and disability could have been missed[50].

Once a vertebral fracture is diagnosed, its cause remains to be determined. Vertebral fractures occurring as a result of osteoporosis should be differentiated from wedging associated with other diseases such Sheurmann's disease, remodeling in osteoarthritis[51], and metastatic bone disease[4].

When a vertebral fracture is caused by osteoporosis, it has to be determined if the fracture is due to primary or secondary osteoporosis. In men in particular, causes of secondary osteoporosis should be carefully assessed, as one in two men with vertebral fracture have secondary osteoporosis (Table 44.5). The incidence of secondary osteoporosis in women in the population has not been established. In women attending an osteoporosis clinic, 11% had a new, unsuspected diagnosis associated with bone loss[121]. The proportion of women with previously undiagnosed conditions may even be higher in osteoporotic women without major risk factors for osteoporosis[81]. In one study, 31% had new diagnoses, such as hypercalciuria, vitamin D deficiency, hyperthyroidism, hyperparathyroidism, gluten-enteropathy, myeloma, Cushing's syndrome and Paget's disease[81]. Thus, a careful history and physical examination are indicated in every patient with osteoporosis. Vigorous pursuit of other diagnoses is appropriate for an osteoporotic woman without major risk factors, with atypical pain or persistence of severe pain for more than 10–12 weeks, or general symptoms (weight loss, diffuse bone pains). In such case, malignant bone diseases, such as osteolytic bone metastases, multiple myeloma and malignant lymphoma of bone, need to be excluded. Further differential diagnoses include osteomalacia, other marrow dysplasias or infiltration, connective tissue diseases, and gastrointestinal and renal disorders. Additional laboratory testing and more sophisticated imaging, such as bone scintigraphy, computer tomography, or magnetic resonance imaging, are then indicated.

REFERENCES

1. World Health Organization. Assessment of fracture risk and its application to screening for postmenopausal osteoporosis. Geneva: World Health Organization Technical Report Series no. 843; 1994.
2. Ross PD. Risk factors for osteoporotic fracture. Endocrinol Metab Clin North Am 1998; 27: 289–301.
3. Parfitt AM. Bone age, mineral density, and fatigue damage. Calcif Tissue Int 1993; 53 (suppl 1): S82–85; discussion S85–86.
4. Cooper C, Atkinson EJ et al. Incidence of clinically diagnosed vertebral fractures: a population-based study in Rochester, Minnesota, 1985–1989. J Bone Miner Res 1992; 7: 221–227.
5. Nevitt MC, Ettinger B et al. The association of radiographically detected vertebral fractures with back pain and function: a prospective study. Ann Intern Med 1998; 128: 793–800.
6. Cooper C, Atkinson EJ et al. Population-based study of survival after osteoporotic fractures. Am J Epidemiol 1993; 137: 1001–1005.
7. Cauley JA, Thompson DE et al. Risk of mortality following clinical fractures. Osteoporos Int 2000; 11: 556–561.
8. Greendale GA, Barrett-Connor E et al. Late physical and functional effects of osteoporotic fracture in women: the Rancho Bernardo Study. J Am Geriatr Soc 1995; 43: 955–961.

9. Greendale GA, DeAmicis TA et al. A prospective study of the effect of fracture on measured physical performance: results from the MacArthur Study–MAC. J Am Geriatr Soc 2000; 48: 546–549.

10. Klotzbuecher CM, Ross PD et al. Patients with prior fractures have an increased risk of future fractures: a summary of the literature and statistical synthesis. J Bone Miner Res 2000; 15: 721–739.

11. Siris E. Alendronate in the treatment of osteoporosis: a review of the clinical trials. J Womens Health Gend Based Med 2000; 9: 599–606.

12. Dequeker J. Prevention and treatment of osteoporosis. Ned Tijdschr Geneesk 1992; 136: 1188–1192.

13. Osteoporosis: review of the evidence for prevention, diagnosis and treatment and cost-effectiveness analysis. Osteoporosis Int 1998 (suppl 4).

14. Kanis JA, Delmas P et al. Guidelines for diagnosis and management of osteoporosis. The European Foundation for Osteoporosis and Bone Disease. Osteoporosis Int 1997; 7: 390–406.

15. Koh LK, Sedrine WB et al. Osteoporosis Self-Assessment Tool for Asians (OSTA) Research Group. A simple tool to identify Asian women at increased risk of osteoporosis. Osteoporos Int 2001; 12: 699–705.

16. van der Voort DJ, Dinant GJ et al. Construction of an algorithm for quick detection of patients with low bone mineral density and its applicability in daily general practice. J Clin Epidemiol 2000; 53: 1095–1103.

17. Pal B. Questionnaire survey of advice given to patients with fractures. Brit Med J 1999; 318: 500–501.

18. Nevitt MC, Thompson DE et al. Effect of alendronate on limited-activity days and bed-disability days caused by back pain in postmenopausal women with existing vertebral fractures. Fracture Intervention Trial Research Group. Arch Intern Med 2000; 160: 77–85.

19. Melton LJ, Cooper C. Magnitude and impact of osteoporosis and fractures. In: Marcus R, Feldman D, Kelsey J, eds. Osteoporosis, 2nd ed. London: Academic Press; 2001.

20. Atkins RM, Duckworth T et al. Features of algodystrophy after Colles' fracture. J Bone Joint Surg 1990; 72: 105–110.

21. Field J, Warwick D et al. Long-term prognosis of displaced Colles' fracture: a 10-year prospective review. Injury 1992; 23: 529–532.

22. Warwick D, Field J et al. Function ten years after Colles' fracture. Clin Orthop 1993; 295: 270–274.

23. Gartland JJ, Werley CW. Evaluation of healed Colles'fractures. J Bone J Surg 1951; 33A: 895–907.

24. Geusens P, Santen M. Algodystrophy. Baillière's Best Pract Res Clin Rheumatol 2000; 14: 499–513.

25. Khan SA, de Geus C et al. Osteoporosis follow-up after wrist fractures following minor trauma. Arch Intern Med 2001; 161: 1309–1312.

26. Schurch MA, Rizzoli R et al. A prospective study on socioeconomic aspects of fracture of the proximal femur. J Bone Miner Res 1996; 11: 1935–1942.

27. Nevitt MC, Cummings SR. Type of fall and risk of hip and wrist fractures: the study of osteoporotic fractures. The Study of Osteoporotic Fractures Research Group. J Am Geriatr Soc 1993; 41: 1226–1234.

28. Martin-Hunyadi C, Heitz D et al. Spontaneous insufficiency fractures of long bones: a prospective epidemiological survey in nursing home subjects. Arch Gerontol Geriatr 2000; 31: 207–214.

29. Obrandt K, ed. Management of fractures in severely osteoporotic bone. Heidelberg: Springer 2000.

30. Koot VC, Peeters PH et al. Functional results after treatment of hip fracture: a multicentre, prospective study in 215 patients. Eur J Surg 2000; 166: 480–485.

31. Baudoin C, Fardellone P et al. Clinical outcomes and mortality after hip fracture: a 2-year follow-up study. Bone 1996; 18(suppl): 149S–157S.

32. Greendale GA, Barrett-Connor E. Outcomes of osteoporotic fractures. In: Marcus R, Feldman D, Kelsey J, eds. Osteoporosis, 2nd ed. London: Academic Press; 2001.

33. Hannan EL, Magaziner J et al. Mortality and locomotion 6 months after hospitalization for hip fracture: risk factors and risk-adjusted hospital outcomes. J Am Med Assoc 2001; 285: 2736–2742.

34. Morrison RS, Siu AL. Survival in end-stage dementia following acute illness. J Am Med Assoc 2000; 284: 47–52.

35. Lippuner K, von Overbeck J et al. Incidence and direct medical costs of hospitalizations due to osteoporotic fractures in Switzerland. Osteoporos Int 1997; 7: 414–425.

36. Haentjens P, Autier P et al. Belgian Hip Fracture Study Group. The economic cost of hip fractures among elderly women. A one-year, prospective, observational cohort study with matched-pair analysis. J Bone Joint Surg Am 2001; 83-A: 493–500.

37. US congress office.

38. Katz S, Heiple K et al. Long-term course of 147 patients with fracture of the hip. Surg Gybecol Obstet 1967; 124: 1219–1230.

39. Marottoli RA, Berkman LF et al. Decline in physical function following hip fracture. J Am Geriatr Soc 1992; 40: 861–866.

40. Michel JP, Hoffmeyer P et al. Prognosis of functional recovery 1 year after hip fracture: typical patient profiles through cluster analysis. J Gerontol A Biol Sci Med Sci 2000; 55: M508–515.

41. Magaziner J, Simonsick EM et al. Predictors of functional recovery one year following hospital discharge for hip fracture: a prospective study. J Gerontol 1990; 45: M101–107.

42. Hall SE, Criddle RA et al. A case-control study of quality of life and functional impairment in women with long-standing vertebral osteoporotic fracture. Osteoporos Int 1999; 9: 508–515.

43. Cummings SR, Phillips SL et al. Recovery of function after hip fracture. The role of social supports. J Am Geriatr Soc 1988; 36: 801–806.

44. Randell AG, Nguyen TV et al. Deterioration in quality of life following hip fracture: a prospective study. Osteoporos Int 2000; 11: 460–466.

45. Adams F. The genuine works of Hippocrates. Baltimore: Williams and Wilkins; 1939: 237–234.

46. Cooper C. Epidemiology of vertebral fractures in Western populations. Spine: State of the Art Reviews 1994; 8: 1–12.

47. Albright F, Smith PH et al. Postmenopausal osteoporosis.J Am Med Assoc 1941; 1116: 2465–2474.

48. Leidig G, Minne HW et al. A study of complaints and their relation to vertebral destruction in patients with osteoporosis. Bone Miner 1990; 8: 217–229.

49. Lyritis GP, Mayasis B et al. The natural history of the osteoporotic vertebral fracture. Clin Rheumatol 1989; 8(Suppl 2): 66–69.

50. Ettinger B, Black DM et al. Contribution of vertebral deformities to chronic back pain and disability. The Study of Osteoporotic Fractures Research Group. J Bone Miner Res 1992; 7: 449–456.

51. Abdel-Hamid Osman A, Bassiouni H et al. Aging of the thoracic spine: distinction between wedging in osteoarthritis and fracture in osteoporosis – a cross-sectional and longitudinal study. Bone 1994; 15: 437–442.

52. Silverman SL. The clinical consequences of vertebral compression fracture. Bone 1992; 13(suppl 2): S27–31.

53. Kanis JA, McCloskey EV. Epidemiology of vertebral osteoporosis. Bone 1992; 13(suppl 2): S1–10.

54. Gold DT. The clinical impact of vertebral fractures: quality of life in women with osteoporosis. Bone 1996; 18(suppl): 185S–189S.

55. Ross PD. Clinical consequences of vertebral fractures. Am J Med 1997; 103(2A): 30S–42S; discussion 42S–43S.

56. Leidig-Bruckner G, Minne HW et al. Clinical grading of spinal osteoporosis: quality of life components and spinal deformity in women with chronic low back pain and women with vertebral osteoporosis. J Bone Miner Res 1997; 12: 663–675.

57. Cook DJ, Guyatt GH et al. Quality of life issues in women with vertebral fractures due to osteoporosis. Arthritis Rheum 1993; 36: 750–756.

58. Lyles KW, Gold DT et al. Association of osteoporotic vertebral compression fractures with impaired functional status. Am J Med 1993; 94: 595–601.

59. Ryan PJ, Blake G et al. A clinical profile of back pain and disability in patients with spinal osteoporosis. Bone 1994; 15: 27–30.

60. Lydick E, Zimmerman SI et al. Development and validation of a discriminative quality of life questionnaire for osteoporosis (the OPTQoL). J Bone Miner Res 1997; 12: 456–463.

61. Lips P, Cooper C et al. Quality of life in patients with vertebral fractures: validation of the Quality of Life Questionnaire of the European Foundation for Osteoporosis (QUALEFFO). Working Party for Quality of Life of the European Foundation for Osteoporosis. Osteoporos Int 1999; 10: 150–160.

62. Cook DJ, Guyatt GH et al. Development and validation of the mini-osteoporosis quality of life questionnaire (OQLQ) in osteoporotic women with back pain due to vertebral fractures. Osteoporosis Quality of Life Study Group. Osteoporos Int 1999; 10: 207–213.

63. Helmes E, Hodsman A et al. A questionnaire to evaluate disability in osteoporotic patients with vertebral compression fractures. J Gerontol A Biol Sci Med Sci 1995; 50: M91–98.

64. Begerow B, Pfeifer M et al. Time since vertebral fracture: an important variable concerning quality of life in patients with postmenopausal osteoporosis. Osteoporos Int 1999; 10: 26–33.

65. Ross PD, Ettinger B et al. Evaluation of adverse health outcomes associated with vertebral fractures. Osteoporos Int 1991; 1: 134–140.

66. Nicholson PH, Haddaway MJ et al. Vertebral deformity, bone mineral density, back pain and height loss in unscreened women over 50 years. Osteoporos Int 1993; 3: 300–307.

67. Chandler JM, Martin AR et al. Reliability of an osteoporosis-targeted quality of life survey instrument for use in the community: OPTQoL. Osteoporos Int 1998; 8: 127–135.

68. Oleksik A, Lips P et al. Health-related quality of life in postmenopausal women with low BMD with or without prevalent vertebral fractures. J Bone Miner Res 200l; 15: 1384–1392.

69. Ross PD, Davis JW et al. Pain and disability associated with new vertebral fractures and other spinal conditions. J Clin Epidemiol 1994; 47: 231–239.

70. Huang C, Ross PD et al. Vertebral fracture and other predictors of physical impairment and health care utilization. Arch Intern Med 1996; 156: 2469–2475.

71. Huang C, Ross PD et al. Vertebral fractures and other predictors of back pain among older women. J Bone Miner Res 1996; 11: 1026–1032.

72. Huang C, Ross PD et al. Contributions of vertebral fractures to stature loss among elderly Japanese-American women in Hawaii. J Bone Miner Res 1996; 11: 408–411.

73. Kado DM, Browner WS et al. Vertebral fractures and mortality in older women: a prospective study. Study of Osteoporotic Fractures Research Group. Arch Intern Med 1999; 159: 1215–1220.

74. Ensrud KE, Thompson DE et al. Prevalent vertebral deformities predict mortality and hospitalization in older women with low bone mass. Fracture Intervention Trial Research Group. J Am Geriatr Soc 2000; 48: 241–249.

75. Ismail AA, Cockerill W et al. Prevalent vertebral deformity predicts incident hip though not distal forearm fracture: results from the European Prospective Osteoporosis Study. Osteoporos Int 2001; 12: 85–90.

76. Johnell O, Oden A et al. Acute and long-term increase in fracture risk after hospitalization for vertebral fracture. Osteoporos Int 2001; 12: 207–214.

77. Ross PD, Davis JW et al. Pre-existing fractures and bone mass predict vertebral fracture incidence in women. Ann Intern Med 1991; 114: 919–923.

78. Lindsay R, Silverman SL et al. Risk of new vertebral fracture in the year following a fracture. J Am Med Assoc 2001; 285: 320–323.

79. Kotowicz MA, Melton LJ 3rd et al. Risk of hip fracture in women with vertebral fracture. J Bone Miner Res 1994; 9: 599–605.

80. Burger H, van Daele PL et al. Vertebral deformities as predictors of non-vertebral fractures. Brit Med J 1994; 309: 991–992.

81. Primer on the metabolic bone disorders of mineral metabolism, 4th ed. Baltimore: Lippincott Williams & Wilkins; 1999.

82. Finsen V. Osteoporosis and back pain among the elderly. Acta Med Scand 1988; 223: 443–449.

83. Spector TD, McCloskey EV et al. Prevalence of vertebral fracture in women and the relationship with bone density and symptoms: the Chingford Study. J Bone Miner Res 1993; 8: 817–822.

84. Gehlbach SH, Bigelow C et al. Recognition of vertebral fracture in a clinical setting. Osteoporos Int 2000; 11: 577–582.

85. Sinaki M, Khosla S et al. Muscle strength in osteoporotic versus normal women. Osteoporos Int 1993; 3: 8–12.

86. Nevitt MC, Cummings SR et al. Risk factors for recurrent nonsyncopal falls. A prospective study. J Am Med Assoc 1989; 261: 2663–2668.

87. Ulivieri FM, Bossi E et al. Quantification by dual photonabsorptiometry of local bone loss after fracture. Clin Orthop 1990; 250: 291–296.

88. Cortet B, Houvenagel E et al. Spinal curvatures and quality of life in women with vertebral fractures secondary to osteoporosis. Spine 1999; 24: 1921–1925.

89. Ensrud KE, Black DM et al. Correlates of kyphosis in older women. The Fracture Intervention Trial Research Group. J Am Geriatr Soc 1997; 45: 682–687.

90. Ettinger B, Black DM et al. Kyphosis in older women and its relation to back pain, disability and osteopenia: the study of osteoporotic fractures. Osteoporos Int 1994; 4: 55–60.

91. Kleerekoper M, Nelson DA et al. Outcome variables in osteoporosis trials. Bone 1992; 13(suppl 1): S29–34.

92. Leech JA, Dulberg C et al. Relationship of lung function to severity of osteoporosis. Am Rev Respir Dis 1990; 141: 68–71.

93. Schlaich C, Minne HW et al. Reduced pulmonary function in patients with spinal osteoporotic fractures. Osteoporos Int 1998; 8: 261–267.

94. Lord SR, Sambrook PN et al. Postural stability, falls and fractures in the elderly: results from the Dubbo Osteoporosis Epidemiology Study. Med J Aust 1994; 160: 684–685, 688–691.

95. Ensrud KE, Nevitt MC et al. Correlates of impaired function in older women. J Am Geriatr Soc 1994; 42: 481–489.

96. Oleksik AM, Ewing SK et al. Three years of health related quality of life in postmenopausal women with osteoporosis: impact of incident vertebral fractures, age and severe adverse events. JBMR 2000; 1: S168.

97. Cook DJ, Guyatt GH et al. Development and validation of the mini-osteoporosis quality of life questionnaire (OQLQ) in osteoporotic women with back pain due to vertebral fractures. Osteoporosis Quality of Life Study Group. Osteoporos Int 1999; 10: 207–213.

98. Rubin SM, Cummings SR. Results of bone densitometry affect women's decisions about taking measures to prevent fractures. Ann Intern Med 1992; 116: 990–995.

99. Gold DT, Bales CW et al. Treatment of osteoporosis: the psychological impact of a medical education program in older patients. JAGS 1989; 37: 417–422.

100. Coelho R, Silva C et al. Bone mineral density and depression: a community study in women. J Psychosom Res 1999; 46: 29–35.

101. Michelson D, Stratakis C, Hill L et al. Bone mineral density in women with depression. N Engl J Med 1996; 335: 1176–1181.

102. Silverman SL, Cranney A. Quality of life measurement in osteoporosis. J Rheumatol 1997; 24: 1218–1221.

103. Lips P, Cooper C et al. Quality of life in patients with vertebral fractures: validation of the Quality of Life Questionnaire of the European Foundation for Osteoporosis (QUALEFFO). Working Party for Quality of Life of the European Foundation for Osteoporosis. Osteoporos Int 1999; 10: 150–160.

104. Cranney A, Tugwell P et al. Osteoporosis clinical trials endpoints: candidate variables and clinimetric properties. J Rheumatol 1997; 24: 1222–1229.

105. Cranney A, Welch V et al. Responsiveness of endpoints in osteoporosis clinical trials – an update. J Rheumatol 1999; 26: 222–228.

106. Cranney A, Welch V et al. Discrimination of changes in osteoporosis outcomes. J Rheumatol 2001; 28: 413–421.

107. Murrell P, Todd CJ et al. Postal administration compared with nurse-supported administration of the QUALEFFO-41 in a population sample: comparison of results and assessment of psychometric properties. Osteoporos Int 2001; 12: 672–679.

108. Cummings SR, Nevitt MC et al. Risk factors for hip fracture in white women. Study of Osteoporotic Fractures Research Group. N Engl J Med 1995; 332: 767–773.

109. Dargent-Molina P, Poitiers F et al. EPIDOS Group. In elderly women weight is the best predictor of a very low bone mineral density: evidence from the EPIDOS study. Osteoporos Int 2000; 11: 881–888.

110. Cadarette SM, Jaglal SB et al. Development and validation of the osteoporosis risk assessment instrument to facilitate selection of women for bone densitometry. CMAJ 2000; 162: 1289–1294.

111. Black DM, Palermo L et al. SOFSURF: A simple, usefull risk factor system can identify the large majority of women with osteoporosis. Bone 1998; 23(suppl): S605.

112. Vanhoof J, Declerck K, Geusens P. Prevalence of rheumatic diseases in a rheumatological outpatient practice. Ann Rheum Dis 2002; 61: 453–455.

113. Nolla JM, Gomez-Vaquero C et al. Osteoporosis diagnosed over a 10 year period. J Rheumatol 2001; 28: 2289–2293. 669 Patients

114. Cummings SR, Black DM et al. Effect of alendronate on risk of fracture in women with low bone density but without vertebral fractures: results from the Fracture Intervention Trial. J Am Med Assoc 1998; 280: 2077–2082.

115. McClung MR, Geusens P et al. Effect of risedronate on the risk of hip fracture in elderly women. Hip Intervention Program Study Group. N Engl J Med 2001; 344: 333–340.

116. Johnell O, O'Neill T et al. Anthropometric measurements and vertebral deformities. European Vertebral Osteoporosis Study (EVOS) Group. Am J Epidemiol 1997; 146: 287–293.

117. Scane AC, Sutcliffe AM, Francis RM. The sequelae of vertebral crush fractures in men. Osteoporos Int 1994; 4: 89–92.

118. Seeman E. Osteoporosis in men. Osteoporos Int 1999; 9(suppl 2): S97–S110.

119. Riggs BL, Melton LJ 3rd. Involutional osteoporosis. N Engl J Med 1986; 314: 1676–1686.

120. Poor G, Atkinson EJ et al. Predictors of hip fractures in elderly men. J Bone Miner Res 1995; 10: 1900–1907.

121. Alonso-Bartolome P, Martinez-Taboada VM, Blanco R, Rodriguez-Valverde V. Insufficiency fractures of the tibia and fibula. Semin Arthritis Rheum 1999; 28: 413–420.

122. Johnson BE, Lucasey B, Robinson RG, Lukert BP. Contributing diagnoses in osteoporosis. The value of a complete medical evaluation. Arch Intern Med 1989; 149: 1069–1072.

METABOLIC BONE DISEASES

45 Management of osteoporosis

Anthony D Woolf and Kristina Åkesson

- Osteoporosis is the structural failure of the skeleton with increased risk of fracture. There is low bone mass and microarchitectural deterioration of bone tissue leading to increased bone fragility. This manifests itself as fracture following low energy trauma
- Fracture is associated with increased mortality and significant short- and long-term morbidity
- The management of osteoporosis must encompass all these components of the condition. Bone mass should be maximized, fractures should be prevented and those who have already sustained a fracture should be rehabilitated to minimize the associated pain, limitation of activities and restriction of participation

INDIVIDUAL VERSUS POPULATION MANAGEMENT

The management of osteoporosis can either be focused on the individual or be targeted at the population. We need to know what the best strategy is for the individuals in the clinic to avoid an osteoporotic fracture in the future, or what to advise the person who has already sustained a low energy fracture to prevent a further fracture and how to rehabilitate them. However, osteoporosis is also a public health issue because of the high incidence and cost of fractures and strategies are needed to reduce the number of osteoporotic fractures in the population. This can be accomplished by reducing the risk for the population as a whole irrespective of their individual risk (primary prevention), or by targeting those who are known to be at high risk of future fracture and who may already have early features of osteoporosis with a low bone mass and may have sustained a fracture (secondary prevention).

Targeting the population as a whole or those at high risk are not mutually exclusive strategies and both approaches are recommended in parallel – general measures to reduce the population risk in conjunction with specific therapies aimed at those who are at most risk of future fracture. There is a move towards the use of specific therapy at a later stage in those at highest risk. This is for two reasons; firstly, there is better identification of those who will gain most because of their high absolute risk of fracture at the time of the treatment effect, and secondly, treatments have an early onset of benefit, with fracture prevention within a year[1]. There are several evidence-based guidelines for the prevention and treatment of osteoporosis[2–5] but the application of them in routine clinical practice still remains a challenge.

WHO TO TREAT?

The main targets for therapy are individuals at increased risk of fracture, in particular if they are likely to have a poor outcome following a fracture. The difficulty is to identify such individuals.

Who is at high risk of future fracture?

The risk of fracture increases with age and is greater in women than men, and the frail elderly have the worst outcome. In addition, the strongest risk factors for fracture include low bone density and falling. There are data on which risk factors can be used to try and identify those who may have low bone density (Table 45.1) or may fall. These

TABLE 45.1 RISK FACTORS FOR FRACTURE RELATED TO LOSS OF BONE MASS		
High risk (RR ≥2)	**Moderate risk (1 <RR <2)**	**No risk (RR ≤1)**
Aging (>70–80 years)	Gender (female)	Consumption of caffeine
Low body weight	Smoking (active)	Consumption of tea
Weight loss	Low sunlight exposure (low or none)	Menopause
Physical inactivity	Family history of osteoporotic fracture	Nulliparity
Corticosteroids	Surgical menopause	Consumption of fluoridated water
Anticonvulsants	Early menopause (<45 years)	Thiazide diuretics
Primary hyperparathyroidism	Short fertile period (<30 years)	
Diabetes mellitus type I	Late menarche (>15 years)	
Anorexia nervosa	No lactation	
Gastrectomy	Low calcium intake (<500–850mg/day)	
Pernicious anemia	Hyperparathyroidism (N/S)	
Prior osteoporotic fracture	Hyperthyroidism	
	Diabetes mellitus (type II or N/S)	
	Rheumatoid arthritis	

(Adapted from Espallargues et al.[9])

various risk factors can be used to aid clinical decision-making about whom to treat.

Bone mineral density (BMD) measured by dual energy X-ray absorptiometry (DXA) accounts for 75–90% of the variance of bone strength[6] and for each decrease of one standard deviation in bone density at the proximal femur or lumbar spine there is a two- to three-fold increase in fracture risk[5]. Nomograms are being developed to estimate absolute fracture risk for any given bone density at any given age over a relative time interval. Measurement of BMD at the total hip is regarded as most reliable because of changes in disc spaces and joints of the lumbar spine with advancing age.

Fracture risk can also be assessed by measurements at other skeletal sites using different techniques. Quantitative ultrasound has a demonstrated role in elderly women[7] but is less established in other age groups and there are problems of standardization of machines and sites of assessment. Forearm densitometry is also used to assess risk[8]. Their specificity is less than DXA of the lumbar spine or proximal femur for predicting fractures at these sites.

Previous fracture of the vertebrae, hip, distal radius and other sites over the age of 40 if a clinical manifestation of existing osteoporosis is an important predictor for future fracture[9]. At present osteoporosis is undiagnosed and untreated in many people who have sustained such fractures. Osteoporosis should thus be suspected following a low energy fracture or in someone who has lost height with kyphosis. A coincidental X-ray of the spine may reveal a vertebral deformity or suggest demineralization.

Fracture is not only a result of bone fragility but also is a consequence of an abnormal force, usually due to a fall. Risk factors for falls thus need to be identified. The best predictors of future falls are a fall in the previous year and abnormality in neuromuscular function, measured simplest as inability to rise unaided from a chair without using the arms.

There are other risk factors for fracture, which are principally mediated either through bone density[9] (Table 45.1) and/or falls[10]. Risk factors identified by systematic review that carry a high risk of osteoporosis, in addition to aging and female gender, include previous low energy fracture, glucocorticosteroid therapy, reduced lifetime estrogen exposure, anorexia nervosa, low body mass index, maternal hip fracture, smoking, low levels of physical activity and certain diseases such as rheumatoid arthritis and diabetes mellitus[9]. Although these factors are associated with increased personal risk, they cannot predict who will fracture and are of limited value alone in deciding who will benefit most from an intervention. They can however be used to identify who should be assessed for their future risk of fracture by bone densitometry[5] and this can form part of a high-risk strategy (see Chapter 44).

Bone loss may be predicted by biochemical markers of high bone turnover. They may be independent measures of future fracture risk but their predictive power for the individual is poor. Used in combination with bone density, biochemical bone markers are more predictive of fracture and may strengthen the indication for treatment[11].

Identification of those at highest risk of fracture

The decision to intervene must consider the balance between the benefits, risks and costs of the intervention, and the level of risk for osteoporosis and future fracture. For example, a well tolerated intervention with additional health benefit outside the skeleton needs only a low level of increased risk of osteoporosis and fracture to justify its recommendation, whereas a treatment that only benefits the skeleton needs greater justification for its use. Any decision by the person around this balance of risk and benefit will be influenced by other factors such as the individual's personal experiences and subsequent anxieties about sustaining a fracture or suffering side effects from treatment. It is not possible to predict for the individual whether they will sustain a fracture or benefit from a treatment but we can estimate probabilities by the

application of knowledge of the above risk factors to the individual. Once the level of risk is estimated, it requires careful explanation to have any meaningful value for the patient.

There are different approaches to identifying those at risk of osteoporosis and fracture at different ages. At the younger ages, predictors of low bone density are the major determinants of future fracture. With a person over 70 years, the prevalence of low bone density is greater and other factors, such as falling, are more important in discriminating those at high risk of fracture.

No method of assessing risk of osteoporosis and fracture has both optimal sensitivity and specificity, and there have to be trade offs in any strategy to identify those at risk. Bone density at the site of a potential fracture is the best predictor of fracture at that site and osteoporosis is defined in terms of bone density. It is generally agreed however that population screening for osteoporosis by bone densitometry is not appropriate. This is because it is not cost-effective, there is poor uptake of the measurements, limited specificity for future fracture and low compliance with the therapeutic recommendations[12]. A two stage process is proposed with the use of the strongest clinical indicators for osteoporosis (Table 45.1) as a first stage with bone densitometry restricted to the second stage, as a more cost-effective approach. The indicators proposed vary between guidelines from just being a women over 65 years[4] to having a variety of known risk factors[5]. Simple self-administered questionnaires can be used to help identify those at potential risk for further assessment. There is a move towards assessing an individual's needs at an older age for bone-specific treatments when the absolute risk of fracture is highest. The 5-year risk of fracture in a 50-year-old women is 3.4%, whereas it is 14.5% in a 75-year-old[13]. Thresholds of bone density T-scores have been recommended for treatment[14]. Clinical indicators for osteoporosis could be used alone to target interventions that are well tolerated, inexpensive or have additional benefits outside the skeleton such as lifestyle changes or estrogen replacement therapy. The presence of multiple vertebral deformities is diagnostic of osteoporosis providing other causes are excluded and treatment with a bone specific agent could be considered. However osteoporosis should ideally be confirmed in most cases by bone density using DXA before using a bone specific treatment. Most intervention studies have specifically shown fracture prevention in the context of low bone mass and/or prevalent vertebral fractures.

Once osteoporosis is confirmed, any underlying cause should be looked for but osteoporosis is idiopathic in most cases, although comorbidities that can affect the outcome are common. If a fracture is the presentation, then other causes of fracture must be considered.

INVESTIGATIONS

Osteoporosis should be assessed and managed in the context of the person's general health. All those with osteoporosis, with or without fracture, should have a diagnostic evaluation including a careful history, physical examination and laboratory investigations to exclude conditions that can mimic osteoporosis, to elucidate secondary causes of osteoporosis and contributory factors, and to identify any comorbidities that will influence outcome. This evaluation also includes an estimate of severity and prognosis to enable the development of an appropriate plan of management. Repeat DXA measurement may be needed to monitor treatment. Much can be learnt from a good history and examination in combination with clinical experience and intuition.

Identifying cause of fracture

If the person presents with sudden onset back pain or loss of height with stoop, then X-ray is first needed to confirm the presence of vertebral deformity. If vertebral deformity is confirmed or if the person presents with a low energy fracture of another site, then causes other than osteoporosis should first be excluded (Tables 45.2 & 45.3).

TABLE 45.2 DIFFERENTIAL DIAGNOSIS OF FRACTURE AND VERTEBRAL DEFORMITY

- Osteoporosis
- Primary malignancy including myeloma
- Metastatic malignancy – breast, prostate, lung and renal most common
- Osteomalacia
- Paget's disease
- Osteomyelitis
- Traumatic vertebral fracture earlier in life
- Scheuermann's osteochondritis of the spine

TABLE 45.3 INVESTIGATION OF FRACTURE OR BONE PAIN

Baseline

- Full examination, in particular breasts or prostate
- X-ray of affected site
- Hematology
  - Full blood count
  - Viscosity or ESR
- Biochemistry
  - Serum calcium, phosphate
  - Serum alkaline phosphatase
  - Serum creatinine
  - Serum albumen
  - Testosterone and SHBG in men

Further assessment

- Further imaging
  - Isotope bone scan – if any concern of metastases
  - CT scan or MRI to characterize lesion
- Biochemistry
  - Liver function tests
  - Serum protein electrophoresis
  - Thyroid function tests
  - Urine Bence-Jones protein
  - PSA in men with possible pathological fractures

Investigations need to be tailored to the individual depending on site of fracture and whether other findings suggest a pathological cause.

TABLE 45.4 CAUSES OF GENERALIZED OSTEOPOROSIS

Cause	Example
Age	
Endocrine	Primary and secondary hypogonadism including early menopause (<45years)
	Hyperparathyroidism
	Hyperthyroidism
	Cushing's syndrome
	Hyperprolactinemia
Specific conditions	Anorexia nervosa
	Over-exercise syndrome
	Osteomalacia
	Pregnancy
	Rheumatoid arthritis
	Chronic obstructive airways disease
	Cystic fibrosis
	Gastrointestinal disease – postgastrectomy, celiac disease, Crohn's disease, ulcerative colitis
	Chronic liver disease
	Chronic renal failure
	Post-transplantation
	Immobility related to paraplegia, multiple sclerosis, etc.
Malignant disease	Metastatic malignancy
	Myeloma
	Leukemia, lymphoma
	Mastocytosis
Drugs	Glucocorticosteroids
	Thyroxine in excess
	Anticonvulsants
	Heparin
Lifestyle factors	Smoking
	Alcohol in excess
	Lack of physical activity
Hereditary connective tissue disorders	Osteogenesis imperfecta
	Marfan's syndrome
	Ehlers–Danlos syndrome
	Homocystinuria

Imaging

Although a plain X-ray cannot be used to diagnose osteoporosis as 30% of bone mass can be lost before it is evident, such imaging should be used to confirm the presence of a vertebral fracture. Vertebrae may show endplate deformities, anterior wedging or crush fractures. The X-ray may reveal bone destruction or lytic lesions and a PA view of the spine may demonstrate pedicles that have been destroyed by metastases. The X-ray of any non-vertebral fracture, including hip fracture, should be carefully viewed for abnormalities to suggest malignancy or osteomalacia. Pathological fractures are however not very likely at some sites such as the distal radius. Stress fractures may not be visible on the plain X-ray and require bone scintigraphy, CT scan, or MRI. Radiographs cannot by themselves tell if the fracture is recent.

Bone density measurement should be considered to confirm underlying osteoporosis. Bone mineral density may be reduced compared to peak bone mass but fractures occur in the presence of bone density within the normal range for their age, particularly in the very old.

Bone scintigraphy will show increased uptake for several weeks after a fracture and can indicate timing of a vertebral fracture but there is rarely reason to obtain such close temporal relationship. Bone scintigraphy,

CT scan or MRI is used when a fracture of non-osteoporotic origin is suspected. Multiple lesions on bone scintigraphy will suggest metastatic disease but it may be normal in myeloma. MRI scan may be necessary to exclude malignancy particularly of the spine, but it is difficult to distinguish myeloma from an osteoporotic vertebral fracture.

Identifying cause of osteoporosis

Osteoporosis is idiopathic in the majority of women but secondary causes are identified in up to 55% of men. The underlying causes of bone loss should be sought (Table 45.4). They often manifest long before presentation with osteoporosis. Comorbidities that affect outcome of osteoporosis and fracture should be identified. These are common in the more elderly and should be treated where present and possible.

Identifying avoidable causes of falls

Fracture usually relates to trauma and causes of that trauma, most often a fall, must also be addressed (Table 45.5). Falls are most effectively prevented by recognizing those most at risk of falling, identifying any intrinsic or extrinsic risk factors and co-ordinating appropriate intervention. Intrinsic risk factors should be sought by a general

TABLE 45.5 CAUSES OF FALLS IN THE ELDERLY

Intrinsic factors

General deterioration associated with aging	Poor postural control
	Defective proprioception
	Reduced walking speed
	Weakness of lower limbs
	Slow reaction time
Balance, gait or mobility problems	Joint disease
	Cerebrovascular disease
	Peripheral neuropathy
	Parkinson's disease
	Alcohol
Multiple drug therapy	Sedatives
	Hypotensive drugs
	Various comorbidities
Visual impairment	Impaired visual acuity
	Cataracts
	Glaucoma
	Retinal degeneration
Impaired cognition or depression	Alzheimer's disease
	Cerebrovascular disease
'Blackouts'	Hypoglycemia
	Postural hypotension
	Cardiac arrhythmia
	TIA, acute onset cerebrovascular attack
	Epilepsy
	Drop attacks ? VBI

Extrinsic factors

Bad lighting
Steep stairs
Slippery floors
Loose rugs
Inappropriate footwear or clothing
Tripping over pets, grandchildren's toys, etc.
Uneven pavements
Bad weather
Lack of safety equipment such as grab rails

examination including checks on pulse, postural blood pressure, vision and neuromuscular function. A careful description of the fall from the patient or an eyewitness is essential. The drug history is important. A formal home assessment for extrinsic risk factors may be necessary, for example by an occupational therapist.

WHAT ARE THE TREATMENT OPTIONS?

Treatments should be evaluated separately for their effect on bone mass and on fracture rate. These effects may be independent for some interventions and the evidence should be considered separately. Primary prevention studies are usually performed in unselected women with normal bone density or in those with osteopenia (bone mineral density T score between −1 and −2.5) and in whom the absolute risk of fracture is low. Subsequently the antifracture efficacy cannot be easily tested, but bone mass is used as an intermediate endpoint. Studies of those at high risk of fracture enable the assessment of anti-fracture efficacy. Such studies are usually of those with osteoporosis (bone mineral density T score below −2.5) with or without a prevalent fracture.

In general pharmacological agents either decrease bone resorption leading to a secondary gain in bone mass or are anabolic with a direct increase of bone mass. Preferably these agents also increase bone strength and quality. Since the turnover of bone is slow, the time from initiating intervention to assessing effect on bone mass or fracture is

extended over years. This has an impact on design of trials – the selection of appropriate subjects (relative risk within duration of study) and duration of study (to ensure intended outcome is measurable within time frame). In addition, few trials assess the duration of effect beyond the treatment period – the offset of effect – which may be either prolonged or be lost soon after termination. This is clearly of clinical importance and influences effectiveness.

Some of these problems are obvious in evaluating intervention studies and hampers their reliability. The reporting of, for example, main outcome as in exact number of fractures or statistical corrections for persons partially completing or non-completers are not always transparent, unfortunately decreasing the quality of a study. A further difficulty is related to the fact that appropriately powered randomized controlled trials have not been made with fracture as end-point for all agents. In the following section the major interventions are briefly described and in some cases the difficulties in interpreting data are pointed out.

PHARMACOLOGICAL INTERVENTIONS

Calcium and vitamin D

Serum calcium levels are tightly regulated as calcium is essential for transmembrane transportation and cell communication for all cell types throughout the body. Bone tissue is the main calcium reservoir, and the bone mineral content is regulated through feedback systems that involve parathyroid hormone (PTH), calcium and vitamin D. PTH initiates bone resorption in response to low serum levels of ionized calcium. Consequently, insufficient calcium intake or absorption may provoke a continuous upregulation of PTH release causing increased bone loss. This low-grade secondary hyperparathyroidism is not uncommon in the elderly. This mechanism provides the rationale for calcium and vitamin D treatment as part of a strategy to prevent bone loss, particularly in the elderly.

Calcium – monotherapy

Calcium is the basic requirement for bone mineralization. The developing skeleton unequivocally needs calcium, while the effectiveness of calcium in the treatment of osteoporosis remains debated, particularly concerning fracture as outcome. Studies using calcium supplement alone as an anti-resorptive agent have shown conflicting results. In a recent Cochrane review[15] that included 15 studies and a total of 1806 women, a small but significant effect on bone density was seen at all measured sites. The anti-fracture effect was estimated at a relative risk of 0.77 (95%CI 0.54–1.09) for vertebral fracture and 0.86 (95%CI 0.43–1.72) for non-vertebral fracture. In an earlier meta-analysis evaluating the association between calcium and hip fracture, the estimates varied between a 3% to 12% fracture risk reduction from an increase in calcium intake of between 300 and 1000mg[16]. Benefits are greatest in those with a low calcium intake[17]. In almost all randomized controlled trials for bone specific anti-resorptive agents, calcium supplementation (400–800mg) is included in the placebo group and typically show a 0.5–2% gain in bone mass at the lumbar spine.

Calcium dietary enrichment or supplementation has also shown beneficial effects on the growing skeleton, with increasing bone density in young girls on additional calcium intake[18].

Vitamin D monotherapy

Vitamin D plays a central role in calcium regulation. It is either provided through food intake or by exposure of the skin to sunlight. Vitamin D, in the ingested form or from dermal conversion of 7-dehydrocholesterol by ultraviolet light, is biologically inactive until metabolized through several stages in the liver and kidneys. Vitamin D insufficiency is common in the elderly, particularly in northern latitude countries with few hours of sunlight.

TABLE 45.6 COMPARING THE FRACTURE EFFECT IN STUDIES OF CALCIUM AND VITAMIN D

Substance	Indication for treatment	Total no. of patients (incl. placebo)	Mean age	Duration (years)	Type fracture	NNT (95% CI)
Calcium[26]	Osteoporosis + fracture	78	58	4	Fractures, various sites	NS
Vitamin D3[27]	Non-specific inclusion criteria	2578	80	3.5	Hip fracture	NS
					Other fractures	NS
Calcium + vitamin D3[24]	Non-specific inclusion criteria: institutionalized patients	1505	84	1.5	Hip fracture	47 (24–429)
					Fracture ≠ vertebra	24 (14–90)

Vitamin D3 supplement of 10μg/day (400IU/day) alone, with the assumption of adequate dietary calcium intake, has not been shown to reduce the incidence of fractures in studies of elderly men and women living in the community[19] or in nursing homes[20]. A recent Cochrane review[21] concluded that the fracture preventive effect from vitamin D supplementation alone was yet to be proven.

Vitamin D has, nevertheless, been shown to increase femoral neck bone density (0.2–2.6%) and reduce the rate of loss in elderly women after 2 years of treatment, while the effect on other skeletal sites remain similar compared to the placebo groups[22,23]. The dose required to obtain a measurable bone effect over this period was between 10–20μg/day.

Duration of treatment in a clinical setting will greatly exceed that of trials, and a long term additive fracture sparing effect directly related to the vitamin D intake cannot be ruled out, in addition to acting as an enhancer of calcium bioavailability.

Combined calcium and vitamin D

Calcium and vitamin D in combination is an accepted baseline treatment for osteoporosis and also as a preventive measure, in particular in the frail elderly. In a large randomized controlled study of elderly French nursing home patients given calcium (1200mg) and vitamin D (20μg, 800IU) there was significant reduction in new hip 0.70 (95% CI 0.62–0.78) and all non-vertebral fractures 0.70 (95% CI 0.51–0.91) after 3 years treatment, with significant benefit at 18 months[24,25] (Table 45.6). A smaller study of community dwelling men and women above age 65 showed a significant reduction in non-vertebral fractures on 17.5μg vitamin D3 and 500mg calcium[28]. It is also possible to give vitamin D as a yearly injection, an advantageous route of administration in institutionalized settings. In a Finnish study, elderly patients were given a yearly dose of 150 000–200 000IU of vitamin D with a significant reduction in fracture risk[29]. Data pooled from epidemiological studies also suggest a small anti-fracture effect of combination treatment[16,30].

These agents have shown an effect on bone mass both in the femoral neck[28], and in the spine in early postmenopausal women[31]. Furthermore in large randomized controlled trials of other agents, calcium and vitamin D supplementation is commonly used in both the placebo with a typical increase of 1–2% on bone density in comparison to baseline after 3–4 years and with a 10–20% decrease in bone turnover markers apparent after 3–6 months of treatment. In a RCT involving men, no effect was seen on spinal bone density after three years with 25μg vitamin D and 1000mg of calcium, but the subjects had a high baseline calcium intake which may obscure the effect or suggests that above a certain intake no additional advantages are evident.

Recommended supplementation

- Calcium 500–1000mg depending on dietary intake to reach a total of 1200–1500mg/day
- Vitamin D 10–20μg (400–800IU) daily – the higher dose is indicated for institutionalized persons or those receiving equivalent care or during the winter in northern latitude countries

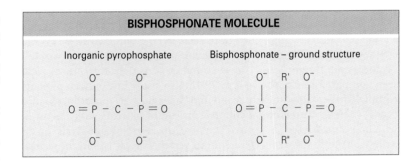

Fig. 45.1 Bisphosphonate molecule.

Calcitriol

The active metabolite calcitriol (1,25 dihydroxyvitamin D) has theoretical therapeutic advantages compared to cholecalciferol, as metabolic activation is surpassed and, for example, an age-dependent decreasing kidney function becomes less important. Side effects include hypercalcemia and nephrolithiasis, which demands close monitoring of serum calcium.

The effectiveness of calcitriol and 1α (OH)-vitamin D is uncertain[4]. The effect on fracture is unclear as only one large one year study, with a much criticized methodology, has been performed[32]. The study was single blinded, included postmenopausal women with one or more vertebral fractures at baseline and it suggested an effect on new vertebral fractures. Other studies have shown inconsistent results, which in part may be related to variable calcium intakes[33,34].

Bisphosphonates

Bisphosphonates are chemically developed from pyrophosphates, compounds that inhibit precipitation of calcium carbonate and have industrial applications. Bisphosphonates are characterized by two C-P bonds (Fig. 45.1). When the bonds are on the same carbon atom as a P-C-P binding structure, it allows for large side chain variation which gives each compound specific physiologic and biochemical properties.

Bisphosphonates have bone anti-resorptive activity with little effect on other organ systems. Bisphosphonates act on bone by binding to the hydroxyapatite and inhibiting osteoclasts. Osteoclast numbers are reduced by inhibition of osteoclast recruitment and increased apoptosis, and osteoclast activity is reduced with decreased ruffled border, alterations of the cytoskeleton, decreased acid production and decreased production of lysosomal enzymes and prostaglandins[35]. Nitrogen-containing bisphosphonates, such as alendronate, risedronate and ibandronate inhibit the mevalonate pathway, while non-nitrogen containing bisphosphonates, such as etidronate, tiludronate or clodronate are metabolized in the cell into cytotoxic ATP analogues.

Bisphosphonates are poorly absorbed from the gastrointestinal tract. Only about 0.5–5% of a given dose is absorbed which is further decreased by food intake (particularly calcium containing foods) or even drinks such as coffee or juice, and is the reason why these drugs must be taken after a food free interval.

The plasma half-life of bisphosphonates is very short and the drug is displaced into bone tissue within 30 min to 2 hours, whereas the half-life of bisphosphonates deposited in bone is probably up to 10 years or more[35].

Side-chain substitution results in different bisphosphonates having up to 1000-fold different potency, which is clinically obviated by giving smaller doses, although variations may also be seen in clinical effects. The following section will therefore describe the main clinical studies related to each compound (see also Hochberg[36]).

Etidronate

Etidronate was the first available bisphosphonate for treatment of osteoporosis. Etidronate is taken cyclically, 400mg for 2 weeks every 3 months, since over dosage may cause mineralization defects.

There are no randomized controlled trials primarily powered to evaluate the effect on fracture. Two trials have been conducted to assess the efficacy of cyclic etidronate treatment in postmenopausal women (Table 45.7). A significantly lower number of vertebral fractures were seen compared to placebo in a small Danish study but only 20 patients completed the study in each group and the validity is questioned, since events (new fractures), were counted instead of patients with fractures, which is considered a statistical violation. *Post-hoc* analysis of an American study showed a reduction in vertebral fractures in those with the most severe osteoporosis[38]. In clinical practice, using prescription data from the British General Practice Research Database, patients on etidronate appear to have fewer non-vertebral fractures compared to patients not treated, however the study also indicates that the treated patients may have a different health situation[39].

Alendronate

Alendronate, a second generation bisphosphonate, was the first bisphosphonate for which a clear anti-fracture effect was seen in large randomized controlled trials. Three major trials have shown a reduction in vertebral deformities of about 50%, and prevention of non-vertebral fractures has been demonstrated.

The first study, which included postmenopausal women with low bone density (T-score ≤ 2.5) with or without prevalent vertebral deformity[40], found the effect was most pronounced in women above age 65 and with at least one vertebral fracture at entry. In the Vertebral Fracture Arm of the Fracture Intervention Trial 1 (FIT 1)[41] 2027 women with at least one prevalent vertebral fracture were included. Alendronate treatment over 3 years gave a highly significant reduction in the number of new radiographic and clinical vertebral fractures ($P = 0.0001$) (Table 45.8) and a significant reduction of hip ($P = 0.0001$) and wrist fractures ($P = 0.0001$), albeit the number of fractures was small. In the Clinical Fracture Arm of FIT (FIT 2) over 4000 women were included on the basis of low BMD (T-score femoral neck < -1.6) in a 4 year trial[42]. The reduction of radiographically verified vertebral deformities was significant, but not for clinically presented vertebral fractures (Table 45.7). In a pre-planned sub-group analysis, all clinical fractures were reduced in women with bone density below the WHO threshold for osteoporosis (T-score of -2.5). In an international multicenter study of alendronate, the number of non-vertebral fractures was reduced in postmenopausal women with a T-score below -2.0[1]. In a randomized placebo controlled study of men with osteoporosis ($n = 241$) treated with alendronate 10mg/day, the incidence of vertebral deformities was lower after two years of treatment (0.8% versus 7.1%, $P = 0.022$)[43] with a corresponding increase in bone mass ($P = 0.001$).

These findings imply that treatment with alendronate is most efficient in reducing fracture in those at highest risk of new fractures by having a prevalent vertebral fracture or bone density confirming osteoporosis (T score of -2.5 or below). Treatment of women at lower risk appears less beneficial with fracture prevention as the end point.

Bone density increases at all sites during alendronate treatment. When comparing with placebo the mean increase over three years is about 6% in the lumbar spine, 4–4.5% in the femoral neck and 4.5–5.0% in the total hip measure. A significant 50–65% decrease of bone markers, particularly resorption markers such as N-telopeptide (NTx), is evident after 6–8 weeks of therapy[44].

Long-term treatment is often recommended, but data is still sparse concerning the continued anti-fracture effect. However, a sustained increase in BMD has been shown at all skeletal sites with 10mg/day of alendronate over 7 years in 235 postmenopausal women, which may suggest a concomitant anti-fracture effect[45]. The off-set of treatment after termination of alendronate therapy is not rapid as with hormone replacement but delayed over several years[46]. With the long-term deposition of alendronate in the skeleton, re-exposure at a site with new cycles of bone turnover is not excluded.

Treatment with alendronate 10mg/day has in clinical practice been linked to gastrointestinal side effects not identified in the randomized controlled trials of which esophageal erosions is the most serious. Side effects and the strict dosing routines for optimal absorption have lowered compliance.

A 70mg once weekly dosing regimen is now available which has been shown to give a similar increase in bone mass as daily or biweekly dosing in a study of 1258 postmenopausal women with osteoporosis. The fracture effect is assumed to be consistent with the reduction seen in earlier studies[47]. No increase in adverse GI events was experienced despite the higher dose, and there may even be a lower risk of serious GI events.

Estrogen and bisphosphonates act through different mechanisms on bone. A possible approach for those failing to gain enough bone on estrogen treatment alone or in those fracturing despite treatment would be to combine estrogen with a bisphosphonate. Two studies suggest an additive effect on BMD when combining estrogen treatment with alendronate in postmenopausal women over 1 or 2 years[48,49], but were not powered to evaluate the effect on fracture.

Risedronate

Risedronate is a third generation bisphosphonate with a 1000-fold higher potency than etidronate that has also been shown to prevent vertebral and non-vertebral fractures.

The number of radiographically diagnosed vertebral fractures was reduced by 41% and non-vertebral fractures reduced by 39% in a 3 year randomized controlled trial of 2458 postmenopausal women with one or more prevalent radiographic vertebral deformities[50] (Table 45.7). The study completion rate was only 55–60% as the 2.5mg group was discontinued prematurely and a high number of patients did not complete for other reasons. However, in the similar European and Australian arm of the trial which included women with two or more vertebral deformities ($n = 1226$), vertebral fractures were reduced by 49% and non-vertebral fractures by 33%[51].

Recently, results of a study to specifically evaluate the effect on hip fractures has been published[52]. Women aged 70–79 with low bone density ($n = 5445$) or women over 80 years with at least one risk factor for hip fracture ($n = 3886$) were randomized to risedronate or placebo. A 49% reduction in hip fracture was evident only in women with low bone density, while no effect was seen in the group of very elderly women aged 80–89 included on risk factors alone. Again this study points out that low bone density is a major determinant for clinical effect of anti-resorptive agents.

The effect on bone density is similar to that of alendronate producing about 4–6% increase in spinal and femoral bone mass after 3 years of treatment.

Risedronate has also become available in a once-weekly formula containing 35mg of active substance to be taken one day a week and thereby simplifying for the patients and enhance adherence to therapy[53].

Risedronate as other bisphosphonates, must be taken according to instructions. It appears to be well tolerated both in the studies and clinically with no serious side effects reported.

TABLE 45.7 THE EFFECT OF PHARMACOLOGICAL TREATMENT ON FRACTURE

Substance (reference)	Indication for treatment	No. of patients; mean age (range)	Duration (years)	Type of fracture; relative risk (95% CI)	NNT (95% CI)	Comments
Alendronate (FIT 1)[41]	Bone mineral density (−2.1) + vertebral fracture	2027; 71 years (55–81)	3	Vertebral fracture (X-ray) ε1; 0.53 (0.41–0.68)	15 (11–25)	A study of adequate design. In patients with prevalent vertebral fracture incident fractures are reduced. Because of small number of other fractures, only one additional hip fracture might have changed the result
				Vertebral fracture (X-ray) ε2; 0.10 (0.05–0.22)	24 (18–35)	
				Hip fracture; 0.49 (0.23–0.99)	90 (43–8949)	
				Vertebral fracture, symptomatic; 0.72 (0.58–0.90)	37 (23–89)	
Alendronate (FIT 2)[42]	Bone mineral density (−1.6) Subgroup: BMD ≤2.5	4432; 68 years (55–81) 266	4	Clinical fractures (all types); 0.86 (0.73–1.01)	NS	A study of adequate design. In patients without earlier fracture, only effect on radiographic vertebral fractures. Subgroup analysis showed effect also on other clinical fractures in women with BMD < −2.5SD. In women with BMD > −2.5SD no fracture reduction
				Vertebral fractures; 0.64 (0.50–0.82)	15 (10–35)	
Risedronate[50]	Osteoporosis + fracture	2458; 69 years (?–84)	3	Vertebral fractures; 0.59 (0.43–0.82)	20 (12–62)	The study is of adequate design, but suffers from a high discontinuation rate
				Non-vertebral fractures; 0.6 (0.39–0.94)	44 (22–640)	
				Hip fracture	NS	
Risedronate[51]	Osteoporosis + fracture	1226; 71 years (?–85)	3	Vertebral fractures; 0.51 (0.36–0.73)	10 (7–24)	The study is of adequate design, but suffers from a high discontinuation rate
				Non-vertebral; 0.67 (0.44–1.04)		
Risedronate[52]	Osteoporosis + fracture	5445; 71 years (?–85)		Hip fracture; 0.6 (0.4–0.9)	99 (52–421)	A study specifically designed to evaluate the effect on hip fracture. Indicates that risk factors alone are insufficient indicators for treatment
	Osteoporosis + risk factor	3886; 83 years	3	Hip fracture; 0.8 (0.6–1.2)	NS	
Etidronate[37]	Osteoporosis + fracture	66; 69 years	≤3	Vertebral fractures	NS	Not significant reduction when analyzed according to intention to treat
Etidronate[38]	Osteoporosis + fracture	378; 65 years	2	Vertebral fractures	NS	Not significant reduction when analyzed according to intention to treat
Raloxifene 60mg[69]	Osteoporosis	3012	3	Vertebral fractures 0.5 (0.4–0.8)	48 (29–120)	A large and well-done study with effect only on vertebral fractures
	Osteoporosis + fracture	1539		Vertebral fractures 0.7 (0.6–0.9)	16 (10–38)	
	Osteoporosis + fracture	7705 67 years (31–80)		Non-vertebral fractures 0.9 (0.8–1.1)	NS	
Estradiol + medroxy-progesterone[54]	Osteoporosis + fracture	75; 65 years	1 year	Vertebral fractures	NS	Limited from small size and short duration
Estradiol + norethisterone or estradiol alone[55]	Post-menopause	1006; 50 years	5 years	All types of fractures	NS	Reduction in wrist fractures when randomized and open label patients were pooled
Calcitonin[71]	Vertebal fracture	1255 70 yrs	5 yrs	Vertebal fractures 0.67 (0.47–0.97)	13 (7–77)	Only effect in the 200IU dose and not the higher dose. The study suffers from a high discontinuation rate
Parathyroid hormone[76]	Vertebal fracture	1637	21 mo	Vertebal fractures 0.31 (0.22–0.55)	11 (8–18)	Fracture reduction in high risk patients.
		70 yrs		Non-vertebral fractures 0.47 (0.25–0.88)		The study was prematurely ended, planned for 24 mo

Summary of major randomized controlled trials with fracture as primary end-point. The table includes number needed to treat (NNT). The interpretation of NNT must consider the specific conditions of the study and the values are therefore not necessarily directly comparable. From the perspective of evidence-based medicine, NNT is nevertheless the best way to obtain an overall comparison.

Sex hormones

In women the balance between bone resorption and bone formation in adulthood is, at least in part dependent on intact estrogen levels. The rapidly decreasing estrogen levels at menopause may lead to increased activation frequency, that is the number of active resorption sites increase while the capacity to refill the site with new bone diminishes causing bone loss. By substituting for estrogen loss or manipulating the estrogen receptor activity, the rate of bone turnover should remain in balance. This is the rationale for the use of ERT and for the development of new drugs that modify the estrogen receptor.

TABLE 45.8 OPTIONS FOR PREVENTING OSTEOPOROSIS AND FRACTURE

For the population	Individuals at high risk of fracture
Health education	**Education**
• Raising awareness	Self management
• General health promotion	Exercise
	Physiotherapy
Promote healthy lifestyle	Rehabilitation
• Encourage physical activity	Calcium and vitamin D supplements
• Dietary calcium and vitamin D	SERMs
• Avoid excess dieting	Fluoride
• Avoid smoking	Calcitonin
• Avoid excess alcohol	Bisphosphonates
	PTH
Avoid premature estrogen deficiency	
• Raising awareness of risks associated	**Fall prevention**
with estrogen deficiency	Targeted at the individual
	Hip protectors
Fall prevention	
• Promote physical activity	
• Reduce environmental hazards	

These can be considered for the population or for the individual.

Estrogen replacement

The initial indication for estrogen substitution to alleviate post-menopausal symptoms related to estrogen withdrawal, with the additional effect on bone turnover and bone mass have led to wide use.

Unfortunately, the effect on fracture by ERT has only been evaluated in two prospective randomized controlled trials[54,55] (Table 45.7) with still inconclusive results and evidence of fracture efficacy relies on epidemiological or case-control studies[30,56–60] in which a 25–50% fracture risk reduction is seen. In the Danish Osteoporosis Prevention study ($n = 2016$) the number of fractures was not significantly reduced in the randomized groups, while pooling with the open label group showed a reduction in wrist fracture. In a meta-analysis identifying 22 studies, data on fractures suggests an overall reduction in non-vertebral fractures, which was more pronounced on women below age 60 (RR 0.67, 95% CI 0.46–0.98) after at least 12 months of HRT[61]. The analysis included both placebo and non-placebo controlled trials, published and unpublished reports and fractures caused by high energy trauma or malignancy, rendering the results less certain but nevertheless indicative.

Numerous studies have indicated the beneficial effect of ERT on bone mass, with an increase of between 2–4% over 3 years in the spine but less in the hip. Even lower doses of estrogen, which may be better tolerated in elderly women, appear to prevent bone loss, particularly in the spine, but there is no fracture data on reduced dosage[62–64].

Estrogen should be given opposed with either cyclic or continuous progestogen to women with intact uterus.

The major concern for most women deciding to start on HRT is regarding the risk of breast cancer. An increase in breast cancer incidence in women taking HRT was seen in a recent large meta-analysis[65]. The relative risk increase was RR 1.023 (95% CI 1.011–1.036) or equal to a 2.3% risk of breast cancer with each year of HRT, but the aggressiveness of identified tumors or mortality was not increased. The findings were recently confirmed in the large randomized controlled trial as part of the Women's Health Initiative, specifically designed to evaluate the overall health benefits and risks of hormone treatment[66]. This trial included 16 608 postmenopausal women randomized to equine estrogen plus progesterone and placebo. At the 5.2-years safely monitoring, the risk estimates for breast cancer and cardiovascular events were significantly increased. On the other hand the study confirmed a risk

reduction for hip fracture (0.66, CI 0.45–0.98) and fracture in total. Duration of HRT should stay within 5–10 years or the risks may outweigh the benefits.

There is no upper age limit for initiating estrogen treatment, although it is better tolerated in recently postmenopausal women, in the elderly dose adjustments are normally necessary. If started in the early postmenopausal years an effect on vertebral fractures is more likely. The mean age for women with hip fracture is about 80 years of age and beginning HRT at later ages may then also confer protection of non-vertebral fractures, but other agents with proven fracture efficacy may be the treatment of choice in this situation. After discontinuation, the bone density effect of HRT rapidly disappears at a loss rate similar to that of normal menopause. Consequently, long-term effects on fracture cannot be assumed. In summary, at present the role of hormone replacement in the prevention and treatment of osteoporosis is questionable. Hormone replacement therapy should primarily be used in early postmenopausal women to alleviate climacteric symptoms during a limited period of time and the beneficial effects on bone and fracture rate regarded as added benefits.

Raloxifene

Selective estrogen receptor modulators (SERM) have been developed related to the identification of estrogen receptors. Binding of raloxifene to the ER blocks the conformational changes of the receptor and by this modulation alters its gene activation and subsequent protein production.

Raloxifene reduces the urinary calcium excretion, conferring a positive calcium balance[67] and decreases bone turnover assessed by bone markers[68].

In the Multiple Outcomes of Raloxifene Effectiveness (MORE) trial that enrolled 7705 osteoporotic women with and without vertebral fractures, there was an overall risk reduction of vertebral fractures (RR 0.70, 95% CI 0.50–0.80) with 60mg/day of raloxifene over 3 years[69] (Table 45.7). No effect was seen on non-vertebral fractures. Bone mass increased with 2.1% in the spine and 2.6% in the femoral neck on 60mg of raloxifene. The side effects were usually mild and mostly short lasting vasomotor symptoms. The more serious side effect was thromboembolic events, both deep vein thrombosis and pulmonary embolism, with a relative risk of 3.1 (95% CI 1.5–6.2) in the MORE trial, which corresponds to the risk with HRT.

New breast cancer cases were lower in the treated groups in the MORE study[70], despite the fact that the study was not powered to study breast cancer and at the 4-year follow up the risk reduction persisted[71]. Among the 5129 women treated with raloxifene 13 new cases were diagnosed, and in the placebo group of 2576 women 27 cases, giving an overall relative risk of 0.24 (95% CI 0.13–0.44). This apparent protective effect on the development of breast cancer is limited to those cancers that are estrogen receptor-positive; no reduction was noted in estrogen receptor-negative tumors.

Tibolone

Tibolone is a synthetic steroid with estrogenic, androgenic and gestagenic properties also exerting its effect by binding to the estrogen receptor. Tibolone relieves climacteric symptoms, without causing menstrual bleeding and with less breast tenderness compared to ERT. Two years of tibolone treatment in early postmenopausal women has shown a bone density response similar to that of ERT, but no data on fracture prevention is available[72,73].

Non-sex hormones
Calcitonin

Calcitonin is a peptide hormone with hypocalcemic and hypophosphatemic properties that acts as a physiologic antagonist to parathyroid hormone. Calcitonin is a 32 amino acid polypeptide synthesized in the parafollicular or C-cells of the thyroid gland, but under little pituitary control. Receptors for calcitonin are primarily present in bone and kidney. Calcitonin reduces bone resorption by acting on osteoclasts, rendering the cells smaller and less mobile, elevated serum calcium levels decrease and the renal excretion of calcium, sodium and phosphate increase. The bone effects have been extensively studied with hopes of obtaining a physiologic anti-resorptive agent. In addition, an analgesic effect from administration has been observed.

Calcitonin is available as subcutaneous or intramuscular injections or as nasal spray, developed from salmon calcitonin. Salmon calcitonin is about 10 times more potent than normally produced human calcitonin with a higher affinity for the receptor. Salmon calcitonin fragments may induce antibody production, a side effect more likely when using the parenteral route of administration. True allergic reactions or resistance are rare, while hot flushes and nausea are common transient side effects.

The potential of preventing vertebral fractures by nasal calcitonin in postmenopausal women is unclear. In a large study ($n = 1255$), postmenopausal women with one or more vertebral deformity were randomized to receive 100IU, 200IU or 400IU of calcitonin for 5 years. Fracture reduction assessed by X-ray was only seen in women treated with 200IU [RR 0.67 (95% CI 0.47–0.97)], while the higher dose 400IU did not significantly affect the fracture rate[74]. Radiographs were available in 88% of the women at one occasion, but only 511 (41%) of the included women completed the 5 year trial. Spinal bone mineral density increased between 1–1.5% from baseline.

In an earlier meta-analysis examining the efficacy of calcitonin in maintaining bone mass, eighteen clinical trials of various length were identified[75]. The mean increase in spinal BMD was 1.97% (CI 1.77–2.17) and in the femoral neck 0.32% (CI 0.27–0.91). The analysis also suggested an effect on vertebral fracture incidence.

In conclusion, present data suggest a relatively smaller effect on bone mineral density from calcitonin treatment compared to other anti-resorptive agents, while a reduction in vertebral fractures may still be induced. It has been speculated that the anti-fracture effect may be related to enhanced bone quality, which is not identified from DEXA measurements.

Parathyroid hormone

The physiological function of parathyroid hormone (PTH) is to maintain extracellular calcium levels. Rapid changes in the plasma calcium levels results from hormonal effects on bone and to a lesser extent on the kidney with change in renal calcium clearance. The effects are either direct on target cells or indirectly mediated through synthesis of 1,25 dihydroxyvitamin D. There is evidence for a dual action on bone and both osteoblasts and osteoclasts are responsive to PTH. Osteoblast differentiation and activity is stimulated as is the recruitment of lining cells and osteoclasts increase in number and activity. The resorptive effect predominates during sustained elevation of PTH, as is also seen in primary or secondary hyperparathyroidism, while an anabolic effect on bone is seen with intermittent dosing.

PTH consists of a single-chain peptide of 84 amino acids. The sequence and structure is well defined and it has been found that the N-terminal 1–34 amino acid residues are essential for the hormonal activity.

Utilizing the anabolic properties of PTH on bone has therefore been an attractive concept in order to obtain larger increases in bone mass than possible with anti-resorptive agents. PTH has been shown to primarily increase the cancellous or trabecular bone, hence the most pronounced effects have been seen in spinal bone density[76]. However, a smaller effect is also seen on the endosteal surface of cortical bone, including increased breaking strength in animal studies[77,78].

Recombinant human PTH (rhPTH) given as subcutaneous injection has been tested in patients with osteoporosis. Postmenopausal women with prevalent vertebral fractures ($n = 1637$) receiving 20 or 40μg of rhPTH 1–34 experienced a 65–69% (95% CI 0.22–0.55 and 0.19–0.50) reduction in new vertebral fractures and 53–54% (95% CI 0.25–0.88 and 0.25–0.86) reduction in non-vertebral fractures over 21 months[79]. There

was a dose dependent increase in spinal and femoral neck BMD of 9–13% and 6–9%, respectively. Other studies have shown marked increases in predominantly spinal BMD and suggested reduction in vertebral fractures, particularly when PTH has been combined with agents reducing bone resorption[80,81].

The availability of PTH, as an anabolic agent, opens up the treatment options for severe cases of osteoporosis, unresponsive to other agents or possibly when side effects prohibits their use. Since PTH needs to be more closely monitored because of risk for hypercalcemia, cyclic combination therapy of PTH with for example a bisphosphonate may be a future alternative for longer term treatment.

Other substances
Fluoride
Fluoride is a potent anabolic agent acting directly on the osteoblast by altering intracellular signal transduction. The effect of fluoride on bone was initially identified as endemic fluorosis in regions of high natural fluoride content in drinking water, causing dental and skeletal deformities and increased bone fragility. Fluoride has been shown to promote incremental increases in bone formation and this anabolic effect can be utilized in the treatment of osteoporosis if the dose is titrated to stay within a therapeutic window. However this is without a demonstrated reduction in fracture rate[82–84]. Further development of fluoride treatment is not anticipated without clear evidence of an anti-fracture effect and the continued suspicion of a detrimental effect on bone quality and bone strength.

Novel therapies
Increasing knowledge of mechanisms regulating bone cell activity provides potential sources for new therapeutic strategies. The unique ability of osteoclasts to dissolve and degrade bone tissue includes production of numerous substances both for mineral dissolution and the enzymatic degradation of matrix. The degradation of matrix is mediated by cathepsin K, an osteoclast protease which appears to specifically act on bone collagen[85]. Animal models confirm the important effect of cathepsin K and deletion of the cathepsin K gene results in an osteopetrotic bone in mice[86]. An inhibitor of cathepsin K may therefore have potential use as an anti-resorptive drug. Recent knowledge on cell differentiation and cell activity shows that cytokines are important regulators on the local level. In addition, molecular biology has provided novel insight about the intracellular signaling and transcellular communication. Most cytokines are implicated as enhancers of osteoclast activity and subsequently bone resorption. Blockage of cytokine activity has already gained success with the anti-TNFα treatment of rheumatoid arthritis (RA), which may have additional effects on bone turnover, since TNFα has been shown to be one of the more important cytokines modifying bone resorption. Bone resorption markers significantly decrease in patients with RA treated with infliximab[87]. This may allow for development of inhibitors to other bone active cytokines, such as IL-1 or IL-6. The relative non-specificity and subsequent effects on other organs may limit the usefulness.

Identification of factors acting on receptors for osteoclast attachment or function, such as the $\alpha_v\beta_3$integrin, RANKL (receptor activator of nuclear factor κB ligand) or the soluble ligand osteoprotegerin may be fertile ground for development of antagonists. Clinical testing of osteoprotegerin indicates a positive effect on bone density in postmenopausal women[88].

NON-PHARMACOLOGICAL INTERVENTION

Physical exercise
Physical activity is of benefit for the well-being and general health of every person. Mechanical loading of the skeleton is one of the mechanisms by which bone remains physiologically intact as it is an important signal for bone remodeling. Bone mass increases in response to increased

load. The question is whether the beneficial effect on bone of physical exercise is maintained beyond active training or through periods of inactivity and if a risk reduction of falls and fracture is measurable.

Evaluating current and lifetime effects on exercise retrospectively indicates higher total and hip BMD in persons exercising[89]. Exercise programs appear to increase bone mass by a few percent in the postmenopausal and elderly women[90]. This is consistent with a meta-analysis which separately estimated the effect from impact and non-impact training in randomized controlled trials[91]. Impact exercise conferred a 0.9–1.6% non-significant net gain in spine or femoral neck bone density in pre- and postmenopausal women. The effect from non-impact exercise was 1.0–1.2% in the spine and not calculable in the femoral neck because of too few trials. Evidence suggests a stronger effect of exercise in childhood prior to sexual maturation and achievement of peak bone mass[92].

Longitudinal and cross-sectional studies suggest a protective effect against fracture in women with a higher physical activity level[93–95]. Since physical activity only gives a small percentage increase in bone mass, it is likely that a significant contribution of an anti-fracture effect is related to improvement of balance, co-ordination and muscle strength. These factors may not only reduce the risk of falls by tripping or misplacing steps, but also reduce the impacts by increased ability to protect and counteract a fall.

Prospective studies indicate that it is possible in the elderly to increase muscle strength[96] and to improve balance with a concomitant decrease in the number of falls[97–99] through exercise programs.

In these studies, as in studies evaluating the effect on bone mass, an effect induced by sampling or participation bias cannot be excluded, and it remains a challenge to determine the full effect of physical activity.

Smoking cessation

Numerous epidemiological studies indicate an independent risk increase of osteoporosis from smoking, the relative risk being between 1.2–1.8[100,101]. Smokers often have additional risk factors and comorbidities such as chronic pulmonary obstruction or emphysema.

The adverse effect of smoking is more pronounced in current smokers and dose dependent with a greater impact in men compared to women[102] with an overall bone mass reduction of 0.1 SD, but most pronounced at the hip and with a positive effect on bone mass with cessation. In addition, an increased risk of hip fracture is seen in both sexes (RR 1.36–1.59), with a higher risk in male smokers[103]. After 5 years male ex-smokers had a decreased risk of hip fracture, while no risk reduction was seen in women, suggesting a longer lasting negative effect of smoking in women.

Hip protectors

Hip fracture, the most debilitating fragility fracture, occurs predominantly in the elderly. An estimated 25% of fracture patients are admitted from institutions or various forms of residential care, indicating the frailty and morbidity of these patients. Hip fractures usually result from a sideways fall with maximum impact on the trochanter to which the faller is unable to take any protective measures. Hip fracture patients are often thin with only minimal cushioning from subcutaneous tissue over the hip. External hip protectors have been developed to reduce the impact on the fall and subsequently the incidence of hip fracture.

An external hip protector has a hard external surface with an underlying soft padding close to the body and it is formed to fit over the trochanter. They are either attached to the underwear or by Velcro belts and worn under clothes.

Studies to evaluate the efficacy of external hip protectors have been made on institutionalized patients of high age (mean 80–85 years), acknowledged frequent fallers and at high risk of hip fracture[104–106] and a Cochrane review concludes that hip protectors reduce the risk of hip fracture in selected populations[107]. One problem has been the low acceptance by the users which has been down to 30–40%.

Fall prevention

The vast numbers of non-vertebral fractures are related to falls, and measures to prevent falls and to reduce the impact of a fall are first line interventions to prevent fractures in those at risk. Fall preventive strategies are aimed at external or environmental factors, both in the home and in society, and at internal or patient related factors. Such factors are described in Table 45.5.

Falls become increasingly common with aging. About 30% of individuals over 65 years fall each year, increasing to 50% over 80 years, most common amongst residents of long-term care institutions. Most falls occur indoors where the majority of hip fractures occur. The likelihood of an elderly person falling is increased if he or she has fallen already. Although not all falls result in fracture, many result in impaired health, hospitalization and permanent disability. There will be an identifiable treatable cause of the fall in 10% of cases; an identifiable environmental cause in a further 10% but the cause of most falls is multifactorial and relates to general ill-health – more specifically, to sensory and musculoskeletal decline with lower limb weakness, unsteadiness and loss of protective mechanisms. The inability to rise unaided from a chair without using the arms is an important risk factor of falls and is common in institutionalized people.

The role of exercise in reducing falls has been discussed above. Interventions to reduce the risk of falling at home are aimed at minimizing known hazards related to falls, such as loose carpets, electrical cords, abundance of furniture or insufficient indoor light. Numerous studies have described the hazards and indicate the attributable risks. Prevention programs, both self-assessed through check-lists or carried out by home care providers, have been developed[10]. The long-term efficacy of fall prevention programs is difficult to evaluate and information is lacking with regards to fracture. Available studies suggest that modification of home hazards particularly in the elderly with a history of falling can reduce the risk of additional falls by 30–40%[108,109], while the evidence is not conclusive in unselected populations.

Preventive steps to reduce hazards in other areas of society should also result in a reduced risk of falls and of fracture, but there is little evidence. Elderly persons sustain falls and fracture in traffic areas without being directly related to traffic accidents for example from slippery or uneven side-walks and curbs, buses starting or breaking abruptly or inadequate snow and ice removal[110].

Rehabilitation following osteoporotic fracture

An important part of the management of osteoporosis is the rehabilitation of subjects following a fracture.

Fracture treatment aims to restore anatomical continuity allowing the patient to regain function or minimize the loss of function and to diminish associated pain. With either conservative or operative treatment the rehabilitation period may last up to a year.

For patients returning to their home a multidisciplinary team-approach often gives a superior result[111]. Hip fracture patients should have a complete assessment of their pre-fracture situation with respect to physical functioning, home and social situation. Based on this assessment an individual rehabilitation plan should be developed including a 'best-outcome' estimate. The plan should be developed with the patient so that he or she has an understanding of the goals, in order to make it successful.

Rehabilitation after hip fracture is often undertaken in the home with support from community health professionals. It is imperative that the care givers are educated in and have an understanding of the different aspects involved in the rehabilitation and healing process after fracture. Walk training, use of walking aids and later adapted exercise programs need to be monitored, but most of all, the patient needs to be encouraged.

The severely disabled elderly women who have previously suffered from multiple fractures including vertebral fractures may need rehabilitative efforts. The main goal should be to preserve the remaining physical function to allow as much independence of self-care as possible. The ability to stand with or without support is an important functional divide in the most frail and the main objective of lower limb fracture treatment. Long periods of non-weight bearing are often detrimental to the standing and walking capability in the elderly, therefore it is equally important to achieve stable fracture fixation in the elderly. With upper extremity fracture early motion training leads to better long term function. Even if full range of motion is not regained the functional impairment may not be perceived as detrimental.

Rehabilitation should also include preventive measures against future fracture. Simple training programs of balance, co-ordination and muscle strength can accomplish improvement even in the eldest[112].

MANAGEMENT STRATEGIES

The principles of fracture prevention are to maximize bone strength and to prevent falls at the age when fracture risk is greatest, that is in later life, and prevention must be considered at all stages of life to achieve this. In addition, those who have already sustained a fracture must be appropriately managed to ensure the best possible outcome.

Strategies will be discussed for the population as a whole and for the individual (Fig. 45.2), relating evidence-based interventions with clinical experience.

Fracture prevention at the population level

Fracture prevention requires addressing all factors that can modify fracture risk throughout life (Fig. 45.2). These recommendations must be supported by raising public awareness of osteoporosis and of what factors should raise their concern about personal risk and the potential health gain to be achieved by its prevention.

Peak bone mass is the major determinant of bone mass in later stages of life. A total of 60–80% of peak bone mass is genetically determined, the rest depending on factors such as nutrition, physical activity and adequate sex hormone levels. The skeleton consolidates in young adults and then turnover is in balance to maintain a relatively stable bone mass. Prevention entails establishing and maintaining a lifestyle that ensures maximum bone mass at all times of life. Exercise increases bone density but the effect is dependent on continued loading so that any activity needs to be sustainable throughout life. Calcium intake influences peak bone mass achieved (Table 45.9). Smoking and excess alcohol are associated with low bone density as is over-exercise and over-dieting leading to hypogonadism and amenorrhea. There needs to be greater awareness of the risk of future osteoporosis associated with reduced exposure to female sex hormones, such as with primary hypogonadism or secondary amenorrhea to encourage early recognition and management.

Bone mass starts to decline in the 5th and 6th decades, slowly in men; however, the menopause marks the onset of rapid bone loss in some women. Regular physical activity, exercise and avoidance of smoking and excess alcohol are recommended. Early postmenopausal rapid bone loss may be slowed down by ERT, however its use is a balance between the individual's risk and the potential benefit and risks from ERT and any decision needs to be made at the level of that individual. Health promotion campaigns should make all women aware of these options and of factors that may influence their own risks of future fracture.

Most fractures occur above the age of 65 years. Over this age there is also the clearest separation between the fit and the unfit aging population. Apart from specific conditions, the level of physical activity is one of the best discriminators of this and much effort needs to be put into trying to encourage people to increase their level of physical activity in a way that is sustainable throughout old age. This will have a small effect on bone mass but the benefit of exercise at this age is more directly related to improving muscle strength, lower limb function, co-ordination and balance with a reduction in risk of falls. At this age bone mass is low in an increasing number and the occurrence of falls is an important discriminator of who does and who does not fracture. Awareness must also be raised of risk factors for falls and environmental causes should be removed. In addition, dietary dairy intake often reduces as age increases and calcium intake must be improved by reversing this trend or by encouraging the use of supplements (Table 45.9). Lack of going outdoors with consequent low sunlight exposure and as well as poor diet can lead to vitamin D insufficiency with secondary hyperparathyroidism, and these trends need reversing.

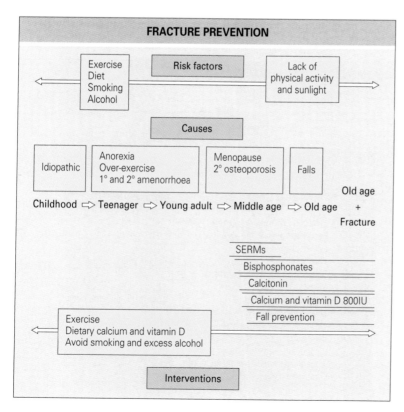

Fig. 45.2 Fracture prevention. Fracture prevention requires addressing all factors that modify fracture risk at all stages of life.

TABLE 45.9 RECOMMENDED DAILY DIETARY ALLOWANCE FOR CALCIUM		
Group	Age (years)	Range (mg)
Newborn	0–0.5	400
Children	1–3	400–600
	4–6	450–600
	7–10	550–700
Men	11–24	900–1000
	25–65	700–800
	65–	700–800
Women	11–24	900–1000
	25–50	700–800
	50–65	800
	65–	700–800
Pregnant		700–900
Lactating		1200

(Adapted from European Community Report[3].)

Fracture prevention in the individual

The prevention of a fracture in an individual requires treating those at highest risk of fracture and addressing all risk factors linked to fracture with low bone mass being one of the most important. It also means preventing fracture in those already with osteoporosis. In addition, any one who has sustained an osteoporotic fracture needs appropriate management to ensure the best outcome.

Who to treat

Those at highest risk of osteoporosis and future fracture need to be recognized at all stages of life.

In childhood and early adulthood the commonest specific cause relates to gonadal hormone deficiency which can affect both sexes. Females with late menarche and secondary amenorrhea need to be identified, the underlying cause found and treated. Anorexia nervosa and over-exercise syndrome are common causes. Infertility is often associated with low estrogen levels that need to be treated beyond the management of infertility. Pregnancy can be rarely associated with osteoporosis with rapid loss of spinal bone mass and fracture. Adequate nutrients during the growth phase are important and lactose intolerance can result in lifelong low calcium intake. Other conditions include celiac disease, causes of prolonged immobility, and steroid treated inflammatory conditions such as juvenile idiopathic arthritis, asthma, inflammatory bowel disease, or rheumatoid arthritis. Cystic fibrosis now has a better prognosis but is often complicated by osteoporosis and may present with fracture. Osteogenesis imperfecta often manifests as childhood fractures. Diagnosis of osteoporosis is difficult by bone density in the growing skeleton as it is dependent on stage of puberty and the relationship of T or Z score with fracture risk is not established at this age.

From mid-life and onwards idiopathic osteoporosis becomes increasingly common. Those who will benefit most from an intervention can be identified by the combination of risk factors (Table 45.1) and bone densitometry. Identification and investigation is only appropriate if the person is prepared to and capable of taking any recommended treatment for long enough to achieve its goal of fracture prevention (Fig. 45.3). Women and men at high risk can either be found by a sys-

tematic approach at a midlife health check or opportunistically when being seen for an intercurrent problem. Risk factors may be documented on health records. A low trauma fracture at this age, such as a Colles fracture, is a strong risk factor for future fracture. Many are however not in routine contact with their family physicians and public awareness campaigns are needed to encourage them to inquire about their individual needs for preventive therapy for osteoporosis.

In the more elderly, it is important to target those who are frail and with an adherent risk of falling, as well as those with other risks for fracture. The benefit from any intervention is greater at this age because of the increased incidence of fractures in the later decades of life. The opportunities for case finding are greater at this age as many will be in contact with health professionals for routine procedures such as flu vaccination or as a result of various intercurrent problems. Indeed, an unique opportunity for case finding is the patient who presents with a low trauma fracture.

The person may present with a low energy fracture of the limb bones or pelvis, a sudden onset of back pain or a gradual loss of height and stoop.

The management of osteoporosis once confirmed

When osteoporosis has been diagnosed the appropriate management must be considered.

Education and support

Osteoporosis must be fully explained to the individual so they understand what the risks are and what they can do to reduce them. They may not have sustained a fracture and one must be careful not to give them a 'disease' when it is a risk they have for a possible future fracture. A bone-healthy lifestyle must be encouraged and unnecessary fear avoided.

Maximize bone strength

Bone mass must be maximized to increase strength and reduce risk of fracture.

In the developing skeleton and younger adults, as these situations are all uncommon, there is little evidence as yet for different interventions, and it is unlikely that fracture prevention data will become readily available. The principles are to treat the underlying condition effectively,

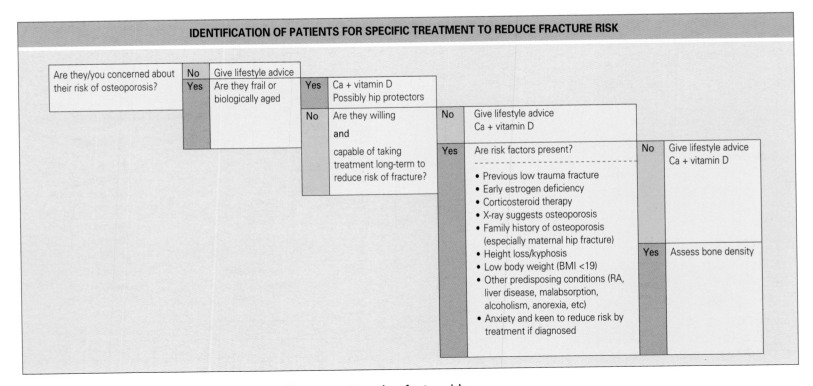

IDENTIFICATION OF PATIENTS FOR SPECIFIC TREATMENT TO REDUCE FRACTURE RISK

Fig. 45.3 A flow chart for identifying patients for specific treatment to reduce fracture risk.

TABLE 45.10 RECOMMENDATIONS FOR MANAGEMENT BASED ON HIP–BONE DENSITY	
T > –1	Lifestyle advice
T –1 to –2.5	Lifestyle advice
T –1 to –2.5 and low-energy fracture	Investigate for causes of fracture Treat <ul><li>Lifestyle advice</li></ul> *and one of* <ul><li>Bisphosphonate</li><li>SERM</li><li>Intranasal calcitonin</li></ul>
T < –2.5	Investigate for causes of osteoporosis Treat <ul><li>Lifestyle advice</li></ul> *and one of* <ul><li>Bisphosphonate</li><li>SERM</li><li>Intranasal calcitonin</li></ul>
T < –2.5 and low-energy fracture	Investigate for causes of osteoporosis Investigate for causes of fracture Treat <ul><li>Lifestyle advice</li></ul> *and one of* <ul><li>Bisphosphonate</li><li>SERM</li><li>Intranasal calcitonin</li></ul>

TABLE 45.11 PRINCIPLES OF FALL PREVENTION

- Identify treatable causes (Table 45.5)
- Maintenance of fitness, balance and alertness
- Maintenance of vision and hearing
- Reduction of environmental hazards
- Reduce impact of falls

TABLE 45.12 PRINCIPLES OF TREATMENT OF ESTABLISHED OSTEOPOROSIS

- Explanation to and education of the patient and partner or care-giver
- Fracture management
- Pain management
- Functional assessment and practical advice
- Physiotherapy advice and exercise regimes
- Prevention of falls and of their impact
- Prevention and attempted reversal of bone loss

---

ensure adequate estrogen levels and avoid any excessive use of corticosteroids where relevant. Specific treatments have to be considered on the merits of the individual case. There is increasing experience of the effective use of bisphosphonates in children and young adults, mainly in the management of osteogenesis imperfecta[113].

At mid-life, in addition to recommending a bone health promoting lifestyle, the interventions chosen and duration of treatment may be based on estimated fracture risk from the T-score measured by bone densitometry (Table 45.10). Because of offset of effect, treatment will have to be taken long-term to prevent fracture at the age they are most prevalent, that is over 70 years. The risks and health economics of this approach have to be considered. From an evidence based point of view the anti-fracture effect is significant only in those with osteoporosis or prevalent vertebral fracture. That is why any specific intervention at this age is targeted at those who are at highest risk of future fracture and why interventions that have broader benefits than just on bone mass and fracture risk should be first considered.

Over 65 years a healthy bone promoting lifestyle is recommended as there is most evidence at this age that correcting calcium deficiency and increasing physical activity are effective. Calcium and vitamin D should be the baseline treatment and have been shown to prevent hip fracture in the institutionalized elderly[24,25]. Bisphosphonates, SERM and calcitonin reduce bone loss and can prevent fracture. There is little comparative data between the different treatment options in this situation. Bisphonates are clearly most effective in those with osteoporosis.

Prevent falls and their impact

Falls can be prevented by identifying those most at risk of falling (Table 45.5) and coordinating appropriate preventive action (Table 45.11). Interventions are most effective that target both the multiple intrinsic risk factors for the individual and environmental hazards[10].

The likelihood of an elderly person falling is increased if he or she has fallen already. It is therefore important to look for the causes of a fall and to try and prevent further falls in future from that or any other correctable cause. Structured home visits can be effective in identifying and modifying both intrinsic and extrinsic causes of the fall. Falls can be reduced by exercise programs that concentrate on improving lower limb strength, co-ordination and balance. Exercises can also improve protective responses.

Hip protectors can prevent fracture of the hip and should be considered in recurrent fallers who have osteoporosis.

The management of established osteoporosis

Once a fracture has occurred in the presence of low bone density, it is called established osteoporosis. Management is directed at the prevention of further fracture and the control of pain and the rehabilitation of the person. Fractures are typically of the distal radius, proximal femur or vertebral bodies, but low bone mineral density is associated with low trauma fractures at all sites except the head.

The aims of treatment are to relieve symptoms, by controlling pain and appropriate fracture treatment, to improve quality of life by tackling functional and practical problems, and to prevent further fractures by prevention of falls and reversal of bone loss (Table 45.12).

Education and support

A patient can cope much better with a chronic painful disabling disease if they have a good understanding of it and know what to expect. Information is available from support organizations and programs that teach self-management but can with advantage be developed locally.

Fracture management

Survival and future independence depends on proper management of the acute fracture. Comorbidity affects outcome and many are frail and confused when they fracture their hip. For the best outcome it is recommended[114] that hip fracture cases should be rapidly transferred to hospital, receive adequate pain relief and pressure area protection, and have surgery if possible within 24 hours. Antibiotic prophylaxis and anticoagulation to prevent thromboembolism are part of routine care. Postoperative pain management, adequate hydration, early mobilization followed by a structured rehabilitation program are important.

Pain management

Pain management is essential for the effective rehabilitation of the person with an acute or previous fracture. Patients tend to avoid analgesics and hence undertreat their pain. Analgesics should be selected according to severity of pain and response to previous treatment.

Acute vertebral fracture may require short-term use of opiate analgesics and bed rest for the first few days to get the pain under control and allow early mobilization. This should be on a background of simple analgesics such as paracetamol, dextropropoxyphene, tramadol or a NSAID. If NSAIDs are used, COX 2 selective inhibitors are recommended in view of age and likely presence of other risk factors for serious upper gastrointestinal complications. It is important to use sufficiently high and regular doses of analgesics to avoid peaks of pain and optimize pain control. If this is inadequate, calcitonin (100IU on alternate days by injection for up to 6 weeks) has some analgesic effects but can be associated with nausea, vomiting, flushing and dizziness. As the pain improves, opiate analgesics should be discontinued. The early introduction of antiresorptive therapy with bisphosphonates will decrease bone fragility and may reduce pain.

Chronic pain may require long-term treatment with analgesics which may need to be used regularly and in combination to gain maximum effect but full pain relief is an optimistic outcome. Tricyclic antidepressants may improve pain control but need to be used with caution to avoid daytime sedation with increased risk of falling. Heat, ultrasound, and massage can help to reduce muscle spasm. Corsets seldom help as they constrict an already compressed abdomen and chest. Surgical vertebroplasty or kyphoplasty, lifting and augmenting the collapsed vertebra, may be a future possibility to decrease pain.

Functional and practical problems and advice

A multidisciplinary approach is needed to assess and discuss problems of everyday life and provide solutions where possible. Many older people lose independence following a limb fracture. Rehabilitation may need to include everything from simple walking aids to home assessment or advanced home care.

Physiotherapy advice and exercise in osteoporosis

The aim of physiotherapy is to reduce symptoms and disability related to the fracture often worsened by comorbidity. Early mobilization is necessary to avoid pressure sores, constipation, venous thromboembolism, disorientation and dependency. Physiotherapy may be used to increase body awareness, encourage pain avoiding behavior, improve balance and coordination and reduce risk and fear of falls. An individualized exercise program is often needed because of pain and comorbidities. Additional benefits of motivation and social interaction can be gained if the program can be performed in a group setting, which also may improve compliance. Any exercise must not increase the risk of falling. Hydrotherapy is especially suitable if in pain and mobility is restricted.

Specific exercises for vertebral osteoporosis should also be encouraged. These should include relaxation to relieve muscle spasm; breathing exercises; and strengthening of postural (legs, back, and abdominals), pelvic floor, shoulder girdle and neck muscles. The exercises should be tried cautiously at first, preferably under supervision, and then performed regularly if they do not aggravate symptoms and are not too exhausting. Height and posture should be monitored. Manipulation should be avoided.

Prevention of further bone loss and fracture

Osteoporosis should be confirmed by bone densitometry, although multiple vertebral fractures are almost always diagnostic of osteoporosis. Bone loss cannot be fully restored at this stage but further bone loss can be slowed or reversed as recommended above with reduction in risk of further fracture. Falls should be prevented where possible by looking for and modifying causes and risk factors. Consideration should be given to the use of hip protectors.

MONITORING TREATMENT

Bone mineral density

Bone mineral density is a surrogate end-point for fracture, but it is the effect measure that is possible to evaluate in the individual patient. Because of the precision error of available bone densitometers and the low rate of change in bone mass even with pharmacological treatment options, reevaluation of the patients is usually not meaningful in clinical practice until after 2 years of anti-resorptive therapy. At the time of remeasurement of bone mass, a change less than 2% in the individual patient is most likely not clinically significant. The estimated rate of loss of 0.5–1.0% per year that might have occurred without any intervention may be considered at reevaluation.

Follow-up measurements by DXA of the hip or spine are validated, while treatment response has not been followed long term by ultrasound of the heel.

Bone markers

Bone markers are extensively studied and used as early markers of effect in pharmaceutical trials. Most therapies act by repressing bone resorption, consequently the major effect is seen on bone resorption markers, such as deoxypyridinoline, N- or C-telopeptide (NTx, CTx,). A 40–60% decrease is commonly observed after 6–12 weeks of specific anti-resorptive therapy with bisphosphonates. The problem in using bone markers is related to the analytical and biological variability, particularly the relatively high intra-individual variability. Part of these problems can be reduced by standardized sampling procedures. If used properly, bone markers have potential in monitoring treatment and evidence suggests that markers can predict the BMD response to treatment for 2–3 years[11].

Quality of life

Osteoporosis with either vertebral or non-vertebral fractures influence quality of life and this should be monitored to ensure optimal management. Pain and loss of physical function, especially mobility, are the common problems with limitation of activities and restricted participation along with anxiety about future fracture. A number of validated instruments are available to measure outcome such as the EFFOQOL[115] which includes questions in the domains pain, physical function, social function, general health perception and mental function. Such instruments are however often too complex to use in regular practice. A simple 4-5-questionnaire would be of advantage for the practising physician to provide a simple, rapid and systematic evaluation of the quality of life that could be used on a regular basis in the clinic. This questionnaire should consider pain that affects function; self care such as washing and dressing; independent activities such as going out; and well-being – are you happy. Suggestions for questions are; (1) "Have you experienced pain that limited your daily activities during the past week?"; (2) "Are you able to wash and dress yourself?"; (3) "Have you walked outside for pleasure or shopping during the past 2 weeks?"; and (4) "Are you satisfied with your current living situation?".

CONCLUSION

- Patients with fracture or with background factors associated with high risk of fracture should be assessed for osteoporosis.
- Patients with high risk of fracture should be considered for specific treatment to reduce the risk of fracturing, dietary assessment and supplementation with calcium and vitamin D.
- Non-pharmacological interventions to prevent falls and to improve bone mass should be encouraged throughout life, emphasizing that the effect is sustained only in those currently training.

REFERENCES

1. Pols HA, Felsenberg D, Hanley DA *et al.* Multinational, placebo-controlled, randomized trial of the effects of alendronate on bone density and fracture risk in postmenopausal women with low bone mass: results of the FOSIT study. Foxamax International Trial Study Group. Osteoporos Int 1999; 9: 461–468.

2. Genant HK, Cooper C, Poor G *et al.* Interim report and recommendations of the World Health Organization Task Force for Osteoporosis. Osteoporos Int 1999; 10: 259–264.

3. Report on osteoporosis in the European Community: action for prevention. Luxembourg: European Communities Report; 1998.

4. National Osteoporosis Foundation. Osteoporosis: review of the evidence for prevention, diagnosis and cost-effectiveness analysis 11. Osteoporos Int 1998; 8: S1–S88.

5. Osteoporosis: clinical guidelines for prevention and treatment. London: Royal College of Physicians; 1999.

6. Lauritzen JB. Hip fractures: incidence, risk factors, energy absorption, and prevention. Bone 1996; 18(suppl): 65S–75S.

7. Hans D, Dargent-Molina P, Schott AM *et al.* Ultrasonographic heel measurements to predict hip fracture in elderly women: the EPIDOS prospective study. Lancet 1996; 348: 511–514.

8. Gardsell P, Johnell O, Nilsson BE, Gullberg B. Predicting various fragility fractures in women by forearm bone densitometry: a follow-up study. Calcif Tissue Int 1993; 52: 348–353.

9. Espallargues M, Sampietro-Colom L, Estrada MD *et al.* Identifying bone-mass-related risk factors for fracture to guide bone densitometry measurements: a systematic review of the literature. Osteoporos Int 2001; 12: 811–822.

10. Department of Health. National service framework for older people. London: DoH; 2001.

11. Ebeling PR, Åkesson K. Role of biochemical markers in the management of osteoporosis. In: Sambrook P, Woolf A, eds. Clinical rheumatology. London: Baillière Tindall, 2001: 385–400.

12. Torgerson DJ, Donaldson C, Reid DM. Bone mineral density measurements: are they worthwhile? J R Soc Med 1996; 89: 457–461.

13. Doherty DA, Sanders KM, Kotowicz MA, Prince RL. Lifetime and five-year age-specific risks of first and subsequent osteoporotic fractures in postmenopausal women. Osteoporos Int 2001; 12(1): 16–23.

14. Osteoporosis: Clinical guidelines for prevention and treatment. Update on pharmacological interventions and an algorithm for management. London: Royal College of Physicians; 2000.

15. Shea B, Rosen CJ, Guyatt GH *et al.* A meta analysis of calcium supplementation for the prevention of postmenopausal osteoporosis. Osteoporos Int 2000; 11(suppl 2): S114.

16. Cumming RG, Nevitt MC. Calcium for prevention of osteoporotic fractures in postmenopausal women. J Bone Miner Res 1997; 12: 1321–1329.

17. Dawson-Hughes B, Dallal GE, Krall EA *et al.* A controlled trial of the effect of calcium supplementation on bone density in postmenopausal women. N Engl J Med 1990; 323: 878–883.

18. Bonjour JP, Carrie AL, Ferrari S *et al.* Calcium-enriched foods and bone mass growth in prepubertal girls: a randomized, double-blind, placebo-controlled trial. J Clin Invest 1997; 99: 1287–1294.

19. Lips P, Graafmans WC, Ooms ME *et al.* Vitamin D supplementation and fracture incidence in elderly persons. A randomized, placebo-controlled clinical trial. Ann Intern Med 1996; 124: 400–406.

20. Meyer HE, Falch JA, Kaavik E *et al.* Can vitamin D supplementation reduce the risk of fracture in the elderly? Osteoporos Int 2000; 11(suppl 2): S114–S115.

21. Gillespie WJ, Henry DA, O'Connell DL, Robertson J. Vitamin D and vitamin D analogues for preventing fractures associated with involutional and post-menopausal osteoporosis. Cochrane Database Syst Rev 2000; CD000227.

22. Ooms ME, Roos JC, Bezemer PD *et al.* Prevention of bone loss by vitamin D supplementation in elderly women: a randomized double-blind trial. J Clin Endocrinol Metab 1995; 80: 1052–1058.

23. Dawson-Hughes B, Harris SS, Krall EA *et al.* Rates of bone loss in postmenopausal women randomly assigned to one of two dosages of vitamin D. Am J Clin Nutr 1995; 61: 1140–1145.

24. Chapuy MC, Arlot ME, Duboeuf F *et al.* Vitamin D3 and calcium to prevent hip fractures in elderly women. N Engl J Med 1992; 327: 1637–1642.

25. Chapuy MC, Arlot ME, Delmas PD, Meunier PJ. Effect of calcium and cholecalciferol treatment for three years on hip fractures in elderly women. Brit Med J 1994; 308: 1081–1082.

26. Reid IR, Ames RW, Evans MC *et al.* Long-term effects of calcium supplementation on bone loss and fractures in postmenopausal women: a randomized controlled trial. Am J Med 1995; 98: 331–335.

27. Lips P. Vitamin D supplementation and fracture incidence in elderly persons. A randomized, placebo-controlled clinical trial. Ann Intern Med 1996; 124: 400–406.

28. Dawson-Hughes B, Harris SS, Krall EA, Dallal GE. Effect of calcium and vitamin D supplementation on bone density in men and women 65 years of age or older. N Engl J Med 1997; 337: 670–676.

29. Heikinheimo RJ, Inkovaara JA, Harju EJ *et al.* Annual injection of vitamin D and fractures of aged bones. Calcif Tissue Int 1992; 51: 105–110.

30. Kanis JA, Johnell O, Gullberg B *et al.* Evidence for efficacy of drugs affecting bone metabolism in preventing hip fracture. Brit Med J 1992; 305: 1124–1128.

31. Baeksgaard L, Andersen KP, Hyldstrup L. Calcium and vitamin D supplementation increases spinal BMD in healthy, postmenopausal women. Osteoporos Int 1998; 8: 255–260.

32. Tilyard MW, Spears GF, Thomson J, Dovey S. Treatment of postmenopausal osteoporosis with calcitriol or calcium. N Engl J Med 1992; 326: 357–362.

33. Aloia JF, Vaswani A, Yeh JK *et al.* Calcitriol in the treatment of postmenopausal osteoporosis. Am J Med 1988; 84: 401–408.

34. Falch JA, Odegaard OR, Finnanger AM, Matheson I. Postmenopausal osteoporosis: no effect of three years treatment with 1,25-dihydroxycholecalciferol. Acta Med Scand 1987; 221: 199–204.

35. Fleisch H. Bisphosphonates in bone disease. From laboratory to man. London: Academic Press; 2000.

36. Hochberg MC. Bisphosphonates. In: Cummings SR, Cosman F, Jamal S, eds. Osteoporosis. Philadelphia: American College of Physicians; 2002, in press.

37. Storm T, Thamsborg G, Steiniche T *et al.* Effect of intermittent cyclical etidronate therapy on bone mass and fracture rate in women with postmenopausal osteoporosis. N Engl J Med 1990; 322: 1265–1271.

38. Watts NB, Harris ST, Genant HK *et al.* Intermittent cyclical etidronate treatment of postmenopausal osteoporosis. N Engl J Med 1990; 323: 73–79.

39. van Staa TP, Abenhaim L, Cooper C. Use of cyclical etidronate and prevention of non-vertebral fractures 2. Br J Rheumatol 1998; 37: 87–94.

40. Liberman UA, Weiss SR, Broll J *et al.* Effect of oral alendronate on bone mineral density and the incidence of fractures in postmenopausal osteoporosis. The Alendronate Phase III Osteoporosis Treatment Study Group. N Engl J Med 1995; 333: 1437–1443.

41. Black DM, Cummings SR, Karpf DB *et al.* Randomised trial of effect of alendronate on risk of fracture in women with existing vertebral fractures. Fracture Intervention Trial Research Group. Lancet 1996; 348: 1535–1541.

42. Cummings SR, Black DM, Thompson DE *et al.* Effect of alendronate on risk of fracture in women with low bone density but without vertebral fractures: results from the Fracture Intervention Trial. J Am Med Assoc 1998; 280: 2077–2082.

43. Orwoll E, Ettinger M, Weiss S *et al.* Alendronate for the treatment of osteoporosis in men. N Engl J Med 2000; 343: 604–610.

44. Greenspan SL, Parker RA, Ferguson L *et al.* Early changes in biochemical markers of bone turnover predict the long-term response to alendronate therapy in representative elderly women: a randomized clinical trial. J Bone Miner Res 1998; 13: 1431–1438.

45. Tonino RP, Meunier PJ, Emkey R *et al.* Skeletal benefits of alendronate: 7–year treatment of postmenopausal osteoporotic women. Phase III Osteoporosis Treatment Study Group. J Clin Endocrinol Metab 2000; 85: 3109–3115.

46. Stock JL, Bell NH, Chesnut CH III *et al.* Increments in bone mineral density of the lumbar spine and hip and suppression of bone turnover are maintained after discontinuation of alendronate in postmenopausal women. Am J Med 1997; 103: 291–297.

47. Schnitzer T, Bone HG, Crepaldi G *et al.* Therapeutic equivalence of alendronate 70mg once-weekly and alendronate 10 mg daily in the treatment of osteoporosis. Alendronate Once-Weekly Study Group. Aging (Milan) 2000; 12: 1–12.

48. Lindsay R, Cosman F, Lobo RA *et al.* Addition of alendronate to ongoing hormone replacement therapy in the treatment of osteoporosis: a randomized, controlled clinical trial. J Clin Endocrinol Metab 1999; 84: 3076–3081.

49. Bone HG, Greenspan SL, McKeever C *et al.* Alendronate and estrogen effects in postmenopausal women with low bone mineral density. Alendronate/Estrogen Study Group. J Clin Endocrinol Metab 2000; 85: 720–726.

50. Harris ST, Watts NB, Genant HK *et al.* Effects of risedronate treatment on vertebral and nonvertebral fractures in women with postmenopausal osteoporosis: a randomized controlled trial. Vertebral Efficacy With Risedronate Therapy (VERT) Study Group. J Am Med Assoc 1999; 282: 1344–1352.

51. Reginster JY, Minne HW, Sorensen OH *et al.* Randomised trial of the effects of risedronate on vertical fractures in women with established postmenopausal osteoporosis. Osteoporos Int 2000; 11: 83–91.

52. McClung MR, Geusens P, Miller PD *et al.* Effect of risedronate on the risk of hip fracture in elderly women. Hip Intervention Program Study Group. N Engl J Med 2001; 344: 333–340.

53. Gordon MS, Gordon MB. Response of bone mineral density to once-weekly administration of risedronate. Endocr Pract 2002 May–Jun; 8(3): 202–207.

54. Lufkin EG, Wahner HW, O'Fallon WM *et al.* Treatment of postmenopausal osteoporosis with transdermal estrogen. Ann Intern Med 1992; 117: 1–9.

55. Mosekilde L, Beck-Nielsen H, Sorensen OH *et al.* Hormonal replacement therapy reduces forearm fracture incidence in recent postmenopausal women – results of the Danish Osteoporosis Prevention Study. Maturitas 2000; 36: 181–193.

56. Maxim P, Ettinger B, Spitalny GM. Fracture protection provided by long-term estrogen treatment. Osteoporos Int 1995; 5: 23–29.

57. Cauley JA, Seeley DG, Ensrud K *et al.* Estrogen replacement therapy and fractures in older women. Study of Osteoporotic Fractures Research Group. Ann Intern Med 1995; 122: 9–16.

58. Kiel DP, Felson DT, Anderson JJ *et al.* Hip fracture and the use of estrogens in postmenopausal women. The Framingham Study. N Engl J Med 1987; 317: 1169–1174.

59. Grady D, Rubin SM, Petitti DB *et al.* Hormone therapy to prevent disease and prolong life in postmenopausal women. Ann Intern Med 1992; 117: 1016–1037.

60. Michaelsson K, Baron JA, Farahmand BY *et al.* Hormone replacement therapy and risk of hip fracture: population based case-control study. The Swedish Hip Fracture Study Group. Brit Med J 1998; 316: 1858–1863.

61. Torgerson DJ, Bell-Syer SE. Hormone replacement therapy and prevention of nonvertebral fractures: a meta-analysis of randomized trials. J Am Med Assoc 2001; 285: 2891–2897.

62. Ettinger B, Genant HK, Cann CE. Postmenopausal bone loss is prevented by treatment with low-dosage estrogen with calcium. Ann Intern Med 1987; 106: 40–45.

63. Genant HK, Lucas J, Weiss S et al. Low-dose esterified estrogen therapy: effects on bone, plasma estradiol concentrations, endometrium, and lipid levels. Estratab/Osteoporosis Study Group. Arch Intern Med 1997; 157: 2609–2615.

64. Recker RR, Davies KM, Dowd RM, Heaney RP. The effect of low-dose continuous estrogen and progesterone therapy with calcium and vitamin D on bone in elderly women. A randomized, controlled trial. Ann Intern Med 1999; 130: 897–904.

65. Beral V, Bull D, Doll R et al. Familial breast cancer: collaborative reanalysis of individual data from 52 epidemiological studies including 58,209 women with breast cancer and 101,986 women without the disease. Lancet 2001; 358: 1389–1399.

66. Rossouw JE, Anderson GL, Prentice RL et al. Writing Group for the Women's Health Initiative Investigators. Risks and benefits of estrogen plus progestin in healthy postmenopausal women: principal results from the Women's Health Initiative randomized controlled trial. JAMA. 2002 Jul 17; 288(3): 321–333.

67. Draper MW, Flowers DE, Huster WJ et al. A controlled trial of raloxifene (LY139481) HCl: impact on bone turnover and serum lipid profile in healthy postmenopausal women. J Bone Miner Res 1996; 11: 835–842.

68. Delmas PD, Bjarnason NH, Mitlak BH et al. Effects of raloxifene on bone mineral density, serum cholesterol concentrations, and uterine endometrium in postmenopausal women. N Engl J Med 1997; 337: 1641–1647.

69. Ettinger B, Black DM, Mitlak BH et al. Reduction of vertebral fracture risk in postmenopausal women with osteoporosis treated with raloxifene: results from a 3-year randomized clinical trial. Multiple Outcomes of Raloxifene Evaluation (MORE) Investigators. J Am Med Assoc 1999; 282: 637–645.

70. Cummings SR, Eckert S, Krueger KA et al. The effect of raloxifene on risk of breast cancer in postmenopausal women: results from the MORE randomized trial. Multiple outcomes of raloxifene evaluation. J Am Med Assoc 1999; 281: 2189–2197.

71. Cauley JA, Norton L, Lippman ME et al. Continued breast cancer risk reduction in postmenopausal women treated with raloxifene: 4-year results from the MORE trial. Multiple outcomes of raloxifene evaluation. Breast Cancer Res Treat 2001; 65: 125–134.

72. Berning B, Kuijk CV, Kuiper JW et al. Effects of two doses of tibolone on trabecular and cortical bone loss in early postmenopausal women: a two-year randomized, placebo-controlled study. Bone 1996; 19: 395–399.

73. Beardsworth SA, Kearney CE, Purdie DW. Prevention of postmenopausal bone loss at lumbar spine and upper femur with tibolone: a two-year randomised controlled trial. Br J Obstet Gynaecol 1999; 106: 678–683.

74. Chesnut CH III, Silverman S, Andriano K et al. A randomized trial of nasal spray salmon calcitonin in postmenopausal women with established osteoporosis: the prevent recurrence of osteoporotic fractures study. PROOF Study Group. Am J Med 2000; 109: 267–276.

75. Cardona JM, Pastor E. Calcitonin versus etidronate for the treatment of postmenopausal osteoporosis: a meta-analysis of published clinical trials. Osteoporos Int 1997; 7: 165–174.

76. Cann CE, Roe EB, Sanchez S et al. PTH effects in the femur: envelope-specific responses by 3DQCT in postmenopausal women. J Bone Miner Res 1999; 14: S137.

77. Mosekilde L, Danielsen CC, Sogaard CH et al. The anabolic effects of parathyroid hormone on cortical bone mass, dimensions and strength-assessed in a sexually mature, ovariectomized rat model. Bone 1995; 16: 223–230.

78. Zanchetta JR, Bogado CE, Ferretti JL et al. Effects of LY333334 recombinant parthyroid hormone (1–34) on cortical bone strength indices as assessed by peripheral quantitative computed tomography. Bone 2001; 28: S86.

79. Neer RM, Arnaud CD, Zanchetta JR et al. Effect of parathyroid hormone (1–34) on fractures and bone mineral density in postmenopausal women with osteoporosis. N Engl J Med 2001; 344: 1434–1441.

80. Lindsay R, Nieves J, Formica C et al. Randomised controlled study of effect of parathyroid hormone on vertebral-bone mass and fracture incidence among postmenopausal women on oestrogen with osteoporosis. Lancet 1997; 350: 550–555.

81. Rittmaster RS, Bolognese M, Ettinger MP et al. Enhancement of bone mass in osteoporotic women with parathyroid hormone followed by alendronate. J Clin Endocrinol Metab 2000; 85: 2129–2134.

82. Riggs BL, Hodgson SF, O'Fallon WM et al. Effect of fluoride treatment on the fracture rate in postmenopausal women with osteoporosis. N Engl J Med 1990; 322: 802–809.

83. Meunier PJ, Sebert JL, Reginster JY et al. Fluoride salts are no better at preventing new vertebral fractures than calcium-vitamin D in postmenopausal osteoporosis: the FAVO Study. Osteoporos Int 1998; 8: 4–12.

84. Pak CY, Sakhaee K, Adams-Huet B et al. Treatment of postmenopausal osteoporosis with slow-release sodium fluoride. Final report of a randomized controlled trial. Ann Intern Med 1995; 123: 401–408.

85. Drake FH, Dodds RA, James IE et al. Cathepsin K, but not cathepsins B, L, or S, is abundantly expressed in human osteoclasts. J Biol Chem 1996; 271: 12511–12516.

86. Gelb BD, Shi GP, Chapman HA, Desnick RJ. Pycnodysostosis, a lysosomal disease caused by cathepsin K deficiency. Science 1996; 273: 1236–1238.

87. Dimai HP, Muller T, Eder S et al. Effects of the TNF-alfa antibody imfliximab on serum markers of bone turnover and mineral metabolism in patients with rheumatoid arthritis. Bone 2001; 28: S179.

88. Bekker PJ, Holloway D, Nakanishi A et al. The effect of a single dose of osteoprotegerin in postmenopausal women. J Bone Miner Res 2001; 16: 348–360.

89. Greendale GA, Barrett-Connor E, Edelstein S et al. Lifetime leisure exercise and osteoporosis. The Rancho Bernardo study. Am J Epidemiol 1995; 141: 951–959.

90. Kelley GA. Aerobic exercise and bone density at the hip in postmenopausal women: a meta-analysis. Prev Med 1998; 27: 798–807.

91. Wallace BA, Cumming RG. Systematic review of randomized trials of the effect of exercise on bone mass in pre- and postmenopausal women. Calcif Tissue Int 2000; 67: 10–18.

92. Karlsson M, Bass S, Seeman E. The evidence that exercise during growth or adulthood reduces the risk of fragility fractures is weak. Baillière's Clin Rheumatol 2001; 15: 429–450.

93. Gregg EW, Cauley JA, Seeley DG et al. Physical activity and osteoporotic fracture risk in older women. Study of Osteoporotic Fractures Research Group. Ann Intern Med 1998; 129: 81–88.

94. Paganini-Hill A, Chao A, Ross RK, Henderson BE. Exercise and other factors in the prevention of hip fracture: the Leisure World study. Epidemiology 1991; 2: 16–25.

95. Johnell O, Gullberg B, Kanis JA et al. Risk factors for hip fracture in European women: the MEDOS Study. Mediterranean Osteoporosis Study. J Bone Miner Res 1995; 10: 1802–1815.

96. Lord SR, Ward JA, Williams P, Strudwick M. The effect of a 12-month exercise trial on balance, strength, and falls in older women: a randomized controlled trial. J Am Geriatr Soc 1995; 43: 1198–1206.

97. Wolf SL, Barnhart HX, Kutner NG et al. Reducing frailty and falls in older persons: an investigation of Tai Chi and computerized balance training. Atlanta FICSIT Group. Frailty and injuries: cooperative studies of intervention techniques. J Am Geriatr Soc 1996; 44: 489–497.

98. Campbell AJ, Robertson MC, Gardner MM et al. Falls prevention over 2 years: a randomized controlled trial in women 80 years and older. Age Ageing 1999; 28: 513–518.

99. Tinetti ME, McAvay G, Claus E. Does multiple risk factor reduction explain the reduction in fall rate in the Yale FICSIT Trial? Frailty and injuries: cooperative studies of intervention techniques. Am J Epidemiol 1996; 144: 389–399.

100. Lunt M, Masaryk P, Scheidt-Nave C et al. The effects of lifestyle, dietary dairy intake and diabetes on bone density and vertebral deformity prevalence: the EVOS study. Osteoporos Int 2001; 12: 688–698.

101. Huopio J, Kroger H, Honkanen R et al. Risk factors for perimenopausal fractures: a prospective study. Osteoporos Int 2000; 11: 219–227.

102. Ward KD, Klesges RC. A meta-analysis of the effects of cigarette smoking on bone mineral density. Calcif Tissue Int 2001; 68: 259–270.

103. Hoidrup S, Prescott E, Sorensen TI et al. Tobacco smoking and risk of hip fracture in men and women. Int J Epidemiol 2000; 29: 253–259.

104. Lauritzen JB, Petersen MM, Lund B. Effect of external hip protectors on hip fractures. Lancet 1993; 341: 11–13.

105. Ekman A, Mallmin H, Michaelsson K, Ljunghall S. External hip protectors to prevent osteoporotic hip fractures. Lancet 1997; 350: 563–564.

106. Kannus P, Parkkari J, Niemi S et al. Prevention of hip fracture in elderly people with use of a hip protector. N Engl J Med 2000; 343: 1506–1513.

107. Parker MJ, Gillespie LD, Gillespie WJ. Hip protectors for preventing hip fractures in the elderly (Cochrane Review). Cochrane Database Syst Rev 2001; 2: CD001255.

108. Cumming RG, Thomas M, Szonyi G et al. Home visits by an occupational therapist for assessment and modification of environmental hazards: a randomized trial of falls prevention. J Am Geriatr Soc 1999; 47: 1397–1402.

109. Gillespie LD, Gillespie WJ, Robertson MC et al. Interventions for preventing falls in elderly people (Cochrane Review). Cochrane Database Syst Rev 2001; 3: CD000340.

110. Ytterstad B. The Harstad injury prevention study: the characteristics and distribution of fractures amongst elders – an eight year study. Int J Circumpolar Health 1999; 58: 84–95.

111. Thorngren KG, Ceder L, Svensson K. Predicting results of rehabilitation after hip fracture. A ten-year follow-up study. Clin Orthop 1993; 287: 76–81.

112. Kronhed AC, Moller M. Effects of physical exercise on bone mass, balance skill and aerobic capacity in women and men with low bone mineral density, after one year of training – a prospective study. Scand J Med Sci Sports 1998; 8: 290–298.

113. Glorieux FH, Bishop NJ, Plotkin H et al. Cyclic administration of pamidronate in children with severe osteogenesis imperfecta. N Engl J Med 1998; 339: 947–952.

114. Prevention and management of hip fracture in older people. A national clinical guideline. Scottish Intercollegiate Guidelines Network 2002.

115. Lips P, Cooper C, Agnusdei D et al. Quality of life in patients with vertebral fractures: validation of the Quality of Life Questionnaire of the European Foundation for Osteoporosis (QUALEFFO). Working Party for Quality of Life of the European Foundation for Osteoporosis. Osteoporos Int 1999; 10(2): 150–160.

METABOLIC BONE DISEASES

46 Glucocorticoid-induced osteoporosis

Philip N Sambrook

- Glucocorticoids are effective agents in many rheumatic diseases but glucocorticoid-induced bone loss is common because of:
  - complex effects of glucocorticoids on gene expression in osteoblasts
  - inhibition by glucocorticoids of bone formation and enhancement of bone resorption
- Glucocorticoids can cause rapid bone loss and increase the risk of fracture throughout the skeleton, but especially in trabecular rich sites such as the spine and ribs
- Glucocorticoid bone loss can be effectively prevented or reversed by therapy with bisphosphonates, PTH and vitamin D metabolites

PATHOPHYSIOLOGY OF GLUCOCORTICOID BONE LOSS

It is currently believed that most of the biological activities of glucocorticoids are mediated via binding to the glucocorticoid receptor (GR). By this classic genomic mechanism, lipophilic glucocorticoid passes across the cell membrane, attaches to the cytosolic GR and after dimerization (Fig. 46.1), the GR binds to conserved sequence motifs (glucocorticoid response elements or GRE) to positively or negatively regulate specific gene transcription[1]. However it is also now recognized certain biological activities of glucocorticoids may be mediated via other transcription factors, such as activated protein (AP)-1 and nuclear factor κB (NFκB), independent of GR binding to DNA but dependent upon interaction with these factors[1].

Glucocorticoids affect bone metabolism through multiple pathways, influencing aspects of both bone formation and bone resorption in the remodeling cycle (Fig. 46.2). However the most important effects of glucocorticoids in relation to bone loss appear to be on bone formation. For the most part, the decreased bone formation is due to direct effects on cells of the osteoblastic lineage although indirect effects related to sex steroid production are also important. Glucocorticoids have complex actions on gene expression in bone cells, dependent on the stage of

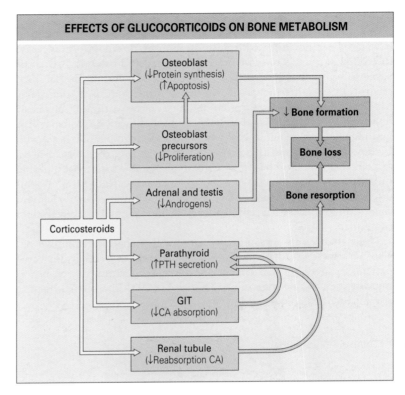

EFFECTS OF GLUCOCORTICOIDS ON BONE METABOLISM

Fig. 46.2 Schematic diagram of effects of glucocorticoids on bone metabolism. The thicker arrows for effects on bone formation indicate this is more important than effects on bone resorption.

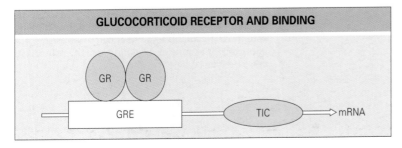

GLUCOCORTICOID RECEPTOR AND BINDING

Fig. 46.1 Schematic diagram of the glucocorticoid receptor and binding. Dimers of GR bind to GRE followed by interaction with the transcriptional initiation complex (TIC) to activate transcription.

osteoblast growth and differentiation[2]. Thus they decrease cell replication and repress type I collagen gene expression by the osteoblast by decreasing the rates of transcription and destabilizing type 1 collagen mRNA. They also have complex and unique effects on collagen degradation and regulate the synthesis of matrix metalloproteinases.

In addition to direct actions on the collagen gene, glucocorticoid effects on skeletal cells may be indirect and involve effects on the synthesis, release, receptor binding or binding proteins of locally produced growth factors. Bone cells synthesize insulin growth factors (IGF) I and II. These molecules are among the most important local regulators of bone cell function because of their abundance and anabolic effects to increase type I collagen synthesis by the osteoblast and bone formation. Glucocorticoids decrease IGF I synthesis in osteoblasts by transcription mechanisms and inhibit IGF II receptor expression in osteoblasts[2]. Glucocorticoids have also been shown to decrease mRNA levels encoding for osteoblast products such as osteocalcin.

Enhanced osteocyte apoptosis has also been implicated as an important mechanism of glucocorticoid osteoporosis[3]. Glucocorticoids have been shown to reduce the birth rate of osteoblasts and osteoclasts and cause earlier death of osteoblasts[3]. The effect of glucocorticoids to promote apoptosis in osteocytes as well as in osteoblasts could account for the rapid increase in fracture susceptibility.

Although there have been many reports that bone resorption is increased in glucocorticoid treated patients, this is probably only true during the first 6 or 12 months of therapy. This early, temporary increase in bone resorption is probably due to increased osteoclast production from the effects of glucocorticoids on osteoprotegerin and its ligand[4]. In addition, osteoclast apoptosis may be postponed, contributing to rapid bone loss. It has been hypothesized that in some patients, secondary hyperparathyroidism increases bone turnover and expands the remodeling space, but this does not usually persist. Indeed with longer term glucocorticoid use, bone turnover is reduced.

The direct inhibitory effects of glucocorticoids on bone formation have also been documented in histomorphometric studies. An increase in eroded surface is observed with glucocorticoid osteoporosis compared to postmenopausal osteoporosis[5]. This does not mean that bone resorption remains increased but rather that there is a long delay between completion of resorption and onset of formation in each basic multicellular unit (BMU) (Fig. 46.3). Indeed activation frequency, the best index of the overall intensity of bone remodeling, is decreased with chronic glucocorticoid therapy. At any time during the lifespan of an osteoid seam the number of osteoblasts depends both on the number initially assembled and the number that have escaped entrapment as osteocytes or death by apoptosis. Even with fewer cycles of remodeling, a significant loss after each remodeling cycle leads to progressively thinner trabeculae.

These changes are not only associated with trabecular thinning, but also perforation and major loss of trabecular connectivity in some patients[6], suggesting that changes in microarchitecture may be just as important as loss of bone mineral density (BMD) in assessing fracture risk in glucocorticoid treated patients (Fig. 46.4).

An additional effect of glucocorticoids is to decrease intestinal absorption of calcium[7]. Glucocorticoids increase urinary phosphate and calcium loss by direct effects on the kidney[8] which, together with impaired calcium absorption, may lead to secondary hyperparathyroidism[8] and increased bone resorption as an early but temporary phenomenon as noted above (Fig. 46.2).

Epidemiology

Glucocorticoids are effective, widely used, agents in rheumatology practice but glucocorticoid-induced osteoporosis is a common associated problem, first recognized by Cushing[9]. The risk of developing osteoporosis with glucocorticoid therapy remains unclear, but has been reported to occur in up to 50% of persons who require long term therapy. Fractures can occur rapidly with a predilection for sites rich in trabecular bone such as the spine and ribs, however prospective epidemiological fracture data in glucocorticoid bone loss is generally lacking. The largest study is a retrospective cohort study of 244 236 subjects on glucocorticoids identified from a general practice registry in the UK matched with 244 235 control patients[10]. The relative risks during oral glucocorticoid therapy for clinical vertebral fracture was 2.6, for hip fracture was 1.6 and for non-vertebral fracture was 1.3 (Fig. 46.5). Fracture risk increased with increasing daily doses of glucocorticoids[10] and on discontinuation, the fracture risk appeared to return to baseline.

The cumulative prevalence of vertebral fracture with glucocorticoids has been derived from cross-sectional studies and rates as high as 28% have been reported[11,12]. Estimates of vertebral fracture incidence with glucocorticoids, derived from the calcium treated control arms of recent randomized trials[13–16] range from 13–22% in the first year of therapy. The incidence appears to be particularly low in premenopausal women, intermediate in men and consequently highest in postmenopausal women.

Fracture risk with glucocorticoids is determined by several factors[17] (Fig. 46.6) including:

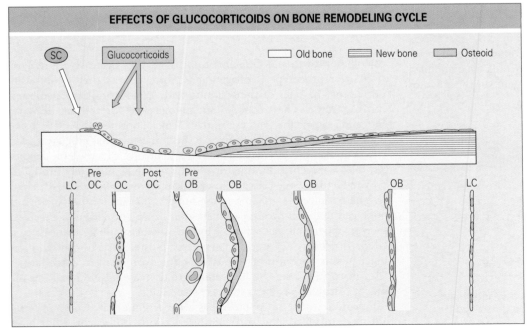

EFFECTS OF GLUCOCORTICOIDS ON BONE REMODELING CYCLE

SC | Glucocorticoids | ▢ Old bone | ▤ New bone | ▢ Osteoid

LC | Pre OC | OC | Post OC | Pre OB | OB | OB | OB | LC

Fig. 46.3 Schematic diagram of the effects of glucocorticoids on bone remodeling cycle. A trabecular BMU is depicted in a longitudinal section (upper panel) and at selected transverse sections (lower panels). Successive stages of quiescence, activation, resorption, formation and quiescence occur. Corticosteroids may enhance activation early, but later delay the interval between completion of resorption and onset of formation. Histomorphometric studies, being cross-sectional in nature, would show an apparent increase in resorptive surfaces, in this situation when resorption is in fact reduced due to decreased recruitment of osteoclast precursors and enhanced osteoblast apoptosis. SC, stem cell; LC, lining cell; OC, osteoclast; OB, osteoblast.

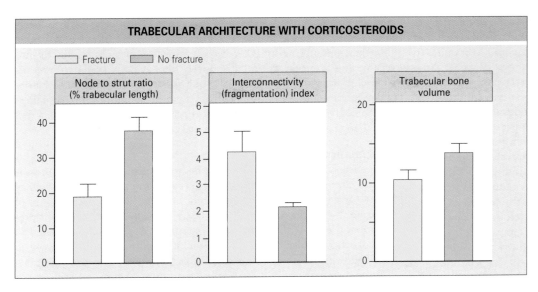

Fig. 46.4 Trabecular architecture with corticosteroids. Histomorphometry of glucocorticoid effects on trabecular connectivity. (Adapted from Chappard et al.[6])

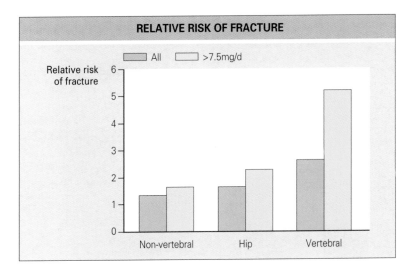

Fig. 46.5 Relative risk of fracture. Relative risk of different types of fracture with glucocorticoids. (Adapted from Van Staa et al.[10])

- age: this is a risk factor for vertebral fracture, independent of bone mineral density (BMD)[12]
- BMD: both the initial value before glucocorticoid therapy and the amount of subsequent glucocorticoid-induced loss are important. Thus bone loss of 10% from a baseline T score of zero (as in a premenopausal woman) has a weaker influence on fracture risk than a similar bone loss from a baseline T score of −2 (as for example in a postmenopausal woman). Indeed the greatest risk of vertebral fracture is in older postmenopausal women
- glucocorticoid dose: bone loss is dependent both on cumulative and mean daily dosage[10]
- duration of exposure, i.e. a short course of glucocorticoids will cause bone loss that is largely reversible on ceasing glucocorticoids, but long term therapy causes a sustained reduction in BMD due to decreased bone formation increasing the likelihood that a fracture will occur eventually
- the underlying disease for which glucocorticoids are prescribed, which may be independently associated with increased fracture risk[18,19].

Bone density and fracture risk

In postmenopausal women, a decrease of one standard deviation in BMD is associated with an approximate doubling of fracture risk.

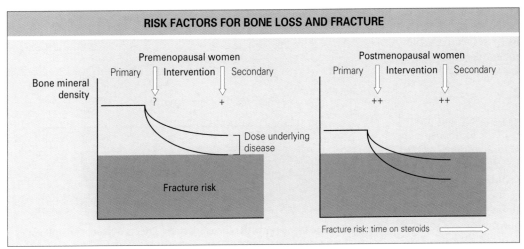

Fig. 46.6 Risk factors for bone loss and fracture. Schematic diagram of how the degree of bone loss and risk of fracture from glucocorticoids varies according to age, dose and underlying disease. The case for early intervention (primary prevention) is strongest in postmenopausal women and older men with low BMD. As fracture risk is a function of time on glucocorticoids, secondary prevention is appropriate to consider in men and pre- and postmenopausal women on long term glucocorticoids with low BMD.

However, this relationship may underestimate fracture risk in patients treated with glucocorticoids. Indeed some studies[11,20] have suggested that vertebral fractures due to glucocorticoids occur at higher BMD values to that observed in other types of osteoporosis. Luengo et al.[20] compared fractured thresholds (determined as the 90th percentile of the mean BMD) between 32 asthma patients with steroid related vertebral fractures and 55 postmenopausal patients with vertebral fractures. Fracture thresholds were 1.17 and 0.98 g/cm^2 respectively, suggesting that glucocorticoid treated patients sustained fractures at significantly higher BMD values. Peel et al.[11] examined vertebral deformity prevalence in patients with rheumatoid arthritis (RA) treated with low dose glucocorticoids, compared to age matched controls. There was a reduction in mean BMD of 0.8 SD in the RA patients. Compared to the overall expected doubling in risk of fracture, the authors found a fivefold increase in the prevalence of vertebral fractures (28 versus 6%). In contrast, Selby et al.[21] observed no increased risk of vertebral fracture in glucocorticoid treated patients compared to other causes of osteoporosis when cumulative fracture prevalence was compared to BMD.

Dose, duration and formulation of therapy and bone loss

Bone loss with glucocorticoids is most rapid in the first 6 to 12 months after starting therapy, followed by a slower decline in patients on chronic glucocorticoids[13–16]. When high dose glucocorticoids are used, rates of spine bone loss range between 5–10% per annum[22]. A serial histomorphometric study of patients treated with prednisone (10–25mg/day) demonstrated a 27% decrease in iliac crest cancellous bone volume by 6 months, however no further decline was observed at re-biopsy after 19 months[23]. In patients on chronic low dose prednisone therapy, bone loss continues at a much slower rate[16]. The overall reduction in BMD and change in microarchitecture with chronic glucocorticoid therapy still increases the likelihood that a fracture will occur eventually. Glucocorticoid bone loss appears reversible at least in part in young patients and recovery in bone density has been reported, for example, following successful treatment of Cushing's syndrome[24].

Although glucocorticoid osteoporosis is dose dependent[10], 'low dose' glucocorticoid may still cause rapid initial bone loss in some patients. A longitudinal study observed loss averaging 9.5% over 20 weeks from spinal trabecular bone in patients receiving a mean dose of 7.5mg prednisone per day[25].

Inhaled steroids are less likely to have systemic effects than oral glucocorticoids, but in higher doses result in adrenal suppression, growth impairment and reduced bone density. Wong et al.[26] reported a large cross-sectional study in patients receiving long term inhaled glucocorticoids for asthma. They found a significant inverse relationship between glucocorticoid dose and duration of glucocorticoid therapy and bone density at the spine and hip. Analysis of 170 818 inhaled glucocorticoid users from the general practice registry in the United Kingdom matched against an equal number of controls observed the relative risk of vertebral, hip and non-vertebral fracture was 1.5, 1.2 and 1.2 respectively but no differences were found between inhaled and bronchodilator groups[27].

Investigations

Bone mineral density

Effects of glucocorticoids on BMD can be measured precisely and accurately using dual energy X-ray absorptiometry (DXA) of the lumbar spine, hip and distal forearm or quantitative computerized tomography (QCT) for the lumbar spine. The earliest changes of glucocorticoid-induced bone loss are seen in the lumbar spine because of its high content of trabecular bone and can be quantitated by QCT or DXA. Since the radiation exposure with QCT is higher than with DXA, it is recommended to obtain a DXA measurement of the lumbar spine (anteroposterior scan) and femoral neck when subjects are initiating glucocorticoid treatment or

soon thereafter. Lateral DXA measurement has also been used to assess glucocorticoid treated patients as it is more sensitive to trabecular bone loss than anteroposterior DXA, however due to positioning issues, its precision and accuracy are much poorer. Repeat DXA scans are recommended at 12 monthly intervals, but should not be repeated before 12 months even in glucocorticoid treated patients because the errors inherent in BMD measurement mean that repeating a scan at a time interval of less than 12 months may not reflect a real change.

Biochemical markers

The effects of glucocorticoids on bone metabolism are reflected in profound changes in biochemical markers of bone turnover. Markers of bone formation such as serum osteocalcin fall within a few hours of treatment with glucocorticoids (Fig. 46.7) to as low as 30% of their pretreatment level[8] with the degree of suppression significantly related to glucocorticoid dose[28]. Markers of bone resorption have been shown to rise following acute glucocorticoid administration[8]. However the exact role of such markers in diagnosis and management remains unclear.

TREATMENT OF GLUCOCORTICOID OSTEOPOROSIS

The most rapid bone loss occurs in the first 6–12 months in patients commencing high dose glucocorticoids. It is thus important to consider two different strategies:

- primary prevention in patients starting glucocorticoids who have not yet lost bone and

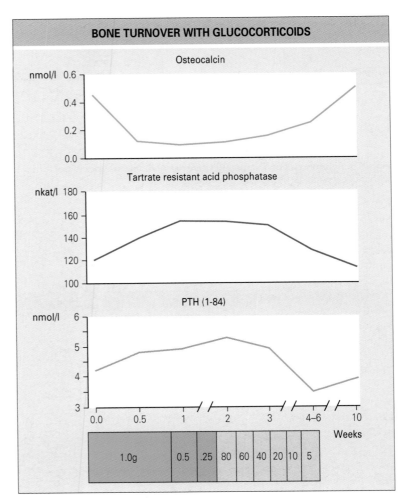

Fig. 46.7 Bone turnover with glucocorticoids. Effects of glucocorticoids on biochemical markers of bone turnover. (Adapted from Cosman et al.[8])

- treatment (or secondary prevention) in patients on chronic glucocorticoids who will almost certainly have some significant degree of existing glucocorticoid related bone loss, with or without fractures.

Current therapeutic approaches to preventing glucocorticoid-induced bone loss include:

- use of the lowest glucocorticoid dose possible
- minimize lifestyle risk factors (e.g. smoking, low dietary calcium intake)
- consider individualized exercise programs with the help of a physical therapist to prevent muscle loss and fall.

In addition there are a number of drugs that have been used both to prevent osteoporosis but also to treat those with established bone loss. A number of agents have been investigated for potential benefit, including calcium, vitamin D and its metabolites, calcitonin, hormone replacement therapy, PTH and bisphosphonates. Agents such as the bisphosphonates have shown most consistent efficacy in clinical trials of glucocorticoid osteoporosis, as discussed below. Although by definition, anti-resorptive therapy should only operate within the bone remodeling envelope (which represents only a small proportion of the bone surface at any given time), their efficacy suggests other effects, such as to reduce osteoblast and osteocyte apoptosis are also important.

Hormone replacement therapy

Hormone replacement therapy is frequently recommended for glucocorticoid treated patients but the evidence supporting its use is limited. There has been only one controlled trial in 15 men receiving chronic glucocorticoids for asthma comparing testosterone 250mg/month with calcium 1000mg in a crossover design. After 12 months, testosterone increased lumbar BMD by 5%, which was significant compared to calcium, but the calcium group had no significant loss[29]. For estrogen there has also been one randomized controlled trial of the effect of estrogen on disease activity and BMD in postmenopausal women with RA. In a small subgroup of patients who were receiving chronic low dose glucocorticoids, lumbar BMD increased by 3.8% over 2 years compared to 0.6% loss in the calcium treated control group[30]. No fracture data are available from these studies. No randomized trials have been performed in glucocorticoid treated premenopausal women.

Calcium and vitamin D

Several studies suggest a benefit of calcium supplementation for secondary prevention in patients receiving chronic low dose glucocorticoids. However primary prevention trials in patients starting glucocorticoids, where calcium alone was used in the control arm, have still observed rapid rates of loss[15,31]. Therefore calcium alone is insufficient to prevent rapid bone loss in patients starting high dose glucocorticoids.

The evidence supporting the use of calcium in combination with vitamin D in glucocorticoid osteoporosis is mostly based upon older studies. One study examined treatment with calcium 500 mg/day and vitamin D 50 000 units per week in patients on chronic glucocorticoids[32]. This showed a significant increase in forearm bone density, but the study was not randomized and the patients were on chronic glucocorticoid treatment. Bone density was also only measured in the radius, whereas the greatest and most rapid bone loss occurs from the spine with glucocorticoids, so the clinical significance of these results is unclear. The only primary prevention study of combination calcium and vitamin D examined the use of 1000mg calcium daily plus 50 000 units vitamin D weekly against placebo over 3 years in 62 patients starting glucocorticoids[33]. Bone loss at the lumbar spine was not significantly different between calcium/vitamin D and placebo. Further, the amount of bone loss observed in the first year with the calcium/vitamin D combination

(4.9%) was similar to that seen in the calcium treated control groups in other primary prevention studies[15,31]. In contrast, a secondary prevention study in patients receiving chronic low dose glucocorticoids for RA[34] observed an annual spinal loss of 2.0% in placebo treated patients compared to 0.7% gain in calcium/vitamin D3 treated patients (1000mg + 500 IU/day respectively). As the patients were on chronic low dose glucocorticoid, the BMD rise may have been a 'remodeling transient' and the results are not necessarily applicable to patients commencing high dose glucocorticoids, i.e. primary prevention.

The term vitamin D covers both the calciferols and active metabolites, but these two groups of agents have quite distinct therapeutic effects. The most commonly used active hormonal forms of vitamin D, are calcitriol (1,25 dihydroxy vitamin D) and alfacalcidol (1α hydroxy vitamin D). Two studies have examined their use in primary prevention of glucocorticoid osteoporosis. One study examined the effect of 12 months of calcium, calcitriol or calcitonin in 103 patients starting glucocorticoids[31]. Patients treated with calcium lost bone rapidly at the lumbar spine (−4.3% in the first year) whereas patients treated with either calcitriol or calcitriol plus calcitonin lost at a much reduced rate (−1.3% and −0.2% per year respectively). The loss in both these latter groups was significantly different from the calcium group. Another randomized double blind controlled trial in 145 patients starting glucocorticoids compared alfacalcidol with calcium[35]. After 12 months, the change in spinal BMD with alfacalcidol was +0.4% compared to −5.7% with calcium. Hypercalcemia occurred in only 6.7% of alfacalcidol treated patients[35] compared to 25% with calcitriol[31]. The exact mechanism of this possible benefit of active metabolites compared to simple vitamin D for primary prevention is unclear, but may relate to reversal of the early temporary secondary hyperparathyroidism.

One secondary prevention study has evaluated the efficacy of active vitamin D metabolites compared with simple vitamin D in patients on chronic glucocorticoids[36]. A total of 85 patients on long-term glucocorticoid therapy were randomized to either 1μg alfacalcidol or 1000IU vitamin D3 with both groups also receiving 500mg calcium. Over 3 years, a small but significant increase was seen in lumbar spine BMD in the alfacalcidol group (+2.0%, $P < 0.0001$) with no significant changes at the femoral neck. In the vitamin D3 group, there were no significant changes at either site. By the end of the study, 12 new vertebral fractures had occurred in 10 patients of the alfacalcidol group and 21 in 17 patients of the vitamin D3 group. The alfacalcidol group showed a significant decrease in back pain ($P < 0.0001$) whereas no change was seen in the vitamin D3 group. This study also suggests active vitamin D metabolites are superior to simple vitamin D in the treatment of established glucocorticoid osteoporosis.

Calcitonin

Calcitonin has been studied both in patients starting glucocorticoids and in those receiving chronic glucocorticoids. In two primary prevention studies, there was no statistically significant evidence of additional benefit of adding calcitonin to calcitriol or cholecalciferol[31,37]. In the latter study, incident vertebral fractures occurred in 11% of calcitonin and 14% of calcium/vitamin D treated controls. No significant spinal bone loss was observed in either group suggesting the high vertebral fracture rate observed was more explained by underlying disease and the largely postmenopausal sample studied rather than the glucocorticoid use.

Bisphosphonates

A number of trials have examined the efficacy of bisphosphonates on glucocorticoid-induced bone loss and vertebral fractures. In 141 patients initiating glucocorticoids (i.e. primary prevention) who received prophylaxis with either cyclical etidronate or 500mg of calcium[13], mean lumbar BMD change with etidronate was +0.6% compared to −3.2% in the calcium group at the end of 12 months. For post menopausal women only, there was a significant reduction in the incidence of new vertebral fractures in the patients treated with etidronate (22 versus 3%).

The combined results of two trials in 477 glucocorticoid treated subjects who received prophylaxis with alendronate or placebo plus calcium/vitamin D (800–1000mg daily plus 250–500 IU daily respectively) have also been reported[14]. Patients were stratified according to the duration of their prior glucocorticoid treatment. Over 12 months of follow up, the mean change in lumbar spine BMD in patients in the primary prevention group (i.e. those who received glucocorticoids for < 4 months) was +3.0% for alendronate 10mg/day compared to –1% in the placebo group. In those who had received chronic glucocorticoids for > 12 months, the increase with alendronate was +2.8% but also +0.2% for calcium. These latter data suggest calcium/vitamin D might be able to prevent further bone loss in patients on chronic low dose glucocorticoids (secondary prevention). Interestingly the spinal bone loss was relatively minor (–1%/year) in patients enrolled within 4 months of initiating glucocorticoids and treated with calcium/vitamin D. These results contrast with the only study with a true untreated control group[35], in which cumulative doses of glucocorticoids were higher and spinal bone loss averaged 4.9%/year despite treatment with calcium with vitamin D. A *post-hoc* analysis of incident vertebral fractures favored alendronate in postmenopausal women (13 versus 4.4%). A 12 month extension of this trial in 212 patients to evaluate the effects of alendronate over 2 years in glucocorticoids osteoporosis has been reported[38]. This showed treatment with either 5 or 10mg of alendronate daily preserved bone mass at all sites compared to placebo over 2 years. No new vertebral fractures occurred in any alendronate treated patients in the second year.

The effects of alendronate on bone histomorphometry has been assessed in 88 patients (52 women and 36 men aged 22–75 years) from the above studies[39]. Iliac bone biopsies were obtained after tetracycline double-labeling at the end of the first year of treatment. Alendronate treatment did not influence osteoblastic activity, which is already low in glucocorticoid-induced osteoporosis. Alendronate also did not impair mineralization at any dose as assessed by mineralization rate. Osteoid thickness and volume were significantly lower in alendronate-treated patients, irrespective of the dose; however, mineral apposition rate was not altered. Significant decreases of mineralizing surfaces, activation frequency and bone formation rate were also noted with alendronate treatment.

Bisphosphonates may act to decrease glucocorticoid-induced apoptosis. Studies have shown etidronate, alendronate and pamidronate can prevent glucocorticoid-induced apoptosis of murine osteocytic cells and alendronate abolished the increased prevalence of apoptosis in vertebral cancellous bone osteocytes and osteoblasts that follows prednisolone administration to mice[40].

The results of primary prevention trial in 224 glucocorticoid treated subjects who received prophylaxis with either risedronate or placebo plus calcium 500mg daily have also been reported[15]. Risedronate 5mg per day prevented spinal bone loss (+0.6%) compared to calcium (–2.8%) over 12 months. Incident vertebral fracture rates were 17.3% with calcium and 5.7% for risedronate 5mg (P = 0.072). Vertebral fractures were only seen in postmenopausal women and men, not in premenopausal women. The effects of risedronate in 290 patients receiving chronic glucocorticoid treatment (prednisone > 7.5mg/day for > 6 months) have also been reported[16]. Approximately one third of patients had vertebral fractures as baseline. The control group, who were treated with calcium (1000mg) plus vitamin D (400IU) daily, showed a stable BMD over 12 months. However treatment with risedronate 5mg/day significantly increased lumbar spine (+2.9%) and femoral neck (+1.8%) BMD. Although not powered to show fracture efficacy, 15% of patients in the control group versus 5% in the risedronate groups sustained new vertebral fractures suggesting a 70% reduction in fracture rate. A combined analysis of 518 patients in these two trials showed risedronate 5mg was associated with a 70% reduction in vertebral fracture risk compared to placebo (P = 0.01)[41].

Intermittent intravenous pamidronate has also been studied as a primary prevention agent in glucocorticoid treated patients[42]. A regimen involving 90mg for the first infusion, then 30mg every 3 months plus calcium 800mg/day found nearly a 4% increase in lumbar spine bone mass and a 3% increase in femoral neck bone mass over 12 months while the placebo group has a –6% at the lumbar spine and –4.1% at the femoral neck.

Parathyroid hormone

Parathyroid hormone is an important hormone in calcium metabolism. Large randomized placebo controlled clinical trials have demonstrated daily low dose injections of human parathyroid hormone (hPTH)(1–34) for 21 months can increase bone density by 14% at the spine[43]. The mechanism for the anabolic effect is not known, however the PTH receptor is located on the bone marrow stromal, preosteoblast cell. In vitro work has found that PTH may increase the lifespan of osteoblasts and osteocytes. It is thought that PTH has the potential to increase osteoblast numbers by increasing both their replication rate and by decreasing apoptosis.

A randomized controlled trial has been performed in postmenopausal women with glucocorticoid-induced osteoporosis[44] comparing hPTH(1–34) and estrogen with estrogen alone. This found that patients treated with hPTH (1–34) and estrogen had significant increases in bone mass (+35% for lumbar spine QCT, +11% by lumbar spine DXA, 1% hip) after 1 year compared to the minimal changes observed in the estrogen alone group. All study patients were followed for an additional year after the hPTH(1–34) was discontinued and total hip and femoral neck bone mass increased about 5% above baseline levels[45]. Treatment with PTH resulted in a dramatic increase in biochemical markers of bone turnover. Osteocalcin increased more than 150% above baseline levels within one month of starting the therapy and remained elevated for the remainder of the treatment period. Bone resorption increased to the same levels as osteocalcin after 6 months of therapy. The study was not powered to determine if hPTH(1–34) could reduce new vertebral fractures in glucocorticoid treated patients.

Based upon the summary evidence reviewed above, an algorithm for the diagnosis and management of glucocorticoid osteoporosis is shown in Figure 46.8.

SUMMARY

Evidence from randomized controlled trials suggests that postmenopausal women receiving glucocorticoids are at the greatest risk of rapid bone loss and consequent vertebral fracture and should be actively considered for prophylactic measures. In men and premenopausal women receiving glucocorticoids, the decision to use anti-osteoporosis prophylaxis is less straightforward and will depend upon a number of factors including BMD, anticipated dose and duration of glucocorticoids and other risk factors. Guidelines for the management of glucocorticoid osteoporosis are continuing to evolve as new evidence from randomized controlled trials become available[46]. Based upon available evidence the rank order of choice for prophylaxis would be a bisphosphonate followed by a vitamin D metabolite or an estrogen type medication. Calcium alone appears unable to prevent rapid bone loss in patients starting glucocorticoids. If an active vitamin D metabolite is used, calcium supplementation should be avoided unless dietary calcium intake is low. HRT should clearly be considered if hypogonadism is present. In patients receiving chronic low dose glucocorticoids, treatment with calcium and vitamin D may be sufficient to prevent further bone loss. However since fracture risk is a function of

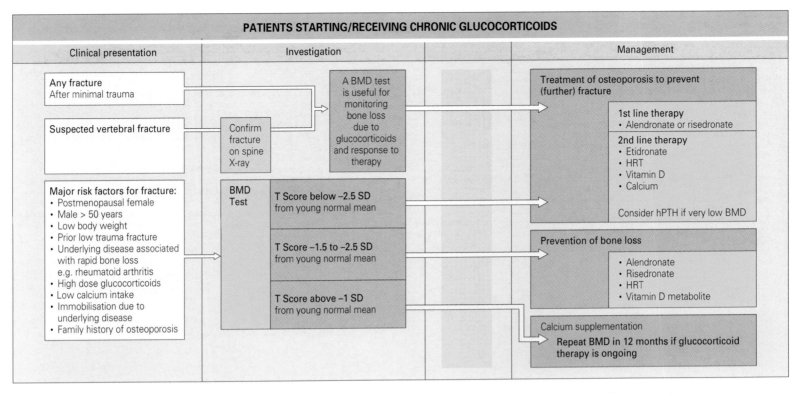

PATIENTS STARTING/RECEIVING CHRONIC GLUCOCORTICOIDS

Fig. 46.8 **Patients starting/receiving chronic glucocorticoids.** Algorithm for the diagnosis and management of glucocorticoid osteoporosis.

multiple factors including the severity of low bone density as well as the duration of exposure, treatment with therapy to increase bone density will further reduce fracture risk in patients receiving chronic low dose glucocorticoids. In patients with severe reductions in bone density, treatment with hPTH (1–34) followed by an anti-resorptive would be appropriate.

REFERENCES

1. Karin M. New twists in gene regulation by glucocorticoid receptor: is DNA binding dispensable? Cell 1998; 93: 487–490.
2. Canalis E. Mechanisms of glucocorticoid action in bone: implications to glucocorticoid induced osteoporosis. J Clin Endocr Metab 1996; 81: 3441–3447.
3. Weinstein RS, Jilka RL, Parfitt AF et al. Inhibition of osteoblastogenesis and promotion of apoptosis of osteoblasts and osteocytes by glucocorticoids. J Clin Invest 1998; 102: 274–282.
4. Hofbauer LC, Gori F, Riggs BL et al. Stimulation of osteoprotegerin ligand and inhibition of osteoprotegerin production by glucocorticoids in human osteoblastic lineage cells: potential paracrine mechanisms of glucocorticoid-induced osteoporosis. Endocrinology 1999; 140: 4382–4389.
5. Carbonare LD, Arlot ME, Chavassieux PM et al. Comparison of trabecular bone microarchitecture and remodeling in glucocorticoid-induced and postmenopausal osteoporosis. J Bone Miner Res 2001; 16: 97–103.
6. Chappard D, Legrand E, Basle MF et al. Altered trabecular architecture induced by glucocorticoids: a bone histomorphometric study. J Bone Miner Res 1996; 11: 676–685.
7. Klein RG, Arnaud SB, Gallagher JC et al. Intestinal calcium absorption in exogenous hypercortisolism. Role of 25-hydroxyvitamin D and glucocorticoid dose. J Clin Invest 1977; 60: 253–259.
8. Cosman F, Nieves J, Herbert J et al. High-dose glucocorticoids in multiple sclerosis patients exert direct effects on the kidney and skeleton. J Bone Miner Res 1994; 9: 1097–1105.
9. Cushing H. The basophil adenomas of the pituitary body and their clinical manifestations. Bull Johns Hopkins Hospital 1932; 50: 137–195.
10. Van Staa TP, Leufkens HGM, Abenhaim L et al. Use of oral glucocorticoids and risk of fractures. J Bone Miner Res 2000; 15: 993–1000.
11. Peel NFA, Moore DJ, Barrington NA et al. Risk of vertebral fracture and relationship to bone mineral density in steroid treated rheumatoid arthritis. Ann Rheum Dis 1995; 54: 801–806.
12. Naganathan V, Jones G, Nash P et al. Vertebral fracture risk with long term glucocorticoids: prevalence, relationship to age, bone density and glucocorticoid use. Arch Int Med 2000; 160: 2917–2922.
13. Adachi JD, Bensen WG, Brown J et al. Intermittent etidronate therapy to prevent glucocorticoid-induced osteoporosis. New Engl J Med 1997; 337: 382–387.
14. Saag K, Emkey R, Schnitzler TJ et al. Alendronate for the prevention and treatment of glucocorticoid induced osteoporosis. New Engl J Med 1998; 339: 292–299.
15. Cohen S, Levy RM, Keller M et al. Residronate therapy prevents glucocorticoid-induced bone loss. Arthritis Rheum 1999; 42: 2309–2318.
16. Reid DM, Hughes RA, Laan RFJM et al. Efficacy and safety of daily risedronate in the treatment of glucocorticoid induced osteoporosis in men and women: a randomised trial. J Bone Miner Res 2000; 15: 1006–1013.
17. Sambrook PN. Glucocorticoid osteoporosis: practical implications of recent trials. J Bone Miner Res 2000; 15: 1645–1649.
18. Gough AK, Lilley J, Eyre S et al. Generalised bone loss in patients with early rheumatoid arthritis. Lancet 1994; 344: 23–27.
19. Pearce G, Ryan PF, Delmas PD et al. The deleterious effects of low-dose corticosteroids on bone density in patients with polymyalgia rheumatica. Brit J Rheumatol 1998; 37: 292–299.
20. Luengo M, Picado C, Del Rio L et al. Vertebral fractures in steroid dependent asthma and involutional osteoporosis: a comparative study. Thorax 1991; 46: 8063–8065.
21. Selby PL, Halsey JP, Adams KRH et al. Glucocorticoids do not alter the threshold for vertebral fractures. J Bone Miner Res 2000; 15: 952–956.
22. Sambrook PN, Kempler S, Birmingham J et al. Glucocorticoid effects on proximal femur bone loss. J Bone Miner Res 1990; 5: 1211–1216.
23. LoCascio V, Bonnucci E, Imbimbo B et al. Bone loss in response to long-term glucocorticoid therapy. Bone Mineral 1992; 8: 39–51.
24. Pocock NA, Eisman JA, Dunstan CR et al. Recovery from steroid-induced osteoporosis. Ann Intern Med 1987; 107: 319–323.
25. Laan RFJM, Van Riel PLCM, Van de Putte LBA et al. Low dose prednisone induces rapid reversible axial bone loss in patients with rheumatoid arthritis. Ann Int Med 1993; 119: 963–968.
26. Wong CA, Walsh LJ, Smith CJP et al. Inhaled glucocorticoid use and bone mineral density in patients with asthma. Lancet 2000; 355: 1399–1403.
27. Van Staa TP, Leufkins HG, Cooper C. Use of inhaled glucocorticoids and risk of fractures. J Bone Miner Res 2001; 16: 581–588.
28. Kotowicz MA, Hall S, Hunder GG et al. Relationship of glucocorticoid dosage to serum bone Gla-protein concentration in patients with rheumatologic disorders. Arthritis Rheum 1990; 33: 1487–1492.
29. Reid IR, Wattie DJ, Evans MC, Stapleton JP. Testosterone therapy in glucocorticoid-treated men. Arch Int Med 1996; 156: 1173–1177.
30. Hall GM, Daniels M, Doyle DV, Spector TD. The effect of hormone replacement therapy on bone mass in rheumatoid arthritis treated with and without steroids. Arthritis Rheum 1994; 37: 1499–1505.

31. Sambrook PN, Birmingham J, Kelly PJ *et al*. Prevention of glucocorticoid osteoporosis; a comparison of calcium, calcitriol and calcitonin. New Engl J Med 1993; 328: 1747–1752.

32. Hahn TJ, Halstead LR, Bran DT *et al*. Effects of short term glucocorticoid administration on intestinal calcium absorption and circulating vitamin D metabolite concentrations in man. J Clin Endocr Metab 1981; 52: 111–115.

33. Adachi J, Bensen W, Bianchi F *et al*. Vitamin D and calcium in the prevention of glucocorticoid-induced osteoporosis: a three year follow up study. J Rheumatol 1996; 23: 995–1000.

34. Buckley LM, Leib ES, Cartularo KS *et al*. Calcium and vitamin D3 supplementation prevents bone loss in the spine secondary to low dose glucocorticoids in patients with rheumatoid arthritis. Ann Intern Med 1996; 125: 961–968.

35. Reginster JY, Kuntz D, Verdicht W *et al*. Prophylactic use of alfacalcidol in glucocorticoid-induced osteoporosis. Osteoporosis Int 1999; 9: 75–81.

36. Ringe JD, Coster A, Meng T *et al*. Treatment of glucocorticoid-induced osteoporosis with alfacalcidol/calcium versus vitamin D/calcium. Calcif Tiss Int 1999; 65: 337–340.

37. Healey J, Paget S, Williams-Russo P *et al*. Randomised trial of salmon calcitonin to prevent bone loss in glucocorticoid treated temporal arteritis and polymyalgia rheumatica. Calcif Tiss Int 1996; 58: 73–80.

38. Adachi JD, Saag KG, Delmas PD *et al*. Two year effects of alendronate on bone mineral density and vertebral fracture in patients receiving glucocorticoids. Arthritis Rheum 2001; 44: 202–211.

39. Chavassieux PM, Arlot ME, Roux JP *et al*. Effects of alendronate on bone quality and remodeling in glucocorticoid-induced osteoporosis: a histomorphometric analysis of transiliac biopsies. J Bone Miner Res 2000; 15: 754–762.

40. Plotkin LI, Weinstein RS, Parfitt AM *et al*. Prevention of osteocyte and osteoblast apoptosis by bisphosphonates and calcitonin. J Clin Invest 1999; 104: 1363–1367.

41. Wallach S, Cohen S, Reid DM *et al*. Effects of risedronate on bone density and vertebral fracture in patients on corticosteroid therapy. Calcif Tissue Int 2000; 67: 277–285.

42. Neer RM, Arnaud CD, Zanchetta JR *et al*. Effect of parathyroid hormone(1–34) on fractures and bone mineral density in postmenopausal women with osteoporosis. N Engl J Med 2001; 344: 1434–1441.

43. Boutsen Y, Jamart J, Esselinckx W *et al*. Primary prevention of glucocorticoid-induced osteoporosis with intermittent intravenous pamidronate: a randomized trial. Calcif Tissue Int 1997; 61: 266–271.

44. Lane NE, Sanchez S, Modin GW *et al*. Parathyroid hormone treatment can reverse glucocorticoid-induced osteoporosis. J Clin Invest 1998; 102: 1627–1633.

45. Lane NE, Pierini E, Modin G *et al*. Bone mass continues to increase after parathyroid hormone treatment is stopped in glucocorticoid-induced osteoporosis. J Bone Min Res 2000; 15: 944–951.

46. American College of Rheumatology Ad Hoc Committee on Glucocorticoid-Induced Osteoporosis. Recommendations for the prevention and treatment of glucocorticoid-induced osteoporosis: 2001 update. Arthritis Rheum 2001; 44: 1496–1503.

APPENDIX
PATIENT SELF-HELP PAGES

A   SELF HELP FOR SHOULDER PAIN

UNDERSTANDING YOUR CONDITION

Shoulder pain most commonly occurs as a result of injury or inflammation to the structures surrounding the shoulder, such as tendons or bursae (cushion-like sacs which allow the tendon to move freely over the bone). Shoulder pain can also originate from various forms of arthritis such as osteoarthritis or rheumatoid arthritis. In addition, disorders of the neck, heart, lungs, or abdominal organs may occasionally present with shoulder pain. Shoulder pain may result in marked limitations of shoulder movement, a condition called frozen shoulder.

EXERCISE

Exercises are *important* in the treatment of shoulder pain.

Basic Exercises

1. Lie on your back holding the ends of a rod in your hands. Swing your arms up overhead, using your good arm to push the affected arm back. Bring your arms down to your side. While sitting, bring the rod above your head and then down behind your neck.
2. Lie on your back. Slide arms to the side and upward overhead, then slide them back down to your side.
3. Lie on your back with your hands clasped behind your neck. Bring elbows forward to touch each other, then push them back as far as possible.
4. Stand and face a wall. Walk the fingers of your affected arm up the wall as far as possible, keeping your elbows straight, and mark the distance you reach. Repeat this exercise ten times, trying to exceed your previous mark each time.

DO

- In most forms of shoulder pain, a combination of range of motion exercises with strengthening exercises should be performed.

DON'T

- Perform exercises that make the shoulder pain worse.

SIMPLE AIDS

- Regular use of warm packs or cold packs applied to the painful area is usually helpful.
- Use clothing that fastens in the front.

MEDICATIONS

- Analgesics (such as acetaminophen/paracetamol) or anti-inflammatory drugs may help to reduce shoulder pain.
- In the treatment of shoulder pain, injection of steroids is sometimes recommended.
- In selected patients surgery may be considered.

DIET

- Diet does not play a role in the treatment of shoulder pain.

Pendulum Exercises
- Bend forward from the waist and hold onto a table with your good arm. Let the affected arm hang loosely with the shoulder relaxed. Use body movement to produce an arm swing;
- Swing the arm forwards and backwards, keeping the elbow straight.
- Swing the arm across your body, right and left. Keep the elbow straight.
- Begin to make circles with your arm. Start with two small circles, then gradually increase their size.
- Do the above exercises holding a one-or two-pound weight in your hand on the affected side.

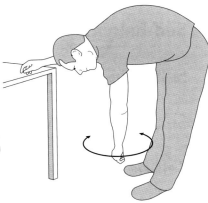

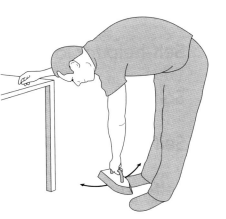

WHERE CAN YOU FIND MORE ON ARTHRITIS?

IN THE USA:
Arthritis Foundation
PO Box 7669
Atlanta
Georgia 30357-0669, USA
Tel: +800 283 78001 +404 872 7100, or call your local chapter (listed in the telephone directory)
Web page address:
http://www.arthritis.org
This is the main voluntary organization devoted to arthritis in the USA. The Foundation publishes free pamphlets on many types of arthritis and a monthly magazine for members that provides up-to-date information on arthritis. The Foundation can also provide physician and clinic referrals.

American College of Rheumatology/Association of Rheumatology Health Professionals
1800 Century Place, Suite 250
Atlanta, Georgia 30345-4300, USA
Tel: +404 633 3777
Fax: +404 633 1870
Web page address:
http://www.rheumatology.org
This association provides referrals to rheumatologists and physical and occupational therapists who have experience of working with people who have rheumatic diseases. The organization also provides educational materials and guidelines about many different rheumatic diseases.

IN THE UK:
Arthritis Research Campaign
Copeman House, St Mary's Court
St Mary's Gate, Chesterfield
Derbyshire S41 7TD, UK
Tel: +1246 558033
Fax: +1246 558007
E-mail address: info@arc.org.uk
Web page address:
http://www.arc.org.uk

Arthritis Care
18 Stephenson Way
London NW1 2HD, UK
Tel: +20 7380 6555 or 0808 800 4050
Fax: +20 7380 6505
Web page address:
http://www.arthritiscare.org.uk

IN CANADA:
The Arthritis Society
393 University Avenue, Suite 1700
Toronto, Ontario M5G 1E6, Canada
Tel: +800 321 1433/+416 979 7228
Fax: +416 979 8366
Web page address:
http://www.arthritis.ca
This organization provides information about many types of arthritis, their treatments, management tips, programs, services and support groups.

Taken from **Practical Rheumatology 3e:** Hochberg, Weinblatt, Silman, Weisman & Smolen (eds) © Copyright 2004 Elsevier Ltd.

B SELF HELP FOR OSTEOARTHRITIS (OA) OF THE KNEE

UNDERSTAND THE CONDITION

Osteoarthritis is the most common cause of knee pain and results from thinning of the cartilage in the knee. The pain is often most marked with weight-bearing activities such as walking. Osteoarthritis can occasionally cause swelling of the knee ('water on the knee').

EXERCISE

Exercise and activity are an important part of the treatment and can help relieve pain. It is important to keep active and not to be overprotective of your knees.

DO

- Keep the joints as mobile as possible – remember to bend and straighten the knee as much as you can once or twice a day.
- Keep the thigh muscles strong by doing exercises daily.
- Keep as generally fit and active as you can – try to do a little more each day, not less; if walking is difficult think about exercises in water (such as aquajogging) or cycling.

DON'T

- Keep your leg bent in the same position for long periods or put pillows under the knees to relieve pain.
- Do things that cause a lot of excessive impact (wear and tear) on the knee joints, like jogging on hard roads.

SIMPLE AIDS

- Use footwear with good cushioning in the heel or wear shock-absorbing insoles; this reduces potentially damaging high-impact forces on the knee.
- Consider using a cane when you walk (in the hand opposite to the side of the worst knee) to reduce the load on the bad knee.
- A simple knee wrap can make the knee feel more secure and relieve the feeling that it might give way.
- Warmth will often help relieve pain. During a flare-up of pain some people also find that a cold pack on the knee helps; if so, keep a packet of frozen peas in the freezer to use in this way.
- Use a handrail on stairs or steps.

MEDICINES

- Simple pain killers such as acetaminophen (paracetamol), as well as non-steroidal anti-inflammatory drugs can help.
- Medicines that you rub on to the knee joint are very safe, may help you, and can be used when you like.

DIET

- If you are overweight you should try to get back to the weight that is right for your height. Being overweight makes the pain worse and probably makes it more likely that the knee will get worse.
- A sensible diet, with plenty of vitamins C, D and E, is advisable but there is no good evidence that any special diets make a difference. Avoid expensive diets or supplements that claim that they may cure arthritis.

EXERCISES

Choose a way of doing exercises so that it is easy for you to do them every day. They can be done sitting or lying down.

You should be able to feel the thigh muscles working when you do these exercises, and you should aim to build them up, doing a little more each day so that the muscles get as strong as possible.

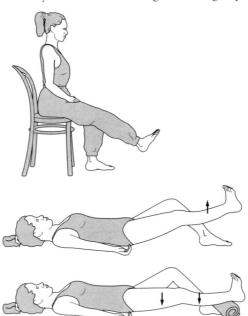

Sitting: Sit well back in the chair, straighten and raise the leg, and hold it up for a slow count of ten, and then slowly lower it again. Repeat several times.

Lying: Place a rolled-up towel under the ankle of the leg to be exercised. With one leg bent at the knee, hold the other leg straight, pull the foot up towards you, and try to push the bad knee down towards the floor. Then slowly raise the straight leg up off the floor, hold for a slow count of five and lower it again. Repeat several times.

WHERE CAN YOU FIND MORE ON ARTHRITIS?

IN THE USA:
Arthritis Foundation
PO Box 7669
Atlanta
Georgia 30357-0669, USA
Tel: +800 283 78001 +404 872 7100, or call your local chapter (listed in the telephone directory)
Web page address:
http://www.arthritis.org
This is the main voluntary organization devoted to arthritis in the USA. The Foundation publishes free pamphlets on many types of arthritis and a monthly magazine for members that provides up-to-date information on arthritis. The Foundation can also provide physician and clinic referrals.

American College of Rheumatology/Association of Rheumatology Health Professionals
1800 Century Place, Suite 250
Atlanta, Georgia 30345-4300, USA
Tel: +404 633 3777
Fax: +404 633 1870
Web page address:
http://www.rheumatology.org
This association provides referrals to rheumatologists and physical and occupational therapists who have experience of working with people who have rheumatic diseases. The organization also provides educational materials and guidelines about many different rheumatic diseases.

IN THE UK:
Arthritis Research Campaign
Copeman House, St Mary's Court
St Mary's Gate, Chesterfield
Derbyshire S41 7TD, UK
Tel: +1246 558033
Fax: +1246 558007
E-mail address: info@arc.org.uk
Web page address:
http://www.arc.org.uk

Arthritis Care
18 Stephenson Way
London NW1 2HD, UK
Tel: +20 7380 6555 or 0808 800 4050
Fax: +20 7380 6505
Web page address:
http://www.arthritiscare.org.uk

IN CANADA:
The Arthritis Society
393 University Avenue, Suite 1700
Toronto, Ontario M5G 1E6,
Canada
Tel: +800 321 1433/+416 979 7228
Fax: +416 979 8366
Web page address:
http://www.arthritis.ca
This organization provides information about many types of arthritis, their treatments, management tips, programs, services and support groups.

Taken from **Practical Rheumatology 3e**: Hochberg, Weinblatt, Silman, Weisman & Smolen (eds) © Copyright 2004 Elsevier Ltd.

C SELF HELP FOR GOUT

UNDERSTAND THE CONDITION

Gout is an abrupt and painful form of arthritis. It usually affects only one joint at a time (typically the big toe, foot, ankle, knee, wrist or elbow); it affects men more commonly than women. The most accurate way to diagnose gout is through removal of fluid from the joint and examination of the fluid under a microscope for the crystals that cause gout. Gout is a very treatable disease but untreated it can cause permanent damage to the joints.

EXERCISE

You will not be able to exercise while your joint is inflamed and you must only resume normal activity when the inflammation has gone down.

DO

- Watch out for early signs of an acute attack. The earlier you start treatment the better.
- Be alert for attacks of gout following minor injury to a joint, other illnesses, or surgery.

DON'T

- Just treat isolated attacks without consulting your physician about continuous treatment for prevention.
- Stop your medicines between attacks if you are on preventative treatment.

SIMPLE AIDS

- Rest your affected joint until the symptoms improve.
- Take your medicines as prescribed.
- Drink plenty of fluids to prevent kidney stones.

MEDICINES

Medicine is important in both the treatment and prevention of attacks. Preventative treatment is necessary in people with tophi (crystals of uric acid appearing under the skin as white pimples), kidney stones and frequent attacks.

- Attacks of gout are usually treated with non-steroidal anti-inflammatory drugs. Other anti-inflammatory agents (such as colchicine, or steroids by injection or as pills) may be recommended.

- Simple pain killers such as acetaminophen (paracetamol) are sometimes added.
- Medicines that are meant to prevent gout attacks such as allopurinol and probenecid may be prescribed, but these medicines are *never* used for an acute attack of gout.
- Medicines must be taken as directed and the treatment should not be shortened unless your physician says so.
- Seek your physician's advice regarding any medicines that might interfere with the effectiveness of the ones you've been told to take.
- Lifetime treatment for prevention of gout may be necessary.

DIET

- The old belief that eating and drinking too much causes gout has now been proven wrong, but over-indulgence in alcohol can make gout attacks more likely.
- Alcohol, aspirin and certain foods (such as liver, sardines and anchovies) may make you more likely to develop gout.

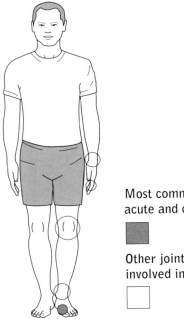

Most common sites of acute and chronic gout

■ Other joints often involved in gout

□

The joints commonly affected by or associated with gout.

WHERE CAN YOU FIND MORE ON ARTHRITIS?

IN THE USA:
Arthritis Foundation
PO Box 7669
Atlanta
Georgia 30357-0669, USA
Tel: +800 283 78001 +404 872 7100, or call your local chapter (listed in the telephone directory)
Web page address:
http://www.arthritis.org
This is the main voluntary organization devoted to arthritis in the USA. The Foundation publishes free pamphlets on many types of arthritis and a monthly magazine for members that provides up-to-date information on arthritis. The Foundation can also provide physician and clinic referrals.

American College of Rheumatology/Association of Rheumatology Health Professionals
1800 Century Place, Suite 250
Atlanta, Georgia 30345-4300, USA
Tel: +404 633 3777
Fax: +404 633 1870
Web page address:
http://www.rheumatology.org
This association provides referrals to rheumatologists and physical and occupational therapists who have experience of working with people who have rheumatic diseases. The organization also provides educational materials and guidelines about many different rheumatic diseases.

IN THE UK:
Arthritis Research Campaign
Copeman House, St Mary's Court
St Mary's Gate, Chesterfield
Derbyshire S41 7TD, UK
Tel: +1246 558033
Fax: +1246 558007
E-mail address: info@arc.org.uk
Web page address:
http://www.arc.org.uk

Arthritis Care
18 Stephenson Way
London NW1 2HD, UK
Tel: +20 7380 6555 or 0808 800 4050
Fax: +20 7380 6505
Web page address:
http://www.arthritiscare.org.uk

IN CANADA:
The Arthritis Society
393 University Avenue, Suite 1700
Toronto, Ontario M5G 1E6,
Canada
Tel: +800 321 1433/+416 979 7228
Fax: +416 979 8366
Web page address:
http://www.arthritis.ca
This organization provides information about many types of arthritis, their treatments, management tips, programs, services and support groups.

Taken from **Practical Rheumatology 3e:** Hochberg, Weinblatt, Silman, Weisman & Smolen (eds) © Copyright 2004 Elsevier Ltd.

D SELF HELP FOR RHEUMATOID ARTHRITIS (RA)

UNDERSTANDING YOUR CONDITION

RA is a disease causing inflammation in the joints of the body, leading to pain, stiffness and swelling. The joints most frequently affected are the hands, wrists, feet and knees. Fatigue can be severe in RA. Rarely, it can cause inflammation in other parts of the body including the lungs, eyes, heart, blood vessels, skin and nerves.

EXERCISE

Exercise plays an important role in the treatment of RA. It is important to strike a balance between resting inflamed joints and keeping them involved in movement so they don't stiffen after the acute inflammation has resolved.

DO

- Take a warm shower or bath first thing in the morning to relieve stiffness.
- Exercise to maintain range of motion and muscle strength in the joint.
- Swim. This is an excellent exercise that places minimal stress on the joints.
- Pace your exercises to prevent fatigue.

DON'T

- Immobilize any joints for long periods of time.

SIMPLE AIDS

- Wear good shoes with shock-absorbing soles.
- Easy access, comfortable seats, automatic transmission and power steering are recommended if you are purchasing a car.
- A cane can be a great help to decrease weight bearing on an inflamed hip or knee.
- Temporary splinting of affected joints can help.

MEDICATIONS

- Non-steroidal anti-inflammatory drugs are often recommended to reduce pain and swelling.
- 'Disease modifying' medications such as hydroxychloroquine, methotrexate or sulfasalazine may be prescribed. You might have to take these drugs for a long time, maybe even for the rest of your life.
- Corticosteroids, such as prednisone, are sometimes prescribed and are given either by injection or as pills when inflammation is severe.
- Multiple medications or combinations of medications may be needed.

DIET

Many diets have been published claiming to cure RA. Nearly always there is no scientific proof that these work.

- Maintain a proper body weight so that you reduce stress on your joints.
- Diets low in saturated fat and supplemented by fish or plant oils are often helpful.

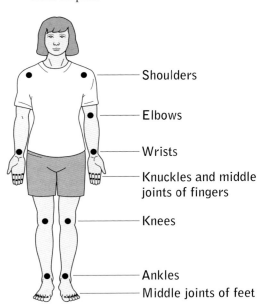

Joints frequently affected by RA; less commonly affected are the elbows, hips and neck.

Shoulders

Elbows

Wrists

Knuckles and middle joints of fingers

Knees

Ankles

Middle joints of feet

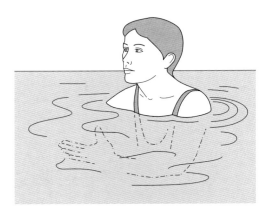

Water exercise is one of the best therapies for rheumatoid arthritis.

WHERE CAN YOU FIND MORE ON ARTHRITIS?

IN THE USA:
Arthritis Foundation
PO Box 7669
Atlanta
Georgia 30357-0669, USA
Tel: +800 283 78001 +404 872 7100, or call your local chapter (listed in the telephone directory)
Web page address:
http://www.arthritis.org
This is the main voluntary organization devoted to arthritis in the USA. The Foundation publishes free pamphlets on many types of arthritis and a monthly magazine for members that provides up-to-date information on arthritis. The Foundation can also provide physician and clinic referrals.

American College of Rheumatology/Association of Rheumatology Health Professionals
1800 Century Place, Suite 250
Atlanta, Georgia 30345-4300, USA
Tel: +404 633 3777
Fax: +404 633 1870
Web page address:
http://www.rheumatology.org
This association provides referrals to rheumatologists and physical and occupational therapists who have experience of working with people who have rheumatic diseases. The organization also provides educational materials and guidelines about many different rheumatic diseases.

IN THE UK:
Arthritis Research Campaign
Copeman House, St Mary's Court
St Mary's Gate, Chesterfield
Derbyshire S41 7TD, UK
Tel: +1246 558033
Fax: +1246 558007
E-mail address: info@arc.org.uk
Web page address:
http://www.arc.org.uk

Arthritis Care
18 Stephenson Way
London NW1 2HD, UK
Tel: +20 7380 6555 or 0808 800 4050
Fax: +20 7380 6505
Web page address:
http://www.arthritiscare.org.uk

IN CANADA:
The Arthritis Society
393 University Avenue, Suite 1700
Toronto, Ontario M5G 1E6,
Canada
Tel: +800 321 1433/+416 979 7228
Fax: +416 979 8366
Web page address:
http://www.arthritis.ca
This organization provides information about many types of arthritis, their treatments, management tips, programs, services and support groups.

Taken from **Practical Rheumatology 3e:** Hochberg, Weinblatt, Silman, Weisman & Smolen (eds) © Copyright 2004 Elsevier Ltd.

E SELF HELP FOR PSORIATIC ARTHRITIS

UNDERSTAND THE CONDITION

Psoriatic arthritis is a type of arthritis that occurs in patients with psoriasis. It can affect any joint, most commonly the tips of the fingers, the knees and spine. The psoriasis can be variable, sometimes involving a large area of skin and sometimes a small one. Psoriatic arthritis occurs equally in men and women, usually beginning between the ages of 30 and 50 years.

EXERCISE

Exercise is important in psoriatic arthritis because it will help maintain joint range of motion and muscle strength.

DO

- Soak in warm water to help reduce morning stiffness.
- Exercise regularly.
- Seek appropriate skin care as management of the psoriasis will often help to control joint symptoms.

DON'T

- Continue to exercise if it is painful to do so.

SIMPLE AIDS

- Try temporary splinting of inflamed joints.
- Wear low-heeled comfortable shoes.

MEDICINES

Medications help to decrease the inflammation that causes pain and swelling in psoriatic arthritis.
- Non-steroidal anti-inflammatory drugs are commonly used.
- If non-steroidals do not control the pain and swelling, then disease-modifying medications such as methotrexate may be recommended.
- Joint replacement surgery may be recommended if you have severe disease.

DIET

There are no specific diets found to be effective in psoriatic arthritis. If you are overweight, it is necessary to lose weight and so reduce the strain put on leg joints.

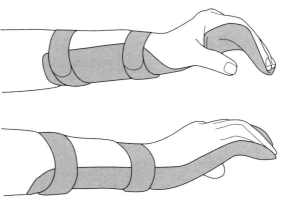

Splinting of the hand in psoriatic arthritis.

WHERE CAN YOU FIND MORE ON ARTHRITIS?

IN THE USA:
Arthritis Foundation
PO Box 7669
Atlanta
Georgia 30357-0669, USA
Tel: +800 283 78001 +404 872 7100, or call your local chapter (listed in the telephone directory)
Web page address:
http://www.arthritis.org
This is the main voluntary organization devoted to arthritis in the USA. The Foundation publishes free pamphlets on many types of arthritis and a monthly magazine for members that provides up-to-date information on arthritis. The Foundation can also provide physician and clinic referrals.

American College of Rheumatology/Association of Rheumatology Health Professionals
1800 Century Place, Suite 250
Atlanta, Georgia 30345-4300, USA
Tel: +404 633 3777
Fax: +404 633 1870
Web page address:
http://www.rheumatology.org
This association provides referrals to rheumatologists and physical and occupational therapists who have experience of working with people who have rheumatic diseases. The organization also provides educational materials and guidelines about many different rheumatic diseases.

IN THE UK:
Arthritis Research Campaign
Copeman House, St Mary's Court
St Mary's Gate, Chesterfield
Derbyshire S41 7TD, UK
Tel: +1246 558033
Fax: +1246 558007
E-mail address: info@arc.org.uk
Web page address:
http://www.arc.org.uk

Arthritis Care
18 Stephenson Way
London NW1 2HD, UK
Tel: +20 7380 6555 or 0808 800 4050
Fax: +20 7380 6505
Web page address:
http://www.arthritiscare.org.uk

IN CANADA:
The Arthritis Society
393 University Avenue, Suite 1700
Toronto, Ontario M5G 1E6,
Canada
Tel: +800 321 1433/+416 979 7228
Fax: +416 979 8366
Web page address:
http://www.arthritis.ca
This organization provides information about many types of arthritis, their treatments, management tips, programs, services and support groups.

Taken from **Practical Rheumatology 3e:** Hochberg, Weinblatt, Silman, Weisman & Smolen (eds) © Copyright 2004 Elsevier Ltd.

F SELF HELP FOR LOW BACK PAIN

UNDERSTANDING YOUR CONDITION

The back is made up of vertebrae (back bones), disks between the vertebrae, and surrounding soft tissues such as muscles and ligaments. If the vertebrae, disks or nerves are damaged, or the muscles and ligaments are strained or torn, back pain will result.

Acute back pain usually results from an injury and lasts 1 to 7 days. Obesity, poor posture and a weak back and abdominal muscles contribute to chronic low back pain. Low back pain can also occur with diseases such as osteoarthritis, ankylosing spondylitis, fibromyalgia, disk problems and Paget's disease.

EXERCISE

Exercise plays an important role in the treatment of back pain. There are various types of exercises; one type may suit one back problem but not another. Your physician may recommend that exercises be carried out under the supervision of a physical therapist.

DO

- Maintain good posture while sitting and walking.
- When sitting for a long time, make a lumbar support by placing a small pillow between your lower back and the seat.
- Stand and walk frequently to reduce low back fatigue and strain.
- Lift heavy objects with the proper straight spine posture. Hold objects close to your body and use your thigh and leg muscles to lift.
- Participate in daily stretching and strengthening exercises.
- Follow a weight loss plan (if you are overweight).
- Report to your doctor if there is numbness or tingling in the legs.

DON'T

- Sit for prolonged periods.
- Lift and twist, push or pull heavy objects.
- Engage in strenuous activity until cleared by your physician.

SIMPLE AIDS

- Massage or deep heat treatments often help to relieve back pain.
- Use a firm mattress or place a board under the mattress.

MEDICINES

- Acetaminophen (paracetamol) or non-steroidal anti-inflammatory drugs are often prescribed to ease back pain.
- With severe pain, narcotic-containing pain medicines may be needed for a short time.

- Muscle relaxants may be prescribed for muscle spasms.
- Injection of steroids by an anaesthesiologist specializing in pain control may be recommended.

DIET

- Excessive weight will aggravate low back conditions.

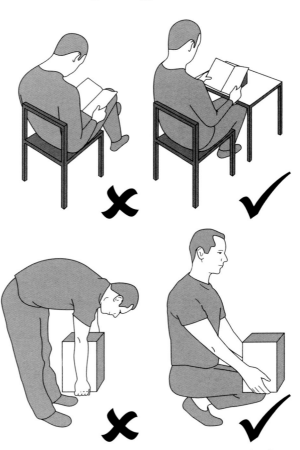

Lifting a weight with the spine bent and knees straight often makes backache worse. Bending your knees when you lift will take the strain off your back. Get as close as possible to whatever you are lifting so that you can keep your back straight.

WHERE CAN YOU FIND MORE ON ARTHRITIS?

IN THE USA:
Arthritis Foundation
PO Box 7669
Atlanta
Georgia 30357-0669, USA
Tel: +800 283 78001 +404 872 7100, or call your local chapter (listed in the telephone directory)
Web page address:
http://www.arthritis.org
This is the main voluntary organization devoted to arthritis in the USA. The Foundation publishes free pamphlets on many types of arthritis and a monthly magazine for members that provides up-to-date information on arthritis. The Foundation can also provide physician and clinic referrals.

American College of Rheumatology/Association of Rheumatology Health Professionals
1800 Century Place, Suite 250
Atlanta, Georgia 30345-4300, USA
Tel: +404 633 3777
Fax: +404 633 1870
Web page address:
http://www.rheumatology.org
This association provides referrals to rheumatologists and physical and occupational therapists who have experience of working with people who have rheumatic diseases. The organization also provides educational materials and guidelines about many different rheumatic diseases.

IN THE UK:
Arthritis Research Campaign
Copeman House, St Mary's Court
St Mary's Gate, Chesterfield
Derbyshire S41 7TD, UK
Tel: +1246 558033
Fax: +1246 558007
E-mail address: info@arc.org.uk
Web page address:
http://www.arc.org.uk

Arthritis Care
18 Stephenson Way
London NW1 2HD, UK
Tel: +20 7380 6555 or 0808 800 4050
Fax: +20 7380 6505
Web page address:
http://www.arthritiscare.org.uk

IN CANADA:
The Arthritis Society
393 University Avenue, Suite 1700
Toronto, Ontario M5G 1E6, Canada
Tel: +800 321 1433/+416 979 7228
Fax: +416 979 8366
Web page address:
http://www.arthritis.ca
This organization provides information about many types of arthritis, their treatments, management tips, programs, services and support groups.

Taken from **Practical Rheumatology 3e:**
Hochberg, Weinblatt, Silman, Weisman & Smolen (eds) © Copyright 2004 Elsevier Ltd.

G SELF HELP FOR NECK PAIN

UNDERSTANDING YOUR CONDITION

The neck is made up of the vertebrae (neck bones), disks between vertebrae, and the surrounding soft tissues such as muscles and ligaments. Neck pain may be caused by an injury or disease process that affects any of these structures.

EXERCISE

Exercise can be an important part of the treatment of neck pain, depending on its cause.

DO

- Practice good posture when sitting and standing.
- Perform neck exercises as indicated by your physician or physical therapist.

DON'T

- Engage in strenuous activities unless cleared with your physicians.

SIMPLE AIDS

- Place a pillow under your head and neck when lying in bed.
- Use a cervical collar to help relieve spasm.
- If your pain is due to injury or if you have muscle spasms, your physician may recommend the use of heat or ice on the area.
- Deep heat or traction by a physical therapist may be recommended.

MEDICATION

- Acetaminophen (paracetamol) or non-steroidal anti-inflammatory drugs may be prescribed to decrease the pain.
- In severe pain, narcotic-containing medicines may be prescribed for a short time.
- If you are having muscle spasms, muscle relaxants may be prescribed.

DIET

Diet does not play a role in the management of neck pain.

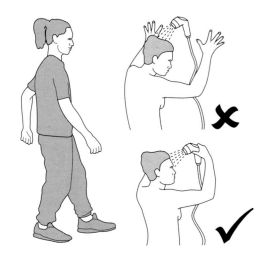

Standing. Slouching can strain your neck. When you're in the shower, bend your knees slightly to get underneath the shower head. When standing or walking, position your head squarely over your body.

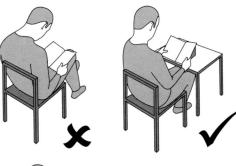

Sitting. Drooping your head forward can stress the muscles in your neck. When reading raise your reading material to eye level using a stack of books or a box. Position your body close to the steering wheel when you drive.

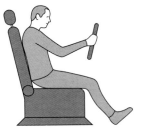

WHERE CAN YOU FIND MORE ON ARTHRITIS?

IN THE USA:
Arthritis Foundation
PO Box 7669
Atlanta
Georgia 30357-0669, USA
Tel: +800 283 78001 +404 872 7100, or call your local chapter (listed in the telephone directory)
Web page address:
http://www.arthritis.org
This is the main voluntary organization devoted to arthritis in the USA. The Foundation publishes free pamphlets on many types of arthritis and a monthly magazine for members that provides up-to-date information on arthritis. The Foundation can also provide physician and clinic referrals.

American College of Rheumatology/Association of Rheumatology/ Health Professionals
1800 Century Place, Suite 250
Atlanta, Georgia 30345-4300, USA
Tel: +404 633 3777
Fax: +404 633 1870
Web page address:
http://www.rheumatology.org
This association provides referrals to rheumatologists and physical and occupational therapists who have experience of working with people who have rheumatic diseases. The organization also provides educational materials and guidelines about many different rheumatic diseases.

IN THE UK:
Arthritis Research Campaign
Copeman House, St Mary's Court
St Mary's Gate, Chesterfield
Derbyshire S41 7TD, UK
Tel: +1246 558033
Fax: +1246 558007
E-mail address: info@arc.org.uk
Web page address:
http://www.arc.org.uk

Arthritis Care
18 Stephenson Way
London NW1 2HD, UK
Tel: +20 7380 6555 or 0808 800 4050
Fax: +20 7380 6505
Web page address:
http://www.arthritiscare.org.uk

IN CANADA:
The Arthritis Society
393 University Avenue, Suite 1700
Toronto, Ontario M5G 1E6,
Canada
Tel: +800 321 1433/+416 979 7228
Fax: +416 979 8366
Web page address:
http://www.arthritis.ca
This organization provides information about many types of arthritis, their treatments, management tips, programs, services and support groups.

Taken from **Practical Rheumatology 3e:** Hochberg, Weinblatt, Silman, Weisman & Smolen (eds) © Copyright 2004 Elsevier Ltd.

H SELF HELP FOR ANKYLOSING SPONDYLITIS

UNDERSTANDING YOUR CONDITION

Ankylosing spondylitis is a form of arthritis mainly affecting the spine, although it may involve the hips and shoulders and other peripheral joints. Ankylosing spondylitis can also produce eye irritation, heart problems and a decreased ability to expand the chest. It usually affects young men.

EXERCISE

Exercise plays a major role in the treatment of ankylosing spondylitis.

DO

- Perform regular exercise.
- Maintain as much motion as possible to prevent stiffness or fusion of the spine in an awkward position.
- Consult a physical therapist regarding therapy, including water therapy.
- Report any back pain following injuries (such as a fall) to your doctor.

DON'T

- Spend long periods in a poor posture, particularly with the head hanging forward.
- Ignore any symptoms of eye discomfort.

SIMPLE AIDS

- Sleep without pillows to prevent the neck from fusing in an abnormally flexed position.
- A wide rear view mirror in the car can help compensate for loss of neck motion.

MEDICATIONS

- Non-steroidal anti-inflammatory drugs are effective in managing the pain.
- Other drugs such as sulfasalazine are sometimes used if conservative treatment is not effective.
- Steroid eye-drops may be recommended if there is associated eye inflammation.

DIET

- Maintain a proper body weight as increased weight will put stress on the spine.

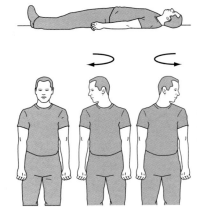

Exercise and range of motion programs will increase spine flexibility. To maintain a straight back and neck, lie flat on the floor and relax gently so that your spine flattens out completely and your head rests on the floor.

To maintain rotation of the neck, twist your neck round each side as far as you can, and repeat a few times.

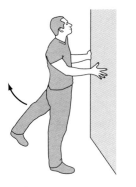

To maintain movement of your hips, stand up against a wall and then push one leg behind you as far as you can.

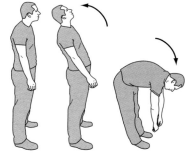

To maintain movement of your lower back, stand straight then arch your spine backwards as far as you can, and then bend forwards as far as you can.

WHERE CAN YOU FIND MORE ON ARTHRITIS?

IN THE USA:
Arthritis Foundation
PO Box 7669
Atlanta
Georgia 30357-0669, USA
Tel: +800 283 78001 +404 872 7100, or call your local chapter (listed in the telephone directory)
Web page address:
http://www.arthritis.org
This is the main voluntary organization devoted to arthritis in the USA. The Foundation publishes free pamphlets on many types of arthritis and a monthly magazine for members that provides up-to-date information on arthritis. The Foundation can also provide physician and clinic referrals.

American College of Rheumatology/Association of Rheumatology Health Professionals
1800 Century Place, Suite 250
Atlanta, Georgia 30345-4300, USA
Tel: +404 633 3777
Fax: +404 633 1870
Web page address:
http://www.rheumatology.org
This association provides referrals to rheumatologists and physical and occupational therapists who have experience of working with people who have rheumatic diseases. The organization also provides educational materials and guidelines about many different rheumatic diseases.

IN THE UK:
Arthritis Research Campaign
Copeman House, St Mary's Court
St Mary's Gate, Chesterfield
Derbyshire S41 7TD, UK
Tel: +1246 558033
Fax: +1246 558007
E-mail address: info@arc.org.uk
Web page address:
http://www.arc.org.uk

Arthritis Care
18 Stephenson Way
London NW1 2HD, UK
Tel: +20 7380 6555 or 0808 800 4050
Fax: +20 7380 6505
Web page address:
http://www.arthritiscare.org.uk

IN CANADA:
The Arthritis Society
393 University Avenue, Suite 1700
Toronto, Ontario M5G 1E6,
Canada
Tel: +800 321 1433/+416 979 7228
Fax: +416 979 8366
Web page address:
http://www.arthritis.ca
This organization provides information about many types of arthritis, their treatments, management tips, programs, services and support groups.

Taken from **Practical Rheumatology 3e:** Hochberg, Weinblatt, Silman, Weisman & Smolen (eds) © Copyright 2004 Elsevier Ltd.

SELF HELP FOR FIBROMYALGIA

UNDERSTAND THE CONDITION

Fibromyalgia is a condition that causes widespread pain in the muscles, tendons and ligaments, and the joints. Most patients have specific areas of tenderness called tender points. Fibromyalgia is often associated with sleep disturbance and profound fatigue.

EXERCISE

Exercise and physical activity are an extremely important part of the treatment of fibromyalgia.

DO

- Begin exercise slowly and increase gradually.
- Stretching exercises should be done every day.
- Endurance or aerobic exercises such as walking, cycling or swimming should be done three or four times a week.

DON'T

- Give up if exercises initially cause pain.
- Be too ambitious.

SIMPLE AIDS

There are a number of simple aids that you can use to reduce pain and decrease fatigue.

- Avoid drugs such as nasal decongestants and don't drink alcohol, tea or coffee late at night as these may disturb your sleep.
- Take time out to relax. Yoga and relaxation techniques are helpful.
- Identify the stresses in your life so that you can learn to cope with them.
- Physiotherapy and massage are sometimes helpful.
- Teach your family about fibromyalgia so that they can be supportive.

MEDICINES

Physicians prescribe medications in fibromyalgia to improve the amount and quality of sleep and to treat pain.

- Medications such as amitriptyline, nortriptyline and cyclobenzaprine in low doses are effective in helping patients sleep better, often leading to improvement in fatigue and pain.

- Pain medication, treatment of associated depression and steroid injections into the affected area may be treatment options.

DIET

- No particular diet has been shown to help, but it is sensible to maintain your ideal body weight.
- At bedtime, avoid drinks containing caffeine.

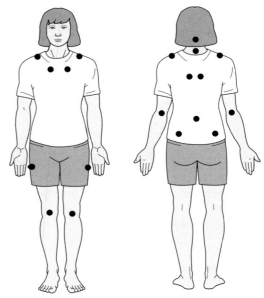

Sites of tenderness in fibromyalgia.

WHERE CAN YOU FIND MORE ON ARTHRITIS?

IN THE USA:
Arthritis Foundation
PO Box 7669
Atlanta
Georgia 30357-0669, USA
Tel: +800 283 78001 +404 872 7100, or call your local chapter (listed in the telephone directory)
Web page address:
http://www.arthritis.org
This is the main voluntary organization devoted to arthritis in the USA. The Foundation publishes free pamphlets on many types of arthritis and a monthly magazine for members that provides up-to-date information on arthritis. The Foundation can also provide physician and clinic referrals.

American College of Rheumatology/Association of Rheumatology Health Professionals
1800 Century Place, Suite 250
Atlanta, Georgia 30345-4300, USA
Tel: +404 633 3777
Fax: +404 633 1870
Web page address:
http://www.rheumatology.org
This association provides referrals to rheumatologists and physical and occupational therapists who have experience of working with people who have rheumatic diseases. The organization also provides educational materials and guidelines about many different rheumatic diseases.

IN THE UK:
Arthritis Research Campaign
Copeman House, St Mary's Court
St Mary's Gate, Chesterfield
Derbyshire S41 7TD, UK
Tel: +1246 558033
Fax: +1246 558007
E-mail address: info@arc.org.uk
Web page address:
http://www.arc.org.uk

Arthritis Care
18 Stephenson Way
London NW1 2HD, UK
Tel: +20 7380 6555 or 0808 800 4050
Fax: +20 7380 6505
Web page address:
http://www.arthritiscare.org.uk

IN CANADA:
The Arthritis Society
393 University Avenue, Suite 1700
Toronto, Ontario M5G 1E6,
Canada
Tel: +800 321 1433/+416 979 7228
Fax: +416 979 8366
Web page address:
http://www.arthritis.ca
This organization provides information about many types of arthritis, their treatments, management tips, programs, services and support groups.

Taken from **Practical Rheumatology 3e:**
Hochberg, Weinblatt, Silman, Weisman & Smolen (eds) © Copyright 2004 Elsevier Ltd.

J SELF HELP FOR LUPUS

UNDERSTANDING YOUR CONDITION

Lupus is a form of arthritis that mainly affects women during their child-bearing years. Lupus usually involves joint pains, especially in the small joints of the hands and feet. Skin rashes are common and these are often made worse when exposed to sunlight. Mouth ulcers can be present and fatigue often occurs. Inflammation of the kidneys, high blood pressure and inflammation of the lining around the heart and lungs can be seen with lupus.

EXERCISE

If your joints are inflamed, exercise will help improve your mobility and help decrease fatigue. If you have lung or heart involvement, you should check with your physician before beginning an exercise program.

DO

- Use a strong sun block when going out in the sun.
- Rest as needed.
- Discuss with your physician if you are thinking about becoming pregnant.
- Get your blood pressure checked frequently.

DON'T

- Ignore headaches, fevers, coughs or abdominal pain.
- Stop your medicines without checking with your physician.

SIMPLE AIDS

- Use a hat to protect you from the sun.
- Use sunglasses to protect your eyes, which may be sensitive to light.

MEDICATIONS

- Joint pains are usually treated with anti-inflammatory drugs.
- Hydroxychloroquine may be recommended for joint and/or skin problems and fatigue.
- Corticosteroids may be prescribed if you have complications such as pleurisy or pericarditis.
- In cases of lupus involving the kidneys or blood, high doses of corticosteroids may be recommended combined with other immunosuppressive drugs (such as azathioprine or cyclophosphamide).
- Corticosteroid creams may be prescribed for rashes.

DIET

There is some evidence to suggest that a diet low in saturated fat and supplemented by fish oil may be helpful.

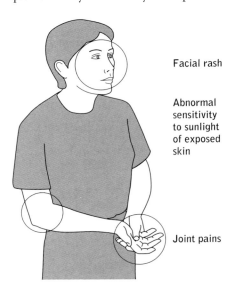

The main symptoms of lupus

Facial rash

Abnormal sensitivity to sunlight of exposed skin

Joint pains

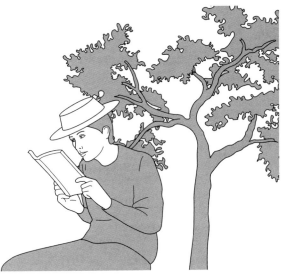

Avoid sun exposure. Too much ultraviolet radiation can flare both the skin rash and sometimes lupus in the internal organs.

WHERE CAN YOU FIND MORE ON ARTHRITIS?

IN THE USA:
Arthritis Foundation
PO Box 7669
Atlanta
Georgia 30357-0669, USA
Tel: +800 283 78001 +404 872 7100, or call your local chapter (listed in the telephone directory)
Web page address:
http://www.arthritis.org
This is the main voluntary organization devoted to arthritis in the USA. The Foundation publishes free pamphlets on many types of arthritis and a monthly magazine for members that provides up-to-date information on arthritis. The Foundation can also provide physician and clinic referrals.

American College of Rheumatology/Association of Rheumatology Health Professionals
1800 Century Place, Suite 250
Atlanta, Georgia 30345-4300, USA
Tel: +404 633 3777
Fax: +404 633 1870
Web page address:
http://www.rheumatology.org
This association provides referrals to rheumatologists and physical and occupational therapists who have experience of working with people who have rheumatic diseases. The organization also provides educational materials and guidelines about many different rheumatic diseases.

IN THE UK:
Arthritis Research Campaign
Copeman House, St Mary's Court
St Mary's Gate, Chesterfield
Derbyshire S41 7TD, UK
Tel: +1246 558033
Fax: +1246 558007
E-mail address: info@arc.org.uk
Web page address:
http://www.arc.org.uk

Arthritis Care
18 Stephenson Way
London NW1 2HD, UK
Tel: +20 7380 6555 or 0808 800 4050
Fax: +20 7380 6505
Web page address:
http://www.arthritiscare.org.uk

IN CANADA:
The Arthritis Society
393 University Avenue, Suite 1700
Toronto, Ontario M5G 1E6,
Canada
Tel: +800 321 1433/+416 979 7228
Fax: +416 979 8366
Web page address:
http://www.arthritis.ca
This organization provides information about many types of arthritis, their treatments, management tips, programs, services and support groups.

Taken from **Practical Rheumatology 3e:** Hochberg, Weinblatt, Silman, Weisman & Smolen (eds) © Copyright 2004 Elsevier Ltd.

K SELF HELP FOR SJOGREN'S SYNDROME

UNDERSTAND THE CONDITION

Sjögren's syndrome is a condition that affects the glands, leading to dry eyes, dry mouth, dry skin and dryness of the vaginal area. It can also be associated with inflammation of the joints, lungs, kidneys, blood vessels, nerves and muscles.

EXERCISE

Exercise is not important in Sjögren's syndrome unless there is associated joint or muscle involvement.

DO

- Ask your doctor about over-the-counter eye-drops (artificial tears) used to decrease dryness.
- Use good dental hygiene and visit your dentist frequently to avoid associated tooth decay.
- Avoid medicines like antihistamines as these have a drying effect.
- Report persistent swelling of the salivary glands or lymph nodes (found in specific areas such as the mouth, neck, lower arm, armpit and groin).

DON'T

- Ignore signs of infection.
- Eat sugary foods that will lead to tooth decay.
- Wear contact lenses.
- Use strong soaps.

SIMPLE AIDS

- Drink liquids frequently throughout the day and at night.
- Vaginal lubricants will decrease vaginal dryness and painful intercourse.
- Creams and ointments for dry skin will help seal in moisture.
- A humidifier at night will prevent dryness of the eyes, mouth and nose.
- Preservative-free eye-drops will help lubricate the eyes.
- Use sugar-free chewing gum or lemon drops to avoid a dry mouth.

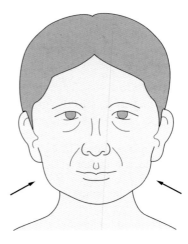

Salivary glands can become swollen in Sjögren's syndrome.

WHERE CAN YOU FIND MORE ON ARTHRITIS?

IN THE USA:
Arthritis Foundation
PO Box 7669
Atlanta
Georgia 30357-0669, USA
Tel: +800 283 78001 +404 872 7100, or call your local chapter (listed in the telephone directory)
Web page address:
http://www.arthritis.org
This is the main voluntary organization devoted to arthritis in the USA. The Foundation publishes free pamphlets on many types of arthritis and a monthly magazine for members that provides up-to-date information on arthritis. The Foundation can also provide physician and clinic referrals.

American College of Rheumatology/Association of Rheumatology Health Professionals
1800 Century Place, Suite 250
Atlanta, Georgia 30345-4300, USA
Tel: +404 633 3777
Fax: +404 633 1870
Web page address:
http://www.rheumatology.org
This association provides referrals to rheumatologists and physical and occupational therapists who have experience of working with people who have rheumatic diseases. The organization also provides educational materials and guidelines about many different rheumatic diseases.

IN THE UK:
Arthritis Research Campaign
Copeman House, St Mary's Court
St Mary's Gate, Chesterfield
Derbyshire S41 7TD, UK
Tel: +1246 558033
Fax: +1246 558007
E-mail address: info@arc.org.uk
Web page address:
http://www.arc.org.uk

Arthritis Care
18 Stephenson Way
London NW1 2HD, UK
Tel: +20 7380 6555 or 0808 800 4050
Fax: +20 7380 6505
Web page address:
http://www.arthritiscare.org.uk

IN CANADA:
The Arthritis Society
393 University Avenue, Suite 1700
Toronto, Ontario M5G 1E6,
Canada
Tel: +800 321 1433/+416 979 7228
Fax: +416 979 8366
Web page address:
http://www.arthritis.ca
This organization provides information about many types of arthritis, their treatments, management tips, programs, services and support groups.

Taken from **Practical Rheumatology 3e:**
Hochberg, Weinblatt, Silman, Weisman & Smolen (eds) © Copyright 2004 Elsevier Ltd.

L SELF HELP FOR RAYNAUD'S PHENOMENON

UNDERSTAND THE CONDITION

Raynaud's phenomenon results from a temporary decreased blood flow (upon exposure to cold temperatures) to one or more of the fingers, toes, ears, and occasionally the tip of the nose. Raynaud's can be associated with other diseases such as scleroderma and lupus.

EXERCISE

Exercise to maintain cardiovascular fitness is recommended, but people with Raynaud's must not exercise the cold.

DO

- Stop smoking. Smoking causes decreased blood flow to the affected areas.
- Seek medical treatment for any sores or infections on your fingers, toes, nose or ears.
- Avoid excessive emotional stress.
- Moisturize the skin to prevent dryness and cracking.

DON'T

- Expose yourself excessively to cold.
- Treat skin infections on your extremities yourself.
- Stop prescribed medicines without checking with your physician.
- Start smoking

SIMPLE AIDS

- Keep yourself warm by dressing in layers, mittens (rather than gloves), hat and scarf.
- If you drive then have someone else warm up your car for you.
- Wear gloves when removing food from the refrigerator and freezer.
- Warm the shower before getting in.
- Avoid second-hand cigarette smoke.
- Learn relaxation techniques.

MEDICINES

Your physician may prescribe a medication such as nifedipine for you if your condition is severe. These medicines improve blood flow to your extremities. The most common side-effects include headaches, light headedness or dizziness, swelling and rash.

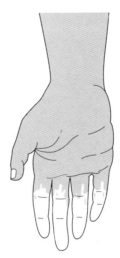

The hand of a patient with Raynaud's phenomenon, showing the typical white appearance of the fingers.

WHERE CAN YOU FIND MORE ON ARTHRITIS?

IN THE USA:
Arthritis Foundation
PO Box 7669
Atlanta
Georgia 30357-0669, USA
Tel: +800 283 78001 +404 872 7100, or call your local chapter (listed in the telephone directory)
Web page address:
http://www.arthritis.org
This is the main voluntary organization devoted to arthritis in the USA. The Foundation publishes free pamphlets on many types of arthritis and a monthly magazine for members that provides up-to-date information on arthritis. The Foundation can also provide physician and clinic referrals.

American College of Rheumatology/Association of Rheumatology Health Professionals
1800 Century Place, Suite 250
Atlanta, Georgia 30345-4300, USA
Tel: +404 633 3777
Fax: +404 633 1870
Web page address:
http://www.rheumatology.org
This association provides referrals to rheumatologists and physical and occupational therapists who have experience of working with people who have rheumatic diseases. The organization also provides educational materials and guidelines about many different rheumatic diseases.

IN THE UK:
Arthritis Research Campaign
Copeman House, St Mary's Court
St Mary's Gate, Chesterfield
Derbyshire S41 7TD, UK
Tel: +1246 558033
Fax: +1246 558007
E-mail address: info@arc.org.uk
Web page address:
http://www.arc.org.uk

Arthritis Care
18 Stephenson Way
London NW1 2HD, UK
Tel: +20 7380 6555 or 0808 800 4050
Fax: +20 7380 6505
Web page address:
http://www.arthritiscare.org.uk

IN CANADA:
The Arthritis Society
393 University Avenue, Suite 1700
Toronto, Ontario M5G 1E6,
Canada
Tel: +800 321 1433/+416 979 7228
Fax: +416 979 8366
Web page address:
http://www.arthritis.ca
This organization provides information about many types of arthritis, their treatments, management tips, programs, services and support groups.

Taken from **Practical Rheumatology 3e:** Hochberg, Weinblatt, Silman, Weisman & Smolen (eds) © Copyright 2004 Elsevier Ltd.

M SELF HELP FOR OSTEOPOROSIS

UNDERSTAND THE CONDITION

Osteoporosis is a condition where a person gradually loses bone mass so that the bones become more fragile. As a result, their bones are more likely to break. There are no warning signs for osteoporosis until a fracture occurs. Osteoporosis is most common in post-menopausal women and is associated with certain risk factors such as low physical activity, smoking, alcohol and treatment with corticosteroid hormones.

EXERCISE

Exercise is an important part of the prevention and treatment of osteoporosis.

DO

- Weight-bearing exercises, such as walking every day.
- Avoid situations that have a risk of your falling.
- Minimize use of sedatives.

DON'T

- Smoke
- Ignore signs of loss of height or curvature of the spine as these can be indicative of osteoporosis.
- Ignore excessive pain after a fall.

SIMPLE AIDS

- Assistive devices such as canes are available if you are unsteady on your feet.
- Use a handrail on stairs.

MEDICINES

In most people, calcium and vitamin D intake is insufficient and they must take nutritional supplements.
- Post-menopausal women should have a measurement of bone mineral density to determine if they have osteoporosis or low bone mass.
- Medicines for prevention and/or treatment include calcitonin and bisphosphonates.
- Surgery may be needed to repair fractured bones.
- Drugs such as phenylhydantoin, corticosteroids or excessive thyroid medicines may contribute to the development of osteoporosis.
- With your physician, discuss the medicines that you take now that may cause balance problems or dizziness.

DIET

- Calcium intake should be between 1000 and 1500 mg of elemental calcium a day. Dairy products are particularly rich in calcium.
- Vitamin D is necessary for the absorption of calcium from the diet, with 400 to 800 international units of vitamin D recommended daily (one or two multivitamins).
- Supplemental calcium is indicated in those who do not get enough in their diet.
- Supplemental vitamin D is necessary for those who do not get it from milk or exposure to the sun.
- Avoid excess caffeine and alcohol.

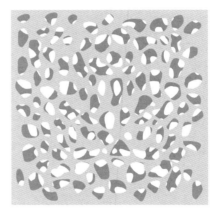

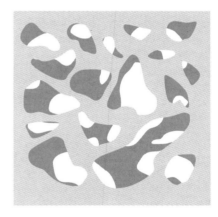

Bone is made of fibers of material called collagen, filled in with minerals (mainly calcium salts) rather like reinforced concrete. The bones of the skeleton have a thick outer shell or 'cortex', inside which there is a meshwork of 'trabecular' bone. The drawings show (above) normal trabecular bone and (below) bone affected by osteoporosis.

WHERE CAN YOU FIND MORE ON ARTHRITIS?

IN THE USA:
Arthritis Foundation
PO Box 7669
Atlanta
Georgia 30357-0669, USA
Tel: +800 283 78001 +404 872 7100, or call your local chapter (listed in the telephone directory)
Web page address:
http://www.arthritis.org
This is the main voluntary organization devoted to arthritis in the USA. The Foundation publishes free pamphlets on many types of arthritis and a monthly magazine for members that provides up-to-date information on arthritis. The Foundation can also provide physician and clinic referrals.

American College of Rheumatology/Association of Rheumatology Health Professionals
1800 Century Place, Suite 250
Atlanta, Georgia 30345-4300, USA
Tel: +404 633 3777
Fax: +404 633 1870
Web page address:
http://www.rheumatology.org
This association provides referrals to rheumatologists and physical and occupational therapists who have experience of working with people who have rheumatic diseases. The organization also provides educational materials and guidelines about many different rheumatic diseases.

IN THE UK:
Arthritis Research Campaign
Copeman House, St Mary's Court
St Mary's Gate, Chesterfield
Derbyshire S41 7TD, UK
Tel: +1246 558033
Fax: +1246 558007
E-mail address: info@arc.org.uk
Web page address:
http://www.arc.org.uk

Arthritis Care
18 Stephenson Way
London NW1 2HD, UK
Tel: +20 7380 6555 or 0808 800 4050
Fax: +20 7380 6505
Web page address:
http://www.arthritiscare.org.uk

IN CANADA:
The Arthritis Society
393 University Avenue, Suite 1700
Toronto, Ontario M5G 1E6, Canada
Tel: +800 321 1433/+416 979 7228
Fax: +416 979 8366
Web page address:
http://www.arthritis.ca
This organization provides information about many types of arthritis, their treatments, management tips, programs, services and support groups.

Taken from **Practical Rheumatology 3e:** Hochberg, Weinblatt, Silman, Weisman & Smolen (eds) © Copyright 2004 Elsevier Ltd.

N SELF HELP FOR JUVENILE IDIOPATHIC ARTHRITIS (JIA)

UNDERSTANDING YOUR CONDITION

JIA refers to various forms of arthritis occurring in children. It is caused by inflammation in the joints causing stiffness, warmth, swelling and pain. It is a chronic disease that may last for many months or years. There are three types of JIA; pauciarticular, polyarticular and systemic. They have different types of problems. Pauciarticular JIA affects only a few joints, starts most commonly in the pre-school years and is more likely to occur in girls. Knees, elbows and ankles are commonly affected, and inflammation in the eyes occurs in about half the children.

Polyarticular JIA affects many joints, often the small joints of the hands and fingers. Joints commonly affected include the neck, knees, ankles, feet, wrists and hands. Girls develop this more commonly. Eye inflammation can develop, but less frequently than in pauciarticular JIA.

Systemic JIA starts with fever, rash, changes in the blood cells, and joint pain. Inflammation of the joints often develops later. Rarely, systemic JIA will involve the heart, lymph nodes, liver and lungs.

EXERCISE

Exercise is very important to maintain joint movement and muscle strength.

DO

- Have children participate in the same activities as other children of their age.
- Have children alternate periods of activity with periods of rest.
- Have children maintain good posture.
- Consider participation in water therapy.
- Arrange regular eye tests even if there are no symptoms.

DON'T

- Continue with an exercise program that causes increased pain.
- Put pillows under the knees as this could lead to permanently bent knees.

SIMPLE AIDS

- Use a firm mattress with one thin pillow.
- Use rest splints if recommended.
- Use a neck collar if recommended.
- Get adequate rest at night.

MEDICATIONS

- Non-steroidal anti-inflammatory drugs are frequently prescribed.
- 'Disease-modifying' medications, including methotrexate are usually prescribed to slow the disease's progress.
- If your child has serious systemic JRA, prednisone may be prescribed.
- Rarely, joint replacement or synovectomy (the removal of joint lining) may be necessary.

DIET

There is no evidence that a special diet plays a part in the care of children with JRA but it is important that children have adequate caloric, protein and calcium intake.

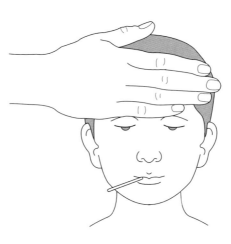

Persistent fevers may be part of JRA. Rest splints hold wrists and knees in a good position.

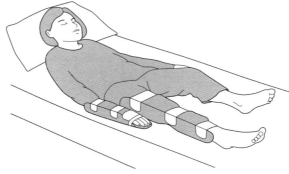

WHERE CAN YOU FIND MORE ON ARTHRITIS?

IN THE USA:
Arthritis Foundation
PO Box 7669
Atlanta
Georgia 30357-0669, USA
Tel: +800 283 78001 +404 872 7100, or call your local chapter (listed in the telephone directory)
Web page address:
http://www.arthritis.org
This is the main voluntary organization devoted to arthritis in the USA. The Foundation publishes free pamphlets on many types of arthritis and a monthly magazine for members that provides up-to-date information on arthritis. The Foundation can also provide physician and clinic referrals.

American College of Rheumatology/Association of Rheumatology Health Professionals
1800 Century Place, Suite 250
Atlanta, Georgia 30345-4300, USA
Tel: +404 633 3777
Fax: +404 633 1870
Web page address:
http://www.rheumatology.org
This association provides referrals to rheumatologists and physical and occupational therapists who have experience of working with people who have rheumatic diseases. The organization also provides educational materials and guidelines about many different rheumatic diseases.

IN THE UK:
Arthritis Research Campaign
Copeman House, St Mary's Court
St Mary's Gate, Chesterfield
Derbyshire S41 7TD, UK
Tel: +1246 558033
Fax: +1246 558007
E-mail address: info@arc.org.uk
Web page address:
http://www.arc.org.uk

Arthritis Care
18 Stephenson Way
London NW1 2HD, UK
Tel: +20 7380 6555 or 0808 800 4050
Fax: +20 7380 6505
Web page address:
http://www.arthritiscare.org.uk

IN CANADA:
The Arthritis Society
393 University Avenue, Suite 1700
Toronto, Ontario M5G 1E6, Canada
Tel: +800 321 1433/+416 979 7228
Fax: +416 979 8366
Web page address:
http://www.arthritis.ca
This organization provides information about many types of arthritis, their treatments, management tips, programs, services and support groups.

Taken from **Practical Rheumatology 3e:** Hochberg, Weinblatt, Silman, Weisman & Smolen (eds) © Copyright 2004 Elsevier Ltd.

INDEX

Page numbers in **bold** refer to major discussions in the text, and usually include aspects such as epidemiology, clinical features, diagnosis, pathology and treatment.
Page numbers in followed by (i) refer to pages on which tables/figures are to be found.
vs denotes *differential diagnosis, or comparisons*
This index is arranged in *letter-by-letter order,* whereby hyphens and spaces between words are ignored in the alphabetization. Terms in brackets are also ignored from initial alphabetization.
Cross-references in *italics* are either general cross-references (e.g. *see also specific drugs*), or refer to subentries within the same main entry .
Readers are advised that the *categorization* inherent in the contents list is not specifically replicated in the index, owing to space constraints.
Owing to divergent views over *juvenile idiopathic arthritis/juvenile rheumatoid arthritis/juvenile inflammatory arthritis,* entries have mostly been kept to the terminology preferred by individual authors. Readers are advised to refer to all variant arthritis forms beginning *juvenile.*
Abbreviations

ACR - American College of Rheumatology
ANCA - antineutrophil cytoplasmic antibodies
AS - ankylosing spondylitis
ARA - American Rheumatism Association
BCP - basic calcium phosphate

CPPD - calcium pyrophosphate dihydrate
ENT - *ear, nose and throat*
ESR - erythrocyte sedimentation rate
GFR - glomerular filtration rate
HBV - hepatitis B virus

HCV - hepatitis C virus
OA - osteoarthritis
RA - rheumatoid arthritis
SLE - systemic lupus erythematosus